# MIDLINE MEDICAL DICTIONARY

(ENGLISH - ENGLISH - HINDI)

## IN MOST EASILY UNDERSTANDABLE LANGUAGE

*Includes*
*Fully Colored Physiology, Illustrations*
*& Anatomy Charts*

### DR. P. S. RAWAT

*Formerly, Editor, The Homeopathic Heritage, Author of
"A Self-study Course in Homeopathy," "Practical Glossary of Medical
Terms," "Homeopathy in Acne & Alopecia," "Homeopathy in Angina
Pectoris," "Select your Dose and Potency," etc.*

**FOURTH IMPROVED EDITION**

### B. JAIN PUBLISHERS (P) LTD.
USA — EUROPE — INDIA

**MIDLINE MEDICAL DICTIONARY**

First Edition: 2005
Second Edition: 1998
Third Edition: 2000
Fourth Edition:
16th impression 2019

All rights reserved. No part of this book may be reproduced, stored in a retrieval system or transmitted, in any form or by any means, mechanical, photocopying, recording or otherwise, without any prior written permission of the publisher.

© with the publisher

*Published by Kuldeep Jain for*
**B. JAIN PUBLISHERS (P) LTD.**
1921/10, Chuna Mandi, Paharganj, New Delhi 110 055 (INDIA)
Tel.: +91-11-4567 1000    Fax: +91-11-4567 1010
Email: info@bjain.com    Website: **www.bjain.com**

*Printed in India*

ISBN: 978-81-319-0353-7

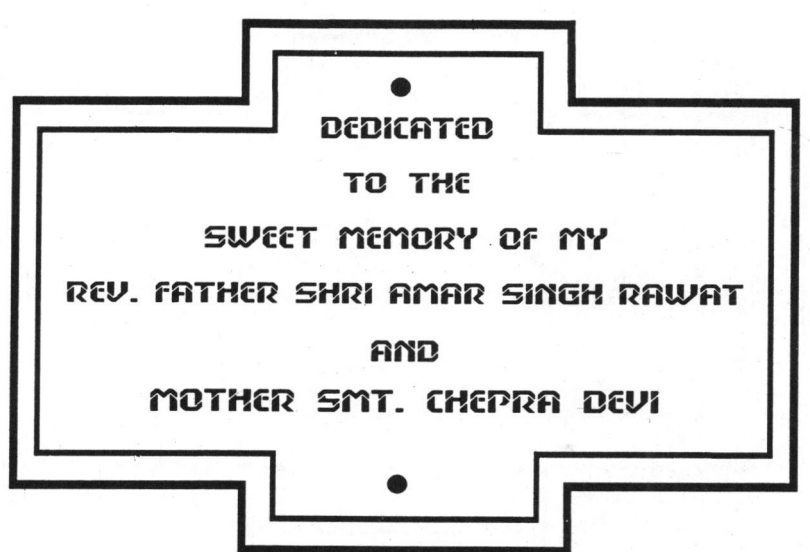

## PREFACE TO THIRD EDITION

I feel proud in presenting the third edition of the "Midline Medical Dictionary" for the benefit of the medical profession by slightly revising, enlarging and trying to do away with the shortcomings of the previous editions. Not only this, but I have also endeavoured to include some of the most important **Charts** relating to the human anatomy at the concluding portion of the "Dictionary" with a view that they may become more and more useful for the medical students and for all those who may have a distinctive liking to broaden their knowledge in the field of medicine.

With this hope that the present edition would prove more fruitful for the medical profession, I would not forget to pay my heartfelt gratitudes to Dr. Vimal Bharadwaj, DHMS, who took great pains in sketching the captioned Charts.

Above all, I feel greatly indebted to the publications' ever - energetic and the most progressive Director - Shri Kuldeep Jain, the genius - for constantly encouraging me to add something more to my writings and translation work.

**P.S. Rawat**

## PREFACE TO SECOND EDITION

A period of more than ten years has elapsed since I had the opportunity to present in the hands of medical world the English-Hindi edition of "Midline Medical Dictionary". No doubt, the profession welcomed the work, but was not, perhaps, satisfied, as it could neither fulfil the desires of English-knowing medical men nor the varnaculars. Hence, there was a hectic demand from all corners of the medical world for making this medical dictionary a more comprehensive and evergreen medical document by incorporating the maximum terms which come in daily use of the medical profession. Really, the work was too tiring to take up, but with the encouragement I had from Mr. Kuldeep Jain, the Director of the publishing house and my utmost hobby to work for the medical world at all times, I started to revise and enlarge the work during these ten years and the same is now in the benevolent hands of the members of the medical profession.

While recompiling the work, my utmost efforts have been to add to my previous work a wide range of terms which are considered so essential, but were lacking in the said compilation. At the same time, I endeavoured to make amends for the errors of the previous work and did my best to explain each term in the most simple and easily understandable language so that the amateurs could also grasp their meanings without experiencing any difficulty.

As in many other works presently available in the market, I have not maintained a separate order for the abbreviated forms of so many terms, but wherever necessary, included them in the same order as has been done in the case of other terms. Simultaneously, I tried my best to give cross references of various terms which I considered most essential and valuable for the present work.

While I am greatly obliged to my pbulishers for encouraging me to recompile the work and to those nears and dears who have greatly helped me, I would not forget to pay my sincere thanks to all those God-gifted masters from whose pens I have borrowed sufficient material to add to the present compilation in the interest of all round knowledge of medical profession and welfare of the mankind.

I shall feel extremely grateful to all my readers and well wishers for any constructive suggestions they may like to give to make the next edition of the work more helping and free from errors.

P.S. Rawat

# PREFACE TO FIRST EDITION

With my growing interest in translating medical books from English to Hindi I often found myself quite handicapped in using the most appropriate words for many a terms to express the exact meanings as set by the original authors. At each such occurrences I felt extreme uneasiness and discomfort, for I had to devote more time in searching out the exact meanings of the given words. In this endeavour I had to consult various medical and other dictionaries available in the market, but the meanings of words given in many cases did not fit to the origin. With the recommendations of my publishers I thought it more advisable to use maximum of the terms given in the Glossary of Medical Sciences published by the Central Hindi Directorate of the Government of India. But when the so translated books reached the market, the members of the profession started criticising me, saying that this sort of Hindi is too difficult to understand by common men. But what to to? This question cropped up my mind at all the times and finally I was compelled to prepare such a dictionary which may be brief in its terminology, explain the English terms in the most easily understandable language and at the same time to make every one understand the Hindi terms with the help of the terms explained in English and the whole work should serve dual purpose. So, I gradually started working on it and with the grace of Almighty succeeded in my humble mission. But while presenting it to the honourable members of the profession, I would not hesitate in admitting the fact that this work does not cover the whole range of medical terminology, but most of those only which we find most frequently in our day-to-day life. None can boast of giving the sum total of every medical term, but the maximum can be done with untiring labour and deep devotion, which is perhaps beyond my capacity.

I hope, the members of the profession would welcome my efforts and give a place to it in their book-shelves. Any suggestion made, will be welcomed from the readers and efforts will be made to carry out the same in the subsequent editions.

With the above, I would not forget to keep on records my earnest thanks to my nephew Shri Pan Singh for assisting me in typing the manuscript, Shri Ashok Jain of Harjeet & Co. for its setting and bringing it out in its present shape.

At the same time, I feel it my utmost duty to pay my sincere thanks to Shri Kuldeep Jain, the publishers. Had he not inspired and encouraged me, I would have never thought of compiling such a tiresome work.

P.S.Rawat

# हृदय
(Heart)

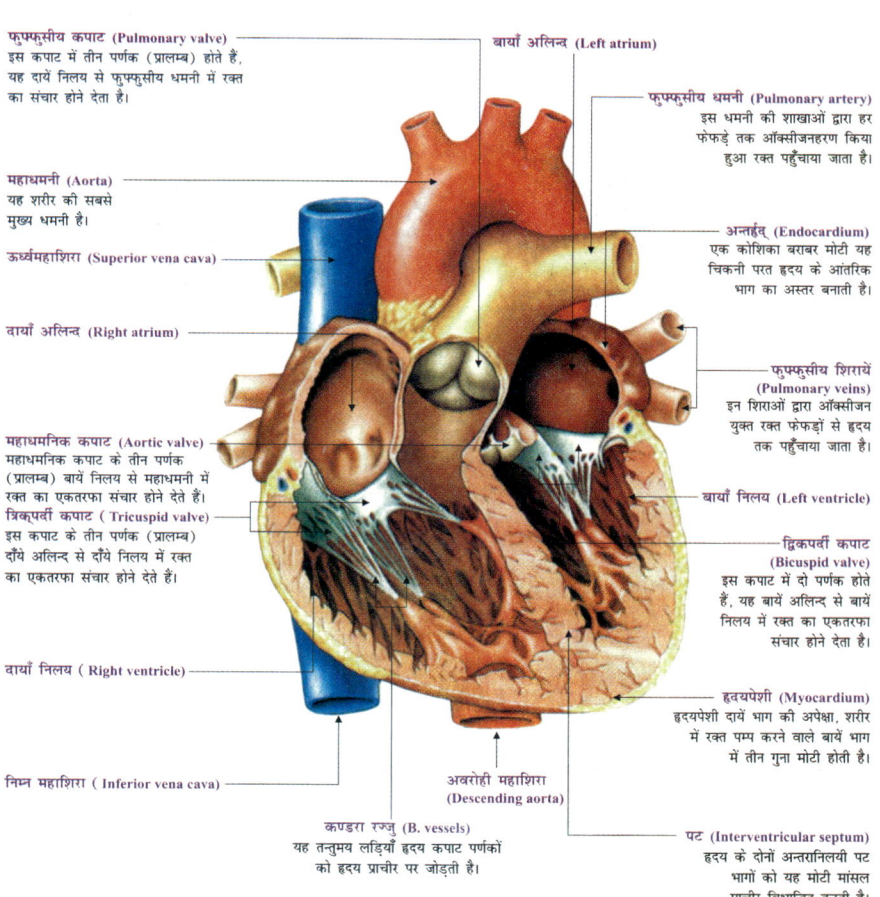

# हृदय कैसे धड़कता है?
## (Cardiac cycle)

### रक्त का मार्ग
### (Passage of blood)

### विद्युतीय सक्रियता
### (Electrical activity)

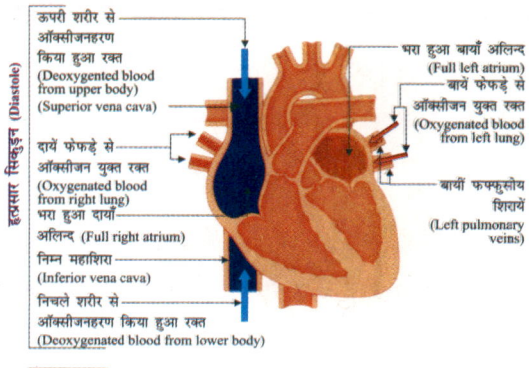
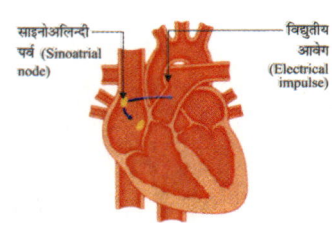

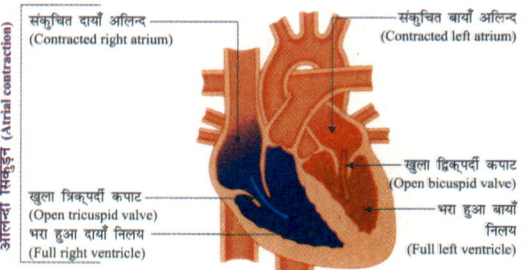
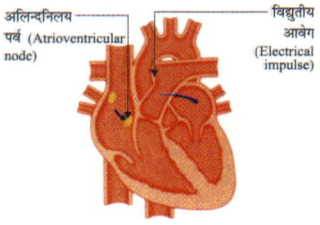

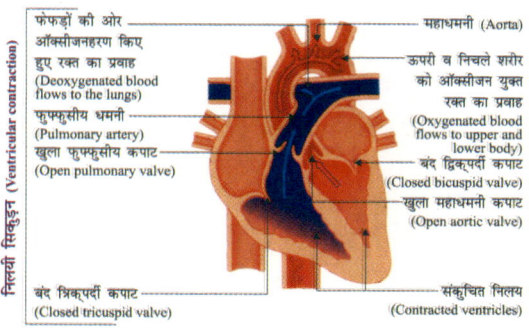
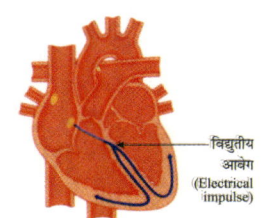

# तंत्रिका तंत्र
## (Nervous system)

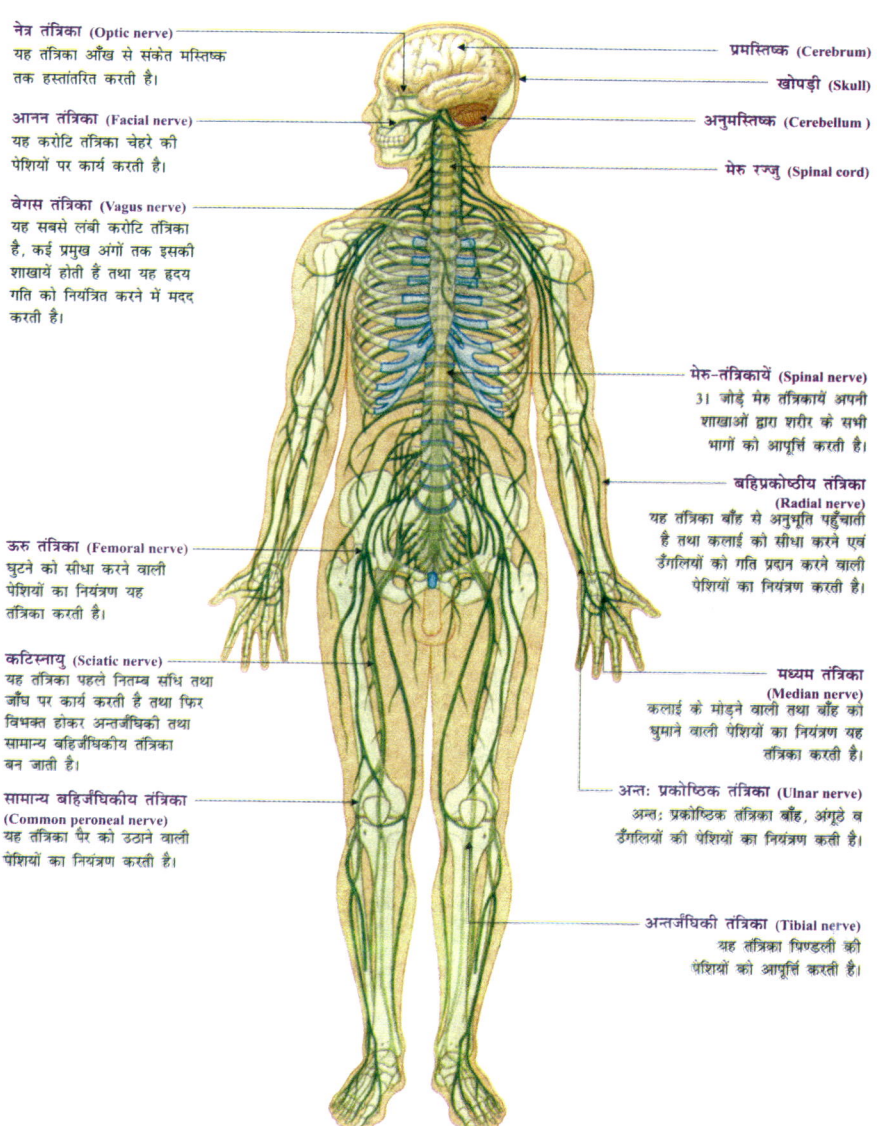

# मस्तिष्क, मेरु रज्जु व तंत्रिकायें
## (Brain, Spinal Cord & Nerves)

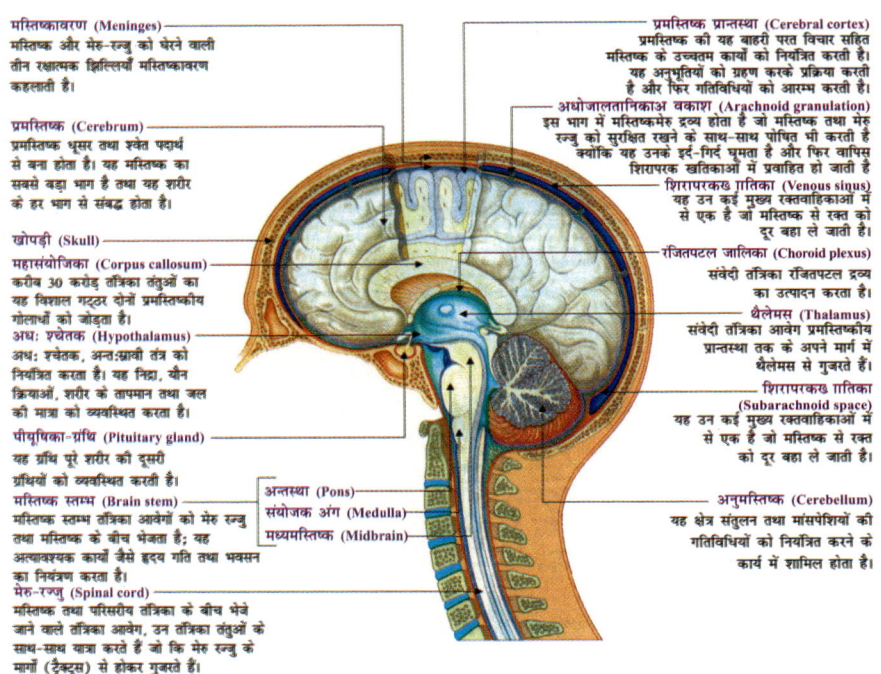

**मस्तिष्कावरण (Meninges)**
मस्तिष्क और मेरु-रज्जु को घेरने वाली तीन रक्षात्मक झिल्लियाँ मस्तिष्कावरण कहलाती है।

**प्रमस्तिष्क (Cerebrum)**
प्रमस्तिष्क धूसर तथा श्वेत पदार्थ से बना होता है। यह मस्तिष्क का सबसे बड़ा भाग है तथा यह शरीर के हर भाग से संबद्ध होता है।

**खोपड़ी (Skull)**

**महासंयोजिका (Corpus callosum)**
करीब 30 करोड़ तंत्रिका तंतुओं का यह विशाल गट्ठर दोनों प्रमस्तिष्कीय गोलार्धों को जोड़ता है।

**अधः श्चेतक (Hypothalamus)**
अधः श्चेतक, अन्तःस्रावी तंत्र को नियंत्रित करता है। यह निद्रा, यौन क्रियाओं, शरीर के तापमान तथा जल की मात्रा को व्यवस्थित करता है।

**पीयूषिका-ग्रंथि (Pituitary gland)**
यह ग्रंथि पूरे शरीर की दूसरी ग्रंथियों को व्यवस्थित करती है।

**मस्तिष्क स्तम्भ (Brain stem)**
मस्तिष्क स्तम्भ तंत्रिका आवेगों को मेरु रज्जु तथा मस्तिष्क के बीच भेजता है; यह अत्यावश्यक कार्यों जैसे हृदय गति तथा श्वसन का नियंत्रण करता है।

**मेरु-रज्जु (Spinal cord)**
मस्तिष्क तथा परिसरीय तंत्रिका के बीच भेजे जाने वाले तंत्रिका आवेग, उन तंत्रिका तंतुओं के साथ-साथ यात्रा करते हैं जो कि मेरु रज्जु के मार्गों (ट्रैक्ट्स) से होकर गुजरते हैं।

**अन्तस्था (Pons)**
**संयोजक अंग (Medulla)**
**मध्यमस्तिष्क (Midbrain)**

**प्रमस्तिष्क प्रान्तस्था (Cerebral cortex)**
प्रमस्तिष्क की यह बाहरी परत विचार सहित मस्तिष्क के उच्चतम कार्यों को नियंत्रित करती है। यह अनुभूतियों को ग्रहण करके प्रक्रिया करती है और फिर गतिविधियों को आरम्भ करती है।

**अधोजालतानिकाअ वकाश (Arachnoid granulation)**
इस भाग में मस्तिष्कमेरु द्रव्य होता है जो मस्तिष्क तथा मेरु रज्जु को सुरक्षित रखने के साथ-साथ पोषित भी करती है क्योंकि यह उनके इर्द-गिर्द घूमता है और फिर वापिस शिरापरक खतिकाओं में प्रवाहित हो जाती है

**शिरापरकछ ातिका (Venous sinus)**
यह उन कई मुख्य रक्तवाहिकाओं में से एक है जो मस्तिष्क से रक्त को दूर बहा ले जाती है।

**रजितपटल जालिका (Choroid plexus)**
संवेदी तंत्रिका रजितपटल द्रव्य का उत्पादन करता है।

**थैलेमस (Thalamus)**
संवेदी तंत्रिका आवेग प्रमस्तिष्कीय प्रान्तस्था तक के अपने मार्ग में थैलेमस से गुजरते हैं।

**शिरापरकछ ातिका (Subarachnoid space)**
यह उन कई मुख्य रक्तवाहिकाओं में से एक है जो मस्तिष्क से रक्त को दूर बहा ले जाती है।

**अनुमस्तिष्क (Cerebellum)**
यह क्षेत्र संतुलन तथा मांसपेशियों की गतिविधियों को नियंत्रित करने के कार्य में शामिल होता है।

# मस्तिष्क
## (Brain)

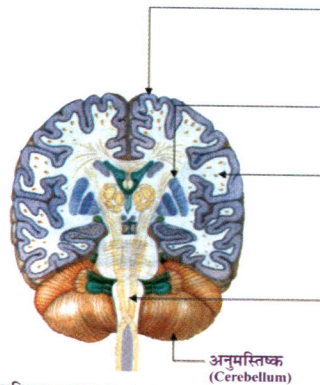

**धूसर पदार्थ (Grey matter)**
धूसर पदार्थ मुख्य रूप से तंत्रिका कोशिकाओं का बना होता है जिनसे तंत्रिका कोशिकाओं का बना होता है जिनसे तंत्रिका आवेग प्रारम्भ होते हैं।

**आधारी गण्डिकायें (Basal ganglia)**
धूसर पदार्थ के ये द्वीप गतिविधियों के समन्वय में मदद करते हैं।

**श्वेत पदार्थ (White matter)**
श्वेत पदार्थ मुख्यत: तंत्रिका तन्तुओं का बना होता है, इसका मुख्य कार्य तंत्रिका आवेगों का सम्प्रेषण करना होता है।

**मस्तिष्क स्तम्भ (Brain stem)**
मुख्य प्रेरक मार्ग, मस्तिष्क स्तम्भ में, मेरु-रज्जु से विपरीत दिशाओं में आर-पार चले जाते हैं।

**अनुमस्तिष्क (Cerebellum)**

**मस्तिष्क ऊतक (Brain tissue)**
मस्तिष्क की बाहरी परत मस्तिष्क प्रान्तस्था, धूसर पदार्थ की बनी होती है। जिसके नीचे श्वेत पदार्थ होता है तथा धूसर पदार्थ के द्वीप होते हैं।

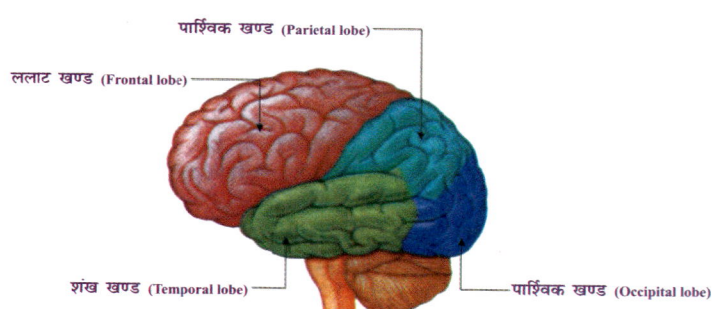

पार्श्विक खण्ड (Parietal lobe)
ललाट खण्ड (Frontal lobe)
शंख खण्ड (Temporal lobe)
पार्श्विक खण्ड (Occipital lobe)

**मस्तिष्क के प्रमुख खण्ड (Major lobes of the brain)**
मस्तिष्क को कई खण्डों में विभाजित किया गया है, जिनके नाम उनको ढाँपने वाली खोपड़ी की हड्डियों के समान है।

# लसीका तंत्र
## (Lymphatic System)

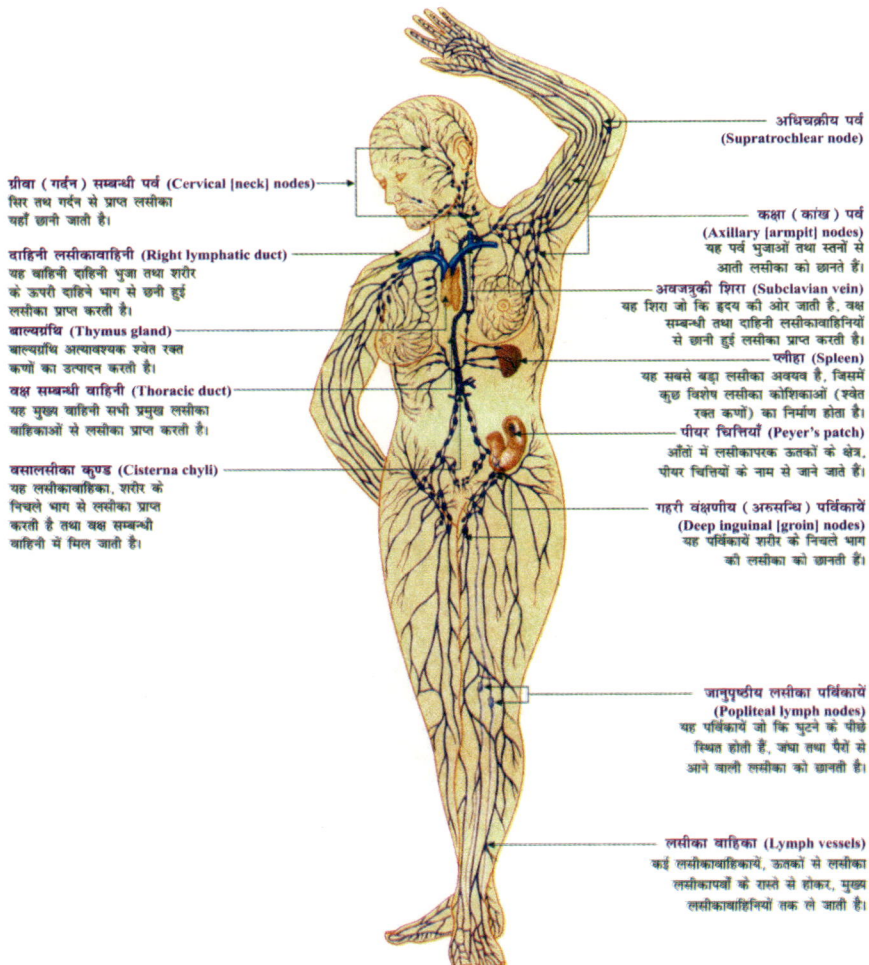

# श्वास तंत्र
## (Respiratory System)

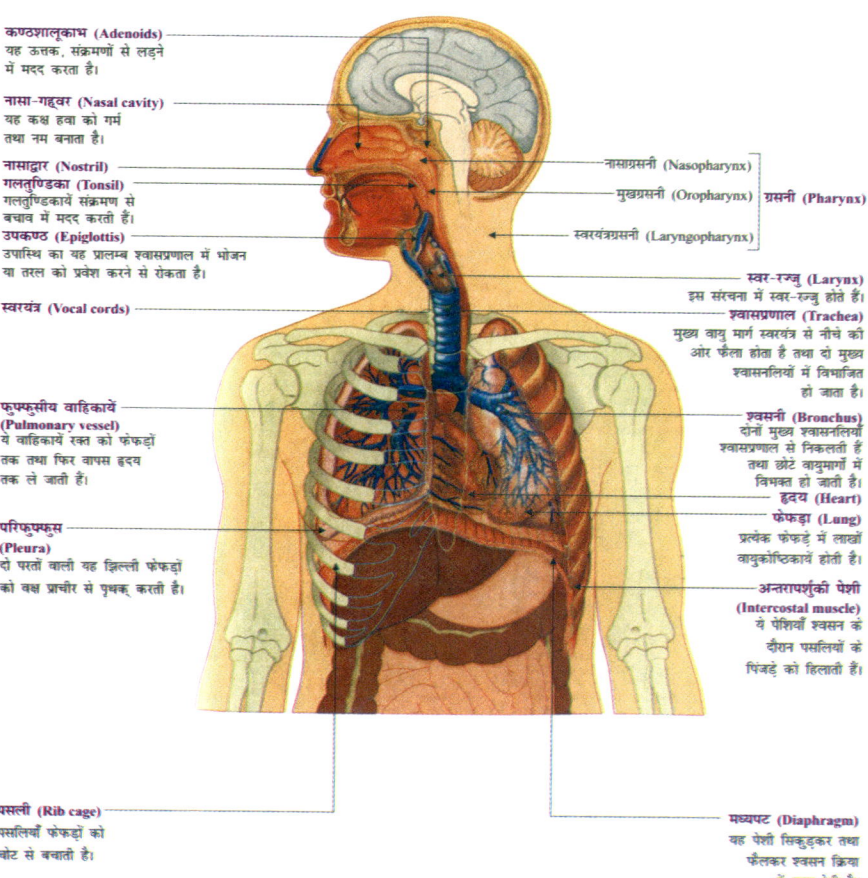

# पाचक तंत्र
## (Digestive System)

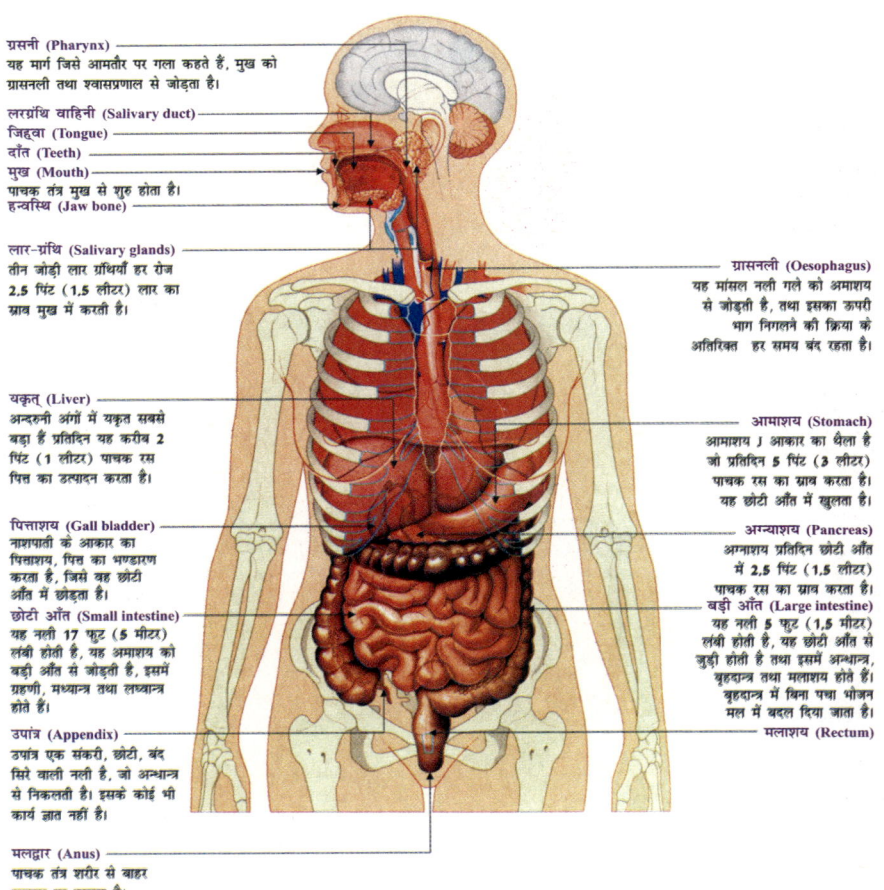

**ग्रसनी (Pharynx)** — यह मार्ग जिसे आमतौर पर गला कहते हैं, मुख को ग्रासनली तथा श्वासप्रणाल से जोड़ता है।

**लरग्रंथि वाहिनी (Salivary duct)**

**जिह्वा (Tongue)**

**दाँत (Teeth)**

**मुख (Mouth)** — पाचक तंत्र मुख से शुरू होता है।

**हन्वस्थि (Jaw bone)**

**लार-ग्रंथि (Salivary glands)** — तीन जोड़ी लार ग्रंथियाँ हर रोज 2.5 पिंट (1.5 लीटर) लार का स्राव मुख में करती हैं।

**यकृत् (Liver)** — अन्दरूनी अंगों में यकृत सबसे बड़ा है प्रतिदिन यह करीब 2 पिंट (1 लीटर) पाचक रस पित्त का उत्पादन करता है।

**पित्ताशय (Gall bladder)** — नाशपाती के आकार का पित्ताशय, पित्त का भण्डारण करता है, जिसे वह छोटी आँत में छोड़ता है।

**छोटी आँत (Small intestine)** — यह नली 17 फुट (5 मीटर) लंबी होती है, यह आमाशय को बड़ी आँत से जोड़ती है, इसमें ग्रहणी, मध्यान्त्र तथा लघ्वान्त्र होते हैं।

**उपांत्र (Appendix)** — उपांत्र एक संकरी, छोटी, बंद सिरे वाली नली है, जो अन्त्रांत्र से निकलती है। इसके कोई भी कार्य ज्ञात नहीं है।

**मलद्वार (Anus)** — पाचक तंत्र शरीर से बाहर मलद्वार पर खुलता है।

**ग्रासनली (Oesophagus)** — यह मांसल नली गले को आमाशय से जोड़ती है, तथा इसका ऊपरी भाग निगलने की क्रिया के अतिरिक्त हर समय बंद रहता है।

**आमाशय (Stomach)** — आमाशय J आकार का थैला है जो प्रतिदिन 5 पिंट (3 लीटर) पाचक रस का स्राव करता है। यह छोटी आँत में खुलता है।

**अग्न्याशय (Pancreas)** — अग्न्याशय प्रतिदिन छोटी आँत में 2.5 पिंट (1.5 लीटर) पाचक रस का स्राव करता है।

**बड़ी आँत (Large intestine)** — यह नली 5 फुट (1.5 मीटर) लंबी होती है, यह छोटी आँत से जुड़ी होती है तथा इसमें अन्धान्त्र, बृहदान्त्र तथा मलाशय होते हैं। बृहदान्त्र में बिना पचा भोजन मल में बदल दिया जाता है।

**मलाशय (Rectum)**

# हॉर्मोन स्रावका ग्रंथियाँ व कोशिकायें
## (Hormone Secreting Glands & Cells)

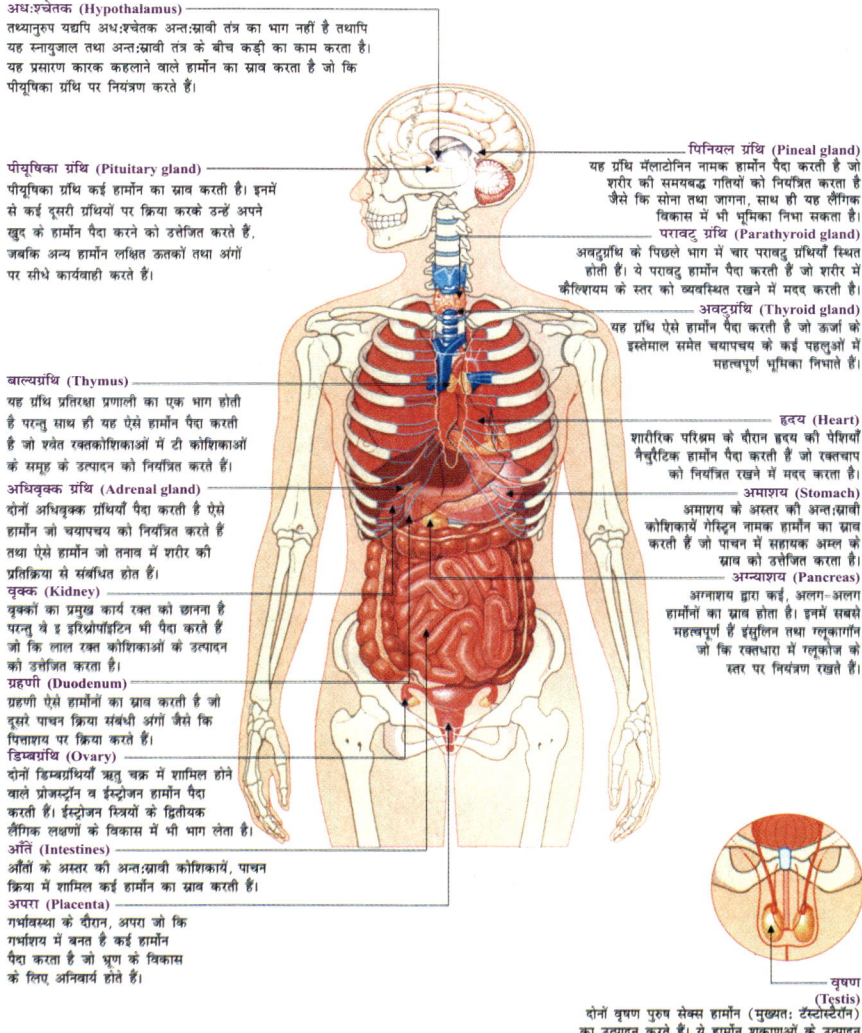

**अध:श्चेतक (Hypothalamus)**
तथ्यानुरुप यद्यपि अध:श्चेतक अन्त:स्रावी तंत्र का भाग नहीं है तथापि यह स्नायुजाल तथा अन्त:स्रावी तंत्र के बीच कड़ी का काम करता है। यह प्रसारण कारक कहलाने वाले हार्मोन का स्राव करता है जो कि पीयूषिका ग्रंथि पर नियंत्रण करते हैं।

**पीयूषिका ग्रंथि (Pituitary gland)**
पीयूषिका ग्रंथि कई हार्मोन का स्राव करती है। इनमें से कई दूसरी ग्रंथियों पर क्रिया करके उन्हें अपने खुद के हार्मोन पैदा करने को उत्तेजित करते हैं, जबकि अन्य हार्मोन लक्षित ऊतकों तथा अंगों पर सीधे कार्यवाही करते हैं।

**बाल्यग्रंथि (Thymus)**
यह ग्रंथि प्रतिरक्षा प्रणाली का एक भाग होती है परन्तु साथ ही यह ऐसे हार्मोन पैदा करती है जो श्वेत रक्तकोशिकाओं में टी कोशिकाओं के समूह के उत्पादन को नियंत्रित करते हैं।

**अधिवृक्क ग्रंथि (Adrenal gland)**
दोनों अधिवृक्क ग्रंथियाँ पैदा करती हैं ऐसे हार्मोन जो चयापचय को नियंत्रित करते हैं तथा ऐसे हार्मोन जो तनाव में शरीर की प्रतिक्रिया से संबन्धित होते हैं।

**वृक्क (Kidney)**
वृक्कों का प्रमुख कार्य रक्त को छानना है परन्तु वे इ इरिश्रोपॉइटिन भी पैदा करते हैं जो कि लाल रक्त कोशिकाओं के उत्पादन को उत्तेजित करते हैं।

**ग्रहणी (Duodenum)**
ग्रहणी ऐसे हार्मोनों का स्राव करती है जी दूसरे पाचन क्रिया संबंधित अंगों जैसे कि पित्ताशय पर क्रिया करते हैं।

**डिम्बग्रंथि (Ovary)**
दोनों डिम्बग्रंथियाँ ऋतु चक्र में शामिल होने वाले प्रोजस्टन व ईस्ट्रोजन हार्मोन पैदा करती हैं। ईस्ट्रोजन स्त्रियों के द्वितीयक लैंगिक लक्षणों के विकास में भी भाग लेता है।

**आंतें (Intestines)**
आंतों के अस्तर की अन्त:स्रावी कोशिकायें, पाचन क्रिया में शामिल कई हार्मोन का स्राव करती हैं।

**अपरा (Placenta)**
गर्भावस्था के दौरान, अपरा जो कि गर्भाशय में बनता है कई हार्मोन पैदा करता है जो भ्रूण के विकास के लिए अनिवार्य होते हैं।

**पिनियल ग्रंथि (Pineal gland)**
यह ग्रंथि मेलाटोनिन नामक हार्मोन पैदा करती है जो शरीर की समयबद्ध गतियों को नियंत्रित करता है जैसे कि सोना तथा जागना, साथ ही यह लैंगिक विकास में भी भूमिका निभा सकता है।

**परावटु ग्रंथि (Parathyroid gland)**
अवटुग्रंथि के पिछले भाग में चार परावटु ग्रंथियाँ स्थित होती हैं। ये परावटु हार्मोन पैदा करती हैं जो शरीर में कैल्शियम के स्तर को व्यवस्थित रखने में मदद करती हैं।

**अवटुग्रंथि (Thyroid gland)**
यह ग्रंथि ऐसे हार्मोन पैदा करती है जो ऊर्जा के इस्तेमाल समेत चयापचय के कई पहलुओं में महत्त्वपूर्ण भूमिका निभाते हैं।

**हृदय (Heart)**
शारीरिक परिश्रम के दौरान हृदय की पेशियाँ नैचुरेटिक हार्मोन पैदा करती हैं जो रक्तचाप को नियंत्रित रखने में मदद करता है।

**आमाशय (Stomach)**
आमाशय के अस्तर की अन्त:स्रावी कोशिकायें गेस्ट्रिन नामक हार्मोन का स्राव करती हैं जो पाचन में सहायक अम्ल के स्राव को उत्तेजित करता है।

**अग्नाशय (Pancreas)**
अग्नाशय द्वारा कई, अलग-अलग हार्मोनों का स्राव होता है। इनमें सबसे महत्त्वपूर्ण हैं इंसुलिन तथा ग्लूकागॉन जो कि रक्तधारा में ग्लूकोज के स्तर पर नियंत्रण रखते हैं।

**वृषण (Testis)**
दोनों वृषण पुरुष सेक्स हार्मोन (मुख्यत: टेस्टोस्टेरॉन) का उत्पादन करते हैं। ये हार्मोन शुक्राणुओं के उत्पादन को उत्तेजित करते हैं तथा पुरुषों के द्वितीयक लैंगिक लक्षणों का विकास करते हैं।

# वृक्क
## (Kidney)

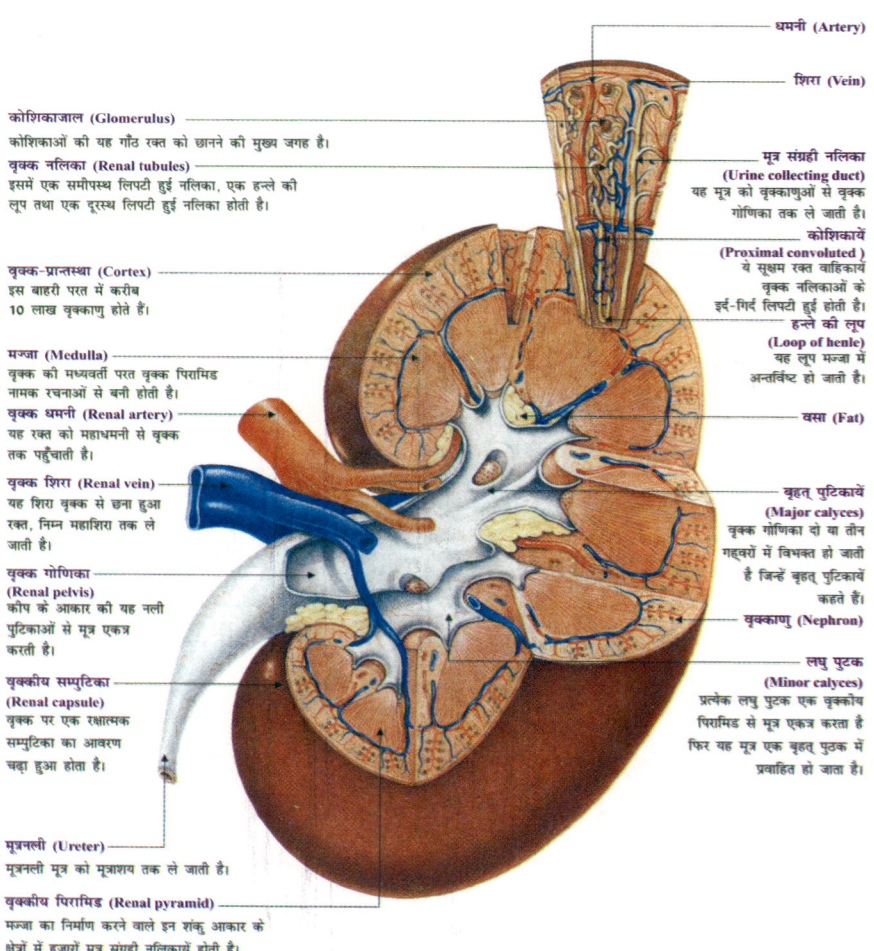

# मूत्र तंत्र
## (Urinary System)

**निम्न महाशिरा (Inferior vena cava)**
यह शिरा शरीर के निचले भाग से खून
लेकर हृदय तक वापिस पहुँचाती है।

**वृक्क धमनी (Renal artery)**
यह महाधमनी की सीधी शाखा
है तथा वृक्क को शुद्ध
धमनि रक्त देती है।

**अधिवृक्क ग्रंथि (संपूर्ण)**
**(Adrenal gland [whole])**
प्रत्येक वृक्क के ऊपर को ओर एक
अधिवृक्क ग्रंथि होती है, जो हार्मोन
का स्राव करता है।

**वृक्क (संपूर्ण) (Kidney [whole])**
शरीर के दाहिने भाग का वृक्क,
बाएँ आर के वृक्क की अपेक्षा
थोड़ा नीचे होता है।

**वृक्क शिरा (Renal vein)**
यह शिरा वृक्क में खून
को निम्न महाशिरा तक
ले जाती है।

**उदरावरण (Peritoneum)**
यह झिल्ली, जिसका यहाँ केवल
एक भाग दिख रहा है, उदर में
अस्तर की तरह ढका है तथा
मूत्राशय की सतह का
ढँकती है।

**मूत्रनली का छिद्र**
**(Opening of ureter)**
यह छिद्र मूत्रनली में मूत्र के
उल्टे बहाव को रोकने में
कपाट का काम करता है।

**मूत्राशय निकास**
**(Bladder outlet)**
मूत्राशय को नीचे के स्थान
जिससे मूत्र का निकास का
निकास होता है।

**पौरुष ग्रंथि**
**(Prostate gland)**
पुरुष में मूत्र पथ चारों ओर
से घेरकर स्थित होती यह
वाहिछिद्रा ग्रंथि है, जिसका
स्राव शुक्राणु का पोषण करता है।

**पुरुष में मूत्र पथ (Male urethra)**
पुरुष में मूत्रमार्ग वृक्षाशय से लिंग
के सिरे तक होता है।

**महाधमनी (Aorta)**
यह शरीर रक्त को हृदय से
हर अंग में ले जाती है।

**अधिवृक्क ग्रंथि (लंबवत् काट)**
**(Adrenal gland [cross section])**

**वृक्क (लंबवत्)**
**(Kidney [cross section])**

**वृक्क-गोणिका (Renal pelvis)**

**वृक्क-प्रान्तस्था**
**(Cortex of the kidney)**
**वृक्क-मज्जा**
**(Medulla of the kidney)**
**मूत्रनली (Ureter)**
प्रत्येक वृक्क से एक मूत्रनली
निकलती है जाकर मूत्र को
मूत्राशय तक पहुँचाती है।

**मूत्राशय**
**(Urinary bladder)**
मूत्र मूत्राशय में एकत्र
होता है, जिसकी भीतरी
मांसल प्राचीर होती है।

**मूत्रनली (Ureter)**
**मूत्रमार्ग (Urethra)**
**मूत्राशय (Bladder)**

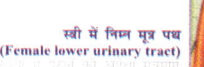

**स्त्री में निम्न मूत्र पथ**
**(Female lower urinary tract)**

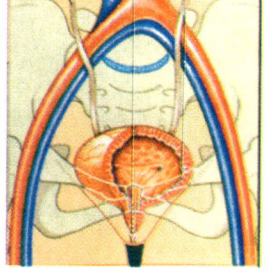

# पुरुष जनन तंत्र
## (Male Reproductive System)

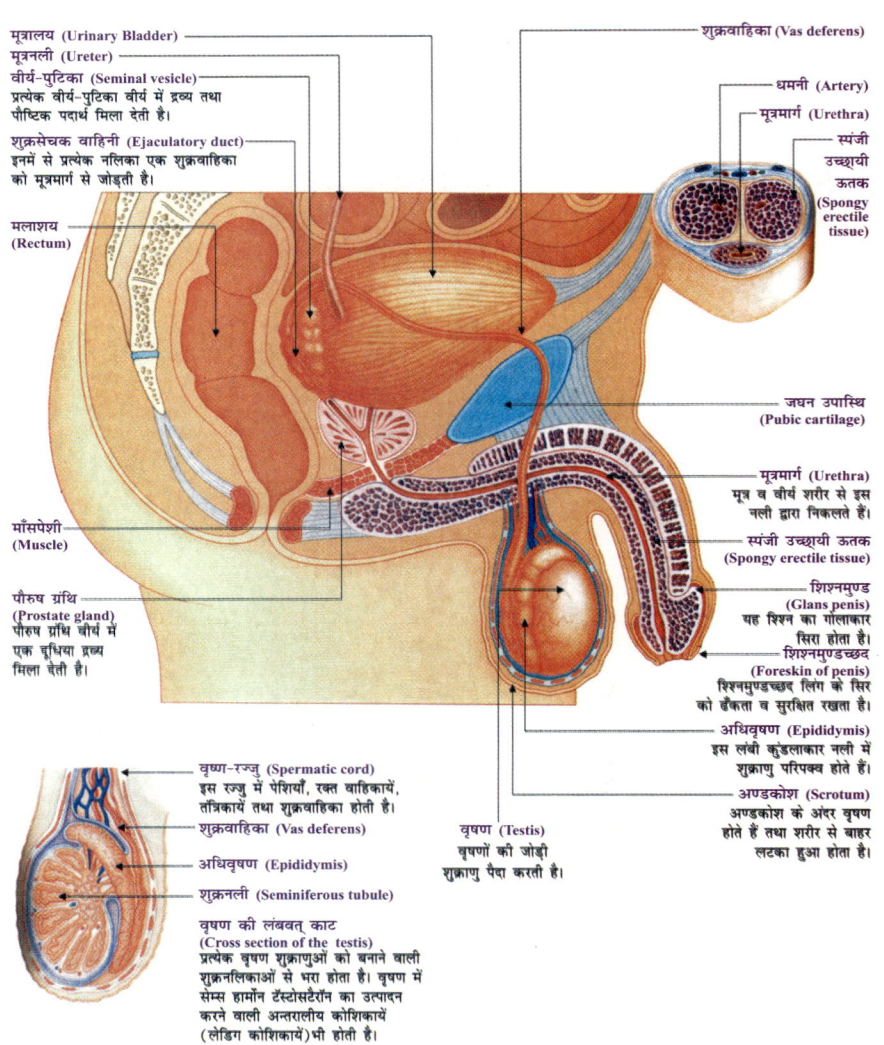

# स्त्री जनन तंत्र
## (Female Reproductive System)

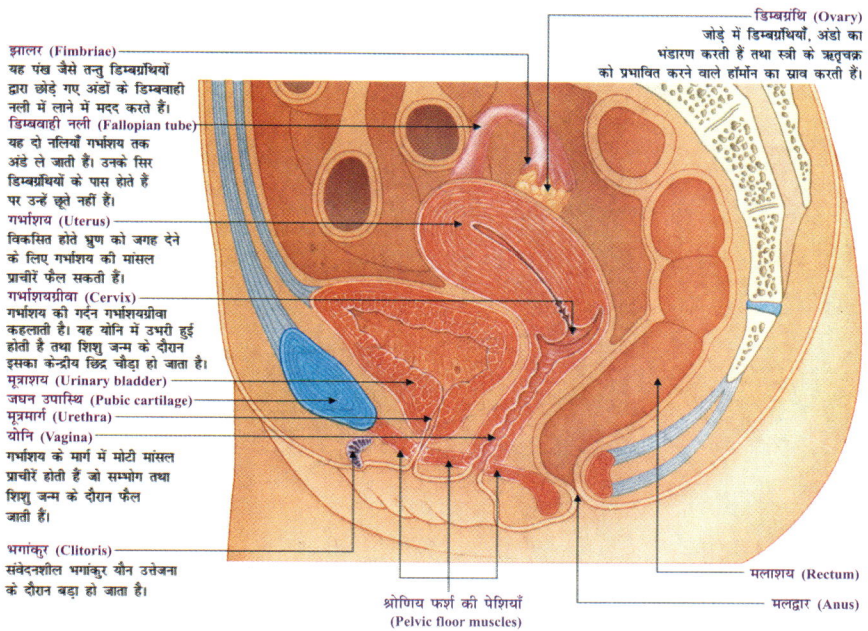

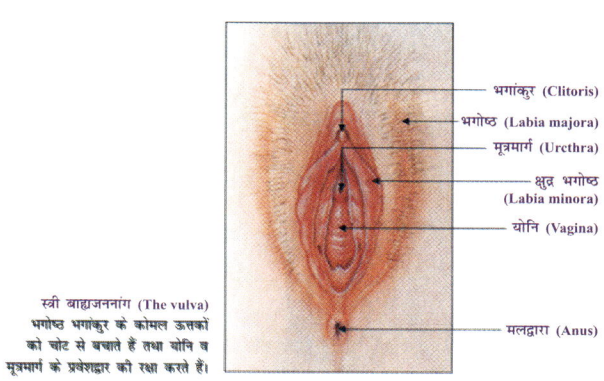

13

# आँख की संरचना
## (Structure of Eye)

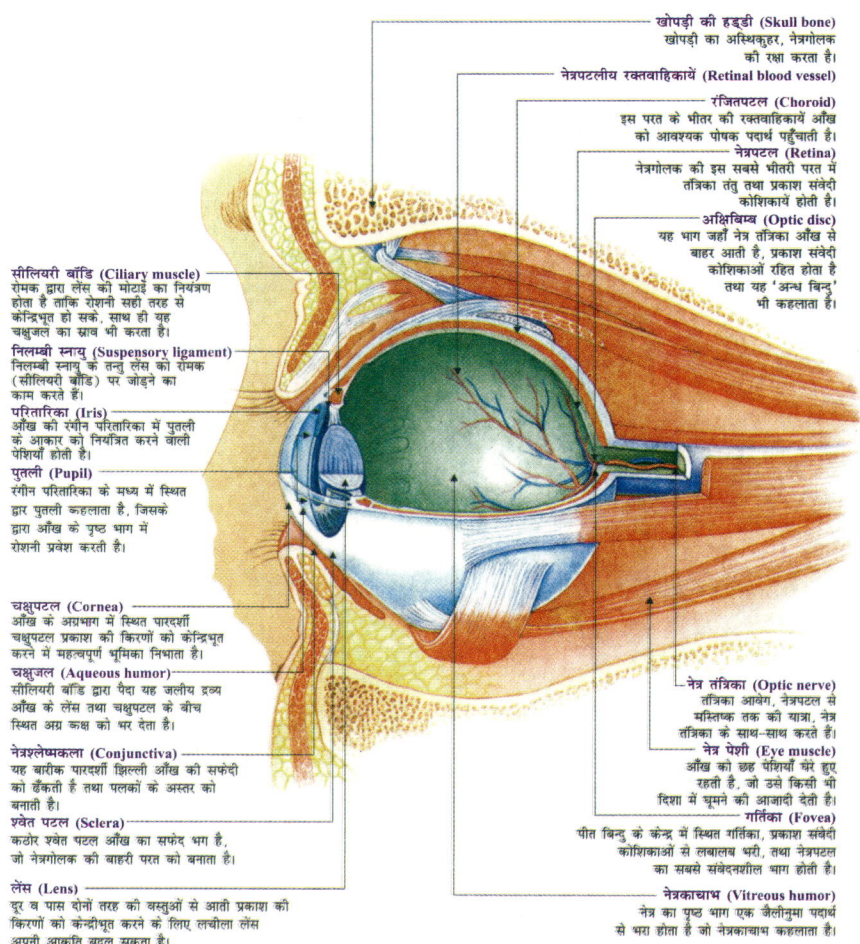

# कान के अवयव
## (Structure of Ear)

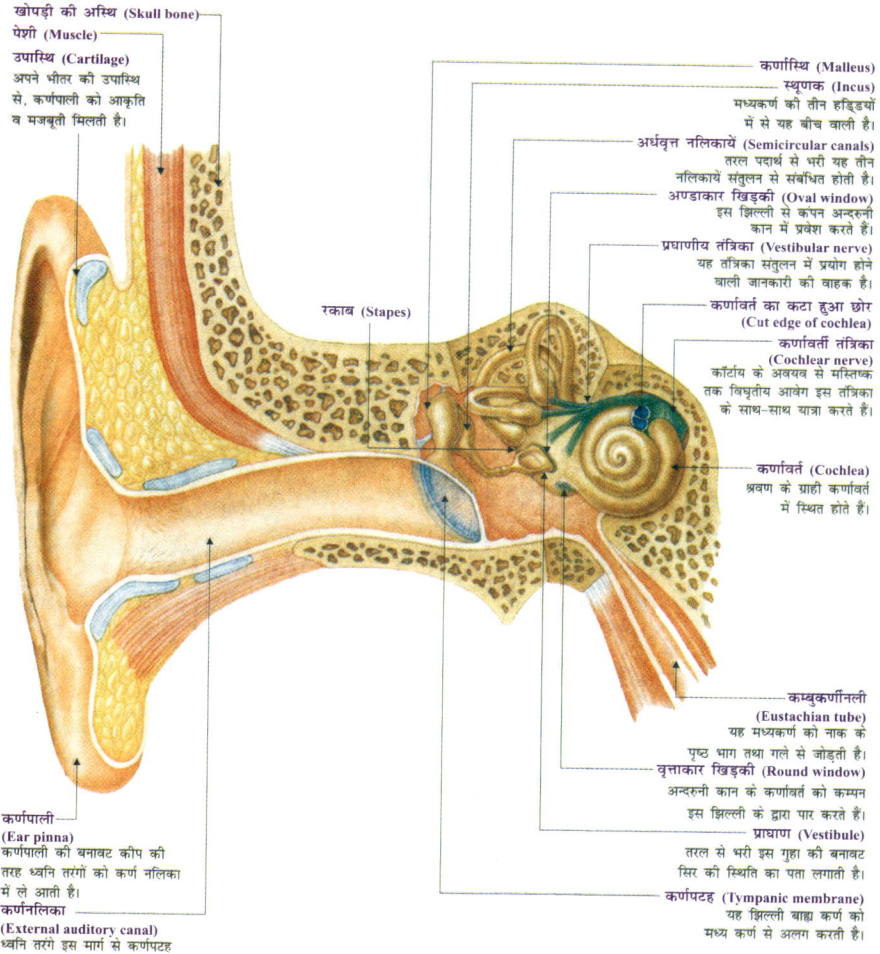

# दाँत व मसूढ़े
## (Teeth & Gums)

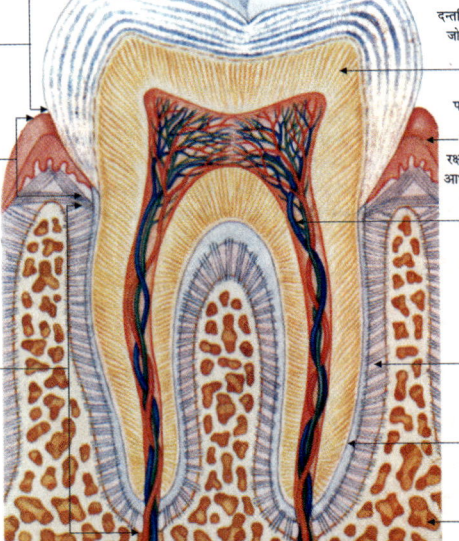

**दन्तवल्क (Enamel)**
दन्तशिखर पर दन्तवल्क की परत होती है, जो कि एक संवेदनहीन, निर्जीवपदार्थ है।

**शिखर (Crown)**
शिखर दाँत का वह भाग है जे कि मसूढ़ों की रेखा से ऊपर दिखाई देता है।

**दन्तधातु (Dentine)**
दन्तधातु हाथी दाँत जैसा एक कठोर पदार्थ है जिसे मज्जा ऊतकों से रक्त व तंत्रिकाओं की आपूर्ति होती है।

**मसूढ़ा (मसूड़ा) (Gum [gingiva])**
रक्षात्मक ऊतकों की यह परत शिखर के आधार के इर्द-गिर्द कसकर जम होती है तथा दाँत की जड़ों को ढँकती है।

**गर्दन (Neck)**
गर्दन दाँत का वह भाग है जो कि मसूढ़ों की रेखा पर थोड़ा सा सँकड़ा हो जाता है।

**मज्जा (Pulp)**
एक दाँत के केन्द्र में नरम मज्जा ऊत्तक होता है जिसमें तंत्रिकायें तथा रक्त वहिकायें होती हैं।

**परिदन्तीय स्नायु (Periodontal ligament)**
यह स्नायु दाँत को जबड़े की हड्डी तथा मसूढ़ों से जोड़ता है।

**जड़ (Root)**
जड़ हन्वस्थि में गढ़े हुए दाँत का लम्बा नुकीला भाग होती है; कृन्तक तथा रदनक में एक जड़ होती है, अग्रचवर्णक में एक या दो तथा चवर्णक में तीन या चार जड़ें होती हैं।

**दन्तबज्र (Cementum)**
सख्त ऊतक की यह परत जड़ को ढँकती है तथा परिदन्तीय स्नायु के तन्तुओं को स्थिरता प्रदान करती है।

**हन्वस्थि (Jaw bone)**
दाँत की जड़ें हन्वस्थि के गहरे गर्त में बन्द रहती है।

**तंत्रिका (Nerve)**
तंत्रिका परिदन्तीय स्नायु, मज्जा, मसूढ़ों तथा जबड़े को आपूर्ति करती है।

**रक्तवाहिनी (Blood vessels)**
यह रक्त वाहिकायें मज्जा ऊतक, अस्थि तथा मसूढ़ों तक पौष्टिक पदार्थ पहुँचाती है।

**तंत्रिका (Blood vessels)**
तंत्रिका परिदन्तीय स्नायु, मज्जा, मसूढ़ों तथा जबड़े को आपूर्ति करती है।

 **कृन्तक (Incisor)**
मुख के अग्रभाग में स्थित धारदार छेनी जैसी कृन्तक भोजन को काटने व पकड़ते हैं।

**रदनक (Canine)**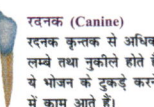
रदनक कृन्तक से अधिक लम्बे तथा नुकीले होते हैं ये भोजन के टुकड़े करने में काम आते हैं।

**अग्रचवर्णक (Premolar)**
अग्रचवर्णक में काटने की सतह पर दो दन्तशिखर होते हैं जो कि भोजन को पीसने का काम करते हैं।

**चवर्णक (Molar)**
सबसे लम्बे दाँत चवर्णक पीसने के काम आते हैं। उनकी चबाने की सतह पर पाँच व छह दन्तशिखर होते हैं।

# त्वचा और बाल
## (Skin & Hair)

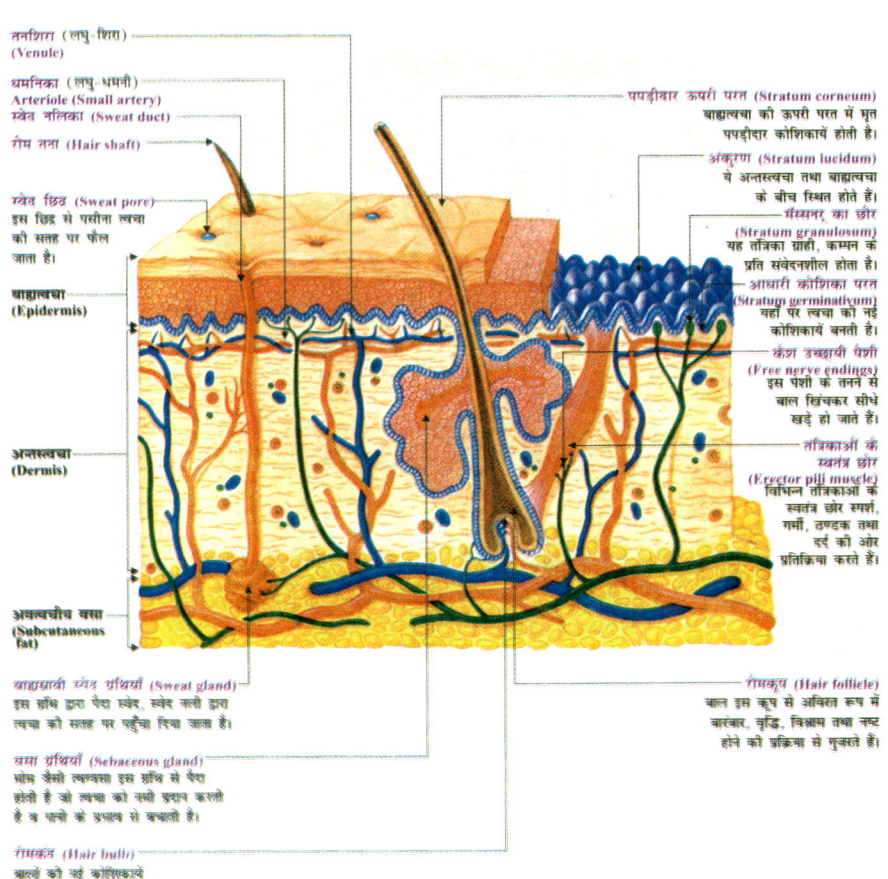

# गर्भावस्था
## (Pregnancy)

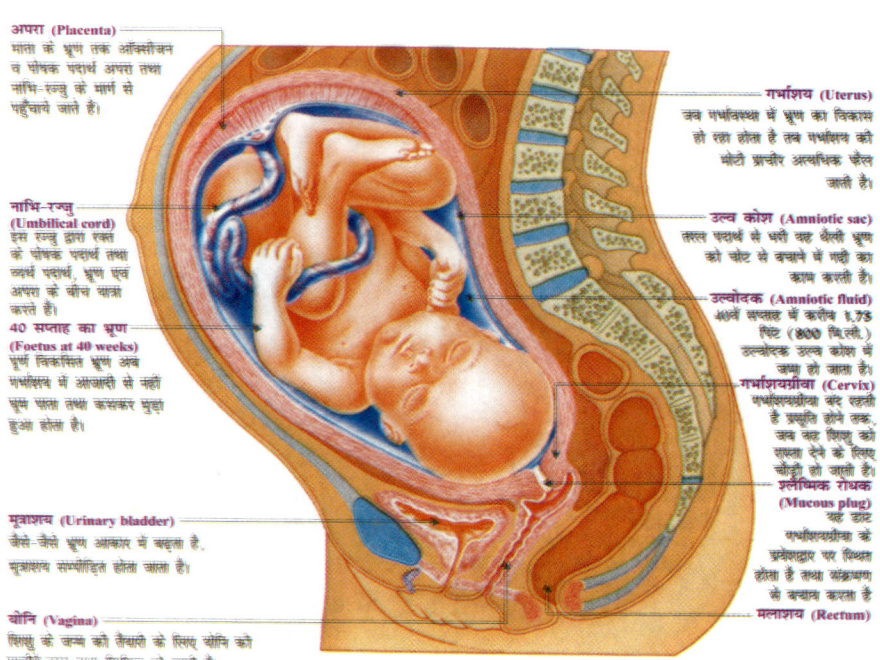

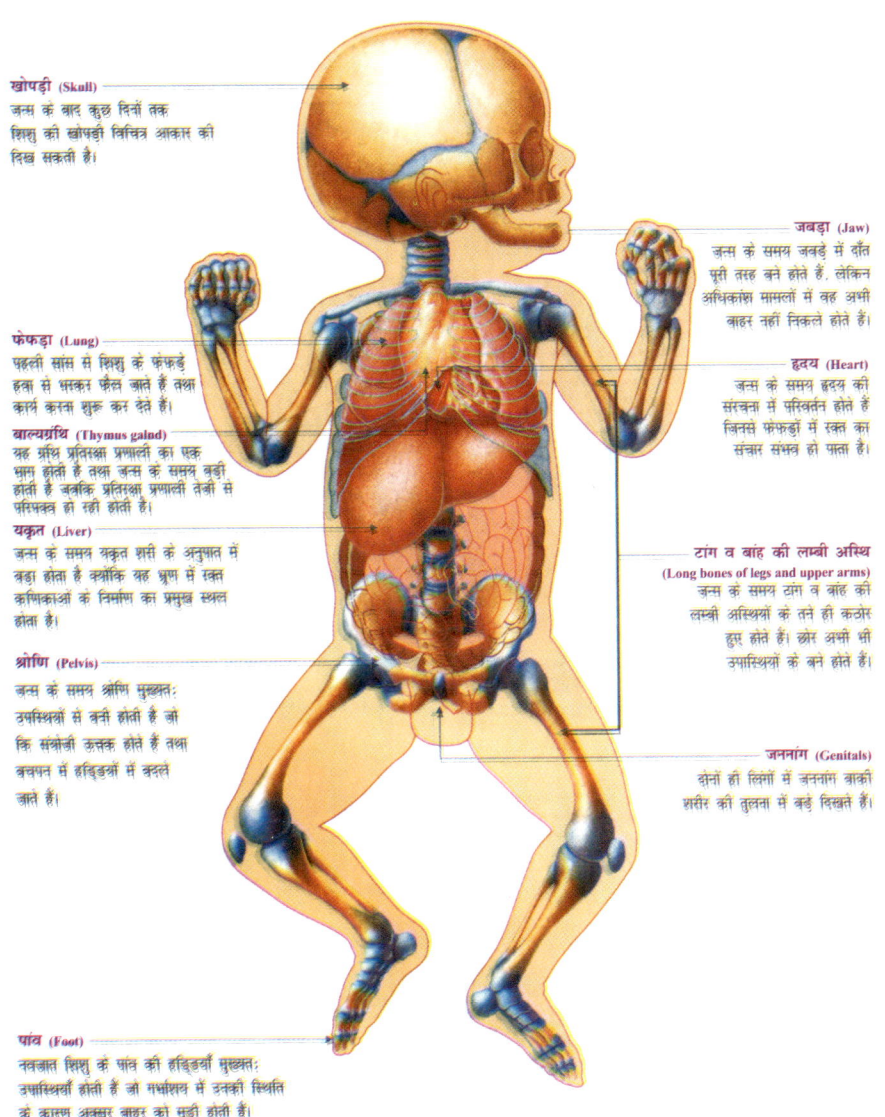# नवजात शिशु
(The Newborn Baby)

# कंकालीय तंत्र
## (Skeletal System)

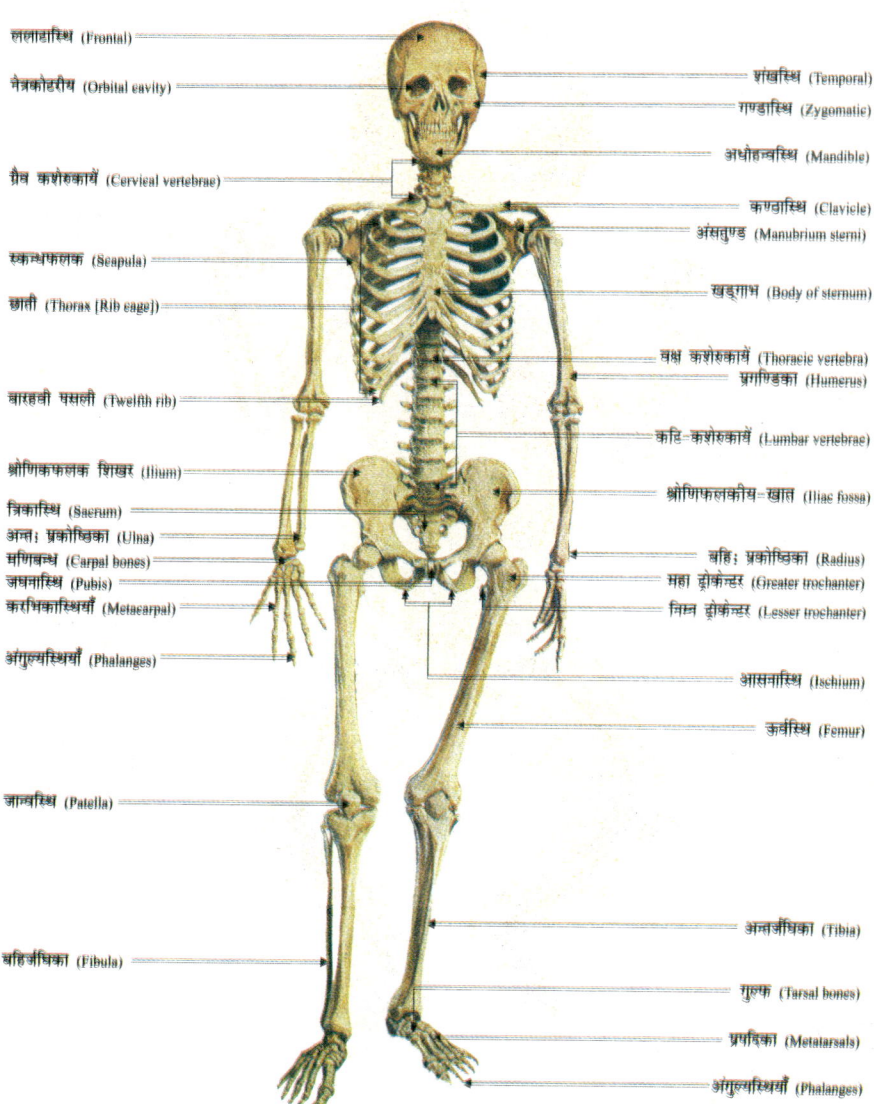

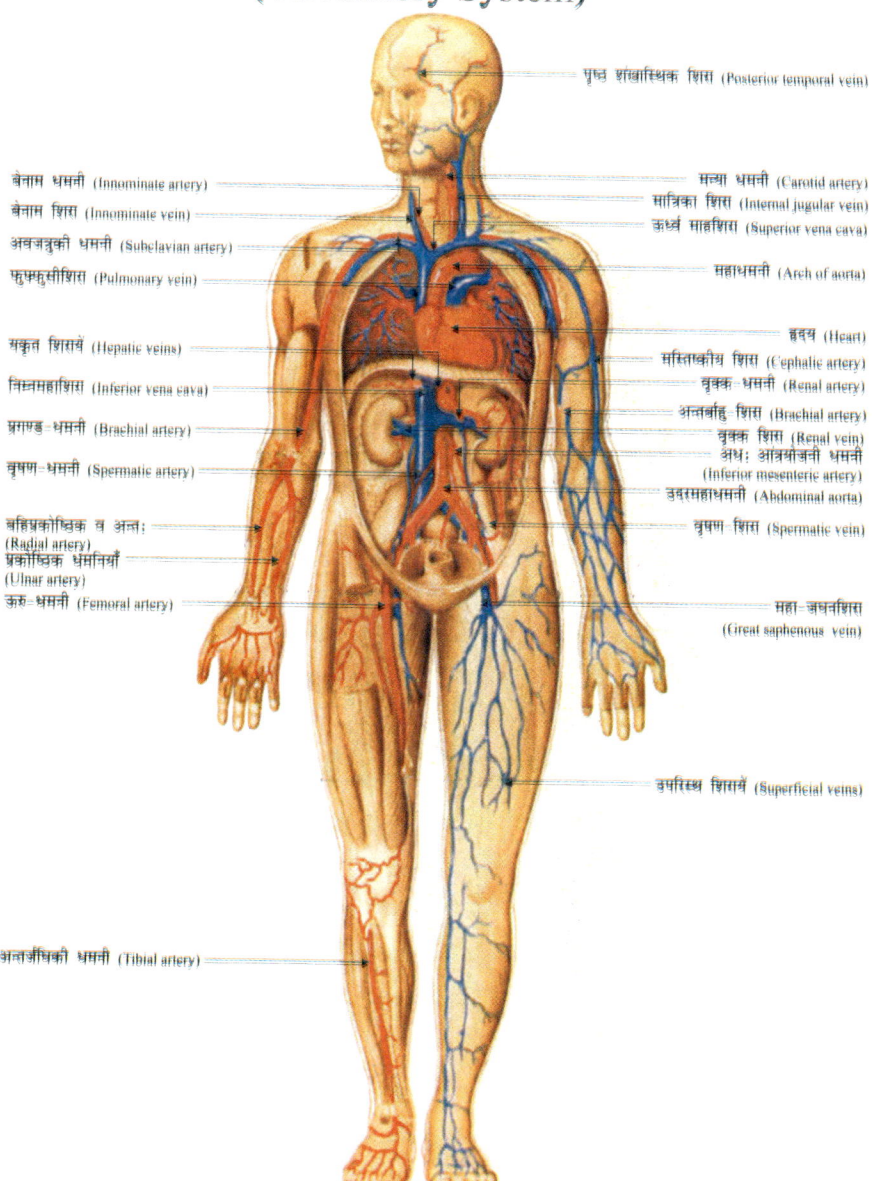

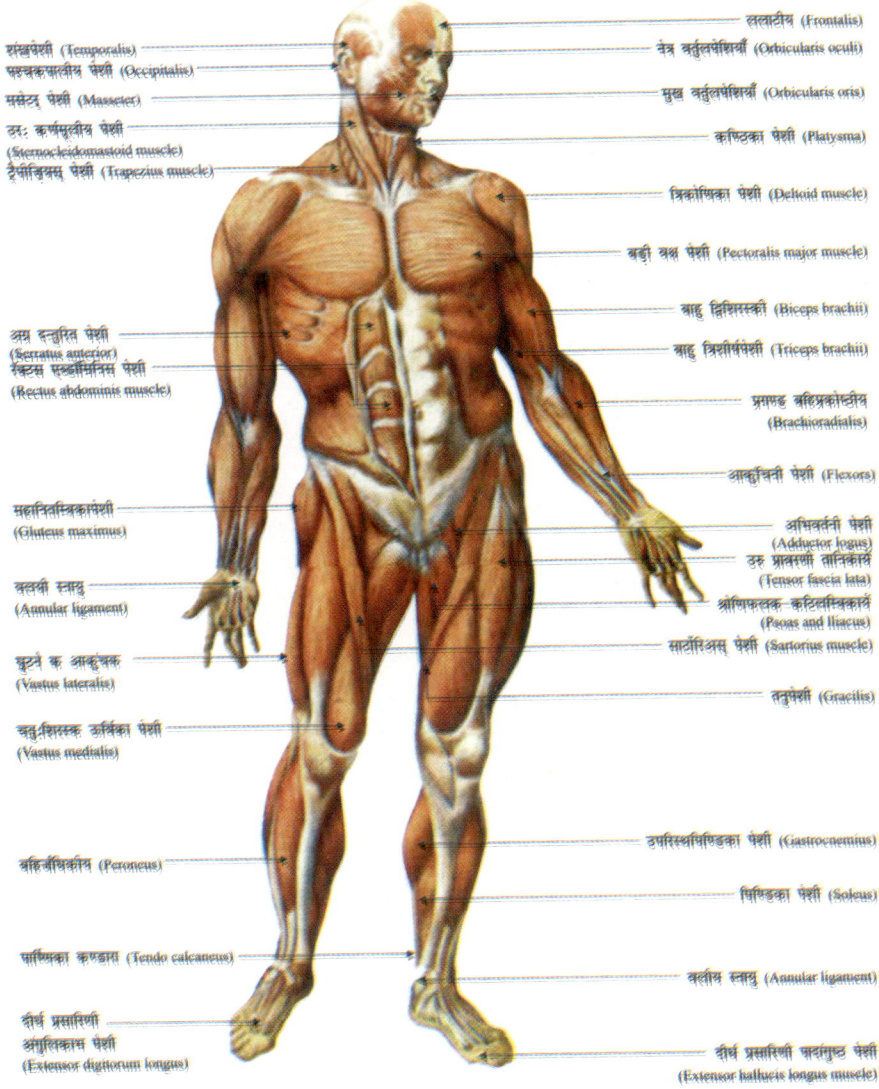

## कपालीय अस्थियाँ (Cranial Bones)

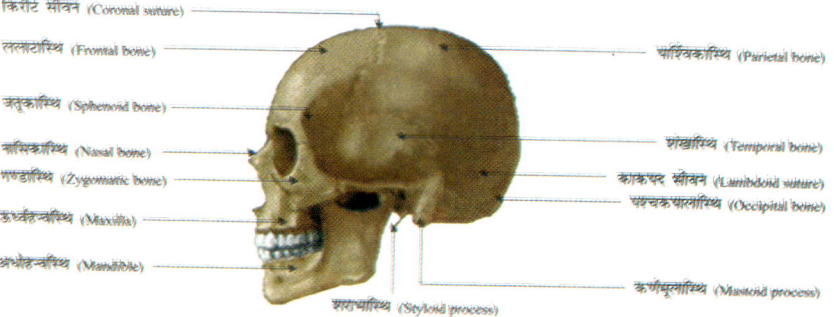

## हाथ की अस्थियाँ (Bones of Hand)

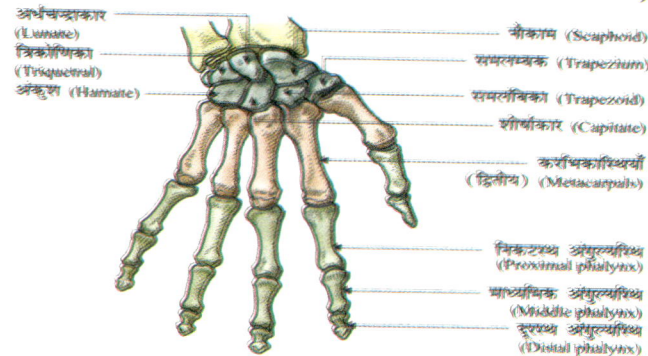

## पैर की अस्थियाँ (Bones of Foot)

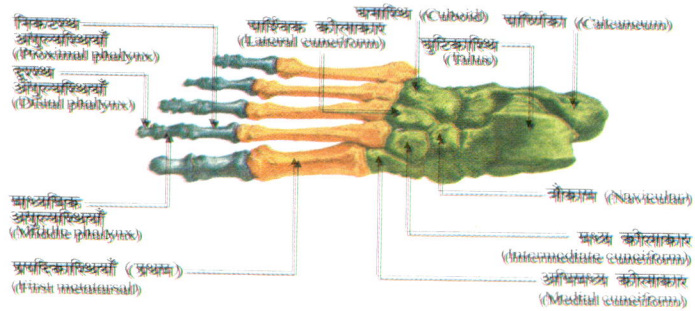

# श्रोणि तथा निम्नांग
## (Lower Limb)

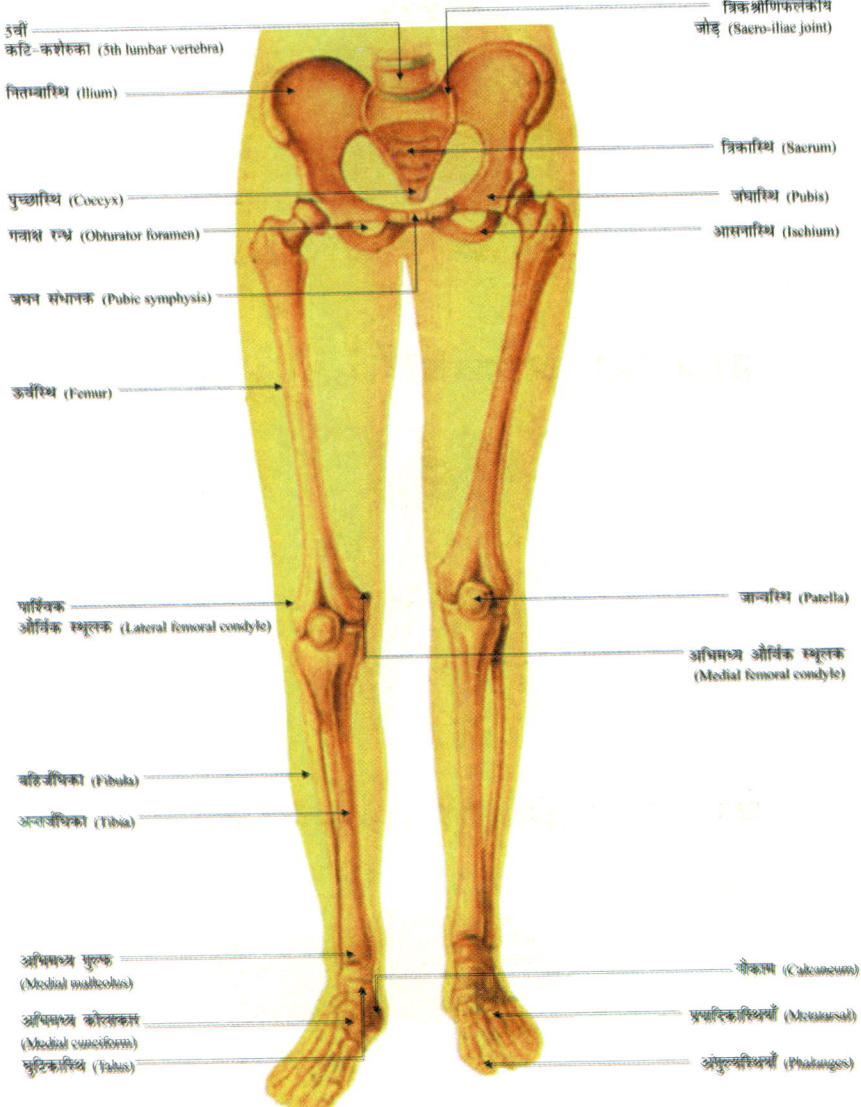

# MIDLINE MEDICAL DICTIONARY

## A

**A-.** Prefix meaning want, or absence of. अभावसूचक उपसर्ग 'अ'

**aa.** Contraction of Greek ana, of each; a term used in prescription, meaning the stated amount of each of the substance to be used in compounding. 'प्रत्येक' का संक्षिप्त रूप, जो नुस्खे में बहुतायत से प्रयुक्त किया जाता है

**Ab-.** Prefix meaning from or away from. 'से' अथवा 'से दूर' के अर्थ में व्यवहृत होने वाला उपसर्ग

**Abacterial.** Without bacteria. अजीवाणुक; जीवाणुहीन; बैक्टीरियाहीन; बिना बैक्टीरिया के; a word used to describe a condition, for instance inflammation, not caused by becteria. एक ऐसा शब्द जो किसी अवस्था का बोध कराता है; उदाहरण के लिये ऐसा शब्द है: 'प्रदाह' अथवा 'शोथ' जिसकी उत्पत्ति जीवाणु द्वारा नहीं होती

**Abactio.** Artificial abortion; Abactus venter. गर्भशातन; प्रचोरित गर्भपात; कृत्रिम गर्भपात

**Abactus Venter.** See **Abactio**.

**Abaissement.** Depression; despondency. विषाद; उदासी

**Abalienation.** Physical or mental decay. शारीरिक अथवा मानसिक शक्ति का ह्रास

**Abalienation mentis.** The mental abalienation. मानसिक विपथन; मनोभ्रंश; मूढ़चित्तता

**Abalone.** A shell known as sea-ear from which the mother of pearl is obtained. कर्णशुक्ति; कनसीपी; मोती का सीप

**Abandon.** To give up to another's control; to forsake. परित्याग करना; परित्यजन करना; छोड़ देना

**Abandoned.** Deserted. परित्यक्त; छोड़ा हुआ; very wicked. दुश्चरित्र; बुरे व्यसनों (आचरण) वाला; अति दुष्ट

**Abandonment.** Renunciation of a claim. परित्याग; परित्यजन; self-surrender. आत्मसमर्पण

**Abanet.** Girdle-shaped bandage. कमरबन्द के आकार जैसी पट्टी या बन्धन; कमरबंद पट्टी

# Abaptiston

**Abaptiston.** A small instrument or saw for the perforation of the skull or cutting out a bone therefrom. करोटि-उच्छेदक; कपालकर्तकयंत्र

**Abarthrosis.** A freely movable joint. चलसन्धि; उन्मुक्त रूप से आगे-पीछे हिलने वाला जोड़

**Abarticular.** Remote from a joint. सन्धिच्युत; किसी सन्धि से दूर; किसी सन्धि से अलग

**Abarticulation.** Dislocation. स्थानच्युति; अपने स्थान से हट जाना; चलसन्धिता

**Abashed.** Ashamed. लज्जित; शर्मिन्दा

**Abasia.** Motor incoordination in walking; want of motor coordination. चलन-अक्षमता; प्रेरक समंजन का अभाव; गति-असमर्थता; गतिभंग;

   **Atactic A.,** see **Abasia Atactica.**

   **Ataxic A.,** see **Abasia Atactica.**

   **Choreic A.,** abasia due to chorea. लास्यज चलन-अक्षमता; नर्तन रोग के कारण चलने-फिरने की अक्षमता;

   **Paralytic A.,** see **Abasia Paralytica.**

   **Spastic A.,** abasia due to rigidity of legs. संस्तम्भी चलन-अक्षमता; टांगों की कठोरता के कारण चलने-फिरने की असमर्थता;

   **Trembling A.,** abasia due to trembling of legs. पदकम्प चलन-अक्षमता; टांगों की कम्पन के कारण चलने-फिरने की असमर्थता;

   **A. Astasia,** loss of standing or walking power. खड़ा रहने या चलने फिरने की अक्षमता;

   **A. Atactica,** abasia distinguished from uncertainty of movement; atactic abasia; ataxic abasia. गतिविभ्रमी चलन-अक्षमता;

   **A. Paralytica,** paralytic abasia; inability to move leg-muscles on account of paralysis. पक्षाघाती (घातज) चलन-अक्षमता; लकवाग्रस्त होने के कारण चलने-फिरने की असमर्थता

**Abasic.** Pertaining to, or denoting abasia; abatic. चलन-अक्षमता सम्बन्धी अथवा चलन-अक्षम

**Abatardissement.** Deterioration of race or breed. जाति अथवा वंश की अपकृष्टता अथवा उसका विनाश

**Abate.** To do away with. उपशमन करना; मुक्त करना

**Abatement.** Decrease of pain or disease. उपशमन; उपशम; ह्रास; दर्द या रोग में आराम या कमी

**Abater.** The palliative agent. उपशामक; आरामदायक पदार्थ

**Abatic.** See **Abasic.**

**Abattoir.** A slaughter house. वधशाला; बूचड़खाना; कसाईखाना

**Abaxial.** Not situated in the axis of the body; abaxile. अपाक्ष; अक्ष-प्रतिमुख; अपाक्षी; शरीर के अक्ष से दूर

**Abaxile.** See **Abaxial.**

**Abbe's Condenser.** A system of lens attached to a microscope for condesing the light upon an object; Abbe's illuminator. अनुवीक्षणयंत्रलेंस; सूक्ष्मदर्शीयंत्र में लगाये जाने वाले परकाले या लेंस, जिनकी सहायता से निर्दिष्ट बिन्दु या वस्तु पर प्रकाश केन्द्रीभूत किया जाता है

**Abbe's Illuminator.** See **Abbe's Condenser.**

**Abbreviation.** Shortening. संक्षेप; संक्षिप्त; छोटा रूप

**Abd.** Abbreviation for Abdomen; abdom. 'उदर', 'पेट', 'कुक्षि', 'जठर', 'उदर-गह्वर' के लिये प्रयुक्त किया जाने वाला संक्षिप्त शब्द

**Abdicate.** To renounce formally or by fault. परित्याग करना; अपत्याग करना; छोड़ देना

**Abdom.** See **Abd.**

**Abdomen.** The belly; the cavity in the body between the thorax and the pelvis. उदर; कुक्षि; जठर; पेट; वक्ष एवं वस्ति का मध्यवर्ती भाग; उदर-गह्वर;

   **Acute A.,** any severe condition within the abdomen needing immediate surgery; surgical abdomen. तीव्र उदर; पेट का ऐसा कोई उग्र रोग जिसमें तुरन्त शल्य चिकित्सा की आवश्यकता पड़ जाती है;

   **Boat-shaped A.,** see **Scaphoid Abdomen.**

   **Navicular A.,** see **Scaphoid Abdomen.**

   **Pendulous A.,** a relaxed condition of the abdominal walls. विलम्बित उदर; उदर-प्राचीरों की ढीली-ढाली अवस्था;

   **Scaphoid A.,** a condition in which the anterior abdominal wall is sunken like a boat; navicular abdomen; boat-shaped abdomen. नौकाभ उदर; पेट का नाव जैसा आकार;

   **Surgical A.,** see **Acute Abdomen.**

   **Tumid A.,** a swollen abdomen. स्फीत-उदर; फूला हुआ पेट

**Abdominal.** Pertaining to the abdomen. उदरीय; औदरीय; औदरिक; कौक्षेय; उदरगह्वरीय; उदर सम्बन्धी;

   **A. Aneurysm,** aneurysm of the abdominal aorta. औदरिक महाधमनी-विस्फार; पेट की बड़ी धमनी का फैल जाना;

   **A. Aorta,** the aorta below the diaphragm. औदरिक महाधमनी; मध्यच्छद के नीचे स्थित पेट की बड़ी धमनी;

## Abdominal

**A. Bandage,** a support for the abdominal walls; abdominal binder. उदर-प्राचीर बन्धन; उदर प्राचीरों को बाँधने के लिये प्रयुक्त की जाने वाली पट्टी;

**A. Binder,** see **Abdominal Bandage.**

**A. Breathing.,** see **Abdominal Respiration.**

**A. Cavity,** the cavity within the peritoneum. उदर-गह्वर; उदरावरण का अन्दरूनी खोल;

**A. Crisis,** severe pain in the abdominal area. तीव्र उदरशूल;

**A. Decompression,** technique used in obstetrics to facilitate child-birth. उदर-सम्पीडन;

**A. Examination,** examination of the abdomen by all means. उदर-जांच;

**A. Gestation,** the lodgement of the developing ovum in the abdominal cavity; abdominal pregnancy; extrauterine pregnancy; abdominocyesis. उदर-गर्भ;

**A. Muscles,** the muscles of the belly-walls. उदर-पेशियां; उदर-प्राचीरों की पेशियां;

**A. Phthisis,** tubercular disease of the bowels or peritoneum. उदर-यक्ष्मा; आन्तों अथवा उदरावरण की क्षयग्रस्तता;

**A. Pregnancy,** see **Abdominal Gestation.**

**A. Reflex,** involuntary spasm of the abdominal muscles. उदर-प्रतिवर्त; उदर-पेशियों की निरंकुश ऐंठन;

**A. Respiration,** that carried on by the diaphragm and the abdominal muscles; abdominal breathing. उदर-श्वास;

**A. Typhus,** typhoid fever. आंत्रिक-ज्वर; मियादी बुखार; टायफाइड (ज्वर);

**A. Viscera,** the organs of the abdomen. उदरांग

**Abdominalgia.** Pain in the abdomen. उदरार्ति; उदरशूल; पेट-दर्द

**Abdominalis.** Located on the abdominal surface. उदरतलस्थित

**Abdominoanterior.** Having the abdomen forward. उदराग्र; अग्रोदर; अग्रवर्ती उदर

**Abdominocentesis.** Perforation or puncturing of abdomen. उदरवेधन; उदरछेदन

**Abdominocyesis.** see **Abdominal Gestation.**

**Abdominocystic.** Relating to the abdomen and the bladder. उदरमूत्राशयिक; उदर तथा मूत्राशय सम्बन्धी

**Abdominogenital.** Relating to the abdomen and the genitals. उदरजननांगी; उदर तथा जननांगों सम्बन्धी

**Abdominopelvic.** Pertaining to the abdomen and the pelvis. उदरगोणिकी; उदर तथा गोणिका सम्बन्धी

**Abdominoperineal.** Pertaining to the abdomen and the perineum. उदरमूलाधारी; उदर तथा मूलाधार सम्बन्धी

**Abdominoplastic.** Relating to abdominoplasty. उदरसंधान सम्बन्धी; उदर-संधानक

**Abdominoplasty.** An operation performed on the abdominal wall. उदरसंधान

**Abdominoposterior.** Having the abdomen backward. उदरपश्च; पश्चोदरी; पश्चाद्वर्ती उदर; पश्चोदर

**Abdominoscopy.** Physical examination of the abdomen; celioscopy. उदरेक्षण; उदरदर्शन; उदरान्तदर्शन; उदर-जांच; उदर-परीक्षा

**Abdominoscrotal.** Relating to the abdomen and the scrotum. उदरवृषणकोषीय; उदर तथा वृषणकोष सम्बन्धी

**Abdominothoracic.** Relating to the abdomen and the chest. उदरवक्षीय; उदर तथा वक्ष सम्बन्धी

**Abdominous.** Corpulent; very fat. स्थूलकाय; मोटा; मोटू; having a large belly. लम्बोदर; महोदर; तुंदिल; तोंदू; बड़े पेट वाला

**Abdominovaginal.** Relating to the abdomen and the vagina. उदर एवं योनि सम्बन्धी

**Abdominovesical.** Relating to the abdomen and the bladder. उदरमूत्राशयी; उदरमूत्राशयिक; उदर तथा मूत्राशय सम्बन्धी

**Abducens.** The sixth pair of the cranial nerves. अपसरणीतंत्रिका; अपवर्तनी अथवा अपकर्षिणी तंत्रिका; शीर्ष अथवा करोटितंत्रिकाओं का षष्टम युगल;

**A. Muscle,** drawing from the median line. अपकर्षिणी पेशी; अपवर्तनी पेशी;

**A. Oculi,** a muscle drawing away the eyeball outward. चक्षुगोलकबहिराकर्षिणी पेशी; नेत्रगोलकों को बाहर की ओर खींचने वाली पेशी;

**A. Oris,** a muscle elevating the angle of the mouth. मुखकोणोत्थापिका पेशी

**Abducent.** Drawing from the centre. अपकर्षिणी; अपवर्तनी; उद्विवर्तनी; अपसरणक;

**A. Muscles,** muscles drawing from the median line. अपकर्षिणी पेशियां; अपवर्तनी पेशियां;

**A. Nerves,** nerves drawing from the median line. अपकर्षिणी तंत्रिकायें; अपवर्तनी तंत्रिकायें

**Abduct.** To draw from the median line. अपावर्तन; अपकर्षण या अपवर्तन करना; मध्याक्ष या केन्द्र से दूर ले जाना

**Abducted.** Drawn from the median line. अपावर्तित; अपवर्तित; अपकर्षित; अपकृष्ट; अपचालित; kidnapped. अपहृत

**Abducting.** Kidnapping; illegal or forcible carrying off. अपहरण करना; गैरकानूनी रूप से या जबरदस्ती उठा कर ले जाना

**Abduction.** To take away by force or fraud. अपहरण; movement from the median line. अपावर्तन; अपकर्षण; अपवर्तन

**Abductor.** An abducent muscle. अपावर्तक (पेशी); अपकर्षी (पेशी); अपवर्ती (पेशी); अपवर्तनी (पेशी); मध्याक्ष या केन्द्र से दूर खींच ले जाने वाली पेशी; a person who abducts another. अपहर्ता; अपहरणकर्ता;

**A. Auris,** the abductor muscle of the ear. कर्णचालक पेशी;

**A. Brevis Brachii,** a small elongated muscle that abducts and rates the humerus. उपवाहचालक पेशी;

**A. Brevis Pollicis,** the short abductor muscle of the thumb. अंगुष्ठचालक पेशी

**Abed.** In bed. शय्यास्थ; शय्या पर; बिस्तरे पर

**Abelmoschus Mostachus.** A species indigenous to Bengal. लताकस्तूरी

**Aberrance.** Deviation from the normal. विपथन; विचलन; विगति; विषमता; सामान्य दशा से हट जाना

**Aberrancy.** The same as **Aberration.**

**Aberrans.** Wandering away. भ्रमणकारी; पथभ्रष्ट; चलायमान

**Aberrant.** Deviating from the normal type. विपथ; पथभ्रष्ट; विपथी; विषम;

**A Arteries,** long, slender vessels connected with the brachial or axillary artery. प्रगण्ड-धमनियां

**Aberratio.** The same as **Aberration.**

**Aberration.** Deviation from the normal; abnormality of action. विपथन; विचलन; अपेरण; भ्रंश; पथभ्रष्टता; imperfect refraction or focalization of a lens. दृष्टि-भ्रम; disordered state of mind or intellect. चित्तविभ्रम; मनोभ्रम;

**Chromatic A.,** an unequal refraction of different coloured rays producing a blurred image. वर्णिक विपथन; वर्णिक विचलन;

विषमकिरण-बक्रता;

**Distantial A.**, indistinct vision due to distance. दूरीविपथन; दूरदृष्टि विचलन;

**Mental A.**, mental derangement that may or may not amount to insanity. मानसिक विपथन; मानसिक विचलन; मनोविचलन; मनोभ्रम;

**Optical A.**, imperfect focus of light rays by a lens. प्रकाश विपथन; दृष्टि विपथन;

**Spheric A.**, unequal refraction of a convex lens; spherical aberration. गोलाकार विपथन; गोलीय (ताल) विचलन;

**Spherical A.**, see **Spheric Aberration**.

**Aberrometer.** An instrument for measuring optical aberration or any error in delicate experiments or observations. विपथनमापी; विचलनमापी (यंत्र)

**Abevacuation.** Incomplete evacuation. अपूर्ण मलोत्सर्ग; अपूर्ण मलविसर्जन

**Abeyance.** Absence. अभाव; suspension. निलम्बन; दुविधा या लटकाव

**Abide.** Remain over; continue. दृढ़ रहना; पालन करना; टिकना

**Abietate.** A salt of abietic acid. एबिएटिक अम्ल का लवण

**Abietite.** A sugar obtained from the leaves of **Abies Pectinata**, the silver fir of Europe. शर्करा; चीनी

**Ability.** Capacity; faculty. सामर्थ्य; योग्यता; सक्षमता; गुण

**Abiogenesis.** The production of living by non-living matter; spontaneous generation. अजीवजनन; अजीवातजीवोत्पत्ति; निर्जीव से सजीव की उत्पत्ति; अजीवातजनन

**Abiogenetic.** Pertaining to abiogenesis; abiogenous. अजीवजनन सम्बन्धी

**Abiogenous.** See **Abiogenetic**.

**Abiologic.** Not related to biology; abiological. अजीवजनन से कोई सम्बन्ध न होना

**Abiological.** See **Abiologic**.

**Abiology.** The study of non-living things; an organology. अजीवविज्ञान; अजैविकी; अजैवी पदार्थों का अध्ययन

**Abiosis.** Death; absence of life; non-viability. अजीवता; अयोनिता; मृत्यु

**Abiotic.** Incompatible with life; non-viable. अजैव; अजीव; अजीवी; निश्चेतन; जड़; मृत

**Abiotrophia.** See **Abiotrophy**.

**Abiotrophy.** Premature loss of vitality; abiotrophia. अजीवीपोषण

**Abirritant.** Allaying irritation. उत्तेजनाहर; उपशमनकारी; उपदाहनाशक; प्रशामक; संतापहर; संतापहारी

**Abirritate.** To sooth; to diminish or ameliorate irritation. शान्त करना; उपशमन करना; उत्तेजना कम करना

**Abirritation.** Diminished irritability. उत्तेजनाहरण; उपशमन

**Ablactation.** Weaning of a child. अपस्तनन; अपस्तन्यन; स्तन्यत्याजन; स्तन्यत्याग; स्तनपान छुड़ाना

**Ablastemic.** Not germinal. अप्रसूकोशिकापुंजी; अंकुरण से सम्बन्ध न रखने वाला

**Ablate.** To cut off. अंशोच्छेदन करना; काट कर अलग करना

**Ablatio.** Ablation; removal; amputation. वियोजन; पृथक्करण; अलग करना या होना;

   **A. Placentae,** detachment of the placenta. अपरा-वियोजन; अपरा-पृथक्करण; अपरा हटा कर अलग कर देना;

   **A. Retinae,** detachment of the retina. दृष्टिपटल वियोजन; दृष्टिपटल का अलग होना या उसे हटा कर अलग कर देना

**Ablation.** Removing of any part of the body by excision or amputation. अंग-उच्छेदन; अंशोच्छेदन; अपकर्तन; अंग काटना; पृथक्करण;

   **Cortical A.,** surgical removal of the cortex; topectomy. प्रान्तस्था-अंशोच्छेदन

**Ablative.** Pertaining to ablation. अंग काट दिये जाने सम्बन्धी; अंशोच्छेदनीय

**Ablepharia.** Congenital absence of eyelids; ablepharon; ablephary. सहजवर्त्महीनता; पलकों का जन्मजात अभाव

**Ablepharon.** See **Ablepharia.**

**Ablepharous.** Without eyelids. वर्त्महीन; पलकविहीन

**Ablephary.** See **Ablepharia.**

**Ablepsia.** Blindness; want of sight; ablepsy. दृष्टिलोप; दृष्टिहीनता; अन्धापन; अन्धता; ज्योतिहीनता

**Ablepsy.** See **Ablepsia.**

**Abluent.** An agent possessing cleansing quality; a detergent. स्वच्छकारी; निर्मलकारी; परिमार्जक; शोधक; प्रक्षालक

**Ablution.** A tepid sitting-bath or bidet occasionally. धावन; परिमार्जन; प्रक्षालन; संक्षालन; स्नान; शोधन

**Abneural.** Distant from the central nervous system. प्रतिपेशीय; केन्द्रीय स्नायुजाल से दूर; उदर सम्पर्कीय; अपकेन्द्रीय तंत्रिकातंत्र

**Abnormal.** Not normal; not according to rule; irregular; unhealthy;

anormal. अपसामान्य; असामान्य; असाधारण; अस्वाभाविक; अस्वस्थ; विभृंखल; नियमविरुद्ध; विकृत

**Abnormality.** An irregularity; a malformation; abnormity. विसामान्यता; अपसामान्यता; अस्वाभाविकता; अनियमितता; विश्रृंखलता; विकृति; विकृतता;

**Congenital A.,** abnormality existing since birth. सहज अपसामान्यता; सहज विसामान्यता; कोई जन्मजात दोष

**Abnormity.** See **Abnormality.**

**Aboiement.** A barking. भोंकना

**Abolition.** Complete suspension, as of a function. विलोपन; उन्मूलन

**Abomasitis.** Inflammation of the abomasum. आमाशयशोथ; जठरान्तशोथ; आमाशय के चतुर्थ कक्ष का प्रदाह

**Abomasum.** The true stomach of the ruminating animals; a rennet; abomasus. जठरान्त; आमाशय का चतुर्थ कक्ष; रोमन्थक जन्तुओं के आमाशय का चतुर्थ कक्ष (जठरान्त)

**Abomasus.** See **Abomasum.**

**Aborad.** Away from the mouth; aboral. अपमुखी; मुख-गह्वर से दूर; मुख से परे

**Aboral.** See **Aborad.**

**Abort.** To arrest the development of a disease. रोग की रोक-थाम करना या उसका विकास न होने देना; premature delivery of a child; to miscarry. गर्भपात होना या करना; गर्भ गिराना या गिरना; गर्भस्राव होना

**Aborticide.** The killing of a foetus within the uterus. गर्भनाशक; गर्भपातक; गर्भपाती; गर्भस्रावक; गर्भस्रावी; गर्भनाशी

**Aborticidium.** The means of killing a foetus. गर्भपातक उपाय

**Abortifacient.** A drug which is used to bring a miscarriage. गर्भपातक; गर्भस्रावक (औषधि या पदार्थ)

**Abortion.** The premature expulsion of a foetus from the womb; miscarriage. गर्भपात; गर्भस्राव;

**Accidental A.,** abortion caused due to an accident. आकस्मिक गर्भपात; दुर्घटनावश गर्भ गिर जाना;

**Artificial A.,** abortion intentionally produced; induced abortion. कृत्रिम गर्भपात; प्रेरित गर्भपात;

**Complete A.,** the entire contents of the uterus are expelled. पूर्ण गर्भपात;

**Criminal A.,** the production of an abortion when not therapeutically indicated; illegal abortion. आपराधिक गर्भपात; अवैध

गर्भपात; पातक गर्भपात; अनावश्यक या दूषित गर्भपात;

**Early A.**, the embryonic abortion. आरम्भिक गर्भपात; गर्भाधान के छः सप्ताह के अन्दर होने वाला गर्भपात;

**Habitual A.**, recurrent abortion. पुनर्पुनर्गर्भपात; पुनरावर्ती गर्भपात;

**Illegal A.**, see **Criminal Abortion.**

**Incomplete A.**, retention of the membranes or placenta after abortion. अपूर्ण गर्भपात; जेररहित गर्भपात; जेरहीन गर्भपात;

**Induced A.**, intentional evacuation of embryo; artificial abortion. प्रेरित गर्भपात; कृत्रिम गर्भपात;

**Inevitable A.**, one which has advanced to a stage where termination of pregnancy cannot be prevented. अपरिहार्य गर्भपात; अनिवार्य गर्भपात; ऐसा गर्भपात जिसे रोका ही न जा सके;

**Missed A.**, the non-expulsion of a dead foetus. लीन गर्भपात; अलक्षित गर्भपात; भ्रष्ट गर्भपात;

**Recurrent A.**, habitual abortion. पुनरावर्ती गर्भपात; बार-बार होने वाला गर्भपात;

**Septic A.**, one associated with uterine infection and rise in body temperature. पूति गर्भपात; गर्भाशय में पीब पड़ने तथा तेज बुखार के कारण होने वाला गर्भपात;

**Spontaneous A.**, abortion not induced artificially. स्वतः गर्भपात; स्वतः प्रवर्तित गर्भपात; सामान्य गर्भपात;

**Therapeutic A.**, abortion induced to save the life of the mother. उपचारक गर्भपात; ऐच्छिक गर्भपात;

**Threatened A.**, slight blood loss per vaginum whilst cervix remains closed. सम्भावित गर्भपात; तर्जित गर्भपात;

**Tubal A.**, a tubal foetus of pregnancy that dies and is expelled from the fimbriated end of the Fallopian tube. डिम्बवाहिनी-गर्भपात; फैलोपी गर्भपात

**Abortionist.** One who makes a practice for producing abortions. गर्भस्रावक अथवा गर्भपातक (चिकित्सक)

**Abortive.** Abortifacient: rudimentary; not reaching full development. गर्भस्रावी; गर्भपातक; गर्भपाती; गर्भनिपाती; prematurely born. अकालप्रसूत

**Abortiveness.** Untimely birth. अकाल-प्रसव; अकाल-उत्पत्ति; गर्भच्युति

**Abortus.** An abortion or the production of an abortion. पतितगर्भ; पतितभ्रूण; गर्भपात; गर्भस्राव

**Aboulia.** A loss or defect of will-power; abulia. मन:शक्तिक्षय; इच्छादौर्बल्य

**Aboulomania.** Mental derangement by weakened willpower; abulomania. मन:शक्तिक्षयोन्माद; इच्छाशक्ति की दुर्बलता के कारण होने वाला मनोविकार; एबूलोमैनिया

**Abrachia.** Congenital absence of the arms. सहज-अप्रगण्डता; बाहों का जन्मजात अभाव; बाहुहीनता

**Abrachiocephalia.** See **Abrachiocephalus.**

**Abrachiocephalus.** Congenital absence of head and arms; abrachiocephalia; abrachiocephaly; acephalobrachia. सहज-अप्रगण्डशीर्षता; प्रगण्डशीर्षहीनता

**Abrachiocephaly.** See **Abrachiocephalus.**

**Abrachius.** Armless; having no arms. प्रगण्डहीन; भुजाविहीन; बाहों से हीन

**Abradant.** See **Abrasive.**

**Abrade.** An abrasion; abrase; abrasio. खरोंच; रगड़न; घर्षण; रगड़

**Abrase.** See **Abrade.**

**Abrasio.** An abrasion; abrase. खरोंच; रगड़न; घर्षण; रगड़;

**A. Corneae,** a scraping of the cornea. कनीनिका की रगड़न; स्वच्छमण्डल की खरोंच

**Abrasion.** A scraping of the skin; excoriation; abrade; abrasio. खरोंच; रगड़न; घर्षण; अपघर्षण

**Abrasive.** That which causes scraping or excoriation; abradant. अपघर्षणक; अपघर्षी; घर्षणकारी; खाल में खरोंच पैदा कर देने वाला या खाल छील देने वाला (पदार्थ या तत्व)

**Abreaction.** An emotional reaction resulting from recall of past painful experiences relived in speech and action during psychoanalysis or under the influence of light anaesthesia. भावविरेचनयुक्ति

**Abreast.** Side by side. पार्श्वानुपार्श्व; पार्श्वत:

**Abridged.** Brief. संक्षिप्त

**Abrin.** The poisonous principle of jequirity. गुंजाविष; एब्रिन

**Abroma Augusta.** A genus of Indian plants, called **Ulat Kambal.** उलट कम्बल

**Abrosia.** A wasting away. क्षय; क्षरण; विनाश; fasting; abstaining from food. निराहार रहना; व्रत रखना

**Abruptio.** See **Abruption.**

**Abruptio**

**A. Placentae,** premature detachment of a normally situated placenta. अपरापृथक्करण

**Abruption.** Abruptio; a tearing asunder. पृथक्करण; transverse fracture of a bone. बक्र-अस्थिभ्रंश; हड्डी का आड़ा-तिरछा या टेढ़ा-मेढ़ा टूटना

**Abrus Precatorius.** Jequirity; the poisonous seeds used in trachoma. गुंजा; घुंघची

**Abscess.** A circumscribed collection of pus in a cavity of the body; a cavity formed by liquefaction necrosis within the solid tissue. विद्रधि; व्रण; फोड़ा;

**Acute A.,** one in the severe form; hot abscess; warm abscess. तीव्र विद्रधि;

**Alveolar A.,** one in the gum or alveolus; tooth abscess. दन्तउलूखल विद्रधि; गर्तिक व्रण; मसूड़े अथवा दन्तकोटर का फोड़ा;

**Amebic A.,** see **Amoebic Abscess.**

**Amoebic A.,** an abscess of the liver following dysentery; amebic abscess; endamebic abscess; tropical abscess. अमीबी विद्रधि; पेचिश के बाद होने वाला जिगर का फोड़ा;

**Anorectal A.,** one surrounding the anus and the rectum. गुदमलाशय विद्रधि; मलद्वार तथा मलाशय के इर्द-गिर्द होने वाला फोड़ा;

**Apical A.,** abscess at the apex of the lung or at the extremity of the root of a tooth. शिखर विद्रधि;

**Appendiceal A.,** see **Appendicular Abscess.**

**Appendicular A.,** an abscess of the appendix; appendiceal abscess. उण्डुकपुच्छ विद्रधि; उपांत्र का फोड़ा;

**Axillary A.,** one or more abscesses of the axilla. कक्षा विद्रधि; कांख या बगल में निकलने वाला फोड़ा;

**Biliary A.,** an abscess of gall-bladder. पैत्तिक विद्रधि; पित्ताशय का फोड़ा;

**Bone A.,** see **Brodie's Abscess.**

**Breast A.,** see **Mammary Abscess.**

**Brodie's A.,** chronic osteomyelitis; bone abscess. जीर्ण अस्थिपेशीशोथ; पर्यस्थि-व्रण; ब्रोडी विद्रधि; रक्तसंक्रमण से उत्पन्न अस्थिव्रण;

**Canalicular A.,** an abscess of the breast communicating with a milk duct. स्तन विद्रधि; दुग्धनलिका विद्रधि;

**Cerebellar A.,** an abscess of the cerebellum. अनुमस्तिष्क विद्रधि; सिर के पिछले भाग में प्रकट होने वाला फोड़ा;

**Chronic A.,** one of the slow developments usually connected with a bone- joint or gland. जीर्ण विद्रधि; चिर विद्रधि;

**Cold A.,** a chronic abscess, usually tuberculous. शीतल विद्रधि; मन्द व्रण;

**Congestive A.,** one in which the pus appears at a point distant from where it is formed. रक्तसंलयी विद्रधि;

**Dental A.,** abscess beside a tooth, usually near the root. दन्त-विद्रधि;

**Embolic A.,** an abscess in the clot of an embolism. आतंची विद्रधि;

**Endamebic A.,** see **Amoebic Abscess.**

**Epidural A.,** one on duramater. अधिदृढ़तानिका-विद्रधि;

**Faecal A.,** one in the rectum or large intestine. आंत्र-विद्रधि; मलाशय अथवा बड़ी आंत का फोड़ा;

**Hot A.,** see **Acute Abscess.**

**Intracranial A.,** one involving the brain and its membranes. अन्त:करोटि-विद्रधि;

**Lacunar A.,** an abscess in the urethral lacunae. मूत्रपथ-विद्रधि;

**Lung A.,** the pulmonary abscess. फुप्फुस-विद्रधि; फेफड़े का फोड़ा;

**Mammary A.,** one in the female breast; breast abscess. स्तन-विद्रधि;

**Metastatic A.,** a secondary embolic abscess. विक्षेपी विद्रधि;

**Milk A.,** one in the mamma during lactation. स्तन-विद्रधि;

**Omental A.,** an abscess of the omentum. वपा-विद्रधि;

**Ovarian A.,** an abscess of the ovary. डिम्बग्रन्थि-विद्रधि;

**Perianal A.,** an abscess about the anus. परिगुदा-विद्रधि;

**Peridental A.,** an abscess about a teeth. परिदन्त-विद्रधि;

**Peridontal A.,** the same as **Peridental Abscess.**

**Peritonsillar A.,** abscess about a tonsil. परिगलतुण्डिका-विद्रधि;

**Phlegmonous A.,** an acute abscess. तीव्र विद्रधि; अधोत्वक्-बन्धन ऊतक-व्रण;

**Pott's A.,** a tuberculous abscess of the spine. यक्ष्मज मेरु-विद्रधि;

**Primary A.,** one arising at the seat of infection. प्रारम्भिक विद्रधि; मूल व्रण; प्रमुख व्रण;

**Psoas A.,** one due to vertebral disease, the pus descending in the sheath of the psoas muscle. कटिलम्बिका-विद्रधि;

**Pulmonary A.**, see **Lung Abscess.**

**Rectal A.**, one in the rectum. मलांत्र-विद्रधि;

**Residual A.**, one occurring in old inflammatory products. अवशिष्ट विद्रधि;

**Scrofulous A.**, one due to tuberculous degeneration of bone or lymphatic gland. कण्ठमाला विद्रधि;

**Secondary A.**, the same as **Embolic Abscess** or **Metastatic Abscess.**

**Tooth A.**, see **Alveolar Abscess.**

**Traumatic A.**, an abscess due to an injury. अभिघातज विद्रधि; चोट आदि लगने के फलस्वरूप होने वाला विद्रधि;

**Tropical A.**, see **Amoebic Abscess.**

**Tubercular A.**, tuberculous abscess; an abscess caused by tubercle bacillus. यक्ष्मज विद्रधि;

**Tuberculous A.**, see **Tubercular Abscess.**

**Tympanitic A.**, an abscess containing gas. वायुपूरित विद्रधि; हवा से परिपूर्ण फोड़ा;

**Warm A.**, see **Acute Abscess.**

**Abscise.** See **Abscission.**

**Abscission.** The removal of a part by excision; abscise. उत्पाटन; विच्छेदन; छेदन; चीर-फाड़; विगलन; किसी अंग को काट कर अलग कर देना

**Absconsio.** A cavity or sinus. गह्वर; गुहिका; विवर; कोटर

**Absence.** Inattention to surroundings. वातावरण से अनभिज्ञता; want. अभाव; कमी; petitmal; पेटीमाल; epilepsy. मिर्गी

**Absente Febre.** Absence of fever. ज्वरहीनता; ज्वराभाव; बुखार का अभाव

**Absentminded.** Not giving attention to. अन्यमनस्क; शून्यमनस्क; भ्रान्तचित्त; खोया-खोया

**Absentmindedness.** The condition of being inattentive. अन्यमनस्कता; शून्यमनस्कता; विमनस्कता; भ्रान्तचित्तता; खोया खोयापन

**Absinth (e).** Wormwood, a bitter plant or its essence; absinthium. चिरायता; कृमिद्रु; नागदौना

**Absinthine.** A poisonous alkaloid of wormwood. चिरायताविष; कृमिद्रुविष

**Ansinthism.** A disease showing mental deterioration and muscular debility due to excessive use of absinthe. चिरायताजन्यविषण्णता; कृमिद्रुविषण्णता; चिरायते से होने वाली विषाक्त अवस्था

**Absinthium.** See **Absinth (e).**

**Absolute.** Pure, perfect or complete. शुद्ध; विशुद्ध; परिशुद्ध; परम; पूर्ण;
  **A. Alcohol,** alcohol as free from water. शुद्ध सुरासार; विशुद्ध सुरासार

**Absorb.** To take away material into the body through lymphatic or blood vessels. शोषना; शोषण करना; अवशोषण करना

**Absorbefacient.** See **Absorbent.**

**Absorbency.** The ability of being absorbed. अवशोषकता; अवशोषणक्षमता

**Absorbent.** Taking up by suction; imbibing; the absorbing agent; absorbefacient; absorber. शोषक; अवशोषक; अवशोषी; अवचूषक;
  **A. Cotton,** cotton freed from oily matters. अवशोषी रुई;
  **A. Vessels,** the lymphatic vessels. लसीका वाहिनियां

**Absorber.** See **Absorbent.**

**Absorptance.** The same as **Absorbency.**

**Absorptimeter.** See **Absorptiometer.**

**Absorptiometer.** An instrument for measuring the thickness of liquid drawn between two glass plates by capillary attraction; absorptimeter. अवशोषणमापी; अवशोषणमापकयंत्र

**Absorption.** Assimilation of one body by another; the act of absorbing or taking up nutritious elements. अवशोषण; शोषण; अवचूषण; सोखना

**Absorptive.** Absorbent. अवशोषी; अवशोषक; शोषक; अवचूषक

**Absorptiveness.** See **Absorptivity.**

**Absorptivity.** Ability to absorb; absorptiveness. अवशोषकता; प्रचूषिता; अवशोषणक्षमता; चूषणशीलता; सोखने की क्षमता

**Abstain.** To keep oneself away; refrain. परिवर्जन करना; परित्याग करना; परहेज करना

**Abstainer.** One who does not drink. परिवर्जक; मद्यत्यागी; शराब न पीने वाला

**Abstemious.** Moderate in matters of diet, etc. मिताहारी; अल्पाहारी

**Abstergent.** A cleansing agent or detergent. शोधक; अपमार्जक; रेचक या मलशोषक (औषधि)

**Abstersion.** The act of purifying. अपमार्जन; शोधन; परिशोधन; रेचन

**Abstersive.** The same as **Abstergent.**

**Abstertion.** The same as **Abstersion.**

**Abstinence.** Voluntary privation or a self-denial in diet, etc. परिवर्जना; परहेज; संयम

# Abstract

**Abstract.** A preparation made by evaporating fluid extract to a powder and trituration with sugar of milk; abstractum. सार; तत्त्व; सारांश

**Abstraction.** Blood-letting. रक्तमोषण; रक्तनिस्सारण; आदान; the process of distillation. शोधन; परिशोधन; सारहरण; पृथक्करण; exclusive attention to an idea. ध्यानमग्नता; ध्यानैकाग्रता; पूर्ण एकाग्रता

**Abstractum.** See **Abstract.**

**Abstuse.** Obstinate; difficult. दुर्गम; जटिल; कठिन

**Absurd.** Unreasonable. असंगत; अनुपयुक्त; विसंगत; अनुचित; अर्थहीन; निरर्थक

**Abulia.** A loss of defect of willpower; aboulia. मन:शक्तिक्षय; इच्छाशक्ति का अभाव या दोष; निर्णय-अक्षमता; कार्य-अक्षमता

**Abulic.** Relating to, or suffering from abulia. इच्छाशक्ति के अभाव से सम्बन्धित या मन:शक्तिक्षयग्रस्त

**Abulomania.** see **Aboulomania.**

**Abundance.** More than a sufficient quantity. प्रचुरता; बहुलता; विपुलता; बाहुल्य

**Abundant.** More than sufficient. प्रचुर; पर्याप्त; विपुल

**Abuse.** Misuse; excessive wrong use of a thing अपव्यवहार; दुरुपयोग

**A.C.** Abbreviation used for Ante cebum, which means before meals. भोजनपूर्व; भोजन से पहले

**Acacia.** A genus of shrubs and trees yielding gum arabic. बबूल; कीकर;

    **A. Arabica,** the babla tree. बबूल-वृक्ष; बबूल अथवा कीकर का पेड़;

    **A. Catechu,** a substance derived from certain bark, called **Katha.** कत्था; खदिर;

    **A. Ferniciana,** gum arabic, derived from the Babla tree. बबूल का गोंद, इरिमेद; दुर्गन्धित खैर;

    **A. Gum,** gum arabic. बबूल या कीकर का गोंद

**Acalculia.** An aphasic condition. परिकलन-अक्षमता

**Acampsia.** Inflexibility of a limb. अकड़न; घनता

**Acantha.** The spine, or the spinal column. मेरुदण्ड; मेरु-प्रवर्ध; रीढ़

**Acanthesthesia.** A sensation, as of a pricking with needles. सूचीवेधी अनुभूति; सुई चुभने जैसी अनुभूति

**Acanthia Lectularia.** Cimex lectularis; the bed-bug. खटमल

**Acanthion.** The base of the anterior nasal spine. नासाग्रकण्टक; नाक की हड्डी का उद्गम स्थल

**Acanthoid** Thorny. कण्टकी; spiny; of a spinous nature. मेरुदण्डवत्; रीढ़ की हड्डी जैसा

**Acanthoma.** A neoplasm or overgrowth of the prickly-layer of the skin. कणिकार्बुद

**Acanthosis.** A disease of the dermic prickle-layer. झुनझुनाहट

**Acanthulus.** An instrument for removing thorns from wounds. सूची; सुई; कांटा निकालने का औजार

**Acapsular.** Not having capsule. सम्पुटहीन

**Acardia.** Absence of heart. अहृदयता; हृदयहीनता

**Acardiac.** Without a heart; the subject of acardia. अहृदय; हृदयहीन

**Acardiacus.** A foetus with no heart. अहृदयभ्रूण; अहृद्गर्भ

**Acardiohemia.** A lack of blood in the heart. रक्ताल्पहृदय; हृदय की रक्ताल्पता

**Acardiotrophia.** Atrophy of the heart. हृद्शोष; हृत्पिण्ड का सूखना

**Acardionervia.** Diminished nervous action of the heart. हृदस्नायुक्रियाल्पता: हृदय की नाड़ियों की मन्द क्रिया

**Acariasis.** A disease due to mites. यूकारोग; जूं पड़ने की बीमारी

**Acaricide.** An agent that destroys the itch-mites. यूकानाशी; जूंमार (औषधि); क्षुद्रकीटनाशक (औषधि); किलनीनाशक (औषधि)

**Acarid.** A mite. यूका; जूं; एक क्षुद्रकीट

**Acaridan.** The same as **Acarid**.

**Acarinosis.** Any disease due to the itch-mites. यूकारोग; जूं पड़ने की बीमारी

**Acarodermatitis.** Dermatitis due to mites. यूकीयत्वक्शोथ; जूं पड़ने के कारण चमड़ी का प्रदाह होना

**Acaroid.** Mite-like. यूकावत्; यूकाभ; जूं जैसा

**Acarophobia.** Morbid fear of itch. कण्डूभीति; खाजभीति; खुजली होने का डर

**Acarpous.** Sterile. बंध्य; बंध्या; बांझ

**Acarus.** Insect infecting the skin, as in itch. चर्मरोगजकीट; चमड़ी की बीमारी पैदा करने वाला कीड़ा;

   A. Scabiei, itch-producing insects. कण्डू-कीट; खाज-कीट

**Acatalepsia,** Uncertainty in diagnosis. अज्ञेयता; नैदानिक अनिश्चितता; dementia. मूढ़चित्तता; unknowingness. बोधहीनता

**Acatalepsy.** The same as **Acatalepsia**.

**Acataleptic.** Mentally deficient; one affected with acatalepsy. मूढ़चित्त; मन्दबुद्धि; suspicious. संशयग्रस्त; शंकालु; शकी

**Acatamathesia.** Inability to comprehend speech; a morbid blunting of perception. अर्थग्रहण-अक्षमता; किसी बात का अर्थ समझने की अयोग्यता

**Acataphasia.** Inability to utter complete sentence, or to correctly formulate a statement. वाक्यरचना-अक्षमता; असम्बद्धवाक्; तुतलाना; किसी वाक्य को पूरी तरह बोलने की असमर्थता

**Acatastasia.** Irregularity; deviation from normal. अनियमितता

**Acatharsia.** A failure to obtain desired purgation. विरेचनाभाव; इच्छानुसार दस्त न होना

**Acathetic.** Unable to retain; diffused. धारण-अक्षम; विसृत;

   **A. Jaundice,** diffused jaundice. विसृत कामला; छितरा या बिखरा हुआ पीलिया

**Acaudal.** Tailless; acaudate. पुच्छहीन; निर्पुच्छ; बिना पूछ का

**Acaudate.** See **Acaudal.**

**Accelerans Nerve.** A nerve that increases the rate and force of the heart's action. हृदयत्वरणतंत्रिका; हृत्त्वरणतंत्रिका; हृत्क्रिया की दर तथा शक्ति बढ़ाने वाली नाड़ी

**Accelerant.** Accelerator. त्वरित्र; त्वरक; गतिवर्धक

**Accelerate.** To put on pace; to make quick. त्वरित करना; द्रुत अथवा तेज गति देना

**Accelerated.** Caused to move quickly. त्वरित

**Acceleration.** An increase of speed. त्वरण; द्रुत गति; तेज चाल

**Accelerative.** Adding to velocity; quickening progression. त्वरक; त्वरित्र; गतिवर्धक

**Accelerator.** That which accelerates. त्वरित्र; त्वरक; गतिवर्धक;

   **A. Nerve,** motor nerve made up of a cranial and a spinal part that supplies the trapezius and sternomastoid muscles and pharynx. गतिवर्धक तंत्रिका

**Accentuation.** Increased distinctness. प्रबलन; उद्दात्तता

**Acceptance.** In the physiological sense, a favourable attitude toward a person. स्वीकृति; स्वीकारोक्ति; प्रतिग्रहण

**Acceptor.** A substance which unites with another substance. स्वीकारक; ग्राहक; ग्राही; प्रतिग्राही

**Access.** The beginning or onset, as of a disease; accession. आरम्भ; शुरुआत

**Accession.** See **Access.**

**Accessorius.** See **Accessory.**

**Accessory.** Auxillary; accessorius; assisting. सहायक; आनुषंगिक; अनुषंगी;

    **A. Nucleus,** the origin of the spinal accessory nerve. अनुषंगी केन्द्रक

**Accident.** A sudden mishappening. दुर्घटना; कोई आकस्मिक दुखद घटना;

    **A. Prone,** said of persons having an unusually high accidents. दुर्घटना-प्रवण

**Accidental.** Due or pertaining to an accident; happening by chance. आकस्मिक दुर्घटना सम्बन्धी;

    **A. Abortion,** that due to accident. आकस्मिक गर्भपात;

    **A. Haemorrhage,** haemorrhage due to premature placental detachment. आकस्मिक रक्तस्राव

**Accipiter.** A facial bandage with tails resembling a hawk's claw. आनन-पट्टिका; बाज के पंजे जैसी चेहरे की पट्टी

**Acclimatation.** See **Acclimatization.**

**Acclimation.** See **Acclimatization.**

**Acclimatization.** Becoming accustomed to a climate; acclimatation; acclimation. दशानुकूलन; पर्यानुकूलन; परिस्थिति-अनुकूलन

**Acclimatize.** To become accustomed to a different environment. दशानुकूलन करना

**Accommodation.** Adaptation, or adjustment, e.g. the power of the eye to alter the convexity of the lens according to the nearness or distance of object so that a distinct image is always retained. समंजन; समायोजन; संधानक्षमता; अवस्थान कौशल; नेत्रों की विविध दूरी की वस्तुयें देखने की एक व्यवस्था;

    **Absolute A.,** accommodation of either eye separately. पूर्ण समंजन;

    **Binocular A.,** accommodation of both eyes jointly. द्विनेत्री समंजन;

    **Excessive A.,** greater-than-needed accommodation of the eye. अतिसमंजन; समंजनाधिक्य;

    **Histologic A.,** changes in the morphology and function of cells, following changed conditions. ऊतिजनक समंजन;

    **Mechanism A.,** method by which curvature of eye lens is changed in order to focus close objects on the retina. यांत्रिक समंजन;

**Negative A.**, the eye passive, at rest. ऋणात्मक समंजन;

**Positive A.**, that for near points produced by contraction of the capillary muscle. धनात्मक समंजन;

**Reflex A.**, loss of the pupil reflex to light; Argyll Robertson pupil. प्रतिवर्त समंजन;

**Relative A.**, quality of accommodation required for single binocular vision for any specified distance, or for any particular degree of convergence. सापेक्ष समंजन;

**Subnormal A.**, insufficient accommodation. अवसामान्य समंजन

**Accommodative.** Relating to, or concerning accommodation. समंजन या समायोजन सम्बन्धी; समायोजनीय;

**A. Iridoplegia,** inability of the iris to respond to accommodative effort. समायोजनीय परितारिकाघात

**Accompaniment.** Appendage. उपांग; आनुषंगिक; सहायक (पदार्थ)

**Accomplish.** To fulfil; to finish entirely. निष्पादन करना; पूरा करना

**Accomplishment.** Attainment; fulfilment. निष्पादन

**Accouchee.** A woman delivered of a child. प्रसूता; सूतिका

**Accouchment.** Child-birth; delivery; lying-in. प्रसव; प्रसूति; शिशुजनन; गर्भमोचन;

**A. Force,** forcible delivery with the hand. शीघ्रप्रसव

**Accoucheur.** An obstetrician; a man-midwife. पुरुष-धातृ; प्रसूतिवैद्य (पुरुष); प्रसावक

**Accoucheuse.** A woman-midwife. धातृ; प्रसाविका; धाय

**Accrescent.** Growing larger after flowering. वर्धनशील; वर्धमान; बढ़ता हुआ

**Accrete.** To grow together. सहवर्धमान; साथ-साथ बढ़ता हुआ

**Accretion.** An increase of substance of deposit around a central object; growth; increase. बृद्धि; अभिबृद्धि; संवर्धन; उपचय

**Accumbent.** Leaning or reclining against anything. प्रतिस्थिति; किसी चीज का सहारा लेकर आराम करने की स्थिति

**Accumulation.** Collection. संचय; संचयन; संग्रह; संग्रहण

**Accumulator.** An instrument that stores up electricity. विद्युत्संचययंत्र; विद्युत्संचायक

**Accuracy.** Exactness. यथार्थता; बिल्कुल सही होने की अवस्था

**Accurate.** Exact. यथार्थ; बिल्कुल सही

**Accuse.** To charge with fault. दोषारोपण करना; अभियोग लगाना

**Accused.** Charged with fault. दोषी; अभियुक्त

**Accustomed.** Customary; familiar. प्रचलित; अभ्यस्त; आदी

**Ace-bandage.** Trade name for an elastic bandage woven of cotton. एस-बैंडेज; सूत के धागे से बुनी हुई एक लचीली पट्टी (का नाम)

**Acecia.** Recovery; cure; acesia. रोगमुक्ति; आरोग्यलाभ; बीमारी से छुटकारा

**Acedia.** Apathy; despondency; listlessness. विरक्ति; अनासक्ति; मतिमन्दता; मन्दबुद्धिता

**Acelious.** Without a belly. अजठर; जठरहीन; आमाशय-विहीन; बिना पेट

**Acellular.** Without cells. अकोशिकीय; कोशिकाहीन; अकोशिक

**Acentric.** Peripheric; not arising in a centre. परिधीय; अकेन्द्री

**Aceology.** Therapeutics. चिकित्साशास्त्र; उपचारविज्ञान; रोगमुक्तिविज्ञान

**Acephal.** Without a head. अशिर; अशीर्ष; शिरोहीन; शीर्षहीन; बेसिरा

**Acephalia.** Congenital absence of the head; acephalism; acephaly. सहज-अशीर्षता; सहजशिरोहीनता; सिर का जन्मजात अभाव

**Acephalism.** See **Acephalia.**

**Acephalobrachia.** Without head and arms; abrachiocephalus. शीर्षप्रगण्डहीन; सिर और बाहों से हीन

**Acephalocardia.** Without head and heart. अशिरहृद्; सिर और हृदय से हीन

**Acephalocheiria.** Without head and hands; acephalochiria. अशिरहस्त; सिर और हाथों से हीन

**Acephalochiria.** See **Acephalocheiria.**

**Acephalogaster.** A foetus without head and stomach. सिर एवं आमाशय विहीन भ्रूण

**Acephalogastria.** Without head and belly. शीर्षजठरहीन; सिर और पेट से हीन

**Acephalopodia.** Without head and feet. अशिरपाद; सिर और पैरों से हीन

**Acephalopodius.** A foetus without head and feet. सिर एवं पैर विहीन भ्रूण; अशिरपादभ्रूण

**Acephalorrhachia.** Without head and spine. शीर्षसुषुम्नाहीन; सिर और रीढ़ की हड्डी से हीन

**Acephalostomia.** Absence of head, with mouth-like opening on superior aspect. अशीर्षता; सिर का अभाव

**Acephalothoracia.** Congenital absence of head and thorax. सहज अशिरवक्ष; सिर एवं वक्ष का जन्मजात अभाव

**Acephalous.** Without a head; headless; acephalus. अशीर्ष; अशिर; शीर्षहीन; शिरोहीन

**Acephalus.** See **Acephalous.**

**Acephaly.** See **Acephalia.**

**Acerate.** Sharp-pointed. नुकीला; तेज नोक वाला

**Aceratosis.** A lack of horny tissues. शृंगोतकहीनता; शृंगी ऊतकों का अभाव

**Acerb.** Acrid. तीक्ष्ण; तीखा; acidic. अम्लज; खट्टा

**Acerbity.** Acridity; acidity combined with astringency. तीक्ष्णता; तीखापन; अम्लता; खट्टापन और कसैलापन

**Acervuline.** Occurring in clusters; aggregated. समुच्चयित; गुच्छित; संग्रहीत

**Acervuloma.** A meningeal tumour containing sandlike material; psammoma. मस्तिष्कावरकार्बुद

**Acervulus.** Gritty; sandy. सिकतामय; रेतीला; बालू या रेत जैसा;
  **A. Cerebri,** concretionary matter near the base of the pineal gland; brain-sand; मस्तिष्क-सिकता; मस्तिष्क-बालुका

**Acescence.** The process of becoming sore. अम्लनिर्माणक प्रक्रिया; slight acidity. हल्का-सा खट्टापन; हल्की-सी खटास

**Acescency.** Mild acidity; moderately sour. मृदु-अम्लता; हल्का-सा खट्टापन

**Acescent.** Slight acid. अल्पाम्ल; हल्का-सा खट्टा

**Acesia.** Recovery; cure; acecia. आरोग्यलाभ; रोगमुक्ति

**Acesodyne.** Anodyne; an agent for relieving pain. वदनाहर; पीड़ाहर

**Acestoma.** Granulation tissue. क्षतांकुर; कणिकी-ऊतक; कणपुंज

**Aceta.** Plural of **Acetum.**

**Acetabula.** Plural of **Acetabulum.**

**Acetabular.** Belonging to the acetabulum. जंघास्थिक; उलूखलीय; उलूखल सम्बन्धी; जांघ की हड्डी सम्बन्धी

**Acetabulectomy.** Excision of the acetabulum. उलूखलोच्छेदन

**Acetabuloplastic.** Relating to acetabuloplasty. उलूखलसंधान सम्बन्धी; उलूखलीय

**Acetabuloplasty.** Plastic operation of acetabulum. उलूखलसंधान

**Acetabulum.** A cup-like socket on the external aspect of the innominate bones, into which the head of the femur fits to form the hip-joint. उलूखल; जंघास्थि; जांघ की हड्डी

**Acetate.** A salt of acetic acid; vinegar. शौक्त; शुक्त; सिरका

**Acetic.** Pertaining to vinegar. शौक्तिक; शौक्तीय; सिरका सम्बन्धी;
   **A. Acid,** the acid present in vinegar. शुक्ताम्ल; असेटिक एसिड

**Acetify.** To produce acetic fermentation or vinegar. शुक्ताम्लोत्पादन; सिरकोत्पादन

**Acetimeter.** An apparatus to determine the amount of acetic acid in a fluid. सिरकामापक (यंत्र); शुक्ताम्लमापी (यंत्र)

**Acetonaemia.** Acetone bodies in the blood; acetonemia. अम्लरक्तता; रक्ताम्लता; रक्त में एसिटोन-पिण्ड विद्यमान रहना

**Acetone.** A substance found in the urine and blood in diabetes. एसिटोन (पदार्थ); बहुमूत्ररोग में पेशाब तथा खून में पाया जाने वाला एक पदार्थ

**Acetonemia.** See **Acetonaemia.**

**Acetonuria.** Excessive acetone bodies in the urine. एसिटोनमेह; पेशाब में एसिटोन पदार्थ जाना

**Acetonuric.** Relating to acetonuria. एसिटोनमेह सम्बन्धी

**Acetum.** Vinegar. सिरका

**Achalasia.** Failure to relax; referring especially to visceral openings or sphincter muscles. अशिथिलता;
   **Cardiac A.,** food fails to pass normally into stomach though there is no obvious obstruction. अभिहृद्-जठर अशिथिलता;
   **Oesophageal A.,** cardiospasm. ग्रासनली-अशिथिलता; हृद्द्वेष्ट;
   **Sphincteral A.,** failure of intestinal sphincter to relax. संवरणी अशिथिलता

**Achalybemia.** A lack of iron in the blood. अलौहरक्तता; खून में लोहे की कमी होना

**Ache.** A continued fixed pain. दुखन; वेदना; कसक; हूक; अविराम पीड़ा

**Acheilia.** Congenital absence of the lips; achilia. सहज-अनोष्ठता; होंठों का जन्मजात अभाव

**Acheilous.** See **Achilous.**

**Acheiria.** Congenital absence of the hands; achiria; सहज-अहस्तता; हाथों का जन्मजात अभाव

**Acheiropodia.** Congenital absence of hands and feet; acheiropody; achiropody. सहज-अहस्तपादता; हाथ-पैरों का जन्मजात अभाव

**Acheiropody.** See **Acheiropodia.**

**Acheirous.** A foetus without hands. हस्तहीन; अहस्तभ्रूण relating to acheiria. हाथ न होने सम्बन्धी; अहस्तपरक; गर्भाशय में पलने वाला ऐसा भ्रूण जिसके हाथ नहीं होते

**Acheirus.** The same as **Acheirous.**

**Achilia.** See **Acheilia.**

**Achilles Jerk.** See **Achilles Tendon Reflex.**

**Achilles Tendon.** The tendinous termination of the gastrocnemius and soleus muscles. कण्डरापेशी; पिण्डिका-कण्डरा; स्नायुजाल; पिण्डली के मांसल भाग के अन्त व जोड़ का निर्माण करने वाला पेशीबन्ध;

**A.T. Reflex,** a contraction of the calf on tapping the tendon of Achilles; Achelles jerk. कण्डरापेशी-प्रतिवर्त

**Achillobursitis.** Inflamiation of the bursa lying over the tendon of the Achilles; retrocalcaneobursitis. कण्डरापेशीपुटीशोथ

**Achillodynia.** Pain in the tendon of Achilles. कण्डरापेशीवेदना; कण्डरापेशीशूल

**Achillorrhaphy.** The operation for stitching the Achilles tendon. पिण्डिका-कण्डरासीवन

**Achillotenotomy.** See **Achillotomy.**

**Achillotomy.** Division of the tendon of the Achilles; achillotenotomy. कण्डरापेशीउच्छेदन; कण्डरापेशीकर्तन

**Achilous.** Without lips; acheilous. ओष्ठहीन; ओष्ठविहीन; ओष्ठरहित; होंठों से हीन

**Aching.** Constant soreness. कसक; दुखन; शूल; हूक; अविराम पीड़ा

**Achiria.** See **Acheiria.**

**Achiropody.** See **Acheiropodia.**

**Achlorhydria.** A lack of hydrochloric acid in the gastric secretions. जठर-अनम्लता; अम्लाभाव; अम्ल का अभाव

**Achloride.** A salt other than a chloride; nonchloride. अनीलेय; क्लोराइडहीन

**Achloropsia.** Green-blindness; a form of colour-blindness in which green colour cannot be distinguished. हरितान्धता; हरा रंग पहचानने की अक्षमता

**Acholia.** Absence or want of bile. अपित्त; पित्त की कमी

**Acholic.** Having no bile; without bile. पित्तहीन; अपित्तज

**Acholous.** Devoid of, or pertaining to acholia; acholus. अपित्तज; पित्ताभाव सम्बन्धी

**Acholuric.** Absence of bile pigment in the urine. अपित्तवर्णकमेह; मूत्र में पित्तवर्णक का अभाव

**Acholuric.** Having no bile pigment in the urine. अपित्तवर्णक (मूत्र)

**Acholus.** See **Acholous.**

**Achondroplasia.** Foetal rickets, resulting in dwarfism. भ्रूणास्थिशोथ; बालास्थिक्षय; उपास्थि-अविकसन

**Achor.** Crusta lactea; a running sore on an infant's head. शिशुकरोटित्वग्वसास्राव; दुग्धनिर्मोक

**Achora.** See **Achroma.**

**Achroa.** See **Achroma.**

**Achroia.** See **Achroma.**

**Achroma.** Pallor; absence of colour; achora; achroa; achroia; achromia. अवर्णता; अरंजकता; अरंज्यता; निर्वर्णता; वर्णहीनता, रंग का अभाव

**Achromacyte.** See **Achromocyte.**

**Achromasia.** Absence of colour; loss of stain from a cell. अवर्णता; निर्वर्णता

**Achromate.** Colour-blind. वर्णान्ध; रंगान्ध (व्यक्ति)

**Achromatic.** Colourless. निर्वर्ण; वर्णहीन; अवर्णी; अरंजित;

A. Lens, one correcting chromatic aberration. अवर्णी लेंस; अरंजित लेंस;

A. Spindle, nuclear spindle; the conelike appearance of the nucleus during certain stages of karyokinesis. अवर्णी तर्कु

**Achromatin.** The substance in the nucleus of a cell prior to division. अरंजक; अरंज्या

**Achromatism.** An absence of colour. वर्णाभाव; रंग का अभाव

**Achromatocyte.** See **Achromocyte.**

**Achromatopia.** See **Achromatopsia.**

**Achromatopsia.** Complete colour-blindness; achromatopia; achromatopsy. पूर्ण वर्णांधता; अरंजित-दृष्टि; धूसर-दृष्टि

**Achromatopsy.** See **Achromatopsia.**

**Achromatosis.** Lack of pigment; albinism; achromia. अवर्णकता; वर्णहीनता; वर्णक का अभाव

**Achromatous.** Without colour. वर्णहीन; रंगहीन; निर्वर्ण

**Achromaturia.** Colourless state of urine. मूत्र-अवर्णता; मूत्रावर्णता; मूत्रवर्णहीनता; रंगहीन पेशाब

**Achromia.** See **Achroma.**

Congenital A., see **Albinism.**

# Achromic

**Achromic.** Belonging to, or affected with achromia; colourless. अवर्णिक; निर्वर्णता सम्बन्धी अथवा निर्वर्णताग्रस्त

**Achromocyte.** A decolourized red blood corpuscle; achromacyte; achromatocyte. अल्पवर्णीकोशिका; वर्णहीनकोशिका; रंगहीनकोशिका

**Achromodermia.** Colourless state of the skin. चर्म-अवर्णता; चर्मवर्णहीनता; चर्मनिर्वर्णता; त्वक्-अवर्णता; त्वक्वर्णहीनता; चमड़ी का स्वाभाविक रंग न होना

**Achromophil.** See **Achromophilic.**

**Achromophilic.** Not being coloured by the histologic or bacteriologic stains; achromophil; achromophilous. अवर्णिक; अरंज्या

**Achromophilous.** See **Achromophilic.**

**Achromotrichia.** Absence of pigment in the hair. केश-अवर्णता; लोम-अवर्णता; रोम-अवर्णता

**Achylia.** Deficient chylification; absence of chyle or gastric juice as well as other digestive secretions; achylosis. स्रवणहीनता; स्रावहीनता; अन्नरसाभाव; पयसाभाव;

　**A. Gastrica,** dysfunction of digestive fluid by atrophy of mucous lining of stomach. जठरस्रवणहीनता; जठरस्रावहीनता;

　**A. Pancreatica,** absence or deficiency of the pacreatic secretion. अग्न्याशयस्रवणहीनता; अग्न्याशयस्रावहीनता

**Achylosis.** See **Achylia.**

**Achylous.** Lacking in gastric juices or other digestive secretions. वसालसीकाहीन; अवसालसीकी; पाचक रसों से हीन

**Achymosis.** Deficient chymification. आहार-रसाभाव; आहार-रस की कमी

**Acicular.** Long and pointed, like a needle. सूच्याकार; सूचीवत्; सुई के आकार जैसा

**Aciculiform.** Of the form of a needle. सूचीरूप; सूचीवत्; सूच्याकार; सुई जैसा

**Acid.** A sour substance, sharp to taste; acidum. एसिड; अम्ल; तेजाब; खट्टा;

　**A. Base Balance,** the mechanism by which the acid and alkanity of the body fluids are kept in a state of equilibrium. अम्लाधार संतुलन;

　**A. Fallout,** see **Acid Rain.**

　**A. Fast,** becteriologically an organism which when stained, does not become discolourized when subjected to dilute acids; acid proof. अम्लस्थाई; अम्लसह; अम्लावरक; अम्ल-अप्रभावी; अम्लदृढ़;

**A. Phosphatase**, enzyme in seminal fluid, secreted by prostate gland; acid phosphate. फास्फेट अम्ल; प्रांगारिक अम्ल;

**A. Phosphates**, see **Acid Phosphatase**.

**A. Poisoning**, ingestion of a toxic acid. अम्ल-विषण्णता;

**A. Proof**, see **Acid Fast**.

**A. Rain**, rain in passing through the atmosphere is contaminated with acid substances; acid fallout. अम्ल वर्षा;

**A. Salt**, a salt formed when only a part of the hydrogen of an acid is replaced by a metal. अम्ल-लवण

**Acidaemia.** See **Acidemia**.

**Acidemia.** A condition of decreased alkanity of the blood; acidaemia. अम्लरक्तता; रुधिराम्लता; रक्त में क्षारक पदार्थों की कमी;

Metabolic A., caused by increased lactic acid production in muscles. चयापचयी अम्लरक्तता; चयापचयी रुधिराम्लता;

Respiratory A., caused by poor ventilation and increasing dioxide. श्वसनअम्लरक्तता; श्वसनरुधिराम्लता

**Acid Fast.** See under **Acid**.

**Acid Proof.** See under **Acid**.

**Acidic.** Sour. अम्लीय; आम्लिक; अम्लज; खट्टा

**Acidifiable.** Susceptible of being made acid. अम्लप्रवण; अम्ल में परिणित किया जाने योग्य

**Acidific.** See **Acidifier**.

**Acidification.** The act of making acid. अम्लीकरण; अम्लीभवन; अम्ल बनाने की क्रिया

**Acidifier.** An agent that makes an acid; acidific; acidulant. अम्लकर; अम्लोत्पादक; अम्ल बनाने वाला पदार्थ

**Acidimeter.** An instrument for determining the purity of acids. अम्लमापी; अम्लमापक (यंत्र)

**Acidimetry.** The determination of free acid in the solution. अम्लमिति; अम्लमापन

**Acidism.** Poisoning caused by acids introduced from outside the body; acidismus. अम्लात्यय

**Acidismus.** See **Acidism**.

**Aciditoxicity.** Poisoning with acids. अम्लविषण्णता; अम्लविषजता

**Acidity.** Sourness; a sign of indigestion. अम्लता; खट्टापन

**Acidocyte.** Eosinophil; eosinophilic leucocyte. इयोसिनरागी; इयोसिनप्रेमी; इयोसिनरागी-श्वेताणु; इयोसिनप्रेमी-श्वेताणु

**Acidocytopenia.** Abnormal reduction in number of eosinophils in the blood. अल्पइयोसिनरागी; अल्पइयोसिनप्रेमी; रक्त में इयोसिनरागी श्वेताणुओं की अस्वाभाविक कमी

**Acidocytosis.** Abnormal increase in number of eosinophils in the blood. अतिइयोसिनरागी; अतिइयोसिनप्रेमी; रक्त में इयोसिनरागी श्वेताणुओं की अस्वाभाविक वृद्धि

**Acidogenic.** Causing acidity. अम्लजन; अम्ल पैदा करने वाला (पदार्थ)

**Acidology.** The study of science of surgical appliances. शल्ययंत्रविज्ञान; शल्ययंत्रों का वैज्ञानिक अध्ययन

**Acidophil.** See **Acidophile.**

**Acidophile.** Capable of being stained readily by acid dyes; acidophil. अम्लरागी; अम्लप्रेमी

**Acidoresistant.** Acid-resisting (said about bacteria). अम्लसह

**Acidosic.** Characterized by acidosis. अम्लरक्तक; अम्लोपचयी; अम्लमय

**Acidosis.** A reduction in the normal alkaline reaction of body tissues; acidaemia. अम्लरक्तता; अम्लमयता; अम्लोपचय; तेजाबी रोग

**Acidotic,** Relating to, or characterized by acidosis. अम्लरक्तक; अम्लरक्तता सम्बन्धी

**Acidulant.** See **Acidifier.**

**Acidulous.** Slightly acid. अल्पाम्ल; हल्का-सा खट्टा

**Acidum.** An acid. अम्ल; एसिड; तेजाब;

 **A. Aceticum,** acetic acid. असेटिक एसिड; सिरका अम्ल;

 **A. Benzoicum,** benzoic acid. बेंजोइक एसिड; लोबान अम्ल;

 **A. Carbolicum,** carbolic acid. कार्बोलिक एसिड;

 **A. Carbonicum,** carbonic acid. कार्बनिक एसिड; अंगाराम्ल;

 **A. Citricum,** citric acid. साइट्रिक एसिड;

 **A. Gallicum,** gallic acid. गैलिक एसिड; माजूफल का तेजाब;

 **A. Hydrochloricum,** hydrochloric acid. हाइड्रोक्लोरिक एसड;

 **A. Hydrocyanicum,** hydrocyanic acid. हाइड्रोस्यानिक एसिड; कड़वे बादाम आदि का तेजाब;

**A. Muriaticum,** muriatic acid. म्यूरिएटिक एसिड; नमक का तेजाब;

**A. Nitricum,** nitric acid. नाइट्रिक एसिड; यवाक्षार; शोराम्ल; शोरे का तेजाब;

**A. Picricum,** picric acid. पिकरिक एसिड;

**A. Prussicum,** prussic acid. प्रूसिक एसिड;

**A. Sulphuricum,** sulphuric acid. सल्प्यूरिक एसिड; गंधक अम्ल; गंधक का तेजाब;

**A. Tannicum,** tannic acid. टैनिक एसिड;

**A. Tartaricum,** tartaric acid. टार्टैरिक एसिड; द्राक्षाम्ल; टाटरी अम्ल

**Aciduria.** The presence of acid in the urine. अम्लमेह; मूत्राम्लता; मूत्र में अम्ल विद्यमान रहना

**Acies.** Margin or border. किनारा

**Aciform.** Like a needle; needle-like; acinic. सूच्याकार; सूचीवत्; सुई जैसा

**Acinar.** Pertaining to an acinus; acinic. कोष्ठकी

**Acinesia.** Loss of motion. गत्याभाव; गति करने की असमर्थता

**Acinesic.** See **Acinetic.**

**Acinetic.** One affected with acinesia; acinesic. गत्याभावग्रस्त

**Acini.** Plural of **Acinus.**

**Acinic.** See **Acinar.**

**Aciniform.** Grape-like. द्राक्षावत्; अंगूर जैसा

**Acinitis.** Inflammation of an acinus. कोष्ठकशोथ

**Acinose.** Containing acini. द्राक्षायुक्त; अंगूरी

**Acinous.** Resembling an acinus or grape-shaped structure. कोष्ठकाकार; द्राक्षाकार; अंगूर की शक्ल जैसा

**Acinus.** Smallest division of a gland. कोष्ठक; खण्ड;

**Liver A.,** a liver-lobule. यकृत् कोष्ठक; यकृत् खण्ड;

**Pulmonary A.,** that part of the airway consising of a terminal bronchiole and all of its branches. फुप्फुस-खण्ड; वायु-कोष्ठक

**Aclastic.** Not refracting. अपवर्तक

**Acme.** The crisis or height of a disease. दारुणावस्था; पराकाष्ठा; पराकोटि; प्रबद्धावस्था; चर्मोत्कर्ष; रोग का प्रचण्ड आवेग

**Acne.** Pimple; comedones. मुहासा; मुहासे; पनसिका; चेहरे की फुन्सी;

**A. Artificialis,** that caused by external irritation. कृत्रिम पनसिका; नकली मुहासे;

# Acne

**A. Atrophica,** a form with the pustules grouped about the forehead and scalp; acne varioliformis; acne frontalis. शोषकर पनसिका;

**A. Ciliaris,** acne of the edges of the eyelids. वर्त्मान्त पनसिका; पलकों के किनारे होने वाली फुन्सी;

**A. Erythematosa,** see **Acne Rosacea.**

**A. Frontalis,** see **Acne Atrophica.**

**A. Generalis,** acne diffused over the whole body. सार्वदैहिक पनसिका;

**A. Indurata,** a variety of acne, marked by chronic, livid indurations. दृढ़ पनसिका; ठोस प्रकार के मुहासे;

**A. Mentagra,** a papular eruption in the beard; barber's itch. चिबुक पनसिका; ठोढ़ी पर निकलने वाले मुहासे;

**A. Neonatorum,** acne in newborn. नवजात पनसिका;

**A. Rosacea,** chronic congestion of the skin of the face; acne erythematosa. रक्तिम पनसिका; चेहरे पर निकलने वाले गुलाबी मुहासे;

**A. Simplex,** see **Acne Vulgaris.**

**A. Varioliformis,** see **Acne Atrophica.**

**A. Vulgaris,** common acne; acne simplex, common in adolescence appearing usually on face, neck and upper part of chest and back. सामान्य पनसिका; सामान्य प्रकार के मुहासे

**Acneiform.** See **Acneform.**

**Acneform.** Resembling acne; acneiform. पनसिकाकार; मुहासाकार; मुहासे जैसा

**Acnegenic.** Producing or causing acne. पनसिकाजनक; मुहासाजनक

**Acnemia.** Wasting of the calves. जंघापिण्डिकाक्षय

**Acnitis.** A papular eruption that becomes pustular, leaving slight scars. पनसिकाशोथ

**Acognosia.** A knowledge of drugs. औषधिज्ञान; भेषजज्ञान

**Acology.** The science of remedies. औषधिविज्ञान; चिकित्साशास्त्र; चिकित्साविज्ञान

**Acomia.** Baldness; alopecia. खल्वाटता; गंजापन; गंज; बाल गिरना

**Aconite.** A drug from the root and leaves of **Aconite Napellus,** containing a powerful and rapid poison, aconitine; aconitum. वत्सनाभ; वच्छनाभ; सिंगिया; मीठा जहर; मीठा तैलिया

**Aconitine.** A very poisonous alkaloid extracted from the dried roots of **Aconitum.** काष्ठविषसार; वत्सनाभ का रस

**Aconitum.** See **Aconite.**

**Aconuresis.** An involuntary voiding of urine. असंयतमूत्रता; निरंकुशमूत्रता; मूत्र का स्वत: निकल जाना

**Acopic.** Allaying the tiredness. श्रमनाशक; थकान दूर करने वाला (वाली)

**Acorea.** A congenital absence of the pupil. सहजपटलाभाव; अक्षिपटल का जन्मजात अभाव

**Acoria.** Canine or insatiable hunger. अतिक्षुधा; बहुत भूख लगना; राक्षसी भूख

**Acorn.** The fruit of oak tree. बांजफल; बंजूफल

**Acorus Calamus.** Sweet flag. वटवृक्ष; उग्रगन्थापादप; वचपादप; बड़ का पेड़

**Acostate.** Having no ribs. अपर्शुक; बिना पसलियों का; पसलीहीन

**Acotyledon.** A plant in which the seed lobes are not present. अबीजफल; अनंकुरक पौधा; बिना बीज का फल

**Acoulation.** An apparatus used in teaching speech to deaf-mutes. ध्वनिविस्तारकयंत्र

**Acoumeter.** An instrument for measuring acuteness of hearing; acouometer. श्रवणध्वनिमापीयंत्र; श्रवणशक्तिमापकयंत्र

**Acouometer.** See **Acoumeter.**

**Acousmatamnesia.** A loss of memory for sounds. ध्वनिस्मृतिलोप

**Acoustic.** Concerned with the function of hearing. शाब्दिक; ध्वनिक; श्रवणेन्द्रिय सम्बन्धी

**Acoustics.** The science concerned with sounds and their perceptions. श्रवणविज्ञान; श्रवणगुणविज्ञान; ध्वनिविज्ञान

**Acquired.** Gained by oneself and for oneself. उपार्जित; अर्जित; जन्मोत्तर; अवंशानुगत

**Acral.** Peripheral parts, such as ears, fingers, toes, etc. परिसरीय अंग, जैसे कान, उंगलियाँ, आदि; अवयवप्रभावी

**Acrania.** Absence of the whole or a part of the cranium. अकपालिता; अकरोटिता; करोटि अर्थात् खोपड़ी का पूर्ण या आंशिक अभाव

**Acranial.** Without a skull. करोटिरहित; करोटिहीन; खोपड़ीहीन

**Acratia.** Failure of strength; weakness. दुर्बलता; कमजोरी; शक्तिह्रास; अजितेन्द्रियता

**Acrid.** Sharp, pungent, irritating or biting to the taste. तीखा; तीक्ष्ण; उग्र; कटु; तिक्त; चरपरा; संतापक

**Acridity.** Sharpness. तीक्ष्णता; तीखापन

**Acriflavine.** A dye; a derivation obtained from coal-tar. एक्रिफ्लैविन; तारकोल से प्राप्त एक रंजक

**Accroaesthesia.** The same as **Acroesthesia**.

**Acroarthritis.** Inflammation of the joints of hands or feet. सन्धिशोथ; जोड़ों का प्रदाह

**Acroasphyxia.** Numbness of fingers. सुन्नांगुलिता; उँगलियों का सुन्नपन

**Acroataxia.** Ataxia affecting the distal portion of the extremities. अंगुलिचलन-अक्षमता

**Acrobiology.** Study of distribution of airborn organisms and their effects. वायुजीवविज्ञान

**Acrocentric.** Pertaining to a chromosome in which the centromere is located near one end. अग्रकेन्द्रिक

**Acrocephalia.** Having a conical head; acrocephaly. शंकुशीर्षता

**Acrocephalosyndactylia.** See **Acrocephalosyndactyly**.

**Acrocephalosyndactyly.** A congenital malformation consisting of a pointed top of head, with webbed hands and feet; acrocephalosyndactylia; acrodysplasia. शंकुशीर्षयुक्तांगुलिता

**Acrocephaly.** See **Acrocephalia**.

**Acrocyanosis.** Coldness and blueness of the extremities due to circulatory disorder. शाखाश्यावता; बाह्यांगों का नीलापन

**Acrodynia.** Painful reddening of the extremities. शाखावेदना; बाह्यांगों की दर्दनाक लाली

**Acrodysplasia.** See **Acrocephalosyndactyly**.

**Acroesthesia.** Hypersensitiveness. अतिसंवेदिता; अतिअनुभूतिता; pain in the extremities. बाह्यांगवेदना; अवयव-पीड़ा

**Acromania.** Incurable insanity. अप्रेरणोन्माद; असाध्य पागलपन

**Acromanial.** Pertaining to the acromania. अप्रेरणोन्मादी; असाध्य पागलपन सम्बन्धी

**Acromastitis.** Inflammation of the nipples. चूचुकशोथ; चूचुकों का प्रदाह

**Acromegalia.** See **Acromegaly**.

**Acromegaly.** A disease in which the bones and soft parts of the face and extremities are abnormally enlarged; acromegalia. अतिकायता; महाकायता; महांगता; शाखा-बृहता

**Acromelalgia.** See **Erythromelalgia.**

**Acromial.** Pertaining to the acromion. अंसकूटी; अंसकूट सम्बन्धी

**Acromicria.** Congenital shortness of the extremities. बाह्यांगलघुता; भुजाओं और टांगों का छोटा रहना

**Acromioclavicular.** Pertaining to the acromion and clavicle. अंसकूट तथा जत्रुक सम्बन्धी;

    **A. Joint**, an arthrodial joint between the acromion and the acromial end of the clavicle. अंसकूट-जत्रुक संधि

**Acromiocoracoid.** Pertaining to the acromion and the coracoid process. अंसकूट तथा अंसतुण्ड सम्बन्धी

**Acromiohumeral.** Pertaining to the acromion and the humerus. अंसकूट तथा प्रगण्ड सम्बन्धी;

    **A. Muscle,** the deltoid muscle. अंसकूट-प्रगण्डपेशी; त्रिकोणिका पेशी

**Acromion.** The projecting process of the scapula. अंसकूट

**Acromioscapular.** Pertaining to the acromion and the scapula. अंसकूट तथा अंसफलक अथवा स्कन्धफलक सम्बन्धी

**Acromiothoracic.** Relating to the acromion and thorax. अंसकूट तथा वक्ष सम्बन्धी

**Acromyotonia.** Myotonia affecting the extremities only; acromyotonus. बाह्यांगपेशीतानता

**Acromyotonus.** See **Acromyotonia.**

**Acronyx.** An ingrowing of nails. अन्तःनख; अन्तर्नख; नाखुनों के अन्दर गुल्मोत्पत्ति होना

**Acropachy.** A thickened state of finger tips. शाखास्थूलता; अंगुलिस्थूलता; उँगलियों का किनारा मोटा हो जाना

**Acroparaesthesia.** Extreme paraesthesia; acroparesthesia. शाखा-अपसंवेदन

**Acroparalysis.** Paralysis of the extremities. शाखाघात; बाह्यांगों अर्थात् हाथ-पैरों का पक्षाघात

**Acroparesthesia.** See **Acroparaesthesia.**

**Acropathology.** Pathology of the extremities. शाखाविकृतिविज्ञान; बाह्यांगविकृतिविज्ञान; भुजाओं तथा टांगों से सम्बन्धित रोगों का विज्ञान

**Acropathy.** Any disease of the extremities. शाखारुग्णता; बाह्यांगविकृति; हाथ-पैरों का कोई रोग

**Acropetal.** Developing from below upward. अग्राभिसारी; ऊर्ध्वगामी; नीचे से ऊपर की ओर बढ़ने वाला

**Acrophobia.** Morbid fear of being at a height. उत्तुंगभीति; ऊँचे स्थानों का डर; ऊँचाई का डर

**Acroposthia.** The prepuce. शिश्नमुण्डच्छद; लिंगाग्रचर्म; लिंगमुण्ड को ढकने वाली चमड़ी

**Acroposthitis.** Inflammation of the prepuce. शिश्नमुण्डच्छदशोथ; लिंगाग्रचर्मशोथ; लिंगमुण्ड को ढकने वाली चमड़ी का प्रदाह

**Acroscleroderma.** See **Acrosclerosis.**

**Acrosclerosis.** Stiffness and tightness of the fingers, with atrophy of the soft tissue and osteoporosis of the distal phalanges of the hands and feet; acroscleroderma. शाखाकाठिन्य

**Acrosome.** The anterior end of the head of the spermatozoon. अग्रपिण्डक

**Acrosphacelus.** Gangrene of the digits. अंगुलिकोथ; उँगलियों का मांस गलना

**Acrotism.** An absence or weakness of the pulse. स्पन्दनाभाव; नाड़ीलोप; नाड़ी-स्पन्द का अभाव; अदृश्य या लुप्त नाड़ी; नाड़ी-विकार

**Acrotismus.** Pulselessness. नाड़ीस्पन्दहीनता; नाड़ीस्पन्द का अभाव

**Act.** To carry out; to perform; to accomplish a function. कार्य करना; काम करना

**Actinic.** Having the power of exciting chemic action. रसायनविकारी; रसायनविकारक; क्रियाशील

**Actino.** X-ray. विकिरण; किरण; क्ष-किरण; एक्स-रे

**Actinodermatitis.** X-ray dermatitis. किरणत्वक्शोथ; प्रकाशविकिरण से उत्पन्न चर्म रोग

**Actinoform.** Of the form of an x-ray. विकिरणरूप

**Actinology.** The science of x-ray. विकिरणशास्त्र; विकिरणविज्ञान; शुप्रभ-ऊर्जाविज्ञान; रसोक्रियकी

**Actinometer.** An instrument for measuring x-ray. किरणक्रियामापी; किरणमापी; प्रकाशरसोक्रियामापी

**Actinomycosis.** A fungus infection acquired from animal contents, characterized by the formation of lumpy tumours on the jaws and tongue. किरणकवकमयता; किरण रोग; विकिरणरुग्णता

**Actinotherapeutics.** The study or science of treatment by violet or ultra-violet rays. विकिरणचिकित्साशास्त्र; विकिरण-चिकित्सा का वैज्ञानिक अध्ययन

**Actinotherapy.** Treatment by violet or ultra-violet rays.

विकिरणचिकित्सा; प्रकाशरसक्रियाचिकित्सा

**Action.** The performance of any of the functions, as of a drug. क्रिया; कार्य; व्यापार; प्रवृत्ति;

**Compulsive A.**, performed by an individual at the supposed instigation at another's dominant will, but against his own. बाध्यताकारी क्रिया;

**Cumulative A.**, suddenly increased action of a drug after several doses have been given. संचयी क्रिया;

**Drug A.**, function of a drug in various body systems. औषध-क्रिया;

**Reflex A.**, an involuntary action of one part of the body due to an impression on some afferent nerve end-organ. प्रतिवर्ती क्रिया; परावर्तित क्रिया;

**Sexual A.**, coition; sexual intercourse. रतिक्रिया; सम्भोग क्रिया;

**Specific A.**, that brought about certain remedial agents in a particular disease. विशिष्ट क्रिया;

**Specific Dynamic. A. (SDA)**, the stimulating effect upon the metabolism produced by the ingestion of food, especially proteins. विशिष्ट गतिशील क्रिया; विशिष्ट गत्यात्मक क्रिया

**Activate.** To render active. सक्रिय करना

**Activated.** Rendered active. सक्रियकृत; सक्रियित

**Activation.** To activate. सक्रियकरण; सक्रियण

**Activator.** The substance which activates. सक्रियकारक; सक्रियकारी; सक्रियक; ऐसा पदार्थ जो दूसरे पदार्थ को सक्रिय करता है

**Active.** Energetic; the reverse of passive. सक्रिय; क्रियाशील; चेतन;

**A. Immunity,** one required during an infectious disease or artificially by vaccination with dead or living organism. सक्रिय रोगक्षमता;

**A. Motion,** active range of motion. सक्रिय गति;

**A. Principle,** an ingredient which gives a complex drug its chief therapeutic value. सक्रिय तत्त्व

**Activity.** The state of being active. सक्रियता

**Actuated.** Put into action. चालित; प्रेरित

**Acu.** See **Acus**.

**Acuity.** Intensity or clearness. तीक्ष्णता; तीखापन; नुकीलापन;

**Auditory A.**, ability to hear clearly and distinctly. श्रवण-तीक्ष्णता;

**Visual A.**, acuteness of vision. दृष्टि-तीक्ष्णता

**Acumeter.** An instrument for testing hearing. श्रवणजांचयंत्र

**Acuminate.** See **Acuminated.**

**Acuminated.** Having a long projecting highly tapering point; acuminate. नोकदार; नुकीला; तीक्ष्णाग्र; आगे से तेज नुकीला

**Acuminatum.** See **Acuminatus.**

**Acuminatus.** Having a pointed apex; acuminatum. नोकदार; नुकीला

**Acuminous.** Possessing sharp wit. कुशाग्रबुद्धि; तेज बुद्धि वाला

**Acupression.** See **Acupressure.**

**Acupressure.** Compression of blood-vessels by means of needles; acupression. सूचीदाब; सुईदाब

**Acupuncture.** Puncture made with long fine needle for diagnostic purpose. सूचीवेध; सूचीभेद;; सूचीभेदन; सूचीवेधी रक्तस्रवण; रोगनिदान की एक पद्धति

**Acus.** Needle, especially a surgical needle; acu. सूची; सुई

**Acusticus.** The auditory nerve. श्रवणतंत्रिका

**Acute.** Rapid; severe; sharp; keen. उग्र; तीव्र; तरुण; नूतन

**Acuteness.** Sharpness; severity; rapidity. उग्रता; तीव्रता; तीक्ष्णता; तेजी

**Acutus.** Of acute course. तरुण रूपी

**Acyanoblepsia.** See **Acyanoblepsy.**

**Acyanoblepsy.** Blue blindness; acyanoblepsia; acyanopsia. नीलवर्णान्धता; नीला रंग पहचानने की असमर्थता

**Acyanopsia.** See **Acyanoblepsy.**

**Acyanosis.** Without cyanosis. अश्याव; नीलिमारहित

**Acyanotic.** Without cyanosis. अश्याव; नीलिमारहित

**Acyclia.** Failure of circulation. संचाररोध; संचार क्रिया रुक जाना

**Acyclic.** Without a cycle. अचक्रक; चक्रहीन

**Acyesis.** Sterility of the female; absence of pregnancy. स्त्री-बंध्यता; स्त्रियों में बांझपन

**Acystia.** A congenital absence of the bladder. सहजमूत्राशयहीनता; अनाशयता; अव्योषिता; मूत्राशय का जन्मजात अभाव

**Acystinervia.** Paralysis of the bladder. मूत्राशयघात; मसाने का पक्षाघात; आशयघात

**Acystonervia.** The same as **Acystinervia.**

**Acystoneuria.** The same as **Acystinervia.**

**A. D.** Auris dextra; right ear. दक्षिण कर्ण; दायां कान

**Ad.** In prescription writing, ad indicates that a substance should be added. नुस्खा लेखन में "तक मिलाओ" का अर्थ देने वाला संकेत चिन्ह

**Adactyl.** Having no toes or fingers. अंगुलिहीन; अनंगुलिक; अंगुलिरहित; उँगलियों से हीन

**Adactylia.** An absence of digits; adactylism. अंगुलिहीनता; अनंगुलिता; उँगलियां न होना

**Adactylism.** See **Adactylia.**

**Adactylous.** Without digits. अंगुलिहीन; अनंगुलिक; अंगुलिरहित; उँगलियों से हीन

**Adamantinoma.** Tumour of the enamel of tooth; adamantoma; ameloblastoma. दन्तवल्क-अर्बुद; दन्तवल्क की रसौली

**Adamantoblast.** An enamel cell; a columnar epithelial cell from which the enamel of teeth is developed. दन्तवल्कप्रसू; दन्तवल्ककोशिका

**Adamantoblastoma.** Overgrowth of an adamantoblast. दन्तवल्कप्रसू-अर्बुद

**Adamantoma.** See **Adamantinoma.**

**Adam's Apple.** The laryngeal prominence in front of the neck, especially in the adult male, formed by the junction of two wings of the thyroid cartilage. स्वरयंत्र-उत्सेध; टेंटुआ; कण्ठमणि

**Adams-Stokes Syndrome.** Altered state of consciousness due to decreased flow of blood to the brain. एडम्स-स्टॉकेस संलक्षण; एडम-स्टॉकेस सिंड्रोम

**Adaptability.** The ability to adjust both mentally and physically to the circumstances. अनुकूलता; अनुकूलनशीलता; अनुकूलनीयता; अनुयोज्यता

**Adaptable.** Capable of being adapted. अनुकूलनीय; अनुयोज्य; उपयुक्त

**Adaptation.** Adjustment, as of pupils and retina to any variation of light. अनुकूलन; अनुवर्तिता; अनुयोजन; अनुकूलता; उपयुक्तता; संधानता;

**Chromatic A.,** a change in hue or saturation or both resulting from pre-exposure to light of other wave-lengths. वर्णानुकूलन; रंगानुकूलन;

**Dark A.,** the adjustment of the eye occurring under reduced illumination in which the sensitivity to light is greatly increased; scotopic adaptation. तमोनुकूलन;

**Light A.,** the adaptation of the eye occurring under increased illumination in which the sansitivity to light is reduced; photopic adaptation. प्रकाशानुकूलन;

**Photopic A.**, see **Light Adaptation**.

**Retinal A.**, adjustment of the eye to the degree of illumination. दृष्टिपटलानुकूलन;

**Scotopic A.**, see **Dark Adaptation**.

**Adapter.** One who adapts. अनुकूलित्र; अनुकूलक; उपायोजक

**Adaptive.** Suitable. अनुकूल; उपयुक्त

**Adaptor.** The same as **Adapter**.

**Add.** See **Addatur**.

**Addatur.** Mix with; add; adde. मिलाइये

**Adde.** See **Addatur**.

**Addict.** One who habitually uses narcotics. व्यसनी; आसक्त; नसेड़ी; आनिसेव; बुरी आदत वाला

**Addiction.** Bad habit. व्यसन; आसक्ति; लत; आसक्तता; अभ्यस्तता;

**Drug A.**, a bad habit of taking drugs frequently. औषध-व्यसन; निरन्तर औषधियों का सेवन करते रहने की आदत

**Addison's Anaemia.** Pernicious anaemia. एडीसन एनीमिया; प्रणाशी अरक्तता; सांघातिक अरक्तता अथवा रक्ताल्पता

**Addison's Disease.** A disease marked by a peculiar bronzed pigmentation of the skin with severe prostration and progressive anaemia. एडीसन रोग; विनाशक अरक्तता; सांघातिक रक्ताल्पता

**Additive.** A substance not essentially part of a material, but is deliberately added to fulfil some specific purpose. योगशील

**Adducent.** Causing adduction. अभिवर्तनकारी; अभिवर्तक

**Adduct.** To draw towards the median line of the body. समीपकर्ष; केन्द्राभिमुखी आकर्षण; अभिवर्तन करना; एक ही केन्द्र की ओर खींचना

**Adduction.** Movement of a limb toward the median line, or beyond it. अभिवर्तन; संव्यूहन; अन्तर्नयन; केन्द्रनयन; समीपकर्षण

**Adductor.** Any muscle which moves a part toward the median axis of the body. अभिवर्तनी; अभिवर्तक; समीपकर्षी; आकर्षणी (पेशी)

**Ademonia.** Mental distress. आत्मनैराश्य; anxiety. अधीरता

**Aden.** A gland; a bubo. ग्रन्थि; गिल्टी; पर्व

**Adenalgia.** Glandular pain; adenodynia. ग्रन्थिशूल; ग्रन्थ्यार्ति; ग्रन्थिवेदना; ग्रन्थिपीड़ा; गिल्टी का दर्द

**Adenasthenia.** Functional weakness of a gland. ग्रन्थिदुर्बलता; ग्रन्थिशैथिल्य; किसी ग्रन्थि की क्रियात्मक दुर्बलता;

**A. Gastrica,** that affecting the gastric gland. जठरग्रन्थिदुर्बलता

**Adenectomy.** The excision of a gland. ग्रन्थ्युच्छेदन; ग्रन्थिकर्तन; किसी ग्रन्थि को काट कर निकाल देना

**Adenectopia.** The dislocation of a gland. ग्रन्थिभ्रंश; ग्रन्थिच्युति; किसी ग्रन्थि का अपने स्थान से हट जाना

**Adenemphraxis.** Glandular obstruction. ग्रन्थिरोध; किसी ग्रन्थि-नली का रुक जाना

**Adenia.** Hodgkin's disease. हॉकिन्स रोग, जिसमें लसीका ऊतक, प्लीहा एवं यकृत् बढ़ जाते हैं

**Adeniform.** Of the shape of a gland. ग्रन्थ्याकार; ग्रन्थिरूप; गिल्टी जैसा

**Adenitis.** Inflammation of a gland or lymph node; glandular inflammation. ग्रन्थिशोथ; ग्रन्थिप्रदाह;

**Cervical A.,** inflammation of the neck glands. ग्रीवाग्रन्थिशोथ; गर्दन की गिल्टियों का प्रदाह;

**Hilar A.,** inflammation of the bronchial lymph nodes. श्वसनिक-लसीकापर्वशोथ

**Adenoblast.** Any active gland cell. ग्रन्थिप्रसू; सक्रियग्रन्थिकोशिका

**Adenocanthoma.** See **Adenocarcinoma.**

**Adenocarcinoma.** A cancer arising from glandular tissue, as in the breast, stomach, etc.; adenocanthoma. ग्रन्थिकैंसर; ग्रन्थिकर्कटता

**Adenocele.** See **Adenoma.**

**Adenochondroma.** A combined adenoma and chondroma. ग्रन्थि-उपास्थिअर्बुद; ग्रंथ्युपास्थ्यबुद

**Adenocystoma.** A cystous adenoma. ग्रन्थिपुटी-अर्बुद

**Adenodynia.** See **Adenalgia.**

**Adenoepithelioma.** Tumour consisting of glandular and epithelial elements. ग्रंथ्युपकलार्बुद

**Adenofibroma.** An adenoma with fibromatous elements. ग्रन्थितन्तु-अर्बुद

**Adenogenous.** Having an origin in glandular tissue. ग्रन्थिजन

**Adenography.** A treatise on the glandular system. ग्रन्थिचित्रण; ग्रन्थिव्याख्या

**Adenohypophysial.** Relating to the adenohypophysis. पीयूषिकाग्रन्थिपरक; पीयूषिकाग्रन्थि सम्बन्धी

**Adenohypophysis.** The pituitary gland. पीयूषिकाग्रन्थि; अग्रपीयूषिकाग्रन्थि

**Adenoid.** Resembling a gland. ग्रन्थ्याभ; लसीकाभ; कण्ठशालूकाभ;

A. **Tumour,** an adenoma. ग्रन्थ्यर्बुद

**Adenoidectomy.** Surgical removal from naso-pharynx of adenoid tissue. कण्ठशालूकोच्छेदन; कण्ठशालूक को काट कर हटा देना

**Adenoids.** Enlarged mass of lymphoid tissue in the naso-pharynx which can obstruct breathing and interfere with hearing. कण्ठशालूक; कण्ठग्रन्थि; गले की गिल्टी

**Adenology.** The doctrine of the glands. ग्रन्थिविज्ञान

**Adenolymphoma.** A combined adenoma and lymphoma. ग्रन्थिलसीकार्बुद

**Adenoma.** An innocent tumour of glandular tissue; adenocele. ग्रन्थ्यर्बुद; ग्रन्थि-अर्बुद;

A. **Destruens,** a destructive form of adenoma. विनाशी ग्रन्थ्यर्बुद;

A. **Sebaceum,** a fatty tumour of face composed of sebaceous glands. त्वग्वसीय ग्रन्थ्यर्बुद

**Adenomalacia.** The softening of a gland. ग्रन्थिमृदुता; किसी ग्रन्थि की कोमलता

**Adenomatoid.** Resembling an adenoma. ग्रन्थ्याभ; गिल्टी जैसा

**Adenomatome.** Instrument for removing adenoids. ग्रन्थ्युच्छेदक

**Adenomatosis.** Development of multiple glandular overgrowths. ग्रन्थ्यर्बुदता

**Adenomyoma.** A tumour composed of muscle and glandular elements. ग्रन्थिपेश्यर्बुद

**Adenomyomata.** Plural of **Adenomyoma.**

**Adenomyosis.** A tumour of the glandular muscles. ग्रन्थिपेशी-अर्बुदता; ग्रन्थिपेश्यर्बुदता; भित्ति-पेशी में ग्रन्थि ऊतकों का अतिक्रमण;

A. **Uteri,** the uterine adenoma. जरायुग्रन्थिपेशी-अर्बुदता

**Adenoncus.** A grandular enlargement. ग्रन्थ्यर्बुद

**Adenopathy.** Any disease of a gland, especially a lymphatic gland; adenosis. ग्रन्थिरोग: गिल्टी की बीमारी

**Adenopharyngitis.** Inflammation of the tonsils and the pharynx. गलतुण्डिकाग्रसनीशोथ; गलतुण्डिका तथा ग्रसनी का प्रदाह

**Adenophthalmia.** Inflammation of the Meibomian gland. नेत्रच्छदग्रन्थिशोथ; मेबोमी अथवा पलकों की ग्रन्थि का प्रदाह

**Adenosclerosis.** Hardening of a gland with or without swelling, usually due to replacement by fibrous tissue or calcification.

ग्रन्थिकाठिन्य; ग्रन्थि की कठोरता

**Adenose.** Gland-like. ग्रन्थ्याभ; गिल्टी जैसा

**Adenosis.** Any chronic abnormality of the glands; adenopathy. ग्रन्थिलता; ग्रन्थिरोग: ग्रन्थियों की कोई पुरानी बीमारी;

**Fibrosing A.**, see **Sclerosing Adenosis.**

**Sclerosing A.**, a nodular benign breast lesion occurring most frequently in relatively young women and consisting of hypoplastic distorted lobules of acinar tissue with increased collagenous stroma; fibrosing adenosis. काठिन्यकर ग्रन्थिलता

**Adenotome.** An instrument for incising gland. ग्रन्थिछेदक; ग्रन्थिकर्तकयंत्र

**Adenotomy.** Incision of a gland. ग्रन्थिछेदन; ग्रन्थिकर्तन; anatomy of the glands. ग्रन्थिरचना; ग्रन्थिसंरचनाज्ञान

**Adenotyphus.** Abdominal typhus fever. औदरिक मोहज्वर

**Adenous.** Like a gland. ग्रन्थिवत्

**Adephagia.** Voracious hunger. अतिक्षुधा; बहुत भूख लगना

**Adeps.** Lard. वसा; चर्बी;

    **A. Anserinus,** goose-grease. हंस-वसा;

    **A. Suillus,** hog's lard. शूकर-वसा

**Adequacy.** Sufficiency. प्रचुरता; प्राचुर्य; पर्याप्तता

**Adequate.** Sufficient. प्रचुर; पर्याप्त

**Adermia.** Congenital absence or defect of the skin. त्वक्दोष; त्वग्दोष; त्वचा की दोषपूर्ण अवस्था

**Adermogenesis.** Imperfect development of the skin. अपूर्णत्वग्विकास; त्वचा का अपूर्ण विकास

**Adermotrophia.** Imperfect development of the skin. अपूर्णत्वग्पोषण; अपूर्णत्वग्विकास; त्वचा का अपूर्ण पोषण या विकास

**Adhere.** To stick fast. चिपकना; चिपकाना; अभिलग्नता

**Adherence.** The quality of being adherent. चिपकाव; संसक्ति

**Adherent.** Sticking. संसक्त; आसंजनशील; अभिलग्न; चिपचिपा

**Adhesio.** Adhesion. आसंजन; आश्लेष; चिपकाव

**Adhesion.** Unnatural union of surfaces, due to inflammation. आसंजन; आसक्ति; आश्लेष; अभिलग्न; चिपकाव; संसक्ति; आसंज;

    **Abdominal A.**, adhesion in abdominal cavity usually involving the intestines. उदर-आसंजन;

**Pericardial A.,** adhesion of the pericardial sac. परिहृद्-आसंजन;

**Primary A.,** healing by first intention. प्राथमिक आसंजन;

**Secondary A.,** healing by granulation, or second intention. गौण आसंजन

**Adhesive.** Sticky; causing adhesion; tenacious. आश्लेषी; आश्लेषक; आसंजी; आसंजक; लेसदार; चिपकने वाला;

**A. Inflammation,** in surgery, the process by which the wounds are united. आसंजी प्रदाह; आश्लेषक प्रदाह;

**A. Plaster,** any plaster which adheres to the skin; resin plaster. आसंजी पलस्तर; आश्लेषक पलस्तर

**Adiactinic.** Impervious to actinic rays. अविघटनाभिक-किरणी; अविघटनाभिक किरणों के लिये अभेद्य

**Adiadochokinesia.** See **Adiadochokinesis.**

**Adiadochokinesis.** Inability to perform rapid alternating movements; adiadochokinesia. शीघ्रपर्यायगतिभंग

**Adiaphoresis.** Deficient perspiration; adiapneustia. अल्पस्वेदन; अस्वेदता; स्वेदाभाव; पसीने की कमी या अभाव

**Adiaphoretic.** Preventing or reducing perspiration. अल्पस्वेदकारी; पसीना रोकने या कम करने वाला

**Adiapneustia.** See **Adiaphoresis.**

**Adiemorrhysis.** Stoppage of the circulation of blood in a certain part. रक्तरोध; रुद्धरक्तता; किसी भाग में रक्त का बहाव रुक जाना

**Adipectomy.** The excision of a mass of adipose tissue. वसोतकोच्छेदन; वसा-ऊतक के किसी पिण्ड को काट कर हटा देना

**Adipescent.** Corpulent; fat. स्थूलकाय; मोटा

**Adipic.** Fatty. वासिक; वसीय; चर्बीयुक्त

**Adipification.** Disposition to fat. वसीयस्ववृत्ति

**Adipo-.** Prefix signifying fats. 'वसा' अथवा 'मेद' के रूप में प्रयुक्त उपसर्ग

**Adipocele.** A hernia containing fat or fatty tissue. मेदोमयबृद्धि

**Adipocere.** Saponification; a greyish fatty substance generated in dead bodies subjected to moisture. वसासिक्थ; शवसिक्थ; मुर्दे की चर्बी; मृत देह से निकली हुई वसा या मोम जैसा पदार्थ

**Adipoceratus.** See **Adipocerous.**

**Adipocerous.** Relating to the adipocere; adipoceratus. शवसिक्थ सम्बन्धी

**Adipocyte.** Fat or adipose cell. वसाकोशिका

**Adipogenesis.** Lipogenesis. वसाजनन

**Adipogenic.** See **Adipogenous.**

**Adipogenous.** That which produces fat; adipogenic. वसोत्पादक; वसाजनक; मेदवर्धक; चर्बी पैदा करने वाला

**Adipolysis.** The hydrolysis or digestion of fats. वसालयन

**Adipolytic.** Effecting the digestion of the fats. वसापाचक; वसाविलयी

**Adipoma.** Lipoma; a fatty tumour. वसार्बुद; लिपोमा

**Adipose.** Pertaining to fat; fatty. वसीय; वसामय; वसायुक्त; मेदोमय; वसा सम्बन्धी;

    A. **Arteries,** arterial branches supplying fats. वसा-धमनियां;

    A. **Tissues,** fat cells united by connective tissues. वसा-ऊतक; वसोतक

**Adiposis.** Corpulence; obesity; fatty degeneration; abnormal accumulation of fat in the body. वसामयता; चर्बीमयता; मेदुरता; मेदुर वसापजनन;

    A. **Dolorosa,** a neurosis characterized by pain and nodular formations. सपीड मेदुरता;

    A. **Hepatica,** fatty degeneration of the liver. यकृत् मेदुरता; यकृत्-वसापजनन

**Adipositas.** Fatness. स्थूलता; मोटापा;

    A. **Cordis,** a fatty condition of the heart. वसाहृद्; हृद्वसामयता; हृत्पिण्ड की मेदपूर्ण अवस्था;

    A. **Universalis,** obesity. स्थूलता; मोटापा

**Adipositis.** Inflammation of the fatty tissues. वसापाक; वसाशोथ; वसा-उतकों का प्रदाह; **वसोतकशोथ**

**Adiposity.** Excessive accumulation of fat in the body. वसामयता; स्थूलता; मेदुरता; चर्बीलापन; चिकनाई; पुष्टता

**Adiposuria.** Fat in the urine. वसामेह; पेशाब में चर्बी विद्यमान रहना

**Adiposus.** The fat level. वसास्तर

**Adipsia.** Absence of thirst; adipsy; thirstlessness. तृष्णाभाव; अपिपासा; प्यास का अभाव; पानी पीने की अनिच्छा

**Adipson.** A beverage relieving thirst. तृष्णाहर-पेय; प्यास बुझाने वाला पेय

**Adipsy.** See **Adipsia.**

**Aditus.** An entrance. प्रवेशपथ; प्रवेशिका; प्रवेशस्थल; छिद्र;

**A. Ad Antrum,** the part of the tympanic cavity above the level of the membrana tympani. कर्णमूलकोटर प्रवेशिका;

**A. Laryngis,** the opening into the larynx. स्वरयंत्र प्रवेशिका

**Adjustment.** The mechanism by which the tube of a microscope is raised or lowered. समायोजन; समंजन

**Adjuvant.** A drug included in a prescription to aid the action of other drugs. सहयोगी; सहौषधि; सह-औषध; गुणवर्धक (औषधि); सहकारिक (औषधि);

**A. Therapy,** supportive measures in addition to main treatment. सहयोगी चिकित्सा; सहायक चिकित्सा; आनुषंगिक चिकित्सा

**Ad-Lib.** Prescription abbreviation for **Ad-Libitum.**

**Ad-Libitum.** As much as desired. यथेच्छ; इच्छानुसार

**Admaxillary.** Connected with or pertaining to the jaw. हनु अर्यात जबड़े सम्बन्धी

**Adminiculum Linea Alba.** The lower thickened portion of the fascia transversalis, which is attached to the spine of the pubis and the ileopectineal eminence. उदरमध्यरेखा-विस्तार

**Administer.** To prescribe. औषधप्रयोग करना; भेषजावधारण करना; दवाई देना

**Adnata.** The conjunctiva covering the eyeball. नेत्रश्लेष्मकला; नेत्रगोलक को ढक कर रखने वाली आँख की श्लैष्मिक झिल्ली

**Adnate.** Growing in or adhering to a part. संलग्न; सह-उत्पन्न

**Adneural.** Situated at or near a nerve. स्नायुस्थित; अभिस्नायु

**Adnexa.** Appendages; sutures which are in close proximity to a part. उपांग: संयुक्तांश; अवयव; सहायी अंग;

**A. Oculi,** the lacrimal apparatus. अश्रुजाल;

**A. Uteri,** the ovaries and Fallopian tubes. जरायुजाल; डिम्बग्रन्थियाँ तथा डिम्बवाही नलियाँ

**Adnexal.** Pertaining to the appendages. उपांगीय; उपांगों सम्बन्धी

**Adnexitis.** Inflammation of the adnexa-uterus. जरायूपांगशोथ; डिम्बग्रन्थियों तथा डिम्बवाही नलियों का प्रदाह

**Adnexum.** Singular of **Adnexa.**

**Adolescence.** Youth; the period between puberty and maturity. कौमार्य; किशोरावस्था; किशोरता; यौवनावस्था; प्रौढ़ता की शुरुआत

**Adolescent.** Advancing to manhood. कुमार; किशोर; कौमार

**Adoral.** Situated at or near the mouth. अभिमुखी; अभिमुखीय; मुख के पास स्थित

**Adosculation.** Impregnation by external contact only. बहिसंम्पर्की गर्भाधान; बाहरी सम्पर्क द्वारा होने वाला गर्भाधान

**Adrenal.** Near the kidney; the suprarenal capsule, one on top of each kidney;adrenal gland. अधिवृक्की; वृक्क के पास ऊपर की ओर स्थित अधिवृक्क सम्पुट; एड्रिनल ग्रन्थि;

A. **Cortex,** controls chemical constitution of the body fluids. अधिवृक्क-प्रान्तस्था;

A. **Gland,** see **Adrenal.**

**Adrenalectomy.** Excision of the adrenal gland. अधिवृक्क-उच्छेदन; अधिवृक्क ग्रन्थि को काट कर बाहर निकाल देना

**Adrenalin.** The trade name of an active principle of the suprarenal gland. एड्रिनैलिन; अधिवृक्कग्रन्थि का हार्मोन

**Adrenaline.** The same as **Adrenalin.**

**Adrenalitis.** Inflammation of the adrenal gland. अधिवृक्कशोथ; अधिवृक्क ग्रन्थि का प्रदाह

**Adrenalopathy.** Any pathologic condition of the adrenal glands; adrenopathy. अधिवृक्कविकृति; अधिवृक्करोग

**Adrenic.** Relating to the adrenal gland. अधिवृक्क सम्बन्धी

**Adrenocortical.** Relating to the suprarenal gland and cortex. अधिवृक्क-प्रान्तस्था सम्बन्धी

**Adrenocorticotrophic.** Having an effect on adrenal cortex; adrenocorticotropic. अधिवृक्कप्रान्तस्थाप्रेरक

**Adrenocorticotropic.** See **Adrenocorticotrophic.**

**Adrenogenic.** Originating in or produced by the adrenal gland; adrenogenous. अधिवृक्कजनक

**Adrenogenital.** Relating to the adrenal gland and the genital organs. अधिवृक्क ग्रन्थि तथा जननांगों सम्बन्धी

**Adrenogenous.** See **Adrenogenic.**

**Adrenomegaly.** Enlargement of the adrenal gland. अतिअधिवृक्कता

**Adrenopathy.** See **Adrenalopathy.**

**Adrenotrophic.** See **Adrenotropic.**

**Adrenotropic.** Nourishing or stimulating to the adrenal gland; adrenotrophic. अधिवृक्कप्रेरक

**Adsorbents.** Solids which attract gases or dissolve substances to their surfaces, as a film. अधिशोषक; अवशोषक; दूसरे पदार्थों को अपनी ओर खींचकर धारण करने वाले पदार्थ

**Adsorption.** The power of a substance to attract and hold to its surface a gas. अधिशोषण; शोषण; अवशोषण; सोखना

**Adspection.** Examination. परीक्षा; जांच

**Adult.** Grown up; mature; arrived at maturity. वयस्क; युवा; प्रौढ़; बालिग

**Adulteration.** The corrupting of pure ingredients with others resembling them, that of inferior value. अपमिश्रण; मिलावट

**Adultery.** Voluntary sexual intercourse of married persons with one of the opposite sex; violation of the marriage bed. व्यभिचार: जारकर्म; परस्त्रीगमन; परपुरुषगमन

**Adultorum.** Occurring in adult years. यौवनकालीन; यौवनकालिक

**Advantage.** Benefit. लाभ; फायदा

**Adventitia.** The external coat of the blood vessels. बाह्यास्तर; बाह्यकंचुक; रक्तवाहिनियों का बाहरी आवरण

**Adventitial.** Relating to the adventitia of an organ or structure. बाह्यास्तर, अथवा किसी अंग या बनावट के बाहरी आवरण सम्बन्धी

**Adventitious.** Accidental. आकस्मिक; foreign. आगंतुक; बाह्य; acquired. उपार्जित; coming from without. अस्वाभाविक; अपस्थानिक

**Adverse.** Undesired. अवांछित; opposite. विरुद्ध; विपरीत

**Adynamia.** Weakness caused by disease. अगतिकता; क्षीणता; दुर्बलता; निर्बलता; कमजोरी; जैवी शक्तियों का अभाव; prostration. अवसन्नता

**Adynamic.** Attended with great debility. अगतिक; क्षीण; निर्बल; दुर्बल; कमजोर; pertaining to adynamia. क्षीणता सम्बन्धी

**Adynatus.** Sickly; weakly. रुग्ण; बीमार

**A.E.G.** Airencephalography. मस्तिष्कवायुचित्रण

**Aeration.** Airing; saturating a fluid with air or gas. वातन; वायुसंचरण

**Aerendocardia.** The presence of gas or air within the heart. वायुहृदयता; हृदय के अन्दर हवा विद्यमान रहना

**Aerenterectasia.** Distension of the intestines with air or gas. वातितांत्रविस्फार; वातपूरितांत्र; वातोच्छ्न; आंतों का हवा से फूल जाना

**Aerial.** Relating to the air. वायवी; वायु सम्बन्धी;

  **A. Roots,** small roots of a plant. वायवी मूल

**Aeriferous.** Carrying air; conducting the air. वायुवाही; वायुयुक्त; वायुवाहक; हवा ले जाने वाला

**Aeriform.** Of the form of air; gaseous. वायुरूप; वाष्पमय; वाष्पाकार; वाष्पीभूत; वायुसदृश; गैसीय

**Aerobe.** One of the aerobia; aerobion. वातापेक्षी; वायुजीवी; हवा पर जीवित रहने वाला

**Aerobia.** Organisms requiring air or oxygen to maintain life. वातापेक्षी; वायुजीवी; हवा पर पलने वाला जीव

**Aerobic.** Unable to live without oxygen; aerophilic; aerophilous. वातापेक्षी; वायुजीवी; ऑक्सीजनजीवी; खुली हवा में जीवित रहने वाला

**Aerobion.** See **Aerobe.**

**Aerobiosis.** Life requiring oxygen. वायुजीवन; जारकजीवन; वातजीवन

**Aerobiotic.** Unable to live without oxygen. वातापेक्षी; वायुजीवी; वातजीवी; relating to aerobiosis. वायुजीवन सम्बन्धी

**Aerocele.** Emphysema; distension of a small natural cavity with gas. वातपुटी; वायुजनिताबुर्द;

  **Cervical A.,** emphysema of the neck due to abnormally large laryngeal ventricles. ग्रैववातपुटी

**Aerocolpos.** Distension of the vagina with air or gas. वातितयोनिविस्फार; गैस से योनि का फूल जाना

**Aerocoly.** Distension of the colon with gas. वातितबृहदांत्रविस्फार; गैस से बृहदांत्र का फूल जाना

**Aerocystoscopy.** Bladder examination with the aero-urethroscope. मूत्राशयदर्शन; मूत्राशयिक जांच

**Aerodermectasia.** Subcutaneous emphysema. अधस्त्वक्वातपुटी

**Aerodontalgia.** Dental pain caused by either increased or reduced atmospheric pressure. वातज दंतार्ति

**Aerodontia.** Branch of dentistry concerned with the effect of changes in atmospheric pressure on teeth. वातज दंतता

**Aerodynamics.** The science of gaseous motion. वायुगतिकीविज्ञान

**Aerogenic.** Gas-forming. वातनिर्माणक; वातजनक; वायुजनक

**Aerogenous.** Gas-producing. वातजनक; वातनिर्माणक; वायुजनक

**Aerogram.** X-ray of tube or hollow viscus after introduction of air or gas. आरोहण–आलेख

**Aerohydropathy.** The treatment of disease by means of air and water. वायुजलचिकित्सा; हवा और पानी से की जाने वाली चिकित्सा

**Aerology.** The science of the atmosphere. वायुमण्डलविज्ञान

**Aeromatic.** Motivated by air or gas. वायुचालित; हवा से चलने वाला

**Aerometer.** An instrument for weighing or estimating the density of air. वायुमापी; वायुघनत्वमापी; गैसघनत्वमापी

**Aeropathy.** Any morbid state induced by a pronounced change in the atmospheric pressure. वायुरुग्णता

**Aeroperitoneum.** See **Aeroperitonia.**

**Aeroperitonia.** Distension of the peritoneal cavity with the gas; aeroperitoneum. वातितउदरावरणविस्फार; गैस से उदरावरक गह्वर का फूल जाना

**Aerophagia.** The swallowing of air; aerophagy. वायुभक्षण; वायुनिगरण; हवा निगलना

**Aerophagy.** See **Aerophagia.**

**Aerophil(e).** Air-loving. वायुप्रेमी; an aerobic organism. वातापेक्षी; वातजीवी

**Aerophilic.** See **Aerobic.**

**Aerophilous.** See **Aerobic.**

**Aerophobia.** A morbid fear of a current of air. वायुभीति; चलती हवा का डर; वायु-आतंक

**Aerophore.** An apparatus for forcing air into the lungs. फुप्फुसवायुप्रवेशयंत्र; फेफड़ों के अन्दर हवा भरने वाला यंत्र

**Aeroplethysmograph.** An instrument for recording the respired air. श्वासप्रश्वासमापीयंत्र; उच्छवासलेखयंत्र

**Aeroscope.** An instrument for examination of air-dust. वायुशुद्धतादर्शी (यंत्र); वायुशुद्धतामापकयंत्र; हवा की शुद्धता मापने वाला यंत्र

**Aeroscopy.** Examination of air-dust. वायुशुद्धतादर्शन

**Aerosis.** The production of gas in the organs of the body. वातोत्पत्ति; शरीर के विभिन्न अंगों में हवा उत्पन्न होना

**Aerotherapeutics.** The mode of treating disease by varying the pressure or composition of the air breathed; aerotherapy. वायुचिकित्साविज्ञान; वायुचिकित्सा; हवा द्वारा बीमारी का इलाज

**Aerotherapy.** See **Aerotherapeutics.**

**Aerothorax.** See **Pneumothorax.**

**Aerotonometer.** An instrument for measuring the tension of oxygen or other gases of the blood. रक्तवायुतानमापी; रक्त में वायु के तनाव को मापने वाला यंत्र

**Aerourethroscope.** An instrument used in aerourethroscopy or aerocystoscopy. वायुमूत्रपथपदर्शी या वायुमूत्राशयदर्शी

**Aerourethroscopy.** Urethral examination by electric light after dilatation with air. वायुमूत्रपथदर्शन

**Aeschynomene Grandiflora.** A plant known as **Agastya.** अगस्त्य बूटी

**Aesculapius.** A physician. चिकित्सक; वैद्य; भिषग्देवता

**Aesthesia.** Sense. बोध; ज्ञान; sensation. सम्वेदना

**Aesthetics.** The science of the beauty in art and nature. कलासौंदर्यविज्ञान; प्रकृतिसौंदर्यविज्ञान

**Aestivalis.** Occurring in the season of summer. ग्रीष्मकालीन; गर्मियों में प्रकट होने वाला

**Aether.** The same as **Ether.**

**Aethiopification.** A discolouration of the skin from the long continued use of drugs, as silver or copper. त्वक्-विवर्णता; त्वचा का स्वाभाविक रंग बदल जाना

**Aetiological.** Relating to aetiology. रोगहेतुविषयक; रोग के कारण से सम्बन्धित

**Aetiology.** The science dealing with the causation of diseases; etiology. रोगहेतुविज्ञान; निदानविद्या; रोगकारणविज्ञान;

**Afeared.** Frightened. भयभीत; भयातुर; डरा हुआ

**Afebrile.** Non-febrile; apyretic; without fever. अज्वर; निर्ज्वर; ज्वरहीन; ज्वराभाव; बिना बुखार के

**Afetal.** Without a foetus. भ्रूणहीन; भ्रूणरहित

**Affect.** A feeling directed towards anything. दुष्प्रभाव पड़ना; भाववृत्ति; अनुभाव

**Affection.** Disease. रोग; बीमारी; विकृति; love. प्रेम; प्यार

**Affective.** Pertaining to motion, feeling, sensibility, or a mental state. गति, अनुभूति, विवेक अथवा मनोदशा सम्बन्धी

**Afferent.** Conveying inward or toward the centre. अन्तर्वहा; अभिवाही; अन्तर्गामी;

  **A. Nerves,** nerves that transmit impulses from the periphery towards the central nervous system. अभिवाही तंत्रिकायें; अन्तर्गामी तंत्रिकायें

**Afferentia.** Any afferent vessel. अभिवाही; अन्तर्वहा; अन्तर्गामी

**Affiliation.** Settling of the paternity of an illegitimate child on the putative father. सम्बन्ध; नाता

**Affinity.** Relationship. सम्बन्ध; नाता; a synonym for attraction. आकर्षण; खिंचाव;

  **Chemic A.,** chemical attraction between two substances. रासायनिक आकर्षण;

**Chemical A.,** see **Chemic Affinity.**

**Residual A.,** the force that associates the components of a chemical reaction. अवशिष्ट आकर्षण

**Afflatus.** A variety of acute erysipelas. विसर्पभेद; तीव्र विसर्प का एक रूप; a current of air. हवा का झोंका

**Afflict.** To distress with bodily or mental suffering. सताना; कष्ट देना; कष्ट पहुँचाना

**Affluence.** See **Afflux.**

**Affluent.** Flowing freely; copious. विपुल; प्रचुर; प्रवाहित

**Afflux.** A flow towards a point; affluence. प्रवाह; बहाव; अभिस्यन्दन

**Affluxion.** Accumulation of fluids or flowing of blood or liquid to a part. द्रवसंचय; रक्तसंचय; जलसंचय; बहाव; किसी भाग की ओर रक्त अथवा किसी अन्य तरल पदार्थ का बहाव

**Affluxus.** The same as **Afflux.**

**Affusion.** A pouring upon, as water on the body. परिषेक; जैसे जलपरिषेक; गीला करना

**Afraid.** Frightened. भयातुर; भयभीत; डरा हुआ

**African Lethargy.** Sleeping sickness among the Africans. निद्रा रोग; अफ्रीकी लोगों की एक बीमारी विशेष

**After-birth.** The placenta and the membrane which are extruded after the birth of a child. अपराकला; जेर; अवरनाल

**After-care.** The care given during convalescence and rehabilitation. अनुरक्षण; उपचारोत्तर देख-भाल

**After-cataract.** A recurring cataract. पुनरावर्ती मोतियाबिन्द

**After-effect.** A response occurring sometime after the original stimulus or condition has produced its primary effect. उत्तर-प्रभाव

**After-image.** Continued retinal sensation after withdrawal of an object. अनुविम्ब; श्वेतपटलीय प्रकाशाकर्षण; उत्तेजना बन्द हो जाने पर भी दृष्टिपटल पर दृष्टिगत पदार्थ की छाप बने रहना

**After-pains.** The pains felt after childbirth, due to contraction and retraction of the uterine muscle fibres. प्रसवोत्तरशूल; अनुदर्द

**After-potential.** Small changes in electrical potential in a stimulated nerve which follow the main potential. अनुविभव

**After-sensation.** A sensation which persists after its original cause has ceased to act. रोगोत्तर सम्वेदना; संवेदना या उत्तेजना बन्द हो जाने

पर भी उसकी अनुभूति होते रहना

**After-sound.** The sensation of sound after the cause of the sound has ceased to act. प्रतिध्वनि; गूंज

**Afunction.** Dysfunction; afunctional. अक्रिया; क्रियाहीन; क्रिया या कार्य की कमी

**Afunctional.** See **Afunction**.

**Agalactia.** Imperfect secretion of milk after child-birth. अपस्तन्यता; प्रसवोत्तर दुग्धाभाव; अस्तन्यता; अल्पदुग्धता; दूध न बनना या बन्द हो जाना

**Agalactious.** Checking the secretion of milk. दुग्धरोधी; दुग्धरोधक; दूध का बहाव रोकने वाला; concerning milk. दुग्ध सम्बन्धी

**Agalorrhea.** See **Agalorrhoea**.

**Agalorrhoea..** Arrest of the flow of milk; agalorrhea. स्तन्यरोध; दुग्धरोध; दूध का बहाव रुकना

**Agamic.** See **Agamous**.

**Agamist.** One who is against marriage. विवाह-विरोधी

**Agamogenesis.** Reproduction without fecundation. अमैथुनजनन; अविवाह-सन्तान; अनिषेकजनन; अलिंगीजनन; अमैथुनी उत्पत्ति

**Agamous.** Without sexual organs; agamic. अयुग्मनी; अविवाही; जननांगों से हीन

**Aganglionic.** Without ganglia. अगण्डिकी

**Aganglionosis.** Absence of ganglia, as those of the distant bowel. सहज-अगण्डिकता; परासंवेदीगण्डिका का जन्मजात अभाव

**Agape.** With mouth open in wonder. भौंचक्का; आश्चर्यचकित

**Agaric.** A term broadly applied to fungi of several genera; agaricus. कुकुरमुत्ता; खुम्भी; छत्रक; शिलीन्ध्र

**Agaricin.** An extract from white agaric. श्वेतछत्रक का सत; एगैरिसिन

**Agaricus.** See **Agaric**.

**Agastric.** Without distinct alimentary canal. जठररहित; पोषणनलीविहीन; जठरहीन; अजठर

**Agave.** A genus of plants, including **American Aloe.** रामबांस

**Age.** Length of life. वय:; आयु; उम्र; वयस; जीवनकाल;
  **Mental A.,** the age of a person with regard to his mental development. मानसिक वय; मनोवय

**Aged.** Old one. वयोवृद्ध; बूढ़ा; बुढ़िया; बृद्ध; बृद्धा; जीर्ण

**Agenesia.** Abnormal or imperfect development. अविकास; अपूर्ण विकास; sterility. बंध्यता; अजनन; impotence. नपुंसकता

**Agenesis.** The same as **Agenesia**.

**Agenosomia.** Poor development of the genitals. जननेन्द्रिय-अविकसन; जननेन्द्रियों का अपूर्ण विकास

**Agent.** A substance that produces changes in the body products. कारक; पदार्थ; माध्यम

**Ageusia.** A defect or loss of taste. विरसता; अस्वाद; स्वाद-अनुभूति का अभाव

**Ageustia.** The same as **Ageusia**.

**Agger-nasi.** An oblique on inner surface of the nasal process of the maxilla. नासा-शिखाग्र; नासाकंटक

**Agglomerated.** Massed together; aggregated. समुच्चयित; पुंजित

**Agglutinant.** Uniting agent; adhesive; a substance with adhesive properties; agglutinative. संयोजक; चिपकाने वाला पदार्थ; गोंद जैसा काम करने वाला पदार्थ; समूहीकृत

**Agglutinate.** To unite with glue. चिपकना; चिपकाना

**Agglutination.** A condition wherein subtance adhere together. संश्लेषण; समूहन; चिपकाव; संयुजता

**Agglutinative.** See **Agglutinant**.

**Agglutinins.** Specific factors present in sera which agglutinate protein matter. संश्लेषक; समूहिका

**Agglutinogen.** A factor which stimulates production of a specific agglutinin, used in the production of immunity. समूहजन

**Aggravate.** To increase the gravity of an ailment. वृद्धि होना; अतिरेक होना; बढ़ना

**Aggravation.** The act of becoming worse. वृद्धि; अतिरेक

**Aggregate.** To group or arrange in clusters. समुच्चय करना

**Aggregated.** See **Agglomerated**.

**Aggregation.** The act of grouping or arranging in clusters. सम्मुच्चय; सम्मुच्चयन; संग्रहणता; पुंजता

**Aggregatus.** Grouped. समुच्चयकृत; समुच्चयित

**Aggressin.** A substance produced in the body by bacteria having the property of weakening the normal protective substances of the body. आक्रामिका; शरीर में उत्पादित एक पदार्थ, जिसमें शरीर के सामान्य रक्षात्मक पदार्थों को दुर्बल करने की क्षमता होती है

**Aggression.** An attack, as of bacteria, resulting in the weakness of the normal protective substances of the body. आक्रमण; हमला

**Aging.** Growing old; maturing. कालप्रभावन; वयोबृद्धि

**Agit. Agita,** means **Shake** or **Stir.** हिलाओ

**Agit. a. us.** Agita ante usum, means "Shake before using". प्रयोग करने से पहले हिलाओ

**Agitated Depression.** Marked restlessness, continual activity, despondency and apprehension. अतिशय व्यग्रता; मानसिक उद्वेलन; भारी बेचैनी

**Agitation.** Violent excitement; a shaking. संघर्ष; व्याकुलता; विक्षोभ; उत्तेजना

**Agitator.** Any apparatus for stirring a mixture. विलोडक

**Agitolalia.** Hasty speech. द्रुतभाषण; तेज बोलना

**Aglobulia.** A decrease in the number of the red blood copuscles. लोहितकोशिकापघटन; लाल रक्तकणों की संख्या कम होना

**Agrophobia.** A morbid frear of pain. पीड़ाभीति; दर्द का भय

**Aglossia.** Congenital absence of the tongue. सहज-जिह्वाभाव; जीभ का जन्मजात अभाव

**Aglutition.** An inability to swallow; dysphagia. निगरण-अक्षमता; निगल न सकने की अयोग्यता

**Aglycosuria.** Absence of carbohydrates in the urine. अश्वेतसारिकमूत्रता

**Aglycosuric.** Relating to aglycosuria. अश्वेतसारिकमूत्रता सम्बन्धी

**Agmatology.** The branch of surgery concerning fractures. अस्थिभंगविज्ञान; हड्डियाँ टूट जाने सम्बन्धी विज्ञान

**Agminated.** Arranged in clusters; grouped. सम्मुच्चययकृत; समुच्चयित; गुच्छित

**Agnail.** Hangnail. छिलौरी; नाखुन की जड़ का मांस उखड़ना

**Agnatha.** See **Agnathia.**

**Agnathia.** Congenital absence of the jaws; agnatha. अहनुता; ठोढ़ी का जन्मजात अभाव

**Agnathus.** Having no jaws. निर्हनु; ठोढ़ीरहित

**Agneithia.** The same as **Agnathia.**

**Agnesia.** Impotence; agnesis. नपुंसकता; नपुंसत्व

**Agnesis.** See **Agnesia.**

**Agnosia.** Inability to understand sensory impressions. अभिज्ञान-अक्षमता; असंबोधिता; अनभिज्ञान; संवेदनालोप

**Agomphiasis.** Looseness of teeth; agomphosis. दान्तों का ढीलापन; दान्त

**Agomphious**

शिथिल पड़ जाना; दन्तदोष

**Agomphious.** Having no teeth. दन्तहीन; दन्तरहित; अदन्ती

**Agomphosis.** See **Agomphiasis.**

**Agonal.** The period just preceding death. अन्तकाल; आसन्नमृत्युकाल; मृत्यु से पूर्व का समय

**Agonia.** Inability to recognise things. वस्तुज्ञान-अक्षमता; distress. अतिनिराशा; sterility. बंध्यता; बांझपन

**Agonise.** To torture; to suffer agony. छटपटाना; तड़पना या तड़पाना

**Agonist.** Muscle that shortens to perform a movement. प्रचालक (पेशी)

**Agony.** Intense pain or anguish of body or mind. छटपटाहट; तड़पन; मनस्ताप; the death struggle. मौत से संघर्ष करना

**Agoraphobia.** A dread of open spaces or places. अवकाशभीति; विवृतिभीति; बहिर्भीति; a dread of crowds. जनातंक; सभाभीति; भीड़-भाड़ से डर

**Agraemia.** See **Agremia.**

**Agrammatism.** An inability to form grammatic sentences. अशुद्धवाक्; अशुद्ध शब्दों का प्रयोग करना

**Agranulocyte.** A non-granular laukoyte. अकणीश्वेतकोशिका

**Agranulocytic.** Relating to agranulocytosis. कणीश्वेतकोशिकाहीनता सम्बन्धी

**Agranulocytopenia.** See **Agranulocytosis.**

**Agranulocytosis.** An aplastic anaemia with an acute febrile course and high mortality; agranulocytopenia. कणीश्वेतकोशिकाहीनता; अकणीश्वेतकोशिकामुखपाक; अकणीकोशिकता

**Agraphia.** An inability to express ideas in writing. लेखन-अक्षमता; अलेखन; अ-आलेखनता; लिखित रूप में विचारों को प्रकट करने की असमर्थता;

   **Absolute A.,** complete incapacity to form a letter. पूर्ण लेखन-अक्षमता; लिखने की पूर्ण अक्षमता;

   **Acoustic A.,** loss of the power of writing when dictated. श्रवणलेखन-अक्षमता; सुनकर लिखने की अक्षमता;

   **Motor A.,** inability to recall the movement of the hands in writing. प्रेरक लेखन-अक्षमता;

   **Verbal A.,** a form in which a number of meaningless words can be written. शाब्दिक लेखन-अक्षमता

**Agraphic.** Relating to agraphia. लेखन-अक्षमता सम्बन्धी

**Agremia.** The gouty diathesis; agraemia. वातरोगप्रवणता; गठिया रोग की प्रवणता

**Agria.** Herpes; any severe pustular eruption. परिसर्प; उग्र सपूय उद्भेद; हर्पीज

**Agriothymia.** Ferocious mania. भीषण उन्माद

**Agrius.** Angry in appearance or malignant in character. अत्युग्र; दुर्दम; बहुत तेज

**Agromania.** A morbid desire for solitude. एकान्तप्रियता

**Agrypnia.** See **Ahypnia**.

**Ague.** Malarial or intermittent fever, marked by chill and sweat. शीतज्वर; विषम ज्वर; मलेरिया; सविराम ज्वर;

> **Quotidian A.,** fever having a daily paroxysm. दैनिक ज्वर; रोज आने वाला बुखार;
>
> **Tertian A.,** fever occurring every third day. तृत्तीयक ज्वर; तीसरे दिन प्रकट होने वाला बुखार;
>
> **A.-brow,** neuralgia frontalis; neuralgia of facial lnerves. आननपेशीतंत्रिकाशूल;
>
> **A.-cake,** malarial enlargement of spleen. शीतज्वरीय प्लीहाबृद्धि;
>
> **A.-face,** facial neuralgia. आननतंत्रिकाशूल;
>
> **A.-root,** aletris. ओक अथवा बांज वृक्ष की जड़

**Agustia.** Loss of taste. विरसता; अस्वाद; स्वाद का लोप

**Ahypnia.** Sleeplessness; insomnia; agrypnia. अनिद्रा; नींद न आना

**A.I.** Artificial insemination. कृत्रिमशुक्रसेचन; कृत्रिम गर्भाधान हेतु वीर्य प्रदान करना

**A.I.D.** Artificial insemination donor. कृत्रिमशुक्रसेचनदाता

**Aid.** Assistance. सहायता

**AIDS.** Acquired immune deficiency syndrome; a disease that compromises the competency of the immune system characterized by persistent lymphadenopathy and various opportunistic infections transmitted by body fluids such as blood (due to transfusion) and semen (due to sexual intercourse with the infected individuals). एड्स; उपार्जित अल्परोगक्षम संलक्षण

**Aidoitis.** Vulvitis; inflammation of the vulva. भगशोथ; भग-प्रदाह

**A.I.H.** Artificial insemination homologous. सहधर्मी कृत्रिम शुक्रसेचन

**Ail.** To trouble with some pain or illness; to suffer. कष्ट देना या होना

**Ailing.** Sick. अस्वस्थ; रुग्ण; बीमार

**Ailment.** An indisposition; sickness. रोग; व्याधि; व्यथा; पीड़ा

**Ailurophobia.** An abnormal fear of cats. विडालभीति; विडालातंक; बिल्लियों का डर

**Air.** The gaseous mixture which makes up the atmosphere surrounding the earth. वायु; पवन; वात; हवा; गैसों का मिश्रण जो आकाश या वायुमण्डल बनाता है;

  **A. Cell,** an air vesicle. वायुकोश; वायुकोशिका;

  **A. Hunger,** dyspnoea on both inspiration and expiration. वायुक्षुधा; श्वासकष्ट;

  **A. Passages,** the mouth, nares, larynx, trachea, bronchi, bronchial tubes, etc.; airways. वायुपथ; वायुमार्ग;

  **A.-ways,** see **Air Passages.**

  **Alveolar A.,** the air in the pulmonary alveoli. कोष्ठिका-वायु;

  **Complemental A.,** the extra air that can be drawn into the lungs by deep inspiration. पूरक वायु;

  **Reserve A.,** air in the chest after a normal expiration. आरक्षित वायु;

  **Residual A.,** that which still remains in the alveoli of the lungs after forced expiration. अवशिष्ट वायु;

  **Tidal A.,** that which passes in and out of the lungs in normal breathing. श्वसन वायु

**Akathisia.** A state in which the patient feels a distressing inner restlessness. मनोव्यथा; अशान्ति और चिन्ता की दशा

**Akeratosis.** Deficiency or absence of horny tissue. शृंगी-ऊतकाल्पता

**Akinesia.** Loss or imperfection of motion; akinesis. अगति; गत्याभाव; गतिशक्तिहीनता

**Akinesis.** See **Akinesia.**

**Akinetic.** Without movement. अगतिक; गतिहीन

**Ala.** A wing. पक्ष; पक्षक; पंख; पक्षनुमा प्रवर्धन;

  **A. Magna,** the great wing of the sphenoid. बृहत्पक्षक;

  **A. Nasi,** the cartilaginous wing of the nose. नासापक्षक; नथुना;

  **A. Parva,** the small wing of the sphenoid. लघुपक्षक

**Alae.** Plural of **Ala.**

 **A. Nasi,** wings of the nose. नासा-पक्षक; नथुने

**Alalia.** Paralytic impairment of speech. वाचाघात; वाक्-अक्षमता; वाचनाक्षयरोग; बोलने की शक्ति का ह्रास

**Alar.** Wing-like; resembling a wing or ala, as of the nose, sphenoid, sacrum, etc. पंखवत्; पक्षवत्; पक्षाभ; पक्षाकार; पक्षोपम; पंख जैसा

**Alarming.** Serious. गम्भीर; खतरनाक; अरिष्ट

**Alastrim.** Milk-pox; variola minor. ऐलास्ट्रम; छोटी माता

**Alate.** Having wings. पक्षपूर्ण; पंखयुक्त; सपंख

**Alb.** Albus; white. श्वेत; सफेद

**Alba.** The white substance of the brain. मस्तिष्क का धवल अर्थात् श्वेत पदार्थ

**Albaras.** A skin disease characterized by the formation of white, shining, anaesthetic patches. श्वित्ररोग; श्वित्र, जिसमें चमड़ी के ऊपर सफेद, चमकते हुए, संवेदना-रहित चकत्ते निकल आते हैं

**Albedo.** Whiteness. धवलता; शुक्लता; सफेदी;

 **A. Retinae,** oedema of the retina. श्वेतपटलशोफ; श्वेतपटल की सजल सूजन

**Albescens.** White. श्वेत; सफेद

**Albicans.** White. श्वेत; सफेद

**Albicantia.** Plural of **Albicans.**

**Albiduria.** See **Albinuria.**

**Albidus.** Of whitish colour. श्वेतवर्ण; सफेद रंग का

**Albiness.** Discolouration; whiteness. वर्णहीनता; अवर्णता; अरंज्यता; धवलता; शुक्लता; सफेदी

**Albinism.** Deficiency of pigment in tissues; achromatosis; congenital achromia. वर्णहीनता; अवर्णता; अरंज्यता; धवलता; शुक्लता; रंगहीनता

**Albino.** White; colourless; a subject of albinism. धवल; वर्णहीन; रंगहीन

**Albinuria.** White urine; albiduria. श्वेतमूत्रता; सफेद पेशाब होना

**Albuginea.** White or whitish. श्वेत; धवल; सफेद या कुछ-कुछ सफेद

**Albugineous.** Whitish. श्वेत

**Albugo.** The white opacity of the cornea. शुक्लार्बुद; श्वितिरोग; अक्षिपुष्प; आँखों की सफेदी का रोग

**Albumen.** An organic element of the blood, e.g. the white of egg

# Albumin

is almost pure albumen. It is an essential constituent of the animal bodies. श्वेतक; शिवति

**Albumin.** A protein widely distributed throughout the tissues and fluids of the plants and animals. It is soluble in water and coagulable by heat. अन्नसार; अण्डे की सफेद जर्दी जैसा पदार्थ

**Albuminate.** A basic compound of albumin. अन्नसार का एक मूल मिश्रण; एल्ब्युमिनेट

**Albuminaturia.** An excess of albumin in the urine. अति-अन्नसारमूत्रता; अत्यन्नसारमेह

**Albuminiferous.** See **Albuminiparous.**

**Albuminimeter.** A graduated test-tube in special stand for estimating the quality of albumin in a fluid. अन्नसारमापी; अन्नसारमापक (यंत्र)

**Albuminiparous.** Secreting albumin; albuminiferous. अन्नसारस्रावी

**Albuminoid.** A substance resembling albumin, or true protein in origin and composition. अन्नसाराभ; अन्नसारवत्; अन्नसार जैसा; प्रोटीन पदार्थ जैसा

**Albuminuria.** Presence of albumin in the urine. अन्नसारमेह; श्वेतकमेह; पेशाब में अन्नसार जाना;

  **Cardiac A.**, that due to chronic valvular disease. हृद्-अन्नसारमेह;

  **Cyclic A.**, albuminuria occurring at stated times in the day; functional albuminuria; paroxysmal albuminuria. चक्रिल अन्नसारमेह; क्रियात्मक अन्नसारमेह; प्रवेगी अन्नसारमेह;

  **False A.**, a mixture of the albumin with the urine during its transit through the urinary passages. कूट अन्नसारमेह;

  **Febrile A.**, that occurring in fever. ज्वर-अन्नसारमेह;

  **Functional A.**, see **Cyclic Albuminuria.**

  **Mixed A.**, true albuminuria combined with false albuminuria. मिश्र अन्नसारमेह;

  **Paroxysmal A.**, see **Cyclic Albuminuria.**

  **True A.**, due to excretion of a part of the albuminous constituents of the blood with the urine. यथार्थ अन्नसारमेह

**Albuminuric.** Pertaining to albuminuria. अन्नसारमेहज; अन्नसारिक; अन्नसारमेह सम्बन्धी

**Albus.** See **Alb.**

**Alcohol.** The pre-or rectified spirit of wine. मद्यसार; सुरासार;

**Absolute A.**, spirit containing no water. शुद्ध सुरासार;

**A.-fast**, a bacteriological term used when alcohol fails to decolourize a stained organism. सुरासारस्थाई

**Alcoholic.** Pertaining to alcohol. मद्यसारिक; मद्यसारीय; सुरासारीय; drunkard. मद्यप; पियक्कड़; शराबी; मद्यसेवी

**Alcoholism.** Drunkenness. मदात्यय; पानात्यय; alcoholic poisoning. मद्यविषण्णता; मद्यविषजता; मदिरोन्मत्तता; मदिरापान से होने वाले रोग

**Alcoholomania.** A morbid craving for alcoholic drinks. मद्योन्माद; मदिरापान की प्रबल इच्छा

**Alcoholometer.** An instrument for measuring the quantity of alcohol in a fluid. सुरासारमापी (यंत्र)

**Alcoholophilia.** A morbid craving for alcoholic drinks. मद्योन्माद; मदिरापान की प्रबल इच्छा

**Alcoholuria.** Alcohol in the urine. मद्यसारमेह; पेशाब में मद्यसार विद्यमान रहना

**Ale.** Liquor made from an infusion of malt by fermentation, flavoured with hops, etc. यवसुरा; जौ की शराब; एल

**Alecithal.** Applied to ova deficient in food yolk. लेसिथिनरहित; योकहीन; अपीतक

**Alembic.** A vessel used for distillation. वक्रयंत्र; कीप; अर्क उतारने का कांच या धातु का भभका

**Aletocyte.** Wandering cell. भ्रमणकोशिका

**Aletris.** Ague-root. ओक वृक्ष की जड़

**Aleukaemia.** A deficiency of white corpuscles in the blood; aleukaemic leukemia. अश्वेतकोशिकारक्तता; ऊनश्वेतकोशिक-श्वेतरक्तता

**Aleukaemic.** Deficient of white corpuscles in the blood; aleukemic. अश्वेतकोशिकारक्तक;

**A. Leukaemia**, see **Aleukaemia.**

**Aleukemia.** See **Aleukaemia.**

**Aleukemic.** See **Aleukaemic.**

**Alexia.** Loss of ability to interpret the significance of the printed or written words, but without loss of visual power; word blindness. लेखान्धता; अक्षरान्धता; शब्दान्धता

**Alexic.** Relating to, or affected with alexia. लेखान्धता सम्बन्धी या लेखान्ध

**Alexin.** Any defensive protein, the complement in the theory of immunity. रोगनिरोधक

**Alexipharmae.** See **Alexipharmic.**

**Alexipharmic.** A medicine neutralizing a poison; alexipharmae; alexiteric. विषरोधी; विषनाशक

**Alexipyretic.** A febrifuge. ज्वरनाशक; ज्वरहर

**Alexiteric.** See **Alexipharmic.**

**Alga.** A sea-weed; scum. शैवाल; काई

**Algae.** Plural of **Alga.**

**Algal.** Resembling or pertaining to alga. शैवालाभ अथवा शैवाल सम्बन्धी

**Algesia.** Excessive or extreme sensitiveness to pain; hyperaesthesia. अत्यार्तिसंवेदिता; पीड़ा या दर्द सहन करने की अक्षमता

**Algesic.** Painful. दर्दनाक; relating to, or causing pain. दर्द सम्बन्धी

**Algesimeter.** An instrument for measuring cutaneous sensitiveness; algometer. आर्तिमापी; पीड़ामापी

**Algentic.** The same as **Algesic.**

**Algia.** A suffix signifying pain, as neuralgia. आर्ति, शूल, पीड़ा, वेदना, आदि के लिये प्रयुक्ति होने वाला शब्दान्त

**Algid.** Chilled with cold; icy cold. शीत; शीतल; ठण्डा; अशिशिर;

  **A. Stage,** the cold stage. शीतावस्था; शरीर का ठण्डापन (प्रमुखतया शक्तिपात अथवा निपातसूचक अवस्था)

**Alginuresis.** Painful micturition. सपीडमूत्रण; कष्टदायक पेशाब होना

**Algogenic.** Causing pain. पीड़ाजनक; दर्दकारी; दर्द पैदा करने वाला; lowering temperture. तापोपशामक; तापन्यूनक; ताप कम करने वाला

**Algometer.** See **Algesimeter.**

**Algophobia.** A morbid fear of pain. पीड़ाभीति; दर्द का भय; पीड़ातंक

**Algor.** An unusual feeling of coldness; a rigor or chill. शीतानुभूति; कम्पकम्पी; शिशिर; ज्वरजनित शीत

**Algoscope.** An instrument for the determination of the freezing-point. हिमांकमापी

**Algoscopy.** The determination of freezing-point. हिमांकमापन

**Algosiogenic.** The same as **Algogenic.**

**Algospasm.** Painful cramp or spasm. दर्दनाक ऐंठन

**Alible.** Nutritive. पोषक

**Alienatio Mentis.** Mental delusion; insanity. मनोभ्रम; विक्षिप्ति; पागलपन

**Alienation.** Mental deragement; insanity. उन्माद; पागलपन; चित्तविभ्रम;

मानसिक विकृति या विकार

**Alienism.** The science of mental disorders. मनोविकृतिविद्या; मनोविकृतिविज्ञान; मनोरोगविज्ञान; मानसिक रोगों का अध्ययन और इलाज

**Alienist.** One who treats mental diseases; psychiatrist. मनोरोगचिकित्सक; मनोरोगविशेषज्ञ; मानसिक रोगों की चिकित्सा करने वाला

**Aliferous.** Having wings. सपंख

**Aliform.** Wing-like; wing-shaped. पक्षोपम; पक्षाकार; पंखवत्

**Alignment.** The act of arranging in a straight line. सरेखण

**Aliment.** Food; any substance which is capable, when introduced into the system, of nourishing it and repairing its losses. अन्न; भोजन; पोषण; खाद्य; पौष्टिक पदार्थ

**Alimentary.** Pertaining to food. पोषण; अन्न अथवा पाचन सम्बन्धी; भोजन-विषयक; having the quality of nourishing. पोषक; पुष्टिकारक; पौष्टिक; शक्तिवर्धक;

A. **Bolus,** the mass of food after mastication. ग्रास; कौर;

A. **Canal,** the musculo-membranous tube through which the food passes. पोषण नली; अन्न नली; भोजन नलिका; पोषिका;

A. **Duct,** the thoracic duct. वक्षनली;

A. **System,** comprising of all organs right from the oral opening to the anus. पाचन प्रणाली; पाचन तंत्र; आहार तंत्र;

A. **Tract,** includes mouth, tongue, gullet, stomach, intestines and rectum upto anus; the tract associated with digestion. पोषण-पथ; अन्न-पथ; पाचन-पथ

**Alimentation.** The act of nourishing with food. पोषण; पुष्टिकरण; भरण-पोषण; पोषण लेना या देना

**Alinasal.** Relating to the nasal wings, or flaring portions of the nostrils. नासापक्षकों सम्बन्धी; नथुनों सम्बन्धी

**Aliphatic.** Relating to a fat; fatty. वसा सम्बन्धी; चर्बी सम्बन्धी

**Alive.** In life; living active. जीवित; सप्राण; सजीव; जीता-जागता; जागृत; सचेत

**Alkalaemia.** Excess of alkali or reduction of acid in the body; alkalemia; alkalosis. क्षाररक्तता; क्षारमयता; क्षारोपचय; रक्त की असाधारण क्षारीयता

**Alkalemia.** See **Alkalaemia.**

**Alkali.** Chemical series of compounds called bases, including soda, potash, ammonia, etc. क्षार; खार; छार; अल्कली; यौगिकों का एक ऐसा

# Alkalies

वर्ग जो अम्ल के साथ मिलकर लवण तथा वसा के साथ मिलकर साबुन बनाते हैं

**Alkalies.** Plural of **Alkali.**

**Alkalimeter.** An instrument to measure the strength of alkalies. क्षारमापी (यंत्र)

**Alkalimetry.** The use of alkalimeter. क्षारमापन; क्षारमिति

**Alkaline.** Possessing the properties of or pertaining to an alkali. क्षारीय पदार्थ; क्षार प्रकृति का पदार्थ; खारीय; क्षार पदार्थ सम्बन्धी

**Alkalinity.** The quality of being alkaline. क्षारीयता; क्षारता; खारापन

**Alkalinuria.** Alkalinity of the urine; alkaluria. क्षारमेह; मूत्र की क्षारीय दशा

**Alkalis.** Plural of **Alkali.**

**Alkaliser.** Rendering alkalinity. क्षारकर; क्षारक; क्षारीयक

**Alkaloid.** Nitrogenous basic substance. क्षारत्व; मूलनेत्रजनीय पदार्थ; resembling alkali. क्षाराभ; क्षारवत्

**Alkalometry.** The method of administering alkaloid in definite doses. क्षारमात्रामिति; क्षारमात्रामापन

**Alkalosis.** See **Alkalaemia.**

**Alkalotic.** Relating to alkalosis. क्षाररक्तता सम्बन्धी

**Alkaluria.** See **Alkalinuria.**

**Allantoic.** Relating to the allantois. अपरापोषिकीय; अपरापोषिक

**Allantois.** A foetal appendage or membrane. अपरापोषिका

**Allay.** To repress; to put down. उपशमन करना; शान्त करना; निराकरण करना

**Allelomorphs.** Hereditary pairs of unit characters, either of which can be exclusively carried to any gamete. युग्मविकल्पी

**Allergen.** A substance capable of producing allergy. प्रत्यूर्जतोत्पादक पदार्थ; एलर्जी पैदा करने वाला तत्व

**Allergenic.** See **Antigenic.**

**Allergies.** Plural of **Allergy.**

**Allergist.** One who specializes in the treatment of allergy. प्रत्यूर्जताविज्ञानी; प्रत्यूर्जता-चिकित्सक

**Allergy.** A sensitivity of the body to substances which in themselves are not irritating to the normal, or an altered or exaggerated susceptibility to various foreign substances or physical agents which are harmless to the great majority of individuals. प्रत्यूर्जता; एलर्जी

**Alleviate.** To relieve; to mitigate. कम करना; धीमा करना; हल्का करना

**Alliaceous.** Resembling garlic. लहसुन जैसा; लहसुन की गंध जैसा

**Allium.** A genus of plants. प्याज या लहसुन का पौधा;

   **A. Cepa,** common onion. प्याज;

   **A. Sativum,** garlic; a diuretic and stimulant. लहसुन; लशुन

**Alloantibody.** An antibody specific for an alloantigen. इतरप्रतिपिण्ड; परप्रतिपिण्ड

**Alloantigen.** An antigen that occurs in some, but not in the other members of the same species. इतरप्रतिजन; परप्रतिजन

**Allochromasia.** Change of colour of the skin or hair. त्वग्विवर्णता; केशविवर्णता; त्वचा अथवा बालों का रंग बदल जाना

**Allodynia.** The distress resulting from painful stimuli. इतरवेदना; परपीड़ा

**Allopath.** One practising allopathy; Allopathist. ऐलोपैथिक चिकित्सक

**Allopathic.** Relating to allopathy. ऐलोपैथिक चिकित्सा सम्बन्धी

**Allopathist.** See **Allopath.**

**Allopathy.** A system of therapeutics in which disease is treated by exciting a morbid process of another kind or in other part; a method of substitution. ऐलोपैथिक चिकित्सा प्रणाली

**Allopsychic.** Denoting the mental processes in their relation to the outer world. परमानसिक

**Allorhythmia.** Variation in the pulse interval or cardiac rhythm. अनियमित-तालता; नाड़ी, हृदय अथवा नब्ज का अक्रमिक या क्रमहीन होना

**Allorhythmic.** Relating to or characterized by allorhythmia. अनियमित-तालता सम्बन्धी अथवा अनियमित तालबद्धता

**Allosome.** One of the chromosomes differing in appearance or behaviour from the ordinary chromosomes. लिंगगुणसूत्र

**Allotrophagy.** A depraved or unnatural appetite. अस्वाभाविक भूख

**Allotropism.** See **Allotropy.**

**Allotropy.** A variation of physical properties without a change in chemic composition; allotropism. अपरूपता

**Alloy.** A combination of two or more metals. मिश्रधातु; दो या दो से अधिक धातुओं का मिश्रण

**Almond.** The kernel of the fruit of Prunus amygdalus. बादाम

**Alochia.** Absence of lochia. सूतिस्राव का अभाव

**Aloe.** A genus of the plants of lily family, with erect spikes of flowers and bitter juice. घीकुँवार; घृतकुमारी; घृतकुमारी रस

**Alogia.** An inability to speak due to nerve lesion. वाक्‌रोध; वाग्रोध; वाक्‌-अक्षमता

**Alopecia.** Baldness; loss of hair. खल्वाटता; गंजापन; खालित्य; केशाभाव;

   A. **Adnata,** the congenital baldnes; alopecia congenita. सहज खालित्य; बालों का जन्मजात अभाव;

   A. **Areata,** baldness appearing in patches. सीमित खालित्य;

   A. **Cicatrisata,** progressive alopecia of the scalp in which tufts of normal hair occur between many bald patches. क्षतांक खालित्य;

   A. **Circumscripta,** the same as **Alopecia Areata.**

   A. **Congenita,** see **Alopecia Adnata.**

   A. **Simplex,** premature baldness. अकाल खालित्य

**Alopecic.** Relating to, or affected with alopecia. खल्वाट (गंजा) अथवा खल्वाटता सम्बन्धी

**A.L.S.** Antilymphocyte serum. प्रतिलसीकाकोशिकारस

**Alstonia.** An antiperiodic and antipyretic. सप्तपर्णछाल; सतोनाछाल

**Alteration.** The state of being altered. परिवर्तन

**Alternately.** In alternation. पर्यायक्रम से; अदल-बदल कर

**Alternating.** Occurring in regular succession, one after the other. परिवर्तनशील; पर्यायक्रमी; पर्याक्रमिक; एकान्तर

**Alternis Horis.** Alt. hor.; every two hours. हर दूसरे घण्टे; दो-दो घण्टे में

**Alt. Hor.** Abbreviation for **Alternis Horis.**

**Alt. Noct.** Abbreviation for **Alternis Nocta.**

**Alternis Nocta.** Alt. noct.; every other night. हर दूसरी रात

**Alum.** A kind of mineral salt; alumen. फिटकरी; फटकड़ी

**Alumen.** See **Alum.**

**Alumina.** Aluminium found in clay and other minerals. स्फटिक-मृदा; एलूमिना

**Aluminated.** Containing or made of alumina. स्फटिकमृदामय; स्फटिकमृदानिर्मित

M.D.F.-2

**Aluminium.** A whitish metal with a low specific gravity; aluminum. एल्मूनियम; एक धातु, जिसके बर्तन बनते हैं

**Aluminum.** See **Aluminium.**

**Alvearium.** The external opening of the ear. कर्णविवर; श्रोत्रगुहा; कान का बाहरी छेद

**Alvei.** Pural of **Alveus.**

**Alveoalgia.** Pain in the alveolus; alveolalgia. दन्तउलूखलार्ति

**Alveolalgia.** See **Alveoalgia.**

**Alveolar.** Pertaining to an alveolus. दन्तउलूखलीय; वायुकोषीय; कोष्ठिक;
   **A. Artery,** the posterior dental artery. दन्तउलूखल-धमनी

**Alveolarium.** The same as **Alvearium.**

**Alveolectomy.** Surgical excision of a portion of the dentoalveolar process. दंतउलूखलोच्छेदन

**Alveoli.** Bony sockets of the teeth. दन्तकोटर; air sacs in lungs at which the blood exchanges carbon-dioxide for fresh supply of oxygen to carry to the body tissues. वायुकोष्ठिका; गर्तिका; फुप्फसवायुगह्वर

**Alveolingual.** Pertaining to an alveolus and the tongue; alveololingual. दन्तउलूखल तथा जिह्वा सम्बन्धी

**Alveolitis.** Inflammation of an alvelous. दन्तउलूखलशोथ; दन्तकोटरशोथ; दन्तकोटर का प्रदाह

**Alveolodental.** Relating to the teeth and alveoli. दान्तों तथा दन्त-कोटरों सम्बन्धी

**Alveololingual.** See **Alveolingual.**

**Alveoloplasty.** Surgical preparation of the alveolar ridges for the reception of dentures; alveoplasty. दन्तउलूखलसंधान

**Alveolotomy.** Incision of an alveolus or a tooth. दन्तउलूखलछेदन

**Alveolus.** The bony socket of the tooth. दन्तउलूखल; दन्तकोटर; दन्तगर्त; one of the small breathing chambers in the lungs. कोष्ठक; वायुकोश; कूपिका

**Alveoplasty.** See **Alveoloplasty.**

**Alveus.** A trough, tube or canal. नली; नलिका; नाली; कुल्या

**Alvine.** Pertaining to the belly or intestines. औदरिक; पेट अथवा आन्तों सम्बन्धी;
   **A. Concretion,** intestinal calculus. आंत्र-अश्मरी; आंत्राश्मरी; आंतों की पथरी;

**A. Discharges,** the faeces. बिष्ठा; मल; पाखाना;

**A. Flux,** diarrhoea. अतिसार; प्रवाहिका; दस्त

**Alvus.** The belly or its contents. पाकाशय तथा पक्वाशय पदार्थ; पेट अथवा उसके पदार्थ

**Alymphia.** An insufficient amount of lymph. लसीकाल्पता; लसीकाहीनता

**A.M.** Ante Meridiem; before noon. पूर्वाह्न; दोपहर से पहले

**A.M.A.** Authorised Medical Attendant. अधिकृत चिकित्सक

**Amaas.** Milk-pox. दुग्ध-मसूरिका

**Amalgam.** Mixture of metal with mercury. पारदमिश्र; पारद धातु योगिक; पारद संसृष्ट धातु; पारदीय खनिज योग

**Amanous.** Having no hands. अहस्तता; हस्तहीनता; हाथों का अभाव

**Amara.** Bitters. तिक्तौषधि; कड़वी दवा

**Amasesis.** Inability to masticate. चर्वण-अशक्तता; चबाने की अयोग्यता

**Amastia.** Congenital absence of the breast; amazia. स्तनहीनता; अस्तनता; स्तन का जन्मजात अभाव

**Amateur.** One who is fond of. शौकीन; शौकिया; अव्यावसायिक

**Amative.** Full of love. प्रणयशील; शृंगारप्रिय; प्रेमासक्त

**Amaurosis.** Partial or total blindness; gutta serena. अन्धता; दृष्टिलोप; दृष्टिहीनता; दृष्टिमांद्य;

   **Albuminuric A.,** that due to renal disease. अन्नसारिक अन्धता;

   **Cerebral A.,** that due to brain lesion. प्रमस्तिष्की अन्धता;

   **Congenital A.,** that existing from birth. सहज अन्धता;

   **Diabetic A.,** that associated with diabetes. मधुमेहज अन्धता;

   **Hysteric A.,** that accompanying hysteria. वातोन्मादी अन्धता;

   **Reflex A.,** that due to reflex action of distant irritation. प्रतिवर्ती अन्धता;

   **Saburral A.,** temporary blindness. अस्थायी अन्धता;

   **Toxic A.,** that caused due to some poisonous effects. विषज अन्धता;

   **Uraemic A.,** that due to uraemia. यूरेमी अन्धता;

   **Uremic A.,** the same as **Uraemic Amaurosis.**

   **A. Fugax,** the momentary blindness. क्षणिक अन्धता

**Amaurotic.** Affected with, or pertaining to amaurosis. मन्ददृष्टिक; दृष्टिमांद्यज; मंददृष्टि अथवा अन्धता सम्बन्धी

**Amaxophobia.** A morbid fear of vehicles. वाहनभीति; वाहनों का डर

**Amazia.** See **Amastia.**

**Ambageusia.** Loss of taste. विरसता; स्वादलोप

**Amber.** A fossil resin from trees now extinct. अम्बर; राल; तृणमणि; कहरुबा

**Ambidexterism.** Ability to use either hand with equal ease; ambidexterity. उभयहस्तता; सव्यसाचिता

**Ambidexterity.** See **Ambidexterism.**

**Ambidextrous.** Equally skilful with both hands. उभयहस्त; सव्यसाची; द्विहत्थी

**Ambilateral.** Relating to both sides. द्विपार्श्विक

**Ambiopia.** Vision with both eyes. उभयदृष्टिता

**Ambivalence.** Co-existence of one person of contradictory and opposing emotions at the same time, e.g. love and hate. उभयवृत्तिता; उभयभाविका; दोहरे विचार वाला

**Ambivalent.** Relating to, or characterized by ambivalence. उभयवृत्तिता संम्बन्धी

**Amblosis.** Abortion; miscarriage. गर्भपात; गर्भस्राव

**Amblotic.** An abortifacient. गर्भपातक; गर्भस्रावक; गर्भपाती; गर्भस्रावी

**Amblyaphia.** A diminution of the sense of touch. स्पर्शज्ञानाल्पता; स्पर्शमन्दता; स्पर्शज्ञान की कमी

**Amblygeustia.** Diminished sense of taste. विरसता; बदला हुआ स्वाद

**Amblyope.** One affected with dimness of sight. मन्ददृष्टिक

**Amblyopia.** Dimness of sight. दृष्टिमांद्य; मंददृष्टि; मन्ददृष्टिता; दृष्टि-न्यूनता; दृष्टि-अल्पता

**Amblyopiatrics.** The study or science dealing with the treatment of amblyopia. मंददृष्टिचिकित्साविज्ञान

**Amblyopic.** Relating to, or affected with amblyopia. मंददृष्टि सम्बन्धी या मंददृष्टिक

**Amblyoscope.** A reflecting stereoscope used for measuring or training binocular vision, or for stimulation of vision in the amblyopic eye. मंददृष्टिदर्शी (यंत्र)

**Amblyosmiosis.** Dullness of hearing. श्रवणाल्पता; कम सुनाई देना

**Amboceptor.** A hypothetical thermostable substance found in blood serum after inoculation. द्विग्राही; उपायन

**Ambrosia.** A genus of plants with styptic properties. पराग; मकरन्द

# Ambulance

**Ambulance.** A vehicle for conveying the sick. एम्बुलैंस; रोगियों को लाने तथा ले जाने वाली गाड़ी; रोगीवाहन

**Ambulant.** Able to walk. चलनक्षम; चलने-फिरने में समर्थ

**Ambulation.** Ability to walk. चलनक्षमता; चलने-फिरने का सामर्थ्य

**Ambulatory.** Mobile, medically applied to a dispensary or the treatment. चल; चलनक्षम

**Ambustial.** Produced by burn. दाहजनित; जलने से उत्पन्न

**Ambusion.** A burn or scald. दाहक्षत; आग, गरम पानी या भाप से जलने के कारण होने वाला घाव

**Ameba.** A minute, one-celled protozoal animal organism; amoeba. अमीबा; एक छोटा-सा, एक-कोशिकी जीवाणु

**Amebae.** Plural of **Ameba.**

**Amebas.** Plural of **Ameba.**

**Amebiasis.** State of being infected by amebas; amebism; amoebiasis. अमीबिकता; अमीबा-रुग्णता

**Amebic.** Relating to an ameba; amoebic. अमीबी; अमीबाजन्य

**Amebicidal.** Destructive to amebas; amoebicidal; amebicide; amoebicide. अमीबाणुनाशी; अमीबाणुनाशक

**Amebicide.** See **Amebicidal.**

**Amebiform.** Of the shape or appearance of an ameba; amoebiform. अमीबारूप

**Amebism.** See **Amebiasis.**

**Ameboid.** Having the movement of an ameba; amoeboid. अमीबागतिक; अमीबागतिज

**Ameburia.** The presence of ameba in the urine; amoeburia. अमीबामेह; मूत्र में अमीबा विद्यमान रहना

**Ametia.** Congenital absence of limb or limbs. सहजअंगहीनता; सहजअनंगता; अंगों का जन्मजात अभाव;

> **Complete A.,** absence of both hands and legs. भुजाओं तथा टांगों का जन्मजात अभाव

**Ameliorate.** To grow better. सुधार होना; सुधार करना

**Amelioration.** Becoming better; improvement in the stages of a disease. सुधार; ह्रास; उपशम

**Ameloblast.** A cell yielding tooth-enamel. दन्तमज्जाप्रसू; दन्तवल्क-कोशिका

**Ameloblastoma.** See **Adamantinoma.**

**Amelus.** A monster without limbs. अनंगजीव; अंगहीन जीव; बिना अंगों का जीव

**Amenable.** Governable. वश्य; परिचलनयोग्य; शास्य

**Amenia.** Amenorrhoea; stoppage of the menses; amenorrhea; amenorrhoea. अनार्तव; ऋतुरोध; रजोरोध; मासिक धर्म का लोप होना

**Amenomania.** Mental disorder of a pleasing character. हास्योन्माद; हँसते रहने का पागलपन

**Amenorrhea.** See **Amenia.**

**Amenorrheic.** See **Amenorrhoeal.**

**Amenorrhoea.** See **Amenia.**

**Amenorrhoeal.** Relating to amenorrhoea; amenorrheic. अनार्तव अथवा ऋतुस्राव नं होने सम्बन्धी

**Ament.** An idiot. जड़मति; बेवकूफ; बुद्धू; क्षीणबुद्धि; मन्दबुद्धि

**Amentia.** Imbecility; the condition of defective intellect. जड़ता; बुद्धिदौर्बल्य; अमनस्कता; क्षीणबुद्धिता; मन्दबुद्धिता

**Ametria.** Congenital absence of the uterus. सहज-अगर्भाशयता; गर्भाशय अर्थात् जरायु का जन्मजात अभाव

**Ametrohemia.** A poor uterine blood supply. जरायु-रक्ताल्पता; अल्पार्तव

**Ametrometer.** An instrument for measuring ametropia; ametropometer. दृष्टिदोषमापी; दृष्टिदोषमापकयंत्र

**Ametrope.** Subject to ametropia. दृष्टिदोषग्रस्त

**Ametropia.** Defective sight due to imperfect power of eye. दृष्टिदोष; अपसामान्य दृष्टि

**Ametropic.** Affected with or pertaining to ametropia. दृष्टिदोषग्रस्त; अपसामान्यदृष्टिक; दृष्टिदोष सम्बन्धी

**Ametropometer.** See **Ametrometer.**

**Ametropometry.** The measurement of ametropia. दृष्टिदोषमिति; दृष्टिदोषमापन

**Amianthinopsy.** Violent blindness. गहनान्धता

**Amimia.** An inability to imitate or gesture correctly. इंगिताभाव

**Amino-acid.** Organic acid in which one or more of the hydrogen atoms are replaced by the ameno group. एमिनो-अम्ल

**Amino-acidemia.** Presence of excessive amino-acids in the blood. एमिनो-अम्लरक्तता; रक्त में एमिनो-अम्ल की अधिकता होना

**Amino-acidopathy.** Disease caused by imbalance of amino-acids. एमिनो-अम्लरुग्णता; एमिनो-अम्लों के असन्तुलन के कारण होने वाला रोग

**Amino-aciduria.** Presence of excessive amino-acids in the urine. एमिनो-अम्लमेह; पेशाब में एमिनो-अम्ल जाना

**Amitosis.** Multiplication of a cell by direct fission. असमसूत्रण; असूत्रीविभाजन; कोशगुणन

**Amitotic.** Not produced by karyokinesis. असूत्रीविभाजक

**Ammonemia.** See **Ammoniemia.**

**Ammonia.** A volatile alkaline gas, soluble in water; ammonium. नरसार; एमोनिया; एक प्रकार का क्षारीय उपादान

**Ammoniac.** Containing or pertaining to ammonia. नरसारयुक्त; नरसार सम्बन्धी

**Ammoniated.** Containing or combined with ammonia. नरसारयुक्त

**Ammoniemia.** Presence of ammonia in the blood; ammonemia. नरसाररक्तता

**Ammonification.** To render ammoniac. नरसारकरण; एमोनियाकरण

**Ammonium.** See **Ammonia.**

**Ammoniuria.** Excess of ammonia in the urine. अतिनरसारमेह; पेशाब में अत्यधिक नरसार जाना

**Ammotherapy.** Treatment by sand-bath. मरुस्नानोपचार; बालुका-स्नान द्वारा की जाने वाली चिकित्सा

**Amnesia.** Loss of memory for words; amestia. शब्दस्मृतिलोप; शब्दस्मृतिभ्रंश; शब्दों को भूल जाना;

    **Anterograde A.,** post-accidental loss of memory. घटनोत्तर स्मृतिलोप;

    **Auditory A.,** word-deafness. शब्द-बधिरता;

    **Retrograde A.,** loss of memory for past events before an accident, etc. घटनापूर्व स्मृतिलोप;

    **Visual A.,** word blindness. शब्दान्धता

**Amnesic.** Affected with, or pertaining to amnesia; amnestic. शब्दस्मृतिलोपग्रस्त अथवा शब्दस्मृतिलोप सम्बन्धी

**Amnestia.** See **Amnesia.**

**Amnestic.** See **Amnesic.**

**Amnial.** See **Amniotic.**

**Amniocentesis.** Aspiration of liquor amnii from its sac. उल्ववेधन

**Amniogenesis.** Formation of the amnion. उल्वजनन

**Amniography.** X-ray of amniotic sac after injection of opaque

medium into the same. उल्वचित्रण
**Amnionic.** See **Amniotic.**
**Amnion.** The thin but strong membrane enclosing the foetus in the womb. उल्व; भ्रूणावरण
**Amnionitis.** Inflammation of the amnion; amniotitis; amnitis. उल्वशोथ; भ्रूणावरणशोथ
**Amniorrhea.** See **Amniorrhoea.**
**Amniorrhexis.** Rupture of the amnion. उल्वभ्रंश
**Amniorrhoea.** A escape of liquor amnii; amniorrhea. उल्वोदकस्राव; गर्भोदकस्राव
**Amniotic.** Pertaining to amnion; amnial; amnionic. उल्व अथवा भ्रूणावरण सम्बन्धी;
   A. **Cavity,** the sac of the amnion. उल्व नलिका;
   A. **Fluid,** liquor amnii. उल्वोदक; गर्भोदक
**Amniotitis.** See **Amnionitis.**
**Amniotome.** An instrument for puncturing the foetal membrane. उल्वछेदक; जरायुकर्तक; भ्रूणावरण में छेद करने का यंत्र
**Amniotomy.** Puncturing of the foetal membrane. उल्वछेदन; उल्वकर्तन
**Amnitis.** See **Amnionitis.**
**Amoeba.** See **Ameba.**
**Amoebae.** Plural of **Amoeba.**
**Amoebas.** Plural of **Amoeba.**
**Amoebiasis.** See **Amebiasis.**
**Amoebic.** See **Amebic.**
**Amoebicidal.** See **Amebicidal.**
**Amoebicide.** See **Amebicidal.**
**Amoebiform.** See **Amebiform.**
**Amoeboid.** See **Ameboid.**
**Amoeburia.** See **Ameburia.**
**Amok.** See **Amoke.**
**Amoke.** A maniacal condition or epileptic insanity; amok; amuck. उन्मत्तावस्था; अपस्मारक विक्षिप्ति
**Amorous.** Inclined to love; lascivious. विलासप्रिय; शृंगारप्रिय; कामुक
**Amorousness.** Lasciviousness. विलासप्रियता; शृंगारप्रियता; कामुकता; प्रेमासक्ति

**Amorphia.** See **Amorphism**.

**Amorphism.** A shapeless state; amorphia. अनाकार स्थिति; अनाकारता

**Amorphous.** Shapeless; formless. अनाकार; अस्प; आकारहीन; रवेहीन; विकृत

**Ampelotherapy.** Treatment by grapes or grape-juice. द्राक्षोपचार; अंगूर या अंगूर-रस द्वारा की जाने वाली चिकित्सा

**Ampere.** The unit of electric-current strength. विद्युत्धारा की इकाई

**Amphiarthrodial.** Relating to amphiarthrosis. अल्पचलसन्धि सम्बन्धी

**Amphiarthrosis.** Articulation by fibrous tissue or strong ligaments, permitting slight motion. अल्पचलसन्धि

**Amphibia.** Animals that live either on land or in water. उभयचर; जल-थलचर; जल-थलवासी

**Amphibious.** Having the characteristics of amphibia. उभयचारी; जल-थलचारी; जल-थलस्थलीय

**Amphicelous.** See **Amphicelus**.

**Amphicelus.** Concave at both ends or sides; amphicelous. उभयउत्तानी; उभयगर्तधारी

**Amphicenteric.** Centering at both ends. उभयकेन्द्रिक

**Amphicrania.** Pain on both sides of the head (opposite of hemicrania). पूर्णशिरोवेदना

**Amphidiarthrosis.** A mixed gliding and hinge articulation. अल्पमुक्तचलसन्धि

**Amphodiplopia.** Double vision with both eyes; amphoterodiplopia. उभयद्विदृष्टिता

**Amphophil (e).** Having affinity for both acids and basic dyes; amphophilic; amphophilous. उभयरागी

**Amphophilic.** See **Amphophil(e)**.

**Amphophilous.** See **Amphophil(e)**.

**Amphoric.** Resembling the sound produced by blow across the mouth of a bottle. प्रणादी (ध्वनि)

**Amphoteric.** Having the power of altering both red and blue test paper. उभयधर्मी

**Amphoterodiplopia.** See **Amphodiplopia**.

**Amplification.** In miscroscopy, an increase of visual area. दृष्टिप्रवर्धन; दृष्टिविस्तार

**Amplifier.** A device for increasing magnification. परिवर्धक; प्रवर्धक; विस्तारक

**Amplitude.** The range or extent, as of the pulse. आयाम; विस्तार

**Ampoule.** A small, hermetically sealed glass phial containing a single sterile dose of a drug; ampule. सम्पुटक; नली

**Ampule.** See **Ampoule.**

**Ampulla.** Any flask-like dilatation. कलशिका; नलिका; तुम्बिका

**Ampullae.** Plural of **Ampulla.**

**Ampullar.** Relating in any sense to an ampulla. कलशिका सम्बन्धी

**Ampullitis.** Inflammation of any ampulla. कलशिकाशोथ; नलिकाशोथ; तुम्बिकाशोथ

**Amputation.** The surgical cutting or removal of a limb or part. विच्छेदन; उच्छेदन; अंगोच्छेदन

**Amrous.** Bitter. तिक्त; कड़वा

**Amuck.** A maniacal condition; amoke. उन्मत्तावस्था; पागलपन

**Amusia.** An inability to distinguish musical sounds. वाद्यध्वनिभेद-अक्षमता; वाद्ययंत्रों का ध्वनिभेद करने की अयोग्यता

**Amyasthenia.** Muscular weakness. पेशीदौर्बल्य; मांस-पेशियों की कमजोरी

**Amyelencephalia.** Congenital absence of the spinal cord and the brain. सहज-मेरुरज्जुमस्तिष्कहीनता; मेरुरज्जु एवं मस्तिष्क का जन्मजात अभाव

**Amyelia.** Congenital absence of the spinal cord. सहज-अमेरुरज्जुता; सहज-मेरुरज्जुहीनता; सहज-सुषुम्नाहीनता; मेरुरज्जु का जन्मजात अभाव

**Amyelic.** See **Amyelous.**

**Amyelotrophy.** Atrophy of the spinal cord. मेरुरज्जुशोष; मेरुरज्जुक्षय; सुषुम्नाक्षीणता

**Amyelous.** Without spinal cord; amyelic. मेरुरज्जुहीन

**Amyelus.** A foetus with no spinal cord. अमेरुरज्जुभ्रूण; सुषुम्नाविहीन भ्रूण

**Amygdala.** A tonsil. गलतुण्डिका; टांसिल; a lobe of the cerebellum. प्रमस्तिष्कखण्ड

**Amygdalitis.** Inflammation of the tonsils; tonsillitis. गलतुण्डिकाशोथ; टांसिल-प्रदाह

**Amygdaloid.** Tonsil-like. गलतुण्डिकाभ; गलतुण्डिका जैसा; resembling an almond. बादाम जैसा या उससे मिलता-जुलता

**Amygdalolith.** A tonsillar calculus. गलतुण्डिकाश्मरी

**Amygdalopathy.** Any disease of the tonsils. गलतुण्डिकारोग; गलतुण्डिकाविकृति

# Amygdalotome 74

**Amygdalotome.** An instrument for excising a tonsil. गलतुण्डिकोच्छेदक

**Amygdalotomy.** Abscission of the tonsils. गलतुण्डिका-उच्छेदन

**Amyl.** A hypothetic radicle. श्वेतसार; माण्ड; स्टार्च

**Amylaceous.** Of a starchy nature. श्वेतसारिक; श्वेतसारमय; मण्डीय; स्टार्च वाला

**Amylase.** An enzyme which converts starches into sugars. एमिलेज; श्वेतसार को शर्करा में बदलने वाला पदार्थ

**Amylnitrite.** Volatile rapid-acting vasodilator, used by inhalation from crushed ampoules. एमिलनाइट्राइट; एक हृदयौषधि

**Amylocardia.** Weakness of the heart-muscles. हृत्पेशी-दौर्बल्य; हृदय की पेशियों की दुर्बलता

**Amylogenesis.** The biosynthesis starch; amylosynthesis. श्वेतसारजनन

**Amylogenic.** Producing starch; amyloplastic. श्वेतसारजनक

**Amylohydrolysis.** See **Amylolysis.**

**Amyloid.** A starch which is wax-like in appearance. श्वेतसाराभ; श्वेतसारिक; मण्डाभ

**Amylolysis.** The conversion of starch into glucose; amylohydrolysis. श्वेतसारलयन; श्वेतसारापघटन

**Amylolytic.** Converting starch into sugar. श्वेतसारलयनिक; श्वेतसार को शर्करा में बदलने वाला

**Amyloplastic.** See **Amylogenic.**

**Amylosuria.** Excretion of the starch in the urine; amyluria. श्वेतसारमेह; पेशाब में माण्ड जाना

**Amylosynthesis.** See **Amylogenesis.**

**Amylum.** Starch; a valuable nutrient. श्वेतसार; मण्ड; माण्ड; स्टार्च

**Amyluria.** See **Amylosuria.**

**Amyocardia.** Cardiac muscular weakness. हृद्पेशीदौर्बल्य; हृदय की पेशियों की दुर्बलता

**Amyoesthesia.** See **Amyoesthesis.**

**Amyoesthesis.** Lack of muscular sense; amyoesthesia. पेशीज्ञानहीनता; पेशीज्ञान का अभाव

**Amyon.** An absence of muscular tissue. पेशीऊतकहीनता; पेशीऊतकों का अभाव

**Amyoplasia.** Insufficient development of muscles. पेशीअविकसन; पेशियों का अपूर्ण विकास

**Amyostasia.** See **Amyostasis.**

**Amyostasis.** Nervous and muscular tremor; amyostasia. स्नायुपेशीकम्प; स्नायु तथा पेशियों की कम्पन

**Amyosthenia.** Deficient muscular power. पेशीदौर्बल्य

**Amyosthenic.** Pertaining to amyosthenia. पेशीदौर्बल्य सम्बन्धी; an agent depressing muscular action. पेशीदुर्बलकारी

**Amyotonia.** Lack of muscular tone. पेशीअतानता

**Amyotrophia.** Muscular atrophy; amyotrophy. पेशीशोष; पेशियों का सूखना

**Amyotrophic.** Pertaining to muscular atrophy. पेशीशोष सम्बन्धी; पेशीशोषी

**Amyotrophy.** See **Amyotrophia.**

**Amyous.** Wanting in muscles. पेशीहीन; पेशियों से हीन

**Amyxia.** Absence or deficiency of mucus. श्लेष्महीनता; अश्लेष्मता; श्लेष्माल्पता; श्लेष्मा का अभाव या कमी

**Ana.** See **aa.**

**Anabiotic.** A restorative or powerful stimulant. स्वास्थ्यवर्धक (पदार्थ या औषधि)

**Anabolic.** Relating to, or promoting anabolism. उपचय सम्बन्धी अथवा उपचय बढ़ाने वाला (तत्व)

**Anabolism.** Constructive metabolism. उपचय; निर्माणिक चयापचय

**Anacamptometer.** An instrument for measuring reflexes. प्रतिवर्तमापी

**Anacardiaceae.** Turpine-producing trees. तारपीन-उत्पादक वृक्ष; देवदारु का पेड़

**Anacardium.** A genus of tropical trees yielding cashew-nut. भिलावा

**Anacatharsis.** Cough with expectoration. कफकास; खाँसी के साथ बलगम; continual vomiting अविराम वमन; निरन्तर वमन होना; लगातार वमन होते रहना

**Anacathartic.** Producing vomiting or expectoration. वामक; वमनकारक; वमनकारी; कफकासोत्पादक; कफकासकारक

**Anacidity.** A lack of acidity. अनम्लता; अम्लाभाव; अम्ल का अभाव

**Anacrotic.** Displaying anacrotism; anadicrotic. विषमारोही

**Anacrotism.** An irregularity of the ascending curve of a sphygmographic tracing; anadicrotism. विषमद्विस्पंदिता

**Anacusis.** Nervous deafness; anakusis. स्नायविक बधिरता

**Anadenia.** Deficiency of glandular action. ग्रन्थि-अल्पक्रियता; ग्रन्थि क्रिया का मन्द पड़ना

**Anadicrotic.** See **Anacrotic.**

**Anadicrotism.** See **Anacrotism.**

**Anadipsia.** Intense thirst. तृषाधिक्य; अत्यधिक प्यास; तीव्र प्यास

**Anadrenalism.** Complete lack of adrenal function. अधिवृक्कक्रियाभाव; अधिवृक्क क्रिया का पूर्ण अभाव

**Anaematosis.** See **Idiopathic Anaemia.**

**Anaemia.** Deficiency of blood or red blood corpuscles; anemia. अरक्तता; रक्ताल्पता; रक्तहीनता; रक्तक्षीणता; खून अथवा लाल रक्तकणों की कमी;

**Addison's A.**, see **Idiopathic Anaemia.**

**Brick-maker's A.**, anaemia caused due to hookworm disease; miner's anaemia; tunnel anaemia. अंकुश-कृमि अरक्तता;

**Essential A.**, see **Idiopathic Anaemia.**

**Haemolytic A.**, associated with destruction of red blood cells and haemolytic jaundice. रक्तसंलायी अरक्तता;

**Idiopathic A.**, primary anaemia, caused due to the disease of the blood or the blood-making organs; anaematosis; anematosis; Addison's anaemia; essential anaemia. प्रारम्भिक अरक्तता;

**Iron Deficiency A.**, that due to blood loss, lack of dietary iron or poor iron absorption. अल्प-अयसी अरक्तता; लौह-अल्पताजन्य अरक्तता;

**Macrocytic A.**, large red cell picture shown by the peripheral blood. बृहत्लोहितकोशिका अरक्तता;

**Malignant A.**, see **Pernicious Anaemia.**

**Megaloblastic A.**, associated with diminished and abnormal production of red blood cells. महालोहितप्रसू अरक्तता;

**Miner's A.**, see **Brick-maker's Anaemia.**

**Pernicious A.**, highly destructive or fatal form of anaemia; malignant anaemia. प्रणाशी अरक्तता, सांघातिक अरक्तता; दुर्दम अरक्तता;

**Primary A.**, see **Idiopathic Anaemia.**

**Secondary A.**, that due to cancer, etc.; symptomatic anaemia. द्वितीयक अरक्तता; गौण अरक्तता; लाक्षणिक अरक्तता;

**Septic A.**, one secondary to septic conditions, usually about the mouth. पूतिज अरक्तता;

**Splenic A.**, that attended by enlarged spleen. प्लीहज अरक्तता;

प्लीहा-विवर्धन के साथ होने वाली अरक्तता;

**Symptomatic A.,** see **Secondary Anaemia.**

**Tropical A.,** the various syndromes, frequently observed in persons in tropical climates. उष्णकटिबन्धीय अरक्तता;

**Tunnel A.,** see **Brick-maker's Anaemia.**

**Anaemic.** One affected with anaemia; anemic. अरक्तक; रक्ताल्प; अल्परक्तक; क्षीणरक्त

**Anaerobe.** A microbe living without air; anaerobion. वातनिरपेक्षी; अवातजीवी; अवायुजीवी; वायु बिना जीवित रहने वाले जीवाणु;

**Facultative A.,** one able to live or grow in the presence or absence of free oxygen. विकल्पी वातनिरपेक्षी; अनाग्रही वातनिरपेक्षी;

**Obligate (Obligatory) A.,** one that will live or grow only in the absence of free oxygen. आग्रही वातनिरपेक्षी

**Anaerobiasis.** See **Anaerobiosis.**

**Anaerobic.** Living without air. वातनिरपेक्षी; अवातजीवी; अवायुजीवी; हवा बिना जीवित रहने वाला; relating to anaerobes. वातनिरपेक्ष जीवाणुओं सम्बन्धी

**Anaerobion.** See **Anaerobe.**

**Anaerobiosis.** The condition of living without air; anaerobiasis. वातनिरपेक्षता; अवायुजीविता; अवातजीविता; वायु बिना जीवित रहना

**Anaeroplasty.** The dressing of wounds with air-exclusion. वातनिरपेक्षीसंधान; वातनिरपेक्षसंधान

**Anaesthesia.** A condition of insensibility to sensations of pains; anesthesia. संज्ञाहरण; संवेदनाहरण; असंवेदनता; निश्चेतना; चेतनालोप;

**Block A.,** see **Regional Anaesthesia.**

**Central A.,** that due to a lesion of the central nerve-system. केन्द्रीय असंवेदनता;

**Cerebral A.,** that due to the lesion of the brain. प्रमस्तिष्क असंवेदनता;

**Conduction A.,** regional anaesthesia in which local anesthetic is injected about nerves to inhibit nerve transmission. क्षेत्रीय संज्ञाहरण; चालन असंवेदनता;

**Dessociated A.,** loss of pain and temperature sensations, the tactile sense being still present. वियोजित असंवेदनता;

**General A.,** one affecting the whole body. सार्वदैहिक संज्ञाहरण; सर्वांगीण असंवेदनता;

**Infiltration A.,** local anaesthesia effected by subscutaneous injections. अन्तःसंचरण संवेदनाहरण;

**Inhalation A.**, general anaesthesia from breathing of anaesthetic gases or vapours. अभिश्वसन संज्ञाहरण;

**Intravenous A.**, general anaesthesia in which venipuncture is used as a means of injecting central nervous system depressants into the circulation. अन्त:शिरासंज्ञाहरण;

**Local A.**, that limited to a part of the body. स्थानिक संवेदनाहरण;

**Muscular A.**, loss of muscle sense. पेशी-अपसंवेदन;

**Olfactory A.**, anosmia. अघ्राणता; घ्राणसंज्ञाहरण; घ्राणसंवेदनाहरण;

**Optic A.**, amaurosis. दृष्टि संज्ञाहरण;

**Rectal A.**, that produced by the injection of an anaesthetic agent into the rectum. गुदा संज्ञाहरण;

**Regional A.**, that limited to the part supplied by an afferent nerve which has been cocainized; block anaesthesia. क्षेत्रीय संज्ञाहरण;

**Segmental A.**, loss of sensation limited to an area supplied by one or more spinal nerve roots. खंडकी असंवेदनता;

**Sexual A.**, anaphrodisia. लैंगिक असंवेदनता;

**Spinal A.**, that due to a lesion of the spinal cord or produced by an anaesthetic injection into the spinal subarachnoid space. सौषुम्निक संवेदनाहरण;

**Stocking A.**, loss of sensation in the area that would be covered by a stocking. पाद संवेदनाहरण;

**Tactile A.**, loss of sense of touch. स्पर्शज्ञानाभाव; स्पर्शअसंवेदनता;

**A. Dolorosa**, painful anaesthesia. सपीड असंवेदनता

**Anaesthesiologist.** One versed in the science of anaesthesia; anesthesiologist. संज्ञाहरणविज्ञानी; निश्चेतनाविज्ञानी

**Anaesthesiology.** The science dealing with the anaesthesia. संज्ञाहरणविज्ञान; निश्चेतनाविज्ञान

**Anaesthetic.** An agent that produces insensibility. संवेदनाहारी; संज्ञाहारी; चेतनालोपी; चेतनाहारी; चेतनाहर; असंवेदनकारी;

**General A.**, a drug which produces general anaesthesia by inhalation or injection. सार्वदैहिक संवेदनाहारी;

**Local A.**, a drug which is injected into the tissues or applied topically causes local insensibility to pain. स्थानिक संवेदनाहारी

**Anaesthetisation.** The act of producing anaesthesia; anaesthetization. संवेदनाहरण; संज्ञाहरण

**Anaesthetised.** Overpowered with anaesthesia. संवेदनाहृत; असंवेदनकृत

**Anaesthetist.** One who administers anaesthetics; anaesthetizer. संवेदनाहारक; संज्ञाहारक; निश्चेतनाविज्ञानी

**Anaesthetization.** See **Anaesthetisation.**

**Anaesthetize.** To produce loss of sensation; anesthetize. संवेदनाहरण करना; निश्चेतन करना

**Anaesthetizer.** See **Anaesthetist.**

**Anakusis.** Nervous deafness. स्नायविक बधिरता

**Anal.** Pertaining to the anus. मलद्वारीय; गुदा अथवा मलद्वार सम्बन्धी

**Analbuminaemia.** Absence of albumin in the blood. अन्नसारहीनरक्तता; रक्त में अन्नसार का अभाव

**Analepsis.** Restoration to health. आरोग्यलाभ

**Analeptic.** An agent restoring strength and health. आरोग्यकारी; संजीवक; शक्ति एवं स्वास्थ्य संचायक

**Analgen.** An antipyretic and analegesic. ज्वर एवं वेदनाहर (औषधि)

**Analgesia.** Insensibility to pain. वेदनाहरण; संवेदनाहरण; वेदना-असंवेदिता; पीड़ा के प्रति संवेदना का अभाव

**Analgesic.** An agent that relieves pain. वेदनाहर; पीड़ाहर; पीड़ानाशक; दर्द से छुटकारा दिलाने वाला पदार्थ

**Analgia.** Painlessness; analgis. वेदनाभाव; वेदनाहीनता; पीड़ा का अभाव

**Analgis.** See **Analgia.**

**Analog.** See **Analogue.**

**Analogous.** Conforming or answering to. अनुधर्मा; समधर्मा; समकार्यक; समवृत्तिक

**Analogue.** A part or organ similar in function to another but different in structure; analog. अनुधर्मी; समधर्मी

**Analogus.** Similar in function, but not in origin. अनुधर्मी; समधर्मी

**Analogy.** Relation which one thing bears to another. अनुरूपता; सादृश्य; संयोग

**Analyser.** See **Analyst.**

**Analyses.** Plural of **Analysis.**

**Analysis.** The resolution of a body into its elements. विश्लेषण; पृथक्करण; किसी पदार्थ के घटक, लक्षण या स्वरूप का निर्धारण;

    **Organic A.,** that of animal and vegetable tissue. जैव या जैवी विश्लेषण;

    **Qualitative A.,** the determination of the nature of the elements of which the body is composed. गुणात्मक विश्लेषण; गुणवत्तात्मक विश्लेषण;

**Quantitative A.**, the determination of the proportionate parts of the elements of a compound. मात्रात्मक विश्लेषण

**Analyst.** A person experienced in analysis; analyser. विश्लेषक; विश्लेषण करने वाला

**Analyte.** Any substance or chemical constituent that is analysed. विश्लेष्य (पदार्थ)

**Analytical.** Relating to analysis. विश्लेषणात्मक; विश्लेषण सम्बन्धी

**Anamnesis.** The past history of a disease. पूर्ववृत्त; रोगी का पूर्व विवरण

**Anamnestic.** Recalling to mind; remembering. स्मरणीय; स्मरण करना; याद करना; concerning anamnesis. पूर्ववृत्त सम्बन्धी

**Anamnia.** Having no amnion; anamniota. उल्वहीनता

**Anamniota.** See **Anamnia**.

**Anamniotic.** Without an amnion. उल्वहीन

**Anamorphous.** Handicapped; disabled. विकलांग; अंगहीन

**Anapeiratic.** Occupational neurosis arising from prolonged muscular exercise. व्यावसायिक मनोविकार; श्रमजनित आक्षेप

**Anaphalantiasis.** Alopecia, especially of the brow. भ्रूखल्वाटता; भ्रूलोप; भौंहें गिर जाना

**Anaphase.** The phenomenon of karyokinesis just before the formation of the daughter-stars (dyasters). पश्चावस्था; गतिस्थिति

**Anaphia.** A deficient sense of touch. स्पर्शशून्यता; स्पर्शज्ञान का अभाव; स्पर्शसंवेदना की कमी

**Anaphoresis.** Insufficient perspiration. स्वेदाल्पता; प्रस्वेदाल्पता; स्वेदनाल्पता; पसीने का अभाव; प्रस्वेदाभाव

**Anaphoretic.** An agent checking perspiration. स्वेदरोधक

**Anaphrodisia.** A diminution of sexual power; sexual anaesthesia. कामाल्पता; सम्भोग की इच्छा कम हो जाना

**Anaphrodisiac.** An agent allaying sexual passion. अवाजीकर

**Anaphylactic.** Oversusceptible. तीव्रग्राही; अतिसुग्राही; relating to anaphylaxis. तीव्रग्राहिता सम्बन्धी

**Anaphylactogenesis.** The production by anaphylaxis. तीव्रग्राहीजनन

**Anaphylactogenic.** Producing anaphylaxis. तीव्रग्राहिताजनक

**Anaphylactoid.** Resembling anaphylaxis. तीव्रग्राहिताभ

**Anaphylaxis.** Oversusceptibility. तीव्रग्राहिता; अतिरंजित प्रतिक्रिया;
  Active A., anaphylaxis resulting from injection of an antigen. सक्रिय तीव्रग्राहिता;
  Antiserum A., see Passive Anaphylaxis.
  Passive A., anaphylaxis induced by injection of serum from a sensitized animal into a normal one; antiserum anaphylaxis. निष्क्रिय तीव्रग्राहिता

**Anaplasia.** The tendency of certain tissues towards reversion to an earlier or embryonal type. प्राक्विकसन; कोशिका-अनुक्रमणीयता

**Anaplastic.** Pertaining to anaplasty. स्वास्थ्यसंधान सम्बन्धी;
  A. Surgery, see Anaplasty.

**Anaplasty.** Restorative surgery; anaplastic surgery. स्वास्थ्यसंस्थापकशल्यकर्म; स्वास्थ्यसंधान; प्लास्टिक सर्जरी

**Anapnometer.** A spirometer. श्वासमापी (यंत्र)

**Anaptic.** Relating to anaphia. स्पर्शशून्यता सम्बन्धी

**Anarthria.** An inability to articulate distinctly. अस्पष्ट उच्चारण;
  A. Literalis, stammering. हकलाहट; हकलाना; अटक-अटक कर बोलना

**Anasarca.** Dropsy of the cellular tissue; a species of dropsy between the skin and the flesh; general dropsy. सर्वांगशोफ; सम्पूर्ण शरीर की शोफज अवस्था

**Anasarcous.** Characterized by, or relating to anasarca. सर्वांगशोफाभ या सर्वांगशोफ सम्बन्धी

**Anastasis.** Convalescence. उल्लाघ; आरोग्यलाभ

**Anastomosis.** The establishment of intercommunication between two vessels, hollow organs or nerves. सम्मिलन; शाखामिलन; शाखामिलनता;
  Crucial A., an arterial anastomosis in the upper part of the thigh; cruciate anastomosis. स्वस्तिकाकार सम्मिलन;
  Cruciate A., see Crucial Anastomosis.
  Intestinal A., the formation of a communication between two parts of the intestine. आंत्र-सम्मिलन

**Anastomotic.** Pertaining to anastomosis. शाखामिलन सम्बन्धी

**Anat.** Brief. संक्षिप्त

**Anatomic.** See Anatomical.

**Anatomical.** Belonging to anatomy; anatomic; structural. शारीरी; शारीरिक; शरीर-रचना सम्बन्धी

**Anatomicoclinical.** Relating to anatomy and diagnosis. शारीरनैदानिक; शरीर-रचना तथा निदान सम्बन्धी

**Anatomist.** One versed in anatomy. शरीर-रचनाविज्ञानी; शरीर-विज्ञानवेत्ता

**Anatomy.** The body structure. शरीर-रचना; शरीर-रचनाविज्ञान; शारीरिकी;

**Dental A.,** one concerning teeth, their location, position and relationship. दंतरचनाविज्ञान;

**Functional A.,** see **Physiologic Anatomy.**

**Physiologic A.,** anatomy studied in its relation to function; functional anatomy. भौतिक शारीरिकी; भौतिक शरीर-रचना;

**Regional A.,** the study of correlated regions of the body. क्षेत्रीय शारीरिकी;

**Veterinary A.,** anatomy of domestic animals. पशु-शरीररचनाविज्ञान; पशु-शारीरिकी

**Anatriptic.** A medicine applied by rubbing. मर्दनौषधि; मालिश की जाने वाली औषधि

**Anbasis.** The first period or accent of a disease. प्रारम्भिक रुग्णता

**Anchylosis.** Formation of stiff joint by consolidation of articulating surfaces; ancylosis; ankylosis. संधिकाठिन्य; जोड़ों की ऐंठन; संसक्ति

**Anchylostoma.** Human hookworm; ancylostoma; ankylostoma. मानवकृमि; अंकुशकृमि;

**A. Duodenale,** hookworm. अंकुशकृमि

**Achylostomiasis.** Hookworm disease. अंकुशकृमिरोग

**Ancillary.** Auxillary. अनुषंगी; सहायक

**Ancipital.** Two-edged. द्विधारी; दो धार या किनारों वाला; two-headed. द्विशिरस्क; दो सिर वाला

**Ancon.** The olecranon; the elbow. कोहनी

**Anconal.** Relating to the elbow; anconeal. कोहनी सम्बन्धी

**Anconeal.** See **Anconal.**

**Anconitis.** Inflammation of the elbow-joint. कोहनीसंधिशोथ; कोहनी के जोड़ का प्रदाह

**Anconoid.** Resembling the elbow. कोहनीवत्; कोहनी से मिलता-जुलता

**Ancylosis.** See **Anchylosis.**

**Ancylostoma.** See **Anchylostoma.**

**Androblastoma.** A tumour of the testes. वृषणार्बुद

**Androgens.** A group of hormones characteristic of the male.

पुल्लिंगी-हॉर्मोन; नृहॉर्मोन; नर-हॉर्मोन; पुंसत्व प्रदान करने वाले हॉर्मोन

**Androgenic.** Relating to an androgen. नर-हॉर्मोन सम्बन्धी

**Andrology.** The science of man. नृविज्ञान; पुरुषविज्ञान; नरविज्ञान

**Andromania.** Nymphomania. स्त्रीकामोन्माद; स्त्रियों में पाया जाने वाला कामोन्माद

**Andromorphous.** Of the form of a man. पुरुषरूपी; नररूपी; नररूप

**Androphobia.** A morbid fear of men. नरातंक; नरभीति; पुरुषभीति; पुरुषों का भय

**Anelectrotonus.** The decreased functional activity in a nerve in the neighbourhood of the anode. धनविद्युत्तान

**Anematosis.** See **Idiopathic Anaemian** under **Anaemia.**

**Anemia.** See **Anaemia.**

**Anemic.** See **Anaemic.**

**Anemometer.** A device that measures the speed of the wind. वायुवेगमापी; वायुवेगमापक यंत्र

**Anemopathy.** Treatment by inhalation. अन्तःश्वसनचिकित्सा; श्वास को अन्दर खींच कर की जाने वाली चिकित्सा

**Anemophobia.** A morbid fear of air. वायुभीति; वायु-आतंक

**Anemoscope.** A device that shows the speed of the wind. वायुवेगमापी; वायुवेगमापकयंत्र

**Anencephalia.** The absence of the brain; anencephaly. अमस्तिष्कता; मस्तिष्कहीनता; मस्तिष्क का अभाव

**Anencephalic.** Having no brain; anencephalous. मस्तिष्कहीन; अमस्तिष्क

**Anencephalous.** See **Anencephalic.**

**Anencephalus.** A foetus having no brain. अमस्तिष्कभ्रूण; मस्तिष्क-विहीन भ्रूण

**Anencephaly.** See **Anencephalia.**

**Anenterous.** Having no intestinal canal. आंत्रविहीन; आंत्ररहित; आंत्रहीन

**Anephric.** Lacking kidneys. वृक्कहीन; गुर्दों से हीन

**Anergastic.** Pertaining to anergasia. अक्रियप्रवृत्ति सम्बन्धी

**Anergasia.** Absence of mental activity. अक्रियप्रवृत्ति

**Anergic.** Inactive. निश्चेष्ट; निष्क्रिय; अनूर्ज; प्रतिक्रियाहीन; relating to anergy. निष्क्रियता सम्बन्धी;

    **A. Stupor,** acute dementia. उग्र जड़िमा; तीव्र जड़िमा

**Anergy.** Inactivity; absence of sensitivity to reaction. निश्चेष्टता; निष्क्रियता; अनूर्जता; प्रतिक्रियाहीनता

**Anesis.** A remission or abatement of a disease. रोगह्रास; रोगोपशम

**Anesthesia.** See **Anaesthesia.**

**Anesthesiologist.** See **Anaesthesiologist.**

**Anesthetic.** The same as **Anaesthetic.**

**Anesthetist.** The same as **Anaesthetizer.**

**Anesthetize.** See **Anaesthetize.**

**Anesthetizer.** One who administers anaesthetics. संवेदनाहारी; बेहोश करने वाला; असंवेदनाकारी; निश्चेतनाकारी

**Anestrum.** See **Anestrus.**

**Anestrus.** The sexual rest period, i.e. the time between the heat periods of animals; anestrum. अमदकाल

**Anetic.** Relieving or assuaging pain; anodyne. वेदनाहर; पीड़ानाशक; दर्दनाशक

**Anetus.** The generic name for intermittent fevers. सविराम ज्वर; एक-एक कर आने वाले बुखार

**Aneuria.** Failure or lack of nervous energy. स्नायुदौर्बल्य; नाड़ीदौर्बल्य; स्नायुशक्ति का अभाव या कमी

**Aneurism.** Morbid enlargement of an artery; aneurysm. धमनीविस्फार; धमनी का असाधारण रूप से बढ़ जाना;

  **Abdominal A.,** aneurysm of the abdominal aorta. उदरधमनीविस्फार;

  **Arteriovenous A.,** the simultaneous rupture of an artery and a vein, the blood being held in the cellular tissue. धमनीशिराविस्फार;

  **Bacterial A.,** caused by growth of bacteria within the vascular wall. रोगाणुज धमनीविस्फार;

  **Cerebral A.,** rupture of the cerebral aorta. प्रमस्तिष्क-धमनीविस्फार;

  **Cirsoid A.,** dilalation of a group of blood vessels due to congenital malformation with arteriovenous shunting; racemose aneurism. कुटिल धमनीविस्फार;

  **Dissecting A.,** one in which the blood forces its way between the coats of an artery. विदारक धमनीविस्फार;

  **False A.,** one due to the rupture of all the coats of an artery and the retention of the blood by the surrounding tissue. कूटधमनीविस्फार; मिथ्याधमनीविस्फार;

  **Fusiform A.,** an elongated spindle-shaped dilatation of an artery. तर्क्वाकार धमनीविस्फार;

  **Mycotic A.,** one due to growth of bacteria in the vessel wall.

पूतिज धमनीविस्फार;

Racemose A., see Cirsoid Aneurism.

Saccular A., a sac-like bulging on one side of an artery; sacculated aneurysm. कोष्ठकी धमनीविस्फार;

Sacculated A., see Saccular Aneurism.

Syphilitic A., one involving the thoracic aorta resulting from tertiary syphilitic aortitis. उपदंशज धमनीविस्फार;

Varicose A., a blood-containing sac, communicating with both an artery and a vein. स्फीतशिरा धमनीविस्फार

Aneurismal. Pertaining to aneurism; aneurysmal. धमनीविस्फार सम्बन्धी

Aneurysm. See Aneurism.

Aneurysmal. See Aneurismal.

Aneurysmoplasty. Restoration of the artery in aneurysm. धमनीसंधान

Anfractuous. Convoluted. कुण्डलित; संवलित; मरोड़ या लपेट वाला

Angi-. Prefix signifying vessel or channel. 'कुल्या', 'प्रणाल', 'वाहिका' का अर्थ देने वाला उपसर्ग

Angiectasia. Abnormal dilatation of the blood vessels; angiectasis. नलिका-विस्फार; वाहिका-विस्फार

Angiectasis. See Angiectasia.

Angiectomy. Excision of a blood vessel. वाहिका-उच्छेदन

Angeitis. See Angiitis.

Angiitis. Vascular inflammation; vasculitis; angeitis. वाहिकाशोथ

Angileucitis. Inflammation of the lymphatics; angioleucitis; angiolymphitis. लसीकाशोथ

Angina. Inflammation of the passage of the throat, causing a sense of suffocation. गलप्रदाह; कण्ठदाह; गलार्ति; pain; neuralgia. शूल;

Agranulocytic A., acute sore-throat and ulceration of the pharynx. अकणिश्वेतकोशिकामुखपाक;

Membranous A., see Angina Membranacea.

A. Acuta, simple sore-throat; acute angina; angina simplex. सामान्य कण्ठदाह;

A. Gangrenosa, putrid sore-throat. सपूय कण्ठदाह;

A. Granulosa, see Clergyman's Sore-throat.

A. Laryngea, see Laryngitis.

A. Maligna, malignant inflammation of the throat. सांघातिक गलप्रदाह;

# Angina

A. **Membranacea,** croup; membranous angina. क्रुप; कलामय गलार्ति;

A. **Parotidea,** mumps; parotitis. कर्णमूलग्रन्थिशोथ; कर्णपूर्वग्रन्थिशोथ; कनफेड़;

A. **Pectoris.,** severe heart-pain; cardiac neuralgia. हृद्शूल; हृच्छूल; हृदयार्ति;

A. **Pharyngea,** inflammation of the mucous membrane of the pharynx. गलकोश-प्रदाह; ग्रसनीशूल;

A. **Simplex,** see **Angina Acuta.**

A. **Tonsillans,** see **Angina Tonsillaris.**

A. **Tonsillaris,** quinsy; angina tonsillans. सपूय गलतुण्डिकाशोथ

**Anginal.** Relating to angina. हृच्छूल, गलप्रदाह, गलार्ति अथवा कण्ठदाह सम्बन्धी

**Anginoid.** Resembling angina, especially angina pectoris. हृच्छूलाभ; हृच्छूल से मिलता-जुलता

**Anginophobia.** A morbid fear of angina pectoris. हृद्शूलभीति; हृच्छूलातंक

**Anginose.** Affected with angina; anginous. गलार्तिग्रस्त; शूलग्रस्त

**Anginous.** See **Anginose.**

**Angio-.** The same as **Angi-.**

**Angioblast.** An embryonic cell developing into vascular tissue. वाहिकाप्रसू; रक्तकोरक; प्रारम्भिक निर्माणकारी ऊतक, जिससे रक्तकोशिकायें तथा रक्तवाहिनियां बनती हैं

**Angioblastoma.** A tumour of the embryonic cell developing into the vascular tissue; hemangioblastoma. वाहिकाप्रसू-अर्बुद

**Angiocardiocinetik.** See **Angiocardiokinetic.**

**Angiocardiogram.** Film demonstrating the heart and great vessels after injection of opaque medium. वाहिकाहृद्चित्र

**Angiocardiography.** Demonstration of heart and great vessels by means of injection of opaque medium into the cardiac circulation. वाहिकाहृद्चित्रण

**Angiocardiokinectic.** A drug which stimulates the vessels of the heart; angiocardiocinetik. हृद्वाहिकाप्रेरक (औषधि)

**Angiocarditis.** Inflammation of the cardiac vessels. हृद्वाहिकाशोथ

**Angiocholitis.** Inflammation of the bile-duct. पित्तनलीशोथ; पित्तनली का प्रदाह

**Angioedema.** See **Angio-oedema.**

**Angiofibroma.** A benign neoplasm of fibrous tissue. वाहिकातंत्वर्बुद

**Angiogenesis.** The development of the vessels. वाहिकाजनन

**Angiogenic.** Relating to angiogenesis. वाहिकाजनक

**Angioglioma.** A vascular tumour of the spinal cord. सुषुम्नावाहिकार्बुद

**Angiogram.** Film demonstrating the arterial system after injection of the opaque medium. वाहिकाचित्र

**Angiograph.** A form of sphygmograph. वाहिकालेखी

**Angiography.** A description of the vessels. वाहिकाचित्रण; वाहिकालेख

**Angioid.** Resembling blood vessels. रक्तवाहिकाभ; रक्तवाहिनी जैसा

**Angioleucitis.** See **Angileucitis**.

**Angiolipoma.** A lipoma that contains an unusually large number of foci of vascular channel. वाहिकावसार्बुद

**Angiolith.** A venous calculus; phlebolith. शिराश्मरी; शिरा की पथरी

**Angiology.** The doctorine of the vascular system. वाहिकाविज्ञान; रक्तनलिकाविज्ञान

**Angiolymphitis.** See **Angileucitis**.

**Angiolymphoma.** A tumour of the lymphatic vessels. लसीकावाहिकार्बुद; लसीकावाहिकाओं की रसौली

**Angiolysis.** Obliteration of blood vessel. वाहिकालयन

**Angioma.** A tumour formed of the blood vessels. वाहिकार्बुद; रक्तवाहिनियों में बनने वाली रसौली

**Angiomata.** Plural of **Angioma**.

**Angiomalacia.** A softening of vessel-wall. वाहिकाप्राचीरमृदुता; रक्तनलिका-भित्तियों की कोमलता

**Angiomatosis.** The formation of a tumour in a blood vessel. वाहिकार्बुदता; किसी रक्तवाहिका में रसौली बनना

**Angiomatoid.** Resembling a tumour of vascular origin. वाहिकार्बुदाभ

**Angiomatous.** Relating to angioma. वाहिकार्बुदीय; वाहिकार्बुद सम्बन्धी

**Angiometer.** An instrument for measuring the diameter and tension of vessels. वाहिकामापी; वाहिकामापकयंत्र; रक्तनलिकाओं के व्यास व तनाव को मापने वाला यंत्र

**Angiomyocardiac.** See **Angiomyocardial**.

**Angiomyocardial.** Pertaining to the muscles of the vessels of the heart; angiomyocardiac. हृद्वाहिकापेशी सम्बन्धी

**Angiomyolipoma.** A benign neoplasm of adipose tissue. वाहिकापेशीवसार्बुद

**Angiomyoma.** A vascular and muscular tumour. धमनीपेश्यर्बुद

**Angiomyosarcoma.** A myosarcoma that has an unusually large number of proliferated and frequently dilated vascular channels. वाहिकापेशी-कर्कटता

**Angiopneumography.** A description of the pulmonary vessels. फुप्फुसवाहिकाचित्रण

**Angioneuroma.** A neuroma of the blood vessels. धमनीतंत्रिकार्बुद; वाहिकातंत्रिकार्बुद

**Angioneurosis.** Neurosis of the blood vessels. वाहिकातंत्रिकता

**Angioneurotic.** Pertaining to angioneurosis. वाहिकातंत्रिकता सम्बन्धी

**Angionoma.** Ulceration of a vessel. वाहिकाव्रण; रक्त नलिकाओं की व्रणग्रस्तता

**Angio-oedema.** A neurosis characterized by the presence of circumscribed noninflammatory swellings; angioedema. वाहिकाशोफ

**Angiopancreatitis.** Inflammation of the vascular tissue of the pancreas. अग्न्याशयवाहिकाऊतकशोथ

**Angioparalysis.** Vasomotor paralysis; vasoparalysis. वाहिकाघात; रक्तवहा-नली का पक्षाघात (फालिज)

**Angiopathic.** Relating to angiopathy. वाहिकारुग्णता सम्बन्धी

**Angiopathy.** Any disease of the vessels. वाहिकारुग्णता; धमनीरोग; रक्त-नलिकाओं का कोई रोग

**Angioplasty.** Plastic surgery upon blood vessels. रक्तवाहिकासंधान

**Angiopneumography.** A description of the pulmonary vessels. फुप्फुसवाहिकाचित्रण

**Angiosarcoma.** A vascular sarcoma, as of the spinal cord. वाहिकासार्कोमा; वाहिकासार्कार्बुद

**Angiosclerosis.** A hardening of the vessel-walls. वाहिकाप्राचीरकाठिन्य; वाहिका प्राचीरों की कठोरता

**Angiosialitis.** Inflammation of a salivary duct. लारनलीशोथ; लारनली का प्रदाह

**Angioses.** Plural of **Angiosis**.

**Angiosis.** Any disease of the blood vessels; angiosus. वाहिकाविकृति; रक्त-नलिकाओं का रोग

**Angiospasm.** A vasomotor spasm. वाहिका-आकर्ष; वाहिका-उद्वेष्ट

**Angiospastic.** Pertaining to angiospasm. वाहिका-आकर्ष सम्बन्धी

**Angiostenosis.** A constriction of the blood-vessels. वाहिकासंकीर्णन; रक्त-नलिकाओं की सिकुड़न

**Angiosus.** See **Angiosis**.

**Angiotelectasia.** See **Angiotelectasis**.

**Angiotelectasis.** Dilatation of the blood vessels; angiotelectasia. वाहिकाविस्फार; रक्त-नलिकाओं का फूलना

**Angiotitis.** Inflammation of the blood vessels of the ear. कर्णवाहिकाशोथ; कान की रक्त-नलिकाओं का प्रदाह

**Angiotomy.** The dissection of blood-vessels. वाहिका-उच्छेदन

**Angitis.** Inflammation of blood or lymph vessels. वाहिकाशोथ; वाहिकास्तरशोथ

**Angle.** The degree of divergence of two lines. कोण

**Angor-animi.** Fear of death. मरणातंक; आसन्नमृत्युभीति; मृत्यु का भय

**Anguish.** Severe bodily or mental pain and restlessness. बेचैनी; छटपटाहट; तड़पन

**Angular.** Pertaining to an angle. कोणीय; कोणिक; कोण सम्बन्धी

**Angulus.** An angle. कोण; corner. किनारा

**Angustation.** A narrowing; constriction. संकीर्णन; संकीर्णता; सिकुड़न

**Anhaphia.** A loss of the sense of touch. स्पर्शज्ञानाभाव; स्पर्श-असंवेदिता; स्पर्शज्ञान का अभाव

**Anhedonia.** Complete loss of the sensation of pleasure. विषय-सुख अथवा आनन्दमयी अनुभूति का पूर्ण लोप

**Anhelation.** Shortness of breath; dyspnoea. श्वासकष्ट; कष्टश्वास; श्वास लेने में कठिनाई

**Anhematosis.** Defective formation of the blood. विषमरक्तता; दूषित रक्तरचना

**Anhidrosis.** A deficiency of sweat. अस्वेदलता; स्वेदाल्पता; पसीने की कमी

**Anhidrotic.** An agent that checks sweating. अस्वेदल; अस्वेदकारी; पसीना रोकने वाला पदार्थ

**Anhistic.** Structureless; shapeless; not organised; anhistous; anidous. आकृतिहीन; अनाकार; आकारहीन

**Anhistous.** Se **Anhistic**.

**Anhydraemia.** Deficient fluid contents of blood; anhydremia.

अजलरक्तता; रक्त में जल का अभाव
**Anhydremia.** See **Anhydraemia**.

**Anhydrous.** Not containing water. जलमुक्त; शुष्क; अजल; निर्जल; निर्जलीय

**Anidous.** See **Anhistic**.

**Anidrosis.** The same as **Anhidrosis**.

**Anidrotic.** The same as **Anhidrotic**.

**Anihydraemia.** The same as **Anhydraemia**.

**Anihydrosis.** The same as **Anhidrosis**.

**Anihydrotic.** The same as **Anhidrotic**.

**Anihydrous.** The same as **Anhydrous**.

**Animal.** An organic being with life and power of motion. जीव; प्राणी; जन्तु; पशु; जीवधारी;

   **A. Heat,** the natural heat of the body. जैवी ताप

**Animalcule.** A microscopic organism. जन्तुक; सूक्ष्मजन्तु

**Animate.** Living; the state of being alive. चेतन; सजीव; सप्राण

**Animation.** Enlivenment;state of being alive or active. चेतन; चैतन्य; सजीवता; प्राण-संचारण

**Anion.** An electronegative element. ऋणायन; विद्युत अपघट्य में धन ध्रुव की ओर आकर्षित करने वाला तत्व

**Anionic.** Pertaining to anion. ऋणायनी; अपक्षालक

**Aniridia.** An absence of the iris. अपरितारकता; श्वेतपटलाभाव; परितारिका का जन्मजात अभाव

**Anischuria.** Enuresis. असंयतमूत्रता; निरंकुशमूत्रता; अनजाने ही पेशाब हो जाना

**Anise.** The herb Pimpinella anisum; the fruit is expectorant and carminative. सौंफ का पौधा

**Aniseeds.** The seeds of anise plant. सौंफ

**Aniseikonia.** Unequal retinal image. असमप्रतिबिम्बता

**Anisochromatic.** Not of uniform colour. विषमवर्णता; विषमवर्णकता

**Anisocoria.** An inequality of the pupils. असमपटलता; विषमपटलता; दोनों आँखों की पुतलियों का भिन्न नाप होना

**Anisocytosis.** Abnormal equality in the size of the red blood cells. असमकोशिकता; विषमकोशिकता; लाल रक्त कोशिकाओं के आकार की असमानता

**Anisodactyly.** Unequal length in corresponding fingers. असमअंगुलिता; विषमअंगुलिता

**Anisomastia.** Asymmetrical breast. विषमस्तनता; असमस्तनता

**Anisomelia.** Unequal length of the limbs. असमांगता; विषमांगता; युगल अंगों की पारस्परिक विषमता

**Anisometropia.** A difference in the refraction of the two eyes. असमदृष्टिता; विषमदृष्टिता

**Anisometropic.** Affected with anisometropia. असमदृष्टि; विषमदृष्टि; चक्षुवर्तनविषमता

**Anisopia.** Inequality of the visual power in the two eyes. असमदृष्टिता; विषमदृष्टिता

**Anisosthenic.** Of unequal power. असमशक्ति; विषमशक्ति

**Anisotonic.** Of an unequal tone. असमतानिक; विषमतानिक

**Anisotropal.** See **Anisotropic.**

**Anisotropic.** Double refractive; anisotropal. असमदिग्वर्ती; विषमदैशिक

**Anisum.** Anise. सौंफ

**Ankle.** The joint between foot and leg. गुल्फ; टखना; पैर तथा टांग की सन्धि के बीच का भाग;

   **A.-bone,** the uppermost bone of the tarsus. गुल्फास्थि; टखने की हड्डी;

   **A.-joint,** tarsus; the joint connecting foot with leg. गुल्फसन्धि; टखने का जोड़

**Ankyloblepharon.** Adhesion of the edges of the eyelids. बद्धवर्त्म; पलकों का परस्पर चिपक जाना

**Ankyloglossia.** Tongue-tie; a congenital shortening of the frenum of the tongue. बद्धजिह्वा; चिपकी हुई जीभ

**Ankyloproctia.** Stricture of the rectum. मलांत्रसंकीर्णता; मलाशय का सिकुड़ जाना

**Ankylosing.** Stiffened or fixed condition of a joint. संधिसायुज्यक; बद्ध

**Ankylosis.** Stiffness or fixation of a joint; anchylosis. अस्थिसमेकन; संधिग्रह;

   **Bony A.,** when the connecting material is bone; true ankylosis. अस्थि-संधिग्रह; यथार्थ संधिग्रह;

   **False A.,** see **Spurious Ankylosis.**

   **Ligamentous A.,** when the medium is fibrous. तंतु संधिग्रह;

   **Spurious A.,** that due to rigidity of the surrounding parts; false ankylosis. कूट संधिग्रह;

   **True A.,** see **Bony Ankylosis.**

**Ankylostoma.** A genus of nematodes of the family *Ankylostomatidae* whose members are intestinal parasites and includes the hookworms; anchylostoma. अंकुशमुखीकृमि; केंचुवा;

   **A. Duodenale,** the hookworm. अंकुशकृमि; कण्टककृमि

**Ankylostomiasis.** Hookworm disease due to ankylostoma duodenale. अंकुशकृमिरोग

**Ankylotic.** Pertaining to, or characterized by ankylosis. संधिग्रह सम्बन्धी या संधिग्राही

**Ankylourethria.** Urethral stricture. मूत्रपथसंकीर्णता; मूत्रमार्गी सिकुड़न

**Ankyroid.** Hook-shaped; ancyroid. कंटकाकार

**Anlage.** The original form. मूलरूप; अनलागे

**Annectent.** Joining; connected with. संयोजक; संयोजी

**Annexa.** The same as **Adnexa.**

**Annexal.** The same as **Adnexal.**

**Annoy.** To irritate. खिझाना; चिढ़ाना; चिढ़ना; उद्विग्न करना या होना

**Annoyance.** Vexation; disgust. खीझ; चिढ़; उद्विग्नता; संतापन; घृणा

**Annular.** Ring-shaped. वलयी; वर्तुलाकार; वृत्ताकार; चक्करदार; छल्लेदार; अंगूठी जैसा; मुद्रोपम; मण्डलाकार;

   **A. Cartilage,** the cricoid cartilage of the larynx. वलयी उपास्थि;

   **A. Ligament,** found surrounding the ankle and proximal and distal ends of radius. वलयी बंधन

**Annuloplasty.** Reconstruction of an incompetent cardiac valve, usually mitral valve. हृत्कपाटसंधान

**Annulus.** The circular opening or margin; anulus. वलय; मुद्राकार घेरे वाला;

   **A. Abdominalis,** one of the abdominal rings. उदर वलय;

   **A. Abdominis,** the inguinal ring. वंक्षण वलय;

   **A. Ciliaris,** the boundary between the iris and the choroid. रोमक वलय;

   **A. Fibrosus,** the fibrous rings or attachments. तन्तु वलय;

   **A. Umbilicus,** the umbilical ring. नाभि वलय

**Anococcygeal.** Pertaining to the anus and the coccyx. गुदा तथा अनुत्रिक सम्बन्धी

**Anodal.** Pertaining to the anode. धनाग्र सम्बन्धी

**Anode.** The positive pole in an electric cell. धनाग्र; विद्युत् धनाग्र; वह

विद्युदग्र जिससे विद्युत्धारा संयंत्र में प्रवेश करती है

**Anodemia.** An absence of the sense of smell. अघ्राणता; घ्राणज्ञानाभाव; सूँघने के ज्ञान का अभाव

**Anodontia.** Absence of the teeth. अदन्तता; दन्तहीनता; दान्तों का अभाव

**Anodyne.** Relieving or assuaging pain; anetic. वेदनाहर; दर्दनाशक; पीड़ाहर; शामक

**Anoesia.** Idiocy; anoia. जड़ता; जड़बुद्धिता; मूर्खता; बेवकूफी

**Anoia.** See **Anoesia**.

**Anomalous.** Deviating from the ordinary; irregular. विषम; असंगत

**Anomaly.** That which is anomalous. असंगति; विसंगति; अनियमितता

**Anonychia.** Congenital absence of the nails. सहजनखाभाव; नाखुनों का जन्मजात अभाव

**Anonymous.** Innominate. अनामी; बिना नाम वाला

**Anoperineal.** Pertaining to the anus and the perineum. गुदा अथवा मलद्वार तथा मूलाधार सम्बन्धी

**Anopheles.** A genus of mosquitoes; the females are the host of the malarial parasite, and their bite is the means of transmitting the disease to man. एनोफ्लीज (नामक मच्छर जिनके काटने से मलेरिया प्रकट होता है)

**Anophthalmia.** An absence of the eyes. अनेत्रता; नेत्रों का अभाव

**Anophthalmos.** A person born without eyes. अनेत्री; अन्धा; दृष्टिहीन

**Anopia.** Blindness; sightlessness. अनेत्रता; अन्धता; दृष्टिहीनता

**Anoplasty.** Reconstructive surgery of the anus. गुदासंधान

**Anopsia.** Disuse of the eyes from certain defects. दृष्टि-अयोग

**Anorchia.** See **Anorchidism**.

**Anorchid.** Without testicles. वृषणहीन

**Anorchidism.** A congenital absence of the testicles; anorchia; anorchism. सहज-अवृषणता; सहज-वृषणहीनता; वृषणों का जन्मजात अभाव

**Anorchism.** See **Anorchidism**.

**Anorchus.** A male with congenital absence of testes in the scrotum. सहजअण्डहीनता; वृषणों का जन्मजात अभाव

**Anorectal.** Pertaining to the anus and the rectum. गुदा एवं मलाशय सम्बन्धी

**Anorectic.** Appetite depressant; anoretic; an agent causing anorexia. भूख कम करने वाला; क्षुधालोपक; अरुचिकारी; अरुचिकर; अरुचिजनक; नीरस;

**Anoretic**

pertaining to anorexia. भूख न लगने अथवा क्षुधालोप सम्बन्धी

**Anoretic.** See **Anorectic**.

**Anorexia.** An absence or loss of appetite. क्षुधालोप; भूख का अभाव; अरुचि; भूख न लगना

**Anorexic.** Relating to, or suffering from anorexia. अरुचि सम्बन्धी या अरुचिग्रस्त

**Anorexigenic.** Promoting or causing anorexia. अरुचिजनक; अरुचिकारी; नीरस

**Anormal.** See **Abnormal**.

**Anorthography.** Agraphia. अलेखन

**Anorthopia.** Obliquity of vision; squinting. नेत्रवक्रता; वक्रदृष्टिता; तिर्यकदृष्टि; बहंगापन; असममित-दृष्टि; विकृत-दृष्टि

**Anosmia.** A loss of the sense of smell; anosphrasia. अघ्राणता; गन्धज्ञानाभाव; घ्राणनाश; सूँघने की शक्ति का ह्रास

**Anosmic.** Relating to anosmia. अघ्राणता सम्बन्धी

**Anosognosia.** Unawareness of one's own disease; anosognosis. स्वरोगज्ञानाभाव; अपना रोग पहचानने की असमर्थता

**Anosognosis.** See **Anosognosia**.

**Anosphrasia.** See **Anosmia**.

**Anospinal.** Relating to the anus and the spine. गुदा एवं रीढ़ की हड्डी सम्बन्धी

**Anosteoplasia.** Imperfect development of bones; anostosis. दुरस्थिविकसन; अस्थियों का अपूर्ण विकास; विकृत अस्थिरचना

**Anostosis.** See **Anosteoplasia**.

**Anotia.** Congenital absence of one or both ears. सहज-अकर्णता; कान (या कानों) का जन्मजात अभाव

**Anotus.** Without ears. अकर्ण; कर्णहीन; बिना कान का

**Anourous.** Without a tail. अपुच्छ; निर्पुच्छ; पुच्छहीन; पूंछविहीन

**Anovesical.** Pertaining to both anus and bladder. गुदा एवं मूत्राशय सम्बन्धी

**Anovular.** Not related to, or coincident with ovulation; anovulatory. डिम्बाक्षरणी

**Anovulatory.** See **Anovular**.

**Anovulation.** Suspension or cessation of ovulation. डिम्बक्षरण

**Anoxaemia.** Insufficient oxygen in the blood; anoxemia; anoxia.

अनॉक्सीरक्तता; रक्त में पर्याप्त ऑक्सीजन की कमी

**Anoxemia.** See **Anoxaemia.**

**Anoxia.** See **Anoxaemia.**

**Ansa.** A loop. पाश; सिक्त;

   **A. Atlantis,** a loop formed by filaments of the first and second cervical nerves. शीर्षधर पाश;

   **A. Cervicalis,** the cervical loop; cervical ansa. ग्रीवा पाश; ग्रैव पाश;

   **A. Hypoglossi,** a loop formed by the descending ramus and the second and third cervical nerves. अधोजिह्वा पाश;

   **A. Intestinalis,** any loop of the small intestines. लघ्वांत्र पाश;

   **A. Lenticularis,** the upper lamina of the ventral stalk of the thalamus. लेंसाभ पाश;

   **A. Lentiformis,** the same as **Ansa Lenticularis.**

   **A. Lumbalis,** a loop made of branches of the lumbar nerves. कटि-पाश;

   **A. Peduncularis,** the ventral stalk of the thalamus. वृन्ताभ पाश;

   **A. Subclavia,** a loop formed by a nerve filament running from middle to the inferior cervical or first thoracic ganglion and passing in front of the subclavian artery. अधोजत्रुक पाश

**Ansae.** Plural of **Ansa.**

**Ansate.** See **Ansiform.**

**Ansiform.** Of the form of a loop; ansate. पाशाकार; पाशरूप

**Antacid.** An alkali that neutralises acidity; antiacid. अम्लघ्न; प्रत्यम्ल; अम्लापकर्षक; अम्लनाशक

**Antacrid.** Correcting acidity; antiacrid. अम्लनिवारक

**Antagonism.** Active opposition; a characteristic of some drugs, muscles and organisms. विरोध; प्रतिद्वन्दिता

**Antagonist.** Rival; a drug neutralizing the effects of another, or a muscle opposing the action of another. विरोधी; प्रतिद्वन्दी; निरोधक; विपरीत-प्रभावी

**Antagonistic.** Acting in an opposite way. विरोधी; प्रतिद्वन्दी; विपरीत

**Antalgesic.** See **Antalgic.**

**Antalgic.** Medicine that relieves pain; antalgesic; analgesic. अनार्तिकर; आर्तिहर; दर्दनाशक (औषधि)

**Antalkaline.** An agent neutralizing alkali. क्षारउदासीनकर; प्रतिक्षारक; क्षारापकर्षक; क्षार या क्षारीयता का प्रतिकार करने वाला पदार्थ

**Antaphrodisiac.** An agent that diminishes sexual desire. रतिदमनकारी; कामनाशक; सम्भोग की उत्तेजना को शान्त करने वाला पदार्थ

**Antarthritic.** Remedies against gout. सन्धिशोथहर; प्रतिसन्धिशोथ; सन्धिवातनाशक

**Antasthenic.** Tending to correct debility. दुर्बलतानाशक; पौष्टिक; कमज़ोरी दूर करने वाला

**Antasthmatic.** A remedy for the relief of asthma. दमाहर; दमानाशक

**Ante-.** Perfix denoting before or in front. 'पूर्व' अथवा 'अग्र' के रूप में प्रयुक्त उपसर्ग

**Antebrachial.** Pertaining to the forearm. भुजा सम्बन्धी

**Antebrachium.** Forearm. भुजा; बांह; बाजू; कोहनी से लेकर कलाई तक का हिस्सा

**Antecebum.** See **Ante cibum.**

**Antecibos.** See **Ante cibum.**

**Ante cibum.** Before meals; antecibos; antecebum; a.c. भोजनपूर्व; भोजन से पहले

**Antedonin.** An animal pigment. पशुवर्णक; ऐंटेडोनिन

**Antefebrile.** See **Antepyretic.**

**Anteflexion.** A bending forward. अग्रकुंचन

**Antejetaculum.** Before breakfast. प्रातराशपूर्व; सुबह का नाश्ता करने से पहले

**Antelocation.** Anterior displacement of an organ. अग्रच्युति

**Antemeridiem.** Before noon; A.M. पूर्वाह्न

**Antemortem.** Before death; opposite of postmortem. मृत्युपूर्व; मरणपूर्व; मृत्यु से पहले

**Antenatal.** Before birth (6th to 9th month of pregnancy); before delivery; antepartal; antepartum. प्रसवपूर्व; प्रसव से पहले

**Antepartal.** See **Antenatal.**

**Antepartum.** See **Antenatal.**

**Antephialtic.** Preventing nightmare. भीतिहर; आतंकहर; भयनाशक

**Anteprandium.** Before dinner; opposite of postprandial. व्यालूपूर्व; निशाहारपूर्व; रात के भोजन से पहले

**Antepyretic.** Prior to the development of a fever; antefebrile. ज्वरपूर्व;

बुखार आने से पहले

**Anterior.** Situated before or in front of. अग्र; अग्रवर्ती; अग्रस्थ; आगे या सामने

**Antero-.** Prefix denoting anterior. 'अग्र' के रूप में प्रयुक्त होने वाला उपसर्ग

**Anterograde.** Proceeding forward. अग्रगामी; आगे की ओर फैला हुआ

**Anterointernal.** Situated in front, to the inner side. अग्रान्तरीय

**Anterolateral.** In front and to the side. अग्रपार्श्विक

**Anteromedian.** In front and to the middle. अग्रमध्य; अग्रमध्यस्थ

**Anteroposterior.** From before backward. अग्रपश्च; अग्रपश्चस्थ

**Anterosuperior.** In front and above. अग्र-ऊर्ध्व; अग्रऊर्ध्वस्थ; अग्रोर्ध्व

**Anteversion.** A turning or bending forward. मुखावर्त्तन; प्रतिवर्त्तन; अग्रनति; अग्रनमन

**Anteverted.** Turned or bent forward. अग्रनत; आगे की ओर झुका हुआ

**Anthaemorrhagic.** See **Antihemorrhagic**.

**Anthelminthic.** See **Anthelmintic**.

**Anthelmintic.** Vermifuge, antidote for worms; anthelminthic; vermifugal; helminthagogue; helminthic. कृमिनाशक; कृमिहर; कृमिघ्न; कीड़े नष्ट करने वाला पदार्थ

**Anther.** The male sexual organ in plants. परागपिटक; परागकोश

**Anthoma.** Fatty enlargement of skin. वसीय त्वग्बृद्धि; चर्बी बढ़ना

**Anthomania.** A morbid desire for flowers. पुष्पोन्माद

**Anthony's Fire, St.** A popular name for erysipelas. विसर्प

**Anthophobia.** A morbid fear of flowers. पुष्पभीति; पुष्पातंक; फूलों से भय

**Anthracaemia.** Anthrax septicaemia. छिद्राबुर्दीय विषरक्तता; asphyxia. श्वासावरोध; श्वासरोध; दम घुटना

**Anthracia.** Disease marked with formation of carbuncle and produced by **Bacillus Anthracis**; anthrax. छिद्राबुर्द; आंगारव्रण; नासूर; दुर्दम पूयस्फोटिका

**Anthracic.** Relating to anthracia or anthrax. आंगारव्रण सम्बन्धी

**Anthracoid.** Resembling anthrax. छिद्राबुर्दाभ; आंगारव्रणाभ; नासूर जैसा

**Anthracosis.** Black pigmentation of lungs due to inhalation of carbon particles. फुप्फुसकालिमा; फेफड़ों का काला पड़ना; carbuncular disease. छिद्राबुर्दता

**Anthrax.** See **Anthracia**.

**Anthropogeny.** The science of the origin of the man. मानवोत्पत्तिविज्ञान; नृमूलविज्ञान; मानवविकासविज्ञान

**Anthropoid.** Resembling a man. नराभ; नृवत्; नृसदृश; मानवाकार; मानव-सदृश; मानव-कल्प

**Anthropologist.** One versed in anthropology. नृविज्ञानी; मानवविज्ञानी

**Anthropology.** The science of man. नृविज्ञान; मानवविज्ञान

**Anthropometer.** An instrument for measuring body. नृमापी; मानवदेहमापी (यंत्र)

**Anthropometric.** Relating to anthropometry. नृमितिक; मानवदेहमिति सम्बन्धी;

A. Instrument, anthropometer. नृमापी; मानवदेहमापी (यंत्र)

**Anthropometry.** The measurement of the human body. नृमिति; मानवदेहमिति; मानवमिति

**Anthropomorphous.** Shaped like a man. नृरूपी; नररूपी

**Anthropophagia.** See **Anthropophagy.**

**Anthropophagy.** Cannibalism; the eating of human flesh. नृमांसभक्षण; नरमांसभक्षण; मनुष्यों का मांस खाना

**Anthropophobia.** Fear of society. मानवभीति; मानव समाज से भय

**Anthroposomatology.** The science of human structure. मानवशरीररचनाविज्ञान; मानवकायसमष्टिविज्ञान

**Anthropotomy.** Human anatomy. मानवशरीररचना (विज्ञान)

**Anthydropic.** Correcting dropsy; antihydropic. जलशोथनिवारक

**Anthypnotic.** Preventing sleep. निद्रारोधक; अनिद्राकारी; निद्रानिवारक; निद्रानाशक

**Anthysteric.** Correcting hysteria. वातोन्मादनिवारक; गुल्मवायुनिवारक

**Anti-.** Prefix meaning against or counteracting. 'रोधक', 'प्रति' अथवा 'रोधी' के अर्थ में प्रयुक्त होने वाला उपसर्ग

**Antiabortifacient.** Preventing abortion. गर्भपातरोधक

**Antiacid.** See **Antacid.**

**Antiacrid.** See **Antacrid.**

**Antiades.** The tonsils. गलतुण्डिकायें; टांसिल्स

**Antiadhesive.** Arresting adhesion. प्रत्यासंजी; चिपकाव रोकने वाला

**Antiaditis.** Tonsillitis. गलतुण्डिकाशोथ; तालुमूल प्रदाह

**Antiallergic.** Preventing or lessening allergy. प्रत्यूर्जतारोधक; प्रत्यूर्जतानाशक

**Antianabolic.** Preventing the synthesis of the body protein. प्रतिचयी

**Antianaphylaxis.** Desensitization. प्रतितीव्रग्राहिता

**Antianaemic.** See **Antianemic.**

**Antianemic.** An agent used to prevent haemorrhage, as Vitamin 'K'; antianaemic. प्रतिअरक्ततकारी; अरक्ततारोधी; रक्ताल्पतारोधी; प्रतिरक्ताल्प

**Antiantibody.** Antibody specific for another antibody. प्रतिप्रतिपिण्ड

**Antiantitoxin.** An antiantibody that inhibits or counteracts the effects of an antitoxin. प्रतिप्रतिविष

**Antiapoplectic.** Correcting apoplexy. रक्ताघातनिरोधी

**Antiarthritic.** A remedy against gout. प्रतिवातौषधि; वातनिरोधक औषधि

**Antibacterial.** Arresting the development of a bacteria. प्रतिजीवाणुक; जीवाणुरोधी; जीवाणुनाशक

**Antibechic.** Relieving cough. कासरोधक; कफशामक; कफ अथवा खाँसी से मुक्ति दिलाने वाला

**Antiberi-beri.** Against beri-beri. बेरी-बेरीरोधक

**Antibilious.** Curative of bilious complaints. पित्तदोषनिवारक

**Antibiosis.** An association between organism which is harmful to one of them. प्रतिजीविता; प्रतिजैवी

**Antibiotics.** Antibacterial substances derived from fungi and bacteria, exemplified by penicillin. प्रतिजीवी; प्रतिजैविक पदार्थ

**Antiblemorrhagic.** Preventing gonorrhoea. सूजाकनाशक; सूजाकरोधी; सूजाक रोकने वाली

**Antibodies.** Plural of **Antibody.**

**Antibody.** Specific substance produced in the blood as a reaction to an antigen. प्रतिपिण्ड; प्रतिरक्षी; प्रतिविष; रोगप्रतिकारक

**Antibrachium.** The forearm. भुजा; बाजू; बाँह; प्रकोष्ठ; अग्रबाहु

**Anticalculus.** Relieving calculus. प्रतिअश्मरी; अश्मरीनिवारक

**Anticardium.** The epigastrium; the pit of the stomach. उदरगर्त

**Anticholerin.** A substance obtained from the cultures of cholera bacillus and used in the treatment of cholera. विसूचिकाणुनाशक; हैजा फैलाने वाले जीवाणुओं को नष्ट करने वाला

**Anticholerine.** The same as **Anticholerin.**

**Anticholinergic.** Antagonistic to the action of parasympathetic or other cholinergic nerve fibres. कोलीनधर्मरोधी

**Anticlinal.** Sloping in opposite direction. अपमत; अपनत; उल्टी दिशा में तिरछा या झुका हुआ

# Anticoagulant

**Anticoagulant.** An agent which prevents or retards clotting of blood. प्रतिस्कन्दी; स्कन्दनरोधी; थक्कारोधी; खून में बनने वाले थक्कों को रोकने वाला

**Anticomplement.** A substance which checks or opposes the action of a complement. प्रतिपूरक; प्रतिसम्पूरक; पूरक का प्रतिकार करने वाला

**Anticomplementary.** The same as **Anticomplement**.

**Anticonvulsant.** Relieving convulsions; anticonvulsive. प्रतिआक्षेपक; आक्षेपरोधी; आक्षेप से मुक्त करने वाली

**Anticonvulsive.** See **Anticonvulsant**.

**Anticus.** Anterior; in front of. अग्रवर्ती; सम्मुखस्थ; आगे की ओर

**Antidepressant.** Name given to drugs that reduce depression. प्रत्यवसादक; अवसादरोधी; अवसादरोधक (औषधि)

**Antidiabetic.** Correcting diabetes; antidiabetin. मधुमेहरोधी; मधुमेहनिवारक

**Antidiabetin.** See **Antidiabetic**.

**Antidinic.** A remedy used in vertigo. भ्रमिरोधी; चक्कर रोकने वाली औषधि

**Antidiphtherin.** A substance derived from the diphtheria bacillus, and used in diptheria; antidiphtheritic. रोहणीरोधक (औषधि); डिफ्थीरिया रोकने वाली औषधि

**Antidiphtheritic.** See **Antidipherin**.

**Antidiuresis.** See **Antidysuric**.

**Antidotal.** Relating to, or acting as an antidote. प्रतिषेधक (औषधि) सम्बन्धी या प्रतिषेधक (औषधि) जैसा कार्य करने वाली

**Antidote.** A remedy which counteracts or neutralizes the action of a poison. प्रतिषेधक; प्रतिषेधी; प्रतिकारक; प्रभावनाशक (औषधि)

**Antidysenteric.** A remedy against dysentery. आमातिसारनिवारक; आमातिसाररोधी; पेचिश रोकने वाली औषधि

**Antidysuric.** A remedy for difficulty in voiding the urine; antidiuresis. प्रतिमूत्रल; मूत्ररोधक; मूत्ररोधी

**Antieczematic.** A preventive to eczema. प्रतिछाजन; छाजनरोधी

**Antiemetic.** That which prevents vomiting. वमनरोधक; वमनरोधी; प्रतिवामक; कै रोकने वाली

**Antienzyme.** A substance neutralizing the digestive enzymes. प्रतिकिण्व; किण्वरोधी; प्रतिएन्जाइम

**Antiepileptic.** Arresting epilepsy. अपस्माररोधी; मिर्गी रोकने वाली औषधि

**Antiexpectorant.** Preventing expectoration. कफरोधी; खमीरणरोधी

**Antifat.** An agent lessening fat. प्रतिवसीय; वसानिवारक

**Antifebrile.** Any agent that allays fever. ज्वररोधी; ज्वरनाशक; बुखार रोकने वाली (औषधि)

**Antifermentative.** Arresting fermentation. किण्वनरोधी; खमीरणरोधी

**Antifibrillatory.** Preventing fibrillation. प्रतिविकम्पी

**Antifungal.** Preventing fungus. कवकरोधी; फंगसरोधी; फफूँदी की वृद्धि को रोकने वाला पदार्थ-विशेष

**Antigalactic.** An agent that diminishes the secretion of milk. दुग्धरोधक; प्रतिदुग्धस्रावक; दुग्धस्राव को कम करने या रोकने वाला पदार्थ

**Antigen.** Substance introduced in the blood to stimulate production of antibodies. प्रतिजन; प्रतिपिण्डों की उत्पत्ति करने वाला पदार्थ

**Antigenic.** Having the properties of an antigen; allergenic; immunogenic. प्रतिजनी; प्रतिजनक

**Antigenicity.** The state of being antigenic. प्रतिजनकता

**Antihaemorrhagic.** See **Antihemorrhagic**.

**Antihelix.** Semicircular ridge of the external ear, opposite the helix. प्रतिकुण्डलिका; प्रतिकर्णशष्कुली

**Antihemorrhagic.** Arresting haemorrhage; anthaemorrhagic; antihaemorrhagic. रक्तस्रावरोधक; रक्तप्रवाह को रोकने वाला पदार्थ

**Antihidrotic.** Lessening the secretion of sweat. प्रतिस्वेदी; स्वेदरोधक; स्वेदरोधी; पसीना रोकने वाली औषधि

**Antihistamines.** Drugs which suppress some of the effect of released histamin. प्रतिहिस्टामिन; हिस्टामिनरोधी

**Antihormone.** Arresting the development of a hormone. प्रतिहॉर्मोनी; हॉर्मोनरोधी; प्रतिअन्त:स्रावी (उद्दीपक)

**Antihydropic.** See **Anthydropic**.

**Antihypertensive.** Any agent which reduces high blood pressure. उच्चरक्तदाबरोधक; उच्चरक्तदाबरोधी

**Antihypnotic.** Preventing sleep. निद्राहर; निद्रारोधक; निद्रारोधी; निद्राहारी

**Antiicteric.** Relieving jaundice. कामलारोधक; कामलारोधी; पीलियारोधी

**Anticrustor.** Preventing crust formation. प्रतिप्रपटीकारक; प्रपटीरोधक; प्रपटीरोधी; पपड़ी रोकने वाला

**Antiinfective.** Any agent which prevents infection. संक्रमणरोधक; संक्रमणरोधी; प्रतिसंक्रमण

**Antiinflammatory.** Any agent which prevents inflammation. शोथरोधक; शोथरोधी; प्रदाहरोधक; प्रदाहरोधी

**Antiketogenesis.** A term applied to the lessening of acidosis through the oxidation in the body of sugars, alcohol, glycerine, and allied bodies. प्रतिकीटोनजनन; कीटोनजननरोधन

**Antiketogenic.** Pertaining to antiketogenesis. कीटोनजननरोधन अथवा प्रतिकीटोनजनन सम्बन्धी

**Antilemic.** Effective against plague. प्लेगरोधक; प्लेगरोधी

**Antileprotic.** Any agent which prevents or cures leprosy. कुष्ठरोधक; कुष्ठरोधी; कुष्ठनाशक

**Antiliming.** Arresting calcification. प्रतिकैल्सीकर; विकैल्सीकर; कैल्सीभवनरोधक; कैल्सीभवनरोधी

**Antilithic.** Preventing the formation of calculi. अश्मरीरोधक; अश्मरीरोधी; पथरीरोधी; पथरीरोधक

**Antiluetic.** Any agent which prevents or cures syphilis. उपदंशरोधक; उपदंशरोधी; उपदंशनिवारक

**Antilysin.** A substance opposed to the activity of a lysin. प्रतिसंलायक

**Antilyssic.** Curative of hydrophobia. अलर्करोधी; जलातंकरोधी

**Antimalarial.** Preventive of malaria. मलेरियारोधी; विषमज्वररोधी

**Antimetabolic.** A substance that prevents metabolism; antimetabolite. प्रतिचयापचयी; प्रतिचयापचयक; चयापचयरोधी

**Antimetabolism.** Preventing metabolism. प्रतिचयापयता; चयापचयरोध

**Antimetabolite.** See **Antimetabolic.**

**Antimiasmatic.** Curative of miasmata. विषदोषनिरोधी; विषदोषनिवारक

**Antimicrobial.** Against microbes; antimicrobic. प्रतिसूक्ष्मजीवाणुक; प्रतिसूक्ष्मजीवी; सूक्ष्मजीवनिवारक

**Antimicrobic.** See **Antimicrobial.**

**Antimitotic.** Any agent which prevents reproduction of a cell by mitosis. समसूत्रणरोधी

**Antimonial.** Relating to antimony. एण्टिमनी सम्बन्धी

**Antimonium.** See **Antimony.**

**Antimony.** A metal commonly found associated with sulphur; antimonium. सीसा; अंजन; एण्टिमनी

**Antimycotic.** Destructive of fungal organism. प्रतिकवकीय; कवकनाशी

**Antinarcotic.** Preventing sleep. प्रतिस्वापक; सुषुप्तिनिवारक; निद्राहारी

**Antinauseant.** A substance that prevents nausea. प्रत्युत्क्लेशक; मितलीरोधी; मिचली या मितली रोकने वाला पदार्थ

**Antineoplastic.** Preventing tumourous growths. अर्बुदरोधक; अर्बुदरोधी; प्रतिदुर्दमकोशिक; दुर्दम कोशिकाओं की परिपक्वता तथा प्रचुरता को रुद्ध करने वाला

**Antinephritic.** Any remedy for preventing renal inflammation. वृक्कशोथरोधक; वृक्कशोथरोधी; वृक्कशोथनाशक

**Antineuralgic.** Relieving neuralgia. तंत्रिकाशोथरोधक; तंत्रिकाशूलरोधी; तंत्रिकाशूलनाशक; स्नायुशूलनाशक

**Antineuritic.** Arresting neuritis. तंत्रिकाशोथरोधक; तंत्रिकाशोथरोधी

**Antinion.** The frontal pole of cranium. करोटिध्रुव

**Antioxidant.** Any substance which delays the process of oxydation. प्रतिउपचायक; ऑक्सीकरणरोधी

**Antiparalytic.** Relieving paralysis. पक्षाघातरोधक; पक्षाघातरोधी; लकवा रोकने वाला

**Antiparasitic.** Any agent that destroys or prevents parasites. प्रतिपरजीवी; परजीवीरोधक; परजीवीरोधी

**Antipathic.** Unlike; opposite; adverse. असम; प्रंतिकूल; विषम; विरोधी; विद्वेषी

**Antipathy.** Aversion; dislike. अरुचि; घृणा

**Antipediculotic.** Destructive of lice. यूकानाशी; यूकानाशक; जूंमार

**Antipellagra.** Curative of pellagra. पेलाग्रारोधी

**Antiperiodic.** A remedy which counteracts periodicity in a disease. सावधिकरोगरोधी; नियतकालिकरोगरोधी; नियतकालिक रोगावस्थाओं का दमन करने वाली औषधि

**Antiperistalsis.** Abnormal movement of bowels towards stomach. प्रतिपुरःसरणी; पुरःसरणरोधी; कृमिकुंचनरोधी

**Antiperistaltic.** Exhibiting or relating to peristalsis. पुरःसरण-प्रदर्शक अथवा पुरःसरण सम्बन्धी; impending or arresting pristalsis. पुरःसरणरोधी; पुरःसरणरोधक

**Antiperspirant.** Correcting perspiration. प्रतिस्वेदक; प्रतिस्वेदी; स्वेदरोधक; स्वेदरोधी

**Antiphlogistic.** Preventive of inflammation; cooling remedy. शोथरोधक; शोथरोधी; शामक औषधि

**Antiphthisic.** An agent checking phthisis. यक्ष्मारोधी

**Antipilus.** Hair destroyer. लोमनाशक; रोमनाशक; बालों को नष्ट करने वाला

**Antiprostatitis.** Inflammation of Cowper's glands. कूपरग्रंथिशोथ; कूपरग्रंथियों का प्रदाह

**Antipruritic.** Relieving itching. कण्डूरोधक; कण्डूरोधी; खाजनाशक; खुजली से मुक्त करने वाली

**Antipsoric.** Opposed to psora, or a tendency to certain form of disease, especially skin affections. कच्छुविषनिवारक; कच्छुविषरोधी

**Antiputrefactive.** Preventing putrefaction. पूतिरोधक; पूतिरोधी; पीब रोकने वाला

**Antipyretic.** Agent reducing temperature; a febrifuge. ज्वरहर; ज्वरनाशक

**Antipyrotic.** An agent curative for burns. दाहनाशक; प्रतिदाह; दाहक्षतों का विरोहण करने वाला पदार्थ

**Antirabic.** Curing hydrophobia. प्रत्यलर्की; अलर्करोधी; जलातंकरोधी

**Antirachitic.** Preventing rickets. रिक्केट्सरोधी

**Antirheumatic.** Correcting rheumatism. आमवातरोधी; आमवातनिवारक; आमवातनाशक

**Antiscorbutic.** A remedy for scurvy. शीतादनाशक; प्रतिस्कर्वी; स्कर्वीरोधी; pertaining to Vitamin C. विटामिन 'सी' सम्बन्धी

**Antisecretory.** Any agent which inhibits secretion. स्रावरोधी; स्रावरोधक

**Antisepsis.** The prevention of sepsis. पूतिरोध; पूतिरोधन; पीब रोकना

**Antiseptic.** Agent counteracting putrefaction. पूतिरोधी; पूतिरोधक; रोगाणुरोधक

**Antiserum.** A serum having the power of agglutinating and precipitating another serum. प्रतिसीरमी; सीरमरोधी

**Antisialagog.** See **Antisialagogue.**

**Antisialagogue.** A substance lessening the secretion of saliva; antisialagog; antisialic. लालास्रावरोधक; लारस्रावरोधक

**Antisialic.** See **Antisialagogue.**

**Antisocial.** Against society. असामाजिक; समाज-विरोधी

**Antispasmodic.** Remedy that relieves spasms; antispastic. उद्वेष्टरोधी; उद्वेष्टरोधक; आक्षेपहर; आक्षेपनाशक

**Antispastic.** See **Antispasmodic.**

**Antisterility.** Against fertility. प्रतिबंध्यता; बंध्यतारोधी; बंध्यतारोधक; बांझपन रोकने वाली औषधि

**Antisudoral.** Diminishing perspiration; antisudorific. स्वेदरोधी; प्रतिस्वेदी; पसीना रोकने वाला

**Antisudorific.** See **Antisudoral**

**Antisyphilitic.** Any measures taken to combat syphilis. उपदंशरोधक; उपदंशरोधी; फिरंगरोधी; उपदंशनिवारक

**Antitetanus Serum.** See **ATS**.

**Antithyroid.** Any agent used to decrease the activity of thyroid gland. प्रत्यवटु; अवटु ग्रंथि की क्रिया मंद करने वाला (तत्व)

**Antitoxic.** Opposed to poisoning. प्रतिजीवविषज

**Antitoxin.** A serum serving to neutralise a toxin. प्रतिजीवविष; जीवविषरोधक; जीवविषरोधी; विषनाशक;

**Artificial A.**, an antitoxin prepared by passing an electric current through a toxic bouillon (liquid nutritive medium). कृत्रिम प्रतिजीवविष

**Antitragus.** The process of the external ear opposite the tragus. प्रतितुंगिका

**Antitubercular.** Any measure used to prevent or cure tuberculosis; antituberculosis; antituberculotic. यक्ष्मारोधी; क्षयरोगनिवारक; क्षयनाशक

**Antituberculosis.** See **Antitubercular**.

**Antituberculotic.** See **Antitubercular**.

**Antitumor.** See **Antitumour**.

**Antitumour.** Preventing tumour; antitumor. अर्बुदरोधी

**Antitussive.** Any measure which relieves cough. कासरोधी; कासरोधक; खाँसी रोकने वाला कोई भी उपाय

**Antivenene.** A substance capable of neutralizing the snake-poison; the blood-serum of animals rendered immune to snake-poison; antivenin; antivenom. सर्पविषरोधी; प्रतिसर्पविष

**Antivenereal.** Antisyphilitic. उपदंशरोधक; उपदंशनाशक

**Antivenin.** See **Antivenene**.

**Antivenom.** See **Antivenene**.

**Antiversion.** A turning or bending forward. अग्रवर्तन; आगे की ओर मुड़ना या झुकना

**Antiviral.** Acting against viruses. प्रतिविषाणुज; वाइरसरोधी

**Antivitamin.** A substance interfering with the absorption or utilization of a vitamin. प्रतिविटामिन; विटामिननाशक

**Antizymic.** That which prevents or arrests fermentation;

**antizymotic.** प्रतिकिण्वक; खमीररोधक

**Antizymotic.** See **Antizymic.**

**Antodontalgic.** Relieving toothache. दन्तार्तिहर; दन्तशूलनाशक; दन्तवेदनाहर; दान्त के दर्द से मुक्त करने वाली (औषधि)

**Antra.** Plural of **Antrum.**

**Antral.** Pertaining to an antrum. कोटरीय; कोटर सम्बन्धी

**Antrectomy.** Excision of the pyloric antrum of stomach. जठरनिर्गमउच्छेदन; जठरनिर्गम को काट कर हटा देना; removal of the walls of an antrum. कोटर-उच्छेदन

**Antritis.** Inflammation of a cavity, as an antum. कोटरशोथ; गह्वरशोथ

**Antrostomy.** An artificial opening from nasal cavity to the antrum of the maxillary sinus. कोटरछेदन; कोटरछिद्रीकरण

**Antrotome.** Instrument for cutting open an antrum. कोटरछेदक; कोटरछिद्रक

**Antrotomy.** Incising an antrum. कोटरछेदन

**Antrotympanitis.** Chronic purulent otitis media. चिरपूतिजमध्यकर्णशोथ

**Antrum.** A cavity, especially in the bone. कोटर, खास तौर से अस्थिकोटर; कोष्ठ; गुहा; गह्वर;

**A. Highmorianum,** a cavity above the teeth in the upper jaw, often liable to inflammation and soreness; the maxillary sinus; antrum of Highmore. ऊर्ध्वदन्तकोटर; ऊपर के जबड़े का गड्ढा;

**A. of Highmore,** see **Antrum Highmorianum.**

**A. Pyloricum,** see **Pyloric Antrum.**

**Pyloric A.,** the portion of the stomach immediately in front of the pylorus; antrum pyloricum. जठरनिर्गम कोटर;

**Tympanic A.,** the cavity of mastoid bone. मध्यकर्णकोटर

**Anulus.** See **Annulus.**

**Anum.** See **Anus.**

**Anuresis.** Defective secretion of urine. विषममूत्रस्राव; असममूत्रता; पेशाब का दोषपूर्ण बहाव

**Anuretic.** Affected with anuria. मूत्राल्पग्रस्त; मूत्ररोधग्रस्त

**Anuria.** An absence or deficiency of urine. अमूत्रता; मूत्राल्पता; suppression of urine. मूत्ररोध; पेशाब दब जाना;

**Calculus A.,** suppression of urine due to renal calculus. अश्मरीजन्य मूत्ररोध

**Anuric.** Relating to anuria. मूत्ररोध अथवा मूत्राल्पता सम्बन्धी
**Anurus.** Wanting the tail. अपुच्छ; निर्पुच्छ; पुच्छविहीन; पूंछरहित
**Anus.** External opening of the rectum; anum. मलद्वार; गुद; गुदा;
    **Artificial A.**, one produced surgically in cases of obstruction through any cause. कृत्रिम गुद;
    **Imperforate A.**, one which has no opening. अछिद्री गुद
**Anvil.** The incus. शूर्मिकास्थि; निहाई के आकार की कान की हड्डी
**Anxiety.** Uneasiness; feeling of fear, apprehension and dread. अधीरता; उद्वेग; उत्सुकता; व्याकुलता; घबराहट
**Aorta.** The great artery of the body; the main arterial trunk. महाधमनी; बड़ी धमनी; बृहद्धमनी;
    **Abdominal A.**, the portion below the diaphragm. उदरमहाधमनी; मध्यच्छद का निचला भाग;
    **Ascending A.**, the first part of the arch of the aorta. आरोही महाधमनी;
    **Thoracic A.**, the part included in the thoracic cavity उरो-महाधमनी; वक्ष-महाधमनी
**Aortal.** See **Aortic.**
**Aortic.** Pertaining to the aorta; aortal. महाधमनिक; महाधमनी सम्बन्धी
**Aorticorenal.** Relating to the aorta and the kidney. महाधमनी तथा वृक्क सम्बन्धी
**Aortitis.** Inflammation of the aorta. महाधमनीशोथ; महाधमनी का प्रदाह
**Aortocoronary.** Relating to the aorta and the coronary arteries. महाधमनी तथा परिहृद्-धमनियों सम्बन्धी
**Aortogram.** See **Arteriogram.**
**Aortography.** A description of the aorta; arteriography. महाधमनीचित्रण
**Aortomalacia.** Softening of the aorta. महाधमनीमृदुता; बड़ी धमनी की कोमलता
**Aortosclerosis.** Hardening of the aorta. महाधमनीकाठिन्य; बड़ी धमनी की कठोरता
**Aortostenosis.** Narrowing of the aorta. महाधमनीसंकीर्णन; महाधमनी की सिकुड़न
**Aortotomy.** Incision of the aorta. महाधमनीछेदन
**Apanthropia.** A morbid love of solitude. एकान्तप्रियता

**Apathetic.** Insensible to emotion. विरक्त; अनासक्त; भावहीन; उदासीन; उदास

**Apathia.** Want of feeling; insensibility to mental or bodily pain; apathy. विरक्ति; अनासक्ति; उदासी; भावहीनता; उदासीनता; भावशून्यता

**Apathy.** See **Apathia.**

**Apepsia.** Imperfect or weak digestion; dyspepsia; apepsy. मंदाग्नि; अजीर्ण; बदहजमी; अग्निमांद्य; मन्द पाचन

**Apepsy.** See **Apepsia.**

**Aperient.** A mild laxative or medicine which opens the bowels gently. मृदुविरेचक; मृदुविरेचन; सारक; हल्की दस्तावर दवाई

**Aperiodic.** Not occurring periodically. अनियतकालिक; अनावधिक

**Aperistalsis.** Cessation or lack of peristalsis. अपुर:सरण; प्रकुंचन किया का अभाव

**Apertura.** An aperture or opening. द्वार; मुख; छिद्र; रन्ध्र

**Aperture.** The same as **Apertura.**

**Apex.** Summit; point; top of anything which is cone-shaped. शिखर; शिखा; शिखाग्र; शीर्ष; चोटी;

  **A.-beat,** the point of maximum impulse of the heart against the chest-wall. हृदुशिखरस्पन्द;

  **A. Murmur,** murmur heard over the apex of the heart. हृदुमर्मर

**Aphacia.** See **Aphakia.**

**Aphacic.** See **Aphakic.**

**Aphagia.** Loss of swallowing power; an inability to swallow; aphagopraxia. निगरण-अक्षमता; किसी पदार्थ को निगलने की असमर्थता

**Aphagopraxia.** See **Aphagia.**

**Aphakia.** Absence of the crystalline lens of the eye; aphacia. लेन्सहीनता

**Aphakic.** Without a crystalline lens; aphacic. लेन्सहीन

**Aphalangia.** Without phalanges. अनंगुलिता; अंगुलिहीनता; उँगलियाँ न होना

**Aphasia.** Inability to speak from a lesion in the brain. वाचाघात; स्वरलोप; अस्वरता; स्वरहानि; वाक्शक्ति का अभाव;

  **Amnesic A.,** want of memory for words; amnestic aphasia. स्मृति वाचाघात;

  **Amnestic A.,** see **Amnesic Aphasia.**

  **Ataxic A.,** inability to articulate words; motor aphasia; aphemia. गतिविभ्रमी वाचाघात;

**Motor A.**, see **Ataxic Aphasia.**

**Sensory A.**, inability to remember or understand words. संवेदी वाचाघात

**Aphasiac.** See **Aphasic.**

**Aphasic.** Resembling or affected with aphasia; aphasiac. वाचाघात सम्बन्धी; वाचाघाती; वाचाघातग्रस्त

**Aphemia.** Motor aphasia; anarthria. वाक्प्रेरणाघात; गतिविभ्रमी वाचाघात

**Aphephobia.** A morbid fear of being touched. स्पर्शभीति; स्पशार्तंक; छुए जाने का डर

**Aphonia.** Inability to use the voice except in a whisper. स्वरलोप; वाणीलोप; स्वरहानि; अस्वरता; गला बैठना; आवाज बिल्कुल बन्द हो जाना;

**A. Clericorum**, see **Clergyman's Sore-throat.**

**A. Paranoica**, stubborn silence in the insane. विक्षिप्तिज स्वरलोप

**Aphoria.** Barrenness; inability to conceive offspring; sterility of the female. बंध्यता; बांझपन; जनन-अक्षमता

**Aphose.** A subjective sensation of shadow. छायानुभूति

**Aphrasia.** Absence of speech. स्वरलोप; वाचाघात; वाणीरोध

**Aphremia.** Unconsciousness. चेतनालोप; मूर्च्छा; बेहोशी; बेसुधी

**Aphrodisia.** Lasciviousness. कामवासना; कामलोलुपता

**Aphrodisiacs.** Drugs that stimulate sexual desire. कामोत्तेजक; कामोद्रेकी; वाजीकर; सम्भोग की इच्छा बढ़ाने वाली औषधियाँ

**Aphtha.** Singular of **Aphthae.**

**Aphthae.** Roundish, whitish vesicles found in the sore mouth; thrush. मुखव्रण; मुखक्षत; छाले

**Aphthoid.** Resembling aphthae. मुखव्रणाभ; मुखक्षताभ

**Aphthosis.** Any condition characterized by the presence of aphthae. मुखव्रणता; मुखक्षतता

**Aphthous.** Belonging to, or complicated with aphthae. मुखक्षतीय; छालेयुक्त; छालों वाला

**Apical.** Pertaining to the apex. शिखरीय; शिखाग्रीय; शिखर सम्बन्धी

**Apicectomy.** Excision of the apex or root-end of a tooth; apicoectomy. शिखरछेदन; दन्तान्तछेदन

**Apices.** Plural of **Apex.**

**Apicitis.** Inflammation of the apex of a structure or organ. शिखरशोथ

**Apicoectomy.** See **Apicectomy.**

**Aplacental. **Without a placenta. अपराहीन; गर्भनालहीन

**Aplasia. **Incomplete development of a tissue. अविकास; विकासरोध; अविकसन

**Aplastic. **Having no definite structure or form; not plastic. अविकासी; अविकसित;

**A. Anaemia, **the result of complete bone-marrow failure. अविकासी अरक्तता;

**A. Lymph, **non-fibrinous lymph. अविकासी लसीका

**Apnea. **A condition wherein the respiratory movements cease for a brief period; apnia; apnoea. श्वासरोध; अश्वसन

**Apneic. **Relating to, or suffering form apnea; apnoeic. श्वासरोध सम्बन्धी अथवा श्वासरोधक

**Apneumia. **Congenital absence of the lungs. सहजफुफ्फुसहीनता; फेफड़ों का जन्मजात अभाव

**Apnia. **See **Apnea.**

**Apnoea. **See **Apnea.**

**Apocenosis. **A discharge; evacuation of stomach contents. स्राव; मलस्राव

**Apochromatic. **Colourless. अवर्णी; वर्णहीन; रंगहीन

**Apocrine. **The modified sweat glands, especially in axillae, genitals and perineal regions. शिखरस्रावी (स्वेद ग्रन्थियाँ)

**Apocynum Cannabinum. **Canadian hemp, the root is emetic and cathartic. कनाडा में पैदा होने वाली हशीश

**Apodal. **Denoting apodia; apodous. पादहीन

**Apodia. **Congenital absence of the feet; apody. सहजअपादता; सहजपादहीनता; पैरों का जन्मजात अभाव

**Apodous. **See **Apodal.**

**Apods. **The footless animals and fishes having no ventral fins. पादहीन; बिना पैर वाले जन्तु तथा मछलियाँ

**Apody. **See **Apodia.**

**Apolar. **Having no pole. ध्रुवहीन; अध्रुवी

**Aponeuroses. **Plural of **Aponeurosis.**

**Aponeurosis. **Fibrous expansion of a tendon. कण्डरातन्तुप्रसार; कण्डराकला के तन्तुओं का फैलाव; कण्डराकला

**Aponeurositis. **Inflammation of an aponeurosis. कण्डराकलाशोथ; कण्डराकला का प्रदाह

**Aponeurotic.** Pertaining to an aponeurosis. कण्डराकला सम्बन्धी
**Aponeurotica Epicranialis.** Epicranial aponeuorosis. अधिकरोटितन्तुप्रसार; अधिकरोटि-कण्डराकला
**Aponeurotica Palatina.** Palatine aponeurosis. तालु-कण्डराकला
**Aponeurotica Plantaris.** Plantar aponeurosis. पदतल-कण्डराकला
**Aponeurotome.** A knife for dividing aponeurosis. कण्डराकलाविभाजक
**Aponeurotomy.** A division of an aponeurosis. कण्डराकलाविभाजन
**Apophraxis.** Amenorrhoea. अनार्तव; ऋतुरोध
**Apophyseal.** Pertaining to an apophysis; apophysial. अस्थिविवर्धन सम्बन्धी; हड्डी बढ़ने सम्बन्धी
**Apophysial.** See **Apophyseal.**
**Apophysis.** An outgrowth or protuberance of bone. विवर्ध; अस्थिविवर्धन; हड्डी बढ़ना
**Apophysitis.** Inflammation of an outgrowth. विवर्धशोथ
**Apoplectic.** One affected with apoplexy. अपसन्यासग्रस्त; रक्ताघातग्रस्त; रक्तमूच्छोग्रस्त; belonging to apoplexy. अपसन्यास, रक्तमूच्छों अथवा रक्ताघात सम्बन्धी
**Apoplectiform.** Of the form of, or resembling apoplexy; apoplectoid. रक्ताघातरूप; रक्ताघातरूपी; अपसन्यासरूपी; अपसन्यासरूप
**Apoplectoid.** See **Apoplectiform.**
**Apoplexia.** Apoplexy. अपसन्यास; रक्ताघात; रक्तमूच्छी; मिर्गी;
  **A. Uteri,** a sudden uterine haemorrhage. गर्भाशयिक रक्ताघात
**Apoplexy.** Sudden rupture of blood vessels in the brain with paralysis and unconsciousness; apoplexia. अपसन्यास; रक्ताघात; रक्तमूच्छी; मिर्गी
**Aporia.** Restlessness caused due to the stoppage of any of the natural secretions; apory. स्रावरोधज व्यग्रता; शरीर के प्राकृतिक स्रावों की रुकावट के कारण होने वाली बेचैनी
**Apory.** See **Aporia.**
**Aposia.** An absence of thirst. तृषाभाव; तृष्णाभाव; प्यास का अभाव
**Apostasis.** An abscess. विद्रधि; फोड़ा; a bony exfoliation. अस्थिसंयोजनाभाव; टूटी हुई हड्डी का न जुड़ना
**Apostaxis.** A slight haemorrhage or bleeding. रक्तस्राव
**Apostema.** An abscess. विद्रधि; फोड़ा
**Aposthia.** Congenital absence of the prepuce. सहजशिश्नमुण्डच्छदाभाव

**Apothica.** An apothecary's shop. औषध-भण्डार; दवाइयों की दुकान

**Apothecary.** One who keeps a store of drugs; druggist. औषधि-विक्रेता; दवा बेचने वाला

**Apparatus.** Instrument for performing a common purpose in medical profession. यंत्र; उपकरण

**Appendage.** That which is attached to an organ as a part of it. उपांग; अवयव; अनुबन्ध; शाखा

**Appendectomy.** Excision of the vermiform appendix; appendicectomy. उपांत्र-उच्छेदन; उण्डुकपुच्छ-उच्छेदन; उण्डुकोच्छेदन; उण्डुकपुच्छोछेदन; अनुबन्धनलिका का उच्छेदन

**Appendical.** See **Appendiceal.**

**Appendiceal.** Relating to an appendix; appendical. उपांत्र सम्बन्धी उपांगीय; उण्डुकीय; उण्डुकपुच्छीय: उपांत्रीय

**Appendicectomy.** See **Appendectomy.**

**Appendices.** Plural of **Appendix.**

**Appendices Epiploicae.** Little masses of fatty tissue, covered with peritoneum, projecting from the large intestine. बृहद्वपा-अनुबन्ध; बृहत्वपानुबन्ध

**Appendicitis.** Inflammation of the appendix. उपांत्रशोथ; उण्डुकपुच्छशोथ; उपांत्र-प्रदाह;

**A. Obliterans,** that obliterating the lumen of appendix. अवलोपक उण्डुकपुच्छशोथ

**Appendicolysis.** Surgical freeing of the appendix from adhesion. उपांत्रलयन; उण्डुकपुच्छलयन

**Appendicosis.** Appendicitis without fever, but with dull pain, local soreness and continuous uneasiness. अज्वर-उपांत्रशोथ; सकष्ट-उपांत्रशोथ

**Appendicostomy.** Incision of the appendix vermiformis for the purpose of irrigating the colon. उण्डुकपुच्छछेदन; उण्डुकपुच्छछिद्रीकरण; उपांत्रछेदन

**Appendicula.** A small appendage. क्षुद्र-उपांग

**Appendicular.** Pertaining to an appendix. उपांगीय; उण्डुकीय; उण्डुकपुच्छीय; उपांत्रीय; उपांत्र सम्बन्धी;

**A. Skeleton,** the arms and hands, legs and feet, shoulders and pelvic bones. उपांगास्थियाँ, जैसे बाहों तथा हाथों की, टांगों तथा पैरों की,

कन्धे की तथा गोणिका की हड्डियाँ

**Appendix.** An appendage; a part attached to an organ. उपांत्र; उण्डुक; उण्डुकपुच्छ; पुच्छ; उपांग;
  **Vermiform A.**, the worm-shaped process of the caecum. उण्डुकपुच्छ; उपांत्र;
  **A. Vermiformis,** the same as **Vermiform Appendix.**

**Apperception.** Clear perception of a sensory stimulus; comprehension. अभिबोध

**Apperceptive.** Capable of apperception. बोधगम्य; relating to apperception. अभिबोध सम्बन्धी

**Appetite.** A desire for food. क्षुधा; बुभुक्षा; भूख; lust. वासना; हवस

**Appetizer.** That which promotes appetite. क्षुधावर्धक

**Applicator.** An instrument for supplying medicines to a part. साधित्र; किसी भाग में दवाई लगाने के लिये प्रयुक्त किया जाने वाला यंत्र; एप्लिकेटर

**Apposition.** The act of fitting together. सन्निधान; पार्श्वस्थापन

**Apprehension.** Grasping of ideas. बोध; ज्ञान; ग्रहण; anxiety. अधीरता; fear. भय; आतंक; डर

**Apprehensive.** Anxious or fearful for future. अधीर; आतंकित; भविष्य के प्रति चिन्तातुर

**Approach.** Access; to come, near to. अभिगम; पहुँच

**Approximation.** Bringing together. सन्निकटन

**Apractic.** See **Apraxic.**

**Apraxia.** Loss of understanding for the uses of things. चेष्टा-अक्षमता; mind-blindness. मनःशक्तिक्षय

**Apraxic.** Marked by, or pertaining to apraxia; apractic. मनःशक्तिक्षयग्रस्त अथवा मनःशक्तिक्षय सम्बन्धी

**Aproctia.** Absence of the anus. गुदाभाव; गुदाहीनता; मलद्वार का अभाव

**Aprosexia.** An inability to fix attention. एकाग्रहीनता; विचार-अक्षमता; मन को एकाग्र करने की अयोग्यता

**Apsychia.** A loss of consciousness. निश्चेतना; चेतनालोप

**Aptitude.** Natural ability and facility in performing tasks, either mental or physical. औचित्य; प्रवणता; रुझान

**Aptyalia.** Lack of saliva; aptyalism; asialism. लालाभाव; लार न बनना

**Aptyalism.** See **Aptyalia.**

**Apyous.** Having no pus. पूयाभाव; पूतिहीनता; अपूतित; पीबरहित

# Apyretic

**Apyretic.** Having no fever. अज्वर; ज्वरहीन; निर्ज्वर

**Apyrexia.** A non-febrile state. अज्वर; ज्वर-विरामकाल; ज्वराभाव

**Aqua.** Water. जल; द्रव्य; पानी;

    A. **Bulientis,** the boiled water. उबला पानी;

    A. **Calcis,** the lime water. चूने का पानी;

    A. **Communis,** the common water. साधारण जल;

    A. **Distillata,** the distilled water. आस्रुत जल;

    A. **Fervens,** hot water. उष्ण जल; गर्म पानी;

    A. **Fontana,** the fountain water. झरने का पानी;

    A. **Fortis,** weak and impure nitric acid. अशक्त एवं अशुद्ध नाइट्रिक एसिड;

    A. **Gelide,** cold water. शीतल जल; ठण्डा पानी;

    A. **Nivialis,** ice water. हिमजल; बरफ का पानी;

    A. **Phobia,** hydrophobia; fear of water. जलातंक; जलभीति;

    A. **Oculi,** the aqueous humour. नेत्रोद;

    A. **Pluvialis,** the rain water. वर्षा जल; बारिश का पानी;

    A. **Potabilis,** the drinking water. पेयजल;

    A. **Pura,** pure water. शुद्ध जल; साफ पानी;

    A. **Putei,** well-water. कूप जल; कुएं का पानी;

    A. **Rosoe,** rose water. गुलाब जल;

    A. **Tepidae,** lukewarm or tepid water. कोसा या हल्का गर्म पानी;

**Aquacapsulitis.** See **Aquocapsulitis.**

**Aquaeduct.** See **Aquaeductus.**

**Aquaeductus.** A canal; aqueduct; aqueductus. कुल्या; नलिका; कृत्रिम जल-प्रणाल;

    A. **Cerebri,** the infundibulum. प्रमस्तिष्क कुल्या

**Aqueductus.** See **Aquaeductus.**

**Aqueous.** Watery. जलाभ; जलीय; पानी जैसा; pertaining to, or containing water. जल सम्बन्धी या जलयुक्त;

    A. **Humour,** the fluid in the anterior chamber of the eye. नेत्रोद; चक्षुजल; जलीय द्रव्य

**Aquocapsulitis.** Serous iritis; aquacapsulitis. सीरमीपरितारिकाशोथ

**Arachis.** Oil expressed from groundnuts. मूंगफली का तेल

**Arachnitis.** Inflammation of the arachnoid membrane.

जालतानिकाशोथ; जालतानिका का प्रदाह

**Arachnodactylia.** Congenital abnormality resulting in spider fingers; arachnodactyly. लूतांगुलिता; दीर्घांगुलिता; दुबली-पतली लम्बी उँगलियों का होना

**Arachnodactyly.** See **Arachnodactylia.**

**Arachnoid.** Resembling a web. जालतानिकाभ; मस्तिष्कावरक झिल्ली, जो मकड़ी के जाल जैसी होती है;

   A. **Cavity,** the space between the arachnoid and dura-mater. जालतानिका-गह्वर;

   A. **Membrane,** the serous membrane of the brain and cord; arachnoidea; arachnoides. जालतानिका-कला; मस्तिष्क-आवरक झिल्ली

**Arachnoidea.** See **Arachnoid Membrane.**

**Arachnoides.** See **Arachnoid Membrane.**

**Arachnoiditis.** Inflammation of the arachnoid membrane. जालतानिकाशोथ; मस्तिष्क-आवरक झिल्ली का प्रदाह

**Aran-Duchenne's Disease.** Progressive muscular atrophy. क्रमिक पेशीशोष

**Arbor Vitae.** The tree-like figure in a section of the cerebellum. शाखिरूपता; वलन; वृक्षोपम अर्थात् वृक्ष जैसी रेखायें, जो प्रमस्तिष्क के मध्यस्थ-काट में दिखाई देती हैं

**Arboresens.** See **Arborescent.**

**Arborescent.** Dendriform; arborescens. प्रशाखी

**Arc.** See **Arch.**

**Arcade.** Arch. चाप; तोरणिका; महराब; वलय; वृत्तांश

**Arch.** A term applied to various curved portions of the body; arc. चाप; वलय; तोरणिका; महराब;

   **Acromio-thoracic A.,** the lower boundary of the front of the thorax. अंसकूट-उरश्चाप;

   **Alveolar A.,** that marking the outlines of the alveolar process of the jaw. दन्तउलूखल चाप;

   **Aortic A.,** one of the vascular arches accompanying the branchial arches. महाधमनी चाप;

   **Branchial A.,** one of the five columns of tissue bordering the gill-clefts; visceral arch. आद्यग्रसनी चाप; गिल चाप;

   **Dental A.,** the curves formed by the cutting-edges of the teeth. दन्त चाप;

**Hyoid A.**, the second branchial arch of the vertebra. कण्ठिका चाप;

**Mandibular A.**, the first branchial arch, developing into the lower jaw. अधोहनुचाप;

**Neural A.**, the superior loop of the typical vertebra. तंत्रिका चाप;

**Palatal A.**, the palatine arch. तालु चाप:

**Palmar A.**, the arch formed by the radial and ulnar arteries in the palm of the hand. करतल चाप;

**Plantar A.**, that made by the external plantar and a branch of the dorsal artery of the foot. पदतल चाप;

**Pharyngeal A.**, the fifth pair of the branchial arches. ग्रसनी चाप;

**Vertebral A.**, the part of the vertebra, formed by two pedicles and two laminas, bounding the spiral foramen dorsally. कशेरुका चाप;

**Visceral A.**, see **Branchial Arch**.

**Zygomatic A.**, that formed by the malar and temporal bones. गण्ड चाप

**Arched.** See **Arcuate**.

**Archenteron.** The cavity formed by the invagination of the blastodermic vesicles. आद्य-आंत्र

**Archeocyte.** A wandering cell. चलकोशिका; भ्रमणकारी कोशिका

**Archetype.** A standard type. आद्य-प्ररूप

**Archipallium.** The rhinencephalon. आद्य-प्रमस्तिष्क प्रावारक

**Architis.** Inflammation of the rectum. मलांत्रशोथ; मलाशय-प्रदाह

**Archnitis.** Inflammation of the brain. मस्तिष्कशोथ; मस्तिष्क-प्रदाह

**Archocele.** Hernia of the rectum. मलांत्र-हर्निया

**Archoptosis.** Prolapse of the rectum. मलाशयभ्रंश; मलांत्रभ्रंश

**Archorrhagia.** Rectal haemorrhage; archorrhea; archorrhoea. मलांत्रजरक्तस्राव

**Archorrhea.** See **Archorrhagia**.

**Archorrhoea.** See **Archorrhagia**.

**Archostenosis.** Rectal constriction. मलाशय-संकीर्णता

**Archosyrin.** Fistula in ano. भगंदर; गुदानालव्रण

**Arciform.** See **Arcuate**.

**Arcin.** Bow-shaped. धनुषाकार

**Arctation.** A narrowing, stricture or constriction. संकीर्णन; सिकुड़न

**Arcuate.** Bent like an arch; arched; arciform. चापाकार; चापी; धनुषाकार; तोरणिका; बक्र; टेढ़ा

**Arcuation.** A bending or curvature. बक्रता; टेढ़ापन

**Arcus.** Arc; arch. चाप; तोरण; धनुषोपम;

   **A. Adiposus,** see **Arcus Senilis.**

   **A. Aortae,** the arch of the aorta. महाधमनी चाप;

   **A. Arteriosus Manus,** the palmar arch. करतल चाप;

   **A. Arteriosus Pedis,** the plantar arch. पदतल चाप;

   **A. Atlantis,** the arch of the atlas. शीर्षधर चाप;

   **A. Corneae,** see **Arcus Senilis.**

   **A. Dentalis,** the dental arch. दन्त चाप;

   **A. Faucicum,** the palatine arch. तालु चाप;

   **A. Juvenilis,** a white ring around the cornea occurring in young individuals and resembling arcus senilis. तारुण्य चाप;

   **A. Palmaris,** the palmar arch; arcus volaris. करतल चाप;

   **A. Senilis,** an opaque ring round the edge of the cornea, seen in old people; arcus adiposus; arcus corneae. जराश्वेतपटल कला;

   **A. Subpubicus,** the pubic arch. जघन चाप;

   **A. Tarseus,** the tarsal arch. गुल्फ चाप;

   **A. Vertebralis,** a vertebral arch. कशेरुका चाप;

   **A. Volaris,** see **Arcus Palmaris.**

   **A. Zygomaticus,** the zygomatic arch. गण्ड चाप

**Ardent.** Burning. ज्वलनकारी; दाहक; feverish. सज्वर; ज्वरवत्; hot. तप्त; गरम; गर्म;

   **A. Spirits,** alcoholic liquors. मदिरा; शराब

**Ardor.** Violent heat; burning. प्रचण्ड ताप; जलन;

   **A. Urinae,** burning urination. ज्वलनकारी मूत्रण

**Area.** Any space with boundaries. क्षेत्र; क्षेत्रफल; स्थल; सीमित स्थल;

   **Auditory A.,** the receptive centre for audition; area acoustica. श्रवण क्षेत्र;

   **Embryonic A.,** the germinating spot of an embryo; area germinativa. भ्रूण क्षेत्र;

   **Frontal A.,** See **Area Facialis.**

   **Motor A.,** the emissive centre for voluntary motion in the precentral convolution. प्रेरक क्षेत्र;

**Occipital A.**, the portion of the brain beneath the occipital bone. पश्चकपाल क्षेत्र;

**Sensorial A.**, see **Sensory Area.**

**Sensory A.**, the general area of the cerebral cortex in which sensation is perceived; sensorial area. संवेदी क्षेत्र;

**Silent A.**, any area of the cerebral or cerebellar surface, lesion of which occasions no definite sensory or motor symptoms. शान्त क्षेत्र;

**Visual A.**, the area of the cortex cerebri. दृष्टि क्षेत्र;

**A. Acoustica**, see **Auditory Area.**

**A. Facialis**, facial or frontal nerve area; frontal area. आननतंत्रिका क्षेत्र; ललाट क्षेत्र;

**A. Germinativa**, see **Embryonic Area.**

**Arefaction.** Dessication; the act of drying. शुष्कीकरण; सुखाना

**Areflexia.** Without any reflex. अप्रतिवर्तता; परावर्तित क्रियाविहीन

**Arenation.** A sand-bath. मरुस्नान; बालुकास्नान

**Arenoid.** Sand-like. बालुसम; बालुसदृश; रेतसम; रेत जैसा

**Areola.** The pigmented area around the nipple of the breast. वृन्त; परिवेश; मण्डल; चक्कर;

**Secondary A.**, see **Areola Mammae.**

**A. Mammae**, a dark circle of pigmentation which surrounds the primary areola in pregnancy; secondary areola. स्तन परिवेश

**Areolar.** Pertaining to, or resembling areola. परिवेशीय; मण्डलीय; सछिद्र; वृन्तवत्;

**A. Tissue**, connective or cellular tissue. संयोजक ऊतक; कोशिका ऊतक

**Areometer.** An instrument for measuring the specific gravity of fluids. द्रवघनत्वमापी

**Areotic.** Medicine promoting perspiration. स्वेदकारी; स्वेदकारक; पसीना लाने वाली दवाई

**A.R.F.** Acute respiratiory failure. तीव्र श्वासरोध

**Argentum.** The silver, a metallic element. रजत; चांदी

**A. Metallicum**, the same as **Argentum.**

**Argyll Robertson Pupil.** Loss of the pupil reflex to light, found in the brain diseases. चक्षुपटलास्थिरता; चक्षुपटलों की अस्थिरता, जो मस्तिष्क

रोगों में पाई जाती है

**Argyria.** Cutaneous staining or discolouration from the continuous use of silver; argyrosis. रजतमयता; चर्मविवर्णता

**Argyrosis.** See **Argyria.**

**Arhinia.** Congenital absence of the nose. सहजनासिकाभाव; नाक का जन्मजात अभाव

**Arhythmia.** See **Arrhythmia.**

**Arhythmic.** See **Arrhythmic.**

**Arithmomania.** A form of insanity in which there is an obsession with number. अंकोन्माद

**Arm.** Upper limb of human body from shoulder to hand. बाहु; भुजा; भुज; बाँह; आस्तीन; कंधे से कलाई तक का भाग

**Armamentarium.** A doctor's outfit of medicines or instruments; armarium; therapeutic armamentarium. चिकित्सीय साधन; उपचारक साधन

**Armarium.** See **Armamentarium.**

**Armilla.** The annular ligament of the wrist. मणिबन्ध; कलाई अथवा बाजूबन्द

**Arnica.** A genus of herbs. आर्निका

**Aroma.** Fragrance. वास; सुवास; गन्ध

**Aromatic.** Fragrant. सुगन्धित; spicy. मसालेदार

**Arrest.** Stoppage; detention. संरोध; रोध; नियंत्रण; नियंत्रित करना;

Cardiac A., a loss of cardiac action. हृद्संरोध;

Epiphyseal A., early and premature fusion between epiphysis and diaphysis. अधिवर्ध रोध

**Arrested.** Checked. संरोधित; नियंत्रित

**Arrhenoblastoma.** A masculinizing tumour of the ovary. पुंसकारी-अर्बुद

**Arrhythmia.** An irregularity of rhythm; arhythmia. अतालता; वितालता;

Cardiac A., an irregularity of the heart's action. हृद्-अतालता

**Arrhythmic.** Without rhythm; arhythmic. अतालता सम्बन्धी

**Arrowroot.** A genus of plant. अराऊट

**Arseniasis.** Poisoning by arsenic; arsenicism. संखिया-विषण्णता

**Arsenic.** A chemical element of greyish white colour; arsenicum. संखिया; श्वेतमल्ल; आर्सेनिक

# Arsenical

**Arsenical.** Belonging to arsenic. श्वेतमल्लीय; संखिया सम्बन्धी

**Arsenicate.** To combine with arsenic. श्वेतमल्लमिश्रित; श्वेतमल्लयुक्त; आर्सेनिकयुक्त

**Arsenicism.** See **Arseniasis.**

**Artefact.** A structure in the cell or tissue brought about by death or use of reagents; artefect; artifact. कृतक; कृत्रिम आकृति; शिल्प-तथ्य

**Artefect.** See **artefact.**

**Artemisia.** A genus of plants. नागदाना; नागदमन

**Arteralgia.** Pain in the artery. धमन्यार्ति; धमनीशूल

**Arterectomy.** See **Arteriectomy.**

**Arteria.** Artery. धमनी; the bronchial tube. श्वासनली

**Arteriae.** Plural of **Arteria.**

**Arteriagra.** Neuralgia of an artery. धमनी-तंत्रिकार्ति

**Arterial.** Pertaining to an artery. धमनीपरक; धमनी सम्बन्धी

**Arteriectomy.** Excision of an artery or more usually part of an artery; arterectomy. धमनी-उच्छेदन; किसी धमनी या उसके किसी भाग को काट कर हटा देना

**Arterioatony.** A relaxed state of the arterial walls. धमनी-अतानता

**Arteriogram.** Film demonstrating arteries after injection of opaque medium; aortogram. धमनीलेख; धमनीचित्र

**Arteriography.** A description of the arteries. धमनीचित्रण

**Arteriola.** See **Arteriole.**

**Arteriolar.** Pertaining to an arteriole. धमनीपरक; धमनिकापरक; धमनिका सम्बन्धी

**Arteriole.** A small artery; arteriola. धमनिका; लघु-धमनी

**Arteriolitis.** Inflammation of an arteriole. धमनिकाशोथ; धमनिका-प्रदाह

**Arteriology.** The science of the arteries. धमनीविज्ञान

**Arteriomalacia.** Abnormal softness of the arterial coats. धमनीअस्तरमृदुता

**Arteriomotor.** Causing changes in the calibre of an artery. धमनीप्रेरक

**Arterionecrosis.** Necrosis of an artery. धमनीपरिगलन; धमनिकाक्षय

**Arteriopathy.** Any disease of the arteries. धमनीविकृति; धमनियों का कोई रोग

**Arterioplasty.** Plastic surgery applied to an artery. धमनीसंधान

**Arterioportal.** Relating to an artery and the portal vein. धमनी तथा प्रतिहारिशिरा सम्बन्धी

**Ateriorrhaphy.** A plastic procedure on an artery. धमनीसीवन; धमनिकासीवन

**Arteriosclerosis.** Thickening of the coats of the arteries promoting blood pressure. धमनीकाठिन्य; धमनी-प्राचीर की कठोरता;

   **Cerebral A.**, a syndrome which may include a shuffling gait, tendency to lean backward, muscular rigidity, loss of memory, mental confusion and incontinence. प्रमस्तिष्क धमनीकाठिन्य;

   **Senile A.**, arteriosclerosis, as a result of advanced age. जराधमनीकाठिन्य

**Arteriosclerotic.** Relating to arteriosclerosis. धमनीकाठिन्यज; धमनीकाठिन्य सम्बन्धी;

   **A. Deafness,** senile deafness. जराबधिरता; बुढ़ापे का बहरापन

**Arteriospasm.** Spasm of one or more arteries. धमनी-उद्वेष्ट

**Arteriostenosis.** Contraction of the lumen of an artery. धमनीसंकीर्णता; धमनीसंकुचन

**Arteriotome.** The knife used in arteriotomy. धमनीछेदक

**Arteriotomy.** Opening of an artery for blood-letting. धमनीछेदन

**Arteriovenous.** Pertaining to the artery and the vein. धमनीशिरापरक; धमनी एवं शिरा सम्बन्धी

**Arterioversion.** A method of arresting haemorrhage by turning the vessel inside out. धमनीवर्तन

**Arterioverter.** An instrument for arterioversion. धमनीवर्तक

**Arteritis.** Inflammation of an artery. धमनीशोथ; धमनी का प्रदाह;

   **Cranial A.**, a collagen disorder. करोटि-धमनीशोथ;

   **Giant Cell A.**, inflammation with possible occlusion, most often in the carotid arteries and branches; temporal arteritis. महाकोशिका धमनीशोथ;

   **Rheumatic A.**, one due to rheumatic fever. आमवाती धमनीशोथ;

   **Temporal A.**, see **Giant Cell Arteritis.**

**Artery.** One of the series of vessels which carry the blood from the heart to the various parts of the body, as distinguished from the veins which carry blood to the heart. धमनी

**Arthragra.** Gout. गठिया; सन्धिवात; जोड़ों का दर्द

**Arthral.** Pertaining to a joint. सन्धिपरक; जोड़ सम्बन्धी

**Arthralgia.** Pain in the joints. सन्धिशूल; सन्धि-आर्ति; जोड़ों का दर्द; gout. गठिया; arthritis. सन्धिशोथ;

**Arthralgic.** Affected with arthralgia. सन्धिशूलग्रस्त; relating to arthralgia. सन्धिशूल सम्बन्धी

**Arthrectomy.** Excision of a joint. सन्धि-उच्छेदन; किसी जोड़ को काट कर हटा देना

**Arthric.** Pertaining to a joint. सन्धिपरक; जोड़ सम्बन्धी

**Arthritic.** Pertaining to artihritis or gout. सन्धिशोथज; सन्धिवात अथवा गठिया सम्बन्धी

**Arthritis.** Inflammation of the joints; gout; arthrosia. सन्धिशोथ; सन्धि-प्रदाह; जोड़ों का प्रदाह; गठिया; सन्धिवात;

   A. **Deformans,** osteoarthritis. विरूपक सन्धिशोथ; अस्थिसन्धिशोथ;

   A. **Nodosa,** gout. गठिया;

   A. **Voga,** erratic gout. चल सन्धिशोथ; चल सन्धिवात

**Arthritides.** Plural of **Arthritis.**

**Arthritism.** The gouty diathesis. सन्धिशोथता; सन्धिवाती प्रवणता

**Arthrocace.** Caries of joints. सन्धि-अस्थिक्षय; जोड़ों की हड्डी गलना

**Arthrochalasis.** Softening of a joint; arthromalacia. सन्धिशैथिल्य; सन्धिमृदुता

**Arthrocleisis.** see **Arthrodesis.**

**Arthrodesis.** The surgical fixation of a joint; arthrocleisis; arthrokleisis. सन्धिस्थिरीकरण; सन्धिसंसक्ति

**Arthrodia.** A joint with a gliding movement. संसर्पी सन्धि; विसर्पण गति करने वाली सन्धि

**Arthrodynia.** The same as **Arthralgia.**

**Arthrodynic.** The same as **Arthralgic.**

**Arthroempyesis.** Suppuration in a joint. सन्धिपूतिता; जोड़ों में पीब पड़ना

**Arthrogram.** An x-ray film demonstrating a joint. सन्धिलेख; सन्धिचित्र

**Arthrography.** A description of the joints. सन्धिचित्रण

**Arthrogryposis.** The unnatural fixture of a joint; persistent contracture of a joint. सन्धिवक्रता; किसी जोड़ का टेढ़ापन

**Arthrokleisis.** See **Arthrodesis.**

**Arthrolithiasis.** Gout. गठिया; सन्धिवात

**Arthrology.** The science which deals with joints, their diseases and treatment. सन्धिप्रकरण; सन्धिविज्ञान; सन्धियों का वैज्ञानिक अध्ययन

**Arthrolysis.** The division or removal of adhesions and bones from an ankylosed joint. सन्धिलयन

**Arthromalacia.** See **Arthrochalasis.**
**Arthromeningitis.** Synovitis. श्लेषककलाशोथ
**Arthrometer.** Goniometer. सन्धिमापक; सन्धिमापी
**Arthrometry.** Measurement of the range of movement in a joint. सन्धिमापन
**Arthroncus.** A swelling or tumour of a joint. सन्धिगुल्म
**Arthroneuralgia.** Pain in a joint. सन्ध्यार्ति; जोड़ का दर्द
**Arthropathy.** Any disease of a joint. सन्धिप्रकरण; सन्धिरोग; जोड़ का कोई रोग
**Arthroplastic.** Relating to arthroplasty. सन्धिसंधान सम्बन्धी
**Arthroplasty.** The formation of an artificial joint. सन्धिसंधान
**Arthropyosis.** Suppuration in a joint. सन्धिपूतिता; किसी जोड़ में पीब बन जाना
**Arthrorheumatism.** Articular rheumatism; rheumatism of a joint. सन्धिवात
**Arthrosclerosis.** Stiffness of the joints. सन्धिकाठिन्य; जोड़ों की अकड़न (कठोरता)
**Arthroscope.** An instrument used for visualization of the interior of a joint cavity. अन्त:सन्धिदर्शक (यंत्र)
**Arthroscopy.** The act of visualizing the interior of a joint. अन्त:सन्धिदर्शन
**Arthrosia.** See **Arthritis.**
**Arthrosis.** An articulation or a joining. सन्धि; a suture. सीवन
**Arthrotomy.** An incision into a joint. सन्धिच्छेदन; सन्धिकर्तन
**Articular.** Pertaining to a joint. सन्धायक; सन्धिपरक; सन्धिस्थ; जोड़ सम्बन्धी
**Articularis.** A small joint. सन्धिका; लघु सन्धि;
   **Processus A.,** articular process. सन्धि-प्रवर्ध; सन्धिका-प्रवर्ध;
   **A. Genu,** the knee-joint. जानु-सन्धि; जानु-सन्धिका; घुटने का जोड़
**Articulata.** Articulate animals. सन्धियुक्त जीव
**Articulate.** To divide into joints. सन्धियों में विभाजित करना
**Articulated.** United by means of a joint. सन्धियुक्त
**Articulatio.** An articulation. सन्धि; जोड़
   **A. Composita,** a joint composed of two or more skeletal elements; compound joint. जटिल सन्धि;

**A. Cubiti,** a compound hinge joint between the humerus and the bones of the foream; cubital articulation of elbow joint. कफोणि सन्धि;

**A. Simplex,** a joint composed of two bones only; simple joint. सरल सन्धि

**Articulation.** The union of bones with each other, as the the joints. सन्धि; जोड़; enunciation of spoken sound, words and sentences. उच्चारण

**Articulatory.** Pertaining to articulation. सन्धि अथवा उच्चारण सम्बन्धी

**Artifact.** See **Artefact.**

**Artificial.** Not natural; made or imitated by art. कृत्रिम; नकली;

**A. Impregnation** see **Artificial Insemination.**

**A. Insemination,** insertion of sperm into uterus using cannula and syringe instead of coitus; artificial impregnation. कृत्रिम शुक्रसेचन;

**A. Respiration,** methods to keep the patient breathing when the moral function has ceased. कृत्रिम श्वसन; कृत्रिम श्वास

**Arum.** Genus of **Monocotyledonous** plants including **Wake-Rabin.** अरुबी; घुइयाँ

**Arytenoid.** Cup-shaped or ladle-shaped. दर्वीकल्प

**Asafetida.** A fetid gum resin with garlic-like odour; asafoetida. हींग

**Asafoetida.** See **Asafetida.**

**Asarum.** A genus of herbs. जंगली अदरक

**Asault.** An attack. आक्रमण; हमला

**Ascariasis.** See **Ascaridiasis.**

**Ascarcide.** A medicine fatal to the ascaris. कृमिनाशक औषधि; कीड़े नष्ट करने वाली औषधि

**Ascarides.** Small intestinal worms; pinworms; threadworms; ascaris. कृमि; त्र्योष्ठ कीट; बारीक कीड़े

**Ascaridiasis.** The existence of ascarides in the bowel; ascariasis. कृमिरुग्णता

**Ascaris.** Singular of **Ascarides.**

**A. Lumbricoides,** the long and round worms. लम्बे व गोल कृमि

**Ascending.** Proceeding towards the superior parts of the body. आरोही; ऊर्ध्वगामी;

**A. Degeneration,** that of nerve-fibers progressing from the periphery to the centre. आरोही अपजनन;

**A. Paralysis,** a paralysis beginning below and extending upward. आरोही पक्षाघात

**Aschheim Zondek Reaction.** See **A.Z.R.**

**Aschheim Zondek Test.** See **A.Z.R.**

**Aschoff's Nodes.** Nodes in the myocardium in rheumatism; Aschoff's nodules. अशोफ पर्व

**Aschoff's Nodules.** See **Aschoff's Nodes.**

**Ascites.** A condition wherein fluids accumulate in the abdominal cavity. जलोदर;

**Chyliform A.,** ascites in which the fluid contains chyle. वसापयसरूपी जलोदर;

**Chylous A.,** the same as **Chyliform Ascites.**

**A. Chylosus,** the same as **Chyliform Ascites.**

**Ascitic.** Affected with ascites. जलोदरग्रस्त; belonging to ascites. जलोदरीय; जलोदर सम्बन्धी

**Asemia.** Inability to comprehend words or signs; asymbolia. शब्दज्ञान-अक्षमता; चिन्हज्ञान-अक्षमता

**Asepsis.** Absence of putrefactive matter or harmful bacteria. अपूतिता; अपूति; पूतिहीनता

**Aseptic.** Absence of septic material. पूतिहीन; पूतिमुक्त; अपूतित; अपूतिज; शुद्ध

**Asepticize.** To render aseptic. पूतिहीन करना

**Asexual.** Having no sex; nonsexual. अलिंगी; अलैंगिक

**Asialia.** A lack of saliva. अलारता; लारहीनता

**Asialism.** See **Aptyalia.**

**Asiatic Cholera.** See under **Cholera.**

**Asitia.** A loss of appetite; a loathing for food. क्षुधाभाव;क्षुधालोप; भूख का अभाव

**Asleep.** Into a state of sleep. सुप्त; सोया हुआ

**Asocial.** Against society. असामाजिक

**Asparagus.** A plant whose vernal shoots are a table delicacy. नागदौन; शतावरी

**Aspect.** The appearance of a thing. अवस्थिति; अभिमुखता; view-point. दृष्टिकोण

**Aspermatism.** See **Aspermia.**

**Aspermia.** Lack of seminal discharge; aspermatism. अशुक्रता; अशुक्राणुता; शुक्राभाव; बीजाभाव; वीर्यहीनता

**Aspersion.** The act of besprinkling. छिड़काव

**Asphyxia.** Suspended animation, attended with an imperceptible pulse and an apparent or real want of action of the lungs, as from drowning, suffocation, etc. श्वासरोध; श्वासावरोध;

Blue A., see Asphyxia Livida.

Pale A., see Asphyxia Pallida.

White A., see Asphyxia Pallida.

**A. Livida,** deep blue appearance of a newborn baby; blue asphyxia. श्याव श्वासावरोध;

**A. Neonatorum,** inability of newlyborn to respire. नवजात श्वासावरोध; शिशु श्वासरोध;

**A. Pallida,** a more severe condition of newborn; pale asphyxia; white asphyxia. श्वेत श्वासावरोध

**Asphyxial.** Marked by asphyxia. श्वासरोधी; श्वासावरोधी; श्वासरोधात्मक; pertaining to asphyxia. श्वासरोधसम्बन्धी

**Aspiration.** Inspiration; imbibition. श्वसन; चूषण

**Aspirator.** An instrument for extracting fluids or air from cavities. चूषित्र; चूषणोपकरण

**Asplenia.** Absence of the spleen. प्लीहाभाव; तिल्ली का अभाव

**Asplenic.** Having no spleen. प्लीहाहीन; तिल्लीरहित

**Assay.** Analysis. विश्लेषण; to subject to analysis. निर्धारण

**Assimilable.** Capable of being assimilated. स्वांगीकरणीय; स्वांगीकरण योग्य

**Assimilate.** To convert nutritious substance furnished by the food into flesh or other tissues of the body. स्वांगीकरण करना; आत्मसात करना

**Assimilation.** Power of absorption of food and of the building up body tissues. स्वांगीकरण; आत्मीकरण; समीकरण

**Astasia.** Motor incoordination for standing, or sitting. स्थिति-असमर्थता; गति-असंगति

**Aster.** The stellate structure surrounding the centrosome. तारक; ताराविन्यास

**Astereognosis.** Loss of the stercognostic sense, or power to recognize the shape and consistency of objects by touch.

विन्यासज्ञानहीनता

**Asterias.** A radiate animal called star-fish. तारकमत्स्य; तारकमीन

**Asterion.** The junction of occipital, parietal and temporal bones. बिन्दुतारक (सन्धि); तारकसन्धि

**Asterionic.** Pertaining to asterion. बिन्दुतारकीय

**Asternal.** Without a sternum. उरोस्थिहीन

**Asternia.** Congenital absence of sternum. उरोस्थि का जन्मजात अभाव; सहज-उरोस्थिहीनता

**Asteroid.** Star-shaped. तारकवत्; तारकरूप; ताराभ; तारोपम; तारकाभ

**Asthenia.** A loss of strength; adynamia. कृशता; अवसाद; अशक्तता; अवसन्नता; दौर्बल्य; दुर्बलता; कमजोरी

**Asthenic.** Extremely weak; applied to diseases of low type or character. कृश; कृशकाय; अवसन्न; दुर्बल; बहुत कमजोर

**Asthenometer.** An instrument for determining asthenia. अवसादमापी (यंत्र)

**Asthenopia.** Weak or painful vision; ophthalmoscopia. नेत्रावसाद; दृष्टिक्षीणता; क्षीणदृष्टिता;

    **Accommodative A.,** that caused by strain of the ciliary muscle. समंजनी नेत्रावसाद;

    **Muscular A.,** that due to strain of the external ocular muscles. पेशीजन्य नेत्रावसाद

**Asthenopic.** Exhibiting asthenopia. नेत्रावसादी; क्षीणदृष्टि

**Asthma.** Violent oppression of breathing; paroxysmal dyspnoea with oppression. दमा; श्वासरोग;

    **Allergic A.,** one due to allergens. प्रत्यूर्जतात्मक दमा;

    **Bronchial A.,** attack of breathlessness associated with bronchial obstruction or spasm. श्वास दमा; श्वसनिका दमा;

    **Cardiac A.,** dyspnoea due to heart disease. हृद्जन्य दमा;

    **Dyspeptic A.,** one due to nervous reflexes through the vagus. अग्निमांद्यज दमा;

    **Renal A.,** that sometimes accompanying Bright's disease. वृक्कज दमा

**Asthmatic.** Affected with, or pertaining to asthma. दमाग्रस्त; दमा का रोगी; दमा या श्वासरोग सम्बन्धी

**Astigmatic.** Affected with astigmatism; astigmic. विषमदृष्टिक; विदृष्टिक; अबिन्दुक

**Astigmatism.** Defective vision caused by inequality of one or more refractive surfaces, usually corneal, so that the light rays do not converge to a point of retina; astigmia. दृष्टिवैषम्य; अबिन्दुकता;
**Compound A.**, when complicated with myopia or hypermetropia. संयुक्त दृष्टिवैषम्य;
**Corneal A.**, due to inequality of curvature of the different meridians of the cornea. स्वच्छपटलीय दृष्टिवैषम्य;
**Irregular A.**, when different parts of a meridian have different refractive powers. अनियमित दृष्टिवैषम्य;
**Lenticular A.**, that due to imperfection of the lens. लेन्सीय दृष्टिवैषम्य;
**Mixed A.**, that in which one principal meridian is myopic, the other hypermetropic. मिश्र-दृष्टिवैषम्य;
**Myopic A.**, astigmatism in which one meridian is myopic and the one or right angle to it is without refractive error. निकट-दृष्टिवैषम्य;
**Regular A.**, when the two principal meridians are at right angle to each other. नियमित दृष्टिवैषम्य;
**Simple A.**, that in which one principal meridian is normal, the other myopic or hyperopic. सरल दृष्टिवैषम्य

**Astigmia.** See **Astigmatism**.

**Astigmic.** See **Astigmatic**.

**Astigmomatometer.** See **Astigmometer**.

**Astigmometer.** An instrument for measuring astigmatism; astigmomatometer. दृष्टिवैषम्यमापी

**Astigmometry.** Determination of the form and measure of the degree of astigmatism. दृष्टिवैषम्यमिति

**Astigmoscope.** An instrument for detecting and measuring the degree of astigmatism. दृष्टिवैषम्यदर्शी

**Astigmoscopy.** The measurement of astigmatism by astigmoscope. दृष्टिवैषम्यदर्शन

**Astomatous.** Without a mouth, or an oral opening; astomous. मुखविहीन

**Astomous.** See **Astomatous**.

**Astomia.** Congenital absence of the mouth. मुखहीनता; अमुखता

**Astragalar.** Relating to the astragalus. घुटिकास्थि अथवा घुटने की हड्डी सम्बन्धी

**Astragalectomy.** Excision of the astragalus; talectomy. घुटिकास्थि-उच्छेदन; घुटने की हड्डी काट कर निकाल देना

**Astragalus.** The ankle-bone or first bone of the foot; talus. घुटिकास्थि; घुटने की हड्डी; गुल्फास्थि

**Astraphobia.** A morbid fear of thunder and lightning; astrapophobia. तूफान और बिजली का भय

**Astrapophobia.** See **Astraphobia.**

**Astriction.** Constipation. मलबद्धता; कब्ज; The action of an astringent. स्तम्भन.

**Astringent.** Medicine used to contract muscular fibres and to construct vessels to retain discharge. स्तम्भक औषधि; स्रावरोधक (औषधि); कषायवर्ग; संकोचक

**Astroblast.** A primitive cell developing into an astrocyte. तारकाणुप्रसू

**Astroblastoma.** A relatively poorly differentiated glioma. तारकाणुप्रसूअर्बुद

**Astrocyte.** A star-shaped bone-corpuscle; astroglia. तारिकाकोशिका; अस्थिकणिका

**Astrocytoma.** A slowly growing tumour of the glial tissue of the brain. तारिकाकोशिकार्बुद

**Astroglia.** See **Astrocyte.**

**Astronomy.** A branch of science which treats the heavenly bodies. खगोलविज्ञान; खगोलिकी; खगोलविद्या

**Astrophobia.** A morbid fear of stars and celestial spaces. खगोलभीति; खगोलातंक

**Asylum.** An institution for the care of the incapables and destitutes. आश्रयस्थल; शरणस्थल; शरणस्थान

**Asymbolia.** See **Asemia.**

**Asymmetric.** See **Asymmetrical.**

**Asymmetrical.** Not having symmetry; asymmetric. असममात्रिक; असममितिक

**Asymmetry.** A want of symmetry or proportion. असममिति

**Asymptomatic.** Symptomless. अलक्षणी; अलाक्षणिक; लक्षणहीन; लक्षणरहित; बिना लक्षण वाला

**Asynclitism.** An oblique presentation of the foetal head at the superior strait of the pelvis. पार्श्विक-तिर्यकता

**Asynergia.** An absence of the coordinate action; asynergy. असहक्रिया; असंगति; विसंगति

**Asynergy.** See **Asynergia.**

**Asynesia.** Stupidity; dementia. जड़ता; विमूढ़ता; मन्दबुद्धिता

**Asynodia.** Impotence for sexual intercourse. ध्वजभंग; रतिशक्तिक्षय

**Asystole.** An imperfect ventricular systole; asystolia. हृद्-अप्रकुंचन; अपूर्ण प्रकुंचन

**Asystolia.** See **Asystole.**

**Asystolic.** Relating to asystole. हृद्-अप्रकुंचन सम्बन्धी; not systole. प्रकुंचनहीन

**Atactic.** Irregular; ataxic; atypic. अनियमित; अरूपी

**Ataractics.** Drugs that without drowsiness, help to relieve anxiety. अधीरताशामक औषधियाँ; बेचैनी कम करने वाली औषधियाँ

**Atavism.** A reversion to ancestral type of structure or function. पूर्वजता; विरासत

**Atavistic.** Relating to atavism. विरासत अथवा पूर्वजता सम्बन्धी

**Atavus.** An ancestor. पूर्वज

**Ataxaphasia.** An inability to arrange words into sentences. वाक्विन्यास-अक्षमता

**Ataxia.** Incoordination of muscular action; ataxy. गतिभंग; गतिविभ्रम;
  **Family A.,** see **Hereditary Ataxia.**
  **Hereditary A.,** sclerosis of posterior and lateral columns of the spinal cord; family ataxia. आनुवंशिक गतिविभ्रम; आनुवंशिक गतिभंग;
  **Locomotor A.,** disease of the posterior columns of spinal cord, marked by fulgurant pains, incoordination, disturbed sensations, etc. प्रेरणज गतिविभ्रम; प्रेरणज गतिभंग;
  **Motor A.,** inability to coordinate the muscles in walking. प्रेरक गतिभंग; चलते समय पेशियों में सामंजस्य रखने की असमर्थता;
  **Static A.,** muscular incoordination in standing. स्थैतिक गतिविभ्रम

**Ataxic.** Pertaining to, or affected with ataxia. गतिविभ्रमी; irregular. अनियमित; विषम
  **A. Fever,** malaria. विषमज्वर; मलेरिया

**Ataxophobia.** An excessive dread of incoordination. गतिभंगभीति

**Ataxy.** See **Ataxia.**

**Atelectasis.** Non-expansion of lungs in newborns. नवजात-श्वासावरोध; श्वासरोध; फुप्फुसपात; फुप्फुस-अनुन्मीलन;

**Congenital A.**, if air has failed to enter lungs immediately after birth. सहजफुप्फुस-अनुन्मीलन;

**Post-operative A.**, obstruction of bronchial tubes with viscid secretion which results in an atelectasis of varying degree. शल्योत्तर श्वासरोध;शल्यकर्मोत्तर श्वासरोध;

**Secondary A.**, pulmonary collapse, particularly of infants. शिशुफुप्फुसपात; गौण फुप्फुस-अनुन्मीलन

**Atelectatic.** Pertaining to atelectasis. अनुन्मीलित; पाती; श्वासरोध सम्बन्धी

**Ateleiosis.** See **Atelia.**

**Atelia.** Persistence of the child's characteristics in the adult; ateleiosis; ateliosis. पीयूषीवामनता; पीयूषीशिशुता

**Ateliosis.** See **Atelia.**

**Atelocardia.** Poor development of the heart. अपूर्णहृदयता; हृदय का अपूर्ण विकास

**Atelocephalosis.** Having an incomplete skull. अपूर्णकरोटिता

**Atelocheilia.** Poor development of the lips. अपूर्णओष्ठता; होंठों का अपूर्ण विकास

**Atelocheiria.** Defective development of hand. अपूर्णहस्तता; हाथ का दोषपूर्ण विकास

**Ateloglossia.** Poor development of the tongue. अपूर्णजिह्वा; जीभ का अपूर्ण विकास

**Atelomyelia.** Poor development of the spinal cord. अपूर्णसुषुम्नता; सुषुम्ना का अपूर्ण विकास

**Atelorrachidia.** Defective development of the spine. अपूर्णमेरुता; मेरुदण्ड का दोषपूर्ण विकास

**Athelia.** Absence of the nipples. अचूचुकता; चूचुकहीनता; चूचुकों का अभाव

**Athermic.** Heatless; no rise in temperature. तापशून्य; तापविहीन; तापहीन

**Atherogenesis.** Formation of an atheroma. मेदार्बुदजनन

**Atherogenic.** Capable of producing atheroma. मेदार्बुदजनक

**Atheroma.** A disease which involves degeneration of blood vessels, chiefly to arteries. मेदार्बुद;

**Cerebral A.**, a fatty degeneration of the cerebellum. प्रमस्तिष्क-मेदार्बुद

**Atheromasia.** Atheromatous degeneration. मेदार्बुदीय अपजनन

**Atheromatous.** Pertaining to, or affected with atheroma. मेदार्बुदीय; मेदार्बुदग्रस्त

**Atherosclerosis.** A disease affecting the lining membranes of the arteries. धमनीकलाकाठिन्य

**Athetosic.** Affected with, or resembling athetosis; athetotic. वलनग्रस्त अथवा वलनवत्

**Athetosis.** Slow, steady movement of the fingers and toes. वलन; हाथ-पैरों की उँगलियों की धीमी, मन्द गति

**Athetotic.** See **Athetosic.**

**Athlete's Foot.** Ringworm of the foot;athletic foot. पाद-दद्रु; पैरों का दाद

**Athlete's Heart.** Aortic incompetence from strain. एथलीट-हाट्; महाधमनी-शैथिल्य

**Athletic.** Vigorous; robust. बलिष्ठ; पुष्टकाय;

  **A. Foot,** ringworm of the foot. पाद-दद्रु; पैरों का दाद

**Athyrea.** The condition due to absence of the thyroid gland or from insufficiency or suppression of its function; athyroidism; hypothyroidism. अवटुअल्पक्रियता

**Athyroidism.** See **Athyrea.**

**Atlantad.** Towards the atlas. शीर्षधरोन्मुख

**Atlantal.** Pertaining to the atlas. शीर्षधर अथवा गर्दन की प्रथम कशेरुका सम्बन्धी

**Atlanto-axial.** Relating to the atlas and the axis. शीर्षधर-अक्षक; शीर्षधर एवं अक्ष सम्बन्धी

**Atlantodidymus.** A foetus with two heads. द्विशिरस्कभ्रूण

**Atlas.** The first cervical vertebra, so called, because it supports the head. एटलस; ग्रीवा की प्रथम कशेरुका; मेरुदण्ड का सबसे ऊपरी अथवा शीर्षस्थ खण्ड

**Atmiatrics.** See **Atmidiatrica.**

**Atmiatry.** See **Atmidiatrica.**

**Atmidiatrica.** The treatment of diseases by vapour; atmiatrics; atmiatry. वाष्प-चिकित्सा; वाष्पोपचार

**Atmosphere.** The air encircling the earth. वायुमण्डल; वातावरण

**Atocia.** Sterility of the females. स्त्री-बंध्यता; औरतों में जननशक्ति का अभाव

**Atom.** The ultimate unit of an element. परमाणु; अणु; कण

**Atomic.** Referring to the atom, the unit of chemical entity. परमाणविक; परमाणवीय; आणविक

**Atomizer.** A spraying instrument. कणित्र; तरल पदार्थों को सूक्ष्म कणों में बदल देने वाला यंत्र

**Atonia.** A want of tone; atony. अतानता; तानाभाव; अशक्तता; शक्तिहीनता

**Atonic.** Without tone; want of tone. अतानिक; अशक्त;

**Atopomenorrhea.** Vicarious menstruation; atopomenorrhoea. अपथप्रवृत्तार्तव; ऋतुस्राव के स्थान पर योनिद्वार के बदले किसी अन्य द्वार से रक्तस्राव होना

**Atopomenorrhoea.** See **Atopomenorrhea.**

**Atremia.** Absence of tremor. कम्पनाभाव

**Atresia.** A blocking of a canal or passage, as the ear. अविवरता; अछिद्रता; नलिकारोध; मार्गरोध;

    A. Ani, imperforate anus; anal atresia. गुद-अविवरता;

    **Anal A.,** see **Atresia Ani.**

    **Biliary A.,** atresia of the major bile ducts. पित्त-अविवरता;

    **Follicular A.,** a normal process affecting the ovarian primordial follicles. कूपिक अविवरता;

    **Intestinal A.,** an obliteration of the lumen of the small intestine involving the jejunum, or duodenum. आंत्र-अविवरता;

    **Mitral A.,** congenital absence of the normal mitral valve orifice. हृत्कपाट-अविवरता;

    **Tricuspid A.,** congenital lack of tricuspid orifice. त्रिकपर्दी अछिद्रता;

    **Vaginal A.,** imperforation or occlusion of the vagina or adhesion of the walls of the vagina. योनि-अविवरता

**Atria.** Plural of **Atrium.**

**Atrial.** Pertaining to atrium. अलिन्दी

**Atrichia.** Baldness; atrichiasis; atrichosis. खालित्य; खल्वाटता; अरोमता; अलोमता; गंजापन

**Atrichiasis.** See **Atrichia.**

**Atrichosis.** See **Atrichia.**

**Atrichous.** Without hair. खल्वाट; गंजा; टकला

**Atriomegaly.** Enlargement of the atrium of the heart. हृदलिन्दविवर्ध

**Atrioventricular.** Pertaining to the atria and ventricles. अलिन्दनिलय सम्बन्धी

**Atrium.** Cavity, entrance or passage; auricle of the heart; part of cavity of tympanum. अलिन्द; परिकोष्ठ

**Atropa Belladonna.** The deadly night-shade. बेलाडौना; साग अंगूर

**Atrophia.** See **Atrophy**.

**Atrophic.** Denoting atrophy. शोषग्रस्त

**Atrophy.** Wasting away of the system from functional disturbances; atrophia. शोष; अपुष्टि; अपकर्ष; क्षय; अपक्षय;

 **Acute Yellow A.,** atrophy of liver with yellow pigmentation; postneurotic cirrhosis. तीव्र पीत-अपुष्टि;

 **Brown A.,** that in which the organ becomes brown. बभ्रु-शोष;

 **Muscular A.,** that affecting muscles. पेशी-शोष;

 **Occular A.,** see Atrophy Bulbi.

 **Progressive Muscular A.,** a chronic disease marked by progressive wasting of muscles associated with paralysis. प्रगामी पेशी-शोष;

 **A. Bulbi,** phthisis bulbi; occular atrophy. नेत्रशोष

**Atropine.** The principal alkaloid of **Belladonna**. ऐट्रोपीन; बेलाडौना; सागअंगूर का प्रमुख क्षार

**ATS.** Antitetanus serum; produces active immunity against tetanus. धनुर्वातरोधी सीरम

**Attack.** Occurrence of some disease or episode often with a dramatic onset. आक्रमण

**Attar of Rose.** Oil of rose. गुलाब तेल; गुलाब का अत्तर

**Attendant.** One who attends a patient. परिचर; परिचारक; सेवक

**Attention.** The direction or the will or thought upon an object or to a particular sensation. ध्यान

**Attenuated.** Thinned; diluted. तनूकृत

**Attenuation.** A thinning; dilution of a medicine in Homoeopathic Pharmacy. तनूकरण

**Attic.** The portion of the tympanum above the atrium. अधिमध्यकर्ण; मध्यकर्णकुहर का एक भाग

**Attitude.** A settled mode of thinking. संस्थिति; वृत्ति; व्यवहार; स्वभाव; रवैया

**Attollens.** Raising up. उत्थापक

**Attraction.** The tendency of particles to draw together. आकर्षण; खिंचाव

**Attrition.** An abrasion or chaffing of the skin. घर्षण; रगड़न; खरोंच

**Atypic.** Erratic; irregulr; having no characteristic symptoms; atypical. अप्ररूपी; अनियमित; चारित्रिक लक्षणों से हीन

**Atypical.** See **Atypic.**

**Audiogram.** A chart of hearing while using an audiometer. श्रवणलेख

**Audiologist.** A specialist in audiology. श्रवणविशेषज्ञ; ध्वनिविज्ञानवेत्ता

**Audiology.** The science dealing with hearing. श्रवणविज्ञान; ध्वनिविज्ञान

**Audiometer.** An instrument for measuring the acuteness of hearing. श्रवणमापी; श्रव्यतामापी

**Audiometrician.** See **Audiometrist.**

**Audiometrist.** One versed in audiometry; audiometrician. श्रवणमितिज्ञ

**Audiometry.** The measurement of the acuteness of hearing. श्रवणमिति; श्रव्यतामिति

**Audiphone.** An instrument for aiding the power of hearing. श्रुतियंत्र; श्रवणयंत्र;

**Audition.** The act of hearing. श्रवण-प्रक्रिया; सुनना; ध्वनिबोध

**Auditory.** Belonging to the sense of hearing. श्रवणीय; श्रवण सम्बन्धी;

   **A. Area,** the cerebral centre for hearing; auditory centre. श्रवण क्षेत्र; श्रवण केन्द्र;

   **A. Centre,** see **Auditory Area.**

   **A. Meatus,** the opening of the ear. कर्णकुहर; कर्णद्वार;

   **A. Nerves,** the eighth pair of the cranial nerves. श्रवण तंत्रिकायें

**Aura.** A sensation as of rising air current preceding an epileptic fit. पूर्वज्ञान; पूर्वाभास;

   **A. Epileptica,** the peculiar sensations experienced before an attack of epilepsy. अपस्मारीय पूर्वज्ञान

**Aurae.** Plural of **Aura.**

**Aural.** Pertaining to the ear. कर्णपरक; कान सम्बन्धी

**Aurantium.** Sweet orange. संतरा; संगतरा; नारंगी

**Aures.** Plural of **Auris.**

**Auric.** Relating to gold. स्वर्ण सम्बन्धी

**Auricles.** The two upper cavities of the heart, one right, the other left; the right receives the blood of the body, the left the blood from the lungs. उत्कोष्ठ; अलिन्द; the external ear. बहिकर्ण; कर्णपाली; कर्णपल्लव

**Auricula.** The auricle or the external ear. अलिन्द; बहिकर्ण; कर्णपाली

**Auriculae.** Plural of **Auricula.**

**Auricular.** Pertaining to the external ear or heart auricle. बहिकर्णीय; हृद्-अलिन्दी

**Auriculocranial.** Pertaining to both ear and the cranium. कर्णकपालीय

**Auriculoventricular.** Pertaining to both ear and the ventricle. अलिन्दनिलयी

**Auriform.** Ear-shaped. कर्णाकार; कर्णरूप; कान जैसा

**Aurigo.** Jaundice. कामला; पीलिया; पाण्डुरोग

**Auris.** The external ear. बहिकर्ण; बाह्यकर्ण; कान का बाहरी हिस्सा

**Auriscalp.** An instrument for cleaning the ear. कर्णशोधकयंत्र

**Auriscope.** An instrument for examining the ear. कर्णदर्शीयंत्र; कर्णपरीक्षक; कान देखने का यंत्र

**Auriscopy.** Examination of the ear with auriscope. कर्णदर्शन

**Aurist.** A specialist in the diseases of the ear. कर्णरोगविशेषज्ञ; कर्णरोगचिकित्सक

**Aurium.** The ear. कर्ण; कान;

A. Sordes, ear-wax; cerumen. कर्णगूथ; कर्णमल;

A. Tinnitus, ringing in the ear. भिनभिनाहट; टनटनाहट

**Aurum.** Gold; the chloride is used in medicine. स्वर्ण; सोना

**Ausculate.** See **Auscult.**

**Ausculatory.** Pertaining to auscultation; auscultatory. परिश्रवणीय; परिश्रवण सम्बन्धी

**Auscult.** To examine by auscultation; ausculate. परिश्रवण करना

**Auscultation.** The art of listening to the sound produced by the heart, lungs, etc. in order to judge the existence or progress of diseases of these organs. परिश्रवण

**Auscultatory.** See **Ausculatory.**

**Autacoids.** Internal secretions. अन्तःस्राव; आन्तरिक स्राव

**Autism.** Morbid or phantastic day-dreaming; schizophrenic syndrome in childhood. स्वपरायणता; स्व-अभिव्यक्तता

**Autistic.** Morbidly self-centred thinking, governed by the wishes of the individual. स्वपरायण; अपने ही विचारों में खोया हुआ

**Auto-.** Prefix meaning self or itself. 'स्व' अथवा 'आत्म' के रूप में प्रयुक्त उपसर्ग

**Autoagglutinin.** An agglutinating autoantibody. स्वसमूहिका

**Autoaudible.** That which can be heard by one's self. स्वश्रवणीय

**Autoantibody.** Substance produced in a reaction, something within the body acting as the stimulus. स्वप्रतिपिण्ड; स्वप्रतिरक्षी

**Autoantigen.** Something within the body capable of initiating the production of autoantibody. स्वप्रतिजन

**Autoclaving.** Sterilizing by steam. वाष्पदावी विसंक्रण

**Autodigestion.** Digestion of the gastric walls, from disease of the stomach. स्वपाचन; अपने ही स्रावों द्वारा ऊतकों का विघटन

**Antoerotic.** Relating to autoeroticism. स्वकामुकता सम्बन्धी

**Autoeroticism.** Self-gratification of the sex instinct. स्वकामुकता

**Autogenesis.** Self-produced; autogenetic; antogenic; autogenous. स्वजात

**Autogenetic.** See **Autogenesis.**

**Antogenic.** See **Autogenesis.**

**Autogenous.** See **Autogenesis.**

**Autohaemotherapy.** Intramuscular injection of a patient using his own blood; autohemotherapy. स्वरक्तचिकित्सा; स्वरक्तोपचार

**Autohemotherapy.** See **Autohaemotherapy.**

**Autoimmunity.** An abnormal immune reaction of unknown cause. स्वक्षमता; स्वरोगक्षमता

**Autoimmunization.** Immunization produced by processes resident in the body. स्वप्रतिरक्षीकरण; स्वरोगक्षमीकरण; स्वप्रतिरक्षण; स्वरोगक्षमता

**Autoinfection.** Self-infection by direct contagion; autoreinfection. स्वोपसर्ग

**Autoinoculation.** Reinoculation by virus from the same person. स्वसंरोपण

**Autointoxication.** A morbid condition produced by poisonous products elaborated within the body. स्वविषाक्तता; शरीर से उत्पन्न विषकारी पदार्थों का पुनर्शोषण

**Autolysin.** A lysin which, produced in an organism, is capable of destroying the cells of that organism. स्वलायिका

**Autolysis.** The process of self-digestion occurring in tissues under pathological conditions. स्वलयन; स्वक्षयता

**Autolytic.** Peraining to, or causing autolysis. स्वलयन सम्बन्धी अथवा स्वलयनजनक

**Automatic.** That which is performed without the influence of will; involuntary acts; spontaneous. स्वचल; स्वचालित; स्वसंचालित; स्वैच्छिक; स्वयम्भू; स्वत:

**Automaticism.** A condition in which actions are performed without consciousness or intention; automatism. स्वचलता; स्वचालिता; स्वचलन

**Automatism.** See **Automaticism.**

**Autonomic.** A term describing the portion of the brain and the nervous system which functions automatically to control over digestion and other activities which sustain life. स्वसंचालित; स्वायत; स्वयंशासी; स्वयंनिर्देशक

**Autonomous.** Independent. स्वायत्त; स्वतंत्र; स्वसंचालित

**Autonomy.** Self-law; not subjected to external law. स्वायत्तता; स्वतंत्रता

**Autopepsia.** Autodigestion. स्वपाचन

**Autophagy.** The act of feeding on one's self. स्वपोषी; स्वायत्तजीवी; स्वभक्षण; स्वत:भोजी

**Autophobia.** A morbid fear of solitude. स्वभीति; एकान्तभीति; स्वातंक

**Autophony.** Hearing one's voice in ear. अपनी आवाज स्वयं अपने ही कानों में गूंजते रहना

**Autoplastic.** Relating to autoplasty. स्वसंधानपरक; स्वसंधान सम्बन्धी

**Autoplasty.** Replacement of tissue from the same body. स्वसंधान; स्वांशसंधान

**Autopsia Cadaveris.** Post-mortem examination by dissection. शवोच्छेदन-जांच; मृतक की चीर-फाड़ करना

**Autopsy.** A post-mortem examination. मरणोत्तर जांच; शवपरीक्षा

**Autoreinfection.** See **Autoinfection**

**Autoscope.** Any instrument for self-examination. स्वदर्शी (यंत्र)

**Autoscopy.** The self-examination. स्वदर्शन

**Autosite.** That portion of a double monster nourishing the other. स्वजीवक्षम-राक्षस

**Autosomal.** Pertaining to autosome. अलिंगसूत्र सम्बन्धी

**Autosome.** A chromosome other than a sex-chromosome. अलिंग; अलिंगसूत्र; कायसूत्र

**Autosuggestion.** A mental state following shock, marked by abatement of will and judgment, and by abnormal responsiveness to suggestion. आत्मसुझाव; स्वसम्मोहन

**Autotherapy.** The spontaneous cure of disease. स्वचिकित्सा; सोपचार
**Autotoxaemia.** Poisoning by one's own secretions; autotoxemia. स्वविषाक्तता
**Autotoxemia.** See **Autotoxaemia.**
**Autotoxicosis.** The symptoms due to self-poisoning. स्वविषाक्तता
**Autotoxin.** Any poisonous substance produced in the body. स्वविष; शरीर में स्वयमेव पैदा होने वाला विष-पदार्थ
**Autotransplantation.** Transplanting an organ from one place to another in the same person. स्वपरारोपण; स्वप्रतिरोपण
**Autotroph.** A micro-organism which uses only inorganic materials as its source of nutrients. स्तपोषी
**Auxesis.** Increase in size or bulk. आकारवृद्धि; आकार बढ़ना
**Auxetic.** Relating to auxesis. आकारवृद्धि सम्बन्धी
**Auxillary.** Helping, aiding or assisting. सहायक; अनुषंगी; आनुषंगिक
**Avascular.** Without blood vessels. अवाहिकी; वाहिकाहीन
**Avascularisation.** Rendering bloodless, as by compression; avascularization. अवाहिकाभवन; अवाहिकाकरण
**Avascularization.** See **Avascularisation.**
**Avena Sativa.** The common oat, a nutritious food. सामान्य यव अथवा जई; आवेना सैटाइवा
**Aversion.** Extreme or intense dislike. अरुचि; अनिच्छा; घृणा
**Avian.** Pertaining to birds. पक्षियों सम्बन्धी
**Avirulent.** Without virulence or infectiousness. अनुग्र; विषाणुहीन; अविषाणुज; असंक्रामक; अप्रचण्डी; अविषाक्त; असांघातिक
**Avitaminosis.** Disease due to lack of vitamins. अविटामिनता; अविटामिनरुग्णता; विटामिनाल्पता; विटामिनाल्परुग्णता
**Avulsion.** The wrenching away of a part. अपदारण; खींचना; चीड़ना; झटका देना
**Axanthopsia.** Yellow-blindness. पीतान्धता; पीला रंग पहचानने की अक्षमता
**Axial.** Pertaining to, or of the shape of an axis; axile. अक्षीय; अक्षाकार;
  **A. Skeleton,** skeletal bones including the spinal column and rib cage. अस्थि-पंजर; head and trunk. सिर तथा धड़
**Axile.** See **Axial.**
**Axilla.** The arm-pit. कक्षा; कांख; बगल
**Axillaris.** See **Axillary.**

**Axillary.** Relating to the axilla or arm-pit; axillaris. कक्षा अथवा कांख सम्बन्धी

**Axin.** A varnish-like substance provided by an insect. एक्सिन; वार्निश जैसा एक कीट-प्रदत्त पदार्थ

**Axes.** Plural of **Axis.**

**Axis.** A line about which any revolving body turns, as second vertebra of the neck on which the head turns. अक्ष; धुरी; द्वितीय ग्रैव कशेरुका;

**A.-cylinder,** the central core of a nerve-fibre. अक्षदण्ड; सूत्राक्ष; स्नायु-मज्जा

**Axon.** The fibre extending from the neuron which is longer than the other fibres; axone. अक्षतंतु; अक्षगात्र; तंत्रिकाक्ष

**Axonal.** Pertaining to an axon. अक्षतंतु सम्बन्धी

**Axone.** See **Axon.**

**Axonotmesis.** Peripheral degeneration as a result of damage to the axons of a nerve. अक्षतंतुविच्छेद

**Axoplasm.** The material surrounding the fibrillas of an axis-cylinder. अक्षतंतुद्रव्य

**Axungia.** Lard; the internal fat of the body. वसा; चर्बी

**Ayurveda.** A system of treatment by plants and drugs indigenous to India; Ayurvedism. आयुर्वेद; यजुर्वेद; प्राचीनतम तथा मूल चिकित्सा-प्रणाली

**Ayurvedic.** Pertaining to Ayurveda. आयुर्वेद सम्बन्धी

**Ayurvedism.** See **Ayurveda.**

**Azoic.** Destitute of living organisms. निष्प्राण; निर्जीव; तन्तुहीन; प्राग्जैविक

**Azoospermia.** An absence of spermatozoa. अशुक्राणुता; शुक्राणुहीनता

**Azote.** Nitrogen. नेत्रजन; नाइट्रोजन

**Azotenesis.** Any disease caused due to excess of nitrogen in the system. नेत्रजनरुग्णता; नाइट्रोजनजनित रुग्णता

**Azoturia.** Pathological excretion of urea in the blood; an increase of urea in the urine. मूत्राम्लमेह; नेत्रजनमेह; पेशाब में यूरिया की अधिकता

**A.Z.R.** Aschheim Zondek Reaction or Test; a test for pregnancy in which the patient's urine is injected subcutaneously into immature female mice. ऐश्चाहइम जोंडिक प्रतिक्रिया; ऐश्चहाइम जोंडिक जांच; गर्भ-ज्ञान के लिये की जाने वाली मूत्र-जांच की एक पद्धति

**Azygos.** See **Azygous.**

**Azygous.** A term applied to single parts; azygos. अयुग्म; एकल (अंग);

ऐसे अंग जो जोड़े के रूप में नहीं रहते
**Azymic.** Not causing fermentation. अकिण्विक; अक्षोभक; अखमीरक
**Azymous.** Unfermented; unleavened. अकिण्वित; अखमीरित
**Azzle Tooth.** A molar tooth. चर्वणक; चर्वण-दन्त

# B

**Babe.** Baby; a newborn child. बाल; शिशु; बच्चा
**Babla.** See **Acacia Arabica.**
**Baby.** See **Babe.**
**Bacca.** A berry or berry-like fruit. बेर; पियारी; रसभरी जैसा एक रसीला फल
**Bacciform.** Shaped like a berry. बेर के आकार का; बेररूप
**Bacillaemia.** The presence of bacilli in the blood; bacillemia. दण्डाणुरक्तता; जीवाणुरक्तता; रक्त में दण्डाणुओं का होना
**Bacillar.** Resembling little rods or bacilli; bacillary. दण्डाणुवत्; दण्डाणु जैसा; जीवाणुवत्;
**Bacillary.** See **Bacillar.**
**Bacillemia.** See **Bacillaemia.**
**Bacilli.** Plural of **Bacillus.**
**Bacillicide.** A substance destroying bacilli. दण्डाणुनाशक; जीवाणुनाशक; दण्डाणुओं को नष्ट करने वाला पदार्थ
**Bacilliform.** Shaped like a bacillus. दण्डाणुरूप; जीवाणुरूप; दण्डाणु जैसी आकृति का
**Bacilliparous.** Producing bacilli. दण्डाणुजनक; जीवाणुजनक; दण्डाणुओं को जन्म देने वाला
**Bacillogenous.** Due to or producing bacillus. दण्डाणुजनक; जीवाणुजनक; दण्डाणु पैदा करने वाला या उसके कारण
**Bacillophobia.** A morbid fear of microbes. दण्डाणुभीति; जीवाणुभीति; दण्डाणुओं का भय
**Bacillum.** A stick; a rod. दण्ड; शलाका; छड़
**Bacilluria.** The presence of bacillus in the urine. दण्डाणुमेह; पेशाब में दण्डाणु जाना

**Bacillus.** Any of a large group of rod-shaped spore-bearing organisms. दण्डाणु; जीवाणु; शलाकाणु;
  **Acid-fast B.** (AFB), those resistant to acids. अम्लसह दण्डाणु;
  **B. Anthracis,** causing anthrax in men and animals. आंगारव्रण-दण्डाणु;
  **B. Leprae,** causing leprosy. कुष्ठाणु; कोढ़ उत्पन्न करने वाला दण्डाणु
**Back.** Hinder surface of the human body. पृष्ठ; पीठ; कमर; पीछे;
  **B.-ache,** pain in the lumbar region; lumbago. पृष्ठवेदना; कटिवेदना; कमरदर्द;
  **B.-bone,** the spinal column. मेरुदण्ड; रीढ़ की हड्डी
**Back-stroke of the heart.** The diastole of the heart. हृद्-अनुशिथिलन
**Backward.** Undeveloped; punny; stunted. अविकसित; मन्द; पिछड़ा हुआ
**Backwardness.** Incomplete development. अविकास; अपूर्ण विकास; मन्दता; पिछड़ापन;
  **Mental B.,** weakness of mind. मन्दबुद्धिता; मानसिक दुर्बलता;
  **Physical B.,** weakness of body. मन्दकायता; शरीरिक दुर्बलता
**Bacteraemia.** The presence of bacteria in the blood; bacteremia; bacteriemia. जीवाणुरक्तता
**Bacteremia.** See **Bacteraemia.**
**Bacteria.** Plural of **Bacterium.**
**Bacterial.** Relating to, or caused by bacteria. जीवाणुज; रोगाणुज; रोगाणुओं अथवा जीवाणुओं द्वारा उत्पत्ति होने सम्बन्धी अथवा उन द्वारा उत्पादित
**Bactericidal.** Destroying bacteria; germicide; bacteriocidal; bactericide. जीवाणुनाशी; जीवाणुनाशक; जीवाणुओं को नष्ट करने वाला
**Bactericide.** See **Bactericidal.**
**Bactericidin.** Antibody which kills bacteria. जीवाणुनाशिका; जीवाणुनाशक; जीवणुनाशी (प्रतिपिण्ड)
**Bacteriemia.** See **Bacteraemia.**
**Bacterin.** Vaccine made from a specific bacterium. जीवाणुविष; जीवाणु-विशेष से तैयार किया गया विष
**Bacteriocidal.** See **Bactericidal.**
**Bacteriogenic.** Caused by bacteria. जीवाणुजनित
**Bacteriogenous.** Producing bacteria. जीवाणुजनक; जीवाणुओं को जन्म देने वाला

**Bacterioid.** Similar to a rod or a bacterium; bacteroid. जीवाणुवत्

**Bacteriologic.** Relating to bacteria or to bacteriology; bacteriological. जीवाणु अथवा जीवाणुविज्ञान सम्बन्धी

**Bacteriological.** See **Bacteriologic.**

**Bacteriologist.** One who is skilled in the science of bacteriology. जीवाणुविज्ञानी; जीवाणुविज्ञानवेत्ता

**Bacteriology.** The science and study of bacteria. जीवाणुविज्ञान; जीवाणुओं का वैज्ञानिक अध्ययन

**Bacteriolysin.** A specific antibody developed in the blood by the action of any one bacterium and capable of causing the disintegration of the same bacterium. जीवाणुलायिका

**Bacteriolysis.** The disintegration of bacteria. जीवाणुलयन; जीवाणुनाश

**Bacteriolytic.** Pertaining to bacteriolysis. जीवाणुलयनी

**Bacteriophage.** Popular term for destruction of bacteria by filterpassing lysins, or by a parasite of parasites ultrasomes. जीवाणुभोजी; जीवाणुभक्षी

**Bacterioscopy.** The microscopic examination of the bacteria. जीवाणुदर्शन

**Bacteriosis.** A localized or generalised bacterial infection. जीवाणुविकृति

**Bacteriostasis.** Arrest or hindrance of bacterial growth. जीवाणुस्तम्भन; जीवाणुरोधन

**Bacteriostat.** An agent which arrests the bacterial growth; bacteristat. जीवाणुस्तम्भक; जीवाणुरोधक

**Bacteriostatic.** Relating to bacteriostasis. जीवाणुस्तम्भन अथवा जीवाणुरोधन सम्बन्धी

**Bacteristat.** See **Bacteriostat.**

**Bacterium.** Microscopic rod-shaped unicellular organisms in decomposing liquids. जीवाणु; दण्डाणु; शलाकाणु

**Bacteriuria.** The presence of bacteria in the urine. जीवाणुमेह; पेशाब में जीवाणुओं का विद्यमान रहना

**Bacteroid.** See **Bacterioid.**

**Baculiform.** Rod-shaped. दण्डाकार; दण्डोपम; शलाकाकार

**Baelz's Disease.** Progressive ulceration and ultimate destruction of the mucous glands of the lips. अधरश्लेष्मग्रन्थिव्रणता; बेल्ज रोग

**Bag.** A sac; a cell. थैली; थैला; कोशिका; कोश; पेटी;

**B. of water,** a sac in the animal bodies containing some fluids; a foetal membrane containing the liquor amnii. जलकोश; पानी की थैली

**Bagnio.** A bath-house. स्नानागार; a house of prostitution. वेश्यालय

**Balance.** An apparatus for weighing substances. तुला; तराजू; harmonious adjustment of the related parts. संतुलन

**Balanic.** Pertaining to the glans penis or the clitoridis. शिश्नमुण्ड अथवा भगशिश्निका सम्बन्धी

**Balanitis.** Inflammation of the glans penis. शिश्नमुण्डशोथ; लिंगाग्रप्रदाह; लिंगमुण्डशोथ

**Balanoblenorrhea.** See **Balanoblenorrhoea.**

**Balanoblenorrhoea.** Gonorrhoeal balanitis; balanoblenorrhea. गोजोजन्य शिश्नमुण्डशोथ; लिंगमुण्ड का सूजाकी प्रदाह

**Balanoplasty.** Plastic surgery of the glans penis. शिश्नमुण्डसंधान; लिंगमुण्डसंधान

**Balanoposthitis.** Inflammation of the prepuce. शिश्नमुण्डच्छदशोथ

**Balanopreputial.** Relating to the glans penis and the prepuce. शिश्नमुण्डच्छदीय; लिंगमुण्डच्छदीय; लिंगमुण्ड एवं लिंगच्छद सम्बन्धी

**Balanorrhagia.** See **Balanorrhoea.**

**Balanorrhea.** See **Balanorrhoea.**

**Balanorrhoea.** False gonorrhoea; purulent balanitis; balanorrhagia; balanorrhea. पूतित शिश्नमुण्डशोथ; सपूय लिंगमुण्डप्रदाह; कूटसूजाक; लिंगमुण्ड का सपूय प्रदाह

**Balanus.** The glans of the penis or clitoridis. शिश्नमुण्ड अथवा भगशिश्निकामुण्ड

**Balbuties.** Stammering. हकलाना; तुतलाना

**Bald.** Without hair; affected with alopecia; alopecic. खल्वाट; केशहीन; गंजा

**Baldness.** Alopecia; absence of hair. खल्वाटता; खालित्य; केशहीनता; गंजापन

**Ball-and-socket joint.** A synovial, free movable joint; diarthrosis. चलसन्धि; स्वच्छन्दगतिक जोड़

**Ballismus.** A tremor. कम्पन; choreic movements. लास्य; नर्तन गतियाँ

**Ballooning.** Distension of a cavity. विस्फार; विस्फारण; फुलाव

**Ballottement.** Testing for a floating object, especially used to diagnose pregnancy. गर्भप्रतिलोठन

**Balm.** A soothing application or ointment. लेप; मरहम; महलम; मल कर आराम पहुँचाने वाली दवा

**Balneation.** The act of bathing. स्नानकार्य

**Balneology.** The science of baths and bathing. स्नानविज्ञान

**Balneotherapy.** The treatment of any disease by baths; water-cure. जल-चिकित्सा; स्नानोपचार; जलोपचार

**Balneum.** A bath. स्नान;

B. Aranae, A sand-bath. मरु-स्नान; बालुकास्नान;

B. Luteum, a mud-bath. मृदा-स्नान

**Balsam.** A compound of an oleoresin with benzoic or cinnamic acid; balsumum. बालसम; सुगन्धित लेप; अर्धठोस घोल

**Balsumum.** See **Balsam.**

**Band.** A strip. बन्धनी; पट्टी; पट्टा; फीता; बन्ध; तस्मा; बांधने की पतली पट्टीनुमा वस्तु

**Bandage.** A piece of cloth or other material for dressing wounds, such as dislocations, etc. पट्टी; पट्टी बांधना; पट्टी करना;

Circular B., that turns about the parts. वृत्ताकार पट्टी;

Compression B., especially used to give support without constriction of vessels. सम्पीडन पट्टी;

Elastic B., especially useful for varicose veins. प्रत्यास्थ पट्टी; लचीली पट्टी;

Oblique B., covering the part by oblique turns. बक्र पट्टी; तिर्यक पट्टी; तिरछी पट्टी;

Roller B., a strip of material, of variable width, rolled into a compact cylinder to facilitate its application. लपेट पट्टी;

Spiral B., each turn covering one-half of the preceding. सर्पिल पट्टी;

Suspensory B., applied so, that it supports and suspends the scrotum. निलम्बी पट्टी;

Triangular B., useful for arm slings. त्रिकोणी पट्टी; त्रिकोणीय पट्टी

**Bandy-leg.** A leg in which the bones are curved outward or inward; bowleg. बक्र-जंघा; धनुर्जंघा; धनुष जैसी आकृति की जांघ या टांग

**Bang.** See **Bhang.**

**Bang's Disease.** Malta fever; an infection causing abortion in animals and a feverish disease in man. माल्टा ज्वर; बैंग रोग

**Bangue.** See **Bhang.**

**Baptorrhea.** Gonorrhoea; baptorrhoea. प्रमेह; सूजाक

**Baptorrhoea.** See **Baptorrhea.**

**Bar.** A rod. दण्ड; छड़; शलाका; सलाख़; डण्डा

**Baragnosis.** Loss of sense of the weight or pressure. भारज्ञानाभाव; दाबज्ञानाभाव; भार अथवा दाब महसूस करने की अक्षमता

**Barber's Itch.** See **Tinea Barbae** and **Sycosis.**

**Barbiturate.** A class of sedative drugs based on barbituric acid. बार्बिटुरेट

**Baresthesia.** Pressure sense. दाबज्ञान

**Baresthesiometer.** An instrument for testing the sense of pressure. दाबज्ञानमापीयंत्र

**Baric.** Pertaining to, or containing barium. बेरियम सम्बन्धी; बेरियमयुक्त

**Barium.** A metal of the alkaline group. बेरियम; क्षारीय वर्ग की एक धातु

**Bark.** The outer cortical cover of the woody parts of a plant, tree or shrub. छाल; वल्क;

    **Jesuits' B.,** cinchona. कुनीन; पेरू;

    **Peruvian B.,** the cinchona bark. कुनीन छाल; पेरू छाल

**Barley.** A cereal used for food. जौ; यव;

    **B. Water,** a nutritious drink made of an infusion of barley. यवरस; जौ का पानी

**Barlow's Disease.** Infant's scurvy which results from exclusive feeding on propriety foods, condensed milk or any food deficient in vitamins. शिशुशीतादरोग

**Baroceptor.** See **Baroreceptor.**

**Baromacrometer.** An instrument for weighing and measuring new-born infants. शिशुमापीयंत्र; नवजातमापीयंत्र

**Barometer.** An instrument for measuring air-pressure. वायुदाबमापी; वायुदाबमापकयंत्र; वायुदाब को मापने का यंत्र

**Barophilic.** Thriving under high environmental pressure. वायुदाबप्रेमी

**Baroreceptor.** A sensory nerve ending that is stimulated by changes in pressure; baroceptor; pressoreceptor. दाबग्राही

**Baroscope.** An instrument for indicating the variations of atmospheric pressure. वायुदाबदर्शीयंत्र; अतिसंवेदी वायुदाबमापी

**Barotaxis.** Reaction of living tissue to changes in pressure. वायुदाबन्यासी

**Barotrauma.** Injury due to trauma in atmospheric or water pressure. दाब-अभिघात

**Barrel-bellied.** Having a large belly. पीपा-उदर; ढोल-उदर; तोंदू

**Barrel-chest.** A globular form of thorax. ढोल-वक्ष

**Barrel-shaped.** Of the form of a barrel. पीपाकार; पीपे जैसा; ढोलाकार

**Barren.** Sterile; incapable of producing offspring; unfruitful. बंध्या; बांझ

**Barrenness.** Sterility; inability to conceive offspring; unfruitfulness. बंध्यता; बांझपन

**Barrier Nursing.** A method of preventing the spread of infection from an infectious patient to others in an open ward. संक्रमणरोधी परिचर्या

**Bartholin's Duct.** The largest of the ducts of the sublingual gland. बार्थोलिन नली

**Bartholin's Glands.** Two small glands situated at each side of the external orifice of the vagina. बार्थोलिन ग्रन्थियाँ

**Bartholinian Abscess.** The abscess of the Bartholin's glands. बार्थोलिन ग्रंथि-विद्रधि

**Bartholinitis.** Inflammation of the Bartholin's glands. बार्थोलिनग्रन्थिशोथ; बार्थोलिनग्रन्थियों का प्रदाह

**Baruria.** High specific gravity of the urine. अतिविशिष्टमूत्रगुरुत्व; मूत्र का प्रवृद्ध आपेक्षिक गुरुत्व

**Baryecoia.** Deafness; dullness of hearing. बधिरता; बहरापन; कम सुनाई देना

**Barylalia.** Thickness of speech. अस्पष्टवाक्

**Baryphonia.** Difficulty of speech. वाग्कष्ट; बोलने में कठिनाई

**Baryta.** Protoxide of barium. हरिजा; बैराइटा; एक विषैला क्षार

**Basal.** Pertaining to, or situated nearer the base of, an organ; basial. आधारी; आधारिक

**Basaloma.** See **Basiloma.**

**Basculation.** The replacement of a retroverted uterus by swinging it into its place. गर्भाशय-पुनर्स्थापन

**Base.** The lower part. आधार; निचला भाग; chief substance of a mixture. प्रमुख औषधि

**Basedow's Disease.** Exophthalmic goitre. नेत्रोत्सेधी गलगण्ड

**Basement.** Base. आधार; निचला भाग

**Basfond.** Fundus; the base of the bladder. मूत्राशयाधार

**Bashful.** Shy; shamefaced. शर्मीला; सलज; लजीला; लज्जाशील

**Basial.** See **Basal.**

**Basiarachnitis.** Inflammation at the base of the skull; basiarachnoiditis. आधारीजालतानिकाशोथ; करोटिमूल का प्रदाह

**Basiarachnoiditis.** See **Basiarachnitis.**

**Basic.** Having properties opposite to acid. सौम्य; अनम्ल; fundamental. आधारी; आधारिक; मूल; relating to a base. आधार सम्बन्धी;

   B. **Salt,** a salt largely basic in nature. आधारी लवण

**Basicranial.** Relating to the base of the skull. कपालाधारीय; कपालाधार सम्बन्धी;

   B. **Axis,** a line from the basin to the middle of the anterior border of the cerebral surface of the shpenoid bone. कपालाधार-अक्ष

**Basil.** A sacred fragrant aromatic plant called Tulsi. तुलसी

**Basilar.** Pertaining to the base, as of the skull. आधारी; आधारिक; मूल;

   B. **Artery,** the artery at the base of the brain. आधारी धमनी;

   B. **Membrane,** the delicate membrane of the cochlea. आधारी कला

**Basilemma.** The basement membrane. आधारी कला

**Basiloma.** A tumour of the basilar cell; basaloma. आधारीकोशिकार्बुद; आधारिक कोशिका की रसौली

**Basin.** A circular desk, wider than its depth. धानी; छिछली रकावी; the pelvis. वस्तिगह्वर; the third ventricle of the brain. मस्तिष्क का तृतीय निलय

**Basioccipital.** The bone forming the central axis of the skull. आधारपश्चकपालीय;

   B. **Bone,** the basilar process. आधारपश्चकपालास्थि

**Basis.** The base. आधार; मूलाधार; the principal remedy. प्रमुख औषधि;

   B. **Cordis,** the base of the heart. हृदाधार;

   B. **Cranii,** the base of the skull. करोटि आधार;

   B. **Pulmonis,** the base of the lung. फुप्फुसाधार

**Basisphenoid.** The base of sphenoid bone. आद्यआधारकजतूक; कपाल की एक अस्थि विशेष

**Basophil.** Readily stained with basic dyes; basophile. क्षाररागी; बेसरागी; क्षार रंगों से शीघ्र रंगी जाने वाली कोशिकायें

**Basophile.** See **Basophil.**

**Basophilia.** Increase of basophils in the blood; basophilism. क्षाररागिता; बेसरागिता; रक्त में क्षाररागियों की अधिकता

**Basophilic.** Relating to basophilia; basophilous. क्षाररागीय; बेसरागीय; क्षाररागिता सम्बन्धी; बेसरागिता सम्बन्धी

**Basophilism.** See **Basophilia.**

**Basophilous.** See **Basophilic.**

**Basophobia.** Emotional inability to walk or stand. चलने-फिरने या खड़े रहने की असमर्थता; abnormal fear of walking. भ्रमणातंक; भ्रमणभीति

**Basophobiac.** One afflicted with basophobia. चलने-फिरने या खड़े रहने में असमर्थ; relating to basophobia. भ्रमणांतक सम्बन्धी

**Bath.** The immersion of the body or any part of it into water or any fluid. स्नान; नहाना; शरीर को जल से साफ करना;

Acid B., one containing nitric acid and hydrochloric acid. अम्लजल-स्नान; अम्लयुक्त जल से नहाना;

Air B., one with free exposure to air and the use of, but little water. वात-स्नान;

Alcohol B., one in dilute alcohol for fever-patients. सुरासार-स्नान; मद्यसार-स्नान;

Alkaline B., a bath containing potassium or sodium. क्षारजल-स्नान;

Bran B., one containing boiled bran. चोकरजल-स्नान;

Cold B., bath water at a temperature of $65°$ F, or $18.3°$c. शीतल जल-स्नान;

Half-b., see **Sitz Bath.**

Hip-b., see **Sitz Bath.**

Mud B., one containing mineral earth. मृदा-स्नान;

Russian B., a vapoured bath. वाष्प-स्नान;

Sand B., immersion in hot sand. बालुका-स्नान;

Sitz B., immersion of the buttocks and hips: half-bath; hip-bath. कटि-स्नान; नितम्ब-स्नान

**Bathophobia.** A morbid fear of depths. अतिगम्यतातंक; गहरे स्थानों का भय

**Bathyanaesthesia.** Loss of deep sensibility; bathyanesthesia. गहन असंवेदनता

**Bathyanesthesia.** See **Bathyanaesthesia.**

**B.C.G.** Bacillus Calmette Guerin, a vaccine prepared from bovine tubercle bacilli. यक्ष्मारोधक टीका; क्षयरोधक टीका

**B.D.** Bis in die; two times a day. दिन में दो बार

**Beaker.** A wide mouthed or lipped cylindrical glass vessel. बीकर; चषक

**Beard.** Hair of the lower face. दाढ़ी

**Beard's Disease.** Neurasthenia; nervous exhaustion. तंत्रिकावसाद; स्नायुदौर्बल्य

**Bearing-down.** Labour-like sensation. प्रवहण-प्रयत्न; प्रसव-तुल्य; प्रसव वेदना जैसी अनुभूति

**Beat.** Rhythm, as of pulse, heart, etc. स्पन्द; स्पन्दन; क्षेप; ताल; धड़कन;

**Apex B.,** the heart-apex stroke against the chest-wall. हृदग्र-स्पन्द;

**Heart B.,** a complete cardiac cycle, including spread of the electrical impulse and the consequent mechanical contraction. हृत्स्पन्द

**Bed.** A couch or support for the body. शय्या; शयन; बिस्तर; बिस्तरा; क्षेत्र; कक्षा; संस्तर;

**B.-bug,** the insect Cimex lectularius, that infests body. खटमल;

**B.-pan,** a vessel for receiving the excreta from bed-patients. शय्यामलपात्र; पलंग पर टट्टी-पेशाब कराने का बर्तन;

**B.-wetting,** involuntary escape of urine during sleep. शय्यामूत्रण; निद्रामूत्रण; नींद में पेशाब कर देना;

**Capillary B.,** the capillaries considered collectively and their volume capacity. केशिका-शय्या;

**Nail B.,** the skin at the tip of digit that lies beneath a nail. नख-शय्या

**Beef.** The flesh of cattle. गोमांस; पशु-मांस;

**B.-tea,** an infusion of beef. गोशोरबा

**Beer's Knife.** A delicate instrument with triangular blade used in cataract operation for incision of cornea. स्वच्छपटलछेदक

**Beeswax.** Cera. मोम; मधुमोम

**Beet.** A carrot-like sweet vegetable.

**Behavior.** See **Behaviour.**

**Behaviour.** In general sense, conduct. As a psychological term, means response to an organism to its situation in relation to its environment; behavior. व्यवहार; आचरण; बर्ताव

**Behavioural.** Pertaining to behaviour. स्वभाव सम्बन्धी

**Behaviourism.** A psychological term which denotes an approach to psychology through the study of responses and reactions. आचरणवाद; व्यवहारशीलता; आचरणशीलता

**Bejel.** Non-venereal syphilis. अरतिज उपदंश

**Belching.** The throwing off, or ejecting of wind from the stomach. डकार; उबकाई

**Belladonna.** A poisonous plant used as an anodyne and antispasmodic; night-shade. बेलाडौना; अंगूरशेफा; सागअंगूर; मकोग

**Bell's Mania.** Acute delirium. उग्र प्रलाप; acute periencephalitis. उग्र प्रमस्तिष्कशोथ

**Bell's Palsy.** See **Bell's Paralysis.**

**Bell's Paralysis.** Peripheral paralysis of the facial nerve; Bell's palsy. आननतंत्रिकाघात; चेहरे की नाड़ी का परिसरीय पक्षाघात

**Belly.** The abdomen; the venter. पेट; उदर; तोंद; पिण्ड;

  **B.-ache,** pain in the abdomen. उदरशूल; पेटदर्द;

  **B.-belt,** see **Abdominal Belt** under **Belt.**

  **B. of a muscle,** fleshy part of a muscle. पेशी-पिण्ड; किसी पेशी का मांसल भाग

**Belonephobia.** Dread of pins, needles or pointed things. नोकभीति; नुकीली चीजों का डर

**Belonoid.** Needle-shaped. सूच्याकार; सुई के आकार जैसा

**Belt.** Encircling strip worn round the waist to support clothes or weapons. पेटी; कटिबन्ध; कमरपट्टा;

  **Abdominal B.,** an elastic support used in pregnancy; belly-belt. उदरपेटी

**Bend.** A curve. मोड़; बंक; झुकाव; घुमाव

**Benedict's Solution.** A solution of copper sulphate which is easily reduced, producing colour changes and used to detect the presence of glucose. बेनीडिक्ट घोल

**Beng.** A name for **Cannabis Indica;** bang; bhang. भांग

**Benign.** Mild; not malignant. सौम्य; सुदम; सुदम्य; मृदु; साध्य; कोमल; हल्का;

  **B. Tumour,** one that has no tendency to recur after removal; benignant; beninus. सुदम अर्बुद; सौम्य अर्बुद; मृदु अर्बुद

**Benignant. See Benign.**

**Beninus. See Benign.**

**Bent-knee.** Knock-knee. बक्रजानु

**Benzene.** A colourless, inflammable liquid obtained from coal-tar and extensively used as a solvent. उदांगर; धूपरस; बेन्जीन

**Benzion.** A resinous substance, dry and brittle, obtained from a large tree of Java, Sumatra, etc. लोबान; धूना; राल; बेंजाइन

**Berberis.** A genus of shrubs called **Daru Haridra.** दारू-हरिद्रा; **B. Asiatica,** the medicinal extract from the root known as Rassout. दारू-हल्दी

**Beri-Beri.** A disease characterized by weakness, anaemia, dropsy, dyspnoea and paraplegia due to lack of vitamins in diet. वात बलासक; बेरी-बेरी; भोजन में विटामिनों, खास तौर से विटामिन B की कमी से होने वाला रोग

**Bernard's Canal.** The accessory duct of the pancreas. अग्न्याशयनली; क्लोमग्रन्थि की सहायक नली

**Bestial Form.** Resembling an animal. पशुरूप; पशुवत्; जानवर से मिलता-जुलता

**Bestiality.** Sexual intercourse with animals. पशुगमन; पशुसम्भोग; तिर्यग्योनिगमन

**Beverage.** Drink. पेय; शराब अथवा शर्बत

**Bhang.** A name of Cannabis Indica; bang; bangue. भांग

**Biarticular.** Relating to two joints; diarthric; diarthicular. द्विसन्धिपरक; दो जोड़ों सम्बन्धी

**Biaxial.** Having two axes. द्विअक्षी; दो अक्ष वाला

**Bibulous.** Having the property of absorbing water. अवशोषी; जलचूषक; जलशोषक

**Bicapitate.** Having two heads. द्विशिरस्क; दो सिर वाला; द्विशिरीय

**Bicapsular.** Having two capsules. द्विसम्पुटी; दो सम्पुट वाला

**Bicaudal. See Bicaudate.**

**Bicaudate.** Having two tails; bicaudal. द्विपुच्छी; दो पूँछ वाला

**Bicellular.** Having two cells. द्विकोशिकी; दो कोशिकाओं वाला

**Bicentric.** Having two centres. द्विकेन्द्रिक; दो केन्द्रों वाला

**Bicephalic. See Bicephalous.**

**Bicephalous.** Having two heads; bicephalic. द्विशिरस्क; द्विशिरीय;

द्विमस्तिष्की; दो सिर वाला

**Biceps.** Two-headed; applied to muscles. द्विशिरस्की; द्विशिरस्क (पेशी); दो निकासों वाली

**Bicipital.** Relating to the biceps muscle. द्विशिरस्कीय; द्विमूलपेशीय

**Bicollis.** Having two necks. द्विग्रीवी; दो गर्दन वाला

**Biconcave.** Concave or hollow on both surfaces. द्विअवतली; उभयावतल; दो कूब वाला

**Biconvex.** Rounded or convex on both surfaces. उभयोत्तल; द्विउत्तल; द्विउन्नत्तोदर

**Bicornate.** See **Bicornuate.**

**Bicornuate.** Having two horns; bicornate; bicornus. द्विशृंगी; दो सींगों वाला

**Bicornus.** See **Bicornuate.**

**Bicuspid.** Having two joints, cusps, points or fangs, as teeth. द्विकस्पी; द्विमूल; द्विकपर्दी; द्विअग्री; द्विवलनी;

   **B. Teeth,** the premolars. द्विकस्पीदंत; अग्रचर्वणक दंत;

   **B. Valve,** the mitral valve between the left atrium and ventricle of the heart. द्विकपर्दी कपाट

**B.I.D.** Bis in die; two times a day; B.D. दिन में दो बार

**Bidactyly.** See **Bidigital.**

**Bidigital.** With two fingers; bidactlyly. द्वयंगुलिता; द्वि-अंगुलिता

**Biennial.** Occurring every two years. द्विवर्षी; द्विवार्षिक; दो वर्ष में प्रकट होने वाला

**Bifid.** Cleft; divided into two; forked; bifida. द्विशाखी; द्विखण्डी; द्विभिद्; द्विशिख; द्विभक्त;

   **B. Spine,** spina bifida; congenital defect in the walls of the spinal canal. द्विमेरुता;

   **B. Tongue,** one cleft longitudinally. द्विजिह्वी

**Bifida.** The same as **Bifid.**

   **Spina B.,** see **Bifid Spine.**

**Bifidous.** The same as **Bifid.**

**Bifocal.** With a double focus, as a lens. द्विकेन्द्रबिन्दुक, जैसे ऐनक का लेंस

**Bifurcate.** See **Bifurcated.**

**Bifurcated.** Divided into two branches; bifurcate. द्विशाखित; द्विशाखी;

# Bifurcation

दो शाखाओं में विभाजित

**Bifurcation.** A forking; a division into two branches. द्विशिखरण; द्विशाखन; द्विविभाजन

**Bigaster.** Having two bellies, as a muscle. द्वितुन्दी

**Bilateral.** Two-sided; having equal sides; pertaining to two sides. द्विपार्श्वी; द्विपार्श्विक; द्विपार्श्वीय; दुतरफा

**Bile.** The yellowish brown or green fluid secreted by the liver. पित्त; यकृत् का वह स्राव जिसका कार्य पाचन तथा विसर्जन दोनों होता है;

B. **Acids,** acids formed in the liver; biliary acids. पित्ताम्ल;

B. **Cyst,** gall-bladder. पित्ताशय;

B. **Ducts,** the hepatic and cystic ducts, which join to form common bile duct. पित्तनलियाँ;

B. **Pigment,** the colouring matter of the bile. पित्तवर्णक

**Bilharzia.** A genus of trematode worms or flukes. बिलहार्जिया; पर्णकृमियों की एक जाति

**Bilharziasis.** Infection by bilharzia; bilharziosis. बिलहार्जियारुग्णता

**Bilharziosis.** See **Bilharziasis.**

**Biliary.** Pertaining to the bile. पैत्तिक; पित्तज; पित्त सम्बन्धी;

B. **Acids,** see **Bile Acids.**

B. **Calculus,** a gall-bladder stone. पित्ताश्मरी; पित्तपथरी;

B. **Colic,** colic from the passage of gall-stone. पित्तशूल;

B. **Duct,** one of the ducts communicating with the liver. पित्तनली;

B. **Fistula,** an abnormal track conveying bile to the suface or to some other organs. पित्तनालव्रण

**Biliation.** Bile-secretion; the excretion of bile. पित्तस्राव

**Bilification.** The formation of bile. पित्तरचना

**Biligenesis.** Bile-production. पित्तजनन; पित्तोत्पादन

**Biligenic.** Bile-producing. पित्तजनक; पित्तोत्पादक

**Bilihumin.** A brown bile-pigment. कपिश-पित्तवर्णक;

**Bilious.** Partaking of the nature of bile. पैत्तिक; पित्तज; पित्तात्मक;

B. **Fever,** fever with vomiting of bile. पित्तज्वर

**Biliousness.** The condition marked by constipation, headache and anorexia due to excess of bile. अतिपित्तता; पित्ताधिक्य; पित्त की बढ़ी हुई मात्रा

**Bilirachia.** Bile in the spinal fluid. मेरुद्रव्यपित्तता

**Bilirubin.** A pigment largely derived from the breakdown of haemoglobin from red blood cells destroyed in the spleen. रक्तिम-पित्तवर्णक; बिलीरुबिन

**Bilirubinaemia.** Bilirubin in the blood; bilirubinemia. रक्तिमपित्तवर्णकता; बिलीरूबिनता

**Bilirubinemia.** See **Bilirubinaemia.**

**Bilirubinuria.** Bilirubin in the urine. रक्तिमपित्तवर्णकमेह; पेशाब में रक्तिमपित्तवर्णक जाना

**Biliuria.** The presence of bile pigments in the urine. पित्तवर्णकमेह; पित्तमेह; पित्तमूत्रण; पेशाब में पित्तवर्णक जाना

**Biliverdin.** The green pigment of the bile; biliverdine. हरित पित्तवर्णक

**Biliverdine.** See **Biliverdin.**

**Bilobate.** Having two lobes; bilobed; bilobete. द्विदली; द्विखण्डी; दो खण्डों वाला

**Bilobed.** See **Bilobate.**

**Bilobete.** See **Bilobate.**

**Bilobular.** Having two little lobes or lobules. द्विखण्डी; द्विखण्डीय; दो छोटे-छोटे खण्डों वाला

**Bilocular.** Having two cells or compartments; biloculate. द्विकोष्ठकीय; द्विकोशिकी; द्विकोशिकीय; द्विकोटरी; द्विकोटरीय; दो कोष्ठों, कोशिकाओं अथवा कोटरों वाला

**Biloculate.** See **Bilocular.**

**Bimana.** Two handed animals. द्विहस्त (जन्तु); दो हाथों वाला जन्तु

**Bimanous.** Having two hands. द्विहस्त; दो हाथों वाला; द्विहस्ती

**Bimanual.** Two-handed; with the help of both the hands; ambidextrous. द्विहस्तक; उभयहस्त; दोनों हाथों से

**Bimastoid.** Relating to the mastoid eminences. द्विकर्णमूलक

**Binary.** Dual or involving pairs; compounded of two elements. द्वियंगी; द्विवर्णी; युग्मक; द्विभागी

**Binaural.** Pertaining to, or having two ears; binotic. द्विश्रोत्री; द्विकर्णी; दो कानों सम्बन्धी अथवा दो कानों वाला

**Binder.** A broad bandage, especially one encircling the abdomen. उदरपट्टी

**Binet's Test.** A series of graded intelligence test in which an individual's level (mental age) is compared with his chronological

**Binocular**

age. बाइनेट जांच; मनःकायविश्लेषण

**Binocular.** Pertaining to, or adapted to both eyes. द्विनेत्री; द्विनेत्रीय; दोनों आँखों सम्बन्धी;

**B. Vision,** normal vision with both eyes. उभय दृष्टि; दोनों आँखों की सामान्य दृष्टि

**Binoculus.** An 'X' shaped bandage for both eyes. 'X' आकार की पट्टी, जिसे आँखों पर लगाया जाता है

**Binotic.** See **Binaural.**

**Binovular.** Derived from two separate ova. द्विडिम्बी; द्विडिम्बज

**Bio-.** Prefix meaning life. 'जैव' तथा 'जीव' के रूप में प्रयुक्त उपसर्ग

**Biochemic.** Pertaining to biochemistry; biochemical. जीवरसायनिक; जीवरसायनशास्त्र सम्बन्धी

**Biochemical.** See **Biochemic.**

**Biochemistry.** The chemistry of living tissues. जीवरसायनशास्त्र; जीवरसायन; जीवरसायनविद्या; जीवरसायनविज्ञान

**Biocidal.** Destructive to life, particularly relating to microorganisms. जीवनाशक; प्राणनाशक; घातक; मारक

**Biodynamics.** The science of vital forces. जीवशक्तिविज्ञान; जैवगतिकी; जीवगतिविज्ञान

**Biogen.** See **Bioplasm.**

**Biogenesis.** Begetting living beings by living beings. जीवात्जीवोत्पत्ति; परतन्त्रोत्पत्ति; जीव जीवों से ही पैदा होते हैं (मत)

**Biogenetic.** Relating to biogenesis. जीवज; जीवात्जीवोत्पत्ति सम्बन्धी

**Biokinetics.** The science treating of the movements of the living organisms. जीवगतिविज्ञान; सजीव प्राणियों की गतियों सम्बन्धी विज्ञान

**Biologic.** See **Biological.**

**Biological.** Pertaining to biology; biologic. जीव; जैवी; जैव; जैविक

**Biologist.** One versed in biology. जीवविज्ञानी

**Biology.** The science of life and living things. जीवविज्ञान; जैविकी

**Biolysis.** The destruction of life. जीवलयन; जैवलयन; जैव-अपघटन; death. मृत्यु

**Biolytic.** Tending to destroy life. जीवलयी; जैवलयी; जीवनाशक

**Biometer.** An instrument for measuring life-sounds. जीवध्वनिमापी; जैवध्वनिमापक यंत्र

**Biometric.** Relating to the measurement of life; biometrical.

जीवमितीय; जीवमितिक
**Biometrical.** See **Biometric**.
**Biometry.** The measurement of life. जीवमिति; जीवमापन (शास्त्र)
**Bionomics.** The science of the laws of life; bionomy. जीवपारिस्थितिकी
**Bionomy.** See **Bionomics**.
**Biophysicist.** One versed in biophysics. जीवभौतिकविज्ञानी
**Biophysics.** The physics of life processes. जीवभौतिकी; जीवनदायी प्रक्रियाओं की भौतिकी
**Bioplasm.** Any living matter; biogen. प्राणी; जीव
**Bioplast.** A cell of bioplasm. जीवकोशिका; जैव-कण
**Diopsy.** Observation of the livings. जीवोति-जांच; जीवित ऊतकों की जांच
**Bioscience.** The science of living beings. जीवशास्त्र; जीवविज्ञान
**Bioscopy.** The examination of the body to see the presence or absence of life. जीवदर्शन; शारीरिक जांच
**Biosocial.** Involving the interplay of biological and social influences. जीवसामाजिक
**Biostatics.** Physics and mechanics of the living bodies. जीवसांख्यिकी
**Biotic.** Pertaining to the life; vital. जैवी; जैविक; जीवनी; जीवन सम्बन्धी
**Biotics.** The science of vital functions and manifestations. जैविकी; सजीवलक्षणविज्ञान
**Biotomy.** Vivisection. अंगोच्छेदन; अंग-उच्छेदन
**Biotoxicology.** The study of poisons produced by living organisms. जीवविषविज्ञान; जीवजनित विषों का वैज्ञानिक अध्ययन
**Biotype.** Individuals with similar fundamental or common characteristics. समयुग्मी; समान गठन वाले व्यक्तियों का समूह
**Biparietal.** Relating to both the parietal bones. द्विपार्श्विकास्थिक; द्विपार्श्विकी
**Biparous.** Producing two offsprings at one birth. युग्मजन; द्विप्रसू; यमलजनक; एक बार में दो बच्चे जनने वाली (स्त्री)
**Bipartite.** Consisting of two portions. द्विभाजित; द्विभागीय; दो भागों में विभाजित
**Biped.** Having two feet. द्विपादी; द्विपाद; दोपाया
**Bipotentiality.** The capability or differentiating along two developmental pathways. द्विविभाविता
**Biramous.** Having two branches. द्विशाखी

**Birefrigence.** Double refraction. द्विगुण-अपवर्तन

**Birth.** Parturition; the delivery of a child. जन्म; प्रसव; प्रजनन;

   **Cross B.,** premature labour with foetus lying transversely. अनुप्रस्थ प्रसव;

   **Dead B.,** one without life; still-birth. मृतजात; मृतप्रसव; मृतजन्म;

   **Live B.,** having taken birth with sound respiration. जीवित जन्म; सप्राण प्रसव;

   **Premature B.,** one occurring after the 7th month of pregnancy but before term. अकाल जन्म; अकाल प्रसव; कालपूर्व जन्म;

   **Still-b.,** see **Dead Birth;**

   **B. Canal,** the cavity or canal of the pelvis through which the baby passes during labour. गर्भनली;

   **B. Certificate,** a legal document given in registration within a specific period of birth. जन्म प्रमाण-पत्र;

   **B. Control,** prevention or regulation of conception by any means; contraception. गर्भ-नियंत्रण; गर्भ-निरोध;

   **B. Defect,** any congenital deformity. जन्म-दोष;

   **B. Injury,** any injury occurring during parturition. जन्म-क्षति; प्रसव-क्षति;

   **B. Mark,** naevus. जन्म-चिन्ह; तिल; न्यच्छ

**Bische.** Endemic dysentery in India. रक्तातिसार; पेचिश; आमातिसार

**Bisection.** The act of cutting into two. द्विविभाजन; दो भागों में काट देना

**Bisexual.** Having the characteristics of both sexes. उभयलिंगी; द्विलिंगी; पुरुष तथा स्त्री दोनों लिंगों की चारित्रिक विशेषताओं से युक्त

**Bis in Die.** See **B.D.** or **B.I.D.**

**Bismuth.** A reddish-white metal whose salts may be found in hair dyes; Bismuthum. बिस्मथ; कसकुट; कांसा

**Bismuthosis.** Chronic bismuth-poisoning. जीर्णविस्मथविषण्णता

**Bismuthum.** See **Bismuth.**

**Bite.** Cut into or nip with the teeth, hence producing a wound. दंश; डंक; काटना; बुड़का मारना;

   **Insect B.,** that of wasps, bees, mosquitoes, etc. कीट-दंश

**Bitemporal.** Belonging to the two temples. द्विशंखी; कनपटियों सम्बन्धी

**Bitter.** Tasting like worm-wood or quinine. तिक्त; कड़वा

**Bitters.** A term for a medicine with a bitter taste. तिक्त-वर्ग; तिक्त-द्रव्य; तिक्तौषधि; कड़वी दवा

**Bitumen.** Mineral pitch. शिलाजीत

**Bivalence.** The state of being bivalent; bivalency. द्विसंयोजकता

**Bivalency.** See **Bivalence**.

**Bivalent.** Having a valence of two. द्विसंयोजक

**Bivalve.** Having two valves or blades. द्विकपाटी; द्विकृपर्दी

**Biventer.** A muscle with two bellies. द्विपिण्डपेशी

**Black.** An absence of light; a colour reflecting no light. श्याम; कृष्ण; काला;

    B. Blood, the venous blood. शिरा-रक्त;

    B. Fever, a bilious fever of Africa. श्याम-ज्वर, पित्त-ज्वर;

    B. Head, a worm-like cast formed of sebum; comedo. त्वक्कील;

    B. Measles, a malignant form of measles. कृष्ण विसर्प; काला खसरा; श्याम रोमांतिका

**Black-out.** A temporary or momentary blindness. अस्थायी-अंधता; क्षणिक-अंधता; संज्ञाशून्यता

**Black Water Fever.** A malignant form of malaria occurring in the tropics. कालामेह ज्वर; मलेरिया का एक सांघातिक रूप

**Bladder.** The membranous sac, situated in the anterior part of the pelvic cavity which serves as a reservoir of urine. आशय; वस्ति; मूत्राशय;

    Atonic B., large, dilated and non-emptying bladder. अतानिक आशय;

    Gall B., a pear-shaped bag on the under-surface of the liver. पित्ताशय;

    Urinary B., a muscular bag situated in the pelvis ; a reservoir for urine. मूत्राशय; मसाना; वस्ति

**Blade.** The leaf, or the flat part of the leaf of any part. फलक

**Blain.** A blister or pustule. फफोला; छाला

**Bland.** Non-irritating; gentle; mild. सौम्य; मृदु; कोमल

**Blastema.** A synonym of protoplasm. प्रसूकोशिकापुंज; a cluster of cells. कोशिकागुच्छ

**Blastemic.** Relating to the blastema. प्रसूकोशिकापुंज अथवा कोशिकागुच्छ सम्बन्धी

**Blastocele.** The cavity of a blastosphore; blastoceloma. बुद्बुदगुहा; फोरकगुहा

**Blastoceloma.** See **Blastocele.**

**Blastocyst.** The germinal vesicle; blastocystinx. बीजगुहा; बीजपुटी

**Blastocystinx.** See **Blastocyst.**

**Blastoderm.** Germinal membrane of an ovum; blastoderma. बीजजनस्तर; कोरकचर्म

**Blastoderma.** See **Blastoderm.**

**Blastoma.** A granular growth due to a micro-organism. प्रसू-अर्बुद; कणिका-गुल्म

**Blastomere.** One of the segments of the ovum after fecundation. प्रसूखण्ड; प्राथमिक कोशिका

**Blastopore.** The orifice of a blastula or a two-layered embryo. आंत्रकन्दराछिद्र; कोरकरन्ध्र

**Blastula.** The two-layered embryo. बुद्बुद; द्वि-अस्तरी भ्रूण; कोरक-कन्दुक

**Blastular.** Pertaining to the blastula. बुद्बुद अथवा द्वि-अस्तरी भ्रूण सम्बन्धी

**Bleaching Powder.** Calcium chloride; a disinfectant mixture. विरंचक चूर्ण; रंगकट चूर्ण; ब्लीचिंग पावडर; कैल्सियम क्लोराइड

**Bleardness.** Blurring. मन्दता; धुँधलापन

**Bleb.** A large blister; bulla. बुलबुला; छाला; फफोला

**Bleeder.** One who lets blood. रक्तस्रावक; रक्तस्रावी; रक्तस्रावशील; one who is suffering from haemophilia; (Bleeder's disease). रक्तस्राव अथवा हीमोफीलिया से पीड़ित

**Bleeder's Disease.** See **Haemophilia.**

**Bleeding.** Haemorrhage. रक्तस्राव; रक्तस्रवण; रक्तप्रवाह; खून बहना

**Blending.** Mixing various sorts of things. मिश्रण

**Blennadenitis.** Inflammation of the mucous follicles. श्लेष्मपुटकशोथ; श्लेष्मग्रन्थिशोथ

**Blennelytria.** Vaginal catarrh; leucorrhoea. प्रदर; श्वेतप्रदर

**Blennenteria.** See **Blennorrhoeria.**

**Blennogenic.** Secreting mucus; blennogenous; muciparous. श्लेष्मस्रावी; श्लेष्मज; श्लेष्मोत्पादी

**Blennogenous.** See **Blennogenic.**

**Blennoid.** Of the form of mucus; muciform. श्लेष्माभ; श्लेष्मवत्

**Blennometritis.** See **Endometritis.**

**Blennophthalmia.** Catarrhal conjunctivitis. प्रतिश्यायी नेत्रश्लेष्मलाशोथ; प्रतिश्यायी नेत्राभिष्यन्द

**Blennoptysis.** Mucous expectoration. श्लेष्मकफ; श्लैष्मिक बतगम

**Blennorrhagia.** Gonorrhoea; copious vaginal discharge. प्रमेह; सूजाक; योनि से होने वाला विपुल स्राव

**Blennorrhea.** Muco-purulent discharge from the eyes or vagina; blenorrhoea. श्लेष्मपूयस्राव; आँखों अथवा योनि से श्लेषमा और पीब बहना

**Blennorrheal.** Gonorrhoeal; blenorrhoeal. प्रमेहज; प्रमेह अथवा सूजाक सम्बन्धी

**Blenorrhoea.** See **Blanhorrhea.**

**Blenorrhoeal.** See **Blenorrheal.**

**Blennorrhoeria.** A mucous flow from the bowels; blennenteria. आमातिसार; आँवयुक्त पाखाना

**Blennuria.** The presence of mucus in the urine. श्लेष्ममेह; पेशाब में श्लेष्मा जाना

**Blephara.** Plural of **Blepharon.**

**Blepharadenitis.** Inflammation of the Meibomian glands; blepharoadenitis. वर्त्मग्रन्थिशोथ; पलकों की ग्रन्थियों का प्रदाह

**Blepharal.** Pertaining to the eyelids. वर्त्म अथवा पलकों सम्बन्धी

**Blepharectomy.** Excision of all or part of an eyelid. पलकोच्छेदन; वर्त्मोच्छेदन

**Blepharism.** Spasm of the eyelids. वर्त्माकर्ष; पलकों की उद्वेष्टता अथवा अकड़न

**Blepharitis.** Inflammation of the eyelids; blepharophthalmia. वर्त्मशोथ; वर्त्मान्तशोथ; पलकान्तशोथ; पलकों का प्रदाह

**Blepharoadenitis.** See **Blepharadenitis.**

**Blepharoadenoma.** Adenoma of the margins of eyelids. वर्त्मग्रन्थिशोथ; पलकों की ग्रन्थियों का प्रदाह

**Blepharochalasis.** Relaxation of the skin of eyelids. वर्त्ममृदुता; पलकों का ढीलापन

**Blepharoclonus.** Thickening of the eyelids. वर्त्मावमोटन; पलकें मोटी होना

**Blepharodiastasis.** Dilatation or protrusion of eyelids. वर्त्मविस्फार; पलकें फैलना

**Blepharon.** The eyelid; palpebra. वर्त्म; पलक; चक्षुपटल; पपोटा; नेत्रच्छद

**Blepharoncus.** A tumour of the eyelids. वर्त्मार्बुद; पलकों की रसौली

**Blepharophimosis.** Abnormal smallness of the palpebral opening. वर्त्मविदरसंकोच

**Blepharophthalmia.** See **Blepharitis.**

**Blepharoplast.** The centrosome in trypanosoma (a genus of parasitic flagellate protozoa). कशामूलक; अधोपिण्ड

**Blepharoplasty.** A plastic operation on the eyelid. वर्त्मसंधान; नेत्रच्छदसंधान; पलकसंधान

**Blepharoplegia.** See **Ptosis.**

**Blepharoptosis.** See **Ptosis.**

**Blepharospasm.** Spasm of the muscles of the eyelid; excessive winking. वर्त्माकर्ष; नेत्रच्छदाकर्ष; पलकों का उद्वेष्ट

**Blepharostenosis.** Narrowing of the interpalpebral opening. वर्त्मसंकीर्णता; पलकों की सिकुड़न

**Blepharotomy.** An incision into the eyelid. वर्त्मछेदन; नेत्रच्छदछेदन; पलकछेदन

**Blind.** Without sight; unable to see. दृष्टिहीन; अंधा; अंध;

   **B. Piles,** piles which do not bleed. वातार्श; सूखी बवासीर

**Blindness.** An absence of vision. दृष्टिहीनता; अन्धता; अन्धापन;

   **Blue B.,** an inability to distinguish a blue colour. नीलवर्णान्धता; नीला रंग पहचाने की असमर्थता;

   **Colour B.,** deficiency of colour perception. वर्णान्धता; रंगज्ञान-अल्पता;

   **Day B.,** partial blindness by day with better vision at night. दिवान्धता; दिनौंधी; दिन में दिखाई न देने का दोष;

   **Mental B.,** see **Psychic Blindness.**

   **Mind B.,** see **Psychic Blindness.**

   **Night B.,** normal vision by day, but subnormal at night; nyctalopia; nocturnal blindness. नक्तान्धता; रतौंधी; रात को न दिखाई देने का रोग;

   **Nocturnal B.,** see **Night Blindness.**

   **Object B.,** apraxia. वस्तु-अन्धता;

   **Psychic B.,** sight without recognition from brain lesion; mental blindness; mind blindness; soul blindness. मानसिक अन्धता; मनो-अन्धता;

   **Snow B.,** conjunctivitis from the glare of sunlight upon the snow. हिमान्धता;

   **Soul B.,** see **Psychic Blindness.**

   **Word B.,** inability to understand written or printed words; alexia. लेखान्धता; शब्दान्धता

**Blinking.** Momentary gleam or glimpses. निमेषण; वर्त्मस्वचलता; पलकों का अपने आप खुलना और बन्द होना

**Blister.** A collection of serum; bloody or watery fluid beneath the epidermis; a vesicle. फफोला; छाला

**Blistering.** Producing blister. फफोला पड़ना; छाला पड़ना

**Bloat.** See **Bloating.**

**Bloated.** Swelled. सूजा हुआ; फूला हुआ; उभरा हुआ

**Bloating.** Distension; swelling; bloat. फुलाव; उभार; सूजन

**Block.** A stoppage. रोध; बाधा; to obstruct. रुकावट डालना

**Blockade.** Arrest of transmission at autonomic synaptic junction, receptor sites or myoneural junctions. अवरोधन

**Blond.** Fair complexioned female; blonde. गौरवर्ण; गोरी; गौरी

**Blonde.** See **Blond.**

**Blood.** The red fluid circulating in the arteries, capillaries and veins. रक्त; खून; रुधिर; शोणित; लहू;

  **B. Bank,** a special refrigerator in which the blood is kept after withdrawal from donors, until required for transfusion. रक्त बैंक;

  **B. Casts,** casts of coagulated red blood corpuscles formed in the renal tubules and found in the urine. रक्तनिर्मोक; खून की पपड़ियाँ;

  **B. Cell,** a blood corpuscle. रक्त कोशिका; रक्त कणिका;

  **B. Clot,** a coagulum. रक्तातंच; खून का थक्का;

  **B. Corpuscles,** the cellular elements of the blood. रक्तकण; रक्तकणिकायें;

  **B. Count,** calculation of the number of red or white cells per cubic millimetre of blood. रक्तगणन;

  **B. Culture,** after withdrawal of blood from a vein it is incubated in suitable medium, at an optimum temperature, so that any contained organisms can multiply and so be isolated and identified under the microscope. रक्तसम्वर्ध;

  **B. Group,** the A.B.O. System. There are four groups A, B, AB and O. The cells of these groups contain the corresponding antigens A, B, AB, except group O cells which contains neither antigen A nor B. For this reason group O blood can be given to any of the other groups and is known as the universal donor. रक्तवर्ग; रुधिरवर्ग; रक्तसमूह;

  **B. Letting,** opening a vein; venesection; a term embracing every artificial discharge of blood. रक्तमोक्षण; खून निकालना;

**B. Plaques,** see **Blood Platelets.**

**B. Plasma,** the fluid portion of the blood. रक्तप्लाविका; रक्तरस;

**B. Platelets,** pale discs found in the blood; blood plaques; blood plates. रक्तबिम्बाणु;

**B. Plates,** see **Blood Platelets.**

**B. Poisoning,** absorption of toxins into the blood. रक्तविषण्णता;

**B. Pressure,** the force exerted by the blood upon the vessel walls. रक्तदाब; रक्तचाप;

**B. Red,** see **Blood Shot.**

**B. Sedimentation Rate,** see **B.S.R.**

**B. Serum,** the fluid which exudes blood clots. It is plasma minus the clotting agents. रक्तसीरम;

**B. Shot,** redness due to turgescence of the blood vessels; blood red. रक्तवर्ण; अत्यधिक लाल;

**B. Stream,** the flowing blood as it is encountered in the organism. रक्तधारा;

**B. Stroke,** apoplexy. रक्ताघात; अपसन्यास;

**B. Sugar,** the amount of glucose in the circulating blood. रक्तशर्करा;

**B. Transfusion,** the intravenous replacement of lost or destroyed blood by compatible citrated human blood. रक्ताधान;

**B. Tube,** see **Blood Vessel.**

**B. Tumour,** haematoma. रक्तार्बुद; खून की गिल्टी या रसौली;

**B. Types,** the O, A, B, AB, four types of blood which are inherited by a child from his parents, especially father. रक्त-प्ररूप; रुधिर-प्ररूप;

**B. Vessel,** an artery or a vein; blood tube. रक्तवाहिनी; रक्तवाहिका; धमनी अथवा शिरा;

**Arterial B.,** blood that is oxygenated in the lungs. धमनी-रक्त; धमनी-रुधिर;

**Ocult B.,** that which is not visible. प्रच्छन्न रुधिर;

**Venous B.,** blood that has passed through the capillaries of various tissues, except the lungs. शिरा-रक्त

**Bloodless.** Without blood. रक्तहीन; अरक्तक;

**Bloody.** Of the nature of, or accompanied by blood. रक्तिम; रक्तवत्; रक्तमिश्रित;

**B. Flux,** dysentery. पेचिश; आमातिसार

**Blotch.** A pustule upon the skin; an eruption usually of large size. स्फोट; व्रण; छाला; फुन्सी; धब्बा

**Blow.** Hard stroke with fist. आघात; चोट; मुष्ठिका-प्रहार

**Blowing.** A whistling sound. सीटी जैसी ध्वनि

**Blue.** A colour. नीला (रंग);

**B. Asphyxia,** see **Blue Baby.**

**B. Baby,** the appearance produced by some congenital heart defects; asphyxia neonatorum; blue asphyxia. शिशु-श्यावता; शिशु-श्वासरोध;

**B. Blindness,** an inability to distinguish a blue colour. नील-वर्णान्धता; नीला रंग पहचानने की अक्षमता;

**B. Vision,** cyanopia. नील-दृष्टि; प्रत्येक वस्तु का नीला दिखाई देना

**Blunt.** Dull, without edge or point. कुन्द; धारहीन; नोकहीन

**Blurring.** Causing imperfection of vision; dimming; darkening. दृष्टिमांद्य; धूमिल दृष्टि

**Blush.** See **Blushing.**

**Blushing.** Sudden reddening of the face due to shame; blush. लज्जारंजन; शर्माना

**B.M.R.** Basal metabolic rate. आधारी चयापचय दर

**Boat-belly.** The sunken appearance of the belly. नौकोदर; नौकाकार पेट; पेट का अन्दर की ओर धँस जाना

**Bodies.** Plural of **Body.**

**Bodily.** Relating to the body. शारीरिक; शरीर सम्बन्धी

**Body.** The trunk of animal frame, with its organs. शरीर; काय; देह; तन; गात; जिस्म; a cadaver. शव; a mass of matter. पिण्ड;

**B. Image,** the image in an individual's mind of his own body. देह-छवि;

**B. Louse,** the pediculus corporis. यूका; जूं;

**B. Wall,** the frame of an animal. अस्थिप्राचीर; अस्थिपंजर; हड्डियों अथवा शरीर का ढांचा

**Boil.** A furuncle; a localized abscess of the skin. फोड़ा; व्रण; बर्रा; फुन्सी; पनसिका

**Boiled.** Subjected to heat in a boiling liquid or water. उबला या उबाला हुआ

**Bole.** Fine clay. चिकनी मिट्टी

**Bolometer.** An instrument used to measure the amount of radiant energy which falls upon it. तेजमापी; सूक्ष्मविकिरक-ऊष्मा को नापने का यंत्र

**Bolus.** A soft, pulpy mass of masticated food. ग्रास; कौर

**Bombus.** Ringing or buzzing in ear. भिनभिनाहट; intestinal rumbling. गुड़गुड़ाहट

**Bone.** The hard tissue forming the framework of the body. अस्थि; हड्डी;

  **Ankle B.**, the talus. गुल्फास्थि; टखने की हड्डी
  **Breast B.**, the sternum. उरोस्थि;
  **Calf B.**, the fibula. बहिर्जंघिकास्थि;
  **Collar B.**, the clavicle. कण्ठास्थि; कालर बोन;
  **Elbow B.**, the ulna. अन्तःप्रकोष्ठिका; कोहनी की हड्डी;
  **Heel B.**, the calcaneus. पार्ष्णिकास्थि; एड़ी की हड्डी;
  **Hip B.**, a large flat bone formed by the fusion of ilium, ischium and pubis, constituting the lateral half of the pelvis. नितम्बास्थि; कूल्हे की हड्डी;
  **Hyoid B.**, see under **Hyoid.**
  **Jaw B.**, the maxilla, especially the mandibula. हन्वस्थि; ठोढ़ी की हड्डी;
  **Shin B.**, the tibia. अंतर्जंघिकास्थि

**Boneache.** Pain in the bone. अस्थिपीड़ा; अस्थिवेदना

**Boneash.** The calcic phosphate and other dry material remaining after the burning of bone. अस्थिभस्म

**Bone-cartilage.** Endochondral bone that develops from cartilage. उपास्थि-अस्थि; उपास्थ्यस्थि

**Bone-conduction.** The transmission of sound through the skull. अस्थि-संवहन

**Bone-corpuscle.** Any connective tissue cell lodged within the laminae of the bone. अस्थि-कण

**Bone-graft.** The transplantation of a piece of bone from one part of the body to another, or from one person to another. अस्थिनिरोप

**Bonelet.** A little bone. लघ्वस्थि; छोटी सी हड्डी

**Bony.** Resembling a bone. अस्थ्याभ; अस्थिवत्; हड्डी जैसी

**Boracic Acid.** The acid of borax; boric acid. बोरेसिक एसिड़; सुहागा अम्ल

**Borax.** Sodium diborate; a transparent crystalline substance of sweetish taste; borate of soda. बोरेक्स; सुहागा

**Borborygmi.** Plural of **Borborygmus.**

**Borborygmus.** Crooking in the bowels and rumbling caused by flatulence. आंत्रकूजन; आटोप; गुड़गुड़हाट

**Border.** Margin; margo; boundary. किनारा; सीमा; धारा

**Boric Acid.** See **Boracic Acid.**

**Born-alive.** Having taken birth with sound respiration. सप्राण-जन्म; सप्राण-प्रसूत

**Boss.** A broad, flat protuberance. उत्सेध; घुण्डी या मूंठ; a lump on the back. कूबड़; कुब्ब; कुब्जता

**Botany.** The science of plants. वनस्पतिविज्ञान; वनस्पतिशास्त्र; पौधों सम्बन्धी विज्ञान

**Bothriocephalus Latus.** The broad tapeworm found in intestines. चौड़े कृमि; स्फीतकृमि; फीताकृमि; पट्टकृमि

**Bottle nose.** Acne rosacea. गुलाबी मुहासे; चेहरे की चमड़ी का जीर्ण रक्तसंलयन

**Bottling.** Filling in the bottle. कूपीभरण; बोतल में भरना

**Bougie.** A slender cylindric instrument for introduction into the urethra, rectum, vagina and oesophagus; bouginaria. बूजी; वर्ति; बत्ती; नम्यशलाका

**Bouginage.** Dilatation by means of a bougie. बूजीप्रवेशन

**Bouginaria.** See **Bougie.**

**Bouillon.** Clear broth made from meat. Used in foods and as a culture medium for bacteria. शोरबा; मांस-रस

**Boulimia.** See **Bulimia.**

**Bovine.** Pertaining to, or derived from the cow or an ox. गोजातीय; गव्य; गाय अथवा बैल सम्बन्धी या उनसे प्राप्त पदार्थ;

    **B. Hunger,** see **Bulimia.**

    **B. Lymphs,** vaccine virus from cow. गोलसीका

**Bow.** Arc. चाप; धनु; धनुष;

    **B.-leg,** arc-like shape of leg; genu varum. धनुर्जंघा; झुकी हुई या मुड़ी हुई टांग

**Bowel.** The intestine; the gut. आंत्र; आंत; अंतड़ी;
    **B. Complaint,** diarrhoea. अतिसार; प्रवाहिका; दस्त
**B.P.** Blood Pressure. रक्तदाब; रक्तचाप; British Pharmacopoea. ब्रिटिश भेषज-संहिता
**B.R.** Breathing reserve. श्वास संचिति
**Brace.** An orthopaedic appliance to hold in the correct position any part of the body. ब्रेस; बर्मा; बरमा
**Brachia.** Plural of **Brachium.**
**Brachial.** Pertaining to the arm. प्रगण्डी; प्रगण्ड सम्बन्धी; भुजा सम्बन्धी;
    **B. Artery,** a continuation of axillary artery. प्रगण्ड धमनी;
    **B. Gland,** one of the lymphatic glands of the arm. प्रगण्ड लसीकाग्रन्थि;
    **B. Plexus,** a plexus of nerves in the neck. ग्रैवस्नायुजाल; गर्दन की नाड़ियों का जाल;
    **B. Vein,** one of the veins of the arms that accompanies the brachial artery. प्रगण्ड शिरा
**Brachialgia.** Pain in the arm. प्रगण्डार्ति; बांह का दर्द
**Brachiocephalic.** Pertaining to both arm and head. प्रगण्ड तथा शीर्ष सम्बन्धी; प्रगण्डशीर्षी
**Brachiocrural.** Pertaining to both arm and leg. बांह तथा टांग सम्बन्धी
**Brachiotomy.** Amputation of the arm. प्रगण्ड-उच्छेदन
**Brachiplex.** The brachial plexus. प्रगण्ड-स्नायुजाल
**Brachium.** The arm from the shoulder to the elbow. बाहु; प्रगण्ड; भुजा का कन्धे से लेकर कोहनी तक का भाग
**Brachycardia.** Slow heart; abnormal infrequency of the pulse; bradycardia. हृद्मन्दता; मन्दस्पन्दन
**Brachycephalic.** Having an egg-shaped skull. पृथुकपाल; पृथुशीर्ष; लघुशीर्ष; लघुशिरस्क; अण्डे की आकृति जैसे सिर वाला
**Brachycephalism.** See **Brachycephaly.**
**Brachycephaly.** The condition of being brachycephalic; brachycephalism. पृथुकपालीयता; लघुशिरस्कता; लघुशीर्षता
**Brachycheilia.** Abnormally short lips; brachichilia. लघुअधरता; ह्रस्वाधरता
**Brachychilia.** See **Brachycheilia.**
**Brachydactylia.** See **Brachydactylism.**

**Brachydactylism.** The condition of being brachydactylous; brachydactylia; brachydactyly. ह्रस्वांगुलिता; हाथ-पांव की उँगलियों का छोटापन

**Brachydactylous.** Having abnormal shortness of the fingers. ह्रस्वांगुलिक

**Brachydactyly.** See **Brachydactylism.**

**Brachydont.** With small teeth. पृथुदन्त; लघुदन्त

**Brachygnathia.** See **Brachygnathous.**

**Brachygnathism.** Abnormal shortness of jaw. पृथुहनुता; लघुहनुता

**Brachygnathous.** With short jaws; brachygnathia. पृथुहनु; लघुहनु

**Brachymetropia.** Myopia. निकटदृष्टिता

**Brachyoesophagus.** Abnormal shortness of oesophagus. लघुग्रासनली; ग्रासनली का अस्वाभाविक रूप से छोटा होना

**Brachyphalangia.** Abnormal shortness of fingers. ह्रस्वांगुलिता; हाथ की उँगलियों का छोटा पड़ना

**Bradyarthria.** A slow and disordered utterance; bradylalia; bradylogia. मन्दवाक्; लघुस्वरता; मन्दवाचालता

**Bradycardia.** See **Brachycardia.**

**Bradycardiac.** Relating to, or affected with bradycardia. हृदमंदता सम्बन्धी अथवा हृदमंदताग्रस्त

**Bradyecoia.** Subnormal acuteness of hearing. मंदश्राव्यता; कम सुनाई देना

**Bradyesthesia.** Dullness of perception. मन्दविवेकशीलता; मन्दसंवेदन

**Bradylalia.** See **Bradyarthria.**

**Bradylogia.** See **Bradyarthria.**

**Bradypepsia.** An abnormally slow digestion. अतिमन्दपाचन; मंदाग्नि की चरम अवस्था

**Bradyphasia.** An abnormal slowness of speech. मन्दवाक्

**Bradypnea.** See **Bradypnoea.**

**Bradypnoea.** Slow respiration; bradypnea. मन्दश्वसन; श्वासोच्छ्वास-वैषम्य

**Bradyspermatism.** A slow emission of semen. मन्दशुक्रता; वीर्य का अत्यधिक मन्द गति से निकलना

**Bradysphygmia.** Slowness of the pulse. मन्दनाड़ीस्पन्द; धीमी नाड़ी

**Bradytosia.** An abnormally slow labour; tedious labour. मन्दप्रसवता; मन्दप्रसवन; प्रसव की अत्यधिक धीमी गति होना

**Bradyuria.** A slow flow of urine. मन्दमूत्रता; मन्दमेहन; पेशाब का अत्यन्त धीमी गति से निकलना

**Brain.** The large mass of nerve tissue within the cranium, including cerebrum, cerebellum, pons and oblongata; the encephalon. मस्तिष्क; भेजा; दिमाग; बुद्धि; मति;

    **B.-fag,** mental fatigue. मनोक्लान्ति;

    **B. Fever,** meningitis. मस्तिष्कावरणशोथ; मस्तिष्क ज्वर;

    **B.-pan,** the cranium. कपाल; खोपड़ी;

    **B.-sick,** idiot. मन्दबुद्धि; मूर्ख;

    **B.-tire,** the same as **Brain-fag.**

**Bran.** The husk or outer covering of grain. धूमशल्क; अनाज का बाहरी छिल्का अथवा आवरण; धान्यशल्क

**Branch.** A division of the main stem, as of a blood vessel. शाखा

**Branchial.** Relating to gills, i.e. fissures or clefts which occur on each side of the neck of the human embryo and which enter into the development of the nose, ears and mouth. गिल अथवा विदर सम्बन्धी; गिली;

    **B. Arches,** the visceral arches; branchial clefts. गिल चाप;

    **B. Clefts,** see **Branchial Arches.**

    **B. Cyst,** a swelling in the neck arising from embryonic remnants. गिल पुटी

**Branchioma.** A tumour developed from remains of the branchial arches. आद्यग्रसनी-अर्बुद

**Branchiomere.** The segment of the lateral mesoderm between each of the two branchial (gill) clefts. गिलखण्ड

**Brandt's Method.** Treatment of affections of the Fallopian tubes by massage in an endeavour to force out their contents into the uterus. ब्रैण्ड पद्धति

**Brandy.** A spiritous liquid distilled from wine. ब्रैण्डी

**Brash.** The acidity in the mouth. मुखाम्लता; मुँह का खट्टापन;

    **Water-b.,** pyrosis. हृद्दाह; अम्लिकोद्गार

**Brassica Alba.** White mustard. सफेद राई; सफेद सरसों

**Brassica Juncea.** Mustard seed. राई अथवा सरसों का बीज

**Brassica Nigra.** Black mustard. काली राई; काली सरसों

**Bread.** A mixture of flour and water baked. रोटी

**Break.** Fracture. भंग; टूट-फूट; तोड़ना;

**Nervous B.-down,** neurasthenia. तंत्रिकावसाद;

**B.-bone Fever,** dengue. डेंगू; अस्थिभंजक ज्वर; हड्डीतोड़ बुखार

**Breast.** The upper anterior part of the body; the mamma. उर; वक्ष; वक्षगह्वर; छाती; स्तन;

**Broken B.,** an abscess of the mammary gland; gathered breast. भंग वक्ष; स्तनग्रन्थ्यर्बुद;

**Chicken B.,** deformity from prominence of the sternum; pigeon breast. कुक्कुट-वक्ष; कपोत-वक्ष;

**Funnel B.,** deformity caused by a marked depression of the lower part of the sternum. कीप-वक्ष;

**Gathered B.,** see **Broken Breast.**

**Pigeon B.,** see **Chicken Breast.**

**B.-bone,** the sternum. उरोस्थि; छाती की हड्डी;

**B.-fed,** being brought up on mother's milk. स्तनपोषित; स्तनपान द्वारा पलने वाला;

**B.-pang,** angina pectoris. हृदशूल; हृच्छूल:

**B.-pump,** an instrument for milking the breast. स्तन-पम्प

**Breath.** The air exhaled from the lungs. श्वास; सांस; श्वसन;

**B.-sound,** the respiratory sound heard upon auscultation. परिश्रवण ध्वनि; श्वास-ध्वनि

**Breathing.** Respiration; taking air into the lungs and expelling it. श्वसन; सांस लेना;

**Abdominal B.,** that which actively engages the abdominal walls and diaphragm. औदरिक श्वसन;

**Interrupting B.,** broken breathing from lung disease or nervousness. रुद्ध श्वसन;

**Puerile B.,** breathing with the respiratory murmur exaggerated as normally heard in children. बाल श्वसन

**Breech.** The hip; buttock. नितम्ब; चूतड़; कूल्हा; underwear. जांघिया; कच्छा; पोतड़ा

**Bregma.** The sinciput or upper part of the head; the anterior fontanelle. ब्रह्मबिन्दु; पूर्वबिन्दु; करोटि; शीर्षस्थान; कपालशीर्ष

**Bregmatic.** Relating to bregma. ब्रह्मबिन्दु सम्बन्धी; ब्रह्मबिन्दुक

**Brevia.** See **Brevis.**

**Brevicollis.** Short-necked. लघुग्रीवा; छोटी गर्दन वाला
**Brevis.** Short; brevia. लघु; छोटा
**Brick-dust Deposit.** A red deposit of urates in the urine. इष्टिकारज-संचय; ईंट के चूरे जैसी परत
**Brick-layers' Itch.** Inflammation or itching of hands caused by contact with lime. राजगीरी खाज; राजगीरों को होने वाली खुजली
**Brick-maker's Anaemia.** Hook-worm disease; brick-makers' disease; dochmiasis. अंकुशकृमिरोग
**Brick-makers' Disease.** See **Brick-makers' Anaemia.**
**Bridge.** A narrow band of the tissues. सेतु; पुल; दो अंगों अथवा आकृतियों को जोड़ने वाले ऊतकों की संकरी पट्टी;
  **B. of the nose,** the ridge formed by the nasal bones. नासिकासेतु; नासासेतु
**Bright's Blindness.** Partial or complete loss of sight. दृष्टिलोप
**Bright's Disease.** Inflammation of the kidney, with a tendency to dropsy; nephritis. वृक्कशोथ; गुर्दे का प्रदाह
**Brightic.** Relating to, or affected with Bright's disease. वृक्कशोथ सम्बन्धी अथवा वृक्कशोथग्रस्त
**Brim.** An edge or margin. पर्यन्त; किनारा;
  **Pelvic B.,** brim of pelvis; boundary of the superior strait of the pelvis. श्रोणि-पर्यन्त
**Brimstone.** Sulphur. गन्धक
**Brine.** The salt-water. लवण-जल; नमकीन पानी;
  **B.-bath,** a salt-water bath. लवण-जलस्नान; नमकीन पानी से नहाना
**Bristle-cells.** Certain cells of the inner ear. अन्तःकर्णकोशिकायें; अन्दरूनी कान की कुछ कोशिकायें
**Brittle.** Apt to break. भंगुर; भुरभुरा; टूटने-फूटने वाला
**Broad.** Wide; extensive. विस्तृत; फैला हुआ;
  **B. Ligaments,** the lateral ligaments. पृथुस्नायु; पृथुशीर्ष; पृष्ठबन्ध
**Broca's Area.** The motor centre for the speech. वाक्प्रेरक केन्द्र
**Brodie's Abscess.** A chronic abscess of bone. जीर्ण अस्थि-विद्रधि; हड्डी का पुराना फोड़ा
**Bromatology.** The science of food and dietetics. खाद्याहारविज्ञान
**Bromatotoxin.** Poisoning by food. खाद्यविषण्णता
**Bromenorrhea.** An offensive menstrual flow; bromenorrhoea.

दुर्गन्धितार्तव; बदबूदार ऋतुस्राव होना

**Bromenorrheal.** Relating to bromenorrhea; bromenorrhoeal. दुर्गन्धितार्तव सम्बन्धी

**Bromenorrhoea.** See **Bromenorrhea.**

**Bromenorrhoeal.** See **Bromenorrheal.**

**Bromhidrosis.** The putrid or foetid perspiration; bromidrosis. दुर्गन्धित पसीना

**Bromidrosis.** See **Bromhidrosis.**

**Bromine.** A liquid non-metallic element obtained from the brines of wells and sea-water. ब्रोमीन

**Bronchadenitis.** See **Bronchoadenitis.**

**Bronchi.** The divisions of the air tubes leading from wind-pipe to lungs. Plural of **Bronchus.** वायुनलियाँ; श्वासनलियाँ

**Bronchia.** Air passages which are smaller than the two bronchi. लघुश्वासनलिकायें; सूक्ष्मश्वासनलिकायें

**Bronchial.** Pertaining to the ramification of air tubes of the lungs. लघु अथवा सूक्ष्म श्वासनलिकाओं सम्बन्धी;

**B. Asthma,** asthma due to bronchial obstructions. श्वासदमा; श्वास-नलिकाओं की अवरुद्ध अवस्था के कारण होने वाला दमा;

**B. Crises,** dyspnoeic paroxysms in locomotor ataxia. श्वासकष्ट; सांस लेने में कठिनाई;

**B. Tubes,** the small ramification of the wind-pipe through the lungs. श्वासनलियाँ

**Bronchiarctia.** Stenosis of the bronchi. श्वासनलिकासंकीर्णन

**Bronchiectasic.** Relating to or affected with bronchiectasis; bronchiectatic. श्वसनिकाविस्फार सम्बन्धी या श्वसनिकाविस्फारग्रस्त

**Bronchiectasis.** Dilatation of the bronchioles. श्वसनीविस्फार; श्वासनलिकाविस्फार; श्वासनलियों का फैलाव

**Bronchiectatic.** See **Bronchiectasic.**

**Bronchiogenic.** See **Bronchogenic.**

**Bronchiolar.** Relating to bronchioles. सूक्ष्मश्वासनलिकाओं सम्बन्धी

**Bronchiole.** A minute bronchial tube; bronchiolus. सूक्ष्मश्वासनलिका; सूक्ष्मश्वासनली; श्वासोपनलिका

**Bronchiolectasis.** Dilatation of the bronchioles. श्वसनीविस्फार; श्वासनलिका-विस्फार; श्वासनलियों का फैलना

**Bronchioli.** Plural of **Bronchiolus.**

**Bronchiolitis.** Inflammation of the bronchioles; capillary bronchitis. श्वासनलिकाशोथ; श्वासनलियों का प्रदाह; वायुनलियों की सूजन

**Bronchiolus.** See **Bronchiole.**

**Bronchitic.** Affected with bronchitis. श्वसनीशोथग्रस्त; वायुनलियों के प्रदाह से पीड़ित (रोगी)

**Bronchitis.** Inflammation of the bronchial tube. श्वसनीशोथ; श्वासनली का प्रदाह; वायुनलिका की सूजन;

**Capillary B.**, inflammation of the finer tubes of the bronchus; bronchiolitis. केशिकाश्वसनीशोथ;

**Catarrhal B.**, a form marked by profuse mucopurulent discharge. प्रतिश्यायी श्वसनीशोथ;

**Chronic B.**, bronchitis characterized by cough, hypersecretion of mucus and expectoration of sputum over a long period of time. जीर्ण श्वसनीशोथ;

**Phthinoid B.**, a consumptive form with foetid sputum. यक्ष्मज श्वसनीशोथ;

**Putrid B.**, a chronic form with foetid sputum. पूतिज श्वसनीशोथ; सपूय श्वसनीशोथ

**Bronchoadenitis.** Inflammation of the bronchial glands; bronchadenitis. श्वसनिकाग्रन्थिशोथ; श्वसनिकाग्रन्थियों का प्रदाह

**Bronchocele.** Goitre; an indolent swelling of the thyroid gland. गलगण्ड; घेंघा; अवटु ग्रन्थि की सूजन

**Bronchoconstrictor.** Causing a reduction in calibre of a bronchus or bronchial tube. श्वसनीसंकीर्णक

**Bronchodilator.** An apparatus for the dilatation of the bronchus. श्वसनीविस्फारक; श्वासनलिकाप्रसारकयंत्र

**Bronchogenic.** Originating from bronchus; bronchiogenic. श्वसनीजन्य; श्वासनलिका से आरम्भ होने वाला

**Bronchogram.** Radiological picture of the bronchi and bronchial tubes rendered radio-opaque. श्वसनीचित्र

**Bronchography.** Preparation of x-ray film after introduction of radio-opaque substance into the bronchi and bronchial tubes. श्वसनीचित्रण

**Broncholite.** See **Broncholith.**

**Broncholith.** A bronchial calculus; broncholite. श्वसनी-अश्मरी; श्वासनलिका की पथरी

**Broncholithiasis.** Formation of bronchial calculi. श्वसनी-अश्मरता; श्वासनली में पथरियां बनना

**Bronchomalacia.** A softening of the bronchus. श्वसनीमृदुता; श्वासनली की कोमलता

**Bronchomotor.** Causing a change in the calibre of dilatation, or contraction of a bronchus or bronchiole. श्वसनीप्रेरक

**Bronchomycosis.** A fungus growth of the bronchi. श्वसनीकवकता

**Bronchopathy.** Any disease of the bronchi. श्वसनीविकृति; श्वासनलियों का कोई रोग

**Bronchophony.** Abnormal resonance of the voice in the bronchial tubes. श्वसनीध्वनि (जो श्रवण यंत्र की सहायता से सुनी जाती है)

**Bronchoplasty.** The operation for closing a tracheal fistula. श्वसनीसंधान

**Bronchopleural.** Relating to the bronchus and the pleura. श्वसनी एवं फुप्फुस सम्बन्धी

**Bronchopleural Fistula.** Pathological communication between the pleural cavity and bronchus. श्वसनीफुप्फुसविदर

**Bronchopneumonia.** Inflammation of the lungs of the bronchial origin. श्वसनीफुप्फुसपाक; श्वसनीफुप्फसशोथ; श्वासनली तथा फेफड़ों का प्रदाह

**Bronchopulmonary.** Pertaining to the bronchi and the lungs. श्वासनलियों तथा फेफड़ों सम्बन्धी

**Bronchorrhagia.** Haemorrhage from or into the bronchi. श्वसनीरक्तस्राव; श्वसनीरक्तस्रवण

**Bronchorrhea.** See **Bronchorrhoea.**

**Bronchorrhoea.** A profuse discharge of mucus from the bronchi; bronchorrhea. श्वसनी-अतिश्लेष्मस्राव; श्वासनलियों से अत्यधिक श्लेष्मा निकलना

**Branchoscope.** An instrument for the direct inspection of the bronchus. श्वसनीदर्शी; श्वासनली की जांच के लिये प्रयुक्त किया जाने वाला यंत्र

**Bronchoscopy.** Inspection of bronchus with bronchoscope. श्वसनीदर्शन; श्वासनली की श्वसनीदर्शीयंत्र द्वारा जांच

**Bronchospasm.** Sudden constriction of the bronchial tubes due to contraction of involuntary plain muscle in their walls. श्वसनी-आकर्ष

**Bronchospirometer.** An instrument for measuring the capacity of the lungs. श्वसनीश्वसनमापकयंत्र; श्वसनीश्वसनमापीयंत्र

**Bronchospirometry.** Measuring of the capacity of the lungs. श्वसनीश्वसनमिति; फेफड़ों की क्षमता का परिमापन करना

**Bronchostenosis.** Narrowing or stenosis of a bronchus. श्वसनीसंकीर्णता; श्वासनली की संकीर्णता

**Bronchotome.** An instrument for bronchotomy. श्वसनिकाछेदक

**Bronchotomy.** Incision of a bronchus. श्वसनिकाछेदन; श्वसनीछेदन

**Bronchus.** One of the main branches of the trachea. श्वसनी; श्वासनली

**Brood Cell.** In cell-division, the mother cell. अंडकोश; मातृकोश; मातृकोशिका

**Broth.** Juice made of flesh. मांसरस; यूष; शोरबा

**Brow.** The region of the supra-orbital ridge. भ्रू; भौंह

**Browache.** The supra-orbital neuralgia. ऊर्ध्वाक्षिक-तंत्रिकार्ति; भ्रूवेदना; भौंह-पीड़ा

**Browague.** Hemicrania. अर्धकपाली; आधासीसी का दर्द

**Brucine.** The alkaloid of Nux vomica. कुचलाविष का उपक्षार; ब्रूसिन

**Bruise.** A discolouration of the skin due to an extravasation of blood into the underlying tissues. नील; कुचलन

**Bruit.** An abnormal sound heard in auscultation. ब्रूई; विरुत; ध्वनि;

   **B.d'airain,** metallic tinkling. पीतल ध्वनि;

   **B. de pot fele,** the cracked-pot sound. भग्नपात्र ध्वनि

**B.S.R.** Blood Sedimentation Rate. रक्त अवसादन दर

**Bubbling.** Making a gurgling sound. बुदबुदाहट

**Bubin.** See **Bubo.**

**Bubo.** Chancre; an inflammation and swelling of the lymphatic gland of the groin; bubin. गिल्टी; ग्रन्थि; गोही; बद; गांठ

**Bubonalgia.** Pain in the groin. वंक्षणार्ति; वंक्षणशूल

**Bubonic.** Pertaining to a bubo or chancre. गिल्टी या शैंकर (कठिनक्षत) सम्बन्धी

**Bubonocele.** An inguinal hernia. वंक्षण हर्निया; आंत्रवृद्धि

**Bucardia.** Extreme hypertrophy of the heart. अतिहृद्वर्धन; हृदय का अत्यधिक बढ़ जाना

**Bucca.** The hollow part of the cheek. मुखगह्वर; कपोल; गाल; the mouth. मुख; मुँह

**Buccae.** Plural of **Bucca.**

**Buccal.** Belonging to the mouth. मुखी; कपोल अथवा गाल सम्बन्धी;
**B. Cavity,** the hollow part inside the mouth surrounded by cheeks and lips. मुखगह्वर

**Buccinator.** A thin, fat muscle of the cheek. कपोलपेशी; कपोल-सम्पीडनी; गालों की पतली, मोटी पेशी

**Bucconasal.** Pertaining to both the mouth and the nose. मुख तथा नाक सम्बन्धी

**Buccopharyngeal.** Pertaining to both the mouth and the pharynx. मुख तथा ग्रसनी सम्बन्धी

**Buccula.** The fleshy part under the chin. चिबुकपेशी; ठोढ़ी का मांसल भाग

**Bucket Fever.** Dengue. डेंगू

**Bucnemia Tropica.** Elephantiasis. श्लीपद; हाथी पैर

**Bud.** A structure that resembles a bud of plants. कलिका; कली

**Budding.** Gemmation; a form of reproduction of cell-division. कोशिकाविभाजन; कलिकोत्पादन, जिसके द्वारा पौधों या जन्तुओं में नये पौधे या जन्तु बनते हैं

**Buerger's Disease.** Thromboangiitis obliterans; an obliterative vascular disease of peripheral vessels. रोधकघनास्रवाहिकाशोथ

**Buffer.** Anything used to reduce shock or jarring due to contact. उभयरोधी; प्रतिरोधक; आघातरोधी

**Bugantia.** A chilblain. शीतदंश; शीतक्षत; फटन

**Buggery.** Sodomy. गुदामैथुन; लौंडेबाजी

**Buginaria.** Bougie. वर्ति; बत्ती; बूजी

**Bulb.** An expansion of a canal or vessel. कन्द; any globular or fusiform structure. कोई गोलाकार वस्तु;
**B. of aorta,** the dilatation of the aorta near its beginning; aortic bulb. महाधमनी कन्द;
**B. of the eye,** the eyeball. नेत्रगोलक; नेत्रकन्द;
**B. of vestibule,** see **Bulbus Vestibuli.**
**Aortic B.,** see **Bulb of aorta.**
**Dental B.,** dental papilla. दन्त कन्द;
**End B.,** one of the oval or rounded bodies in which the sensory fibres terminate in mucous membrane. अन्त्य कन्द;
**Hair B.,** expanded portion at the lower end of the hair-root; bulbus pili. रोम कन्द; लोम कन्द;

**Olfactory B.,** the anterior enlargement of the olfactory track; bulbus olfactorius. घ्राण कन्द

**Bulbar.** Pertaining to the medulla oblongata. मेरुशीर्ष सम्बन्धी; कन्दी

**Bulbi.** Plural of **Bulbus.**

**Bulbiform.** Of the form of a bulb. कन्दोपम; कन्दाकार; कन्दरूप

**Bulbocavernosus.** The accelator urinae or sphincter vaginae. कन्दगह्वरिका

**Bulbospinal.** Pertaining to the medulla oblongata and the spine. मेरुशीर्ष तथा मेरुदण्ड सम्बन्धी

**Bulbourethral.** Relating to the bulb of the urethra. मूत्रपथीय कन्द सम्बन्धी

**Bulbous.** Having bulbs. कन्दिल; कन्दीय; कन्दयुक्त; सकन्द; round. गोलाकार; गोल

**Bulbus.** A bulb. कन्द;

   **B. Arteriosus,** the enlargement of the bulb of the aorta. धमनी कन्द;

   **B. Cordis,** the cardiac bulb. हृत्कन्द;

   **B. Oculi,** the eyeball. नेत्रगोलक; नेत्रकन्द;

   **B. Olfactorius,** see **Olfactory Bulb.**

   **B. Penis,** the bulb of penis or urethra. शिश्नकन्द;

   **B. Pili,** see **Hair Bulb.**

   **B. Vestibuli,** bulb of the vestibule. प्रघाण कन्द

**Bulging.** Distension. उभार; फुलाव

**Bulimia.** Excessive, morbid hunger; boulimia; bulimy; bovine hunger. अतिक्षुधा; अतिबुभुक्षा; अत्यधिक भूख लगना; भस्मक रोग

**Bulimic.** Affected with bulimia. अतिक्षुधाग्रस्त; भस्मक रोग से पीड़ित

**Bulimy.** See **Bulimia.**

**Bulla.** A large bleb or blister. जलस्फोट; छाला; फफोला; बुलबुला; बुद्बुद्

**Bullae.** Plural of **Bulla.**

**Bullous.** Marked by the presence of bullae. जलस्फोटी; फफोलेदार; छालेदार

**Bundle.** A collection or group of fibres; a fasciculus. पूलिका; पोटली; तन्तुसंग्रह; पुलिन्दा; गठरी

**Bunion.** Inflammation of the bursa mucosa, at the ball of the toe. अंगुलबेढ़ा; पैर के अंगूठे की सूजन

**Bunionectomy.** Excision of a bunion. अंगुलबेढ़ाकर्तन; अंगुलबेढ़ा-उच्छेदन

**Bunodont.** With curved teeth. बक्रदन्त; टेढ़े-मेढ़े दान्तों वाला

**Buphthalmia.** See **Buphthalmos.**

**Buphthalmos.** Congenital glaucoma; ox-eye; buphthalmia; buphthalmus. वृषभाक्षि

**Buphthalmus.** See **Buphthalmos.**

**Bur.** A rotatory cutting instrument used in dentistry; burr. बर्र

**Burn.** To consume with fire, chemicals, dry heat, electricity, friction or radiation, etc. दाह; जलना; जल जाना; a wound caused due to burning with fire. दाहक्षत; जलने से होने वाला घाव

**Burner.** A name for a lamp or heating apparatus used in laboratories. ज्वालक; बर्नर

**Burning.** Being affected with a sensation of heat. दाह; जलन; ज्वलनकारी; ज्वलनशील

**Burn's Amaurosis.** Impaired vision caused by masturbation or sexual excesses. रतिज दृष्टिमांद्य

**Burnt.** Scorched. दग्ध; जला हुआ

**Burr.** See **Bur.**

**Bursa.** A fibrous sac lined with synovial membrane and containing a small quantity of synovial fluid. पुटी, जैसे श्लेषपुटी, स्नेहपुटी;

**Adventitious B.,** a cystic formation due to some mechanical injury, such as friction. आगंतुक श्लेषपुटी;

**Omental B.,** see **Bursa Omentalis.**

**Synovial B.,** see **Bursa Mucosa.**

**B. Mucosa,** a membranous sac secreting synovial fluid; synovial bursa. श्लेष्मल श्लेषपुटी;

**B. Omentalis,** the cavity of the great omentum; omental bursa. वपा-श्लेषपुटी;

**B. Pharyngeae,** one in the dorsal wall of the nasopharynx. ग्रसनी गर्तिका; ग्रसनी श्लेषपुटी

**Bursae.** Plural of **Bursa.**

**Bursal.** Pertaining to a bursa or sac. श्लेषपुटी अथवा स्नेहपुटी सम्बन्धी

**Bursalis Musculus.** A small flat muscle situated at the upper and anterior part of the thigh. लघुजघनपेशी; जांघ की छोटी पेशी

**Bursectomy.** Excision of a bursa. श्लेषपुटी-उच्छेदन; स्नेहपुटी-उच्छेदन

**Bursitis.** Inflammation of a bursa. श्लेषपुटीशोथ; स्नेहपुटीशोथ; श्लेष अथवा स्नेहपुटी का प्रदाह;

# Bursitis

**Prepatellar B.,** the housemaid's knee. पुरोजानुकाश्लेषपुटीशोथ

**Bursolith.** A calculus formed in a bursa. पुटी-अश्मरी

**Bursopathy.** Any disease of a bursa. पुटीरोग

**Bursotomy.** Incision through the wall of a bursa. पुटीछेदन

**Butter.** The fatty portion of milk; butter-fat. स्नेह; मक्खन; नवनीत

**Butter-fat.** See **Butter.**

**Butter-fly.** A winged insect called **Titli.** तितली;

    **B. Patch,** lupus of cheeks and nose. कपोल-चर्म तथा नासिकाचर्म का क्षय

**Butter-milk.** The liquid left after extracting the butter from cream. छाछ; मट्ठा; तक्र

**Buttocks.** The two projections posterior to the hip joints; the nates, rumps, or gluteal region. नितम्ब; कूल्हे

**Butyric Acid.** One of the common organic acids. ब्यूटाइरिक अम्ल

**Buzzing.** Humming. भिनभिनाहट; गुंजन

**Bypass.** A surgically created shunt or auxillary flow through a diversionary channel. बाइपास; उपमार्ग

**Byssinosis.** A pulmonary affection caused due to the inhalation of cotton dust. फुफ्फुसकार्पासता

**Byssophthisis.** Phthisis produced by inhaling the dust of cotton. फुफ्फुसक्षय; सांस के साथ रुई की धूल जाने के फलस्वरूप होने वाला फेफड़ों का रोग

**Byssus.** Charpie, lint or cotton. सूत्रगुच्छ; क्षौमसूत्र; धज्जियाँ

# C

**C.** Symbol for carbon, celseus, centesimal (hundred), congius (gallon), etc. कार्बन, सेल्सियस, सेण्टिसिमल (शतमलव), गैलन, (कॉंजियस), आदि के लिये प्रयुक्त किया जाने वाला चिन्ह

**Ca.** Symbol for calcium, cathode, etc. कैल्शियम, कैथोड, आदि के लिये प्रयुक्त किया जाने वाला चिन्ह

**Cacaerometer.** An apparatus for determining the impurity of the air. वायुदूषणमापी (यंत्र)

**Cacanthrax.** Contagious anthrax. सांसर्गिक आंगारव्रण

**Cacation.** Defecation. मलोत्सरण; मलोत्सर्जन; मलत्याग

**Cacemia.** A depraved condition of the blood. रक्तदोष

**Cacethesia.** A morbid sensation. रोगानुभूति; रुग्णानुभूति; अक्रमिक संवेदनशीलता; रुग्णसंवेदना

**Cachaemia.** Septicaemia; cachemia. रुधिरविषाक्तता; रक्तविषण्णता

**Cachectic.** See **Cachetic**

**Cachelcoma.** A malignant ulcer. दुर्दम-व्रण; सांघातिक फोड़ा

**Cachemia.** See **Cachaemia.**

**Cachet.** A flat capsule for carrying medicines. पुटक; कैशे; दवाई रखने का चपटा केप्सूल

**Cachetic.** In a state of exhaustion and weakness or characterized by cachexia; cachectic; chacheticle. कृशकाय; क्षीणकाय; दुर्बल; कमजोर

**Cacheticle.** See **Cachetic.**

**Cachexia.** A depraved condition of nutritions, characterized by bodily emaciation, sallow unhealthy skin and heavy lustreless eyes; cachexy. क्षीणता; दुर्बलता; कृशता; कमजोरी;

   **Cancerous C.**, due to poisoning from malignant tumours. कैंसर-कृशता;

   **Lymphatic C.**, Hodgkin's disease. हॉज्किन रोग; कैंसर; गण्डमाला; लसीकापर्वार्बुद;

   **Malarial C.**, chronic malaria. जीर्ण विषम-ज्वर; चिरकारी मलेरिया;

   **Miner's C.**, dochmiasis. अंकुशकृमिरोग;

   **Pachydermic C.**, myxedema. श्लेष्मशोफ;

   **Thyroid C.**, exophthalmic goitre. नेत्रोत्सेधी गलगण्ड;

   **C. Strumipriva**, a cretinoid state following the extirpation of the thyroid gland; cachexia thyreopriva. अनवटुक्षीणता;

   **C. Thyreopriva**, see **Cachexia Strumipriva.**

**Cachexy.** See **Cachexia.**

**Cachochylia.** Indigestion. मन्दाग्नि; अजीर्ण; अपच

**Cacocolpia.** Gangrene of the vulva. भगकोथ

**Cacodorous.** Having a bad smell. दुर्गन्धित; बदबूदार

**Cacoethes.** Any bad habit, propensity or disorder. बुरी आदत (दुर्व्यसन), प्रवृत्ति अथवा दोष

**Cacogastric.** Dyspeptic. मन्दाग्निग्रस्त; अग्निमांद्य से पीड़ित

**Cacogeusia.** Bad taste. विरसता; भद्दा स्वाद

**Cacomelia.** Congenital deformity of one or more limbs. सहज-अंगदोष; एक अथवा एक से अधिक अंगों की दोषपूर्ण अवस्था

**Cacopathy.** Malignant condition or disease. सांघातिक रुग्णता

**Cacosmia.** A bad odour. दुर्गन्ध; बदबू

**Cacosomium.** A hospital for incurables. असाध्यरोगीगृह; लाइलाज रोगियों का अस्पताल

**Cacospermia.** A bad condition of the semen. विकृतशुक्राणुता; वीर्य की दोषपूर्ण अवस्था

**Cacosphyxia.** An abnormal state of the pulse. नाड़ीदोष, नाड़ीविकार

**Cacosplanchnia.** Emaciation due to indigestion. अपचकृशता; अपच के कारण होने वाली कमजोरी

**Cacothanasia.** Painful, miserable death. दारुण-मृत्यु; दर्दनाक मौत

**Cacothymia.** A disordered state of mind. मनोविशृंखिलता; रुग्ण मानसिक स्थिति; विशृंखिलमनोदशा

**Cactus.** A genus of cactaceous plants. नागफनी; कैक्टस;

    **C. Grandiflorus,** a cardiac stimulating medicine. कैक्टस ग्रैण्डिफ्लोरस; एक हृद्बलवर्धक औषधि

**Cacumen.** The top or apex; cacumena. शिखर; शीर्ष

**Cacumena.** See **Cacumen.**

**Cacumenal.** Relating to cacumen. शिखर सम्बन्धी

**Cadaver.** Corpse; the dead body. शव; लोथ; लाश; मुर्दा; मृत शरीर

**Cadaveric.** Pertaining to a cadaver. शव अथवा लाश सम्बन्धी; like a dead body or corpse; cadaverous. शव अथवा लाश जैसा; शवतुल्य

**Cadaverous.** Corpse-like; resembling a dead body. शवतुल्य; शववत्; शव जैसा

**Cadmium.** A bluish-white metal, resembling tin in appearance and zinc in chemical relations. कैड्मियम; अरगजी; एक नीलश्वेत धातु, जो यशद की खानों में पाई जाती है

**Caduca.** The deciduous membrane of the uterus. जरायुपातिकला; गर्भाशयपातककला

**Caducous.** Dropping off early. आशुपाती; शीघ्रपाती

**Caeca.** Plural of **Caecum.**

**Caecal.** Belonging to the caecum; cecal. उण्डुकीय; उण्डुक अथवा अन्धान्त्र सम्बन्धी

**Caecitis.** Inflammation of the caecum; cecitis. अन्धान्त्रशोथ; उण्डुकशोथ; अन्धान्त्र अथवा उण्डुक का प्रदाह

**Caecocolostomy.** Surgical anastomosis between caecum and colon; cecocolostomy. अन्धान्त्रबृहदान्त्रसम्मिलन

**Caecoptosis.** Prolapse of appendix; cecoptosis. अन्धान्त्रच्युति; उण्डुकभ्रंश; अन्धान्त्र का अपने स्थान से हट जाना

**Caecorrhaphy.** A suturing of the appendix. उण्डुकसीवन; उपान्त्रसीवन

**Caecostomy.** Surgical formation of a caecal fistula; cecostomy; typhlostomy. अन्धान्त्र-सम्मिलन

**Caecotomy.** Incision into the caecum; cecotomy. अन्धान्त्रछेदन; उण्डुकछेदन

**Caecum.** The blind pouch at the head of the large intestine; cecum. अन्धान्त्र; उण्डुक

**Caenogenesis.** A new growth; cenogenesis. नवोत्पत्ति; गुल्म

**Caesarean Operation.** See **Caesarean Section.**

**Caesarean Section.** The operation by which the foetus is taken out of the uterus; caesarean operation; caesarotomy; cesarean operation; cesarean section; cesarotomy. शल्यजनन; शल्यक्रिया द्वारा प्रसव कराना

**Caesarotomy.** See **Caesarean Section.**

**Caffea.** Coffee. कॉफी

**Caffein.** The central nervous system stimulant, present in tea and coffee; caffeine. कॉफी-सार; कैफीन; केन्द्रीय स्नायु-प्रणाली को उत्तेजित करने वाला पदार्थ

**Caffeine.** See **Caffein.**

**Caisson Disease.** The group of symptoms due to working under increased atmospheric pressure; compression illness. सम्पीडित वायुव्याधि; वातमंजूषा रोग

**Calcaneal.** Relating to calcaneum; calcanean. पार्ष्णिकीय; पार्ष्णिका अथवा एड़ी की हड्डी सम्बन्धी

**Calcanean.** See **Calcaneal.**

**Calcanei.** Plural of **Calcaneum** or **Calcaneus.**

**Calcaneitis.** Inflammation of the calcaneum. पार्ष्णिकाशोथ; एड़ी की हड्डी का प्रदाह

**Calcaneocuboid.** Relating to the calcaneus and the cuboid bone. पार्ष्णिकाघनास्थिज

**Calcaneodynia.** Painful heel; calcodynia. पार्ष्णिकार्ति; दर्दनाक एड़ी

**Calcaneum.** The heel bone; os calcis; calcaneus. पार्ष्णिका; एड़ी की हड्डी

**Calcaneus.** See **Calcaneum.**

**Calcar.** A spur. प्रसर; उत्सेध;

  **C. Avis,** Hippocampus minor; an elevation in the posterior cornu of the lateral ventricle. शूक-उत्सेध;

  **C. Pedis,** the heel bone. पार्ष्णिका; एड़ी की हड्डी

**Calcarea.** Lime. कल्केरिया; कैल्सियम; चूना

**Calcareous.** Containing lime; having the nature of lime, or chalk. कैल्सियममय; कैल्सियमयुक्त; चूनेदार; चूने का

**Calcariuria.** Excretion of calcium in the urine. कैल्सियममेह; पेशाब में चूना जाना

**Calces.** Plural of **Calx.**

**Calcic.** Relating to lime, or calcium. कैल्सियम सम्बन्धी

**Calcicosis.** See **Pneumoconiosis.**

**Calcification.** The deposition of calcium salts in the tissue. कैल्सीकरण; कैल्सीभवन; खरिकोत्पादन; खरिकसंचय

**Calcigerous.** Containing lime. कैल्सियमयुक्त; चूनामय

**Calcination.** The process of expelling by heat the volatile elements of a substance. निस्तापन

**Calcinosis.** Condition marked by abnormal deposition of lime salts in tissues. कैल्सियममयता; कैल्सियमता

**Calcis, os.** The heel bone; os calcis. गुल्फास्थि; एड़ी की हड्डी

**Calcium.** The basic element of lime. कैल्सियम; चूना; चूने का सार

**Calcodynia.** See **Calcaneodynia.**

**Calcoid.** A tumour of the tooth-pulp. दन्तगुहार्बुद; दन्तमज्जार्बुद

**Calculary.** Relating to bladder-stone disease; calculous. वृक्काश्मरीय; गुर्दे की पथरी सम्बन्धी

**Calculi.** Plural of **Calculus.**

**Calculifragous.** Having the power of dissolving calculi. अश्मविलेय; अश्मरीविलेय; पथरी घोलने की शक्ति से सम्पन्न

**Calculosis.** The tendency to form calculi or stones. अश्मप्रवणता;

अश्मरियां अथवा पथरियां बनने की प्रवृत्ति

**Calculous.** See **Calculary.**

**Calculus.** Gravel; a stone; a collection of mineral matter either in bile duct, kidney or bladder. अश्म; अश्मरी; पथरी;

**Biliary C.,** a gall-stone. पित्त-पथरी; पित्ताश्मरी;

**Coral C.,** see **Stag-horn Calculus.**

**Dental C.,** calcified deposits formed around the teeth. दंताश्मरी; दंत-पथरी;

**Dendritic C.,** see **Stag-horn Calculus.**

**Mulberry C.,** the oxalate of lime variety, like a mulberry in form and colour. तूत-अश्मरी;

**Prostate C.,** one in the prostate gland. पुरःस्थ-अश्मरी;

**Pulmonary C.,** one in the lungs. फुप्फुस-अश्मरी; फेफड़े की पथरी;

**Renal C.,** urinary calculus; a stone formed in the kidney. वृक्क-अश्मरी; वृक्काश्म; मूत्राश्मरी; मूत्र-पथरी;

**Salivary C.,** one in the duct of a salivary gland. लालाश्मरी; लाराश्मरी; लार-पथरी;

**Stag-horn C.,** a calculus occurring in the renal pelvis, with branches extending into the infundibula and calices; coral calculus; dendritic calculus. वृक्कगोणिकाश्मरी;

**Urinary C.,** see **Renal Calculus.**

**Vaginal C.,** one in the vagina. योनि-अश्मरी; योनि-पथरी

**Caldarium.** A hot-bath. ऊष्मा-प्रक्षालन; ऊष्मास्नान; गरम पानी से नहाना

**Calefacient.** Exciting warmth; causing a sense of warmth. उत्तापक; गरमाई देने वाला

**Calendula.** A genus of plants. गेंदा; गेंदुक;

**C. Officinalis,** marigold; it is used in sprains and bruises. गेन्दुक पुष्प; गेंदे का फूल

**Calenture.** Sun-stroke. लू लगना

**Calf.** The fleshy mass on the back of leg, below the knee. जघनपिण्डिका; पिण्डली; टांग के पीछे की ओर घुटने के नीचे का मांस-पिण्ड

**Caliber.** Cavity or hollow vessels. विवर; नलिका; छेद; the diameter of a tube. कैलीबर; किसी नली का व्यास; अन्तर्व्यास

**Caliceal.** Relating to calix. आलवाल अथवा बाह्यदलपुंज सम्बन्धी

**Calicectasis.** Dilatation of calices; caliectasis. आलवालविस्फार

**Calicectomy.** Excision of calix; caliectomy. आलवाल-उच्छेदन

**Calices.** Plural of **Calix.**

**Calicoplasty.** Surgical repair of calix. आलवालसंधान

**Calicotomy.** Incision into a calix. आलवालछेदन

**Caliculus.** A bud-shaped or cup-shaped structure. चषक

**Caliectasis.** See **Calicectasis.**

**Caliectomy.** See **Calicectomy.**

**Caligo.** Dimness of vision. दृष्टिमांद्य; मन्द-दृष्टिता; loss of sight. दृष्टिलोप; अन्धापन; अन्धता

**Caliper.** A two-pronged instrument with sharp points which are inserted into the lower end of a fractured long bone. कैलीपर

**Calisthenics.** The science of developing by regulated movements, grace and vigour of the body. विकासविद्या

**Calix.** See **Calyx.**

**Callomania.** Mania in which the patient believes herself endowed with beauty. स्वरूपोन्माद; स्वसौन्दर्योन्माद; पागलपन की वह अवस्था जिसमें रोगिणी स्वयं को अतीव सुन्दरी महसूस करती है

**Callosal.** Pertaining to the corpus callosum. महासंयोजिका सम्बन्धी

**Callosity.** A hardness of the skin, caused by intermittent pressure or friction; a corn. किण; किणता; कृन्तिता; कील; घट्टा

**Callosum.** The bridge of white nerve substance joining the hemisphere of the brain. महासंयोजिका; मस्तिष्क के अर्धगोलकों को जोड़ने वाला श्वेत स्नायु-पदार्थ का सेतु

**Callous.** Hardened, indurated, as the edges of an ulcer. कठोर; दृढ़; ठोस; relating to a callus or callosity. किण अथवा घट्टा सम्बन्धी

**Callus.** A callosity. किण; घट्टा; a new bony deposit about a fracture. टूटी हुई हड्डी केआस-पास बनने वाली नई हड्डी

**Calmant.** A sedative; calmative. वेदनाहर; पीड़ानाशक; प्रशमनकारी; उत्तेजनाहर

**Calmative.** See **Calmant.**

**Calomel.** Mild chloride of mercury; a purgative. रसकर्पूर; रसकपूर; पारद का एक सौम्य रूप नीलेय, जिसका प्रयोग विरेचक के रूप में किया जाता है

**Calor.** Heat; one of the four classic local signs of inflammation (calor, rubor, tumour, dolour). ताप; ऊष्मा; गर्मी; गरमाई;

   **C. Animalis,** animal heat. जैवी ताप

**Calorescence.** The conversion of non-luminous heat-rays into luminous heat-rays. ताप-दीप्ति

**Caloric.** Pertaining to heat or its principal calory. ऊष्मा अथवा ताप सम्बन्धी

**Caloricity.** A unity of heat. ऊष्माशक्ति; ताप की एक इकाई

**Caloricrescent.** An agent producing heat in the body. देहतापवर्धक; देहतापवर्धी; शरीर के तापमान को बढ़ाने वाला पदार्थ

**Calorie.** See **Calory**.

**Calories.** Plural of **Calory**.

**Calorifacient.** See **Calorific**.

**Calorific.** Heat-producing; calorifacient; calorigenic. तापवर्धक; तापजनक; ऊष्माजनक; ऊष्माकर; गर्माई उत्पन्न करने वाला

**Calorigenic.** See **Calorific**.

**Calorimeter.** An instrument for measuring the heat of bodies. ऊष्मामापी; तापमापकयंत्र; ऊष्मामापकयंत्र

**Calorimetric.** Belonging to calorimetry. ऊष्मामितीय; ऊष्मामितिय; तापमिति; तापमितिक

**Colorimetry.** Measurement of heat. ऊष्मामापन; ऊष्मामिति; तापमिति; तापमापन

**Calory.** Heat; the amount of heat necessary to raise the temperature of one kilogram of water 10c; also called a large calorie. ऊष्मा; ताप; कैलोरी

**Calva.** The vertex; skull-cap; roof of the skull; the upper domelike portion of the skull. करोटिशीर्ष; कपालशीर्ष

**Calvaria.** The skull-cap; calvarium; the vault of the skull. कपाल; ब्रह्मरन्ध्र; कपालगुम्बद; कपालोर्ध्व

**Calvariae.** Plural of **Calvaria**.

**Calvarial.** Belonging to the calvarium. कपाल अथवा ब्रह्मरन्ध्र सम्बन्धी

**Calvarium.** See **Calvaria**.

**Calves.** Plural of **Calf**.

**Calvities.** Diffused or general baldness. खल्वाटता; खालित्य; गंजापन

**Calx.** The heel; the posterior rounded extremity of the foot. गुल्फ; एड़ी

**Calyces.** Plural of **Calyx**.

**Calyx.** A cup-like ensheathing structure, as one of the funnel-shaped tissues surrounding the renal pyramids; calix. आलवाल; बाह्यदलपुंज; पुटक

**Camera.** A chamber or vaulted structure. कक्ष; प्रकोष्ठ; कोष्ठ; कैमरा;
   **C. Cordis,** the enveloping membrane of the heart; the pericardium. हृदयावरण; परिहृद्; हृद्कक्ष;
   **C. Oculi,** the chamber of the eye. चक्षु-प्रकोष्ठ; नेत्र-कक्ष

**Camerae.** Plural of **Camera.**

**Camp Fever.** Typhus fever. मोहज्वर; शिविर ज्वर; कैम्प ज्वर, जिसमें शरीर पर लाल-लाल चित्तियाँ निकल आती हैं

**Camphol.** Oil of camphor. कर्पूर तेल; कपूर का तेल

**Camphor.** A solid volatile oil from the Cinnamomum camphora. कर्पूर; कपूर

**Camphora.** The same as **Camphor.**

**Camphoraceous.** Resembling or containing camphor. कर्पूरवत्; कपूर जैसा; कर्पूरित; कपूरयुक्त

**Camphorated.** Impregnated with camphor. कर्पूरित; कर्पूरयुक्त

**Campimeter.** A portable, hand-held type of tangent screen used to measure the central visual field. दृष्टिकेन्द्रक्षेत्रमापी

**Campimetry.** Investigation of the visual field by means of a campimeter. दृष्टिकेन्द्रक्षेत्रमापन

**Campsis.** An abnormal curving of a limb. अग्रवक्रता; किसी अंग का असाधारण रूप से टेढ़ा पड़ जाना

**Camptocormia.** A conversion reaction or hysterical condition in which the patient is completely bent forward and is unable to straighten up. अग्रकुब्जता

**Camptodactylia.** See **Campylodactyly.**

**Camptodactyly.** See **Campylodactyly.**

**Campylodactyly.** Permanent flexion of interphallangeal joints of one or more fingers; camptodactylia; camptodactyly. वक्रांगुलिता; उँगलियों का ढेढ़ा-मेढ़ा हो जाना

**Campylotropous.** Curved. वक्र; टेढ़ा

**Canal.** A tube, narrow passage or channel carrying the body fluids; canalis. नलिका; नली; नाली; नाल; खातिका; कुल्या; विशाखा;
   **Alimentary C.,** the whole digestive tube from the mouth to the anus. पोषण नली; पाचन नली; भोजन नली;
   **Anal C.,** the third part of the rectum, or space between the rectum proper and the anus. गुद-नाल; गुदा-नाल;
   **Bile C.,** see **Biliary Canal.**

**Biliary C.**, one of the intracellular channels that occurs between liver cells; bile canal. पित्त नली;

**Birth C.**, the cavity of the uterus and the vagina through which the foetus passes; parturient canal. जननमार्ग; जन्म नली;

**Carotid C.**, one in the petrous (stone-like) bone which transmits the internal carotid artery. मन्या नाल; मन्या नलिका;

**Cervical C.**, the part of the uterine canal between the internal and external os; canal of cervix uteri. गर्भाशयग्रीवा नलिका;

**Cochlear C.**, see **Spiral Canal**.

**Ethmoidal C.**, formed by articulation of the ethmoid and frontal bones. झर्झरिका नलिका;

**Femoral C.**, the inner compartment of the sheath of the femoral vessel. औवीं नलिका;

**Inguinal C.**, the passage from the internal to the exteral abdominal ring. वंक्षण नाल;

**Lachrymal C.**, see **Lacrimal Canal**.

**Lacrimal C.**, the bony canal in which the nasal duct is lodged; lachrymal canal. अश्रु-नली;

**Parturient C.**, see **Birth Canal**.

**Sacral C.**, the continuation of the vertebral canal in the sacrum. त्रिक-नाल;

**Semicircular C.'s**, the three bony canals of the labyrinth of the ear. अर्धवृत्त नलिकायें;

**Spiral C.**, the spiral cavity of the cochlea; cochlear canal. सर्पिल नलिका;

**Uterine C.**, the whole cavity of the uterus. जरायु नाल

**Canales.** Plural of **Canalis.**

**Canalicular.** Relating to canaliculus. सूक्ष्मनलिका सम्बन्धी

**Canaliculi.** Plural of **Canaliculus.**

**Canaliculitis.** Inflammation of the lacrimal duct. अश्रुनलीशोथ; अश्रुनली का प्रदाह

**Canaliculization.** Formation of small canals or channels in the tissue; canalisation. सूक्ष्मनलिकाभवन

**Canaliculus.** A small canal or groove; canalis; canal. सूक्ष्मनलिका

**Canalis.** See **Canal.**

**Canalisation.** The formation of a channel or canal, as in a clot;

**Canalization**

canaliculization; canalization. नलिकाकरण; नलिकाभवन
**Canalization.** See **Canalisation.**
**Cancellate.** See **Cancellous.**
**Cancellated.** See **Cancellous.**
**Cancellous.** Resembling lattice-work; cancellate; cancellated. सुषिर; जालीदार; जालीनुमा; झर्झरीनुमा
**Cancer.** A scirrhus, livid tumour, intersected by firm whitish divergent bands. कर्कट; कैंसर
**Canceroid.** Having the appearance of a cancer. कर्कटाभ; कैंसराभ; कैंसर जैसा
**Cancerophobia.** Extreme fear of cancer; carcinophobia. कर्कटभीति; कैंसरभीति; कैंसर हो जाने का भय
**Cancerous.** Of the nature of a cancer. कर्कटाभ; कर्कटाकार; कैंसरवत्; कैंसर जैसा; pertaining to cancer. कैंसरीय; कैंसर सम्बन्धी
**Cancra.** Plural of **Cancrum.**
**Cancriform.** Like a cancer. कर्कटाकार; कर्कटाभ; कैंसराभ; कैंसर जैसा
**Cancroid.** Having the appearance of a cancer. कर्कटाभ; कर्कटाकार; कैंसराभ; कैंसर जैसा
**Cancrum.** Gangrenous, ulcerative, inflammatory lesion. कोथज; व्रणोद्भवी; प्रदाहक विक्षति; कंकर
**Cancrum Oris.** Mortification or gangrene of the teeth or mouth; noma. मुखकोथ; कोथज मुखपाक; मुँह का नासूर
**Canine.** Pertaining to, or like that which belongs to a dog. रदनक; भेदक; श्वान सम्बन्धी;

  C. **Appetite,** excessive hunger; canine hunger. अतृप्त क्षुधा; अतिक्षुधा; अत्यधिक भूख; श्वान-क्षुधा;

  C. **Hunger,** the same as **Canine Appetite.**

  C. **Madness,** hydrophobia. अलर्क; जलातंक; जलभीति;

  C. **Teeth,** the cuspid or dog-teeth. भेदक दन्त; रदनक दन्त
**Canities.** Blanching, greyness or whiteness of the hair. पालित्य; बाल सफेद हो जाना
**Canker.** Ulcer of the mouth or throat of unknown cause; canker oris; canker sores. मुखकर्कट; कर्कटव्रण; कण्ठव्रण
**Canker Oris.** See **Canker.**
**Canker Sores.** See **Canker.**

**Cannabis.** Hemp; a genus of narcotic, antispasmodic and aphrodisiac plants. भांग;गांजा;

**C. Indica,** Indian hemp. भारतीय भांग का पौधा;

**C. Sativa,** the common hemp. भांग का पौधा

**Cannabism.** Poisoning by preparation of Cannabis. भांगात्यय; भांगविषण्णता

**Cannula.** A surgical tube for withdrawal of fluid from the body; canula. प्रवेशिनी; शल्यक्रिया में प्रयुक्त एक नली, जिससे शरीर के द्रव्यों को निकाला जाता है

**Cantani's Diet.** An exclusive meat diet in diabetes. मांसाहार

**Canthal.** Pertaining to the canthus. नेत्रकोण सम्बन्धी

**Catharides.** Plural of **Cantharis.**

**Cantharis.** A blistering agent prepared from the dried Spanish beetle. हरिभृंग; तेलनी; फफोलाजनक मक्षिका; स्पेन देश की एक सूखी मक्खी

**Canthectomy.** Excision of the canthus. नेत्रकोण-उच्छेदन

**Canthi.** Plural of **Canthus.**

**Canthitis.** Inflammation of the canthus. नेत्रकोणशोथ; कनीनिकाशोथ; चक्षुकोण-प्रदाह

**Cantholysis.** The surgical division of a canthus. नेत्रकोणवियोजन; कनीनिकावियोजन

**Canthoplasty.** A plastic operation on the canthus. नेत्रकोणसंधान; कनीनिकासंधान

**Canthorrhaphy.** Suture of the eyelids at either canthus. नेत्रकोणसीवन

**Canthotomy.** Division of the canthus. नेत्रकोणविभाजन; नेत्रकोण-उच्छेदन; कनीनिका-उच्छेदन

**Canthus.** The palpebral angle formed by the junction of the eyelids. नेत्रकोण; चक्षुकोण; कनीनिका;

Inner C., the internal junction of the eyelids. आन्तर नेत्रकोण;

Outer C., the external junction of the eyelids. बाह्य नेत्रकोण

**Canula.** See **Cannula.**

**Cap.** Any structure that resembles a protective covering for the head. छादन; कपालिका; कैप;

Knee-c., the patella. जानुका

**Capacitation.** See **Capacity.**

**Capacity.** Ability; cubic extent; capacitation. क्षमता; सामर्थ्य

# Capillaceous

**Capillaceous.** Resembling a hair. केशाभ; रोमाभ; लोमवत्; बाल जैसा

**Capillarectasia.** Dilatation of the capillaries. केशिकाविस्फार; केशिकाविस्तारण

**Capillaries.** Plural of **Capillary**.

**Capillariomotor.** Vasomotor, with special reference to the capillaries. केशिकाप्रेरक

**Capillaritis.** Inflammation of a capillary or capillaries. केशिकाशोथ

**Capillaropathy.** Any disease of the capillaries. केशिकाविकृति

**Capillary.** A minute blood vessel. केशिका; एक सूक्ष्म रक्त-वाहिका

**Capilli.** Plural of **Capillus**.

**Capillus.** Hair. रोम; लोम; बाल; केश

**Capistration.** See **Phimosis**.

**Capita.** Plural of **Caput**.

**Capitate.** Head-shaped; having a rounded extremity. शीर्षाकार

**Capiti.** In the head. सिर में

**Capitis.** The head. शीर्ष; सिर

**Capitium.** A bandage for the head. शीर्षपट्टिका

**Capitula.** Plural of **Capitulum**.

**Capitulum.** Knobbed end of part of an organ. मुण्डक

**Capping.** A covering. छद; आवरण

**Capricious.** Whimsical. अस्थिरचित्त; चंचल; मौजी

**Caprizant.** Of irregular motion. असमगतिक; विषमगतिक

**Capsicum.** A genus of **Solanaceous Plants** of various species; African pepper. लाल मिर्च का पौधा;
    C. Annum, the red pepper. लाल मिर्च

**Capsid Fructus.** The red peppers. लाल मिर्च

**Capsitis.** See **Capsulitis**.

**Capsotomy.** See **Capsulotomy**.

**Capsula.** Capsule. सम्पुट; कैप्सूल

**Capsulae.** Plural of **Capsula**.

**Capsular.** Pertaining to a capsule. सम्पुटीय; सम्पुट सम्बन्धी

**Capsulation.** Inclosing in capsules, as drugs. सम्पुटन

**Capsule.** Membranous sac. सम्पुट; सम्पुटिका; एक झिलीदार नली या थैली; the ligament which surrounds a joint. जोड़ों का एक बन्धन; a gelatinous paper container for noxious drugs. कैप्सूल

**Capsulectomy.** See **Capsulotomy.**
**Capsulitis.** Inflammation of a capsule; capsitis. सम्पुटशोथ; सम्पुट-प्रदाह
**Capsuloplasty.** Plastic operation of a capsule. सम्पुटसन्धान
**Capsulotome.** An instrument for performing capsulotomy; cystotome. सम्पुटछेदक
**Capsulotomy.** An incision of the capsule of the crystalline lens; capsotomy; capsulectomy; cystotomy. सम्पुटछेदन
**Caput.** The head; the chief part of an organ. शीर्ष; मुण्ड; मस्तक; सिर;

   **C. Coli,** the head of the colon; cecum. बृहदान्त्रशीर्ष

   **C. Medusae,** a venous dilatation around the navel. शिराछत्रक; नाभिशीर्ष;

   **C. Obstipum.** wry-neck; torticollis. बक्र-ग्रीवास्तम्भ;

   **C. Succedaneum,** a serosanguineous tumour on the presenting part of the foetus. प्रसवशीर्षशोफ

**Caramel.** Anhydrous or burnt sugar. दुग्धशर्करा; शुष्कशर्करा
**Caraway.** A genus of plants; the seeds are carminative. शाहजीरा; कालाजीरा
**Carbamid.** Urea. मूत्रक्षार; यूरिया
**Carbasus.** Lint. पट्टी
**Carbo.** Charcoal; carbon. चारकोल; कार्बन; प्रांगार; आंगार;

   **C. Animalis,** the animal charcoal. जन्तु-प्रांगार; एनिमल कार्बन;

   **C. Ligni,** wood charcoal; charcoal. काष्ठांगार;

   **C. Vegetabilis,** the vegetable carbon. वनस्पत्यांगार; शाक् कार्बन

**Carbohydrate.** An organic compound containing carbon, hydrogen and oxygen. श्वेतसार; कार्बोहाइड्रेट
**Carbohydraturia.** An excess of carbohydrates in the urine. श्वेतसारमेह; पेशाब में श्वेतसार जाना
**Carbolic Acid.** Phenol. प्रांगारिक अम्ल; कार्बोलिक एसिड
**Carbolism.** Carbolic acid poisoning. प्रांगारिक अम्ल-विषण्णता; कार्बोलिक एसिड से होने वाली विषाक्तता
**Carboluria.** Carbolic acid in the urine. प्रांगारिक अम्लमेह; पेशाब में कार्बोलिक एसिड जाना
**Carbon.** A non-metallic element present in all organic compounds. प्रांगार; हीरे या कोयले के रूप में पाया जाने वाला पदार्थ;

   **C. Dioxide,** a gas; a waste product of many forms of combustion and metabolism excreted *via* the lungs. कार्बनडाइआक्साइड;

**C. Monoxide,** poisonous gas which forms a stable compound with haemoglobin, thus robbing the body of its oxygen carrying mechanism. कार्बनमोनोक्साइड $C_2O$; कार्बन के अपूर्ण दहन से बनने वाली गैस जो रक्तकणरंजकद्रव्य के साथ एक स्थाई यौगिक बनाती है

**Carbonaceous.** Containing carbon. प्रांगारिक; कार्बनमय; कार्बनयुक्त

**Carbonate.** Any salt of carbonic acid. कार्बोनेट; प्रांगारिक अम्ल का लवण

**Carbonation.** Conversion into carbon; carbonization. कार्बनीकरण; कार्बनीभवन

**Carbonic Acid.** A heavy colourless gas; a compound of oxygen gas. कार्बनिक अम्ल; कार्बनिक एसिड

**Carbonization.** See **Carbonation.**

**Carbuncle.** An acute circumscribed inflammation involving several hair follicles and surrounding subcutaneous tissue; carbunculus; anthrax. छिद्राबुंद; नासूर; आंगारक्षण

**Carbunculus.** See **Carbuncle.**

**Carcase.** The dead body of an animal; carcass. शव; पशुशव; किसी पशु अथवा जन्तु की मृत देह अथवा लाश

**Carcass.** See **Carcase.**

**Carcinelcosis.** Malignant or cancerous ulceration. दुर्दम व्रणता; कर्कट-व्रणता

**Carcinogen.** Any cancer-producing agent or substance. कर्कटजन; कैंसरजन; कैंसरज; कैंसर पैदा करने वाला पदार्थ

**Carcinogenesis.** The production of cancer. कर्कटजनन; कैंसरजनन

**Carcinogenetic.** See **Carcinogenic.**

**Carcinogenic.** An agent producing cancer; carcinogenetic. कर्कटजनक; कैंसरजनक; कैंसर पैदा करने वाला पदार्थ

**Carcinogenicity.** An ability to produce cancer. कर्कटजननशीलता; कैंसरजननशीलता; कार्सिनोमाजननक्षमता

**Carcinoid.** Resembling a cancer or a crab. कर्कटाभ; कैंसराभ; कैंसर जैसा

**Carcinology.** The study of cancerous diathesis. कर्कटविद्या; कैंसरविद्या

**Carcinoma.** A cancer that arises from the cells of the skin or lining cells of the inner organs. कर्कट; कैंसर; कार्सिनोमा;

**Bronchogenic C.,** squamous cell or lung carcinoma which arises in the mucosa of the large bronchi and produces a persistent productive cough or haemoptysis. श्वसनीजन्य कार्सिनोमा;

**Chimney-Sweeper's C.,** scrotal epithelioma. अण्डकोशीय कैंसर ;

**Epidermoid C.,** see **Squamous Cell Carcinoma.**

**Squamous Cell C.,** a maligant neoplasm that is derived from the squamous cells; epidermoid carcinoma. दुर्दम कोशिका कार्सिनोमा

**Carcinomatosis.** A condition in which carcinoma is widely disseminated; carcinosis. कर्कटमयता; कर्कटार्बुदता; कार्सिनोमामयता

**Carcinomatous.** Pertaining to, or of the nature of carcinoma. कर्कटार्बुदीय; कर्कटार्बुदाभ

**Carcinomelcosis.** Cancerous ulceration. कर्कट-व्रणता; कर्कटार्बुदीय व्रणता

**Carcinophobia.** See **Cancerophobia.**

**Carcinosarcoma.** A mixed tumour having the characters of carcinoma and sarcoma; it usually affects the thyroid. अवटुकर्कटता

**Carcinosis.** A cancerous diathesis; the production and development of cancer; carcinomatosis. कैंसर; कर्कट; कर्कट-वृद्धि; कैंसर-प्रवणता; कर्कट-प्रवणता

**Cardamom.** The fruit of **Eletharia Cardamomum.** इलायची

**Cardia.** The heart; an orifice of the stomach. हृद्; हृदय; हृत्पिण्ड; अभिहृद्; उठरागम; आमाशय का एक प्रवेश पथ

**Cardiac.** Pertaining to the heart or cardia. हृदय अथवा हृत्पिण्ड सम्बन्धी;

  **C. Accelerator,** increasing the rate of the heart-beat. हृद्त्वरक; हृत्त्वरक; हृत्त्वरित्र; हृत्स्पन्दवर्धक;

  **C. Arrest,** complete cessation of the heart's activity. पूर्णहृद्रोध;

  **C. Oedema,** gravitational dropsy. हृद्शोफ;

  **C. Calculus.,** see **Cardiolith.**

  **C. Neurosis;** see **Cardioneurosis.**

  **C. Plexus,** a network formed by cardiac nerves at the back part of the aorta, near the heart. हृद्स्नायुजाल;

  **C. Puncture,** cardiopuncture. हृद्वेधन;

  **C. Temponade,** compression of heart. हृत्सम्पीडन

**Cardiagra.** Gout of the heart. हृद्वात; हृदय का गठिया

**Cardialgia.** Pain in the heart; heat-burn; cardiodynia. हृदयार्ति; हृद्शूल; हृच्छूल; हृद्वेदना

**Cardiant.** A remedy that affects the heart; a heart remedy. हृदयौषधि; हृदय को प्रभावित करने वाली औषधि

**Cardiasthenia.** Weakness in the action of the heart. हृद्दौर्बल्य

**Cardiatrophia.** Artophy of the heart. हृद्शोष; हृत्पिण्ड का सूखना

**Cardiectasia.** See **Cardiectasis.**

**Cardiectasis.** Dilatation of the heart; cardiectasia. हृत्विस्फार; हृदय का फैलना

**Cardinal.** Chief; principal. प्रमुख; प्रधान

**Cardioacceleration.** The act of increasing the rate of the heart-beat. हृद्त्वरण; हृत्स्पन्दवर्धन

**Cardioaccelerator.** An agent increasing the rate of heart-beat. हृत्वरक; हृत्वरित्र; हृत्स्पन्दवर्धक; हृदय की धड़कन बढ़ाने वाला

**Cardioactive.** Influencing the heart. हृत्वरक; हृत्वरित्र; हृदय की क्रिया को प्रभावित करने वाला

**Cardioangiology.** The science concerned with the heart and blood vessels. हृद्वाहिकाविज्ञान

**Cordioaortic.** Relating to the heart and the aorta. हृदय तथा महाधमनी सम्बन्धी

**Cardioarterial.** Relating to the heart and the arteries. हृदय तथा धमनियों सम्बन्धी

**Cardiocele.** Hernia of the heart. हृद्पुटी; हृद्संस; हृद्हर्निया

**Cardiocentesis.** See **Cardiopuncture.**

**Cardiodynia.** Pain in the heart; cardialgia; heart-burn. हृत्पीड़ा; हृद्वेदना; हृद्शूल; हृच्छूल; हृद्दाह; हृदय-पीड़ा

**Cardiogenic.** Originating from the heart. हृद्जन्य; हृदयजनित

**Cardiogmus.** Cardialgia; angina pectoris. हृद्शूल; हृत्पीड़ा; aneurysm of the heart. हृद्धमनीविस्फार; हृदय की बड़ी धमनी का फैलना

**Cardiogram.** Tracing made by cardiograph. हृद्लेख; हृद्गतिलेख; हृत्स्पन्दलेख

**Cardiograph.** An instrument for recording the heart-motion. हृद्गतिलेखी; हृत्स्पन्दमापी (यंत्र)

**Cardiography.** A description of the heart. हृद्लेख; हृत्स्पन्दलेख; हृद्गतिलेख;

**Ultrasound C.,** use of ultrasound in the diagnosis of the cardiovascular lesions and recording of the size, motion and composition of various cardiac structures; echocardiography. पराध्वनि हृद्लेख; प्रतिध्वनि हृद्लेख

**Cardioinhibitory.** Controlling the heart's action. हृद्संदमी; हृदय की क्रिया को नियंत्रित करने वाला

**Cardiolith.** A concretion in the heart, or an area of calcareous degeneration in its walls or valves; cardiac calculus. हृदश्मरी; हृत्पिण्ड की पथरी

**Cardiologist.** A specialist in the study of cardiology. हृद्विज्ञानी; हृदयरोग विशेषज्ञ

**Cardiology.** The science of the heart. हृद्रोगविज्ञान; हृद्विज्ञान; हृदयरोगविज्ञान

**Cardiolysis.** Resection of the ribs and sternum over the pericardium to free the latter from its adhesions to the anterior chest wall in adhesive mediastinopericarditis. परिहृद्वियोजन; हृदयलयन

**Cardiomalacia.** A softening of the heart-substance. हृद्मृदुता; हृत्पिण्ड की कोमलता

**Cardiomegaly.** Enlargement of the heart. हृद्बृहत्ता; हृदय की बढ़ी हुई अवस्था

**Cardiomotility.** Movement of the heart. हृद्गति

**Cardiomyoliposis.** Fatty degeneration of the myocardium. हृत्पेशी-वसापजनन

**Cardiomyopathy.** Any disease of the muscles of the heart. हृत्पेशीविकृति; हृदय की पेशियों का रोग

**Cardiomyotomy.** Incision of the muscles of the openings of the heart. जठरागमपेशीछेदन; हृदय की मुखीपेशियों को छेदना

**Cardionephric.** See **Cardiorenal.**

**Cardioneurosis.** Anxiety concerning the state of the heart as a result of palpitation, chest pain, or other symptoms not due to heart disease; cardiac neurosis. हृद्विक्षिप्ति

**Cardio-omentopexy.** Surgical attachment of omentum of the heart to improve its blood supply. हृद्वपास्थिरीकरण

**Cardiopalmus.** Palpitation of the heart. हृत्स्पन्दन; हृदय की धड़कन

**Cardiopathy.** Any heart-disease. हृद्-विकृति; हृदय का कोई रोग

**Cardiopericarditis.** Inflammation of the heart and pericardium. हृद्परिहृद्शोथ; हृदय तथा हृदयावरण का प्रदाह

**Cardiophobia.** Morbid fear of heart-disease. हृद्रोगभीति; हृदय रोग होने का भय

**Cardiophone.** A microphone or stethoscope for listening to sound of the heart. हृद्ध्वनिक; हृद्फोन; हृद्ध्वनि को सुनने योग्य बनाने वाला यंत्र

**Cardioplasty.** Plastic operation of the cardiac sphincter. हृद्संधान;

हृत्संधान; जठरागमसंधान
**Cardioplegia.** Paralysis of the heart. हृद्घात; हृदय का पक्षाघात
**Cardiopneumatic.** See **Cardiopulmonary.**
**Cardiopulmonary.** Pertaining to the heart and the lungs; cardiopneumatic. हृदय तथा फेफड़ों सम्बन्धी; हृत्फुप्फुसीय;
   **C. Bypass,** used in open heart surgery. हृद्फुप्फुस पार्श्वपथ
**Cardiopuncture.** Cardiocentesis; surgical incision of the heart. हृद्छिद्रण; हृद्वेधन
**Cardiorator.** Apparatus for visual recording of the heart-beat. हृत्स्पन्ददृष्टिलेखयंत्र
**Cardiorenal.** Pertaining to the heart and kidney; cardionephric. हृदय तथा वृक्क सम्बन्धी
**Cardiorespiratory.** Pertaining to the heart and the respiratory system. हृदय तथा श्वास सम्बन्धी
**Cardiorrhaphy.** Stitching or suturing of the heart wall. हृद्प्राचीरसंधान; हृत्प्राचीररसीवन
**Cardiorrhexis.** Rupture of the heart-wall. हृद्प्राचीरखंस
**Cardiosclerosis.** Induration of the heart. हृत्तन्तुकाठिन्य; हृत्पिण्ड की कठोरता
**Cardioscope.** An instrument fitted with a lens and illumination for examining the inside of the heart. हृत्कपाटदर्शी; हृद्लेखदर्शी
**Cardioscopy.** A microscopic examination of the inside of the heart. हृत्कपाटदर्शन; हृद्लेखदर्शन
**Cardiospasm.** A spasmodic contraction of the cardiac end of the stomach. अभिहृद्जठराकर्ष; अभिहृद्जठर-अशिथिलता
**Cardiostenosis.** Stenosis of the heart-valve. हृत्कपाटसंकोच; हृत्कपाट की सिकुड़न
**Cardiotachometer.** An instrument for measuring the rapidity of the heart-beat. हृद्स्पन्दमापी
**Cardiothoracic.** Pertaining to the heart and the thoracic cavity. हृदय तथा वक्ष-गह्वर सम्बन्धी
**Cardiotomy.** Dissection of the heart. हृदुच्छेदन; हृदय की चीर-फाड़ करना
**Cardiotonics.** Tonics which invigorate the heart. हृद्बल्यवर्ग; हृद्यवर्ग; हृदय को ताकत देने वाले पौष्टिक पदार्थ
**Cardiovascular.** Pertaining to the heart and blood vessels. हृदय तथा रक्तवाहिकाओं सम्बन्धी

**Cardioversion.** Use of electrical countershock for restoring heart-rhythm to normal. हृत्तालवर्धन

**Cardioverter.** An agent which increases the rhythms of the heart. हृत्तालवर्धक

**Carditis.** Inflammation of the heart. हृद्शोथ; हृत्पिण्ड अथवा हृदयपिण्ड का प्रदाह

**Care.** Look-after. रक्षण; अवेक्षा; देख-भाल; देख-रेख

**Caries.** Ulceration, wasting, usually associated with pus formation. क्षरण; क्षय; यक्ष्मा; परिगलन;

   **C. of spine,** spinal tuberculosis; Pott's spine; spinal caries. मेरु-क्षय; मेरु-क्षरण; रीढ़ की हड्डी का गलना;

   **C. of teeth,** decaying of teeth. दन्तक्षय; दन्तक्षरण;

   **Spinal C.,** see **Caries of spine.**

**Carious.** Affected with caries. क्षरणग्रस्त; क्षयग्रस्त; परिगलित

**Carminative.** A medicine which expels wind from the body. वातानुलोमक; वायुनाशक; वातसारी

**Carneous.** Fleshy. मांसल

**Carnia.** The spine. मेरुदण्ड; रीढ़

**Carniform.** Having the appearance of the flesh. मांसाभ ; मांसवत्; मांस जैसा; गोश्त जैसा

**Carnivore.** See **Carnivorous.**

**Carnivorous.** Flesh-eating animals. मांसाहारी; मांसभक्षी; मांस खाने वाला

**Carnophobia.** Morbid fear of eating flesh. मांसाहारभीति; गोश्त खाने का डर

**Carotid.** The principal artery of the neck. मन्या; ग्रैव; ग्रीवापरक;

   **C. Artery,** one of the two large arteries of the neck. मन्या धमनी; गर्दन की नाड़ी;

   **C. Gland,** the neck gland. मन्या-ग्रन्थि; ग्रीवा-ग्रन्थि;

**Carpagra.** Pain in the wrist. मणिबन्धार्ति; कलाई का दर्द

**Carpal.** Belonging to the carpus, or wrist. मणिबन्धीय; कलाई सम्बन्धी

**Carpectomy.** Excision of a portion of carpus. मणिबन्धउच्छेदन

**Carphology.** Involuntary picking at the bed-clothes. शय्यालुंचन; वस्त्रलुंचनोन्माद

**Carpi.** The wrist. मणिबन्ध; कलाई; बाजूबन्द

**Carpometacarpal.** Pertaining to the carpus and metacarpus. मणिबन्ध तथा करभ सम्बन्धी

**Carpoptosia.** See **Carpoptosis.**

**Carpoptosis.** Wrist-drop; carpoptosia. मणिबन्धस्रंस

**Carpus.** The wrist, or the wrist-joint; carpi. मणिबन्ध; कलाई अथवा कलाई का जोड़

**Carrier.** A healthy animal or human host who harbours pathogenic organism and passes it to his environment. वाहक; वाहित्र; रोगाणुओं को अपने साथ ले जाना वाला

**Car-sickness.** Sickness produced by travelling in a car, rail, etc. वाहन-रुग्णता; मोटरकार, रेलगाड़ी की सवारी, आदि करने के कारण होने वाली बीमारी

**Cartilage.** A tissue less hard and more elastic than bone, found in joints and elsewhere. उपास्थि;

  **Arytenoid C.**, one of cup-shaped or ladle-shaped cartilages of the larynx; cartilago arytenoidea. दर्वीकल्प उपास्थि;

  **Costal C.**, that lying between the true ribs and the sternum; cartilago costalis. पर्शुका उपास्थि;

  **Cricoid C.**, the ring like cartilage of the larynx; cartilago basilaris; cartilago cricoidea. मुद्रिका उपास्थि;

  **Cuneiform C.**, a wedge-shaped cartilage of the larynx; cartilago cuneiformis. कीलक उपास्थि;

  **Permanent C.**, cartilage that remains as such and does not become converted into bone. स्थायी उपास्थि;

  **Precursory C.**, see **Temporary Cartilage.**

  **Temporary C.**, cartilage that normally becomes replaced by bone to form part of skeleton; precursory cartilage. अस्थायी उपास्थि;

  **Thyroid C.**, see **Cartilago Thyreoidea.**

**Cartilaginification.** Conversion into cartilage. उपास्थिभवन

**Cartilaginiform.** Resembling a cartilage; cartilaginoid. उपास्थिवत्; उपास्थिरूप; उपास्थि से मिलता-जुलता

**Cartilaginoid.** See **Cartilaginiform.**

**Cartilaginous.** Pertaining to, or consisting of a cartilage. उपास्थिपरक अथवा उपास्थिमय

**Cartilago.** A cartilage. उपास्थि;

  **C. Arytenoidea.**, see **Arytenoid Cartilage.**

  **C. Basilaris**, see **Cricoid Cartilage.**

  **C. Costalis**, see **Costal Catilage.**

C. **Corniculata,** the horny cartilage of the larynx. शृंगी उपास्थि;

C. **Cricoidea,** see **Cricoid Cartilage.**

C. **Cuneiformis,** see **Cuneiform Cartilage.**

C. **Septinasi,** the cartilage of the nasal septum. नासापट-उपास्थि;

C. **Thyreoidea,** the thyroid cartilage. अवटु-उपास्थि; अवटूपास्थि;

C. **Triticea,** a cartilage in the thyroid ligament. उपास्थिकण;

C. **Wrisbergii,** the same as **Cartilago Cuneiformis.**

**Caruncle.** A red, fleshy projection; caruncula; carunculus. मांसांकुर; बीजचोलक; अधिमांस; मांस का बढ़ा हुआ भाग

**Caruncula.** See **Caruncle.**

**Carunculae.** Plural of **Caruncula.**

**Carunculae Hymenales.** The remains of the hymen after rupture during coitus. योनिच्छदशेष; फटने के बाद योनिच्छद के अवशिष्ट भाग

**Carunculae Myrtiformis.** The same as **Carunculae Hymenales.**

**Carunculus.** See **Caruncle.**

**Carus.** The last degree of coma; profound stupor; complete insensibility. गहन मूर्च्छा; जड़िमा; सन्यास

**Cascara.** A purgative bark used for constipation. कसकरा; कसकरा नामक पेड़ की छाल से प्राप्त एक रेचक पदार्थ

**Case.** The patient. रोगी;

C. **History,** see **Case Taking.**

C. **Record,** see **Case Sheet.**

C. **Sheet,** the document containing the particulars of the patient as well as the description of the disease, treatment, etc.; case record. रोग आलेख;

C. **Taking,** the collection of memoranda and preservation of records of clinical cases; case history. रोगवृत्त; रोगी का विवरण

**Caseation.** Precipitation of casein during coagulation of milk. किलाटीभवन; पनीरीभवन

**Casein.** The clotted protein of milk; cheese. पनीर; केसीन; दूध में पाया जाने वाला थक्केदार प्रोटीन

**Caseous.** Having the nature of cheese. किलाटीरूप; पनीरी; पनीर जैसा;

C. **Degeneration,** caseation. किलाटीभवन; पनीरीभवन; पनीरी-अपजनन; पनीरी-व्यपजनन

**Cast.** A mass of plastic matter having the cavity in which it has been molded and it is named according to its source of constituents. निर्मोक; पपड़ी;

**Blood C.**, a urinary cast composed principally of red blood cells. रक्त-निर्मोक;

**Body C.**, cast used to immobilize the spine which may extend from the thorax to the groin. पिण्ड-निर्मोक;

**Epithelial C.**, a cast containing cells from inner lining of uriniferous tubules, seen in acute nephritis. उपकला-निर्मोक;

**Fatty C.**, any cast made of fat globules. वसा-निर्मोक;

**Pus C.**, leukocyte cast found in urine in suppuration of kidney. पूति-निर्मोक;

**Uterine C.**, cast from the uterus passed in exfoliative endomentritis or membranous dysmenorrhoea. जरायु-निर्मोक; गर्भाशयिक निर्मोक;

**Waxy C.**, light yellowish well-defined urinary cast with tendency to split transversally. मोमी निर्मोक

**Castor Oil.** A purgative; the oil extracted from the seeds of the **Ricinus communis.** कैस्टर आयल; एरंड का तेल

**Castration.** Sterilization. बन्ध्याकरण; बन्ध्यीकरण; बीजग्रन्थिनाशन; बीजग्रन्थि-उच्छेदन

**Casualty.** Accidental injury. आहत; अत्याहत; हताहत; घायल

**Catabasis.** The decline of a disease. रोगावरोहरण; रोग-ह्रास

**Catabolic.** Pertaining to catabolism. अपचयी; अपचयज; उपचयी; अपचय सम्बन्धी

**Catabolin.** See **Catabolite.**

**Catabolism.** The series of chemical reaction in the living body; katabolism. अपचय; उपचय; शरीर में रासायनिक प्रतिक्रिया की क्रमिकता

**Catabolite.** A product of catabolism; catabolin. अपचयज; अपचयी; अपचय-उत्पाद

**Catacrotic.** Elevations in the down-stroke of the sphygmogram. विषमावरोही

**Catacrotism.** The condition of being catacrotic. विषमावरोहिता

**Catadicrotic.** Having one secondary expansion. अवद्विस्पन्दी

**Catadicrotism.** A divided or double pulsation in the down-stroke of the sphygmograph. अवद्विस्पन्दिता

**Catagenesis.** Involution or retrogression. प्रत्यावर्तन अथवा प्रतिगमन

**Catagma.** An acute fracture. तीव्र अस्थिभ्रंश; तरुण अस्थिभंग

**Catalepsy.** A peculiar form of nervous disease allied to hysteria, occurring in paroxysms. पेशीप्रतिष्टम्भ; निस्पन्दवात

**Cataleptic.** Affected with catalepsy. पेशीप्रतिष्टम्भग्रस्त; निस्पन्दवातग्रस्त

**Catalysis.** A chemical reaction promoted by the presence of a third unaffected substance. उत्प्रेरण; परमाणुओं का संयोग-वियोग करने वाली शक्ति

**Catalyst.** Substance which induces or speeds up a reaction by its presence, but itself remains intact. उत्प्रेरक; आवेजक

**Catalytic.** Produced by or pertaining to catalysis. उत्प्रेरकीय; रक्तदोषनाशक; उत्प्रेरण सम्बन्धी; alternate medicine. विकल्पी अथवा वैकल्पिक औषधि

**Catalyze.** To act as a catalyser. उत्प्रेरक तुल्य कार्य करना

**Catamenia.** The menses, or monthly discharge of women. आर्तव; ऋतुस्राव; रजोधर्म; मासिक धर्म; रज:स्राव

**Catamenial.** Relating to monthly period of women. आर्तव अथवा ऋतुस्राव सम्बन्धी

**Catamnesis.** The medical history of a patient after an illness. रोगवृत्त

**Catamnestic.** Relating to catamnesis. रोगवृत्त सम्बन्धी

**Cataphasia.** A disturbance of speech in which there is a constant repetition of the same word or words. मुहुर्मुहुर्वाक्; वाक्-असंगतता; शब्दों को बार-बार दोहराते रहने की आदत

**Cataphora.** Semicoma. अर्धसन्यास; अर्धचेतन

**Cataphoresis.** The anodal diffusion of medicament to deep-seated tissues. वैद्युत्कणसंचलन; विद्युत्धारा द्वारा गहन-ऊतकों में औषधि का प्रवेश करना

**Cataphoria.** An inclination of the visual axis below the horizontal plane; catatopia. उभयनेत्र-अध:चलनप्रवृत्ति

**Cataphylaxis.** Weakening of the infection defenses of the body. रोगक्षमतानाश; रोगप्रतिरक्षीकरण का ह्रास

**Cataplasm.** See **Cataplasma.**

**Cataplasma.** A poultice; cataplasm. उपनाह; पुल्टिस

**Cataplectic.** Relating to cataplexy. मरणानुभूति-पेशीप्रतिष्टम्भ सम्बन्धी

**Cataplexy.** A condition of muscular rigidity induced by severe mental shock, fear and in which the patient remains conscious. मरणानुभूति-पेशीप्रतिष्टम्भ; पेशीतान का अचानक लोप हो जाना (फलस्वरूप रोगी निर्जीव-सा हो जाता है)

**Cataract.** A clouding of the crystalline lens in the eye obscuring vision. मोतियाबिंद; मोतियाबिन्दु; मुक्ताबिंद; मोतिया;

**Annular C.,** a congenital cataract in which the central white membrane replaces the nucleus. वलयी मोतियाबिंद;

**Black C.,** a cataract in which the lens is hardened and turns dark brown. श्याम मोतियाबिंद; काला मोतिया;

**Capsular C.,** one from deposits on the inner surface of the capsule. सम्पुटी मोतियाबिंद;

**Cortical C.,** loss of transparency of the outer layers of the lens. प्रान्तस्था मोतियाबिंद;

**Glaucomatous C.,** a nuclear opacity usually seen in absolute glaucoma. अधिमंथज मोतियाबिंद;

**Grey C.,** a cataract of grey colour, usually seen in senile, mature or cortical cataract. धूसर मोतियाबिंद;

**Immature C.,** one in which only a part of the lens-substance is cataractous. अपक्व मोतियाबिंद;

**Incipient C.,** one in an early stage. आरभमाण मोतियाबिंद;

**Lamellar C.,** one due to opacity of certain nucleus; zonular cataract. पटलित मोतियाबिंद;

**Mature C.,** one in which the whole lens-substance is cataractous; ripe cataract. पक्व मोतियाबिंद; पका मोतियाबिन्द;

**Ripe C.,** see **Mature Cataract.**

**Senile C.,** cataract spontaneously occurring in old age. जराजन्य मोतियाबिंद;

**Zonular C.,** see **Lamellar Cataract.**

**Cataracta Brunescence.** The grey cataract. धूसर मोतियाबिंद; भूरा मोतिया

**Cataracta Coerulea.** The blue cataract. नीला मोतियाबिंद; आसमानी मोतियाबिंद

**Cataractogenic.** Cataract-producing. मोतियाबिंदजनक

**Cataractous.** Having the nature of a cataract. मोतियाबिंदाभ; मोतियाबिन्द की प्रकृति का या मोतियाबिंद जैसा

**Catarrh.** Inflammation of the mucous membrane. प्रतिश्याय; सर्दी-जुकाम; सर्दी; अभिष्यन्द;

**Epidemic C.,** influenza. इन्फ्लुएंजा; श्लेम-ज्वर; श्लैष्मिक ज्वर;

**Gastric C.,** gastritis. जठरशोथ; पेट का प्रदाह; पेट की सर्दी;

**Intestinal C.**, enteritis. आंत्रशोथ; आंतों का प्रदाह; आंतों की सर्दी;
**Nasal C.**, coryza. नासा-प्रतिश्याय; नजला; नाक की सर्दी;
**Pulmonary C.**, bronchitis. श्वसनीशोथ; श्वासनली का प्रदाह;
**Spring C.**, see **Vernal Catarrh.**
**Uterine C.**, endometritis. अंतर्गर्भाशयकलाशोथ;
**Vernal C.**, that coming on with the spring; spring catarrh. वासंती अभिष्यंद

**Catarrhal.** Belonging to, or of the nature of catarrh. प्रतिश्यायी; श्लेष्मस्रावी; प्रतिश्याय अथवा श्लेष्मस्राव सबन्धी;
**C. Ophthalmia**, an inflammation of the first covering of the eyeball, produced by, or associated with cold. प्रतिश्यायी नेत्राभिष्यंद; सर्दी-जुकाम के कारण आँखें आना

**Catastaltic.** Inhibitory; restricting; restraining. रोधक; रोधी

**Catastasis.** Constitution, state or condition. गठन; स्थिति; अवस्था; extension and displacement of a dislocated limb. अतिरिक्तपुर:सरण

**Catatonia.** A form of insanity progressing to imbecility; catatony. तानप्रतिष्टम्भ; विक्षिप्ति का एक रूप

**Catatonic.** Stuporous; relating to catatonia. तानप्रतिष्टम्भी

**Catatony.** See **Catatonia.**

**Catatopia.** see **Cataphoria.**

**Catch cold.** Affected with cold. सर्दी-जुकाम लगना

**Catechu.** An extract prepared from the wood of **Acacia catechu,** used in medicine as an astringent. कत्था; खादिर

**Caternating.** Connecting; linking. संयोजी; जोड़ने वाला

**Catgut.** A ligature substance made from sheep's intestines. आन्त्रतन्ति; भेड़ की आन्तों से तैयार किया जाने वाला एक धागा या बन्धन

**Catharsis.** Purgation. दस्त; अतिसार; प्रवाहिका; रेचन

**Cathartic.** A drug that stimulates bowel action. रेचक; विरेचक; सारक; भेदक; दस्तावर दवाई

**Catheter.** A flexible rubber tube used for draining the bladder or its cavities. मूत्रशलाका; नालशलाका; मूत्रनिस्सारक नली; पेशाब कराने वाली नली

**Catheterisation.** Insertion of a catheter; catheterization. नालशलाका-प्रवेशन

**Catheterization.** See **Catheterisation.**

**Cathode.** The negative pole of an electric current; Kathode. ऋणाग्र;

**Cation** 206

विद्युत्धारा का ऋण ध्रुव

**Cation.** An electropositive element. धनायन; धनविद्युत्तत्व

**Catnep.** Stimulant and tonic. उद्दीपक एवं पौष्टिक

**Cat's ear.** A deformed ear similar to that of a cat. विडाल कर्ण; बिल्ली जैसे कान

**Cauda.** A tail, or tail-like appendage. पुच्छ; पूंछ; पुच्छांग

**Caudae.** Plural of **Cauda.**

**Caudal.** Pertaining to tail. पुच्छ अथवा पूंछ सम्बन्धी

**Caudage.** Having a tail. पुच्छक; पूंछ वाला

**Caudicle.** A short tail or appendage. पुच्छ; पूंछ

**Caul.** The great omentum. बृहत् वपा; the membrane capping the head of the baby when born. सावरण जन्म

**Caulophyllum.** A genus of herbs. राजचम्पा

**Causal.** Pertaining to a cause. हेतुक; कारण और कार्य सम्बन्धी

**Causalgia.** Neuralgia with intense burning. चोष; दाहार्ति; जलन के साथ दर्द

**Cause.** That which produces or effects a result. हेतु; कारण

**Caustic.** Burning or corrosive; pyrotic. दाहक; ज्वलनकारी; संक्षारक

**Causticity.** Capability to burn. दाहकता; संक्षारकता

**Cauterant.** A caustic. दाहक (पदार्थ)

**Cauterization.** The application of a cautery. दहन; दहनकर्म; दागना; क्षारकर्म करना

**Cauterize.** To burn or otherwise act on a diseased part by heat, caustic, etc. दहनकर्म करना; दागना; क्षारकर्म करना;

**Cautery.** Any caustic agent. दाहक; दह्य; प्रदाहक; कोई जलाने वाला पदार्थ

**Cava.** Either of the large veins which open directly in the right auricle. बृहत् शिरायें; बड़ी शिरायें;

  **Vena C.,** see under **Vena.**

**Cave.** A cavity. गुहा; गह्वर; कोटर; विवर; छिद्र

**Cavernitis.** Inflammation of the hollow tissues of the penis; cavernositis. शिश्नगह्वरशोथ

**Cavernositis.** See **Cavernitis.**

**Cavernous.** Having hollow places. गह्वरी; गह्वरीय; गह्वरयुक्त; छिद्रिल;

  **C. Rale,** breathing sound by passage of air through a small cavity with flaccid walls. गह्वर-ध्वनि

**Cavitary.** Relating to, or having a body-cavity or many cavities. गह्वरीय; गह्वर सम्बन्धी; of intestinal tract. आंत्रपथीय

**Cavitas.** See **Cavity.**

**Cavitates.** Plural of **Cavitas.**

**Cavitation.** The formation of a cavity, as in the pulmonary tuberculosis. गह्वरण; गुहिकायन; कोटरण

**Cavity.** A hollow part in the body; cavitas; cavum. गह्वर; गुहिका; कोटर; विवर; गुहा; गर्त;

    **Abdominal C.,** that below the diaphragm. उदर-गह्वर; उदर-गुहा;

    **Buccal C.,** the mouth. मुख; मुख-गह्वर; मुख-गुहा;

    **Cerebral C.,** the ventricles of the brain. मस्तिष्क-गह्वर; मस्तिष्क-गुहा;

    **Cranial C.,** the brain-box formed by the bones. कपाल-गह्वर; कपाल-गुहा;

    **Peritoneal C.,** potential space between the parietal and visceral layers of the peritoneum. उदरावरण गुहा; उदरावरण गह्वर;

    **Pleural C.,** the potential space between the pulmonary and the parietal pleurae which in health are in contact in all phases of respiration. फुप्फुस-गह्वर; फुप्फुस-गुहा;

    **Synovial C.,** the potential space in a joint. श्लेष-गह्वर; श्लेष-गुहा;

    **Uterine C.,** that of the uterus. जरायु-गह्वर; जरायु-गुहा; गर्भाशय-गह्वर; गर्भाशय-गुहा

**Cavum.** A cavity; cavus. गुहा; गह्वर;

    **C. Abdominis,** the abdominal cavity. उदर-गुहा; उदर-गह्वर;

    **C. Dentis,** the pulp cavity of a tooth. दन्त-गुहा; दन्त-गह्वर;

    **C. Laryngis,** the laryngeal cavity. स्वरयंत्र-गुहा; स्वरयंत्र-गह्वर; कण्ठगुहा;

    **C. Oris Proprius,** the cavity of the mouth proper. मुख-गुहा; मुख-गह्वर;

    **C. Pericardii,** the pericardial cavity. परिहृद्-गुहा; परिहृद्-गह्वर

    **C. Pleurae,** the pleural cavity. फुप्फुस-गुहा; फुप्फुस-गह्वर;

    **C. Uteri,** the cavity of the uterus. जरायु-गुहा; गर्भाशय-गुहा; जरायु-गह्वर; गर्भाशय-गह्वर

**Ceca.** Plural of **Cecum.**

**Cecal.** See **Caecal.**

**Cecectomy.** Excision of a part of cecum. अन्धान्त्र-उच्छेदन

**Cecitis.** See **Caecitis.**

**Cecocolostomy.** See **Caecocolostomy.**

**Cecoptosis.** See **Caecoptosis.**

**Cecostomy.** See **Caecostomy.**

**Cecotomy.** See **Caecotomy.**

**Cecum.** See **Caecum.**

**Celia.** The belly. कुक्षि; उदर; पेट

**Celiac.** Belonging to the belly. उदरीय; औदरीय; औदरिक; उदर सम्बन्धी

**Celialgia.** Abdominal pain. कुक्षिशूल; उदरशूल; पेट का दर्द

**Celibacy.** Unmarried life. कौमार्य; ब्रह्मचर्य; कुंआरापन; अविवाहित जीवन

**Celiomyositis.** Inflammation of the abdominal muscles. उदरपेशीशोथ; उदर पेशियों का प्रदाह

**Celipathy.** Any abdominal disease. उदररोग

**Celiorrhaphy.** Suture of a wound in the abdominal wall; laparorrhaphy. उदरप्राचीरसंधान; उदरसीवन

**Celioscopy.** Examination of the contents of abdomin with a peritoneoscope; laparoscopy; ventroscopy. उदरदर्शन

**Celiotomy.** Abdominal section; transabdominal incision into the peritoneal cavity; laparotomy; ventrotomy. उदरछेदन

**Celitis.** Inflammation of the abdominal organs. कुक्षिशोथ; उदरशोथ; पेट का प्रदाह

**Cell.** The building block of the body; the structural unit of any living being. कोशिका; कोष; कोषाणु; कोष्ठिका;

    **Acinar C.,** any secreting cell lining an acinous; acinous cell. कोष्ठकी कोशिका;

    **Acinous C.,** see **Acinar Cell.**

    **Adipose C.,** see **Fat Cell.**

    **Basal C.,** a cell of the deepest layer of an epithelium. आधार कोशिका; आधारी कोशिका;

    **Decidual C.,** a proliferation of young connective tissue cells above the uterine glands taking place after the ovum is impregnated. पतनिका कोशिका;

    **Endothelial C.,** one of the cells composing endothelium. उपकला कोशिका;

**Fat C.**, a connective tissue cell containing oil; adipose cell. वसा कोशिका;

**Follicular C.**, an epithelial cell lining a follicle, such as thyroid or ovary. कूपिका कोशिका;

**Ganglion C.**, those of the grey matter of the brain or spinal cord. गण्डिका कोशिका;

**Germ C.**, see **Sex Cell**.

**Germinal C.**, the epiblastic cell from which a neurone is derived. बीज कोशिका;

**Giant C.**, one of the large multinuclear cells in the bone. महाकोशिका;

**Goblet C.**, an epithelial cell buldged out like a globlet by the mucin within. चषक कोशिका;

**Gustatory C.**, a taste cell. स्वाद कोशिका;

**Hair C.**, an epithelial cell with a hair-like process. लोम कोशिका; रोम कोशिका;

**Mother C.**, a multiplying cell. मातृ कोशिका;

**Mucous C.**, a cell that secretes mucus. श्लेष्म कोशिका;

**Prickle C.**, an epidermal cell furnished with radiating processes which connect with similar cells. शूक कोशिका;

**Red Blood C. (RBC)**, erythrocyte; red cell. लोहित कोशिका; लाल रक्त कोशिका;

**Red C.**, see **Red Blood Cell**.

**Sex C.**, a spermatozoon or an ovum; germ cell. शुक्राणु अथवा डिम्बाणु; लिंग कोशिका; बीज कोशिका;

**Taste C.**, a spindle-shaped cell in taste-buds. स्वाद कोशिका;

**White Blood C. (WBC)**, leucocyte. श्वेत रुधिर कोशिका;

**C.-body**, the mass of a cell. कोशिका-पिण्ड;

**C.-capsule**, thick, strong cell-wall. कोशिका-सम्पुट;

**C.-division**, indirect nuclear division. कोशिका-विभाजन;

**C.-plate**, the forerunner of the partition wall in dividing plant-cell. कोशिका-पट्ट;

**C.-sap**, the more fluid part of the cell-contents. कोशिका-रस;

**C.-theory**, the doctorine that cell-formation is the essential biogenetic element. कोशिका-सिद्धान्त;

**C.-wall,** the membrane surrounding a cell. कोशिका-प्राचीर

**Cellar.** An underground room. तहखाना; भूमिगत कक्ष

**Cellula.** A little cell; cullule. सूक्ष्मकोशिका; क्षुद्रकोष; क्षुद्रकोशिका; क्षुद्रगुहा

**Cellulae.** Plural of **Cellula.**

**Cellular.** Pertaining to, or composed of cells. कोशीय; कोशिकीय; कोशमय; कोशिक;

 **C. Inflammation,** see **Cellulitis.**

 **C. Tissue,** tissue consisting of cells. कोशोतक; कोशिका-ऊतक

**Cellule.** See **Cellula.**

**Cellulicidal.** Destructive to cells. कोशिकाघाती

**Cellulitis.** Cellular inflammation; inflammation of cellular or connective tissue. कोशिकाशोथ; कोशिका-प्रदाह; संयोजकऊतिशोथ; संयोजीऊतकशोथ;

 **Orbital C.,** inflammation of a connective tissue of the eyeball. नेत्रगोलक-संयोजकऊतिशोथ;

 **Pelvic C.,** parametritis. श्रोणि-संयोजकऊतिशोथ

**Celluloneuritis.** Inflammation of a nerve-cell. तंत्रिकाकोशिकाशोथ; स्नायुकोशिका का प्रदाह

**Cellulose.** The principal ingredient of the cellular substance of the plants. कोशिकारस; सेलूलोज

**Celom.** The embryonic body-cavity; celoma; coelom. भ्रूणदेहगह्वर; भ्रूणदेहविवर

**Celoma.** see **Celom.**

**Cementoblast.** A cell concerned with the formation of the cementum of teeth. संयोजीकोशिकाप्रसू

**Cementoma.** A tumour of the cementum of a tooth. दन्तबज्ञ-अर्बुद; दन्तबज्ञार्बुद

**Cementum.** The vitreous substance covering the root of the tooth; cement. दन्तबज्ञ; सीमेंट

**Cenesthesia.** A sense of existence, painful or pleasurable; cenesthesis. अस्तित्वज्ञान; चेतना का आभास अथवा अनुभव होना

**Cenesthesis.** See **Cenesthesia.**

**Cenogenesis.** See **Caenogenesis.**

**Cenotica.** Diseases of the fluids. द्रव्यव्याधि; द्रवविकार; द्रवविकृति

**Census.** An official numbering of population. जनगणना

**Centaur.** A mythological figure; half-man and half-horse. किन्नर

**Center.** See **Centre.**

**Centesimal.** Relating to the division into hundredth, i.e. proportion of 1 to 100; centisimal. शतमलव; सौ हिस्सों में बँटा हुआ

**Centesis.** Puncture; perforation. छिद्र; छेद; विवर

**Centi-.** Prefix denoting hundred. 'शत' अथवा 'सौ' का अर्थ देने वाला उपसर्ग

**Centigrade.** Having one hundred degrees of grades. सेंटीग्रेड

**Centigram.** The hundredth part of a gram. सेंटीग्राम; ग्राम का सौवाँ भाग

**Centimeter.** The hundredth part of a meter. सेंटीमीटर; मीटर का सौवाँ भाग

**Centisimal.** See **Centesimal.**

**Centra.** Plural of **Centrum.**

**Central.** Pertaining to the centre. केन्द्रीय; केन्द्रक;

    **C. Canal,** the canal of the vertebral column. केन्द्र-नलिका;

    **C. Nervous System,** the brain and the spinal cord. केन्द्रीय स्नायुजाल; केन्द्रीय स्नायुतंत्र; केन्द्रीय स्नायु-प्रणाली

**Centre.** The centre or the middle part of a body; center; centrum. केन्द्र;

    **Auditory C.,** the cerebral centre for hearing. श्रवण केन्द्र;

    **Broca's C.,** a small posterior part of the inferior frontal gyrus of the left hemisphere, identified as an essential component of the motor mechanism, governing articulated speech; Broca's area; motor speech centre. ब्रोका केन्द्र; ब्रोका क्षेत्र; वाक्प्रेरक केन्द्र;

    **Cardioinhibitory C.,** one in the oblongata, efferent impulses being carried by the vagus. हृद्बाधक केन्द्र;

    **Motor C.,** a nervous centre controlling motion. प्रेरक केन्द्र;

    **Motor Speech C.,** see **Broca's Centre.**

    **Nerve C.,** a group of nerve-cells acting for the performance of some function. स्नायु केन्द्र; तंत्रिका केन्द्र;

    **Optic C.,** the point in the lens of the eye where light rays cross each other in proceeding from the cornea to the retina. दृष्टि केन्द्र;

    **Respiratory C.,** in the oblongata, between the nuclei of the vagus and accessorius. श्वास केन्द्र; श्वसन केन्द्र

**Centric.** Pertaining to a centre. केन्द्रीय; केन्द्रिक; केन्द्र सम्बन्धी; केन्द्र से सम्बन्धित

**Centrifugal.** Flying from the centre. केन्द्रापसारी; अपकेन्द्री; केन्द्र से दूर हटने वाला

**Centrifuge.** A centrifugal machine, or the apparatus that rotates, thereby increasing the force of gravity so that substances of different densities are separated. अपकेन्द्रित्र; केन्द्रापसारी (यंत्र)

**Centrilobular.** At or near the centre of a lobule. केन्द्र-खण्डकी

**Centriole.** A term given to a minute granule in the centrosome when this granule is simple. तारककेन्द्रक

**Centripetal.** Tending to move towards the centre. केन्द्राभिसारी; अभिकेन्द्री; केन्द्राभिमुखी

**Centromere.** The nonstaining primary constriction of a chromosome which in the point of attachment of the spindle fibre, is concerned with chromosome movement during cell division, divides the chromosome into two arms, and is constant for a specific chromosome. गुणसूत्रबिंदु

**Centrosome.** A rounded body along side the nucleus of a cell that is undergoing karyokinesis. तारककाय; केन्द्रपिण्ड

**Centrum.** See **Centre.**

**Cephalagra.** Gout in the head. शिरोवात; सिर का गठिया

**Cephalalgia.** Headache, usually symptomatic of some other affection; cephalgia. शीर्षार्ति; शिरोवेदना; मस्तिष्कशूल; सिरदर्द

**Cephaledema.** Oedema of the head; cephaloedema. शिरोशोफ; सिर की शोफमयी सूजन

**Cephalemia.** Congestion of the brain. मस्तिष्कीय रक्तसंलयन; मस्तिष्करक्तसंलयन

**Cephalgia.** See **Cephalalgia.**

**Cephalhaematoma.** A bloody tumour beneath the pericranium; cephalhematoma; cephalohaematoma; cephalohematoma. शीर्षरक्तसंग्रह; सिर में खून जमा हो जाना

**Cephalhematoma.** See **Cephalhaematoma.**

**Cephalic.** Pertaining to the head; cranial. शीर्षी; मस्तिष्कीय; कपालीय; सिर सम्बन्धी

**Cephalitis.** Inflammation of the brain; encephalitis. मस्तिष्कशोथ; मस्तिष्क का प्रदाह

**Cephaloauricular.** Pertaining to the brain and ear. शिरोकर्णी; मस्तिष्क अथवा सिर तथा कान सम्बन्धी

**Cephalocele.** Hernia of the brain; encephalocele. मस्तिष्कपुटी; मस्तिष्क-हर्निया; मस्तिष्क-बहि:सरण
**Cephalodynia.** Pain in the head. शिरोवेदना; सिरदर्द
**Cephaloedema.** See **Cephaledema.**
**Cephalography.** A description of the head. शीर्षलेख; मस्तिष्कलेख
**Cephalohaematoma.** See **Cephalhaematoma.**
**Cephalohematoma.** See **Cephalhaematoma.**
**Cephaloid.** Resembling the head. शीर्षाभ; सिर जैसा
**Cephaloma.** A soft carcinoma. मृदुकर्कट; मृदुकैंसर
**Cephalomegaly.** Enlargement of the head. बृहत्तशीर्षता; शीर्षबृहत्तता; सिर का आकार बढ़ जाना
**Cephalomenia.** Aberration of the menses to the head. शिरोन्मुखार्तव
**Cephalomeningitis.** Inflammation of the brain membranes. शीर्षमस्तिष्कावरणशोथ; सिर और उसकी झिल्ली का प्रदाह
**Cephalometer.** An instrument for measuring the head; cephalostat. शीर्षमापी (यंत्र)
**Cephalometry.** The art of measuring the head. शीर्षमिति; शीर्षमापन
**Cephalomotor.** Relating to movements of the head. मस्तिष्कप्रेरक; सिर की गतियों से सम्बन्धित
**Cephalomyelitis.** Inflammation of the head-muscles. शीर्षपेशीशोथ; सिर की पेशियों का प्रदाह
**Cephalon.** The head. शीर्ष; सिर; शिर
**Cephalopagus.** Double monster with the heads united at the top. बद्धकपालयमल; सिर से जुड़े हुये; जुड़वाँ
**Cephalopathy.** Any disease of the head. शिरोव्याधि; सिर का कोई रोग
**Cephaloplegia.** Paralysis of the head-muscle. शीर्षपेशीघात; सिर की पेशी का पक्षाघात
**Cephalostat.** See **Cephalometer.**
**Cephalothoracic.** Relating to the head and the chest. सिर एवं वक्ष सम्बन्धी
**Cephalothoracopagus.** A double-headed monster with united thoraces. बद्धशिरोवक्ष
**Cephalotome.** An instrument for performing cephalotomy. शिरोछिद्रक; कपालकर्तक
**Cephalotomy.** The crushing of the foetal head. शिरोछेदन; कपालकर्तन

**Cephalotribe. **An instrument to crush the foetal head. शीर्षप्रवलक्; कपालविदारक; भ्रूण के सिर को कुचलने का यंत्र

**Cephalotripsy.** The crushing of the foetal head. कपालविदारण; शीर्षप्रवलन; भ्रूण का सिर कुचलना

**Cera.** Wax. मोम;

 **C. Alba,** white wax. सफेद मोम;

 **C. Flava,** beeswax. पीला मोम

**Ceraceous.** Waxy. मोमी; मोम जैसा

**Cerate.** A composition having wax as a basis. सिक्थ; दृढ़ मरहम;

 **Simple C.,** an excellent vehicle for any external remedy, made of 1 oz. of white wax to 1 oz. of the lard. सामान्य सिक्थ

**Ceratitis.** See **Keratitis.**

**Cerea.** Waxy. मोमी; मोम जैसा

**Cereals.** The grain-plants used for food; also the grains of plants. धान्य

**Cerebella.** Plural of **Cerebellum.**

**Cerebellar.** Pertaining to the cerebellum. अनुमस्तिष्कीय; अनुमस्तिष्क सम्बन्धी

**Cerebellectomy.** Excision of the cerebellum. अनुमस्तिष्क-उच्छेदन

**Cerebellitis.** Inflammation of the cerebellum. अनुमस्तिष्कशोथ

**Cerebellum.** The posterior brain mass lying behind the pons and medulla and beneath the posterior portion of the cerebrum. अनुमस्तिष्क; पश्चमस्तिष्कपिण्ड

**Cerebra.** Plural of **Cerebrum.**

**Cerebral.** Pertaining to the brain, or more specifically the forebrain, where conscious controls the centre. प्रमस्तिष्कीय;

 **C. Cortex,** the surface of the brain. प्रमस्तिष्क-प्रान्तस्था

**Cerebrasthenia.** Weakness of mind. मस्तिष्कदौर्बल्य; बुद्धिदौर्बल्य; दिमागी कमजोरी

**Cerebration.** Mental activity. प्रमस्तिष्कव्यापार; प्रमस्तिष्कक्रिया; मानसिक सक्रियता

**Cerebriform.** Resembling the external fissures and convolution of the brain. प्रमस्तिष्करूप

**Cerebritis.** Inflammation of the brain. प्रमस्तिष्कशोथ; मस्तिष्क का प्रदाह

**Cerebrology.** The science of the brain. प्रमस्तिष्कविज्ञान

**Cerebroma.** Herniation of the brain substance; encephaloma. प्रमस्तिष्कार्बुद; मस्तिष्कार्बुद

**Cerebromalacia.** Softening of the brain. प्रमस्तिष्कमृदुता; मस्तिष्क की कोमलता

**Cerebromeningitis.** Inflammation of the brain and its membranes; encephalomeningitis; meningoencephalitis. प्रमस्तिष्कमस्तिष्कावरणशोथ

**Cerebropathy.** Any brain disease; cerebrosis. प्रमस्तिष्कविकृति; प्रमस्तिष्करोग

**Cerebropontile.** See **Cerebropontine.**

**Cerebropontine.** Relating to the cerebrum and pons; cerebropontile. प्रमस्तिष्कसेतुक

**Cerebrosclerosis.** Hardening of the brain. प्रमस्तिष्ककाठिन्य; मास्तक की कठोरता

**Cerebrosis.** See **Cerebropathy.**

**Cerebrospinal.** Pertaining to the brain and the spinal cord. सौषुम्निक; प्रमस्तिष्कमेरु सम्बन्धी;

  **C. Fluid,** the fluid of the brain and cord-spaces. मस्तिष्कमेरु-द्रव्य;

  **C. Meningitis,** inflammation of the brain and cord. मस्तिष्कमेरुशोथ;

  **C. Sclerosis,** multiple sclerosis of the brain and cord. मस्तिष्कमेरुकाठिन्य

**Cerebrovascular.** Pertaining to the blood vessels of the brain. प्रमस्तिष्कवाहिकीय; मस्तिष्क और रक्तवाहिनियों सम्बन्धी

**Cerebrum.** Upper and front part of the brain. प्रमस्तिष्क; मस्तिष्क का ऊपरी और अगला भाग

**Cerin.** The wax. सिक्थ; मोम

**Cerous.** Wax-like. मोमवत्; मोमी; सिक्थरूप

**Certificate.** Testimony in writing, voucher, acquirement, etc. प्रमाण-पत्र; सैर्टिफिकेट;

  **Birth C.,** a legal written certificate containing the date of birth of a child or person. जन्म प्रमाण-पत्र;

  **Death C.,** a certificate containing the date of death of a person. मृत्यु प्रमाण-पत्र;

  **Medical C.,** a certificate containing the description of the illness of the patient issued by the attending physician or any other medical authority. चिकित्सा प्रमाण-पत्र

**Cerumen.** The ear-wax in outer canal. कर्णगूथ; कर्णशिक्थ; कर्णमल; कान का मैल

**Ceruminosis.** An excessive secretion of cerumen. अतिकर्णगूथता; कानों से अत्यधिक मैल निकलना

**Ceruminous.** Relating to the cerumen. कर्णशूथज; कर्णगूथ सम्बन्धी

**Cervical.** Relating to the neck or a cervix. ग्रैव; ग्रीवा सम्बन्धी; गर्दन सम्बन्धी;

    **C. Adenitis,** inflammation of the cervical glands. ग्रीवाग्रन्थिशोथ; गर्दन की ग्रन्थियों का प्रदाह;

    **C. Rib,** a supernumerary rib in the cervical region. ग्रैव पर्शुका; गर्दन की पसली;

    **C. Spondylitis,** see **Cervical Spondylosis.**

    **C. Spondylosis,** inflammation of the cervical vertebras; cervical spondylitis. ग्रैवकशेरुकाशोथ; गर्दन की कशेरुकाओं का प्रदाह

**Cervicectomy.** Amputation of the cervix uteri. जरायुग्रीवा-उच्छेदन; गर्भाशयग्रीवा-उच्छेदन

**Cervices.** Plural of **Cervix.**

**Cervicitis.** Inflammation of the neck of the womb. जरायुग्रीवाशोथ; गर्भाशयग्रीवाशोथ; गर्भाशयग्रीवा का प्रदाह

**Cervicobrachial.** Relating to the neck and arm. गर्दन तथा बाजू सम्बन्धी

**Cervicodynia.** Pain in the neck. ग्रीवार्ति; गर्दन मे दर्द होना

**Cervicotomy.** Incision of the cervix uteri. जरायुग्रीवाछेदन; गर्भाशयग्रीवाछेदन

**Cervix.** The neck; any neck-part. ग्रीवा; गर्दन जैसी आकृति वाला कोई भी भाग;

    **C. Uteri,** the neck of the uterus. जरायुग्रीवा; गर्भाशयग्रीवा;

    **C. Vesicae,** the neck of the bladder. मूत्राशयग्रीवा

**Cesarean Operation.** Surgical removal of the baby from the uterus; cesarean section; cesarotomy. शल्यक्रियात्मक प्रजनन; सिजेरियन ऑपरेशन

**Cesarean Section.** See **Cesarean Operation.**

**Cesarotomy.** See **Cesarean Operation.**

**Cesspool.** A well sunk. मलिनजलकुण्ड

**Cestoda.** See **Cestode.**

**Cestode.** Tapeworm; cestoda; cestoidea. स्फीतकृमि; फीताकृमि

**Cestoid.** Like intestinal or tapeworm. स्फीतकृम्याभ; फीताकृमि जैसा

**Cestoidea.** See **Cestode.**

**Chafing.** A fret or gall of the skin. शल्कन; विशल्कन; पपड़ियाना

**Chagrin.** Vexation; acute disappointment. असन्तोष; घोर निराशा; व्यथा; क्लेश; खीझ

**Chain.** A connected series. शृंखला; माला; श्रेणी

**Chalaza.** A twisted cord binding the yolk-bag of an egg to the lining membrane. कुन्तलिका; निभाग

**Chalazia.** Plural of **Chalazion.**

**Chalazion.** A cyst on the edge of the eyelid from retained secretion of the Meibomian glands. नेत्रवर्त्मग्रन्थि; पलकों की गिल्टी

**Chalazonephritis.** Granular inflammation of the kindney. वृक्ककणिकाशोथ; गुर्दे का कणिकीय प्रदाह

**Chalcosis.** Chronic copper poisoning. ताम्रविषण्णता; ताम्ररुणता

**Chalicosis.** Lung-disease due to inhalation of stone-dust. फुप्फुसताम्ररुग्णता

**Chalk.** Carbonate of lime. खड़िया; चाक

**Chalybeate.** Containing iron in solution, as occurring in mineral springs. लौहयुक्त; लौहमिश्रित; अयसयुक्त

**Chamber.** A compartment or closed space; a hollow. कोष्ठ; कक्ष; कुण्ड;

**Anterior C.,** the space between the cornea and iris. अग्र-कक्ष;

**Aqueous C.,** the space between the cornea and the lens of the eye. नेत्रोद-कक्ष;

**Inspection C.,** a compartment for examining the patients. निरीक्षण कक्ष;

**Posterior C.,** the space between the iris and the lens of the eye. पश्च-कक्ष;

**Vitreous C. (of the eye),** the large space between the lens and the retina. नेत्रकाचाभद्रव कक्ष; विट्रियस कक्ष

**Champacol.** Camphor. कर्पूर; कपूर

**Chancre.** The primary lesion of syphilis; also called the hard chancre. शैंकर; कठिनक्षत; उपदंश का प्रारम्भिक घाव; उपदंशक्षत;

**Hard C.,** see **Chancre.**

**Soft C.,** a nonsyphilitic venereal ulcer; simple chancre. मृदुक्षत

**Chancriform.** Of the form of chancre. शैंकररूप; कठिनक्षत जैसा

**Chancroid.** Resembling a chancre. शैंकराभ; कठिनक्षताभ; the soft chancre. मृदुक्षत;

**Phagedenic C.,** a form with a tendency to erosion. विनाशी मृदुक्षत;

**Serpiginous C.**, phagedenic chancroid spreading in curves. सर्पिल मृदुक्षत

**Chancroidal.** Pertaining to a chancre. उपदंशक्षत सम्बन्धी

**Chancrous.** Of the nature of a chancre. उपदंशक्षतरूप; उपदंश के घाव जैसा

**Change of life.** The menopause. रजोनिवृत्ति; वय:सन्धिकाल

**Chap.** A slight fissure of the skin. दरार; फटन; विदर

**Chapped.** Cracked. दरारयुक्त; विदरित; विफटित; कटा-फटा; फटा हुआ

**Character.** The sum total of the known and the predictable mental characteristics of an individual, particularly his conduct. चरित्र; गुण; लक्षण; स्वभाव; किसी व्यक्ति द्वारा प्रदर्शित स्पष्ट चिन्ह अथवा भाव-विशेष

**Acquired C.**, a character developed as a result of environment. उपार्जित गुण;

**Dominant C.**, an inherited character determined by a dominant gene. प्रभावी गुण;

**Inherited C.**, a single attribute of an animal or plant that is transmitted from generation to generation. आनुवंशिक गुण;

**Recessive C.**, an inherited character determined by a recessive gene. अप्रभावी गुण

**Characteristics.** The features or marks which serve to distinguish one thing from another. चारित्रिकतायें; अभिलक्षण; लक्षण; विशेषतायें

**Charbon.** Malingnant pustule or anthrax. दुर्दम पूयस्फोटिका; आंगाररक्षण

**Charcoal.** The residue after burning organic substances at a high temperature in an enclosed vessel. कोयला; जैवी पदार्थों के जलने से प्राप्त प्रांगार

**Charcot's Fever.** A septic fever occurring in cases of jaundice due to impacted gall-stone. पूतिज्वर; विष-ज्वर

**Charcot's Pain.** Hysteric pain in ovarian region. जरायुशूल; गर्भाशयशूल

**Charlatan.** A quack; empty boaster. कुवैद्य; नीम-हकीम

**Charlatanary.** Quackery. कुवैद्यकी; नीम-हकीमी

**Charpie.** Linen shreds for dressing the wounds. व्रणतूलिपट; घाव पर बांधने की सूती या रेशमी धज्जी

**Chasma.** A yawn; chasmus. जम्भाई; जम्हाई

**Chasmus.** See **Chasma**.

**Chastisment.** Punishment; penalty. दण्ड; सजा; जुर्माना;

**Corporeal C.**, physical punishment. शारीरिक दण्ड
**Chaude Pissue.** Gonorrhoea. प्रमेह; सूजाक
**Check-up.** Examination. जांच; परीक्षण; परीक्षा;
    **Health C.**, physical examination; medical check-up. स्वास्थ्य परीक्षण; शारीरिक जांच
    **Medical C.**, see **Health Check-up.**
**Cheek.** The side of the face. कपोल; गाल; गण्ड
**Cheese.** The coagulum of milk compressed into a solid mass. पनीर
**Cheesy.** Resembling cheese. पनीरवत्; पनीराभ
**Cheilalgia.** Pain in lip; chilalgia. ओष्ठार्ति; ओष्ठवेदना; सृक्कवेदना
**Cheilectomy.** Excision of the lips; chilectomy. ओष्ठोच्छेदन; ओष्ठकर्तन
**Cheilitis.** Inflammation of the lip; chilitis. ओष्ठशोथ; ओष्ठ-प्रदाह; अधरशोथ; होंठों का प्रदाह; सृक्कशोथ
**Cheiloid.** Lip-like; applied to a skin disease. ओष्ठाभ; ओष्ठवत्; सृक्काभ
**Cheiloplasty.** Plastic operation upon the lips. ओष्ठसंधान; सृक्कसंधान
**Cheilorrhaphy.** A suturing of the lips. ओष्ठसीवन
**Cheilochisis.** Hare-lip; cleft-lip; chiloschisis. खण्डोष्ठ
**Cheilosis.** Maceration at angles of the mouth; chilosis. ओष्ठविदरण; ओष्ठविदरता
**Cheilostomatoplasty.** Plastic restoration of the mouth. ओष्ठमुखसंधानकर्म
**Cheilotomy.** Incision into the lip; chilotomy. ओष्ठछेदन
**Cheiragra.** Gout in the hand. हस्तसंधिवात; हाथों का गठिया
**Cheiromegaly.** Abnormally large hands; chiromegaly. बृहद्हस्तता
**Cheiroplasty.** A plastic operation upon the hand; chiroplasty. हस्तसंधान
**Cheiropodalgia.** Pain in the hands and feet; chiropodalgia. हस्तपादार्ति; हाथ-पैरों में दर्द होना
**Cheirospasm.** Spasm of muscles of hand, as in writer's cramp; chirospasm. हस्ताकर्ष; हाथ की पेशियों की ऐंठन
**Chemic.** See **Chemical.**
**Chemical.** Relating to chemistry; chemic. रसायन; रासायनिक; रसायनविज्ञान सम्बन्धी
**Chemist.** One versed in chemistry. रसायनज्ञ; रसायनविज्ञानी; रसायनशास्त्री

# Chemistry

**Chemistry.** The science which treats of the elements and atomic relations of matter and of various compounds of the elements. रसायनविज्ञान; रसायनशास्त्र;

**Inorganic C.,** chemistry of compounds not containing carbon. अकार्बनिक रसायनशास्त्र;

**Organic C.,** chemistry of carbon compounds. कार्बनिक रसायनशास्त्र

**Chemopallidectomy.** The destruction of a predetermined section of a lump by chemicals. रसायनीपाण्डुपिण्डोच्छेदन

**Chemoprophylaxis.** Prevention of diseases by administration of chemicals. रसायनरोगनिरोध; रासायनिक पदार्थों द्वारा रोगों की रोक-थाम

**Chemoreceptor.** A chemical linkage in a living cell having an affinity for, and capable of combining with certain other chemical substances; a sensory end-organ capable of reacting a chemical stimulus. रसायनग्राही; रसवेदनाग्राही

**Chemosis.** Inflammatory swelling of the conjunctiva. नेत्रश्लेष्मलाशोफ; श्लेष्मलाशोथ; अर्जुनरोग; नेत्रों की श्लैष्मिक झिल्ली की प्रदाहक सूजन

**Chemotactic.** Relating to chemotaxis. रसायन-अनुचलन सम्बन्धी

**Chemotaxis.** Response of organisms to chemical stimuli; chemotropism. रसायन-अनुचलन; कोशिकाओं या स्वतंत्रगामी जीवों की रासायनिक उत्तेजनाओं से उत्पन्न प्रतिक्रिया

**Chemotherapeutics.** See **Chemotherapy.**

**Chemotherapy.** Treatment with chemical means; chemotherapeutics. रसायन-चिकित्सा; रसायनोपचार; केमोथेरापी

**Chemotic.** Affected with chemosis. श्लेष्मलाशोफग्रस्त; अर्जुनरोग से पीड़ित; relating to chemosis. श्लेष्मलाशोफ सम्बन्धी;

**Chemotropism.** See **Chemotaxis**.

**Chenopodium Oil.** An anthelmintic. बथुये का तेल

**Chest.** The thorax. वक्ष; उर; छाती;

**Barrel C.,** a chest presenting the shape of a barrel during full inspiration. ढोल वक्ष;

**Flail C.,** flapping chest wall. शिथिल वक्ष;

**Flat C.,** a chest in which the anteroposterior diameter is less than the average. सपाट वक्ष;

**Funnel C.,** a hollow at the lower part of the chest caused by displacement of xiphoid cartilage; funnel breast. कीप वक्ष;

**Pigeon C.,** condition of the chest in which sides are considerably flattened and sternum prominent. कपोत वक्ष

**Cheyne Stoke's Asthma.** Dyspnoea due to pulmonary congestion in an advanced stage of chronic myocarditis. फुप्फुसरक्तसंलयी श्वासकष्ट

**Cheyne Stoke's Respiration.** Arhythmic breathing of a periodical type occurring in certain grave affections of the central nervous system, heart and lungs and certain intoxications. अताल-श्वसन

**Chiasm.** See **Chiasma.**

**Chiasma.** X-shaped crossing or decussation; chiasm; chiasmaticus. व्यत्यासिका;

    **Optic C.**, the meeting of the optic nerves. अक्षि-व्यत्यासिका;

    **C. Opticum,** the same as **Optic chiasma.**

**Chiasmaticus.** See **Chiasma.**

**Chickenfat Clot.** A yellowish blood clot. पीतरक्तकण; रक्त का पीला-सा थक्का

**Chicken-pox.** A vesicular eruption of the body, almost peculiar to the young; varicella. लघुमसूरिका; छोटी माता

**Chiggers.** Small biting and burrowing insects common in many areas where vegetation occurs. मांसपिस्सू; मांसपिशु

**Chilalgia.** See **Cheilalgia.**

**Chilblain.** An inflammatory swelling of the toes, feet or fingers due to the influence of cold. शीतशोथ; शीतदंश; शीतक्षत; बिवाई फटना

**Child-bearing.** Pregnancy and parturition. गर्भ एवं प्रसव

**Child-bed.** The condition during and after labour. सूतिका; सूतिकावस्था;

    **C.-b. fever,** puerperal fever. सूतिका ज्वर; प्रसूति ज्वर

**Childhood.** The period of life between infancy and puberty. बचपन; बाल्यकाल

**Chilectomy.** See **Cheilectomy.**

**Chilitis.** See **Cheilitis.**

**Chill.** A feeling of cold with shivering and pallor. शीतकम्प; ठण्ड लगने के साथ कंपकंपी होना

**Chiloschisis.** See **Cheiloschisis.**

**Chilosis.** See **Cheilosis.**

**Chilotomy.** See **Cheilotomy.**

**Chimney Sweeper's Cancer.** Scrotal epithelioma. अण्डकोषीय कैंसर

**Chin.** The mentum; the prominence formed by the anterior projection of mandible or lower jaw. हनु; चिबुक; ठोढ़ी;

**C. Cough,** whooping cough. कूकर कास; काली खाँसी

**China.** Cinchona; a drug made of peruvian bark. कुनीन; सिंकोना

**Chiragra.** Gout in the hands. हस्तसन्धिवात; हाथों का गठिया

**Chirarthritis.** Articular inflammation of the hand. हस्तसन्धिशोथ; हाथ के जोड़ का प्रदाह

**Chiromegaly.** See **Cheiromegaly.**

**Chiroplasty.** See **Cheiroplasty.**

**Chiropodalgia.** See **Cheiropodalgia.**

**Chiropodist.** One who is versed in the treatment of the diseases of the hands and feet. हस्तपाद-चिकित्सक; हाथों तथा पैरों को प्रभावित करने वाले रोगों की चिकित्सा करने वाला

**Chirospasm.** See **Cheirospasm.**

**Chirurgia.** Surgery. शल्य-चिकित्सा; शल्यकर्म

**Chirurgiacal.** Relating to surgery; surgical. शल्य-चिकित्सा अथवा शल्यकर्म सम्बन्धी

**Chliasma.** A poultice. उपनाह; प्रलेप; पुल्टिस

**Chloasma.** Pigmentation of the skin. विवर्णलांछन; चम्बल; त्वक्-विवर्णता;
   **C. Gravidarum,** the brown discolouration of pregnancy; chloasma uterinum. गर्भिणी विवर्णलांछन;
   **C. Uterinum,** see **Chloasma Gravidarum.**

**Chloral.** A colourless crystalline solid; hypnotic. क्लोरल; एक तेज गंध वाला वर्णहीन स्निग्ध द्रव्य;
   **C. Hydrate,** a rapid active sedative and hypnotic of great value in nervous insomnia. क्लोरल हाइड्रेट; एक रवेदार यौगिक, जिसका प्रयोग नींद लाने वाली औषधि के रूप में किया जाता है

**Chloramin.** An organic compound that slowly liberates chlorine in solution; chloramine. क्लोरामिन

**Chloramine.** See **Chloramin.**

**Chloranemia.** See **Chloroanaemia.**

**Chloremia.** Chlorosis. हरित्पाण्डुरोग; हरिद्रक्तता

**Chloride.** A binary compound containing chlorine; chloruret. क्लोराइड; नीलेय

**Chlorinated.** Containing chlorine. क्लोरीनयुक्त

**Chlorine.** A non-metallic gaseous element; chlorum. क्लोरीन; नीरजी; हरिद

**Chloroanaemia.** Chlorosis; chloranemia. हरित्पाण्डुरोग; हरिद्रक्तता

**Chloroform.** A heavy, colourless liquid used as an anaesthetic and internally as a narcotic. क्लोरोफॉर्म; मूर्च्छक; बेहोशी लाने वाला एक भारी, रंगहीन तरल पदार्थ

**Chloroleukemia.** Leukemia with chlorosis. श्वेतहरितरक्तता; श्वेतहरित्पाण्डुता

**Chloroma.** A tumour having greenish colour; chloromyeloma. हरितार्बुद; हरे रंग की गूमड़ी या रसौली

**Chloromyeloma.** See **Chloroma.**

**Chlolrophill.** See **Chlorophyll.**

**Chlorophyll.** The green colouring matter of leaves; chlorophill. क्लोरोफिल; पर्णहरित; पौधों अथवा पत्तों में पाया जाने वाला एक रसायन

**Chloropia.** Green vision; chloropsia. हरित-दृष्टि; ऐसा दृष्टिदोष जिसमें प्रत्येक वस्तु हरी दिखाई देती है

**Chloropsia.** See **Chloropia.**

**Chloroquin.** A patent antimalarial remedy, effective in the treatment and suppression of the disease. क्लोरोक्विन; कुनीन-निर्मित एक औषधि

**Chloroquine.** The same as **Chloroquin.**

**Chlorosis.** A disease affecting young females, more particularly those who have not menstruated. हरित्पाण्डुरोग; हरित्पाण्डुता

**Chlorotic.** Exhibiting chlorosis. हरित्पाण्डुर; relating to chlorosis. हरितपाण्डुरोग सम्बन्धी

**Chlorum.** See **Chlorine.**

**Chloruret.** See **Chloride.**

**Choana.** The posterior nare. पश्चनासाद्वार; पश्चनासारन्ध्र; अन्तर्नासाछिद्र

**Choanae.** Plural of **Choana.**

**Cholaemia.** The presence of bile-pigment in the blood. पित्तरक्तता; पित्तप्रकोपरुजा; रक्त में पित्तवर्णक विद्यमान रहना

**Cholagog.** See **Cholagogue.**

**Cholagogue.** A medicine that promotes the flow of bile; cholagog. पित्तवर्धी; पित्त का बहाव बढ़ाने वाली औषधि

**Cholangeitis.** See **Cholangitis.**

**Cholangiectasis.** Dilatation of the bile-duct. पित्तवाहिनीविस्फार; पित्तनली का फैलना

**Cholangioadenoma.** A tumour of the bile-duct. पित्तवाहिनीग्रन्थ्यर्बुद; पित्तनली का अर्बुद

**Cholangioenterostomy.** Surgical anastomosis of bile-duct to intestine. पित्तनलीआंत्रसम्मिलन

**Chalangiofibrosis.** Fibrosis of the bile-duct. पित्तवाहिनीतन्तुमयता

**Cholangiogram.** Film demonstrating hepatic, cystic and bile-ducts; choledochogram. पित्तवाहिनीचित्र

**Cholangiography.** Radiographic examination of hepatic, cystic and bile-ducts; choledochography. पित्तवाहिनीचित्रण

**Cholangiohepatitis.** Inflammation of the liver and bile-duct. पित्तवाहिनीयकृत्शोथ; यकृत् तथा पित्तनली का प्रदाह

**Cholangioma.** A tumour of the bile-duct. पित्तवाहिकार्बुद; पित्तवाहिनीअर्बुद; पित्तनली का अर्बुद

**Cholangiotomy.** Incision into a bile-duct. पित्तवाहिनीछेदन

**Cholangitis.** Inflammation of a bile-duct; cholangeitis. पित्तवाहिनीशोथ; पित्तनली का प्रदाह

**Chole.** The bile. पित्त

**Cholecyst.** The gall-bladder; cholecystis. पित्ताशय; पित्तकोष

**Cholecystalgia.** Biliary colic. पित्तशूल

**Cholecystangiogram.** Film demonstrating gall-bladder, cystic and common bile-ducts after administration of opaque medium. पित्ताशयवाहिकाचित्र

**Cholecystangiography.** Radiographic examination of the gall-bladder, cystic and common bile-ducts after administration of opaque medium. पित्ताशयवाहिकाचित्रण

**Cholecystatony.** An atonic condition of the gall-bladder. पित्ताशय-अतानता; पित्ताशय की अतानिक अवस्था

**Cholecystic.** Pertaining to the gall-bladder. पित्ताशयशोथ अथवा पित्तकोष के प्रदाह से सम्बन्धित

**Cholecystenterostomy.** Formation of a direct communication between the gall-bladder and the intestine. पित्ताशयआंत्रछिद्रीकरण; पित्ताशयबृहदांत्रसम्मिलन

**Cholecystis.** See **Cholecyst.**

**Cholecystoduodenostomy.** Establishment of a communication between the gall-bladder and the duodenum. पित्ताशयग्रहणीछिद्रीकरण; पित्ताशयग्रहणीसम्मिलन

**Cholecystogastrostomy.** Establishment of a communication between the gall-bladder and the stomach. पित्ताशयजठरसम्मिलन

**Cholecystogram.** Film demonstrating gall-bladder after administration of opaque medium. पित्ताशयचित्रण

**Cholecystolithiasis.** The presence of stone or stones in the gall-bladder. पित्ताशयाश्मरता; पित्ताशय में पथरियाँ विद्यमान रहना

**Cholecystopathy.** Any disease of the gall-bladder. पित्ताशयविकृति; पित्ताशय का कोई रोग

**Cholecystostomy.** The formation of a fistula into the gall-bladder. पित्ताशयछिद्रीकरण

**Cholecystotomy.** Incision of the gall-bladder. पित्ताशयछेदन

**Choledochectomy.** Excision of a part of the common bile-duct. पित्ताशय-उच्छेदन; पित्तनली का आंशिक उच्छेदन

**Choledochitis.** Inflammation of the bile-duct. पित्तवाहिनीशोथ; पित्तनली का प्रदाह

**Choledochoduodenostomy.** The formation of a fistula between the duodenum and the common bile-duct. सामान्यपित्तवाहिनीआंत्रसम्मिलन

**Choledochojejunostomy.** Anastomosis between the common bile-duct and the jejunum. पित्ताशयमध्यांत्रसम्मिलन

**Choledochogram.** See **Cholangiogram.**

**Choledochography.** See **Cholangiography.**

**Choledocholithiasis.** The presence of a stone or stones in the bile-duct. पित्तवाहिनी-अश्मरता; पित्तनली में पथरियाँ विद्यमान रहना

**Choledocholithotomy.** The incision of the common bile-duct for removal of a gall-stone. पित्तवाहिनी-अश्मरीहरण

**Choledochoplasty.** Plastic surgery on the common bile-duct. पित्तवाहिनीसंधान

**Choledochostomy.** Establishment of a fistula in the common bile-duct. पित्तवाहिनीछिद्रीकरण

**Choledochotomy.** An incision into the common bile-duct. पित्तवाहिनीछेदन

**Choledochous.** Receiving or holding bile. पित्तग्राही

**Choleic.** Pertaining to the bile; cholic. पैत्तिक; पित्तज; पित्त सम्बन्धी

**Cholelith.** Gall-stone. पित्तपथरी

**Cholelithiasis.** The formation of calculi within the gall-bladder; gall-stone. पित्ताश्मरता; पित्तपथरी

**Cholelithotomy.** An incision into the bile-duct for the removal of the gall-stones. पित्ताश्मरीहरण; पित्त-पथरियाँ निकालने के लिये पित्ताशय

के अन्दर छेद करना

**Cholemesia.** See **Cholemesis.**

**Cholemesis.** The vomiting of bile; cholemesia. पित्तवमन; पित्तयुक्त कै होना

**Cholemia.** The presence of bile pigment in the blood. पित्तरक्तता; रक्त में पित्त की अधिकता

**Cholepoiesis.** The production or increase of bile. पित्तोत्पादन; पित्तवर्धन; पित्त बढ़ना

**Cholepoietic.** Producing bile. पित्तोत्पादक; पित्त पैदा करने वाला

**Choleprasin.** The bile pigment. पित्तवर्णक

**Cholera.** An acute disease characterized by copious watery stools, vomiting, cramps, prostration and suppression of urine. विसूचिका; हैजा;

C. **Asiatica,** a malignant form of cholera; Asiatic cholera. सांघातिक विसूचिका; दुर्दमरूप विसूचिका;

C. **Infantum,** summer complaints of the children; infantile cholera. शिशु-विसूचिका; बच्चों को होने वाली हैजा;

C. **Morbus,** sporadic or summer cholera; cholera rostras; sporadic cholera; summer cholera. ग्रीष्मकालीन विसूचिका; सामान्य विसूचिका;

C. **Rostras,** see **Cholera Morbus.**

C. **Sicca,** a form of cholera in which vomiting and diarrhoea are absent. शुष्क विसूचिका;

**Asiatic C.,** see **Cholera Asiatica.**

**Infantile C.,** see **Cholera Infantum.**

**Sporadic C.,** see **Cholera Morbus.**

**Summer C.,** see **Cholera Morbus.**

**Choleraic.** Pertaining to cholera. विसूचिका अथवा हैजा सम्बन्धी

**Choleratic.** An agent which increases the bile. पित्तवर्धी; पित्तवर्धक; पित्त बढ़ाने वाला

**Choleriform.** Resembling cholera; choleroid. पित्ताभ; पित्तवत्; पित्तरूप; पित्त से मिलता-जुलता

**Cholerine.** A mild form of cholera. सौम्य विसूचिका; सुदम विसूचिका; resembling cholera. विसूचिकाभ; हैजा जैसा

**Choleroid.** See **Choleriform.**

**Choleromania.** Madness occasionally seen in cholera. विसूचिकोन्माद; हैजे के दौरान होने वाला पागलपन

**Cholerophobia.** A morbid fear of cholera. विसूचिकाभीति; हैजा होने का डर

**Cholestasis.** Diminution or arrest of the flow of bile. पित्तस्थिरता; **Intrahepatic C.**, syndrome comprising jaundice of an obstructive type. अन्तर्यकृत्-पित्तस्थिरता

**Cholesterin.** A substance derived from bile and the principal ingredient of gall-stone. कोलेस्ट्रीन; रक्त और पित्त में पाया जाने वाला एक स्वादहीन, गन्धहीन, स्निग्ध, श्वेत पदार्थ

**Cholesterine.** The same as **Cholesterin.**

**Cholesterol.** The most abundant steroid in animal tissues, especially in bile and gall-stone. कोलेस्ट्रॉल; रक्तवसा

**Choleuria.** See **Choluria.**

**Cholic.** See **Choleic.**

**Cholicele.** A tumour of the gall-bladder. पित्तकोषार्बुद; पित्ताशयार्बुद

**Chololith.** A biliary calculus. पित्ताश्मरी; पित्तपथरी

**Cholorrhea.** An excessive discharge of bile; cholorrhoea. अतिपित्तस्राव; अत्यधिक पित्तस्राव होना

**Cholorrhoea.** See **Cholorrhea.**

**Choluria.** The presence of bile in the urine; choleuria; biliuria. पित्तमेह; मूत्र में पित्त जाना

**Chondral.** Pertaining to a cartilage. उपास्थिपरक; उपास्थि सम्बन्धी

**Chondralgia.** Pain of the cartilage; chondrodynia. उपास्थिशूल; उपास्थि-वेदना

**Chondrectomy.** Excision of a cartilage. उपास्थि-उच्छेदन

**Chondric.** Pertaining to a cartilage. उपास्थि सम्बन्धी

**Chondrification.** The formation of cartilage. उपास्थीभवन; उपास्थि बनना

**Chondritis.** Inflammation of cartilage. उपास्थिशोथ; उपास्थि का प्रदाह

**Chondroarthritis.** Inflammation of the cartilaginous part of a joint. उपास्थिसन्धिशोथ

**Chondroblast.** An embryonic cell of the tissue which becomes a cartilage; chondroplast. उपास्थिप्रसू

**Chondroblastoma.** A tumour of an embryonic cell forming cartilage. उपास्थिप्रसू-अर्बुद

**Chondrocranium.** A cartilaginous cranium, as of the embryo. उपास्थिकरोटि

**Chondrocyte.** A connective tissue cell that occupies a lacuna within the cartilage matrix. उपास्थिकोशिका

**Chondrodynia.** Pain in the cartilage. उपास्थिवेदना; उपास्थिशूल

**Chondrodysplasia.** See **Chondrodystrophia.**

**Chondrodystrophia.** Foetal rickets; chondrodystrophy; chondrodysplasia. उपास्थिदुष्पोषण

**Chondrodystrophy.** See **Chondrodystrophia.**

**Chondrogenesis.** The formation of cartilage; chondrosis. उपास्थिजनन; उपास्थि बनना

**Chondroid.** Resembling a cartilage. उपास्थिसम; उपास्थि-सदृश; उपास्थिवत्; उपास्थि जैसा

**Chondrology.** The science of cartilages. उपास्थिरचनाविज्ञान

**Chondrolysis.** Disappearance of articular cartilage as the result of dissolution of a cartilage. उपास्थिलयन

**Chondroma.** A benign tumour of the cartilage. उपास्थि-अर्बुद; उपास्थ्यर्बुद

**Chondromalacia.** A morbid softening of the cartilage; chondromalacosis. उपास्थिमृदुता; उपास्थि की अस्वाभाविक कोमलता

**Chondromalacosis.** See **Chondromalacia.**

**Chondromatosis.** Presence of multiple tumour-like foci in a cartilage. उपास्थि-अर्बुदता

**Chondromucoid.** A mucin present in the interstitial substance of a cartilage. उपास्थिश्लेष्मा

**Chondronecrosis.** Necrosis of a cartilage. उपास्थि-परिगलन

**Chondropathy.** Any disease of the cartilage. उपास्थिरोग

**Chondroplast.** See **Chondroblast.**

**Chondroplasty.** Reparative or plastic surgery of cartilage. उपास्थिसंधान

**Chondrosis.** See **Chondrogenesis.**

**Chorda.** A collection of fibres forming a cord, tendon or filament. बन्धन; तन्तु; दण्ड; रज्जु;

**C. Dorsalis,** the primitive back-bone; chorda vertebralis. मेरुदण्ड; पृष्ठरज्जु; पृष्ठदण्ड;

**C. Saliva,** the saliva produced by stimulation of the tympanic nerve. लालारज्जु;

**C. Tendineae,** the tendinous strings stretching from the papillary muscles to the auriculoventricular valves. कण्डरा-रज्जु;

**C. Tympani,** the tympanic nerve. कर्णपटहतंत्रिका;

**C. Umbilicalis,** the umbilical cord. नाभिरज्जु;

**C. Vertebralis,** see **Chorda Dorsalis.**

**C. Vocalis,** vocal cord. स्वररज्जु

**Chordae.** Plural of **Chorda.**

**Chordee.** Painful and persistent erection of the penis in gonorrhoea. कॉर्डी; कष्टदायक तथा अविराम लिंगोद्रेक

**Chorditis.** Inflammation of the spermatic or vocal cord. रज्जुशोथ; रज्जुप्रदाह; वृषणरज्जुशोथ; स्वररज्जुशोथ

**Chordotomy.** Division of anterolateral nerve pathways in the spinal cord; cordotomy. सुषुम्ना-उच्छेदन

**Chorea.** An involuntary dancing state while walking; St. Vitus' dance. लास्य; नर्तनरोग; कोरिया;

**Electric C.,** dancing mania. लास्योन्माद; नाचने का पागलपन;

**C. Sancti Viti,** St. Vitus' Dance. लास्य; नर्तनरोग

**Choreal.** Pertaining to chorea; choreic. लास्य अथवा नर्तन रोग सम्बन्धी

**Choreic.** See **Choreal.**

**Choreiform.** Resembling chorea; choreoiod. लास्यरूप; लास्य से मिलता-जुलता

**Choreoiod.** See **Choreiform.**

**Corial.** Pertaining to the uterus. जरायु अथवा गर्भाशय सम्बन्धी

**Chorioadenoma.** A glandular tumour of the uterus. जरायुग्रन्थ्यर्बुद; गर्भाशयग्रन्थि का अर्बुद

**Chorioangioma.** A benign tumour of placental blood vessels, usually of no clinical significance. जरायुवाहिकार्बुद

**Choriocapillaris.** The capillary layer of the choroid coat. रंजितपटलकोशिका

**Choriocarcinoma.** A highly malignant tumour arising from the chorionic cells. जरायुकर्कट; जरायुकैंसर; गर्भाशयकर्कट

**Chorioepithelioma.** A tumour arising from the epithelial covering of the vascular tufts on the surface of the chorion; chorion epithelioma. दुर्दमजरायु-उपकलार्बुद

**Chorioiod.** See **Choroid.**

**Chorioioditis.** See **Choroiditis.**

**Chorion.** The outer envelope of the foetus. जरायु; गर्भाशय; भ्रूण की बाहरी झिल्ली;

**C. Epithelioma,** see **Chorioepithelioma.**

**C. Frondosum,** the part covered by the vascular tufts on the surface of the chorion. परिअंकुरी जरायु;

**C. Leave,** the membranous part of the chorion. निरंकुर जरायु

**Chorionic.** Relating to the chorion. जरायु सम्बन्धी

**Chorionitis.** Inflammation of the chorion. जरायुशोथ; गर्भाशयशोथ; जरायु-प्रदाह; गर्भाशय-प्रदाह

**Choroid.** A structure of the deeper parts of the eye; chorioiod. रंजितपटल

**Choroideremia.** Absence of the choroid. अरंजितपटलता

**Choroiditis.** Chorioioditis; inflammation of the choroid. रंजितपटलशोथ; degeneration of the choroid. रंजितपटल-व्यपजनन; रंजितपटलापजनन

**Choroidoiritis.** Inflammation of the choroid coat and the iris. रंजितपटलपरितारिकाशोथ

**Choroidopathy.** Non-inflammatory degeneration of the choroid. रंजितपटलविकृति; रंजितपटल का प्रदाहहीन अपजनन

**Choromania.** A hysteric disease, causing dancing mania. लास्योन्माद; नर्तनोन्माद

**Chromaffine.** Pertaining to the cells which take on a peculiar yellow colour when treated with chromic acid salts. वर्णरागी; वर्णग्राही; रंगग्राही; रंगप्रेमी

**Chromatic.** Relating to, or possessing colour. वर्णक; वर्ण सम्बन्धी

**Chromatin.** Colour. वर्ण; रंग

**Chromatism.** Abnormal pigmentation. विषमवर्णकता

**Chromatogenous.** Chromatin-producing; causing pigmentation. वर्णोत्पादक; वर्णजनक

**Chromatogram.** Tracing produced by chromatography. वर्णलस

**Chromatography.** Consists of the separation of substances on a chromatography column. वर्णलेखन

**Chromatometer.** An instrument for measuring colour perception or the intensity of the colour. वर्णमापी; वर्णमापकयंत्र

**Chromatometry.** Measuring the intensity of the colour. वर्णमिति; वर्णमापन

**Chromatophore.** Any coloured cell-plastid found in certain forms of protozoa. वर्णधरकोशिका; वर्णयुक्तकोशिका

**Chromatoplasm.** Any substance forming the colour for nerve-cells. रंज्य-द्रव्य

**Chromatopsia.** Abnormal sensation of colour. रंजित-दृष्टि; किसी रंग-विशेष की अस्वाभाविक अनुभूति

**Chromatoptometer.** An instrument for testing the colour-perception. वर्णविभेदनमितिक; वर्णविभेदनमापी

**Chromatoptometry.** Testing the power of colour-perception. वर्णविभेदनमापन; वर्णविभेदनमिति

**Chromatosis.** An abnormal pigmentation of the skin. रंजितचर्मता; त्वचा की अस्वाभाविक रंजकता

**Chrome.** See **Chromium.**

**Chromhidrosis.** See **Chromidrosis.**

**Chromidrosis.** The secretion of coloured sweat; chromhidrosis. रंजितस्वेदलता; रंगीन पसीना होना

**Chromium.** A very hard metallic element, which is a source of pigment; chrome. क्रोमियम; एक ठोस धातु जिससे वर्णक प्राप्त होता है

**Chromocyte.** Any coloured cell. रंजितकोशिका

**Chromogen.** A colourless body producing pigment. वर्णजन

**Chromogenesis.** The production of pigment. वर्णजननता; वर्णोत्पादकता

**Chromogenic.** Producing pigment. वर्णजनक; वर्णजनीय; वर्णोत्पादक;

**Chromomere.** A granule of a chromosome. वर्णसूत्र

**Chromosomal.** Pertaining to the chromosome. गुणसूत्री; केन्द्रकीय

**Chromosome.** Any one of the thread-like bodies into which the cell nucleus divides during mitosis and which splits longitudinally in that process. गुणसूत्र; परम्परासूत्र

**Chromotherapy.** The treatment of disease by coloured light. रंजित-प्रकाशचिकित्सा

**Chronic.** Inveterate or requiring long treatment; indistinctive or the reverse of acute. चिरकारी; जीर्ण; पुराना

**Chronicity.** The condition of being chronic. जीर्णता; चिरकारिता

**Chronothermal.** Relating to time and temperature. समय तथा तापमान सम्बन्धी

**Chrysotherapy.** Treatment of disease by the administration of gold salts. स्वर्णचिकित्सा

**Chyle.** A nutritive fluid of milky whiteness. अन्नरस; वसालसीका; पायस

**Chylification.** The process by which the chyme is converted into chile; chyle-formation; chylopoiesis; chylosis. अन्नरस-निर्माण प्रक्रिया; वसालसीकाभवन

**Chyliform.** Of the form of chyle. अन्नरसाभ; वसालसीकाभ

**Chylocele.** An effusion of chylous fluid in the cavity of the tunica vaginalis testis. वसालसीकावृषण

**Chylopericardium.** An effusion of chyle within the pericardium. वसालसीकापरिहृद्

**Chyloperitoneum.** The effusion of chyle in the peritoneal cavity. वसालसीकापर्युदर्या

**Chylopoiesis.** See **Chylification.**

**Chylopoietic.** Chyle-producing. वसालसीकोत्पादक; अन्नरसोत्पादक; relating to chylopoeisis. वसालसीकाभवन सम्बन्धी

**Chylorrhea.** See **Chylorrhoea.**

**Chylorrhoea.** An excessive flow of chyle; chylorrhea. अतिवसालसीकामयता

**Chylosis.** See **Chylification.**

**Chylothorax.** The presence of chyle in the pleural cavity. वसालसीकावक्ष

**Chylous.** Consisting of chyle; of the nature of chyle. वसालसीकी; अन्नरसाभ; relating to chyle. वसालसीका सम्बन्धी

**Chyluria.** The presence of chyle in the urine. वसालसीकामेह; पेशाब में अन्नरस जाना

**Chyme.** The mass into which the food is reduced after being subjected to the action of the stomach and gastric juice; the food that has undergone gastric but not intestinal digestion. काइम; आमरस; अर्धपक्वान्न

**Chymification.** The process of digestion converting the food into chyme; chymopoeisis. पाचन-प्रक्रिया; काइमीकरण

**Chymopoeisis.** See **Chymification.**

**Cibus.** Food. भोजन

**Cicatrectomy.** Excision of a scar. क्षतांक-उच्छेदन

**Cicatrices.** Plural of **Cicatrix.**

**Cicatricial.** Pertaining to the cicatrix. क्षतांक सम्बन्धी

**Cicatrix.** Scar left from a healed wound. क्षतांकन; क्षतचिन्ह; व्रणचिन्ह; घाव का निशान

**Cicatrizant.** Causing or favouring cicatrization. क्षतांकनजनक

**Cicatrization.** The process of healing. क्षतांकन; विरोहण

**Cilia.** The hair of the eyelids; eyelashes; plural of **Cilium**. रोमक; पक्ष्माभिकायें; पलकें; पक्ष्म; बरौनियां; पपनियां

**Ciliary.** Pertaining to cilia or eyebrows. पलकों अथवा भौहों सम्बन्धी; रोमक

**Ciliated.** Having cilia, as certain cells. रोमक

**Ciliectomy.** Excision of a portion of the ciliary body; cyclectomy. रोमकपिण्ड-उच्छेदन

**Cilium.** Eyelash; the edge of eyelid. रोमक; वर्त्म; पक्ष्म; पलक; बरोनी; पपनी

**Cillosis.** A spasmodic trembling of the upper eyelid. ऊर्ध्ववर्त्मकम्प; ऊपरी पलकों की ऐंठनयुक्त कम्पन

**Cimex Lectularius.** The common bedbug. खटमल

**Cinchona.** A genus of trees, the bark of which yields quinine. सिन्कोना; कुनीन वृक्ष

**Cinchonism.** Quininism; the systemic effect of quinine in overdose. कुनीनात्यय; कुनीनविषजता; कुनीनविषण्णता

**Cinder.** Ash. भस्म; राख

**Cineangiocardiography.** Motion picture of passage of contrast medium through the heart and blood vessels. चलवाहिकाहृद्चित्रण

**Cineradiography.** Moving picture radiography. चल-एक्सरेचित्रण

**Cinerea.** The grey matter of the brain and other parts of the nervous system. धूसर पदार्थ; स्नायुमण्डल का धूमिल अंश

**Cingulectomy.** See **Cingulotomy**.

**Cingulotomy.** Excision of a cingulum; cingulectomy. मेखला-उच्छेदन

**Cingulum.** The waist. मेखला; परिबंध; कमरबंध

**Cinnabar.** Red mercuric sulphide. सिंगरफ; हिंगुल

**Cinnamomum.** An aromatic bark with carminative mild astringent properties; cinnamon. तेजपात; दालचीनी

**Cinnamon.** See **Cinnamomum**.

**Cionitis.** Inflammation of the uvula. काकलकशोथ; उपजिह्वा अथवा अलिजिह्वा का प्रदाह

**Circinate.** In the form of a circle or segment of a circle; circinatus;

**Circinatus**

circular; ring-shaped. कुण्डलित; वृत्ताकार; अग्रवलित; कुण्डलाकार
**Circinatus.** See **Circinate.**
**Circle.** A round-shaped ring. वृत्त; मण्डल; गोलाकार छल्ला
**Circoid.** See **Cirsoid.**
**Circuit.** The path of galvanic current. चक्र; परिपथ; सर्किट
**Circular.** Pertaining to, or like a circle. वृत्ताकार; वर्तुल; मण्डलाकार
**Circulation.** The passage of the blood to and from the heart through the body, by means of the arteries and veins. परिसंचरण; संचार;

**Blood C.**, the circulation of the blood from the heart, through the arteries, capillaries and veins and back again to the heart. रक्त-परिसंचरण; रक्तसंचार;

**Collateral C.**, that taking place through secondary channels after stoppage of the principal route. समपार्श्वी परिसंचरण; समपार्श्वी संचार;

**Compensatory C.**, circulation establised in dilated collateral vessels when the main artery of the part in obstructed. क्षतिपूरक परिसंचरण;

**Coronary C.**, that of blood through the heart-walls. हृद्धमनी परिसंचरण;

**Enterohepatic C.**, circulation of substances, such as bile salts, which are absorbed by the intestine and carried to the liver, where they are secreted into the bile and again enter the intestine. आंत्रयकृत् परिसंचरण;

**Extracorporeal C.**, when the blood is taken from the body, directed through a machine and returned to the general circulation. शरीर बाह्य-परिसंचरण;

**Foetal C.**, that of the foetus, including that through the placenta and umbilical cord; placental circulation. गर्भरक्तपरिसंचरण;

**Placental C.**, see **Foetal Circulation.**

**Portal C.**, the passage of the blood from the gastro-intestinal tract and spleen through the liver and its exist by the hepatic vein. प्रतिहारपरिसंचरण;

**Pulmonary C.**, that of the blood through the lungs for purification. फुप्फुस-रक्त परिसंचरण

**Circulatory.** Pertaining to the circulation. संचार सम्बन्धी; sanguiferous. रक्तवाही;

**C. System,** the system of the animal body, consisting of the heart, arteries, veins, etc., through which blood circulates. संचार प्रणाली

**Circulus.** A circle; any ring-like structure. वृत्त;
  **C. Arteriosus,** the arterial circle. धमनी वृत्त;
  **C. Arteriosus Iridis Major,** an arterial circle around the circumference of the iris. बृहत्-परितारिका धमनीवृत्त;
  **C. Arteriosus Iridis Minor,** one around the free margin of the iris. लघुपरितारिका धमनीवृत्त
**Circumcise.** To perform circumcision. सुन्नत अथवा खतना करना
**Circumcision.** Excision of the prepuce, or foreskin. सुन्नत; खतना; लिंगाग्रचर्म-उच्छेदन; शिश्न के आगे की चमड़ी काटना
**Circumcorneal.** Around the cornea. परिस्वच्छमण्डलीय; स्वच्छमण्डल के चारों ओर
**Circumduction.** Continuous circular movement of limbs. पर्यावर्तन; अंगों की अविराम गोलाकार गति
**Circumflex.** Surrounding, as a vessel or nerve; winding. परिवेष्टक; गोलमोल
**Circumscribed.** Clearly defined, as an abscess. परिगत; परिसीमित
**Circumvallate.** Surrounded by a wall. परिवृत्त; परिखावृत्त
**Cirrhosis.** Hardening due to an increase in the connective tissue of an organ. सिरोसिस; अधितन्तुरुजा;
  **C. of liver,** cirrhosis due to infiltration of fibrous tissue and nodule formation accompanied by impaired liver function. यकृद्दाल्युदर; यकृत् का सूत्रण रोग;
  **Biliary C.,** that due to chronic retention of bile, or biliary obstruction. पैत्तिक सिरोसिस;
  **Cardiac C.,** an excessive fibrotic reaction within the liver as a result of prolonged congestive heart failure. हृद्जन्य सिरोसिस;
  **Hypertrophic C.,** that associated with hypertrophy. अतिबृद्ध सिरोसिस
**Cirrhotic.** Pertaining to cirrhosis. सिरोसी; सूत्रण रोग सम्बन्धी; affected with cirrhosis. सूत्रणरोगग्रस्त; सिरोसिसग्रस्त
**Cirsectomy.** Excision of a varicose vein. स्फीतशिरा-उच्छेदन
**Cirsocele.** A varicocele. शिरार्बुद
**Cirsoid.** Resembling a varix; circoid; varicoid. स्फीतशिराभ
**Cirsomphalos.** The presence of varicose vein around the umbilicus. नाभिशिरास्फीति; नाभिशिरा का फूल जाना

**Cirsophthalmia.** Varicose ophthalmia. नेत्रशिराविस्फार; नेत्रशिरा का फूल जाना

**Cistern.** A dilatation. विस्फार; फैलाव; a reservoir. कुण्ड; जलाशय

**Cisterna.** The same as **Cistern.**

**C. Magna,** is a subarachnoid space in the cleft between the carebellum and medulla oblongata. महाकुण्ड

**Cisternal.** Relating to a cisterna. कुण्ड सम्बन्धी

**Citrus Aurantium.** An orange tree. संतरे का पेड़; नारंगी का पेड़

**Citrus Limonia.** A lemon tree. नीम्बू का पेड़

**Citrus Medica.** A lemon tree. नीम्बू का पेड़

**Cl.** Symbol for chlorine. क्लोरीन के लिये प्रयुक्त किया जाने वाला संक्षिप्त चिन्ह

**Clairvoyance.** The extra sensory perception of objective events. दूरद्रष्टा; दूर की सोचने वाला

**Clammy.** Adhesive; glutinous; sticky. चिपचिपा; चेपदार; लेसदार

**Clamp.** An instrument for compressing vessels. संधर; शिकंजा; कीलक

**Clap.** A slang term for gonorrhoea. प्रमेह अर्थात् सूजाक के लिये प्रयुक्त एक शब्द

**Clarificant.** A substance for clearing a solution. शोधक; शोषक

**Clarification.** The process of purifying or refining. शोधन; शोषण

**Clasmatocyte.** A large cell with a tendency to break into pieces. भंजककोशिका

**Clasmatocytosis.** The breaking up of clasmatocytes. कोशिकांशभंजन

**Classification.** Systemic arrangement. वर्गीकरण

**Claudication.** Lameness. खंजता; लुंजता; लंगड़ापन

**Claudicatory.** Relating to claudication. खंजता सम्बन्धी

**Claustra.** Plural of **Claustrum.**

**Claustrophobia.** A morbid dread of an inclosed space. संवृतिभीति; किसी घिरे हुए स्थान का आतंक

**Claustrum.** A grey layer between the insula and lenticula. रोधपट

**Clavicle.** Collar-bone. जत्रुक; कण्ठास्थि; हँसुली

**Clavicotomy.** Surgical division of the clavicle. जत्रुक-उच्छेदन

**Clavicular.** Pertaining to clavicle. जत्रुकीय; जत्रुक, कण्ठास्थि अथवा हँसली सम्बधी

**Clavipectoral.** Pertaining to clavicle and the chest. जत्रुक तथा वक्ष सम्बधी

**Clavipedis.** Corn. घट्टा; चण्डी; कील

**Clavus.** A nail. नखर; नाखुन; नख; a corn; heloma. घट्टा; कील;
   **C. Hystericus,** a severe headache found in the hysterical subjects. वातोन्मादी सिरदर्द; माथे में कील ठोके जाने जैसा दर्द

**Claw-foot.** A deformity and atrophy of the foot; pes cavus. नखर-पाद

**Claw-hand.** A condition in atrophy of interosseous muscles of hand. नखरहस्त

**Clearance.** Removal of a substance from the blood plasma by the kidney. उत्सर्जन

**Cleavage.** Splitting a complex molecule into two or more simpler ones; segmentation. विदलन;
   **C. Cell,** the blastomere. विदलन कोशिका

**Cleft.** A fissure; crevice; rima. विदर; दरार; नासूर;
   **C. Lip,** hare-lip; a congenital cleft or separation of the upper lip; cheiloschisis. खण्डोष्ठ;
   **C. Palate,** a congenital palatine fissure. खण्डतालु;
   **C. Tongue,** a bifid tongue. द्विभिद्जिह्वा

**Cleidotomy.** Operative division of the clavicle. अक्षकछेदन; अक्षककर्तन

**Clergyman's Sore-throat.** A granular form of pharyngitis; angina granulosa; aphonia clericorum. कणिकीय ग्रासनलीशोथ

**Client.** The patient of a health-care professional. रोगी; ग्राहक

**Climacteric.** A critical period in life; the menopause. लैंगिक क्षीणताकाल; जननिवृत्तिकाल; रजोनिवृत्तिकाल; वय:सन्धिकाल

**Climax.** The crisis of a disease or its utmost violence. चरमति; रोग की अत्युन्नत अवस्था

**Clinic.** The doctor's chamber. निदानशाला; क्लीनिक; चिकित्सालय; औषधालय

**Clinical.** Concerned with disease in its practical aspects. नैदानिक; निदानालयी; लाक्षणिक; रोगविषयक; अनुभूत;
   **C. Medicine,** the part of medicine which is occupied with the investigation of diseases at bed-side. अनुभूत औषधि; अनुभूत चिकित्सा

**Clinician.** A physician skilled in clinical work; clinicist. चिकित्सक; वैद्य; हकीम

**Clinicideus.** See **Clinoid.**

**Clinicist.** See **Clinician.**

**Clinocephaly.** Concavity of the upper suface of the skull presenting a saddle-shaped appearance in profile. बक्रमस्तिष्कता

**Clinodactyly.** An abnormal flexure of fingers or toes. बक्रांगुलिता; उँगलियों का अस्वाभाविक टेढ़ापन

**Clinoid.** Resembling a bed; clinicideus. स्याणुक

**Clitoridectomy.** Excision of the clitoris. भगशिश्निका-उच्छेदन; भगांकुर-उच्छेदन

**Clitorides.** Plural of **Clitoris.**

**Clitoriditis.** Inflammation of the clitoris; clitoritis. भगशिश्निकाशोथ; भगांकुर-प्रदाह

**Clitoris.** An organ of the female homologous with the penis in the male; clitoridis. भगशिश्निका; भगांकुर

**Clitorism.** Prolonged and usually painful erection of the clitoris. भग्नशिश्निका की दीर्घकालीन तथा दर्दनाक उत्तानता

**Clitorismus.** Morbid enlargement of the clitoris. भगशिश्निका-विवर्धन; भगांकुर-विवर्धन

**Clitoritis.** See **Clitoriditis.**

**Clivus.** A slope or downward sloping surface. जतूक-प्रवण

**Cloaca.** An opening in the diseased bone; a cavity containing pus. अवस्करगुहा

**Cloacal.** Pertaining to the cloaca. अवस्करगुहा सम्बन्धी

**Clonic.** Pertaining to, or of the nature of clonus. अवमोटनीय; पेशियों की अनियमित सिकुड़न सम्बन्धी अथवा सिकुड़न जैसी;

    **C. Spasm,** not permanently rigid; lent with alternation of relaxation. झटका; अवमोटन-उद्वेष्ट

**Clonicity.** The state of being clonic. अवमोटनता

**Clonospasm.** See **Clonus.**

**Clonus.** Spasm in which rigidity and relaxation succeed each other; clonospasm. अवमोटन; पेशियों की अनियमित सिकुड़न

**Clot.** A mass of thickened blood. थक्का; आतंच; स्कन्द

**Clotting.** Formation of a mass of blood. आतंचन; स्कन्दन

**Cloudy Swelling.** Parenchymatous degeneration of cells. धूमिल सूजन

**Clownism.** The hysteric display of contortions and poses. आक्षेप; अकड़न

**Clubbed-finger.** Swelling of the soft tissue at the extremities and often occurs in heart and lung diseases. मुद्गरांगुलिकता; उँगली के कोमल ऊतक की सूजन

**Club-foot.** A deformity of the foot; talipes. मुद्गरपाद; सहजपादबक्रता

**Club-hand.** A deformity of the hand similar to that of club-foot. मुद्गरहस्त; सहजहस्तबक्रता

**Club-shaped.** Shaped like a heavy staff or piece of wood. मुद्गररूप; मुद्गराकार; मूसली जैसा

**Clyster.** An injection into the bowels for promoting an evacuation and relieving costiveness. गुदवस्ति; एनीमा; मलाशयी अन्तःक्षेपण

**C.M.** Cras Mane; tomorrow morning. कल सुबह; chirurgiae magister, which means Master in Surgery (M.S.). शल्याचार्य

**CM.** Symbol for centimeter. सेण्टिमीटर के लिये प्रयुक्त चिन्ह

**C.M.O.** Chief Medical Officer. मुख्य चिकित्सा अधिकारी

**C.N.** Cras Nocte; tomorrow night. कल रात को

**Cnidosis.** Urticaria. शीतपित्त; छपाकी; जुलपित्ती

**Co-.** Prefix meaning together. 'सह' के रूप में प्रयुक्त उपसर्ग

**Coagula.** Plural of **Coagulum.**

**Coagulable.** Capable of being coagulated or clotted. आतंचनशील; स्कन्दनशील

**Coagulant.** Causing stimulating or accelerating coagulation. स्कन्दक

**Coagulation.** A change from a fluid to a solid condition, as in the coagulation of blood. आतंचन; स्कन्दन; जमना; गाढ़ा होना

**Coagulative.** Promoting a process of coagulation. आतंची; स्कन्दी

**Coagulometer.** An instrument for studying the coagulability of the blood. स्कन्दनमापी; आतंचमापी

**Coagulum.** A clot or mass of the thickened blood. आतंच; रक्तातंच; रक्तकण; स्कन्द; थक्का; खून का जमा हुआ कण

**Coalescence.** The union of two or more parts. संश्लेष; दो या दो से अधिक अंगों का मेल

**Coaltar.** A viscid liquid from dry distillation of mineral pitch-coal. अलकतरा; कोलतार

**Coaptation.** The adjustment of the edges of fractures. सन्धान

**Coarctation.** The compression of the walls of a vessel. सम्पीडन; निकुंचन

**Coarctotomy.** The division of an urethral stricture. मूत्रपथ-उच्छेदन

**Coarse.** Not fine; gross; rough. खर्बर; खुरदरा

**Coat.** The membrane covering a part. कला; आवरण; लेप; कंचुक; परत; झिल्ली; पटल; तह; अस्तर

**Cobalamin.** A general term for compounds containing vitamin $B_{12}$. कोबालामिन; विटामिन बी$_{12}$ युक्त यौगिक

**Cobalt.** A metal capable of radioactivity, useful in treating cancer. कोबाल्ट; निकिल जैसी एक धातु

**Coca.** A genus of plant; several alkaloids including cocaine, are derived from the dried leaves of the shrub. कोका; प्राचेतपर्णी; दक्षिण अमेरिका में पाई जाने वाली एक बूटी जिसकी पत्तियों से कोकीन बनाई जाती है

**Cocaine.** A drug derived from coca leaves used as a local anaesthetic; also habit forming narcotic. कोकीन; प्राचेतनी; कोका का सत

**Cocainomania.** Mania for excessive use of cocaine. कोकीनोन्माद;

**Cocci.** Plural of **Coccus.**

**Coccoid.** Resembling a coccus. गोलाणुवत्; कोशिका तथा सम्पुट जैसा

**Cocculus Indicus.** Indian cockle. As a homoeopathic agent, it affects the cerebrum. गुडूची; काक्कूलस इण्डिकस

**Coccus.** A bacterium of round, spherical or ovoid form. गोलाणु

**Coccyalgia.** Pain in the coccyx; coccydynia. त्रिकास्थिशूल; अनुत्रिकार्ति; गुदास्थिशूल; पुच्छास्थिशूल

**Coccydynia.** Neuralgia of coccyx; coccygodynia; coccyodynia. अनुत्रिकवेदना; अनुत्रिकार्ति; गुदास्थि-पीड़ा; पुच्छास्थि-पीड़ा

**Coccygeal.** Pertaining to the coccyx. अनुत्रिकीय; गुदास्थिक; अनुत्रिक अथवा गुदास्थि सम्बन्धी

**Coccygectomy.** Excision of the coccyx; coccygotomy. अनुत्रिक-उच्छेदन; गुदास्थि-उच्छेदन

**Coccyges.** Plural of **Cocyx.**

**Coccygis.** See **Coccyx.**

**Coccygodynia.** See **Coccydynia.**

**Coccygotomy.** See **Coccygectomy.**

**Coccyodynia.** See **Coccydynia.**

**Coccyx.** Extremity of the vertebral column; tail-bone; coccygis. अनुत्रिक; गुदास्थि; पुच्छास्थि

**Cochin-leg.** Elephantiasis. श्लीपद; हाथी-पैर

**Cochlea.** Cavity of the internal ear. कर्णावर्त; अन्तःकर्णगह्वर; कम्बु; कान की अन्दरूनी गुहा

**Cochleae.** Plural of **Cochlea.**

**Cochlear.** Relating to the cochlea. कर्णावर्ती; अन्तःकर्णगह्वर सम्बन्धी

**Cochlearaeformis.** Of the form of the cochlea. कर्णावर्तरूपी; अन्तःकर्णगह्वर जैसे आकार का

**Cochleare.** A spoonful. चम्मच भर;
   C. Amplum, a table spoonful. बड़ा चम्मच भर;
   C. Magnum, a dessert spoonful. मझला चम्मच भर;
   C. Medium, a dessert spoonful. मझला चम्मच भर;
   C. Minimum, a teaspoonful. छोटा चम्मच भर

**Cochleariform.** Spoon-shaped. चम्मचाकार; चम्मचवत्

**Cochleitis.** See **Cochlitis.**

**Cochlitis.** Inflammation of cochlea; cochleitis. कर्णावर्तशोथ; अन्तःकर्णगह्वरशोथ

**Cocoa.** A genus of plant called **Theobroma.** The seeds of **Theobroma cocao** furnish chocolate and coca. कोको;
   C. Oil, coconut oil; the oil from the fruit of the palm. नारियल तेल

**Coconut Oil.** See **Cocoa Oil.**

**Codein.** See **Codeine.**

**Codeine.** A pain-dulling drug derived from opium; codein. कोडीन; अफीम से प्राप्त एक दर्दनाशक औषधि

**Coefficient.** Expression of the degree of amount or degree of any quality possessed by a substance. गुणांक

**Codex.** The French Pharmacopoeia. फ्रांसीसी भेषज-संहिता

**Coeliac.** Relating to the abdominal cavity; celiac. कुक्षि अथवा उदर गह्वर सम्बन्धी

**Coelom.** See **Celom.**

**Coffea.** See **Coffee.**

**Coffee.** Berries of **Coffea Arabica,** used as stimulants; coffea. कॉफी

**Cognition.** Perception. बोध; ज्ञान

**Cohabitation.** Coition; copulation. सहवास; संगम; मैथुन; रति; सम्भोग; समागम

**Cohesion.** The "attraction of aggregation". संसक्ति; आकर्षण; विनियोग;

**Cohesiveness**

संयुजता; पृथक कणों का परस्पर मिल जाना

**Cohesiveness.** The ability of cohesion. ससंजनशीलता; संयुजनशीलता

**Cohobation.** The redistilling of a substance in the distilled water. पुनर्पुनरासवन

**Coil.** A spiral. कुण्डली; कुटिल;

   **C. Gland,** a sweat gland. स्वेद ग्रन्थि; कुटिल ग्रन्थि

**Coition.** See **Coitus.**

**Coitophobia.** Morbid dread of coitus. संगमभीति; मैथुनातंक

**Coitus.** Act of venery; copulation; coition. सहवास; संगम; मैथुन; रति; सम्भोग; समागम

**Colation.** The operation of staining. स्थूलनिस्यंदन

**Colauxe.** The dilatation of the colon. बृहदांत्रविस्फार; बड़ी आन्त का फैलना

**Colchicum Autumnale.** Meadow saffron; is an emetic and a drastic cathartic. It is used in gout and other rheumatic affections. हिरण्यतुत्थ; हरिणतूतिया; सुरिंजन

**Cold.** Coryza; the common name for the catarrh of the respiratory tract. प्रतिश्याय; सर्दी-जुकाम; ठण्ड; ठण्डा; शीत; शीतल;

   **C. Abscess,** a chronic abscess, usually tuberculous. शीतल विद्रधि;

   **C. Bath,** a bath with the temperature below 70 ° F. शीतल स्नान;

   **C. Blooded,** adapting body temperature to environment. अनियमिततापी; असमतापी; शीत रक्तक;

   **C. Pack,** the cold-water sheet wrapped around a patient to reduce temperature. शीतल परिवेष्टन;

   **Rose C.,** a hay-fever. परागज ज्वर

**Colectomy.** The excision of a portion of colon. बृहदांत्र-उच्छेदन; बड़ी आन्त के किसी भाग को काट कर निकाल देना

**Coleocele.** Vaginal hernia. योनिहर्निया; योनिबहि:सरण

**Coleocystitis.** Inflammation of the vagina and bladder. योनिमूत्राशयशोथ; योनि एवं मूत्राशय का प्रदाह

**Colic.** Abdominal distress due to the spasm or obstruction of intestines, due to the spasm or obstruction of intestines, gall-bladder, or ureter. शूल; उदरशूल; पीड़ा; relating to the colon. बृहदांत्र सम्बन्धी;

   **Biliary C.,** that due to the passage of gall-stone through the gall-ducts; hepatic colic. पित्ताश्मशूल; पित्त-पथरी के कारण होने वाला दर्द;

   **Hepatic C.,** see **Biliary Colic.**

**Intestinal C.**, abnormal peristaltic movement of an irritated gut. आंत्रशूल;

**Lead C.**, intestinal colic due to lead-poisoning; painter's colic; saturnine colic. सीसक-शूल; सीसक-विषण्णता के कारण होने वाला आन्त्रशूल;

**Menstrual C.**, the pain of menstruation. ऋतुशूल; आर्तवपीड़ा;

**Painter's C.**, see **Lead Colic**.

**Renal C.**, due to a calculus in the ureter. वृक्कशूल; गुर्दे का दर्द;

**Saturnine C.**, see **Lead Colic**.

**Uteric C.**, see **Uterine Colic**.

**Uterine C.**, paroxysmal pains at the menstrual period; uteric colic. जरायुशूल; गर्भाशयशूल;

**Vesical C.**, pain in the bladder. मूत्राशयशूल

**Colica Pictonum.** Painters' colic due to lead-absorption. रंगसाजों का उदरशूल; सीसक-विषण्णता

**Colicky.** Relating to colic. शूल अथवा उदरशूल सम्बन्धी

**Colicystitis.** Cystitis from the colon-bacillus. पित्ताशयशोथ; पित्ताशय का प्रदाह

**Colitis.** Inflammation of large bowel, or colon; colonitis. बृहदान्त्रशोथ; बड़ी आंत का प्रदाह;

**Amoebic C.**, inflammation of the colon in amoebiasis. अमीबी बृहदांत्रशोथ;

**Ulcerative C.**, an inflammatory and ulcerative condition of the colon. सव्रण बृहदान्त्रशोथ; बड़ी आन्त की प्रदाहक एवं व्रणग्रस्त अवस्था

**Colla.** Plural of **Collum**.

**Collagen.** A general term referring to the structural tissues of the body other than bone, cartilage, membrane, tendon, etc. कोलेजन; श्लेषजन; मज्जा

**Collagenic.** See **Collagenous**.

**Collagenous.** Producing or containing collagen; collagenic. कोलेजनउत्पादी; श्लेषजनउत्पादी

**Collapse.** Physical or nervous prostration; sudden failure of the vital functions. निपात; निपातावस्था; पतनावस्था

**Collar-bone.** The clavicle. जत्रुक; कण्ठास्थि; हँसुली

**Collateral.** Subsidiary or accessory to the main thing; side by side; secondary; accessory. समपार्श्वी; सहायक; गौण

**Collect**. To bring together. संग्रह करना

**Colleculectomy**. Excision of a colliculus seminalis. शुक्रवप्र-उच्छेदन

**Colleculi**. Plural of **Colliculus**.

**Colliculus**. A small eminence. वप्र; छोटा-सा उभार;

   **C. Facialis**, a rounded eminence on the floor of the fourth ventricle. आनन वप्र;

   **C. Seminalis**, the longitudinal ridge in the floor of the male urethra. शुक्र वप्र

**Collilongus**. The long muscle of the neck. बृहत्ग्रीवापेशी; गर्दन की बड़ी पेशी

**Colliquation**. A liquidification of the tissues. द्रवण; ऊतकद्रवण; द्रवणशीलता; excessive विपुल; प्रचुर

**Colliquative**. Profuse; excessive. विपुल; प्रचुर; capable of being liquidificated. द्रवणशील

**Colloid**. A semi-solid non-crystalline substance jelly, rubber, glue, albumen, etc. कोलाइड; लेसदार; कलिल; सरेस जैसा पदार्थ

**Collum**. The neck. ग्रीवा; गर्दन;

   **C. Distortum**, torticollis. मन्यास्तम्भ;

   **C. Femoris**, the neck of the femur. ऊरु-अस्थि ग्रीवा; ऊर्वस्थि ग्रीवा;

   **C. Uteri**, the cervix uteri. गर्भाशय ग्रीवा; जरायु ग्रीवा

**Collutorium**. A nose-wash; a gargle; collutory. नासा-धावन; कोलूटोरियम

**Collutory**. See **Collutorium**.

**Collyrium**. The medical lotion for the eyes. नेत्रबिन्दु; कोलीरियम

**Coloboma**. A fissure, especially of the parts of the eye. नेत्रविदर

**Colocentesis**. Surgical puncture of the colon; colopuncture. बृहदान्त्रछिद्रण; बृहदान्त्रछेदन

**Colocynth**. The peeled papo of **Citrulus colocynthis;** it is a drastic hydragog cathartic; colocynthis. इन्द्रायण; इन्द्रवारुणी

**Colocynthis**. See **Colocynth**.

**Colocystoplasty**. Operation to increase urinary bladder by using part of the colon. बृहदांत्रमूत्राशयसंधान

**Colon**. The large bowel; the part of large intestine from the cecum to the rectum. बृहदान्त्र; बड़ी आंत;

   **Ascending C.**, the portion of the colon in the right side, going cephalad from the cecum. आरोही बृहदान्त्र;

**Descending C.**, the part of the colon on the left side, between the transverse colon and the sigmoid flexure. अवरोही बृहदान्त्र;

**Sigmoid C.**, the part of the colon describing an S-shaped curve between the pelvic brim and the third sacral segment, continuous with the rectum. अवग्रह बृहदांत्र;

**Transverse C.**, the part of the colon which goes transversely across the upper part of the abdomen from right to left. अनुप्रस्थ बृहदान्त्र

**Colonalgia.** Pain in the colon. बृहदांत्रशूल

**Colonic.** Relating to the colon. बृहदान्त्र सम्बन्धी

**Colonitis.** See **Colitis**.

**Colonopathy.** Any disease of the colon; colopathy. बृहदान्त्र-विकृति; बड़ी आन्त का कोई रोग

**Colonoscope.** An instrument for examining the colon. बृहदान्त्रदर्शी (यंत्र)

**Colonoscopy.** Examination by means of a colonoscope. बृहदान्त्रदर्शन

**Calopathy.** See **Colonopathy**.

**Coloproctitis.** Inflammation of the colon and rectum; colorectitis. बृहदान्त्र-मलान्त्रशोथ; बड़ी आन्त और मलाशय का प्रदाह

**Coloproctosia.** See **Coloptosis**.

**Coloptosis.** A displacement of the colon; coloproctosia. बृहदान्त्रभ्रंश; बड़ी आन्त की स्थानच्युति

**Colopuncture.** See **Colocentesis**.

**Color.** The tint or hue of any object; colour. वर्ण; रंग;

**C. Blindness,** deficiency of color-perception. वर्णान्धता; रंग-बोध की अक्षमता

**Colorectitis.** See **Coloproctitis**.

**Colorimeter.** An instrument for estimating colouring matter. वर्णमापी; वर्णमापक (यंत्र)

**Colorimetry.** Estimation of colouring matter with the help of colorimeter. वर्णमिति

**Colorrhaphy.** Suture of the colon. बृहदांत्रसीवन

**Coloscopy.** Visual examination of the colon during laparotomy by use of a sterlized endoscope. बृहदांत्रदर्शन

**Colostomy.** The formation of a colonic fistula. बृहदान्त्रसम्मिलन; बृहदान्त्रछिद्रीकरण

**Colostrum.** The first milk secreted by the breasts. प्रथमस्तन्य; खीस; स्तनों से पहले-पहल निकलने वाला दूध
**Colotomy.** Cutting into colon. बृहादान्त्र-उच्छेदन; बड़ी आन्त को काटना
**Colour.** See **Color.**
**Colpalgia.** Pain in the vagina; colpodynia. योनिशूल; योनिवेदना; योनिपीड़ा
**Colpectasia.** Distension of the vagina; colpectasis. योनिविस्फार; योनि का फैल जाना
**Colpectasis.** See **Colpectasia.**
**Colpectomy.** Incision of vagina. योनिछेदन
**Colpeurysis.** Vaginal dilatation. योनिविस्फार
**Colpitis.** Inflammation of vagina. योनिशोथ; योनि का प्रदाह
**Colpocele.** A hernia or tumour in the vagina. योनि-हर्निया; योनि-अर्बुद
**Colpocystitis.** Inflammation of both the bladder and the vagina. मूत्राशययोनिशोथ; मूत्राशय तथा योनि का प्रदाह
**Colpocystocele.** See **Cystocele.**
**Colpocystoplasty.** Plastic surgery to repair the vesicovaginal wall. मूत्राशययोनिभित्तिसंधान
**Colpodynia.** See **Colpalgia.**
**Colpoperineoplasty.** Plastic surgery for repair of an injury of the perineum involving the vagina; vaginoperineoplasty. योनिमूलाधारसंधान
**Colpoperineorrhaphy.** The surgical repair of an injured vaginal and deficient perineum. मूलाधारयोनिभित्तिसीवन
**Colpopexy.** Suture of a relaxed and prolapsed vagina to the abominal wall; vaginofixation; vaginopexy. योनिस्थिरीकरण
**Colpoplasty.** Any plastic operation of the vagina. योनिसंधान
**Colpoptosis.** Any prolapse of the vagina. योनिभ्रंश
**Colporrhaphy.** Suturing of the vagina. योनिभित्तिसीवन
**Colporrhexis.** Rupture or laceration of the vagina. योनिभित्तिविदर
**Colposcope.** An instrument for the visual examination of the vagina. योनिभित्तिदर्शी
**Colposcopy.** A visual examination of the vagina with the help of a colposcope. योनिभित्तिदर्शन
**Colpospasm.** The vaginal spasm. योनि-उद्वेष्ट; योनि की जकड़न या ऐंठन
**Colpostenosis.** Narrowing of the vagina. योनिसंकीर्णता
**Colpostenotomy.** Surgical correction of colpostenosis. योनिसंकीर्णता हटाना
**Colpotomy.** Any incision of the vagina. योनिभित्तिछेदन; योनिभित्तिकर्तन

**Columella.** A small column; columnella. स्तम्भिका; खण्ड;
   **C. Nasi,** the nasal septum. नासा-स्तम्भिका
**Column.** A pillar or pillar-like part; columna. स्तम्भ; वली; खण्ड; दण्ड
**Columna.** See **Column.**
**Columnae.** Plural of **Columna.**
**Columnar.** Shaped like a column. स्तम्भिकाकार; स्तम्भाकार; खण्डाकार
**Columnella.** See **Columella.**
**Coma.** Lethargy; unnatural propensity to sleep. सन्यास; गहन मूर्च्छा; जड़िमा;
   **Alcoholic C.,** due to alcoholism. मद्यविषज सन्यास;
   **Diabetic C.,** due to diabetes. मधुमेहज सन्यास; .
   **C. Vigil,** delirious lethargy with open eyes. सजग सन्यास; प्रलाप और तन्द्रा
**Comatose.** Affected with or in a condition of coma. सन्यस्त; मूर्च्छित; बेहोश
**Combination.** Mixture. मिश्रण; योगिक; संयोजन
**Cimbined.** Mixed. मिश्रित; मिलाया हुआ
**Combustible.** Capable of being burnt. दह्य; जलाया जाने योग्य
**Combustion.** The process of oxidation. दहन; जलना
**Comedo.** Black-head; a worm-like mass in an obstructed sebaceous duct. त्वक्कील
**Comedones.** Plural of **Comedo.**
**Coma Bacillus.** The spirillum of **Asiatic cholera.** विसूचिकाणु; हैजा फैलाने वाला जीवाणु
**Commensal.** Harmonious living together of two or more dissimilar organisms. सहभोजी; अन्य प्रकार के जीवों के साथ रहने और भोजन करने वाला प्राणी
**Commensalism.** The stage of being commensal. सहभोजिता
**Comminute.** To break into pieces. विखण्डन (होना); विचूर्णन (होना); टूट-फूट होना
**Comminuted.** Broken to pieces. विखण्डित; विचूर्णित; टुकड़े-टुकड़े होना
**Comminution.** The process of breaking into pieces. विखण्डन; विचूर्णन
**Commissura.** See **Commissure.**
**Commissural.** Relating to commissure. संयोजिका सम्बन्धी
**Commissure.** A joining or uniting; commissura. संयोजिका; संयोग;

Grey C., the transverse band of grey matter uniting the masses of grey matter of the two halves of the spinal cord. धूसर संयोजिका

**Commissurotomy.** Incision of commissura. संयोजिकाछेदन

**Common Cold.** A virus infection of the upper breathing organ. प्रतिश्याय; जुकाम

**Commotio.** Concussion. संघट्ट; संघात; विकम्पन; motion. गति;

C. **Cerebri,** the cerebral concussion. प्रमस्तिष्क संघट्ट;

C. **Retinae,** impairment of vision following a blow upon or near the eye. संघट्ट दृष्टिपटलशोफ

**Communicable.** Transmissible, directly or indirectly, from one person to another. संचारी; संचरणशील

**Communicans.** Communicating. संचारी

**Communicating.** Connecting. संयोजी

**Communication.** In anatomy, a joining or connecting, said of fibres, solid structures, etc., e.g. tendons and nerves. संचार; संयोजन

**Communis.** Common. सामान्य

**Commutator.** An instrument for reversing electric current. द्विक्परिवर्तक

**Comose.** Having much hair. अतिरोमिल

**Compact.** Dense; having a dense structure. सघन; गठीला

**Comparative.** Relating to comparison. तुलनीय; तुलनात्मक

**Compatibility.** The power of a substance to mix with another without unfavourable results. संगतता; संयोज्यता; अनुकूलता

**Compatible.** Capable of existing together. संगत; संयोज्य; अनुकूल; अनुगुण;

C. **Blood,** blood from the individuals of the same blood group that can be easily given in transfusion. संयोज्य रक्त; अनुगुण रक्त

**Compensating.** Making amends for. क्षतिपूरक; पूरक; प्रतिकारी

**Compensation.** The state of counterbalancing a defect of structure or function. क्षतिपूर्ति; सम्पूर्ति; प्रतिकार; मुआवजा; हर्जाना

**Compensatory.** Relating to, or characterized by compensation. क्षतिपूर्ति सम्बन्धी; क्षतिपूर्तिज

**Competence.** The quality of being competent or capable of performing an allotted function. दक्षता; पूर्ण सक्षमता

**Complaint.** Any morbid state. रुग्णता; बीमारी; कष्ट

**Complement.** Assisting each other. पूरक; अनुपूरक; सहायक

**Complemental.** See **Complementary.**

**Complementary.** Accessory; complemental. पूरक; अनुपूरक; सहायक

**Complex.** Complicated; intricate. संकर; सम्मिश्र; जटिल; उलझा हुआ

**Complexion.** Countenance, i.e. colour, texture and general appearance of the face. वर्ण; रूप; रंग-रूप; हाव-भाव; भाव-भंगिमा

**Complexus.** The totality of symptoms of a disease. रोगलक्षणसमष्टि;
C. Muscle, the broad muscle of the back of the neck. ग्रीवापश्चपेशी; गर्दन के पीछे की चौड़ी पेशी

**Complicated.** Complex. जटिल; उलझनपूर्ण; उलझा हुआ; संकर

**Complication.** A morbid process or event occurring during a disease which is not an essential part of the disease, although it may result from it or from independent causes. उपद्रव; जटिलता

**Component.** Constituent. अवयव; घटक

**Composition.** The constituents of a mixture. रचना; संघटन; संगठन; मिश्रण

**Compos Mentis.** Of sound mind; sane. बुद्धिमान; प्रबुद्ध

**Compound.** Mixture; composed of several parts. सम्मिश्र; मिश्रण; योगिक; to mix. मिलाना

**Compounder.** A dispensar of medicine. कम्पाउण्डर

**Comprehension.** Mental grasp of meaning and relationship. अभिबोध; ज्ञान; समझ

**Compress.** Folded cloth for local pressure and dressing the wounds. सम्पीड; सेक; दाब; तह की हुई पट्टी;
Cold C., a wet compress to be kept on the forehead to relieve headache. शीत सेक; ठण्डा सेक

**Compressibility.** Ability to compress. सम्पीड्यता; सम्पीडनशीलता

**Compressible.** Capable of being compressed. सम्पीडनशील; सम्पीड्य; दवाब योग्य

**Compression.** The state of being compressed. सम्पीडन; दबाव;
C. Illness, see **Caisson Disease.**
Cerebral C., arises from any space-occupying intracranial lesion. प्रमस्तिष्क सम्पीडन

**Compressor.** An instrument for compressing a vessel. सम्पीडक; सम्पीडिका; सम्पीडित्र; दबाव डालने वाला; a muscle, contraction of which

**Compulsion**

causes compression of any structure. सम्पीडक पेशी

**Compulsion.** Uncontrollable thoughts or impulses to perform an act. बाध्यता; अनिवार्यता

**Conarium.** The pineal gland of the brain. बालग्रन्थि

**Concave.** Presenting a hollow incurvation; having a depressed or hollowed surface. नतोदर; खोखला; अवतल; अन्दर की ओर दबा हुआ या घुसा हुआ

**Concavity.** A depression or fossa. नतोदरता; खोखलापन; खात

**Concavo-concave.** Concave on two opposing surfaces. नतोदर-उन्नतोदर

**Concavo-convex.** One side concave, the other side convex, or concave on one surface and convex on the opposite surface. अवतलोत्तल; उत्तलावतल

**Concealed.** Not disclosed or open. गुप्त

**Concentrate.** To make a liquid more stronger or purer. सान्द्र; सान्द्रित करना; गाढ़ा

**Concentrated.** Made stronger or purer. सान्द्रित; समाहृत

**Concentration.** The act of rendering a liquid or medicine stronger by evaporation. सान्द्रण; सान्द्रता

**Concentric.** Having a common centre. संकेन्द्रिक; एककेन्द्रिक

**Concept.** An abstract generalization resulting from the mental process of abstracting and recombining certain qualities or characteristics of a number of ideas. धारणा; संकल्पना

**Conception.** Impregnation of the ovum or the male sperm, when results a new being. गर्भाधान; गर्भधारण; concept. संकल्पना

**Conch.** A marine cell. शंख; शुक्तिका

**Concha.** The turbinated bone; a ridge on the upper part of the nasal surface of the maxilla. नासा-शुक्तिका; conchalis. शंख; शुक्तिका; the outer ear. बाह्यकर्ण;

   **C. Labyrinthi,** the cochlea. कर्णावर्त; कर्णशुक्तिका; कर्णकुहर;

   **C. Nasalis,** the nasal concha; paired ossicles of pyramidal shape, the bases forming the roof of the nasal cavity. नासा-शुक्तिका

   **C. Sphenoidalis,** the sphenoidal concha. जतूक शुक्तिका

**Conchalis.** See **Concha.**

**Conchitis.** Inflammation of any concha. शंखशोथ; शुक्तिकाशोथ;

बाह्यकर्णशोथ

**Conchoidal.** Shaped like a concha. शुक्तिकाभ; शंखाभ; शुक्तिकाकार

**Conchoscope.** An instrument for examining the nasal cavity. नासागह्वरदर्शी; नासा-गह्वर की जांच के लिये प्रयुक्त किया जाने वाला यंत्र

**Conchotome.** An instrument for excising the middle turbinated bone. शुक्तिकाउच्छेदक; शुक्तिकाछेदक

**Concoction.** The digestive process. पाचन; पाचन-क्रिया

**Concomitant.** Accompanying; accessory. आनुषंगिक; सहवर्ती

**Concrete.** Condensed or solidified. ठोस; मूर्त; पिण्डीभूत

**Concretion.** A hard substance gradually formed in any part of the body; a calculus; an osseous deposit. कणिकाश्मरी

**Concubitus.** Copulation; sexual intercourse. मैथुन; सम्भोग; संगम; सहवास

**Concussion.** A violent shock or shaking. संघट्टन; विकम्पन; आघात;
**C. of brain,** shock or agitation of the brain. मस्तिष्क संघट्टन; मस्तिष्क विकम्पन;
**Spinal C.,** sudden transient loss of function of the spinal cord, caused by trauma, but without permanent gross damage. मेरु-संघट्टन

**Condensation.** The act of making denser; condensing. संघनन; घनीकरण; संक्षेपण

**Condensed.** Reduced into a denser form. संघनित; घनीकृत

**Condenser.** A device for condensing gas or light. संघनित्र; द्रवणित्र

**Condensing.** See **Condensation.**

**Condition.** State; position. स्थिति; अवस्था; दशा; हालत

**Conditioning.** A process of acquiring, developing, educating, establishing, learning, or training new responses in both respondant and operant behaviour. अनुकूलन

**Condom.** A rubber sheath of penis worn during coitus to prevent infection or impregnation. निरोध; संगम के दौरान शिश्न पर लगाई जाने वाली रबड़ की थैली

**Conductance.** The ratio of an electric current through a conductor to the electromotive force; a measure of conductivity. चालकता; चालकत्व; संवाहकता; संवाहकत्व

**Conducting.** The act of transmitting energies through suitable media. चालन; संवहन; संचार

**Conduction.** The transmission of heat, light or sound waves through suitable media. चालन; संवहन; संचार

**Conductivity.** The capacity for conducting. चालकता; संचारिता; संवाहकता

**Conductor.** Applied to body which can transmit heat or electric influence; the transmitter of a force, as an electric current. चालक; संचारक; संवाहक

**Conduit.** A channel for passage of fluids. वाहकनलिका

**Condylar.** Pertaining to a condyle. स्थूलक सम्बन्धी

**Condyle.** A rounded eminence at the articular end of a bone; condylus. स्थूलक; किसी सन्धि पर हड्डी का उभार

**Condylectomy.** Excision of a condyle. स्थूलक-उच्छेदन

**Condyloid.** Resembling a condyle. स्थूलकाय; स्थूलकवत्

**Condyloma.** A soft, fleshy, indolent excrescence. मांसगुल्म; कांडिलोमा; कीलाबुंद

**Condylomata.** Wart-like excrescences on the pudenda or anus, or on face; condyloma. मांसगुल्म; क्रांडिलोमेटा; कीलाबुंद

**Condylomatous.** Relating to a condyloma. मांसगुल्म सम्बन्धी

**Condylotomy.** Division, without removal of a condyle. मांसगुल्म-विभाजन

**Condylus.** See **Condyle.**

**Cone.** Singular of **Cones.**

**Cones.** Specialized cells in the retina of th eye which are able to distinguish colour. शंकु

**Confabulation.** A symptom common in confusional state when there is impairment of memory for recent events. गल्पन

**Confectio.** See **Confection.**

**Confection.** Anything made into a pulpy mass with sugar or honey; confectio. पाक; अवलेह

**Confertus.** Confluent; closed together. सम्प्रवाही; सहगामी; सम्मिलित

**Configuration.** The general form of the body and its parts. विन्यास

**Confinement.** The period of parturition. प्रसव; प्रसवता; प्रसवकाल; प्रसूतिकाल

**Conflict.** In psychiatry, presence in the unconsciousness of two incompatible and contrasting wishes or emotions. संघर्ष

**Confluence.** A flowing or running together. सम्प्रवाह; a joining. संगम; सम्मिलन

**Confluent.** Running together; spreading over a large surface, as confluent small-pox. सम्प्रवाही; सहगामी; सम्मिलित

**Conformation.** The natural shape. प्राकृतिक आकार; रचना; बनावट

**Confusion.** Used to describe the mental state which is out of touch with reality and associated with a clouding of consciousness. सम्भ्रम; भ्रम; भ्रान्ति; उलझन

**Congealing Point.** The freezing point. संघनांक; प्रशीतनांक

**Congelation.** Frost-bite or freezing. शीतदंश अथवा प्रशीतन

**Congenital.** Existing right from birth; hereditary; innate. सहज; जन्मजात; आनुवंशिक; पैत्रिक; आजन्म;

**C. Defect,** a birth deficiency. सहज दोष; जन्मजात दोष; आजन्म दोष;

**C. Syphilis,** is acquired by the foetus from the infected mother just after the 4th month of intrauterine life. सहज उपदंश; सहमति संबन्धी

**Congested.** Hyperaemic; denoting congestion. रक्तसंकुलित; संकुलित; रक्ताधिक्ययुक्त

**Congestion.** Overfulness of the blood vessel; accumulation of blood in a part; hyperaemia. रक्ताधिक्य; द्रवाधिक्य; रक्तसंकुलन; रक्तसंलयन;

**C. of lung,** pneumonia. फुप्फुसपाक; निमोनिया

**Congestive.** Pertaining to congestion. रक्तसंलयी; रक्तसंकुलन सम्बन्धी

**Congius.** A gallon; the symbol is C. गैलन

**Conglomerate.** Heaped or massed together. संगुटित

**Conglutinant.** Glueing together. अपलगनशील; योजक; संलगन

**Conglutination.** A sticking together. अपलगनशीलता; संलगन

**Coni.** Plural of **Conus.**

**Conic.** See **Conical.**

**Conical.** Cone-shaped; conic. शंकुरूप; शंखाकार

**Conium.** Poison hemlock. विषगर्जर; विषैला वृक्ष-रस; कोनियम

**Conization.** Removal of a cone-shaped part of the cervix by the knife or cautery. शंकु-उच्छेदन

**Conjoined.** United in close connection. संयुक्त; सम्मिलित

**Conjugate.** Coupled; joined or paired; conjugated. संयुग्म; संयुग्मी; संयुग्मित; अनुबद्ध; a measurement of the bony pelvis. संयुग्मी व्यास,

**Diagonal C.,** the clinical measurement taken in pelvic

assessment from the lower border of the symphysis pubis to the sacral promontory. विकर्ण संयुग्मी व्यास;

**Obstetric C.**, the available space for the foetal head; obstetrical. प्रासूतिक संयुग्मी व्यास;

**Obstetrical C.**, see **Obstetric Conjugate.**

**True C.**, the distance from sacral promontory to the summit of the symphysis pubis. वास्तविक अथवा यथार्थ संयुग्मी व्यास;

**C. Diameter**, the anteroposterior diameter of the inlet. संयुग्मी व्यास

**Conjugated.** See **Conjugate.**

**Conjugation.** A form of reproduction or cell-division. संयुग्मन; संयुजता; अनुबद्धता; संगम

**Conjunctiva.** The membrane which covers the eyeballs and lines the eyelids. नेत्रश्लेष्मला; नेत्रश्लेष्मकला; आँखों की श्लैष्मिक झिल्ली

**Conjunctivae.** Plural of **Conjunctiva.**

**Conjunctival.** Relating to the conjunctiva. नेत्रश्लेष्मल; नेत्रश्लेष्मला सम्बन्धी

**Conjunctivitis.** Inflammation of the conjunctiva. नेत्रश्लेष्मलाशोथ; नेत्रश्लेष्मकलाशोथ; आँखों की श्लैष्मिक झिल्ली का प्रदाह;

**Allergic C.**, a conjunctival reaction to a substance producing an allergic response, either immediate or delayed. एलर्जिक नेत्रश्लेष्मलाशोथ; प्रत्यूर्जित नेत्रश्लेष्मलाशोथ;

**Catarrhal C.**, that due to cold or irritation. प्रतिश्यायी नेत्रश्लेष्मलाशोथ;

**Contagious C.**, one due to contact. सांसर्गिक नेत्रश्लेष्मलाशोथ; trachoma. रोहें; ट्रैकोमा

**Follicular C.**, formed by the presence of follicles. पुटकी नेत्रश्लेष्मलाशोथ;

**Gonococcal C.**, see **Gonorrhoeal Conjunctivitis.**

**Gonorrhoeal C.**, a severe purulent form due to infection by gonococci; gonococcal conjuntivitis. प्रमेहज नेत्रश्लेष्मलाशोथ;

**Purulent C.**, that marked by a thick creamy discharge. सपूय नेत्रश्लेष्मलाशोथ

**Conjunctivoplasty.** Plastic operation on the conjunctiva. नेत्रश्लेष्मलासंधान

**Connate.** Congenital. सहज; जन्मजात; आजन्म; confluent. सम्प्रवाही; united. सम्मिलित; संयुक्त

**Connecting.** Binding; uniting. संयोजी; संयोजक

**Connection.** Union. संयोजन; relation. सम्बन्ध

**Connective.** Connecting; binding. संयोजी; संयोजक;
  **C. Tissue,** the binding tissue of the body holding other tissues together or in proper relation of each other. संयोजी ऊतक

**Conoid.** Resembling a cone; conic. शंकुक; शंखाकार; शंकुरूप; शंकुवत्

**Consanguinity.** Blood-relationship; kinship, because of common ancestry. समोद्भवता; खून का सम्बन्ध

**Conscience.** The intense sense of feeling. अन्तर्ज्ञान; विवेक

**Conscious.** Having the sense of feeling; aware. चेतन; जागृत; सचेत; ज्ञानशक्ति से सम्पन्न; विवेक से परिपूर्ण

**Consciousness.** The state of being conscious or aware of one's own existence. चेतना; संज्ञा; जागृतावस्था; विवेकशीलता

**Consensual.** Of the nature of reflex action involving sensation, but not volition. सहवेदी

**Conservative.** Denoting treatment by gradual, limited or well-established procedure, as opposed to radical. संरक्षी

**Consistency.** The density of hardness. घनत्व; घनता; कठोरता

**Consolidation.** Solidification; becoming solid. संघनन; घनीभवन; दृढ़ीकरण; ठोस बनना या बनाना

**Constant.** Not changing; fixed. स्थिर; अविच्छिन्न; अविरल; अचल; अपरिवर्तनशील

**Constipant.** An agent causing constipation; constipating. मलबन्धकर; मलबद्धताकारी; कब्ज पैदा करने वाला; मलावरोधक; मलावरोधी

**Constipating.** See **Constipant.**

**Constipation.** Inability to perform normal bowel elimination function; obstipation; costiveness. मलबद्धता; मलबन्धता; कोष्ठबद्धता; कब्ज

**Constituent.** Applied to substances introduced into medicinal combination. गठन; संघटन; घटक

**Constitutional.** Inherited. पैत्रिक; वंशगत; temperamental. प्रकृति या स्वभाव सम्बन्धी; relating to the consititution. गठन अथवा संघटन सम्बन्धी; general. सार्वदैहिक
  **C. Disease,** inherited disease, pervading the whole system. पैत्रिक अथवा वंशगत रोग

**Constricted.** Drawn together in a part. आकुंचित; संकीर्ण; संकुचित; सिकुड़ा हुआ

**Constrictes.** The contracting muscle. आकुंचक पेशी

**Constriction.** Contraction or drawing together of a part; binding. आकुंचन; संकीर्णन; संकुचन; सिकुड़न

**Constrictur.** A contracting or compressing muscle. संकीर्णक पेशी; सिकोड़ने या दबाव देने वाली पेशी

**Constrigent.** Any agent causing bowel obstruction. मलरोधक; मलावरोधक; कब्जियत करने वाला पदार्थ

**Constructive.** Formative. रचनात्मक

**Consultant.** A consulting physician. परामर्शदाता अथवा सलाहकार चिकित्सक

**Consultation.** Deliberation of physicians concerning a patient. परामर्श; सलाह; मशविरा

**Consumption.** Phthisis; tuberculosis; क्षय; यक्ष्मा; क्षय रोग; wasting disease; atrophy. अपक्षय; शोष; क्षीणता

**Contact.** Direct or indirect exposure to an infection. सम्पर्क; संसर्ग; रोग से प्रत्यक्ष या परोक्ष रूप में प्रभावित होना; touching or apposition of two bodies. स्पर्श; संस्पर्श;
  **C. Receptors,** nerves which transmit stimuli only on contact, as touch. आग्रही तंत्रिकायें

**Contagion.** The communication of diseases by contact. संसर्ग; रोग-संक्रमण; छूत से फैलने वाला रोगों का संचार

**Contagious.** Infection of diseases by contact; contagius. संक्रामक; सांसर्गिक; communicable. संचारी; relating to contagion. रोग-संक्रमण सम्बन्धी

**Contagium.** The septic matter or germ of specific disease. संक्रामक अथवा संक्रमणकारी पदार्थ

**Contagius.** See **Contagious.**

**Contaminant.** Any polluting agent; that which causes contamination. संदूषक; प्रदूषक; दूषित करने वाला

**Contamination.** The act of contaminating. संदूषण; दूषण

**Contiguity.** Contact without actual continuity. सन्निधि

**Continence.** Restraint of passions, self-command, temperateness, chastity. संयम; आत्मनियंत्रण; इन्द्रियदमन; अव्यभिचार

**Continued.** Continuous. सतत; अविराम; अविच्छिन्न;

**C. Fever,** a fever which runs its course without decided remissions, intermissions, etc. सतत् ज्वर; अविराम ज्वर

**Continuity.** Uninterrupted connection. सततता; अविरामता; अविच्छिन्नता

**Continuous.** Uninterrupted. सतत्; अविराम; अविच्छिन्न

**Contorted.** Twisted. व्यावृत्त; व्यावर्तित; मोड़ा हुआ

**Contra-.** Prefix signifying opposition. 'प्रतिकूल', 'विपरीत', 'के विरुद्ध', आदि का अर्थ देने वाला उपसर्ग

**Contraception.** Prevention of conception. निरोध; गर्भनिरोध; गर्भरोध

**Contraceptive.** Anything used to prevent contraception. गर्भनिरोधक; गर्भरोधक; गर्भ रोकने वाला कोई भी उपाय;

   **Intrauterine C.,** a device used to prevent pregnancy. आन्तर्जरायु गर्भरोधक (यंत्र);

   **Oral C.,** any orally effective preparation to prevent conception. मुखी गर्भरोधक (औषधि)

**Contract.** To draw the parts together; to shrink. आकुंचित करना; सिकोड़ना; to acquire by contagion. संसर्ग; संक्रमण

**Contracted.** Constricted. आकुंचित; संकुचित; सिकुड़ा हुआ या सिकोड़ा हुआ

**Contractile.** Having the power to contraction. आकुंचनशील; संकुचनशील

**Contractility.** The inherent quality by which body shrinks or contracts. आकुंचनशीलता; संकुचनशीलता

**Contraction.** Shortening, especially applied to muscle fibre. आकुंचन; संकुचन; संकोच; सिकुड़न;

   **Hourglass C.,** constriction of the middle portion of a hollow organ, such as the stomach, or gravid uterus. डमरूवत् संकोच;

   **Isotonic C.,** contraction of a muscle, its tension remaining the same throughout the act. समतानी संकुचन;

   **Uterine C.,** rhythmic activity of the myometrium with menstruation, pregnancy or labour. जरायु-संकोच

**Contracture.** A state of permanent rigidity. अवकुंचन; निकोचन; स्थाई कठोरता की अवस्था

**Contraindicated.** Opposed to the nature of a disease. प्रतिनिर्दिष्ट; निषिद्ध

**Contraindication.** Circumstances which suggest avoidance of certain medical or surgical procedure. प्रतिनिर्देश; निषेध

**Contralateral.** Pertaining to objects situated on the opposite side. प्रतिपक्षी

**Contrecoup.** A fracture or injury in a part opposite to that which receives the blow. विपरीतांगपात

**Contributory.** Accessory; auxillary; concomitant. योगदत्त; अंशदायी; सहायक

**Control.** To check by observations and test their correctness. नियंत्रण करना; नियंत्रित करना; नियंत्रण रखना;

**Birth C.,** restriction of the number of offspring by means of contraceptive measures or other methods. जन्म नियंत्रण;

**Quality C.,** control of laboratory analytical errors by monitoring analytical performance. गुण नियंत्रण; गुणता नियंत्रण; गुणवत्ता नियंत्रण

**Controlled.** Checked. नियंत्रित

**Contuse.** To bruise. मर्दन करना; कुचलना; गुप्त या अन्दरूनी मार करना

**Contused.** Bruised. मर्दित; कुचला हुआ;

**C. Wound,** a wound produced by a blunt instrument or body. मर्दित घाव; नील

**Contusion.** A bruise; an injury of the external part of the body. नील; कुचलन; गुमचोट; a short of abrasion. एक प्रकार की रगड़न या खरोंच

**Conus.** A cone. शंकु;

**C. Arteriosus,** the upper anterior angle of the right cardiac ventricle or infundibulum of right ventricle. दक्षिण निलय शंकु;

**C. Elasticus,** the cricothyroid membrane, i.e. the membrane connecting the thyroid and cricoid cartilages of the larynx. प्रत्यास्थ शंकु;

**C. Medullaris,** the lower conic termination of the spinal cord. मेरु-अंत्य शंकु

**Convalescence.** The stage of recovery from illness. उल्लाघ; पुनर्स्वास्थ्यसंचय; रोगनिवृत्ति

**Convalescent.** Gradual return to health after disease; gaining strength. उल्लाघ; रोगनिवृत्ति के बाद शक्तिसंचय करने की अवस्था; pertaining to convalescence. उल्लाघ अथवा रोगनिवृत्ति सम्बन्धी

**Convection.** Transfer of heat from the hotter to the colder part. संवहन; प्रमुख रूप से ताप का किसी अधिक तप्त भाग से अधिक शीतल भाग पर स्थानान्तरित होना

**Convergence.** The tending of two or more objects toward a common point; a coming together. समानीकरण; अभिसरण; संसरण

**Conversion.** Transformation of an embryo into a physical

manifestation; transmutation; change. रूपान्तरण; एक स्थिति से दूसरी स्थिति में लाने की अवस्था; **परिवर्तन**

**Convex.** Curved outward on the external surface. उत्तल; उन्नतोदर; किनारों पर दबा हुआ, लेकिन बीच में उभरा हुआ

**Convexoconcave.** Both convex and concave. उत्तलावतल

**Convexoconvex.** Convex on both surfaces. उभयोत्तल; उत्तलोत्तल; दोनों ओर से उभरा हुआ

**Convolution.** Twist or coil of any organ, especially one of the prominent convex parts of the brain. संवलन; लहरिका; लपेट; तह

**Convulsant.** A medicine causing spasms. आक्षेपक; आक्षेपकारी

**Convulsions.** Unconsciousness accompanied by muscular twitching. आक्षेप; पेशी-स्फुरण के साथ बेहोशी और ऐंठन;

  Clonic C., slow alternating contraction and relaxation of muscle groups. अवमोटनी आक्षेप; पेशी-समूहों का पर्यायक्रम से सिकुड़ना और ढीला पड़ना;

  Epileptiform C., one marked by total loss of consciousness. अपस्मारक आक्षेप; पूर्ण चेतनालोप के साथ पड़ने वाला दौरा;

  Facial C., see Mimetic Convulsions.

  Febrile C., a convulsion in infancy or early childhood, associated with fever. ज्वरीय आक्षेप; ज्वर के साथ शरीर का अकड़ना;

  Hysterical C., apparent loss of consciousness due to hysteria. वातोन्मादी आक्षेप;

  Mimetic C., a facial convulsion. आनन आक्षेप; ललाटीय आक्षेप;

  Puerperal C., eclampsia during parturition. प्रासूतिक आक्षेप; प्रसव के दौरान पड़ने वाला दौरा;

  Tetanic C., tonic convulsion, without loss of consciousness. धनुस्तम्भी आक्षेप; धनुर्वाती आक्षेप, जिसमें रोगी बेहोश नहीं होता;

  Tonic C., reveals sustained rigidity. तानिक आक्षेप;

  Uraemic C., a convulsion due to renal disease; uremic convulsions. यूरेमी आक्षेप; मिहेयी आक्षेप; वृक्क रोग के कारण पड़ने वाला दौरा;

  Uremic C., see Uraemic Convulsions.

**Convulsive.** One of the nature of convulsions. आक्षेपिक; आक्षेपरूप; marked by or producing convulsions. आक्षेपमय अथवा आक्षेपजनक; relating to convulsions. आक्षेप सम्बन्धी

**Coordination.** Harmonious action, as of a muscle, or group of muscles. समन्वय; सामंजस्य;

**Muscular C.,** harmonious action of muscles. पेशी-समन्वय

**Cophosis.** Loss of hearing; deafness. बधिरता; बहरापन

**Copiopia.** A fatigued condition of the eyes. नेत्रावसाद; आँखों की थकान

**Copious.** Profuse; excessive. विपुल; अत्यधिक; प्रचुर

**Copper.** A reddish-brown metal. ताम्र; ताम्बा

**Copremesis.** Faecal vomiting. मलवमन

**Coprolalia.** Filthy or obscene speech. मलवाच्यता; गन्दी भाषा का प्रयोग करना

**Coprolith.** A hard mass consisting of inspissated faeces; faecalith; stercolith. मलाश्मरी; मलपथरी

**Coprology.** The study of the faeces or dung; scatology. मलविज्ञान; मलप्रकरण

**Coproma.** Accumulation of inspissated faeces in the colon or rectum giving the appearance of an abdominal tumour; faecaloma; stercoroma. मलार्बुद; पाखाने की रसौली

**Coprophagia.** See **Coprophagy.**

**Coprophagy.** The eating of dung; coprophagia. मलभक्षण

**Coprophobia.** Morbid abhorrance of defaecation and faeces. मलभीति

**Copulation.** Sexual intercourse; coition; coitus. संगम; रति; मैथुन; सम्भोग

**Cor.** The heart; cordis. हृदय; हृद्; दिल;

**C. Adiposum,** a fatty heart. वसाहृद्;

**C. Villosum,** a hairy heart. लोमहृद्

**Coracoacromial.** Relating to the coracoid process of acromion. तुण्ड-अंसकूटी

**Coracoclavicular.** Attached to coracoid process and clavicle. तुण्ड-जत्रुकी

**Coracohumeral.** Relating to the coracoid process and clavicle. तुण्ड-प्रगण्डीय

**Coracoid.** Shaped like a crow's beak. अंसतुण्ड; तुण्ड; कौए की चोंच जैसी

**Cord.** Ligature. रज्जु; बन्ध; बन्धन;

**Spermatic C.,** that which suspends the testicles in the scrotum. वृषण-रज्जु;

**Spinal C.,** a cord-like structure which lies in the spinal column.

मेरु-रज्जु;

**Umbilical C.**, the naval string. नाभि-रज्जु

**Cordate.** Heart-shaped; cordiform. हृदयाकार; हृद्सम; हृदय जैसी आकृति का

**Cordectomy.** Excision of a part or whole of a cord, as of a vocal cord. रज्जु-उच्छेदन

**Cordial.** Stimulating the heart; invigorating. हृद्बलकारी; बलवर्धक

**Cordiform.** Heart-shaped. हृत्पिण्डाकार; हृदयपिण्ड जैसी आकृति का

**Cordis.** The heart; the cardia; cor. हृदय; हृद्; दिल

**Cordopexy.** Surgical fixation of a cord. रज्जु-स्थिरीकरण

**Cordotomy.** Chordotomy. सुषुम्ना-उच्छेदन

**Core.** The central portion, usually applied to the slough in the centre of a boil. अन्त:करण; अभ्यान्तर; कोर

**Corecleisis.** See **Coreclisis.**

**Coreclisis.** An obliteration of the pupil of the eye; corecleisis. चक्षुपटलक्षय; ताराक्षय

**Corectasia.** See **Corectasis.**

**Corectasis.** Dilatation of the pupil; corectasia; corediastasis. चक्षुपटलविस्फार; ताराविस्फार; नेत्रपटल का फैल जाना

**Corectopia.** A displacement of the pupil. ताराविस्थिति; नेत्रपटल की स्थानच्युति; ताराभ्रंश

**Corediastasis.** See **Corectasis.**

**Coreometry.** Measurement of the pupil. चक्षुपटलमिति; तारामापन

**Coreoplasty.** Connection of a deformed or occluded pupil; coroplasty. तारासंधान; पटलसंधान

**Coria.** Plural of **Corium.**

**Corium.** The derma; the deep layer of the cutis. अन्तस्त्वचा; अन्तर्त्वचा; यथार्थ त्वचा

**Corm.** A bulb-like, solid, fleshy, subterranean stem. घनकन्द

**Corn.** A horny hardness of the skin; clavus. घट्टा; मस्सा; किण

**Cornea.** The transparent coat of front part of the eyeball. स्वच्छमण्डल; कनीनिका; चक्षुपटल; नेत्रपटल

**Corneal.** Pertaining to the cornea. स्वच्छमण्डलीय; चक्षुपटलीय; नेत्रपटलीय; कनीनिका सम्बन्धी;

**C. Graft,** see **Corneoplasty.**

**Corneitis.** See **Cornitis.**

**Corneoplasty.** Plastic operation of cornea; corneal graft. कनीनिकासंधान

**Corneous.** Horny; corneus; corniculata. शृंगी; शृंगाकार; नुकीला

**Corneus.** See **Corneous.**

**Corniculata.** See **Corneous.**

**Corniculate.** Resembling a horn or having horn-shaped appendages. शृंगाभ; शृंगवत्

**Cornification.** The process of making hard or horny. शृंगीभवन; शल्कीभवन; शृंगीकरण

**Cornified.** Made horny. शृंगित; शल्कित

**Cornitis.** Inflammation of the cornea; corneitis. स्वच्छमण्डलशोथ; चक्षुपटलशोथ; कनीनिकाशोथ

**Cornu.** A horn or horn-shaped structure; cornus. शृंग

**Cornua.** Plural of **Cornu.**

**Cornual.** Relating to a cornu. शृंग सम्बन्धी

**Cornus.** See **Cornu.**

**Corolla.** The internal envelope of a stema of a flower. दलपुंज; फूल का अन्दरूनी आवरण

**Corona.** A crown, as of the head. किरीट; शिखर;

   **C. Dentis,** the crown of a tooth. दन्तकिरीट; दन्तशिखर;

   **C. Glandis,** the prominent margin of the glans penis. शिश्नमुण्ड किरीट; लिंगमुण्ड किरीट;

   **C. Radiata,** the fibres radiating from the optic thalamus. अरीय किरीट;

   **C. Veneris,** syphilitic blotches in the head. रति किरीट; उपदंशज किरीट

**Coronal.** Pertaining to a crown. किरीटी; किरीट सम्बन्धी

**Coronarium.** See **Coronary.**

**Coronary.** The blood vessels that nourish the heart structure; coronarium. हृद्धमनी; रक्तवाहिनी;

   **C. Artery,** that which is around the heart and lips. परिहृद्-धमनी;

   **C. Sinus,** a passage of the blood into the right auricle. महाहार्दिकी शिरा; दायें ग्राहक कोष्ठ में रक्त आने का एक पथ;

   **C. Thrombosis,** occlusion of a coronary vessel by a clot of blood. हृद्धमनी-घनास्त्रता

**Coroner.** An officer who holds inquests on those dead from violence. अपमृत्युमीमांसक; आकस्मिक अथवा अपघात-सम्भूत मृत्यु के कारणों की जांच करने वाला अधिकारी

**Coronoid.** Crown-shaped. किरीटाकार; मुण्डाकार

**Coroplasty.** See **Coreoplasty.**

**Corpora.** Plural of **Corpus.**

  **C. Albicantia,** two rounded masses of white matter forming the bulbs of the fornix. श्वेत पिण्ड;

  **C. Quadrigemina,** the optic lobe of the brain. पिण्ड-चतुष्टि

**Corporeal.** Material, as opposed to spiritual. दैहिक; कायिक; शारीरिक; pertaining to a body or to a corpus. शरीर अथवा शव सम्बन्धी

**Corporis.** The body. काय; शरीर; देह; पिण्ड

**Corpse.** A dead body; a cadaver. शव; मृतदेह; मृतकाय; निष्प्राण शरीर

**Corpulence.** See **Corpulency.**

**Corpulency.** Obesity; an unusual development of fat or flesh in proportion to the build of the body; corpulence; corpulense. स्थूलता; स्थूलकायता; मोटापा .

**Corpulense.** See **Corpulency.**

**Corpulent.** Having a superfluity of flesh, or fat; obese. स्थूलकाय; मोटा

**Corpulmonale.** Heart disease following any disease of lung, which strains the right ventricle. फुप्फुसजन्य हृद्रोग; फेफड़े सम्बन्धी किसी रोग के बाद होने वाला हृदय रोग

**Corpus.** The human body. मानवशरीर; शरीर; देह; काय; a body, or mass. पिण्ड;

  **C. Adiposus,** a mass of adipose tissues. वसापिण्ड; वसा-ऊतकों का पिण्ड अथवा झुण्ड;

  **C. Albicans,** two rounded masses of white matter forming the bulbs of the fornix; corpus albicantes. श्वेत पिण्ड;

  **C. Albicantes,** see **Corpus Albicans.**

  **C. Callosum,** hard cerebral substance uniting the cerebral hemisphere of the base. महासंयोजिका; महासंयोजन पिण्ड;

  **C. Cavernosum,** the body of the penis. रक्तधर पिण्ड; सगुह-पिण्ड;

  **C. Delecti,** the dead-body of an injured person. हतव्यक्तिशव; आहत व्यक्ति की मृत देह;

  **C. Luteum,** a small yellow body formed in the ovary within a ruptured follicle. पीत-पिण्ड;

**C. Mammilare,** the mammilary body. चूचुक पिण्ड;

**C. Quadrigemina,** the optic lobes of the brain. चतुष्टय पिण्ड; पिण्ड-चतुष्टि;

**C. Spongiosum Penis,** the spongy body of the penis. स्पंजी पिण्ड;

**C. Striatum,** two grey bodies in the lateral ventricles of the brain. रेखित पिण्ड;

**C. Ventriculi,** body of the stomach; the part of the stomach that lies between the fundus above and the pyloric antrum below. निलय पिण्ड

**Corpuscle.** A minute body. कणिका; क्षुद्र पिण्ड; a cell. कोशिका;

**Blood C.,** the cellular element of the blood. रक्त-कणिका; रक्त का कोशिका-तत्व;

**Genital C.,** special nerve-endings in the external genitalia. जननेन्द्रिय कणिका;

**Nerve C.,** the nerve-cell. तंत्रिका-कोशिका;

**Red C.,** erythrocyte. लोहित कणिका;

**White C.,** any type of leukocyte. श्वेत कणिका

**Corpuscula.** Plural of **Corpusculum.**

**Corpuscular.** Composed of corpuscles. कणिकीय

**Corpusculum.** The same as **Corpuscle.**

**Corrective.** Modifying favourably; corrigent. शोधक; दोषनिवारक

**Correlation.** Interdependence; reciprocal relation. सह-सम्बन्ध; अन्योन्य सम्बन्ध; पारस्परिक सम्बन्ध

**Corrigent.** See **Corrective.**

**Corroborant.** A tonic invigorating remedy. पौष्टिक अथवा बलवर्धक (औषधि)

**Corroding.** Eating away. संक्षारक; तीक्ष्ण; तीखा; तीखी

**Corrosive.** Having the power to eat away or destroy the tissues. संक्षारक; तीक्ष्ण; तीखा; तीखी;

**C. Sublimate,** the bichloride of mercury. कोरोसिव सब्लीमेट; एक पारद विष; रस-कर्पूर

**Corrugation.** Wrinkling. वलि; झुर्री

**Corrugator.** A muscle that wrinkles. संकोचक (पेशी); वलयी (पेशी)

**Cortectomy.** Excision of the cortex of the brain.

मस्तिष्कप्रान्तस्था-उच्छेदन; मस्तिष्कप्रान्तस्था को काट कर हटा देना

**Cortex.** Surface of the brain. प्रान्तस्था; the bark of an exogenous plant. बाह्यस्तर; वल्क; किसी पौधे का बाहरी या ऊपरी छिलका;

**Adrenal C.**, a flattened, roughly triangular body upon the upper end of each kidney. अधिवृक्क प्रान्तस्था;

**Cerebellar C.**, the thin grey surface-layer of the cerebellum. अनुमस्तिष्क प्रान्तस्था;

**Cerebral C.**, the layer of grey matter covering the entire surface of the cerebral hemisphere. मस्तिष्क प्रान्तस्था;

**Renal C.**, the part of the kidney containing the glomeruli and the proximal and distal convoluted tubules. वृक्क प्रान्तस्था

**Cortical.** Concerned with the cortex or surface of the brain. मस्तिष्कप्रान्तस्था सम्बन्धी

**Cortices.** Plural of **Cortex.**

**Corticofugal.** Conducting from the cortex cerebri. मस्तिष्कप्रान्तस्थापवाही

**Corticospinal.** Pertaining to cortex cerebri and spinal cord. मस्तिष्कप्रान्तस्था एवं सुषुम्ना सम्बन्धी

**Cortin.** A hormone from the adrenal cortex which prolongs the life of animals with impaired adrenals. कॉर्टिन

**Cortisis.** The same as **Cortex.**

**Cortisone.** See **Cortizone.**

**Cortizone.** A hormone of the adrenal cortex; cortisone. कॉर्टिजोन; वृक्क-प्रान्तस्था का एक हॉर्मोन

**Coryza.** Catarrhal inflammation of the nose; acute rhinitis. प्रतिश्याय; सर्दी-जुकाम

**Cosmesis.** A concern in therapeutics, especially in surgical operation for the appearance of the patient. अंगरागता; सौंदर्यप्रसाधनता; सौंदर्यवर्धन

**Cosmetic.** A beautifying substance. सौंदर्यप्रसाधक पदार्थ; सौंदर्यवर्धक पदार्थ

**Cosmetitian.** A cosmetic practitioner. सौंदर्यप्रसाधक; शृंगारप्रसाधक; अंगरागविज्ञानी

**Cosmetics.** That which is done to improve the appearance or prevent disfigurement. शृंगारप्रसाधन; the science of beautifying substances. अंगरागविज्ञान

**Costa.** A rib; a border or side of the scapula; costalis. पर्शुका; पसली;

**C. Cervicalis,** cervical rib. ग्रैव पर्शुका; गर्दन की पसली

**Costal.** Relating to a rib. पर्शुका अर्थात् पसली सम्बन्धी;

**Costal.** Relating to a rib. पर्शुका अर्थात् पसली सम्बन्धी;
  **C. Cartilage,** the anterior cartilaginous extremity of a rib. उपपर्शुका; किसी पसली की अगली उपास्थि
**Costalgia.** Neuralgia of the rib. पर्शुकार्ति; पसली का दर्द; pleurodynia. परिफुप्फुस वेदना
**Costalis.** See **Costa.**
**Costectomy.** Excision of a rib. पर्शुका-उच्छेदन
**Costicartilage.** The cartilage lying between the two ribs and sternum. उपपर्शुका; दो पसलियों तथा उरोस्थि के बीच स्थित उपास्थि
**Costive.** Abnormal digestion marked by hardness and retention of the faeces. अवरोधी; मलावरोधी; कब्ज करने वाली
**Costiveness.** Difficulty in having evacuating from the bowels; constipation. मलबद्धता; कोष्ठबद्धता; कब्ज; कब्जियत
**Costocentral.** Relating to a rib and vertebra. पर्शुका और कशेरुका सम्बन्धी
**Costocervical.** Pertaining to a rib and the neck. पर्शुका एवं ग्रीवा सम्बन्धी; पसली तथा गर्दन सम्बन्धी
**Costochondritis.** Inflammation of one or more costal cartilages. पर्शुकोपास्थिशोथ
**Costoinferior.** Pertaining to the lower ribs. अवपर्शुकी; निचली पसलियों सम्बन्धी
**Costosternoplasty.** A plastic operation of the sternum. उरोस्थिसंधान
**Costosuperior.** Pertaining to the upper ribs. अधोपर्शुकी; ऊपरी पसलियों सम्बन्धी
**Costotomy.** Division of a rib. पर्शुकाविच्छेदन
**Costotransversectomy.** Excision of a proximal portion of a rib and the articulating transverse process. पर्शुका-अनुप्रस्थप्रवर्ध-उच्छेदन
**Costovertebral.** Relating to a rib and vertebra. पर्शुका एवं कशेरुका सम्बन्धी
**Cotton.** The seed-hair of many species of **Gossypium.** कपास; रुई
**Cotyledon.** One of the subdivisions of the uterine surfaces of the placenta. दल; अपरादल; बीजपत्र; ग्राहकगुच्छ
**Couching.** An outmoded operation for cataract. काउचिंग
**Cough.** A sudden noisy explosion of air from the lungs through glottis. कास; खाँसी;
  **Whooping C.,** pertussis; barking cough. कूकर-कास; काली-खाँसी
**Count.** An account. गणन
**Countenance.** Complexion; appearance. रूप; आकृति; मुखाकृति
**Counter.** A device that counts. गणक

**Counteraction.** Contrary action. प्रतिकर्म; रोकथाम

**Counterextension.** The opposing traction upon the proximal extremity of a fractured limb to hold the ends in place; countertraction. प्रतिप्रसार

**Counterirritation.** Irritation produced in one part of the body, with a view of lessening that existing in another part. प्रतिक्षोभण

**Counterpoison.** A poison given to counteract another poison. प्रतिविष

**Coutershock.** An electric shock applied to the heart to terminate a disturbance of its rhythm. प्रति-आघात; प्रत्याघात

**Counterstain.** A stain used to bring into contrast parts of tissue coloured by another stain. प्रतिरंजन; प्रतिरंजक

**Countertraction.** See **Counterextension.**

**Coup De Souleil.** Sun-stroke. लू लगना

**Courses.** Menses. आर्तव; ऋतुस्राव; माहवारी

**Cover- glass.** A thin glass plate over the object on a microscopic slide. आवरण-काच; ढक्कन; ढकना

**Cowper's Glands.** Two compound tubular glands situated between two layers of the triangular ligament, anteriorly to the prostate glands. कूपर ग्रन्थियाँ; शिश्नमूल ग्रन्थियाँ

**Cowperitis.** Inflammation of the Cowper's glands. कूपरग्रन्थिशोथ; शिश्नमूल ग्रन्थिशोथ

**Cow-pox.** Virus-disease of the cow. गोमसूरिका; गोशीतला; लघुमसूरिका; छोटी माता

**Coxa.** The hip or hip-joint; femur. नितम्बसन्धि; नितम्ब; ऊरु; कक्षांग;

   **C. Plana,** the normal condition of the hip-joints. समतल नितम्ब;

   **C. Valga,** a deformity in which the angle made by the neck and shaft of the femur is greater than normal. बहिर्नत नितम्ब;

   **C. Vara,** one in which the said angle is less than normal. अन्तर्नत नितम्ब

**Coxae.** Plural of **Coxa.**

**Coxagra.** Sciatica; gout in the hip. गृध्रसी; पृथुस्नायुशूल; नितम्बसन्धि का गठिया

**Coxalgia.** Pain in the hip-joint; coxodynia. नितम्बार्ति; नितम्बसन्धिशूल; श्रोणिपीड़ा; कूल्हे के जोड़ का दर्द

**Coxarius Morbus.** Hip-joint disease. नितम्बसन्धि रोग

**Coxarthritis.** See **Coxitis.**

**Coxitis.** Inflammation of the hip-joint; coxarthritis. नितम्बसन्धिशोथ; नितम्बसन्धि का प्रदाह

**Coxodynia.** See **Coxlagia.**

**Coxotuberculosis.** Tuberculous hip-joint disease. यक्ष्मज नितम्बसन्धिरोग

**Crab.** The thigh. जघन; जांघ; ऊरु;

   **C. Louse,** a louse infesting the genital hair. जघन यूका

**Cradle.** A semicircle of thin wood, or strips of wood and wire. दोला; पालना; झूला

**Cramp.** Sudden and violent contraction of the muscles; spasms. उद्वेष्टन; उद्वेष्ट; ऐंठन; मरोड़; बाँयटा; पेशियों का आकस्मिक एवं प्रबल रूप से सिकुड़ना व दर्द करना;

   **Occupational C.,** spasm of the certain groups of muscles from continuous use in daily occupation. व्यवसायज उद्वेष्ट; व्यावसायिक ऐंठन; दैनिक व्यवसाय के कारण कतिपय पेशी-समूहों का ऐंठ जाना;

   **Piano-player's C.,** spasms caused due to piano-playing. पियानो-वादक उद्वेष्ट; पियानो बजाने के कारण होने वाली अकड़न;

   **Writer's C.,** spasm caused due to constant writing. लिपिक उद्वेष्ट; लेखकों की उँगलियों में बांयटेदार दर्द होना

**Crania.** Plural of **Cranium.**

**Cranial.** Pertaining to the cranium. करोटीय; कपालीय; करोटि सम्बन्धी;

   **C. Nerve,** one of the 12 nerves of the cranium arising directly from the brain and exiting through an opening in the skull. करोटि-तंत्रिका

**Craniectomy.** A partial excision of the skull. कपालोच्छेदन; करोटि-उच्छेन

**Craniocele.** Encephalocele. मस्तिष्कहर्निया

**Craniocerebral.** Relating to the cranium and the brain. करोटि तथा मस्तिष्क सम्बन्धी

**Cranioclast.** An instrument used in cranioclasty. कपालध्वंसी; करोटिध्वंसक यंत्र

**Cranioclasty.** The crushing of the foetal head. कपालध्वंसन; करोटिध्वंसन

**Craniofacial.** Pertaining to the cranium and face. कपालाननीय; कपाल एवं आनन सम्बन्धी

**Craniological.** Relating to the craniology. कपालविज्ञान सम्बन्धी; करोटिविज्ञान सम्बन्धी

**Craniologist.** One versed in craniology. कपालविज्ञानी; करोटिविज्ञानी

**Craniology.** The study of cranium of the skull. कपालविज्ञान; करोटिविज्ञान; खोपड़ी का वैज्ञानिक अध्ययन

**Craniomalacia.** A softening of the skull. करोटिमृदुता; कपालमृदुता; खोपड़ी की कोमलता

**Craniometer.** An instrument for measuring skull. कपालमापी; करोटिमापी

**Craniometry.** The measurement of the skull. करोटिमापन; करोटिमिति; कपालमापन

**Craniopagus.** Twins with adherent heads. बद्धकपालयमल; ऐसे जुड़वे जिनके सिर आपस में मिले रहते हैं

**Craniopathy.** Any disease of the skull. कपालविकृति; खोपड़ी का कोई रोग

**Cranioplasty.** Plastic operation on the skull. कपालसंधानकर्म

**Craniopuncture.** Surgical puncture of the skull. करोटिछिद्रण

**Craniorrhachischisis.** Congenital fissure of the skull and spine. कपालमेरुदण्डविदर; खोपड़ी और रीढ़ का जन्मजात विदर

**Cranioschisis.** Congenital fissure of the cranium. कपालविदर; सहज करोटिविदर; खोपड़ी का आजन्म विदर

**Craniosclerosis.** A hardening of the cranium. कपालकाठिन्य; खोपड़ी की कठोरता

**Craniostenosis.** Stenosis of the skull. कपालसंकीर्णता; खोपड़ी की सिकुड़न

**Craniostosis.** Congenital ossification of the cranial sutures. कालपूर्वकपालसीवनी-अस्थीभवन

**Craniotabes.** Rachitic thinning of the skull. कपालशोष; खोपड़ी की हड्डियों का पतला पड़ना

**Craniotomy.** The excision of a part of the skull. कपाल-उच्छेदन; करोटि-उच्छेदन

**Cranium.** The skull, comprising of the bones which inclose the brain and form the head. कपाल; करोटि; खोपड़ी; मस्तिष्क-कोटर

**Cras.** Tomorrow. कल;

   **C. Mane(CM),** tomorrow morning. कल सुबह; कल प्रात:;

   **C. Nocte (CN),** tomorrow night. कल रात;

   **C. Vespere (CV),** tomorrow evening. कल शाम

**Crasis.** Normal individual condition of the blood. रक्त की सामान्य

दशा; constitution. गठन; temperament. स्वभाव; प्रकृति
**Crassamentum.** A clot, as of blood. थक्का; आतंच
**Crater.** A fossa; a sinus. विवर; गर्त; खात; कोटर
**Crateriform.** Of the form of a sinus. कोटराकार; विवररूप
**Cravat Bandage.** A bandage made from a triangular cloth. त्रिकोण पट्टी; क्रैव पट्टिका
**Craving.** A morbid desire for a thing. ललक; लालसा; उत्कट इच्छा
**Crawling.** See **Creeping.**
**Crazy.** Mad; insane. विक्षिप्त; पागल; उद्भ्रांत
**Creaking.** Making a sharp, harsh, grating sound. चिरमिराहट; चरमराहट
**Cream.** The rich, fatty part of milk. क्रीम; वसायुक्त मलाई; दूध से निकाला जाने वाला स्नेह तथा तैलयुक्त पदार्थ
**Crease.** A line made by folding. ऊर्मिका; शिकन; सिकुड़न; पुटचिन्ह
**Creasote.** See **Creosote.**
**Creeping.** Moving along on the ground or any other surface; crawling. विसर्पण
**Cremation.** Burning of the dead-body. शवदाह; शवदहन-क्रिया
**Crematorium.** A place for burning the dead-bodies. शवदाहगृह
**Crena.** A notch or cleft. विदर; दरार; नासूर
**Crenate.** See **Crenated.**
**Crenated.** Notched; crenate; indented. दन्तुर; दन्तिल
**Crenocyte.** A red blood cell with serrated, notched edges. दन्तुर लालरक्त-कोशिका
**Creosote.** A phenolic antiseptic obtained from beech-wood; creasote; kreosote. क्रियोजोट; एक रासायनिक तेल
**Crepitant.** Crackling; applied to pneumonic rales. करकरी; कर्कर; चरचराती हुई;
C. Rale, fine rubbing noise of air passing through the obstructed tube. कर्कर ध्वनि; चरचराती ध्वनि
**Crepitatio.** See **Crepitation.**
**Crepitation.** A cracking sound heard by the stethoscope in certain affections of the lungs; crepitatio. करकराहट; चरचराहट; पटपटाहट; चटचटाहट
**Crepitus.** The peculiar rattle of pneumonia. करकर (ध्वनि); crepitation. करकराहट; चरचराहट

**Crescent.** Having the shape of a new moon. चन्द्रार्ध; अर्धचन्द्र; नालचन्द्र; नवचन्द्र

**Crescentic.** Shaped like a new moon. अर्धचन्द्राकार; नवचन्द्राकार; नालचन्द्राकार

**Crest.** A ridge, especially on bone, forming its principal border; crista. शिखा; किरीट; शीर्ष; शृंग; शिखर; उभरा हुआ भाग;

  **Ampullary C.**, an elevation on the inner surface of the ampulla of each semicircular duct; crista ampullaris. कलशिका शिखा; कलशिका शिखर;

  **Ethmoidal C.**, see **Crista Ethmoidalis.**

  **Frontal C.**, a ridge along the middle line of the internal surface of the frontal bone; crista frontalis. ललाट शिखा; ललाट शिखर;

  **Iliac C.**, the expanded upper border of the ilium; crista iliaca. श्रोणिफलक शिखा; श्रोणिफलक शिखर;

  **Lacrimal C.**, a vertical ridge dividing the external surface of the lacrimal bone; crista lacrimalis. अश्रु शिखा; अश्रु शिखर;

  **Nasal C.**, one on the internal border of the nasal bone, forming a part of the nasal septum; crista nasalis. नासा शिखा; नासा शिखर;

  **Neural C.**, a ridge found on either side of the neural tube in the embryo. तंत्रिका शिखा; तंत्रिका शिखर;

  **Occipital C.**, a vertical ridge on the external surface of the occipital bone; crista occipitalis. पश्चकपाल शिखा; पश्चकपाल शिखर;

  **Pubic C.**, crest extending from the spine to the inner extremity of the pubis; crista pubica. जघन शिखा; जघन शिखर;

  **Urethral C.**, the crest of the urethra; crista urethralis. मूत्रमार्ग शिखा; मूत्रमार्ग शिखर;

  **Vestibular C.**, a prominence on the floor of the vestibule of the ear; crista vestibuli. प्रघाण शिखा; प्रघाण शिखर

**Creta.** Chalk. खड़िया

**Cretin.** One affected with cretinism. अवटुवामन; बौना

**Cretinism.** A condition of arrested development due to insufficiency of the thyroid gland. अवटुवामनता; जड़वामनता; बौनापन

**Crevice.** A crack or small fissure. क्षुद्रविदर; लघुविदर; लघुरन्ध्र; छोटी-सी दरार

**Cribriform.** Perforated; like a sieve. चालनीरूप; चालनी जैसा छिद्रित;

  **C. Plate,** the upper perforated plate of the ethmoid bone; cribrum. चालनी-पटल

**Cribrose.** Like a sieve. चालनीवत्; चालनी जैसा
**Cribrum.** See **Cribriform Plate.**
**Crick.** Any painful spasmodic affection. अकड़न; ऐंठन; झटका; मरोड़; कोई दर्दनाक तथा ऐंठनयुक्त रोग;
   **C. in the neck,** a spasmodic affection of the muscles of the neck. गर्दन की मरोड़; ग्रीवा-पेशियों का उद्वेष्ट
**Cricoarytenoid.** Pertaining to the cricoid and arytenoid cartilages. मुद्रिकादर्विकी
**Cricoid.** Ring-like; ring-shaped. मुद्रिकाभ; मुद्राकार; छल्ले जैसा;
   **C. Cartilage,** cartilage of the larynx. मुद्रिका-उपास्थि; स्वरयंत्रोपास्थि; स्वरयंत्र की छल्ले जैसी गोल उपास्थि
**Cricoidectomy.** Excision of the cricoid cartilage. मुद्रिकाउपास्थि-उच्छेदन
**Cricothyroid.** Pertaining to the cricoid and the thyroid cartilages. मुद्रिकावटुउपास्थिज; मुद्रिका-उपास्थि एवं अवटु-उपास्थि सम्बन्धी
**Cricotomy.** Any incision into the cricoid cartilage. मुद्रिका-उपास्थिछेदन
**Criminal Malpractice.** See **Criminal Practice.**
**Criminal Practice.** The unlawful production of abortion; criminal malpractice. अवैध गर्भपात; अपराधिक गर्भपात
**Criminology.** The study of crimes. अपराधविज्ञान; अपराधप्रकरण
**Crinogenic.** Causing secretion. स्रावकारी; स्रावजनक; स्रावी
**Crippled.** Handicapped; disabled. अपंग; विकलांग; अशक्त
**Crises.** Plural of **Crisis.**
**Crisis.** The culmination of the symptoms of a disease, either for recovery or death. चरमति; चरमोत्कर्ष; संघर्षपूर्ण; संकटपूर्ण; संकटापन्न स्थिति
**Crista.** A crest, ridge, or elevated line. शिखा; शिखर; चोटी;
   **C. Ampullaris,** see **Ampullary Crest.**
   **C. Collicostae,** a crest on the superior border of the neck of the rib. पर्शुकाग्रीवा शिखा;
   **C. Conchalis,** the inferior turbinated crest of the maxilla and palate bone. शुक्तिका शिखा;
   **C. Ethmoidalis,** the superior turbinated crest of the maxilla and palate-bone; ethmoidal crest. झर्झरिका शिखा; झर्झरिका शिखर;
   **C. Frontalis,** see **Frontal Crest.**
   **C. Galli,** the superior triangular process of the ethmoid bone. शिखंडिका शिखा;

**C. Iliaca**, see **Iliac Crest**.

**C. Lacrimalis**, see **Lacrimal Crest**.

**C. Nasalis**, see **Nasal Crest**.

**C. Occipitalis**, see **Occipital Crest**.

**C. Pubica**, see **Pubic Crest**.

**C. Urethralis**, see **Urethral Crest**.

**C. Vestibuli**, see **Vestibular Crest**.

**Critical.** Pertaining to a crisis; applied especially to days in fevers and to symptoms. संकटापन्न; नाजुक

**Crocated.** Containing saffron. केशरमिश्रित

**Crocus Sativus.** Saffron. केसर; जाफ़रान

**Cross.** Any structure or figure in the shape of a cross; crux. तिर्यक; व्यत्यस; पारगामी; स्वस्ति चिन्ह; क्रूस

**Crossed.** Cross-shaped; applied to alternate sides of the body. विपक्ष; विपरीतांग; व्यत्यस्त

**Crotalus.** The rattle snake, and also its virus. क्रोटेलस; रेंगने वाला सांप और उसका विष

**Crotaphion.** The point at the tip of the great sphenoid wing. जतूकपक्षबिन्दु

**Croton.** A genus of trees furnishing cascarilla and croton oil. जमालगोटा

**Croup.** Laryngeal obstruction due to inflammation of the larynx and trachea, with dyspnoea and membranous deposit. क्रुप; स्वरयंत्र की अवरुद्धता के कारण होने वाली अविराम खाँसी

**Croupous.** Pertaining to croup. क्रुपी; क्रुप सम्बन्धी

**Croupy.** Of the nature of croup. क्रुपी; क्रुपवत्

**Crown.** Corona. शीर्ष; किरीट; शिखर; ऊपरी भाग;

   **Dental C.**, crown of tooth, i.e. the part of tooth above gums. दन्त-शिखर

**Cruces.** Plural of **Crux**.

**Crucial.** Resembling a cross; cross-like. स्वास्तिक; क्रूसाकार

**Cruciate.** Shaped like a cross. स्वास्तिक; resembling a cross. स्वस्ति-चिन्ह से मिलता-जुलता

**Crucible.** A vessel for exposing substances to intense heat. मूषा; कुठाली

**Cruciform.** Shaped like a cross; crucial. स्वास्तिकाकार
**Crude.** In the natural form; raw; unripe. अपरिष्कृत; कच्चा; स्थूल
**Crumpling.** Wrinkling. विवलन; तोड़-मरोड़; झुर्रियां पड़ना
**Cruor.** Coagulated blood. आतंचित रक्त; जमा हुआ खून
**Cruorin.** Haemoglobin. रक्तकणरंजकद्रव्य
**Crura.** Plural of **Crus**.
**Crural.** Pertaining to the crura. पादविषयक; स्तम्भविषयक;
    **C. Cerebri,** the peduncles of the cerebrum. मस्तिष्कस्तम्भ
**Cruris.** The same as **Crus**.
**Crurum.** Foot. पाद; पैर
**Crus.** The leg. टांग; अग्रजंघा; अधोजानु; a leg-like structure. क्रस; टांग जैसी बनावट का
**Crust.** A dried mass of exudate on the skin; a scab. निर्मोक; पपड़ी
    **Milk C.,** see **Crusta Lactea**.
**Crusta.** A crust. निर्मोक; पपड़ी;
    **C. Lactea,** seborrhea of the scalp in infants; milk crust. दुग्ध-निर्मोक; बच्चों की खोपड़ी से होने वाला त्वग्वसास्राव
**Crutch.** A device used singly or in pairs to assist in walking when the act is impaired by transferring weight-bearing to the upper extremity. बैसाखी
**Crux.** See **Cross**.
**Cryaesthesia.** See **Cryesthesia**.
**Cryalgesia.** Pain from the application of cold. शीतवेदना; शीतप्रयोग से दर्द होना
**Cryesthesia.** Abnormal sensitiveness to cold; cryaesthesia. अतिसंवेदनशीलता
**Crymophylactic.** Resistant to cold; cryophylactic. शीतप्रतिरोधी; शीतप्रतिरोधक
**Crymotherapy.** Therapeutic use of cold; cryotherapy. शीतोपचार; शीत-चिकित्सा
**Cryopathy.** A condition in which exposure to cold is an important factor. शीतरुग्णता
**Cryophylactic.** See **Crymophylactic**.
**Cryoscope.** An instrument for the dertermination of the freezing point. हिमांकमापी

**Cryoscopic.** Pertaining to the cryoscopy. हिमांकमापीय; हिमांकमापन सम्बन्धी

**Cryoscopy.** The dertermination of the freezing-point of liquids. हिमांकमापन

**Cryotherapy.** See **Crymotherapy.**

**Crypt.** A small sac or follicle. क्षुद्रनली; क्षुद्रपुटक; a glandular cavity. ग्रन्थि-गह्वर; ग्रन्थिल गह्वर; a pit-like depression or tubular recess. दरी; hidden; occult; secret. गुप्त; प्रच्छन्न

**Cryptamenorrhoea.** See **Cryptomenorrhea.**

**Cryptitis.** Inflammation of the crypt. पुटकशोथ; ग्रन्थिगह्वरशोथ

**Cryptogam.** A flowerless plant. अपुष्पीपादपवर्ग; ऐसे पौधे जिनमें फूल नहीं लगते

**Cryptogamic.** Relating to the flowerless plants. अपुष्पीपादपवर्गीय; अपुष्पीपादपवर्ग सम्बन्धी

**Cryptogenic.** Obscure in origin. प्रच्छन्न; अज्ञातोत्पन्न

**Cryptomenorrhea.** Retention of the menses due to a congenital obstruction, such as an imperforate hymen or atresia of the vagina; cryptamenorrhoea; cryptomenorrhoea. प्रच्छन्नार्तव; प्रच्छन्न-ऋतुस्राव

**Cryptomenorrhoea.** See **Cryptomenorrhea.**

**Cryptomnesia.** Subconscious memory. अर्धचेतनस्मृति

**Cryptorchid.** An individual with undescended testes; cryptorchis. गुप्तवृषण; प्रच्छन्न अण्डग्रन्थि

**Cryptorchidism.** A retention of the testes in the abdomen or the inguinal canal; cryptorchism. गुप्तवृषणता; प्रच्छन्न-अण्डग्रन्थिता

**Cryptorchis.** See **Cryptorchid.**

**Cryptorchism.** See **Cryptorchidism.**

**Crystal.** A regular solid mineral with smooth planes of faeces. रवा; क्रिस्टल; स्फट

**Crystalline.** Like a crystal. क्रिस्टलाभ; मणिभ; स्फटिकाभ; स्फटाभ;
  **C. Lens,** the lens of the eye situated immediately behind the pupil, and surrounded by the ciliary process. स्फट-वीक्ष; स्फट-लेंस

**Crystallization.** The formation of crystals. मणिभीकरण; क्रिस्टलीभवन

**Crystalloid.** Having a crystalline structure. क्रिस्टलाभ; स्फटिकाभ

**Cubeb.** Unripe fruit of piper cubeba. कबाब चीनी
**Cubical.** Pertaining to, or shaped like a cube; cubic. घनीय; घनाकृतिक
**Cubit.** The same as **Cubitus**.
**Cubital.** Pertaining to the forearm. प्रकोष्ठीय; प्रकोष्ठ सम्बन्धी
**Cubiti.** Plural of **Cubitus**.
**Cubitus.** The forearm. भुजा; अग्रबाहु; elbow. कफोणि; कोहनी; ulna. अन्त:प्रकोष्ठिका
**Cuboid.** Like a cube; cuboidal. घनाभ; घनरूप; घनोपम;
   **C. Bone,** a small bone of the foot. घनास्थि
**Cuboidal.** See **Cuboid**.
**Cucumis Sativus.** Cuccumber. ककड़ी; खीरा
**Cuirass Cancer.** A large cancer of the chest. वक्ष कर्कट; छाती का कैंसर
**Cul-de-sac.** A passage without an outlet. अन्ध-घानी; अन्ध-थैली
**Culdoplasty.** A surgical procedure to remedy relaxation of the posterior fornix of the vagina. योनिभित्तिसंधान
**Culdoscope.** An endoscopic instrument used in culdoscopy. योनिभित्तिदर्शी
**Culdoscopy.** Introduction of an endoscope through the posterior vaginal wall to view the rectovaginal pouch and pelvic viscera. योनिभित्तिदर्शन
**Culex.** A genus of mosquitoes. क्यूलेक्स
**Culicide.** An agent that kills mosquitoes. मशकनाशी; मच्छरों को नष्ट करने वाला पदार्थ
**Culicifuge.** An agent to drive away mosquitoes. मशकनिवारक; मच्छरों को नष्ट करने वाला पदार्थ
**Cultivation.** See **Culture**.
**Cultural.** Relating to the culture, as of bacteria. सम्वर्धन सम्बन्धी
**Culture.** The preparation of micro-organism on, or in artificial media of various kinds; cultivation. सम्वर्ध; सम्वर्धन;
   **Pure C.,** culture of a single micro-organism. शुद्ध सम्वर्ध;
   **Tissue C.,** maintenance of live tissue after removal from the body by placing in a vessel with a sterile nutritive medium. ऊतक सम्वर्ध;
   **C. Media,** substances used for cultivating. सम्वर्ध माध्यम
**Cumulative.** Increasing by successive additions. संचयी
**Cuneate.** See **Cuneiform**.

**Cunei.** Plural of **Cuneus.**

**Cuneiform.** Wedge-shaped; cuneate. कीलाकार; फानाकार; नोकदार

**Cuneocuboid.** Pertaining to both cuneiform and cuboid bones. कीलक-घन सम्बन्धी

**Cuneus.** A wedge-shaped convolution in the occipital lobe of the brain. कीलक

**Cunnilinction.** See **Cunnilingus.**

**Cunnilinctus.** See **Cunnilingus.**

**Cunnilingus.** Licking or kissing of the vulva, or clitoris as a type of oral genital sexual activity; cunnilinction; cunnilinctus. योनिचूषण

**Cunnus.** The vulva. भग

**Cup.** A cupping glass. चषक; गर्त; कप; प्याला

**Cupola.** A dome-shaped extremity of the cochlear canal; cupula. कम्बु-शिखर; गुम्बद-छतरी

**Cupping.** Blood-abstraction by means of a cupping glass. चषकन; सींगी द्वारा रक्त निकालना; application of a cupping glass. चषक-प्रयोग

**Cupric.** Pertaining to copper. ताम्र सम्बन्धी

**Cuprum.** Copper; a reddish-brown metal; also called **Cuprum metallicum.** ताम्र; ताम्बा

**Cupula.** See **Cupola.**

**Cupulae.** Plural of **Cupula.**

**Curare.** An extract of poisonous plants. कुरारी; अमरीकी पौधों से प्राप्त होने वाला एक पेशीघातक विष

**Curareform.** Denoting a drug having an action like curare. कुरारीरूप; कुरारीवत्

**Curative.** Tending to restore health. रोगहर; रोगनिवारक; रोगमुक्तिकारक; रोगसाध्य

**Curd.** The coagulum of milk. दधि; दही

**Curdy.** Curd-like. दधिवत्; दही जैसा

**Cure.** Restoration to health. रोगमुक्ति; रोगनिवारण; आरोग्य; a special method or course of treatment. उपचार

**Curet.** A spoon-shaped instrument for scrapping; curette. आखुरी; खुरचनी; घर्षणी; to use a curette. खुरचनी का व्यवहार करना; खुरचना

**Curetage.** See **Curettage.**

**Curettage.** The use of the curet; curetage; curettement. आखुरण करना; खुरचना

**Curette.** See **Curet.**

**Curettement.** See **Curettage.**

**Current.** The passage of a liquid, electricity, etc. प्रवाह; धारा

**Curvature.** Bending; curving. बक्रता; बक्रिमा; आनति; घुमाव; टेढ़ापन; बक्र;

   **C. of spine,** a bending of the axis of the spine due to diseases, or to muscular action. मेरु-बक्रता

**Curve.** A bending. बक्र; टेढ़ापन; बक्रता; आनति; मोड़; घुमाव

   **C. of carus,** the curved pelvis axis. केरस बक्र; गोणिकाक्षि बक्र

**Curvoccipital.** The occipital curve. पश्चकपाल बक्र

**Cushingoid.** Resembling the signs and symptoms of Cushing's disease or syndrome. कुशिंग रोग अथवा कुशिंग संलक्षण से मिलता-जुलता

**Cushion.** Any structure resembling a pad or custion. उपधानी

**Cushing's Disease.** A rare disorder, mainly of females, characterized principally by virilism, obesity, hyperglycaemia, glycosuria and hypertension. कुशिंग रोग

**Cushing's Syndrome.** A disorder clinically similar to Cushing's disease, but commoner, in which excessive hormonal activity of the adrenal cortex is due to intrinsic hyperplasia or tumour of the adrenal cortex. कुशिंग संलक्षण

**Cushion.** Any structure resembling a pad or cusion. उपधानी

**Cusp.** The pointed crown of a teeth. कर्पर्दिका; दन्तशिखर; दन्ताग्र; नोक; शिखर; शीर्ष; सिरा; a leaflet of the heart's valve. हृत्पाटशिखर; हृत्कर्पर्दिका

**Cuspal.** Relating to a cusp. कर्पर्दिकी; कर्पर्दिका सम्बन्धी

**Cuspid.** Furnished with a cusp; cuspidate. नुकीला; नोकदार

**Cuspidate.** See **Cuspid.**

**Custodia Vaginitatis.** The hymen. योनिच्छद

**Cut.** A division of the skin and flesh by a sharp cutting instrument. घाव; क्षत

**Cutaneous.** Belonging to the skin, as a cutaneous disease. त्वचीय; त्वचा सम्बन्धी; चर्म सम्बन्धी

**Cuticle.** Outer skin; epidermis; cuticula. उपत्वचा; उपचर्म; अध:स्त्वक; बाह्यचर्म

**Cuticula.** See **Cuticle.**

**C. Dentis**, the cuticle of a tooth. दन्तचर्म

**Cuticularization.** Cutification or the formation of the skin. चर्मनिर्माण; चर्मोत्पत्ति; त्वक्निर्माण

**Cutification.** The formation of skin. त्वक्निर्माण; चर्मनिर्माण; चर्मोत्पत्ति

**Cutis.** The true skin. त्वक्; त्वचा; चर्म; शरीर का बाह्य-आवरण;
   **A. Anserina,** goose-flesh. लोमत्वगुत्तानता;
   **C. Vera,** the true skin under the epidermis. अन्तःत्वचा; यथार्थ त्वचा

**Cutisector.** An instrument for cutting small pieces of skin for grafting or to remove a section of skin for microscopic examination. त्वगुच्छेदक; क्यूटिसेक्टर

**Cutitis.** Dermatitis. त्वग्शोथ

**C.V.** Cras vespere; tomorrow evening. कल शाम

**Cyanemia.** A blue colour of the blood due to imperfect oxygenation. रक्तश्यावता; खून का नीला पड़ना

**Cyanhidrosis.** Blue sweat. श्यावस्वेद; नीला पसीना

**Cyanoderm.** See **Cyanosis.**

**Cyanopathy.** See **Cyanosis.**

**Cyanopia.** A perverted state of the vision rendering all objects blue; cyanopsia. नीलदृष्टि; नीलवर्णता; प्रत्येक वस्तु नीली दिखाई देना

**Cyanopsia.** See **Cyanopia.**

**Cyanosed.** Affected with cyanosis. श्यावग्रस्त; नीलरोग से पीड़ित

**Cyanosis.** Blue discolouration of the skin from non-oxidation of the blood; cyanoderm; cyanopathy. श्यावता; नीलरोग; नीलिमा; नील-पाण्डु

**Cyanotic.** Pertaining to cyanosis. श्यावता अथवा नीलरोग सम्बन्धी

**Cyath.** Abbreviated form of **Cyathus.**

**Cyathus.** A glassfull. गिलास भर;
   **C. Amplus,** a big glassfull; cyathus magnus. बड़ा गिलास भर;
   **C. Magnus,** see **Cyathus Amplus.**
   **C. Medicus,** a medium glassfull. मझला गिलास भर
   **C. Vinarius,** a small glassfull; cyathus vinosus. छोटा गिलास भर;
   **C. Vinosus,** see **Cyathus Vinarius.**

**Cycle.** A regular series of movements or events. चक्र; आवर्तन;
   **Cardiac C.,** the process or complete round of diastole and systole. हृद्-चक्र;

**Menstrual C.**, the periodically recurring series of changes in breasts, ovaries and uterus culminating in menstruation. आर्तवचक्र; ऋतुचक्र

**Cyclectomy.** See **Ciliectomy.**

**Cyclic.** See **Cyclical.**

**Cyclical.** Occurring in cycles; cyclic. चक्रिल; चक्रिक; चक्रीय;

**C. Syndrome,** used for premenstrual symptom-complex. चक्रिल संलक्षण;

**C. Vomiting,** periodic attacks of vomiting. चक्रिल वमन

**Cyclicotomy.** See **Cyclotomy.**

**Cyclitis.** Inflammation of the ciliary body of the eye. रोमकपिण्डशोथ; पलकों का प्रदाह

**Cyclodialysis.** Detachment of the ciliary body from the sclera. रोमकपिण्डविलयन

**Cyclodiathermy.** Destruction by diathermy of the ciliary body. रोमकपिण्डनाशन

**Cyclokeratitis.** Inflammation of both the ciliary body and the cornea. रोकमपिण्डकनीनिकाशोथ; रोमकपिण्ड तथा कनीनिका का प्रदाह

**Cyclopia.** Fusion of the orbits; synophthalmia; synopsia. मध्यनेत्रता

**Cycloplegia.** Paralysis of the ciliary muscles. रोमकपेशीघात; चक्षुपटलों का पक्षाघात

**Cycloplegics.** Drugs which cause paralysis of the ciliary muscles. रोमकपेशीघातक औषधियाँ

**Cyclothemia.** A tendency to alternating mood swings between elation and depression; cyclothymia. चक्रविक्षिप्ति; उत्तेजनाविषाद

**Cyclothymia.** See **Cyclothemia.**

**Cyclotomy.** Cutting the ciliary muscle; cyclicotomy. रोमकपेशी-उच्छेदन

**Cyema.** The product of conception. गर्भ भ्रूण

**Cyemology.** Embryology. भ्रूणविज्ञान

**Cyesis.** Pregnancy. सगर्भता; गर्भावस्था; गर्भ

**Cyetic.** Relating to pregnancy. सगर्भता अथवा गर्भ सम्बन्धी

**Cylinder.** A hollow, tube-shaped body. सिलिंडर

**Cylindric.** See **Cylindrical.**

**Cylindrical.** Having the form of a cylinder; cylindric. बेलनाकार

**Cylindroadenoma.** See **Cylindroma.**

**Cylindroma.** A tumour composed of cylindric hyaline processes; cylindroadenoma. बेलनार्बुद

**Cylindruria.** Presence of renal casts in the urine. निर्मोकमूत्रता; निर्मोकमेह

**Cynanche.** An inflammatory disease of the throat. गलशोथ; कण्ठशोथ;
   **C. Parotidia,** mumps. कनफेड़; कर्णमूलग्रन्थिशोथ; कर्णपूर्वग्रन्थिशोथ;
   **C. Tonsillaris,** quinsy. गलतुण्डिकाशोथ;
   **C. Trachealis,** croup. क्रुप

**Cynic.** Relating to a dog. श्वान सम्बन्धी

**Cynophobia.** Morbid dread of dogs. श्वानातंक; कुत्तों का भय

**Cyophoria.** The period of pregnancy. गर्भकाल

**Cypriphobia.** A morbid fear of coitus. रतिभीति; संगमभीति

**Cyst.** A bag or membranous sac containing matter or other fluids. पुटक; पुटी; पुटिका; कोशिका; bladder. आशय; मूत्राशय;
   **Bartholin's C.,** a cyst arising from the major vestibular gland or its ducts. बार्थोलिन पुटी;
   **Blood C.,** a cyst containing blood; haemorrhagic cyst; haematocyst; haematocele. रक्त पुटी;
   **Branchial C.,** one resulting from the incomplete closure of a branchial cleft. गिल पुटी;
   **Daughter C.,** one developed by secondary growth from the walls of a large one. अपत्य पुटी;
   **Dentigerous C.,** one containing teeth. दन्तधर पुटी;
   **Dermoid C.,** a congenital cyst containing bone, hair, teeth, etc. त्वग्-पुटी;
   **Extravasation C.,** one formed by the encapsulation of a haemorrhage into the tissue. परिस्रवण पुटी;
   **Follicular C.,** one due to the occlusion of the duct of a small follicle or gland. कूपिक पुटी (या पुटक); पुटकीय पुटी;
   **Haemorrhagic C.,** see **Blood Cyst.**
   **Mucous C.,** a retention cyst containing mucus. श्लेष्म पुटी;
   **Ovarian C.,** a cystic tumour of the ovary. डिम्ब पुटी;
   **Parasitic C.,** a cyst formed by the larva of a parasite. परजीवी पुटिका; परजीवीपुटी; परजीवीपुटक;
   **Pilar C.,** see **Sebaceous Cyst.**

**Sebaceous C.,** a retention cyst of a sebaceous gland; pilar cyst. वसा-पुटी

**Cystadenoma.** Adenoma of the bladder; a cystic adenoma. पुटीग्रन्थि-अर्बुद; पुटीग्रन्थ्यर्बुद

**Cystalgia.** Pain in the bladder. पुटीशूल; वस्तिशूल; मूत्राशयशूल

**Cystaptosis.** A rupture of the bladder. मूत्राशयस्त्रंस; मूत्राशय का फटना

**Cystatrophia.** Atrophy of the bladder. मूत्राशयशोष; मूत्राशय का सूखना

**Cystectasia.** Dilatation of the bladder; cystectasis; cystectasy. मूत्राशयविस्फार; मूत्राशय का फैलना

**Cystectasis.** See **Cystectasia.**

**Cystectasy.** See **Cystectasia.**

**Cystectomy.** Excision of the cystic duct, or removal of a duct. पुटी-उच्छेदन; वस्ति-उच्छेदन; मूत्राशय-उच्छेदन

**Cystelcosis.** Ulceration of the bladder. मूत्राशय-व्रणता

**Cystic.** Pertaining to a cyst or bladder. पुटीय; मूत्राशयी; मूत्राशयिक; containing cysts. पुटीयुक्त

**Cystiform.** Of the form of a cyst; cystoid. पुटीरूप

**Cystirrhagia.** Haemorrhage from the bladder. मूत्राशयरक्तता; मूत्राशय से रक्तस्राव होना

**Cystirrhea.** See **Cystirrhoea.**

**Cystirrhoea.** Catarrh of the bladder; cystirrhea. मूत्राशय-प्रतिश्याय;

   **C. Cystica,** a cystic inflammation of the bladder. पुटीमूत्राशयशोथ;

   **C. Glandularis,** a glandular inflammation of the bladder. ग्रन्थिल मूत्राशयशोथ

**Cystis.** A cyst. पुटी

**Cystitis.** Inflammation of the urinary bladder. मूत्राशयशोथ; मूत्राशय का प्रदाह

**Cystitome.** See **Cystotome.**

**Cystitomy.** See **Cystotomy.**

**Cystocele.** Hernia or rupture of the urinary bladder; colpocystocele; vesicocele. मूत्राशय-हर्निया

**Cystodynia.** Pain in the bladder. मूत्राशयशूल; मूत्राशय-पीड़ा

**Cystoenterocele.** A hernia of the urinary bladder and the intestine. मूत्राशय-आंत्रहर्निया

**Cystogram.** An x-ray film demonstrating the urinary bladder.

वस्तिचित्र; मूत्राशयचित्र

**Cystography.** Radiographic examination of the urinary bladder, after it has been rendered radio-opaque. मूत्राशयचित्रण; वस्तिचित्रण

**Cystoid.** A tumour resembling a cyst; cystiform; cystomorphous; bladder-like. पुटीवत्; पुटी जैसा; आशयाभ; आशयवत्

**Cystolith.** A urinary or vesical calculus. मूत्राशय-अश्मरी; मूत्र-पथरी

**Cystolithectomy.** See **Cystolithotomy.**

**Cystolithiasis.** The formation of a stone in the bladder. मूत्राशय अश्मरता

**Cystolithotomy.** Removal of stone from the bladder; cystolithectomy. मूत्रपथरी-उच्छेदन

**Cystoma.** A tumour containing cysts. पुटी-अर्बुद

**Cystometer.** A device for studying bladder function by measuring capacity, sensation, intravesical pressure and residual urine. मूत्राशयदाबमापी

**Cystometrography.** See **Cystometry.**

**Cystometry.** The study of pressure changes wihtin the urinary bladder; cystometrogaphy. मूत्राशयदाबमिति

**Cystomorphous.** See **Cystoid.**

**Cystoparalysis.** See **Cystoplegia.**

**Cystopexia.** See **Cystopexy.**

**Cystopexy.** Suspension of the bladder; cystopexia. मूत्राशय स्थिरीकरण

**Cystoplasm.** The living material of the cell external to the nucleus. कोशरस; कोशिकासार; कोशिकाद्रव्य

**Cystoplasty.** Surgical repair of the bladder. मूत्राशयसंधान

**Cystoplegia.** Paralysis of the bladder; cystoparalysis. मूत्राशयघात; मूत्राशय का पक्षाघात

**Cystopyelitis.** Inflammation of both the bladder and the pelvis of the kidney. मूत्राशयवृक्कगोणिकाशोथ

**Cystorrhagia.** Haemorrhage from the bladder. मूत्राशयरक्तता; मूत्राशय से रक्तस्राव होना

**Cystorrhaphy.** Suture of a wound or defect of the urinary bladder. मूत्राशयसीवन

**Cystorrhea.** Catarrh of the bladder; cystorrhoea. मूत्राशय प्रतिश्याय

**Cystorrhoea.** See **Cystorrhea.**

**Cystoscope.** An instrument for examining interior of the bladder. मूत्राशयदर्शी

**Cystoscopy.** Examination of the interior of the bladder. मूत्राशयदर्शन

**Cystospasm.** Spasm of the bladder. मूत्राशयोद्वेष्ट; मूत्राशय की ऐंठन

**Cystotome.** A knife used in cystotomy; cystitome; capsulotome. मूत्राशयछेदक

**Cystotomy.** An incision of the bladder; cystitomy; capsulotomy; vesicotomy. मूत्राशयछेदन; मूत्राशयछिद्रीकरण;

  **Suprapubic C.**, opening into the bladder through an incision above the symphysis pubis; epicystotomy. अधिजघन मूत्राशयछिद्रीकरण

**Cystourethritis.** Inflamation of the urinary bladder and the urethra. वस्तिमूत्रमार्गशोथ; मूत्राशय तथा मूत्रमार्ग का प्रदाह

**Cystourethrogram.** An x-ray film demonstrating the urinary bladder and urethra. मूत्राशयपथचित्र; वस्तिमूत्रमार्गचित्र

**Cystourethrography.** Radiographic examination of the urinary bladder and urethra, after they have been rendered radio-opaque. मूत्राशयपथचित्रण; वस्तिमूत्रमार्गचित्रण

**Cystourethropexy.** Forward fixation of the bladder and upper urethra in an attempt to combat incontinence of urine. वस्तिमूत्रपथ-स्थिरीकरण

**Cystourethroscope.** An instrument for examining the interior of urinary bladder and urethra. वस्तिमूत्रपथदर्शी

**Cystourethroscopy.** Examination of the interior of the urinary bladder and urethra. वस्तिमूत्रपथदर्शन

**Cytoblast.** The cellular strands of the trophoblast. कोशिकाप्रसू

**Cytocidal.** Causing the death of cell. कोशिकामारक; कोशिकाघाती

**Cytocide.** An agent that is destructive to cell. कोशिकानाशक

**Cytodiagnosis.** The microscopic study of the cellular elements in fluids as an aid in diagnosis. कोशिकानिदान

**Cytogenesis.** The development of cells. कोशिकाजनन

**Cytogenetics.** Laboratory examination of a person's chromosomes by culture technique, using either lymphocytes or a piece of tissue, such as skin. कोशिकानुवंशिकी; कोशिकाजननप्रकरण

**Cytogenous.** Cell forming. कोशिका-निर्माण

**Cytoid.** Resembling a cell. कोशिकाभ; कोशिकोपम

**Cytologic.** See **Cytological.**

**Cytological.** Pertaining to cytology; cytologic. कोशिकीय; कोशिका सम्बन्धी

**Cytologist.** A specialist in cytology. कोशिकाविज्ञानवेत्ता

**Cytology.** The science of cell-formation and cell-life. कोशिका-प्रकरण; कोशिकाविज्ञान

**Cytolysin.** A substance produced in the body through the injection of foriegn cells of any kind. कोशिकालायिका

**Cytolysis.** Cell-disintegration. कोशिकालयन; कोशिका-विघटन

**Cytoma.** A cell-tumour. कोशिकार्बुद

**Cytometer.** An instrument for counting cells. कोशिकामापी

**Cytometry.** Counting of the cells with the help of a cytometer. कोशिकामिति

**Cytopathic.** Pertaining to the diseased condition of a cell. कोशिकाविकृति सम्बन्धी

**Cytopathogenic.** Pertaining to an agent or substance that causes a diseased condition in cells. कोशिकाविकृतिजनक

**Cytopathologic.** See **Cytopathological.**

**Cytopathological.** Relating to cytopathologic. कोशिकाविकृतिविज्ञान सम्बन्धी

**Cytopathologist.** A physician skilled in cytopathology. कोशिकाविकृतिविज्ञानी

**Cytopathology.** The science concerned with studies and diagnosis of health and disease by microscopic examination and evaluation of cellular specimen. कोशिकाविकृतिविज्ञान

**Cytophagous.** Destructive of cells. कोशिकानाशी; कोशिकाओं को नष्ट करने वाला

**Cytoplasm.** The living material of the cell external to the nucleus. कोशिकाद्रव्य

**Cytospasm.** Spasm of the bladder. मूत्राशय-आकर्ष; मूत्राशय-उद्वेष्ट

**Cytotoxic.** Any substance which is toxic to cells. कोशिकाविषी; कोशिकाओं को विषाक्त करने वाला पदार्थ

**Cytotrophoblast.** The inner layer of the trophoblast. कोशिकापोषकप्रसू

**Cytula.** The impregnated ovum. अनुप्राणित बिम्बाणु; निषिक्त डिम्ब

# D

**D. Symbol for Decimal.** दशमलव के चिन्ह के रूप में प्रयुक्त किया जाने वाला वर्ण

**Dacosta's Syndrome.** A syndrome of functional, nervous and circulatory disorders marked by increased susceptibility to fatigue, palpitation of heart, dyspnoea, rapid pulse, precordial pain and anxiety; cardiac neurosis. हृदक्षिप्रता; डाकोस्टा संलक्षण

**Dacrocyst.** See **Dacryocyst.**

**Dacrocystectomy.** See **Dacryocystectomy.**

**Dacrocystitis.** See **Dacryocystitis.**

**Dacrocystography.** See **Dacryocystography.**

**Dacryadenalgia.** Pain in the lacrimal gland; dacryoadenalgia. अश्रुग्रन्थिशूल; अश्रुग्रन्थ्यार्ति; अश्रुग्रन्थि में पीड़ा

**Dacryadenitis.** See **Dacryoadenitis.**

**Dacryagog.** See **Dacryagogue.**

**Dacryagogue.** An agent causing a flow of tears; dacryagog. अश्रु-उत्पादी; अश्रुजन्य पदार्थ; आँसू उत्पन्न करने वाला पदार्थ

**Dacryoadenalgia.** See **Dacryadenalgia.**

**Dacryoadenitis.** Inflammation of a lacrimal gland; dacryadenitis. अश्रुग्रन्थिशोथ; अश्रुकोश का प्रदाह

**Dacryocyst.** The lacrimal sac; dacrocyst. अश्रुकोश; आँसू की थैली; अश्रुनली

**Dacryocystalgia.** Pain in the lacrimal sac. अश्रुकोशार्ति; अश्रुनली का दर्द

**Dacryocystectomy.** Excision of any part of the lacrimal sac; dacrocystectomy. अश्रुकोशोच्छेदन; अश्रुकोश-उच्छेदन

**Dacryocystitis.** Inflammation of the lacrimal sac; dacrocystitis. अश्रुकोशशोथ; अश्रुकोश का प्रदाह

**Dacryocystography.** Radiographic examination of the tear drainage; dacrocystography. अश्रुकोशचित्रण

**Dacryocystorhinostomy.** An operation to establish drainage from the lacrimal sac into the nose when there is obstruction of the nasolacrimal duct. अश्रुकोशनासायोजीछिद्रीकरण; अश्रुनली तथा नाक की निकास नली को जोड़ने के लिये किया जाने वाला ऑपरेशन

**Dacryocystotomy.** Incision of the lacrimal sac. अश्रुकोशछेदन

**Dacryolith.** The lacrimal calculus; a concretion in the lacrimal passage. अश्रुकोशाश्मरी; अश्रुकोश की पथरी

**Dacryolithiasis.** The formation of lacrimal calculi. अश्रुकोशाश्मरता; अश्रुकोश में पथरी बनना

**Dacryoma.** A tumour of the lacrimal apparatus. अश्रुकोशार्बुद; a cyst formed by accumulation of tears in an obstructed duct. अश्रुकोशपुटिका

**Dacryon.** The point of the junction of the frontal, lacrimal and superior maxillary bones; dakryon. अश्रुकोण; अश्रुपीठास्थिबिन्दु

**Dacryops.** Excess of tears in the eye. अतिअश्रुता; अत्यधिक अश्रुपात होना

**Dacryopyorrhea.** Discharge of tears containing pus; dacryopyorhoea. पूतिअश्रुता; पीबयुक्त आँसू बहना

**Dacryopyorrhoea.** See **Dacryopyorrhea**.

**Dacryosolenitis.** Inflammation of a lacrimal or nasal duct. अश्रुकोश अथवा नासाकोश का प्रदाह; अश्रुकोशशोथ; नासाकोशशोथ

**Dacryostenosis.** Stricture of a lacrimal or nasal duct. अश्रुकोशसंकीर्णता अथवा नासाकोशसंकीर्णता

**Dactyl.** A digit, finger or toe; dactyle. अंगुलि; उँगली

**Dactylar.** Relating to a digit, finger or toe. आंगुलिक; उँगली सम्बन्धी

**Dactylate.** Like a digit, finger or toe. अंगुलिसम; अंगुलिवत्; उँगली जैसा

**Dactyle.** See **Dactyl**.

**Dactyli.** Plural of **Dactylus**.

**Dactylic.** Of the form of a digit, finger or toe. अंगुल्याकार; उँगली जैसी आकृति का

**Dactylion.** Webbed finger. जालित उँगली

**Dactylitis.** Inflammation of a digit, finger or toe. अंगुलिशोथ; उँगली का प्रदाह

**Dactylogryposis.** Contraction of the fingers. अंगुलिसंकीर्णन

**Dactylogy.** The finger-sign method of communication with deaf and dumb people. अंगुलिइंगितविद्या; अंगुलिसंकेतविज्ञान

**Dactyloscope.** An instrument for performing dactyloscopy. अंगुलिवीक्षक; अंगुलिदर्शी

**Dactyloscopy.** Classifying and identifying finger prints. अंगुलिवीक्षिकी; अंगुलिदर्शन

**Dactylose.** Of the form of a finger or toe. अंगुलिरूप; उँगली जैसे आकार का

**Dactylus.** Digit; digitus; finger. अंगुलि; उँगली

**Daft.** Insane. उन्मत्त; विक्षिप्त; सनकी; पागल

**Dakryon.** See **Dacryon.**

**Daltonism.** Colour blindness. वर्णान्धता; रंग पहचानने की अयोग्यता

**Damage.** Loss. क्षति; हानि; नुकसान

**Damp.** Moist. आर्द्र; नम

**Danders.** The skin particles of animals which may cause allergy when breathed. उत्सर्ग; निर्मोक; पपड़ियाँ

**Dandruff.** Cast of cells from the outer layers of skin mainly noted in the scalp. रूसी; फास; खौस; बालों की जड़ों तथा त्वचा पर जमने वाली पपड़ी

**Dandy Fever.** Dengue. दण्डक-ज्वर; अस्थिभंजक-ज्वर; हड्डीतोड़ बुखार; डेंगू

**Danielssen's Disease.** Hansen's disease; leprosy. कुष्ठ; कोढ़

**Dartos.** A contractile fibrous layer which corrugates the scrotum; tunica dartos. वृषणकोशकला; अण्डकोश की झिल्ली;

**Tunica D.,** see **Dartos.**

**Dartre.** Herpes. परिसर्प

**Darwinian.** Relating to, or described by Charles Darwin. डार्विनवाद सम्बन्धी अथवा चार्ल्स डार्विन द्वारा वर्णित

**Darwinism.** The theory of descent by evolution. डार्विनता; डार्विनवाद

**Datura Stramonium.** Jamestown weed; Jimson weed; the seeds and leaves are narcotic and antispasmodic. काला धतूरा

**Daturism.** Stramonium-poisoning. धतूरात्यय; धतूरा-विषण्णता

**Day Blindness.** Subnormal vision in the day-light. दिवसान्धता; दिनान्धता; दिवान्धता; दिनौंधी; दिन में न दिखाई देना

**Debrisoquine.** Hypotensive agent. रक्तदाबवर्धक पदार्थ अथवा औषधि; डेब्रिसोक्विन

**Dead.** Deprived of life. मृत; निष्प्राण; मरा हुआ

**Deaf.** One who does not possess the quality of hearing. बधिर; बहरा;

**D.-mutism,** deafness, with loss of speech. बधिर-मूकता; बहरेपन के साथ गूंगापन

**Deafness.** Loss of hearing. बधिरता; बहरापन;

**Conductive D.,** hearing loss due to inability of the ear to transmit sounds to the nerves ending in the inner ear. चालनरोधी बधिरता;

**Nerve D.**, inability of the hearing nerves to transmit sound stimuli to the brain. तंत्रिका बधिरता;

**Word D.**, inability to recognize or understand the sound heard. शब्द बधिरता

**Death.** Extinction or cessation of life. मृत्यु; मौत; स्वर्गवास; जीवन के समस्त लक्षणों का लोप होना;

**D. Rate,** the number of deaths per 100 unit of population or other frame of reference. मृत्यु-दर;

**D. Rattle,** the gurgling in the throat of a moribund person. मृत्यु-घर्घर; कण्ठ की मृत्युकालीन घर्घराहट

**Debilitant.** An agent allaying excitement; weakening. उत्तेजनाहर; दुर्बलकारी; दुर्बल करने वाला; कमजोरी लाने वाली या वाला

**Debilitated.** Weak. दुर्बल; कमजोर

**Debilitating.** Weakening; causing weakness. दुर्बलकारी; कमजोरी लाने वाली

**Debility.** Weakness. दुर्बलता; कमजोरी; prostration. अवसाद; अवसन्नता

**Debouchee.** Visciously sexual person. व्यसनी; कामुक; दुराचारी; व्यभिचारी

**Debouchery.** Habitual lewdness. व्यसन; कामुकता; दुराचार; व्यभिचार

**Debridement.** Enlarging a wound in operating and removing the damaged or infected tissue. क्षतशोधन; घाव का शोधन

**Debt.** That which is owed; a liability to be rendered. ऋण; कर्ज; कर्जा

**Decalcification.** Removal of calcareous matter from the bones. विकैल्सीभवनं; विकैल्सीकरण; हड्डियों से कैल्सियम पदार्थ निकाल देना

**Decalcifying.** That which causes decalcification. विकैल्सीकारक

**Decalvant.** Destroying hair. केशनाशक; रोमनाशक; लोमनाशक; बालों को नष्ट करने वाला

**Decameter.** Ten meters or 32.8 feet. डेकामीटर; दस मीटर अथवा ३२.८ फीट

**Decannulation.** A term currently in use for the introduction of decreasingly smaller tubes to wean an infant from reliance on the original tracheostomy tube. नलिकानिष्कासन

**Decantation.** The operation for removing the supernatant fluid from a sediment. निस्तारण करना; नितारना; नियारना

**Decapitation.** Surgical removal of head or a capsule. शीर्षोच्छेदन; सम्पुट-उच्छेदन

**Decay.** To deteriorate. क्षय; नष्ट होना

**Decayed.** Deteriorated; putrified. दूषित; नष्ट; गला-सड़ा

**Decaying.** Deteriorating. विनाशशील; गलने-सड़ने लगना

**Decentering.** Removal from a centre; decentration. विकेन्द्रण; केन्द्र से हटाना

**Decentration.** See **Decentering.**

**Decerebrate.** Without cerebral function; a state of deep unconsciousness. विप्रमस्तिष्क; गहन निश्चेतना; मस्तिष्क-क्रिया से हीन

**Decerebration.** The removal of the brain. विप्रमस्तिष्कन; प्रमस्तिष्कवियोजन

**Decidua.** The altered mucous membrane of the pregnant uterus, forming an envelope of the foetus. पतनिका; पत्या; आँवल; गर्भाशय की पतनशील झिल्ली जो प्रसव के साथ निकल जाती है;

  **D. Basalis,** that part which lies under the embedded ovum and forms the maternal part of the placenta; decidua scrotina. आधार पतनिका;

  **D. Capsularis,** the part that lies over the developing ovum; decidua reflexa. सम्पुट पतनिका;

  **D. Menstrualis,** the succulent mucous membrane of the non-pregnant uterus at the menstrual period. आर्तव पतनिका;

  **D. Parietalis,** see **Decidua Vera.**

  **D. Reflexa,** see **Decidua Capsularis.**

  **D. Scrotina,** see **Decidua Basalis.**

  **D. Vera,** the decidua lining the rest of the uterus; decidua parietalis. यथार्थ पतनिका

**Deciduitis.** Inflammation of the decidual membrane of the gravid uterus. पतनिकाशोथ; गर्भाशय की पतनिका कला का प्रदाह

**Deciduic.** Plural of **Deciduous.**

**Deciduoma.** The intrauterine tumour containing decidual relics. पतनिकार्बुद; अन्तर्जरायु-अर्बुद, जिसमें पतनिका के भग्नावशेष मिले रहते हैं;

  **D. Malignum,** chorionepithelioma, i.e. very malignant neoplasm, usually of uterus. दुर्दम पतनिकार्बुद

**Deciduous.** Shedding; not permanent. पाती; अचिर; पतनशील;

  **D. Teeth,** the twenty baby teeth. पाती दन्त; अचिर दन्त; दूध के २० दान्त

**Decimal.** In the proportion of 1 : 10. दशमलव; १ और १० के अनुपात में

**Decimus.** One-tenth of any measurement. दशमांश; दसवाँ भाग

**Decipara.** A woman pregnant for the tenth time. दशमगर्भा; दसवीं बार गर्भवती होने वाली स्त्री

**Decline.** That period of a disorder or paroxysm when the symptoms begin to abate; a gradual decrease or wasting away. अपक्षय प्रावस्था; रोगोपशमन; रोगह्रास; उतार

**Declivus Cerebelli.** The sloping posterior aspect of the monticulus. अनुमस्तिष्कनतांश

**Decoction.** The act or process of boiling; decoctum. क्वाथ; काढ़ा

**Decoctum.** See **Decoction.**

**Decoloration.** See **Decolouration.**

**Decolorization.** see **Decolouration.**

**Decolouration.** The removing of colour; decoloration; decolorization. विवर्णीभवन; विवर्णीकरण; निर्वर्णीकरण; निर्वर्णीभवन

**Decompensation.** A failure of compensation. क्षति-अपूर्ति; क्षतिपूर्ति न कर सकना

**Decompose.** To dissolve a compound into its component parts; to disintegrate. विघटन करना; अपघटन करना; to decay. नष्ट होना

**Decomposed.** Decayed; putrified. विघटित; अपघटित; गला-सड़ा

**Decomposition.** Putrefaction. विघटन; अपघटन; पूतीभवन; analysis of the body. शरीर-विश्लेषण

**Decompression.** Removal of pressure or a compressing force. विसम्पीडन; दाबरहित करना या अधिक दबाव को कम करना

**Decongestant.** A drug that reduces tissue swelling; decongestive. विसंकुलक; रक्ताधिक्यहारी; ऊतकों की सूजन कम करने वाली औषधि

**Decongestion.** Relief of congestion. विसंकुलन; रक्ताधिक्यहरण

**Decongestive.** See **Decongestant.**

**Decortication.** Surgical removal of the cortex or outer covering of an organ. प्रान्तस्था-उच्छेदन; प्रान्तस्थाहरण; प्रान्तस्था अथवा किसी अंग के आवरण को शल्य-क्रिया द्वारा हटा देना

**Decrement.** The decrease or proportion in which anything is lessened. न्यूनता; कमी; अल्पता

**Decubital.** Relating to a bed-sore, or to decubitus. शय्याक्षत अथवा क्षैतिज-स्थिति सम्बन्धी

**Decubitus.** The recumbent position; lying down. क्षैतिज-स्थिति; a bed-sore. शय्याक्षत

**Decurrent.** Running or extending downward. अधोवर्धी; निम्नाभिमुखी

**Decussate.** To intersect; to interlace; to cross. काटना; crossed like the arms of an X. क्रासित

**Decussatio.** A decussation. व्यत्यास

**Decussation.** Intersection; chiasma; crossing of nerve fibres at a point beyond their origin, as in the optic and pyramidal tracts. व्यत्यास; व्यत्यासिका

**Decussationes.** Plural of **Decussation.**

**Dedentition.** The shedding of the teeth. दन्तोत्पाटन; दान्तों का गिरना

**Deep.** Neither superficial nor near the surface; profundus. गभीर; गहरा

**Deerfly Fever.** See **Tularaemia.**

**Defaecate.** To perform defaecation; defecate. मलोत्सर्जन करना; मलत्याग करना; पाखाना करना

**Defaecation.** Stool alvine evacuation; voiding of faeces per anum; defecation. मलोत्सर्जन; मलोत्सर्ग; मलविसर्जन; पाखाना करना

**Defecate.** See **Defaecate.**

**Defecation.** See **Defaecation.**

**Defect.** Deformity; an imperfection. दोष; विकार; अपूर्णता; त्रुटि

**Defective.** Deformed; imperfect. सदोष; दोषपूर्ण; विकारयुक्त; त्रुटिपूर्ण; अपूर्ण

**Defense.** Resistance to disease. रोग-प्रतिरोध; to protect one from any harm or injury. रक्षा करना

**Deferent.** Carrying away. प्रवाही; वाहक;

**D. Duct,** vas deferens. प्रवाहीनली; वाहकनली; केन्द्र से परे ले जाने वाली नली

**Deferentectomy.** Excision of segment of the vas deferens; vasectomy. प्रवाहीनली-खण्डोच्छेदन

**Deferential.** Relating to the deferent duct. प्रवाहीनली सम्बन्धी

**Deferentitis.** Inflammation of the deferent duct. प्रवाहीनलीशोथ; वाहकनली का प्रदाह

**Defervescence.** Decrease or abatement of a fever. तापाभाव; ज्वरमोक्ष

**Defibrillation.** The arrest of fibrillation of the cardiac muscle and restoration of normal cycle. तन्तुविकम्पहरण

**Defibrillator.** Any agent, e.g. an electric shock, which arrests ventricular fibrillation and restores normal rhythm. वितन्तुविकम्प्नित्र

**Defibrination.** Removal of fibrin from the blood. फाइब्रिनहरण; रक्त से फाइब्रिन हटा देना

**Deficiency.** Defect. दोष; त्रुटि; an imperfection. अपूर्णता; decrease. हीनता; कमी; न्यूनता; अल्पता;

    **D. Disease,** disease resulting from dietary deficiency or any substance essential for good health, especially the vitamins. हीनताजन्यरोग; खान-पान की कमी के कारण होने वाला रोग

**Deficient.** Below par. हीन; अपूर्ण; त्रुटियुक्त; त्रुटिपूर्ण

**Definitive.** Limiting the extent; final. निश्चित; मुख्य; अन्तिम

**Deflagration.** A rapid explosive combustion. उद्दहन

**Deflection.** Bending from a straight course; deviation. विपथन

**Defloration.** The act of depriving of virginity. बलात्कार; कौमार्यभंग; शीलभंग

**Deflovium Capillorum.** Alopecia; baldness. खल्वाटता; खालित्य; गंजापन

**Defluxio.** Diarrhoea. अतिसार; प्रवाहिका; दस्त

**Defluxion.** Catarrh. प्रतिश्याय; सर्दी-जुकाम; congestion. रक्तसंलयन; रक्तसंकुलन; रक्तसंचय

**Deformans.** The disfiguring agents. विरूपक; विद्रूपक

**Deformation.** See **Deformity.**

**Deforming.** Disfiguring. विरूपण; विद्रूपण

**Deformity.** Physical malformation or distortion; deformation. विरूपता; विरूपांगता; रचना-विकार

**Defunction.** Inactivity. अक्रिया; क्रियाहीनता; निष्क्रियता

**Degeneration.** Deterioration in structure of a tissue or organ. अपजनन; व्यपजनन;

    Adipose D., see **Fatty Degeneration.**

    Cystic D., degeneration with cyst formation. पुटीय व्यपजनन;

    Fatty D., the conversion of an organ into oil; adipose degeneration. वसापजनन; वसाव्यपजनन;

    Glossy D., see **Hyaline Degeneration.**

    Hyaline D., the disorganised tissue becomes shining and translucent; glossy degeneration. काचाभ व्यपजनन; काचाभ अपजनन;

**Waxy D.,** infiltration of amyloid between cells and fibres of tissues and organs. मोमी अपजनन

**Degenerative.** Relating to, or marked by degeneration. अपजननात्मक; अपजनन सम्बन्धी

**Deglutination.** See **Deglutition.**

**Deglutition.** The act or power of swallowing; deglutination. निगरण; निगलना; गले से नीचे उतारना

**Degradation.** The change of a chemical compound into a less complex compound. अध:पतन

**Degree.** Position in a graded series. वर्गस्थिति; an interval in thermometric scale. अंश; a title conferred by a University. उपाधि

**Dehiscence.** The formation of a fissure. विदरण; विदलनशीलता; स्फुटन; चटकना

**Dehydration.** Loss or removal of fluid. निर्जलीकरण; निर्जलीभवन; निर्जलन

**Dejecta.** Evacuation; faeces. बिष्ठा; मल; विसर्जित पदार्थ

**Dejection.** Despondency. खिन्नता; उदासी; निराशा; depression. हताशा; discharge of faecal matter. मलोत्सर्जन; मलविसर्जन; मलत्याग

**Delacrimation.** Excessive secretion of tears. अतिअश्रुता; प्रचुर अश्रुपात होना

**Delactation.** The act of weaning. अस्तन्यता; दूध छुड़ाना; स्तनपान छुड़ाना

**Deleterious.** Injurious; noxious; harmful. हानिकारक; हानिकर; हानिप्रद; नुकसानदायक

**Deliquescent.** Capable of absorption, thus becoming fluid. प्रस्वेदी; अवशोष्य; अवशोषण के योग्य

**Deliriant.** An agent causing delirium. प्रलापक; प्रलापकारी; प्रलापजनक

**Delirious.** Affected with delirium. प्रलापी; प्रलापग्रस्त

**Deliritous.** A condition in which the patient has confused ideas of past and present circumstances. भ्रमित; उद्भ्रान्त

**Delirium.** A condition of mental confusion and excitement, marked by defective perception and belief in non-existence circumstances, usually with illusions and hallucinations. प्रलाप; चित्तविपर्यय; उन्माद;

**D. Tremens,** the horrors; mania a potu; delirium due to alcoholism. कम्पोन्माद; अधिक मदिरा पीने के कारण होने वाला प्रलाप

**Delivery.** Child-birth; parturition. प्रसव; प्रसूति; बच्चा जनना;

**Forceps D.,** assisted birth of child by an instrument designed to grasp the head of the child. संदंश प्रसव; फोर्सेप डिलिवरी;

**Postmortem D.,** extraction of the foetus after the death of the mother. मरणोत्तर प्रसव;

**Premature D.,** birth of a foetus before its proper time. कालपूर्व प्रसव; अकाल प्रसव

**Deltoid.** Delta-shaped. त्रिकोणीय; त्रिकोणिका; डेल्टाकार;

**D. Muscle,** the triangular muscle of the shoulder. त्रिकोणिका पेशी; कंधे की त्रिकोणक पेशी

**Delusion.** A false belief which cannot be altered by argument or reasoning. विभ्रम; भ्रान्ति; मिथ्याभ्रम; भ्रम

**Delusional.** Relating to delusion; of the nature of a delusion. भ्रान्तिमय

**Demarcation.** A term applied to medicines which have a softening or nullifying effect; an outlining of the junction of the diseased and healthy tissue. सीमानिर्धारण; औषध-सीमानिर्धारण

**Dement.** An insane person. उन्मत्त; विक्षिप्त; पागल

**Dementia.** Insanity; idiocy; mental decay; acatalepsy; irreversible organic deterioration of mental faculties. उन्माद; विक्षिप्ति; पागलपन; मनोभ्रंश;

**D. Neonatorum,** the infantile mental decay; infantile dementia. शिशु-मनोभ्रंश; शिशुओं के मानसिक गुणों का ह्रास;

**D. Paralytica,** general paralysis of the insane; paralytic dementia. पागल का व्यापक अंगघात;

**D. Praecox,** any one of the group of psychotic disorders known as the schizophrenia; dementia precox. कालपूर्व मनोभ्रंश; अन्तराबंध मनोभ्रंश;

**D. Precox,** see **Dementia Praecox.**

**D. Presenilis,** dementia developing before old age; presenile dementia. जरापूर्व मनोभ्रंश;

**Infantile D.,** see **Dementia Neonatorum.**

**Paralytic D.,** see **Dementia Paralytica.**

**Presenile D.,** see **Dementia Presenilis.**

**Demilune.** Semilunar. अर्धचन्द्राकार; नवचन्द्राकार

**Demineralization.** A loss or decrease of mineral constituents of the body or individual tissues, especially of bone. विखनिजीकरण

**Demography. Social science, including vital statistics. जनपदविज्ञान्; जनसांख्यिकी

**Demonomania.** A kind of madness in which the patient fancies himself a devil. स्वप्रेतानुभूति; स्वप्रेतोन्माद; स्वयं को भूत-प्रेत महसूस करने का पागलपन

**Demonophobia.** Morbid dread of the devil. प्रेतभीति; भूत-प्रेत का भय; प्रेतातंक

**Demonstrator.** An assistanr or subordinate teacher. संसाधक; प्रदर्शक

**Demulcent.** See **Demulscent.**

**Demulscent.** Soothing; allaying the irritation; demulcent. प्रशामक; उपशामक; शामक; स्निग्धकारक; तापहर औषधि

**Denatured.** Made unnatural or changed from the normal in any of its charateristics. विकृत

**Dendriform.** Tree-shaped; dendroid. वृक्षिकाभ; वृक्षाकार; पेड़ की आकृति का

**Dendrite.** Fibre extending from the nerve cell (neuron), other than the axon; dendron. पार्श्वतन्तु; वृक्षिका

**Dendritic.** Tree-like. वृक्षवत्; पेड़ जैसा

**Dendroid.** See **Dendriform.**

**Dendron.** See **Dendrite.**

**Denervate.** To cut off the nerve supply of a part by incision, excision or local anaesthesia. वितंत्रीकरण करना

**Denervation.** The means by which a nerve supply is cut off. वितंत्रिकीकरण; वितंत्रीकरण; वितंत्रीभवन; वितंत्रिकीभवन; निस्तेजन

**Dengue.** Break-bone fever; dandy fever; a zymotic disease. डेंगू; अस्थिभंजक ज्वर; हड्डीतोड़ बुख़ार

**Dens.** A tooth. दन्त; दान्त

**Densimeter.** An instrument for determining densities; densiometer. घनत्वमापी; घनत्वमापकयंत्र

**Densimetry.** Determination of densities; densiometry. घनत्वमापन; घनत्वमिति

**Densiometer.** See **Densimeter.**

**Densiometry.** See **Densimetry.**

**Density.** Compactness of a substance. घनत्व; घनता; ठोसपन; दृढ़ता

**Dentagra.** Toothache. दन्तशूल; दन्तवेदना; दान्त का दर्द

**Dental.** Pertaining to the teeth. दन्तज; दान्तों सम्बन्धी;
    **D. Arch,** the arch of the alveolar process. दन्त-चाप;
    **D. Bulb,** the dental papilla. दन्त-कन्द;
    **D. Caries,** decaying of the teeth. दन्त-क्षरण; दन्त-क्षय;
    **D. Papilla,** dental pulp. दन्त-अंकुरक; दन्तांकुर; दन्त-मज्जा;
    **D. Pulp,** the inner substance of a tooth, including the nerve. दन्त-मज्जा; दन्त-अंकुरक
**Dentalgia.** Neuralgia of the teeth. दन्तार्ति; दन्तशूल; दान्तों का दर्द
**Dentate.** Toothed; notched; cogged. दन्तुर; दन्ती; दन्ताल
**Dentes Canini.** The cuspid or canine teeth. भेदक दन्त; कूकर दन्त
**Dentes Deciduii.** Deciduous, or mild teeth. दुग्ध-दन्त; दूध के दांत
**Dentes Sapiantiae.** Wisdom teeth; the third molar teeth. तृत्तीय चर्वणक दन्त
**Denticle.** A small tooth or projection. दन्तिका; क्षुद्रदन्त; छोटा-सा दान्त या सदृश प्रवर्धन
**Denticulate.** Furnished with minute teeth. दन्तिकी
**Dentifrice.** A preparation useful in cleaning the teeth. दन्तमंजन
**Dentigerous.** Bearing teeth. दन्तधर; arising from a teeth. दन्तजनित; दन्तोत्पादित
**Dentilabial.** Relating to the teeth and lips. दन्तोष्ठीय; दान्तों तथा होंठों सम्बन्धी
**Dentilingual.** Relating to the teeth and the tongue. दन्तजिह्वीय; दान्तों तथा जीभ सम्बन्धी
**Dentin.** The bony structure of the teeth; dentine; dentinum. दन्तधातु; दान्तों को बनाने वाला एक कठोर पदार्थ-विशेष
**Dentinal.** Pertaining to dentin. दन्तधात्विक; दन्तधातु सम्बन्धी
**Dentine.** See **Dentin.**
**Dentinification.** The formation of dentin. दन्तधातुरचना
**Dentinitis.** Inflammation of the dentinal tubules. दन्तधातुशोथ; दन्तधातु का प्रदाह
**Dentinogenesis.** The process of dentin formation in the development of teeth. दन्तधातुजनन; दन्तुरजनन
**Dentinoid.** Resembling dentin. दन्तुराभ; दन्तधातु जैसा
**Dentinum.** See **Dentin.**

**Dentiparous.** Teeth-bearing. दन्तधारक

**Dentist.** A dental surgeon. दन्तचिकित्सक; दान्तों का डाक्टर

**Dentistry.** The science of dental surgery. दन्तचिकित्साविज्ञान

**Dentition.** The cutting off of the teeth; teething. दन्तोद्गम; दन्तोद्भवन; दन्तोद्भेदन

**Dentoid.** Tooth-like; resembling or shaped like a tooth. दन्ताभ; दान्त जैसा

**Dentrition.** The wearing or wasting of a part. अंगक्षय; अंगदौर्बल्य

**Denture.** A set of artificial teeth. कृत्रिमदन्तावली; नकली दान्त

**Denudation.** Laying any part bare. नग्नांग; किसी भाग को नंगा करना

**Denutrition.** A want of nutrition. पोषणाभाव; कुपोषण

**Deodorant.** Preparation which masks or diminishes any unpleasant odour; a deodorizer. गन्धहर; दुर्गन्धहर; गन्धहारक; निर्गन्धकारक; दुर्गन्ध दूर करने वाला पदार्थ

**Deodorise.** To remove foul odours; to free from odour. दुर्गन्ध दूर करना; निर्गन्धीकरण करना; बदबू हटाना

**Deodorizer.** See **Deodorant.**

**Deoxidation.** The driving off of oxygen from any substance; deoxidization. विजारण; ऑक्सीजनहरण-क्रिया

**Deoxidization.** see **Deoxidation.**

**Deoxidizer.** A deodorizing substance; deoxydizer. विउपचायक; विजारक

**Deoxigenation.** The removal of oxygen; deoxygenation. ऑक्सीजनहरण

**Deoxydizer.** See **Deoxidizer.**

**Deoxygenation.** See **Deoxigenation.**

**Depancreatisation.** Removal of the pancreas. अग्न्याशयहरण; क्लोमग्रन्थि हटाना

**Dependence.** The quality or condition of lacking independence by relying upon, being influenced by a person or object reflecting a particular need. पराश्रयता; पराश्रित रहना; दूसरे पर निर्भर रहना; आश्रितता; निर्भरता

**Dependent.** One who relies on another for support or favour. आश्रित; पराश्रित

**Depersonalisation.** A state in which a person loses the feeling of his own identity in relation to others in his family. अवैयक्तिकीकरण

**Dephlegmation.** Concentration by distillation. आंशिक संघनन; प्रभाजी आसवन

**Depigmentation.** Loss of partial or complete pigmentation. विरंजनता; विवर्णकता

**Depilate.** To remove the hair. विलोमन करना; लोमशातन करना; बाल हटाना या काटना

**Depilation.** Removal or loss of hair. लोमशातन; बाल झड़ना

**Depilatory.** An agent which removes the hair; epilatory. लोमशातक; केशहर; लोमनाशक; रोमनाशक

**Depilous.** Without hair. लोमहीन; रोमहीन; केशहीन

**Deplete.** To reduce; to lessen; to empty. आरेचन करना; रिक्त करना

**Depletion.** Diminution of a fluid of the body, as the blood. निःशेषण

**Depolarisation.** See **Depolarization.**

**Depolarization.** A destruction of polarity; depolarisation. विध्रुवण

**Deposit.** A sediment; a collection of morbid particles in a body. तलछट; मवाद; निक्षेप

**Depravation.** A depraved condition or morbid change. विकार; दोष

**Depraved.** Perverted; deteriorated; viciated. विकृत; दूषित

**Depressant.** An agent diminishing functional activity. अवसादक; क्रियात्मक शक्ति घटाने वाला पदार्थ

**Depressed.** Flattened from above. अवनमित; अवनत; दबा हुआ; dejected. निराश; हताश

**Depression.** A mental state of deep sadness and self-accusation beyond the normal reaction to grief or other adverse circumstances; a depressed condition. अवदाब; अवसाद; अवनमन; उदासी; ग्लानि; हताशा; a hollow or fossa. गर्त; खात;

  **Agitated D.**, depression with excitement and restlessness. सोद्वेग अवसाद;

  **Reactive D.**, a psychotic state occasioned directly by an intensely sad external situation. प्रतिक्रियात्मक अवसाद

**Depressor.** A muscle or an instrument that depresses. अवदाबी; अवसादी; अवनमनी; विपर्यय; अधःकर्षक; दबाने वाला; डेपरेशर

**Deprival.** See **Deprivation.**

**Deprivation.** Absence or loss; deprival; deprivement. अभाव; कमी

**Deprivement.** See **Deprivation.**

**Depth.** Distance from the surface downward. गहराई

**Depurant.** See **Depurative.**

**Depuration.** Purification; a cleansing process. विशोधन; शोधन; शुद्धीकरण की एक प्रक्रिया

**Depurative.** Cleansing; removing impurities; depurant. विशोधक; शोधक

**Depurator.** A drug or device for aiding a cleansing process. स्वच्छकारी; साफ करने वाला

**Deradenitis.** Inflammation of the cervical glands. ग्रीवाग्रन्थिशोथ; गर्दन की गिल्टियों का प्रदाह

**Derangement.** Disorder, especially of intellect; insanity. विपर्यय; अपविन्यास; दोष; गड़बड़, विशेष रूप से मानसिक

**Derbyshire Neck.** Goitre; bronchocele. गलगण्ड; घेंघा

**Derealisation.** Feelings of unreality, such as occur to normal people during dream. अयथार्थ अनुभूति

**Derivant.** See **Derivative.**

**Derivative.** Counter-irritant; repulsive remedy; derivant. प्रत्युत्तेजक औषधि

**Derm.** The true skin; derma; dermis. त्वचा; त्वक्; उपत्वचा; बाहरी खाल के नीचे वाला अस्तर

**Derma.** See **Derm.**

**Dermal.** Pertaining to the skin; dermatic; dermic. त्वचीय; त्वचा सम्बन्धी;
  **D. Armour,** covering of the skin. त्वचावरण; त्वगावरण; त्वकावरण; त्वचा का आवरण

**Dermalaxia.** Morbid softening of the skin. त्वग्मृदुता; चर्ममृदुता; त्वचा की असाधारण कोमलता

**Dermalgia.** Neuralgia of the skin; dermatodynia. त्वकार्ति; त्वचार्ति; त्वक्शूल; त्वक्-पीड़ा

**Dermatergosis.** Any occupational disease of the skin. व्यावसायिक त्वग्विकार

**Dermatic.** See **Dermal.**

**Dermatitis.** Inflammation of the skin; dermitis. त्वक्शोथ; त्वचा का प्रदाह

**Dermatodynia.** See **Dermalgia.**

**Dermatoglyphics.** Study of rigid patterns of the skin of the fingertips, palms and soles to discover developmental anomalies.

चर्मरेखाशास्त्र; अंगुलिचिन्ह-विद्या; अंगुलिचिन्ह-विज्ञान
**Dermatography.** A description of the skin. चर्मलेख; त्वक्लेख
**Dermatoid.** See Dermoid.
**Dermatologist.** One who is skilled in the diseases of the skin. त्वचाविज्ञानी; चर्मरोगविशेषज्ञ; चर्मरोगविज्ञानी
**Dermatology.** The science which deals with the skin, its structure, functions, diseases and their treatment. त्वचाविज्ञान; चर्मरोगविज्ञान
**Dermatolysis.** Loosening of the skin or atrophy of the skin by disease. त्वग्लयन
**Dermatoma.** A tumour of the skin. चर्मार्बुद; त्वचार्बुद; चमड़ी की रसौली
**Dermatome.** An instrument for cutting slices of the skin of varying thickness, usually for grafting. त्वक्-उच्छेदक; चर्म-उच्छेदक
**Dermatomegaly.** A congenital defect in which the skin hangs in folds. अतिचर्मता
**Dermatomycosis.** Fungal infection of the skin; ringworm. चर्मकवकता; त्वक्कवकता; त्वचाकवकता; त्वचाकवकरोग; दद्रु
**Dermatomyoma.** Myoma involving the skin. त्वक्पेशी-अर्बुद
**Dermatomyositis.** An acute inflammation of the skin and muscles which presents with oedema and muscular weakness. त्वक्पेशीशोथ; त्वग्पेशी-प्रदाह
**Dermatoneurosis.** Any cutaneous eruption due to emotional stimuli. त्वग्विक्षति
**Dermatonosus.** Any disease of the skin. चर्मरोग; त्वग्विकृति
**Dermatopathic.** Relating to the diseases of the skin. त्वग्विकृतिक; चर्मरोग सम्बन्धी
**Dermatopathology.** Histopathology of skin lesions; any disease of the skin. चर्मरोगविज्ञान; त्वग्विकृतिविज्ञान
**Dermatopathy.** Any disease of the skin; dermopathy. त्वग्विकृति; चर्मरोग
**Dermatophytes.** A group of the fungi which invades the superficial skin. त्वक्विकारीकवक
**Dermatoplastic.** Relating to dermatoplasty. चर्मसंधान सम्बन्धी
**Dermatoplasty.** Any plastic operation on the skin; dermoplasty. चर्मसंधान; त्वक्संधान
**Dermatorrhagia.** Hamorrhage from or into the skin. त्वग्रक्तस्राव; त्वचा से अथवा त्वचा के अन्दर होने वाला रक्तस्राव

**Dermatorrhea.** See **Dermatorrhoea.**

**Dematorrhoea.** An excessive secretion from the sebaceous or sweat glands of the skin; dermatorrhea. अतित्वग्स्राव; वसा या स्वेद ग्रन्थियों से अत्यधिक स्राव होना

**Dermatosis.** Generic term for skin disease. त्वग्रोग; त्वग्रुग्णता; त्वग्विकार

**Dermatrophia.** Atrophy of the skin. चर्मक्षय; त्वक्क्षय; त्वक्शोष

**Dermic.** Pertaining to the skin; dermal. त्वक्परक; त्वचा सम्बन्धी;

**D. Graft,** the skin-graft. त्वग्रोपण

**Dermis.** Derma; cutis vera; the true skin; corium. त्वचा; त्वक्; यथार्थ त्वचा; अन्तस्त्वचा; चमड़ी की बाहरी झिल्ली के नीचे का अस्तर

**Dermitis.** See **Dermatitis.**

**Dermoblast.** One of the mesodermal cells from which the corium is developed. त्वग्प्रसू

**Dermoid.** Resembling or pertaining to the skin; dermatoid. त्वचाभ; त्वग्वत्; त्वचा सम्बन्धी;

**D. Cyst,** dermatoid tumour. त्वग्बुद; त्वग्पुटी

**Dermoidectomy.** Surgical removal of the dermoid cyst. त्वग्पुटी-उच्छेदन

**Dermolipoma.** The fatty tumour of the skin. त्वग्वसार्बुद; चमड़ी की चर्बीमय रसौली

**Dermomycosis.** A skin disease from the fungi; dermatomycosis. कवकचर्मता; त्वक्कवकता

**Dermopathy.** see **Dermatopathy.**

**Dermoplasty.** see **Dermatoplasty.**

**Dermorrhagia.** Haemorrhage from the skin. त्वग्रक्तस्राव; त्वचा से खून बहना

**Dermostenosis.** Constriction of the skin. त्वक्संकीर्णन; त्वचा का सिकुड़ना

**Desanimania.** Amentia; dementia. बुद्धिह्रास; मनोभ्रंश; उन्माद

**Desaturation.** The act or the result of making something less completely saturated. विसंतृप्तीकरण

**Descending.** Proceeding downward. अवरोही

**Descensus.** Descent; a falling. भ्रंश; च्युति;

**D. Uteri,** falling of the womb. जरायुभ्रंश; गर्भाशयभ्रंश; गर्भाशयच्युति

**Descent.** In obstetrics, the passage of the presenting part of the foetus into and through the birth canal. अवरोहण; descensus; a falling. भ्रंश; च्युति

**Desensitization.** The act of removing an emotional complex or abolition of allergic sensitivity or reactions to the specific allergen. विसुग्राहीकरण

**Desiccant.** The drying agent; desiccative. शोषक; अवशोषक; सुखाने वाला पदार्थ

**Desiccate.** To dry absolutely; to render free from moisture. शुष्क करना; सुखाना

**Desiccation.** The process of drying. शुष्कन; निर्जलीकरण; सुखाना

**Desiccative.** See **Desiccant.**

**Desmalgia.** Pain in the ligament. स्नायुशूल; बन्धार्ति

**Desmitis.** Inflammation of a ligament. स्नायुशोथ; स्नायुप्रदाह; बन्धशोथ

**Desmoid.** Resembling a bundle. सौत्रिक; गट्ठर जैसा;

**D. Tumour,** a hard fibrous tumour. सौत्रिकार्बुद; तन्तु-अर्बुद; तन्त्वर्बुद; तान्तवार्बुद;

**Desmopathy.** Any disease of the ligaments. स्नायुविकृति; स्नायुविकार; बन्धविकार

**Desmosis.** Any disease of the connective tissue. संयोजीऊतकविकृति; संयोजी ऊतक का कोई रोग

**Despondency.** Dejection. हताशा; उदासी; नैराश्य; निराशा

**Desquamation.** Scaling off or separation of the outlayer of the skin called epidermis, in small scales. विशल्कन; खाल उतरना

**Destructive.** Having a tendency to destroy. विनाशकारी

**Desudation.** Profuse or morbid sweating. स्वेदाधिक्य; पसीने की अधिकता

**Detachment.** The act of separating or detaching. वियोजन; विलगन; अलग करना

**Detection.** The results of the application of a chemical test. पद्धति; निरूपण; अभिज्ञान; खोज

**Detergent.** A cleaning or purging agent; cleansing. अपमार्जक; शोधक; विरेचक

**Deterioration.** Progressive destruction, as of the tissues of the body. क्रमिकविनाश; अवनति; अपकर्ष; बिगाड़

**Determination.** Direction to a part or an organ. दिशानिर्धारण; निर्धारण;

**D. of blood,** excessive flow of blood to a part. रक्त-निर्धारण

**Detonation.** An explosive combustion. विस्फोटन; विस्फोट; धमाका; धड़ाका

**Detoxication.** The process of removing the poisonous property of

a substance; detoxification. निर्विषीकरण; अविषीकरण; विषहीन करना
**Detoxification.** See **Detoxication.**
**Detrition.** A wearing away of a part by use of friction. अपरदन
**Detritus.** Matter produced by detrition; waste matter from disintegration. अपरद; कंकड़
**Detrusor.** The muscle of the urinary bladder. निस्सारिका (पेशी); मूत्राशयपेशी;

   **D. Urinae,** the longitudinal muscle-fibre of the bladder; detrusor vesicae. मूत्रनिस्सारिका;

   **D. Vesicae,** see **Detrusor Urinae.**

**Dettol.** A non-caustic antiseptic agent. डेटॉल
**Detumescence.** Subsidence of a swelling. विफुल्लता
**Deuteranomalopia.** Partial green-blindness; deuteranomaly. आंशिकहरितान्धता; आंशिकहरितवर्णान्धता
**Deuteranomaly.** See **Deuteranomalopia.**
**Deuteranopia.** A defect in second constituent essential for colour vision, as in green-blindness. हरितवर्णान्धता; हरा रंग पहचानने की अक्षमता अथवा अयोग्यता
**Deuteroplasm.** See **Deutoplasm.**
**Deutoplasm.** A store of nutrient material in the ovum, from which the embryo draws to support its growth; deuteroplasm. पोषक उपद्रव्य
**Devascularization.** Occlusion of all or most of the blood vessels to any part or organ. निर्वाहिकाकरण; निर्वाहिकाभवन
**Development.** Growth; advancement; progression towards maturity. विकास; परिवर्धन; वर्धन; बृद्धि; उन्नति
**Developmental.** Evolutionary. परिवर्धनकारी; परिवर्धनीय
**Deviance.** See **Deviation.**
**Deviation.** A turning aside from the normal; deflection; deviance. विचलन; विपथन
**Device.** A design; any means, usually of a specific function. युक्ति; साधन
**Devil's Dung.** Asafoetida. हींग
**Devitalize.** To destroy vitality. अशक्त बनाना; जीवनीशक्ति को नष्ट करना
**Devitalized.** Devoid of life; dead. मृत; निष्प्राण

**Devolution.** The reverse of evolution, प्रतिविकास; degeneration. अपजनन; व्यपजनन; अवक्रमण

**Devonshire Colic.** Lead-poisoning. सीसाविष; सीसाविषण्णता; सीसजविषण्णता; सीसजविषाक्तता

**Dew-point.** The temperature at which the dew forms. ओसांक

**Dexter.** Right; upon the right side. दक्षिण; दक्षिणवर्त; दायाँ

**Dextrad.** Pertaining to, or toward the right side; dextral. दक्षिणवर्ती; दायीं ओर; दाहिनी तरफ

**Dextral.** See **Dextrad.**

**Dextrality.** Right-handedness. दक्षिणहस्तता

**Dextrocardia.** Transposition of the heart to the right side of the thorax. दक्षिण-हृदयता

**Dextrocular.** Right-eyed. दक्षिणाक्षिक; दाईं आँख का; दाईं आँख वाला; relating to right eye. दाईं आँख सम्बन्धी

**Dextropedal.** Right-footed. दक्षिणपाद; दायें पैर का; दायें पैर वाला; relating to right foot. दायें पैर सम्बन्धी

**Dextrose.** A sugar of glucose group. द्रक्षौज; द्राक्ष-शर्करा

**Dextroversion.** A turning to the right. दक्षिणवर्तन

**Dhobie-itch.** A skin disease transmitted by clothing; tinea cruris. वंक्षण-दद्रु; धोबियों को होने वाला चर्म रोग

**Diabetes.** A disease characterized by excessive flow of urine called polyuria; without qualification it means **Diabetes Mellitus, Diabetes Innocens** or **Renal Glycosuria.** बहुमूत्र; मूत्रमेह;

**D. Insipidus,** polyuria; the chronic excretion of very large amounts of pale urine of low specific gravity, accompanied by extreme thirst. उदकमेह; मूत्रमेह; बहुमूत्ररोग;

**D. Mellitus,** an excessive flow of urine containing sugar. मधुमेह

**Diabetic.** Pertaining to diabetes. मधुमेहज; मधुमेह सम्बन्धी; a person afflicted with diabetes. मधुमेहग्रस्त (रोगी)

**Diabetogenic.** Causing diabetes; diabetogenous. मधुमेहजनक

**Diabetogenous.** See **Diabetogenic.**

**Diabrotic.** A corrosive. तीक्ष्ण; संक्षारक; दाहक

**Diacele.** The third cavity of the brain. तृतीय मस्तिष्क-गह्वर

**Diachorema.** Excrement; faeces. स्राव; मल; बिष्ठा

**Diachoresis.** Defecation. मलविसर्जन; मलोत्सर्जन; मलोत्सरण

**Diacid.** Having an acidity of two. द्विआम्लिक; द्विअम्लज

**Diaclasia.** Breaking of bone before removing a limb or amputation; diaclasis. अस्थिभंजन, जो किसी अंग की चीर-फाड़ से पहले किया जाता है

**Diaclasis.** See **Diaclasia.**

**Diaclast.** An instrument for breaking up the foetal head. भ्रूणशीर्षभंजक; डायाक्लास्ट

**Diad.** See **Dyad.**

**Diadochokinesia.** The normal power of alternately bringing a limb into opposite position; diadokinesis. शीघ्रपर्यायगति

**Diadochokinesis.** See **Diadochokinesia.**

**Diagnose.** To determine the nature of the disease. निदान करना

**Diagnosis.** The act of distinguishing diseases by symptoms. निदान; रोगनिदान; रोगनिर्णय;

**Differential D.**, arriving at a correct decision between presenting a similar clinical picture. सापेक्ष निदान; विभेदक रोगनिदान

**Diagnost.** See **Diagnostician.**

**Diagnostic.** Pertaining to diagnosis, serving as evidence in diagnosis. नैदानिक; निदानकारी

**Diagnostician.** One skilled in diagnosing; diagnost. निदानज्ञ; निदानकर्ता

**Diagram.** A figure giving the outlines or general plan of an object. आरेख; चित्र; डायाग्राम

**Diagraph.** An apparatus for recording the outlines of crania. आकारलेखी

**Dialysate.** Any product taken from a solution by dialysis. अपोहित; विलगित

**Dialyser.** An instrument for performing dialysis; dialyzer. अपोहक; अपोहन यंत्र

**Dialysis.** A separation of parts in general; the separation of crystalline from colloid substances by means of a porous diaphragm. अपोहन; विलगन; a loss of strength. शक्तिक्षय; अशक्तता;

**Peritoneal D.**, a method of irrigating the peritoneum. पर्युदर्या अपोहन

**Dialyzer.** See **Dialyser.**

**Diamagnetic.** Repelled by the magnet. प्रतिचुम्बकीय

**Diameter.** A straight line passing through the centre of a body or figure. व्यास

**Diapedesis.** The passage of blood cells through the vessel walls into the tissues. कोशिकापारण; रक्तवाहिनियों की भित्तियों से श्वेताणुओं का पारगमन

**Diaper.** Underwear. पोतड़ा; कच्छा; कच्छी

**Diaphanoscope.** The instrument used in diaphanoscopy. पारप्रदीपक; पारप्रदीपन के निमित्त प्रयुक्त किया जाने वाला यंत्र

**Diaphanoscopy.** Examining body cavities by electric light. पारप्रदीपन

**Diaphanous.** Transmitting light. पारभासी

**Diaphoresis.** Perspiration; sweating. स्वेदलता; स्वेदन; स्वेद; पसीना

**Diaphoretic.** An agent producing perspiration. स्वेदल; स्वेदकारी; पसीने लाने वाला पदार्थ

**Diaphragm.** The sheet of muscle and tendon separating the chest from the abdomen; the mid-riff; any partitioning membrane or septum. मध्यच्छद; मध्यपट; डायाफ़्राम

**Diaphragmalgia.** Pain in the diaphragm. मध्यच्छदार्ति; मध्यच्छद-पीड़ा

**Diaphragmatic.** Belonging to the diaphragm. मध्यच्छदीय; मध्यपटीय; मध्यच्छद सम्बन्धी

**Diaphragmatitis.** Inflammation of the diaphragm; diaphragmitis. मध्यच्छदशोथ; मध्यपटशोथ; मध्यच्छद का प्रदाह

**Diaphragmitis.** See **Diaphragmatitis.**

**Diaphragmodynia.** Pain in the diaphragm. मध्यच्छदपीड़ा; मध्यपटवेदना

**Diaphyseal.** See **Diaphysial.**

**Diaphyses.** Plural of **Diaphysis.**

**Diaphysial.** Relating to the diaphysis; diaphyseal. अस्थिवर्ध सम्बन्धी; अस्थिदण्ड सम्बन्धी

**Diaphysis.** The shaft of a long bone. अस्थिवर्ध; अस्थिदण्ड

**Diaphysitis.** Inflammation of the diaphysis. अस्थिवर्धशोथ

**Diaplacental.** Through the placenta. अपरा द्वारा; अपरा के माध्यम से

**Diaplasis.** Setting of a fracture. अस्थिसंयोजन; टूटी हुई हड्डी को ठीक जगह बिठाना

**Diapne.** Perspiration. स्वेद; स्वेदन; पसीना

**Diapyetic.** Promoting suppuration. पूतिजनक; पूतिजन्य; पीब पैदा करने वाला

**Diarrhea.** See **Diarrhoea.**

**Diarrheal.** See **Diarrhoeic.**

**Diarrheic.** See **Diarrhoeic.**

**Diarrhoea.** Frequent, loose watery stools; diarrhea. अतिसार; प्रवाहिका; संग्रहणी; दस्त;

   **Colliquative D.,** the type of diarrhoea which produces rapid exhaustion. क्षयकर प्रवाहिका;

   **Summer D.,** an acute form in children during the heat of summer. ग्रीष्म प्रवाहिका;

   **D. Hectica,** a dangerous diarrhoea of India, seriously affecting the constitution. सांघातिक प्रवाहिका; दुर्दम प्रवाहिका

**Diarrhoeal.** See **Diarrhoeic.**

**Diarrhoeic.** Producing diarrhoea; diarrheal; diarrheic; diarrhoeal; diarrhoeitic. अतिसारजनक; दस्तावर

**Diarrhoeitic.** See **Diarrhoeic.**

**Diarthroses.** Plural of **Diarthrosis.**

**Diarthrosis.** A synovial, free movable joint; ball-and-socket joint. चलसन्धि; स्वच्छन्दगतिक जोड़

**Diastasis.** A separation of bones without fracture; dislocation. अनुशिथिलता; विस्थिति; स्थानच्युति

**Diastasuria.** Amylasuria; the excretion of amylase in the urine. एमिलेजमेह

**Diastatic.** Relating to diastasis. अनुशिथिलता सम्बन्धी

**Diastema.** A space or cleft, as between teeth. दन्तांतराल; दन्तावकाश

**Diastemata.** Plural of **Diastema.**

**Diastole.** Relaxation period of cardiac cycle, as opposed to systole. अनुशिथिलन; हृत्प्रसार

**Diastolic.** Pertaining to the diastole. हृत्प्रसार सम्बन्धी; अनुशिथिलनीय

**Diathermal.** Permeable by radiant heat; diathermic. पारतापनीय; विद्युत्तापनीय

**Diathermia.** See **Diathermy.**

**Diathermic.** See **Diathermal.**

**Diathermy.** The passage of a high frequency electric current through the tissues whereby heat is produced; diathermia. पारतापन; विद्युत्तापन; डायाथर्मी; शरीर की गहरी स्नायुओं में गर्मी पैदा करने के लिए प्रयुक्त विद्युत्धारा का प्रयोग

**Diathesis.** A tendency of the individual to certain disease manifestations. प्रवृत्ति; प्रवणता; धातुदोष;

**Haemorrhagic D.,** haemophilia. रक्तस्रावी प्रवृत्ति; रक्तस्रावी प्रवणता; रक्तस्रावी स्वभाव

**Diathetic.** Relating to diathesis. प्रवणता अथवा प्रवृत्ति सम्बन्धी

**Diazoreaction.** The urinary test for phthisis and typhoid fever. डायजोप्रतिक्रिया; यक्ष्मा तथा आंत्रिक ज्वर के निदानार्थ की जाने वाली मूत्र जांच

**Dicephalous.** See **Dicephalus.**

**Dicephalus.** Two-headed; diacephalous. द्विशीर्ष; द्विशीर्षी; दो सिर वाला

**Dichotomy.** Division. विभाजन; भाजन; द्विभाजन

**Dicoria.** See **Diplocoria.**

**Dicrotic.** Pertaining to, or having a double beat; dicrotous; dicrotus. द्विस्पन्दी

**Dicrotism.** The condition of being dicrotic. द्विस्पन्दिता

**Dicrotous.** See **Dicrotic.**

**Dicrotus.** See **Dicrotic.**

**Didactylism.** Having only two digits on hand or foot. द्विअंगुलिता

**Didymalgia.** Pain in the testicle. वृषणकोशार्ति; अण्डकोशार्ति; अण्डकोश में पीड़ा

**Didymitis.** Orchitis; inflammation of the testis. वृषणकोशशोथ; वृषणकोशप्रदाह; अण्डकोशशोथ; अण्डकोशप्रदाह

**Didymus.** Testicle. वृषण

**Diencephala.** Plural of **Diencephalon.**

**Diencephalon.** The middle brain, including the thalami and the third ventricle. आन्तर-अग्रमस्तिष्क; अन्तर्मस्तिष्क

**Diet.** Food; a system of aliment. आहार; भोजन; पथ्य;

**Balanced D.,** a diet that furnishes in proper proportions all of the nutrients necessary for adequate nutrition. संतुलित आहार;

**Bland D.,** a regular diet omitting foods that irritate the gastrointestinal tract. सौम्य आहार;

**Diabetic D.,** a diet suitable for a diabetic patient. मधुमेहरोगी आहार;

**Salt-free D.,** a diet devoid of salt. लवणहीन आहार

**Dietary.** Pertaining to diet; dietetic. आहार अथवा पथ्यापथ्य सम्बन्धी

**Dietetic.** See **Dietary.**

**Dietetics.** The interpretation and application of the scientific principle of nutrition to feeding in health and disease. आहारिकी; आहारविज्ञान; पोषणविज्ञान

**Dietitian.** One who applies the principles of nutrition to the feeding of an individual or a group of individuals in a heterogenous setting of economy or health; a diet expert. आहारिकीविद; आहारविज्ञानी; आहारवेत्ता

**Differential Blood Count.** The estimation of the relative proportion of the different leucocyte cells in the blood. The differential count is : polymorphs 50% to 90%; lymphocytes 20% to 40%; monocytes 4% to 8%; neutrophils 40% to 60%; eosinophils 0 to 3%; basophils 0.5% to 1%. सापेक्ष रक्त गणन; विभेदक रक्त गणन; विभेदी रक्त गणन

**Differentiation.** The specialization of tissues, organs or functions. विभेदन; विभेदीकरण

**Diffraction.** The deflection of a ray of light on passing through a small opening. विवर्तन; प्रकाश-किरण को उसके घटकों में तोड़ना

**Diffuse.** Widely spread. विसरित; विसृत; विसारित; विस्तीर्ण; छितरा या बिखरा हुआ;

**D. Inflammation,** inflammation affecting all parts of an organ. विसरित प्रदाह; विसृत प्रदाह

**Diffused.** Widely spread. विसरित; विसृत; विसारित; विस्तीर्ण; छितरा या बिखरा हुआ

**Diffusible.** Capable of being spread rapidly. विसरणशील

**Diffusion.** The process whereby gases and liquids of different densities intermingle when brought into contact until the density is equal throughout dialysis. विसरण; विसार; विस्तार; प्रसारण; फैलाव

**Digastric.** Double bellied; biventral. द्विपिण्डी; द्वितुन्दी; द्विआमाशयिक; दो पेटों वाला; relating to the gastric muscle. आमाशय-पेशी सम्बन्धी

**Digerant.** A digestant. पाचक; पाचन में सहायक

**Digest.** To prepare for absorption, e.g. food. पाचन; पचाना; पचना

**Digestant.** Ferment aiding solution of food in alimentary canal; digestive. पाचक; पाचन में सहायक

**Digestible.** Capable of being digested. सुपाच्य; पाचन योग्य; पचाने या पचने योग्य

**Digestion.** The conversion of food into proper condition to supply nourishment for the body. पाचन

**Digestive.** Pertaining to digestion. पाचन सम्बन्धी; adding digestion; digestant. पाचक; पाचनयोग्य

**Digit.** A finger or toe; digitas; digitus; dactylus. अंगुलि; उँगली

**Digital.** Belonging to fingers. आंगुलिक; उँगलियों सम्बन्धी; resembling a digit or digits. अंगुलिकाभ; उँगली या उँगलियों जैसा

**Digitalis.** The botanical name for the fox-glove; a basic drug for use in certain heart diseases. डिजिटैलिस; नागफनी का रस; हृदय रोगों की एक मूल औषधि

**Digitas.** A finger or toe; digit. अंगुलि; उँगली

**Digitate.** Branched like the fingers. अंगुल्याकार; प्रांगुलित; उँगलियों जैसा शाखित

**Digitation.** A finger-like process. प्रांगुलन; कोई उँगलियों जैसी प्रक्रिया

**Digiti.** Plural of **Digitus.**

**Digitus.** A finger or toe; digit; digitas; dactylus. अंगुलि; उँगली

**Diglossia.** Having double tongue. द्विजिह्वी; दो जीभों वाला

**Dignathus.** Having two lower jaws. द्विअवहनुक; दो ठोढ़ियों वाला

**Dilaceration.** A tearing apart, as of a cataract. विदरण

**Dilatant.** A drug causing dilatation. विस्फारक; विस्फारण करने वाली औषधि

**Dilatation.** The act of spreading or expanding in all directions; dilation. स्फारण; विस्फारण; फैलाव

**Dilatation and Curettage (D&C).** Dilatation of the cervix and curettement of the endometrium. विस्फारण एवं आखुरण

**Dilatation and Evacuation (D&E).** Dilatation of the cervix and removal of the early product of conception. विस्फारण एवं उत्सरण

**Dilatator.** See **Dilator.**

**Dilation.** See **Dilatation.**

**Dilator.** An instrument for stretching a cavity or opening; dilatator. विस्फारक; स्फारक; फैलाने वाला;

   **D. Iridis,** the set of muscular fibres dilating the pupil. तारा-विस्फारक

**Dildo.** An artificial penis; dildoe. कृत्रिम-शिश्न

**Dildoe.** See **Dildo.**

**Diluent.** An agent for diluting concentrated fluid; diluting. तनूकर; पतला या दुर्बल करने वाला पदार्थ

**Diluting.** See **Diluent.**

**Dilution.** A weakening with water. तनुता; पानी में मिलाकर पतला या कमजोर करना; a weakned solution. तनूकरण;

   **Lower D.,** in homoeopathy, from mother tincture to 6th potency. निम्न तनूकरण

**Dimelia.** Congenital duplication of all or part of a limb. द्विअंगता

**Dimetria.** The state of having double uterus. द्विजरायुता; द्विगुणजरायुता; द्विगर्भाशयता; दो गर्भाशय होने की अवस्था

**Dimidium.** Half. अर्ध; आधा

**Dimorphic.** See **Dimorphous.**

**Dimorphism.** Existence in two shapes or forms. द्विरूपता

**Dimorphous.** Existing in two forms; dimorphic. द्विरूपी; दो रूपों में प्रकट होने वाला

**Dimple.** An identation or depression, usually circular and small in the chin, cheek, or sacral region. गर्तिका; वलय; झुर्री

**Dinomania.** Dancing mania. नृत्योन्माद; लास्योन्माद; नाचने का पागलपन

**Dinus.** Vertigo. भ्रमि; शिरोघूर्णन; चक्कर

**Diobus Alternis.** Alternate or every other day. एक दिन छोड़ कर

**Diovular.** See **Diovulatory.**

**Diovulatory.** Releasing two ova in one ovarian cycle; diovular. द्विडिम्बज

**Dioxide.** Oxide formed by combination of two atoms of oxygen with one of the metal or non-metal. द्विजारेय; द्विऑक्साइड; डाईऑक्साइड

**Diphallus.** Bifid penis. द्विशाखी-शिश्न

**Diphasic.** Occurring in or referring to two phases or stages. द्विप्रावस्थिक

**Diphtheria.** An infectious disease of the throat and glands in which false membranes are formed; diphtheritis. डिफ्थीरिया; रोहिणी; गलझिल्ली का प्रदाह

**Diphtherial.** See **Diphtheritic.**

**Diphtheric.** See **Diphtheritic.**

**Diphtheritic.** Relating to, or accompanying diphtheria; diphtherial; diphtheric. डिफ्थीरिया अथवा रोहिणी सम्बन्धी; रोहिणीयुक्त

**Diphtheritis.** See **Diphtheria.**

**Diplacusis.** A double voice from disease of the larynx. ध्वनिभेदश्रवण; द्विगुणध्वनि; एक ही ध्वनि को दो ध्वनियों के रूप में सुनना

**Diplegia.** Double symmetrical paralysis of legs, usually associated with cerebral damage. द्विपार्श्वघात; द्विपार्श्वअंगघात; द्विपार्श्वीअंगघात; शरीर के दोनों ओर के समान भागों का पक्षाघात

**Diplocoria.** Double pupil; dicoria. द्विपटलता; द्वितारकता

**Diploe.** The cellular bony tissue between the cranial tables. द्विपत्रक-मध्या; सच्छिद्रास्तर; कपाल-पटों के मध्य कोशिकीय अस्थि-ऊतक

**Diploic.** Relating to the diploe. द्विपत्रकमध्यापरक; सच्छिद्रास्तर सम्बन्धी

**Diplomyelia.** A congenital doubling of the spinal cord. द्विमेरुरज्जुता; द्विखण्डी-सुषुम्ना; सुषुम्ना की सहज द्विखण्डी अवस्था

**Diplopia.** Double vision. द्विगुणदृष्टि; द्विदृष्टिता; दोहरा दिखाई देना;

    **Binocular D.**, due to a derangement of the muscular balance; the images of the object being thus thrown upon non-identical points of the retina. द्विनेत्री द्विदृष्टिता;

    **Crossed D.**, see **Heteronymous Diplopia.**

    **Direct D.**, see **Homonymous Diplopia.**

    **Heteronymous D.**, that wherein the image of the right eye appears upon the left side and that of the left eye upon the right side; crossed diplopia. विषमदिक् द्विदृष्टिता;

    **Homonymous D.**, the reverse of crossed diplopia; direct diplopia. समदिक् द्विदृष्टिता;

    **Monocular D.**, diplopia with a single eye; uniocular diplopia; monodiplopia. एकनेत्री द्विदृष्टिता;

    **Uniocular D.**, see **Monocular Diplopia.**

**Diplopiometer.** A device for measuring diplopia. द्विगुणदृष्टिमापी

**Dipsesis.** Abnormal or excessive thirst; dipsosis. अतिपिपासा; अत्यधिक प्यास लगना

**Dipsia.** Thirst. प्यास; पिपासा

**Dipsogen.** A thirst-provoking agent. पिपासाजन; प्यास लगाने वाला (पदार्थ)

**Dipsomania.** Inordinate craving for alcoholic stimulants. मद्योन्माद; शराब पीने की अदम्य इच्छा

**Dipsopathy.** See **Dipsotherapy.**

**Dipsotherapy.** Treatment of certain diseases by abstaining from liquids; thirst-cure; dipsopathy. पिपासोपचार; प्यासोपचार

**Dipsosis.** Morbid thirst; dipsesis. अतिपिपासा; अत्यधिक प्यास लगना

**Direct.** In a right or straight line. प्रत्यक्ष; ऋजु

**Director.** A grooved instrument to direct a knife. डाइरेक्टर; शल्यकर्म के दौरान चाकू को सीधा रखने वाला यंत्र

**Dirt-eating.** Geophagia; the practice of eating dirt or clay. मृदा-भक्षण; धूल-मिट्टी खाना

**Disability.** Handicap. वैकल्य; अशक्तता; विकलांगता

**Disabled.** Handicapped; crippled. विकलांग; विकलीभूत

**Disablement.** Medicolegal term signifying loss of function without loss of earning power. विकलांगता

**Disarticulation.** Amputation at a joint; exarticulation. सन्धिविच्छेदन; किसी अंग को जोड़ से काटना

**Disassimilation.** Failure or loss of assimilative power. असमीकरण; असात्मीकरण

**Disassociation.** Separation of the parts of a compound. असाहचर्य; सम्बन्धविच्छेदन

**Disc.** A flat circular part or plate-like structure; disk. चक्र; चक्रिका; बिम्ब;

   **Articular D.**, see **Discus Articularis.**
   **Blood D.**, a.blood-corpuscle. रक्तकण; रक्तबिम्ब;
   **Choked D.**, papillitis; papilledema. अक्षिबिम्बशोथ; अक्षिबिम्बशोफ; रुद्धबिम्ब;
   **Optic D.**, entrance of the optic nerve into the retina. अक्षिबिम्ब

**Discectomy.** Surgical removal of a disc; discotomy. चक्रिका-उच्छेदन

**Discharge.** An excretion or evacuation of substance. स्राव; आस्राव; विसर्जन

**Discharging.** Flowing out, e.g. pus. निर्वहण; स्राव (होना)

**Disciform.** Of the form of a disc; disc-shaped. चक्राकार; बिम्बाकार; चक्रिकारूप; चक्ररूप; बिम्बरूप

**Dyscinesia.** Inability to perform voluntary movements. ऐच्छिकगत्यक्षमता; ऐच्छिक गतियाँ करने की असमर्थता

**Discission.** Rupturing of lens capsule to allow absorption of lens substance in the condition of cataract. विपाटन; कोंचना; छेदना

**Discogenic.** Arising in or produced by a disc, usually an intervertebral disc. बिम्बजनक; चक्रिकाजनक

**Discogram.** See **Discography.**

**Discography.** X-ray of an intervertebral disc after it has been rendered radio-opaque; discogram; diskogram. चक्रिकाचित्रण; बिम्बचित्रण

**Discoid.** Shaped like a disc. चक्रिकाभ; चक्राभ; बिम्ब जैसा; बिम्बोपम

**Discopathy.** Any disease of a disc. चक्रविकृति; बिम्बविकृति

**Discotomy.** See **Discectomy.**

**Disc-shaped.** See **Disciform.**

**Discus.** A disc. चक्र; चक्रिका; बिम्ब;

   **D. Articularis,** a plate or ring of fibrocartilage attached to the joint capsule for separating the articular surface of the bones; articular disc. सन्धायक चक्र;

**D. Proligerus,** the mass of the cells of the membrana granulosa of the Graafian vesicle that surrounds the ovum. परिडिम्ब चक्रिका; सन्तति बिम्ब; संतान उत्पन्न करने वाले कोशिका-पुंजों से बना बिम्ब

**Discutient.** An agent capable of dispersing a swelling or effusion. शोथविम्लापक; सूजन नष्ट करने वाली औषधि

**Disease.** Sickness; a pathological condition of any part or organ of the body or of the mind. रोग; व्याधि; बीमारी;

**Acute D.,** disease marked by rapid onset and course. तरुण रोग; उग्र रोग;

**Addison's D.,** chronic adrenocortical insufficiency. जीर्ण अधिवृक्कप्रान्तस्था-अपर्याप्तता; एडीसन रोग;

**Barlow's D.,** infantile scurvy. शिशु-शीताद; बार्लो रोग;

**Basedow's D.,** see **Grave's Disease.**

**Blue D.,** cyanosis. श्यावता; नीलिमा; नीलापन; नील रोग;

**Bright's D.,** nephritis. वृक्कशोथ; ब्राइट रोग;

**Caisson's D.,** decompression sickness. विसम्पीडन रुग्णता; केसन रोग;

**Chronic D.,** one that is slow in its course. जीर्ण रोग; चिरकारी रोग; चिर रोग;

**Communicable D.,** any disease that is transmissible by infection or contagion; contagious disease. संक्रामक रोग; सांसर्गिक रोग;

**Constitutional D.,** one that affects a system of organs or the whole body. वंशगत रोग; पैत्रिक रोग;

**Contagious D.,** see **Communicable Disease.**

**Deficiency D.,** a condition caused by the absence of certain food elements in the diet. हीनताजन्य रोग; खान-पान की कमी के कारण होने वाला रोग;

**Grave's D.,** toxic goitre, characterized by hyperplasia of thyroid gland; Basedow's disease. विषण्ण गलगण्ड; ग्रैव रोग; बेसडोव रोग;

**Hansen's D.,** leprosy. कुष्ठ; कोढ़;

**Hodgkin's D.,** a disease marked by chronic enlargement of lymph nodes, spleen and often liver, by anaemia and fever. हॉजकिन रोग;

**Notifiable D.,** a disease that by statutory requirements must be reported to public health anthorities at diagnosis because of its

**Disease**

importance to human or animal health. विज्ञाप्य रोग;

**Organic D.**, a disease in which there is anatomical change in some tissue or organ. आंगिक रोग;

**Raynaud's D.**, idiopathic paroxysmal bilateral cyanosis of the digits due to arterial and arteriolar contraction caused by cold or emotion. रेनाड रोग;

**Specific D.**, one due to a specific virus or poison within the body. विशिष्ट रोग; किसी विशिष्ट विषाणु अथवा विष के कारण होने वाला रोग;

**Sub-acute D.**, a condition tending towards chronicity. अर्धजीर्ण रोग; अर्धचिरकारी रोग; अर्धचिर रोग

**Venereal D.**, one contracted in sexual intercourse. रतिज रोग

**Disinfect.** To free from infection. रोगाणुनाशन करना; संक्रमणनाश करना

**Disinfectant.** A germ destroyer; disinfector. निःसंक्रामक; विसंक्रामक; संक्रमणहारी; रोगाणुनाशक

**Disinfection.** The destruction of all micro-organisms except spores, and can refer to the action of antiseptics as well as disinfectants. विसंक्रमण; संक्रमणहरण; रोगाणुनाशन

**Disinfector.** See **Disinfectant.**

**Disinfestation.** Extermination of infesting agents, especially lice. पीड़कजन्तुनाशन; यूकानाशन; जूं नष्ट करना

**Disinsertion.** Detachment of retina at its periphery; retinodylisis. निर्निवेश

**Disintegration.** The product of catabolism; the falling apart of the constituents of a substance. अवखण्डन; वियोजन

**Disk.** See **Disc.**

**Diskogram.** See **Discography.**

**Dislocated.** Displaced. विस्थापित; च्युत; भ्रंश; स्थान से हटा हुआ

**Dislocation.** The displacement of organs or articular surfaces. स्थानच्युति; संधिच्युति; भ्रंश; विस्थापन;

**Complete D.**, the bones entirely separated. पूर्ण सन्धिच्युति;

**Incomplete D.**, see **Partial Dislocation.**

**Open D.**, a dislocation complicated by a wound opening from the surface down to the affected joint. विवृत्त संधिच्युति;

**Partial D.**, the articulating surfaces remain in partial contact; incomplete dislocation. अपूर्ण सन्धिच्युति;

**Pathologic D.**, due to diseased joint or paralysis of the controlling muscles. वैकृत सन्धिच्युति

**Disorder.** Sickness; disease. विकार; रोग; defect. दोष

**Disorientation.** Loss of orientation. स्थितिभ्रान्ति

**Dispensary.** A place where the drugs are dispensed. औषधालय; डिस्पेंसरी; दवाखाना

**Dispensatory.** A book describing drugs, their composition, effects and uses. औषधयोगसंग्रह; ऐसा ग्रन्थ जिसमें औषधियों के निर्माण, प्रभाव तथा प्रयोग का वर्णन रहता है

**Dispense.** To give out drugs and other necessities to the sick. औषधि-योजन करना

**Displaced.** Dislocated. विस्थापित; च्युत; भ्रंश; स्थान से हटा हुआ

**Displacement.** A removal from the normal position. विस्थापन; च्युति; अपगमन; सामान्य स्थिति से हटा हुआ

**Disruptive.** Bursting; rending. विदारक; विध्वंसक; विनाशक

**Dissect.** To separate the parts of. विच्छेदन करना; चीर-फाड़ करना

**Dissecting.** Performing dissection. विच्छेदक; विच्छेदन; विदारक;
  **D. Instruments,** instruments used in dissection. विदारक यंत्र

**Dissection.** The cutting off of a part of tissues. व्यच्छेदन; व्यवच्छेदन; चीर-फाड़

**Disseminated.** Widely scattered through an organ, tissue or the body. प्रसृत; विकीर्ण; बिखरा हुआ

**Dessemination.** A scattering, as of disease germs. प्रसार; विकीर्णन

**Dissimilation.** Failure to convert into a like substance; disassimilation. विषमीकरण; असमीकरण; निर्स्वांगीकरण; अपचयन

**Dissipate.** To separate or disperse. अलग-थलग कर देना या तितर-बितर कर देना

**Dissipation.** Disassociation; separation. विसरण; विलगन

**Dissociation.** Separation of parts of a compound. वियोजन

**Dissolution.** Process of dissolving. विलोपन; प्रविलयन; विघटन; विसर्जन; death. मृत्यु

**Dissolve.** To make solution of. विलय करना; घोलना; द्रवीभूत करना

**Dissolvent.** Capable of dissolving substance. विलायक; घुलनकारी

**Distal.** Peripheral; away from the centre; fartherest from the head or source; distalis. दूरस्थ; दूरवर्ती; केन्द्र से दूर

**Distalis.** See **Distal**.

**Distance.** The measure of space between two objects. दूरी

**Distention.** The act or state of being distended or stretched. आध्मान; अफारा; फुलाव

**Distichia.** See **Distichiasis.**

**Distichiasis.** An extra row of eyelashes at the inner lid border, which is turned inward against the eye; distichia. द्विपक्ष्मराजिता; द्विपंक्तिकपक्ष्म; पलकों के अन्दर आँख की बरौनियों की एक अलग कतार रहना

**Distillation.** Vaporization, then condensing a liquid. आसवन; वाष्पन-क्रिया द्वारा किसी तरल पदार्थ का संचयन करना

**Distilled.** Vaporized by heat and condensing. आसुत

**Distinct.** Not united by growth. सुस्पष्ट; स्वतन्त्र; स्वछन्द

**Distoma.** A genus of trematode worms having two mouths; distomum. द्विमुख कृमि; दो मुँह वाला कृमि

**Distomia.** The condition of having two mouths. द्विमुखता; द्विमुख; दो मुँह होने की अवस्था

**Distomiasis.** The presence of distoma in the body. द्विमुखकृमिरोग

**Distomum.** See **Distoma.**

**Distortion.** A twisting out of normal shape or form; a deformity in which the part or structure is altered in a shape. विरूपण

**Distractibility.** A psychiatric term applied to a disorder of the power of attention when it can only be applied momentarily. ध्यानान्तरण

**Distress.** Physical or mental trouble or suffering. कष्ट; वेदना

**Distribution.** Dividing or spreading the branches of arteries or nerves to the tissues or organs. वितरण; the area in which the branch of an artery or nerve terminates, or the area is supplied by such artery or nerve. प्रसार; फैलाव

**Ditch.** Fossa. खात

**Diuresis.** An abundant secretion of urine. मूत्रलता; मूत्राधिक्य; अधिक पेशाब होना

**Diuretics.** Drugs causing increased secretion of urine. मूत्रल; मूत्रस्राववर्धक औषधियाँ

**Diurnal.** Pertaining to the daylight, or happening in the daytime; opposite of nocturnal. दिवाकालीन; दिवाकाल सम्बन्धी

**Div.** Divide. विभाजन करो

**Divagation.** Delirium. प्रलाप; disconnected speech. असम्बद्ध-वाक्; वाणी-असन्तुलन

**Divalent.** The same as **Bivalent.**

**Divergence.** A separation. विच्छिन्नता; अपसरण; अपसारिता

**Divergent.** Moving in different directions from a common point. विच्छिन्न; छितराया हुआ

**Diverticula.** Plural of **Diverticulum.**

**Diverticular.** Pertaining to a diverticulum. विपुटीय; अन्धवर्धी

**Diverticulectomy.** Excision of a diverticulum. विपुटी-उच्छेदन

**Diverticulitis.** Inflammation of a diverticulum. विपुटीशोथ; विपुटीप्रदाह

**Diverticulosis.** A condition in which there are many diverticula, especially in the intestines. विपुटिता

**Diverticulum.** A pouch or sac protruding from the wall of a tube or a hollow organ. विपुटी; अन्धवर्ध; गुप्तमार्ग; छेद; अन्धनली; अन्धनलिका

**Divided.** Separated. विभाजित

**Division.** Separation. विभाजन; the unit of an organisation. विभाग; भाग; प्रभाग

**Dizygotic.** Double birth. द्वियुग्मजन; द्विनिषिक्त डिम्ब

**Dizziness.** Vertigo; giddiness. भ्रमि; घुमरी; चक्कर

**Dochmiasis.** Hook-worm disease; miner's cachexia. अंकुशकृमिरोग

**Doctor.** A licensed medical practitioner. चिकित्सक; डॉक्टर

**Dog Button.** Nux vomica. कुचला; नक्स वौमिका

**Dolichocephalic.** Long-headed. दीर्घकपालिक; दीर्घकपाली; लम्बे या बड़े सिर वाला

**Dolichocephalism.** Long-headedness. दीर्घकपालिकता; दीर्घकपालिता

**Dolichocephalus.** See **Dolichocephaly.**

**Dolichocephaly.** Long-headed; dolichocephalus. दीर्घकपालिक; दीर्घकपाली; दीर्घशीर्ष; लम्बे या बड़े सिर वाला

**Dolomol.** See **Dolor.**

**Dolor.** Pain; a classical sign of inflammation; dolomol. वेदना; दर्द; पीड़ा

**Dolorific.** Producing pain. वेदनाकर; पीड़ाजनक; पीड़ाकारी

**Dolorimetry.** The measurement of pain. पीड़ामिति; वेदनामिति

**Dolorous.** Painful. वेदनाशील; पीड़ाप्रद; दर्दनाक; दर्दभरा

**Dominant.** Ruling or controlling. प्रभावी; प्रबल

**Donor.** An individual from whom blood, tissue or an organ is taken for transplantation. दाता; डोनर;

**Donor**

    **Universal D.,** one whose blood is of Group O, which is compatible with most other blood types. यूनिवर्सल डोनर

**Dormant.** Sleeping. प्रसुप्त; सुप्त; सोया हुआ

**Dorsa.** Plural of **Dorsum.**

**Dorsad.** Toward the back. पृष्ठाभिमुख; पीठ की ओर

**Dorsal.** Pertaining to the back or the posterior part of an organ. अभिपृष्ठ; पश्चांगी; पृष्ठस्थ; पृष्ठीय;

    **D. Region,** the back region. अभिपृष्ठ प्रदेश; पश्चप्रदेश

**Dorsalgia.** Pain in the back. पृष्ठार्ति; पीठ में दर्द

**Dorsi.** See **Dorsum.**

**Dorsiflexion.** Bending backward. अभिपृष्ठ-आकुंचन; पीछे की ओर मुड़ना

**Dorsocentral.** At the back and in the centre. अभिपृष्ठ-अन्तःकेन्द्रक; पीछे और केन्द्र में

**Dorsolateral.** Pertaining to the back and side of an object. अभिपृष्ठ-पार्श्विक; पृष्ठपार्श्विक

**Dorsolumbar.** The lumbar region of the back. अभिपृष्ठ-कटिक

**Dorsum.** Dorsi; the back of the body; the upper or posterior side, surface, or the back of any part. पृष्ठतल; पीछे कमर वाला भाग; पृष्ठ; अभिपृष्ठ; पीठ

    **D. Nasi,** the posterior side of the nose. नासापृष्ठ; नाक का पिछला भाग

**Dosage.** The determination of the proper remedy. मात्रा-निर्धारण; मात्रा-व्यवस्था; the giving of medicine or other therapeutic agent in prescribed amount. मात्रा

**Dose.** The quantity of medicine taken at a time. मात्रा; अंश; खूराक; डोज;

    **Booster D.,** a dose given at some time after an initial dose to enhance its effect. अनुवर्धक मात्रा;

    **Divided D.,** one taken in fractional portions at short intervals. विभाजित मात्रा;

    **Effective D.,** the dose which produces the desired effect. प्रभावी मात्रा;

    **Lethal D.,** a fatal dose. घातक मात्रा;

    **Maximum D.,** the largest dose consistent with safety. महत्तम मात्रा;

    **Minimum D.,** the smallest effective dose. अल्पतम मात्रा;

Single D., not more than one dose. एक मात्रा; एकल मात्रा

**Dosimeter.** Apparatus for measuring minute doses. मात्रामापी

**Dosimetry.** The acurate and systematic measurement of medicinal doses. मात्रामिति

**Dot.** A small spot. बिन्दु

**Double.** Two-fold; in pairs. द्विगुण; दुगुना; द्वि;

   **D. Hearing,** sounds heard doubly. द्विगुण श्राव्यता;

   **D. Vision,** seeing things double. द्विगुण दृष्टि

**Douche.** A stream of fluid directed against the body externally or into a body cavity. डूश

**Dozing.** Sleeping slightly. झपकी; हल्की नींद; तन्द्रा; ऊँघ

**D.P.T.** Diptheria, poliomyelitis and tetanus. रोहिणी-पोलियो-धनुर्वात

**Dr.** Abbreviation for **Dram, Drachm,** or **Doctor.** ड्राम अथवा डाक्टर का संक्षिप्त रूप

**Drachm.** Dram; 60 grains; one-eighth of an ounce. ड्राम; ६० ग्रेन; एक औंस का आठवां भाग

**Dracontiasis.** Infestation with **Dracunculus Medinensis,** i.e. guinea-worm, a nematode parasite; dracunculiasis; dracunculosis. नारू रोग

**Dracunculiasis.** See **Dracontiasis.**

**Dracunculosis.** See **Dracontiasis.**

**Dracunculus Medinensis.** Nematode parasite responsible for dracontiasis. नारूरोग परजीवी

**Draft.** A quantity of liquid medicine taken at one time; draught. घूंट

**Drain.** A passage or channel of exist for discharges from an abscess, etc. निकासिका; नाली; नली; to draw off fluid from a cavity as it forms. निकालना

**Drainage.** The gradual removal of the contents of a suppurating cavity. निकास; अपवहन

**Dram.** See **Drachm.**

**Drastic.** Violent purgative. उग्र विरेचक; तेज दस्तावर दवाई

**Draught.** See **Draft.**

**Dream.** Ideas or images formed in the mind during sleep. स्वप्न

**Dresser.** One whose office is to dress wounds. ड्रेसर; व्रणबन्धक;

**Dressing**

मरहम-पट्टी करने वाला

**Dressing.** The material applied to a wound for healing purposes. ड्रेसिंग; व्रणोपचार; मरहमपट्टी

**Drinker.** An alcoholic. मद्यप; शराबी; पियक्कड़

**Drivelling.** An involuntary flow of saliva. निरंकुश-लारमयता; निरंकुशलारता

**Drop.** A globule of liquid. बिन्दु; पात; बून्द

**Dropper.** A bottle or pipe to emit a fluid by drops. ड्रॉपर; बिन्दुपातक; बिन्दुपाती

**Dropsical.** Pertaining to dropsy. शोफज; शोफमय; शोफ सम्बन्धी

**Dropsy.** An effusion of fluid into the tissues or cavities of the body. शोफ; जलशोथ; जलशोफ

**Drug.** A substance used as medicine. औषधि; औषध; भेषज

**Drum.** The membrana tympani; the tympanic membrane. कर्णपटह; कान का पर्दा

**Drunkard.** An alcoholic; drinker. मद्यप; शराबी; पियक्कड़

**Druse.** Rupture of the tissues. स्फुटगुच्छ; ऊतकविदारण

**Dry.** Not moist. शुष्क; रूक्ष; रूखा

**Dualism.** The concept that blood cells have two origins, viz. lymphogenous and myelogenous. द्विमूलता

**Ducrey's Bacillus.** Gram-negative rod-shaped organism. ग्राम-ऋण दण्डाणु

**Duct.** A tube giving exist to secretion of a gland or conducting any fluid; ductus. नली; नलिका; वाहिनी;

**Alveolar D.,** the smallest of the intralobular ducts in the mammary glands; ductus alveolaris. वायुकोष्ठकी वाहिनी;

**Bile D.,** one formed by the junction of the cystic and hepatic ducts coveying the bile to the duodenum; biliary duct; gall duct. पित्तनली; पित्तवाहिनी;

**Biliary D.,** see **Bile Duct.**

**Cystic D.,** the excretory duct of the gall-bladder. पित्ताशय वाहिनी;

**Ejaculatory D.,** a duct formed by the union of the vas and the duct of the seminal vesicle, conveying semen into the urethra. शुक्रसेचक वाहिनी;

**Galactophorous D.,** one of the milk-ducts of the lobes of the mammary glands. दुग्ध वाहिनी;

**Gall D.**, see **Bile Duct**.

**Hepatic D.**, the duct receiving the bile from the liver. यकृत् वाहिनी;

**Parotid D.**, that conveying the secretion of the parotid gland into the mouth. कर्णपूर्व वाहिनी;

**Salivary D.**, a duct of any salivary gland. लारग्रन्थि वाहिनी; लालावाहिनी;

**Urogenital D.**, one that receives the urine and the genital products. मूत्रजनन वाहिनी;

**Ductal.** Relating to a duct. वाहिनीपरक; नलीपरक

**Ductless.** Without any duct. नलीहीन; नलीविहीन; अन्तःस्रावी; स्रोतहीन

**Ductless Gland.** Endocrine gland; organs without duct. स्रोतहीन ग्रन्थि; अन्तःस्रावी ग्रन्थि

**Ductule.** A small duct; ductulus. वाहिनिका; क्षुद्रनलिका

**Ductuli.** Plural of **Ductule**.

**Ductulus.** See **Ductule**.

**Ductus.** A duct or canal. वाहिनी; नली; नलिका;

**D. Alveolaris**, see **Alveolar Duct**.

**D. Arteriosus**, a short duct in the foetus connecting the pulmonary artery with the aorta. धमनी वाहिनी;

**D. Ovaricus**, the ovarian duct. डिम्ब-वाहिनी;

**D. Venosus**, a foetal blood vessel joining the umbilical vein and the ascending large vein. शिरा वाहिनी

**Dulcamara.** Bitter sweet. कट्वामधु; एक कड़वा और मीठा फल

**Dull.** Not resonant on percussion; blunt; slow of perception. अननुनादी; मन्द; कुन्द; सुस्त; कुण्ठित

**Dullness.** A non-resonant percussion; dulness. अननुनाद; मन्दता; मन्दस्वरता

**Dulness.** See **Dullness**.

**Dumb.** Unable to speak; mute. मूक; गूंगा

**Dumbness.** Muteness; silence. मूकता; गूंगापन

**Duodena.** Plural of **Duodenum**.

**Duodenal.** Pertaining to, or situated in duodenum. ग्रहणी सम्बन्धी; ग्रहणी-स्थित

**Duodenectomy.** Excision of the duodenum. ग्रहणी-उच्छेदन

**Duodeni.** See **Duodenum**.

**Duodenitis.** Inflammation of the duodenum. ग्रहणीशोथ

**Duodenocholecystostomy.** Formation of fistula between duodenum and gall-bladder; duodenocystostomy. ग्रहणीपित्ताशयसम्मिलन

**Duodenocholedochotomy.** Incision into the common bile-duct by way of a cut through the duodenum. ग्रहणीपित्तवाहिनीछेदन

**Duodenocystostomy.** See **Duodenocholecystostomy.**

**Duodenoenterostomy.** The formation of a fistula between the duodenum and the small intestine. ग्रहणीलघ्वांत्रसम्मिलन

**Duodenojejunal.** Pertaining to duodenum and jejunum. ग्रहणी तथा मध्यांत्र सम्बन्धी

**Duodenojejunum.** The duodenum and the jejunum. ग्रहणीमध्यांत्र; ग्रहणी तथा मध्यांत्र

**Duodenolysis.** Incision of adhesions to the duodenum. ग्रहणीलयन

**Duodenopancreactomy.** Surgical excision of the duodenum and part of the pancreas. ग्रहणी-अग्न्याशयोच्छेदन

**Duodenoplasty.** A plastic operation on the duodenum. ग्रहणीसंधान

**Duodenorrhaphy.** Suture of a tear of incision in the duodenum. ग्रहणीसीवन

**Duodenoscopy.** Inspection of the interior of the duodenum through an endoscope. ग्रहणीदर्शन

**Duodenostomy.** The formation of an opening through the abdominal wall into the duodenum. ग्रहणीछिद्रीकरण; ग्रहणीसम्मिलन

**Duodenotomy.** Incision of the duodenum. ग्रहणीछेदन

**Duodenum.** The first part of the bowel, next to stomach; upper part of the small intestine; duodeni. ग्रहणी; लघ्वांत्राग्र; पक्वाशय; पाचनान्त्र

**Duplication.** A doubling. द्विगुनन; द्विगुणीकरण; अनुलिपिकरण; आवृत्ति

**Dupuytren's Contraction.** Contraction of the palmar aponeurosis. करतलप्रावरणी-आकुंचन

**Dura.** See **Duramater.**

**Dural.** Relating to dura. दृढ़तानिका सम्बन्धी

**Duramater.** The tough fibrous semitransparent outer membrane lining the skull and covering the brain; dura. दृढ़तानिका; मस्तिष्क की बाहरी झिल्ली

**Duration.** Continuance in time. अवधि; काल; मियाद; समय

**Duritis.** Inflammation of the dura. दृढ़तानिकाशोथ; मस्तिष्क की बाहरी झिल्ली का प्रदाह

**Dusting Powder.** Any fine powder to be sprinkled upon the affected surface. बुकनी

**D.V.M.** Doctor of Veterinery Medicine. पशुरोग चिकित्सक

**D.V.T.** Deep vein thrombosis. गहन शिरा घनास्रता

**Dwarf.** An abnormally underdeveloped person. वामन; बौना; ठिगना; नाटा

**Dwarfism.** The condition of being a dwarf. वामनता; बौनापन; ठिगनापन; नाटापन

**Dyad.** Pair; diad. द्वि; युगल; जोड़ा

**Dye.** A stain or colouring matter. रंजक

**Dynamia.** Vital strength or energy. जीवनीशक्ति; प्राणशक्ति

**Dynamic.** Pertaining to, or manifesting force. गतिक; गतिशील; सक्रिय

**Dynamics.** The science of motion and laws of force. गतिविज्ञान; बलनियम; गतिकी

**Dynamisation.** The hypothetical increase of the active virtues of a medicine by agitation; act of making drugs effective by dilutions. गतिकरण; होम्योपैथी में औषध-निर्माण का एक तरीका; प्रबलीकरण; शक्तिकरण

**Dynamogenesis.** Production of force, especially of muscular or nervous energy. शक्तिजनन

**Dynamogenic.** Generating force. शक्तिजनक; शक्ति पैदा करने वाला; relating to dynamogenesis. शक्तिजनन सम्बन्धी

**Dynamometer.** Apparatus to test the strength of grip; ergometer. शक्तिमापी

**Dys-.** Prefix meaning bad, difficult or painful. 'दु':; 'दुर्' अथवा 'दुस्' के रूप में प्रयुक्त उपसर्ग

**Dysaphe.** Disordered sense of touch; dysaphia. स्पर्शज्ञानदोष; स्पर्शसंवेदना की गड़बड़ी

**Dysaphia.** See **Dysaphe.**

**Dysarthria.** See **Dyslalia.**

**Dysarthrosis.** Dyslalia. वाक्विकार; malformation of a joint. अयुक्तसंधि; वियुक्तसन्धि; a false joint. कूटसन्धि; dysarthria. दुरुच्चारण

**Dysautonomia.** Abnormal functioning of the autonomic nervous system. दु:स्वायत्तता

**Dysbasia.** Difficulty in walking. कष्टचलन; सकष्टगति; चलने में कठिनाई

**Dyschesia.** Painful and difficult defaecation. सकष्टमलत्याग;

सकष्टमलोत्सर्ग

**Dyschondroplasia.** Underdevelopment of cartilages. उपास्थिदुर्विकसन; उपास्थियों का अपूर्ण विकास

**Dyschromia.** Discolouration, as of the skin. विवर्णता

**Dyscoia.** Deafness. बधिरता; बहरापन

**Dyscoria.** Abnormality of the pupil. दृष्टिपटलदोष

**Dyscrasia.** Any abnormal state, especially of the blood. विकृति; दोष

**Dysenteric.** Pertaining to dysentery. आमातिसार सम्बन्धी; पेचिश सम्बन्धी

**Dysentery.** A disease of the intestines attended with frequent bloody and mucous stools; bloody-flux. आमातिसार; रक्तातिसार; पेचिश;
  **Amebic D.,** see **Amoebic Dysentery.**
  **Amoebic D.,** that due to the presence of amoeba; amebic dysentery. अमीबातिसार; अमीबी पेचिश;
  **Bacillary D.,** that caused by infection with **Shigella dysenteriae** or other organisms. दण्डाणुज अतिसार

**Dysesthesia.** Dullness of sensation. अपसंवेदन

**Dysfunction.** See **Dysfunctioning.**

**Dysfunctioning.** Abnormal functioning of any organ or part; dysfunction. दुष्क्रिया; शरीर के किसी अंग या भाग की अस्वाभाविक क्रिया

**Dysgenesis.** Malformation during embryonic development. दुर्विकास; bad breeding. अपजनन; कुजनन; sterility. बंध्यता; बांझपन

**Dysgenic.** Relating to bad breeding or sterility. कुजनन अथवा बंध्यता सम्बन्धी

**Dysgerminoma.** A tumour of the ovary of low malignancy. डिम्बग्रन्थ्यर्बुद; डिम्बग्रन्थि की रसौली

**Dysgnosia.** Any mental disorder or disease. मनोविकृति

**Dyshidrosis.** Abnormal sweating. दुस्वेदलता; अस्वाभाविक रूप से पसीना होना

**Dyskinesia.** Impairment of voluntary movement; diskinesis. अपगति; स्वच्छन्द अथवा ऐच्छिक गति की दोषपूर्ण अवस्था

**Dyskinesis.** See **Dyskinesia.**

**Dyslalia.** Difficulty in talking due to defect of speech organ; dysarthria; dysarthrosis. वाक्विकार; सकष्टवाक्; दुरुच्चारण

**Dyslexia.** Impairment of reading ability. अपपठन; वाक्विकार; पढ़ने में किसी प्रकार का दोष होना

**Dysmasesis.** Impairment of masticating ability. कष्टचर्वण; चर्वणदोष;

चबाने में किसी प्रकार का दोष होना

**Dysmelia.** Limb deficiency. अंगाल्पता; अंगदोष

**Dysmenorrhea.** See **Dysmenorrhoea.**

**Dysmenorrhoea.** Painful menstruation; dysmenorrhea. कष्टार्तव; कृच्छ्रार्तव; दर्दनाक ऋतुस्राव होना

**Dysmetria.** Lack of harmonious action of muscular movements. दुर्मिति; अपमिति

**Dysopia.** Defective or painful vision; dysopsia. दृष्टिदोष; दोषपूर्ण दृष्टि होना

**Dysopsia.** See **Dysopia.**

**Dysorexia.** Abnormal hunger; unnatural appetite. क्षुधादोष; अस्वाभाविक भूख लगना

**Dysosmia.** Perverted sense of smell. घ्राणेन्द्रिय विकार; सूंघने में किसी प्रकार की अस्वाभाविकता होना

**Dysosteogenesis.** Defective bone formation; dysotosis. दुरस्थिता

**Dysostosis.** See **Dysosteogenesis.**

**Dyspareunia.** Painful or difficult coition. कृच्छ्रमैथुन; सकष्टसंगम; दर्दनाक संगम होना

**Dyspepsia.** Weakness of digestion; indigestion. अग्निमांद्य; मंदाग्नि; दुष्पचन; अजीर्ण; अपच; पाचन-दौर्बल्य

**Dyspeptic.** Relating to dyspepsia. मंदाग्नि सम्बन्धी; suffering from dyspepsia. मंदाग्निग्रस्त

**Dyspermatism.** Defective secretion of semen. शुक्रदोष; दोषपूर्ण वीर्यपात होना

**Dysphagia.** Difficulty of swallowing; dysphagy. निगरणकष्ट; निगलने में कठिनाई

**Dysphagy.** See **Disphagia.**

**Dysphasia.** See **Dysphrasia.**

**Dysphemia.** Stammering; disorder of phonation or articulation due to emotional or intellectual deficiency. तुतलाना; हकलाना; अटक-अटक कर बोलना

**Dysphonia.** Difficulty in producing sounds; dysphrasia. वाक्कृच्छ्रता; दु:स्वरता; वाग्वैकल्य

**Dysphoria.** Restlessness; a feeling of unpleasantness or discomfort. व्यग्रता; व्याकुलता; बेचैनी

**Dysphrasia.** Imperfect speech; stammering; dysphasia. वाग्दोष; हकलाना

**Dysplasia.** Formation of abnormal tissue. दुर्विकसन; वर्धन असंगति

**Dyspnea.** Laboured breathing; dyspnoea. श्वासकष्ट; कृच्छ्श्वसन

**Dyspneic.** Affected with dyspnoea; dyspnoeic. श्वासकृच्छ्रूरोगी; श्वासकष्ट से पीड़ित रोगी

**Dyspnoea.** See **Dyspnea.**

**Dyspnoeic.** See **Dyspneic.**

**Dyspragia.** Difficult and painful functioning in any organ; dyspraxia. दुष्क्रिया; कठिन अथवा दर्दनाक क्रिया होना

**Dyspraxia.** See **Dispragia.**

**Dysrhythmia.** Disordered rhythm. दुस्तालता; ताल बदल जाना

**Dyssynergia.** Ataxia; failure of muscular coordination; dyssynergy. अपसहक्रिया

**Dyssynergy.** See **Dyssynergia.**

**Dystaxia.** Difficulty in controlling the voluntary muscles; partial ataxia. आंशिक गतिभंग

**Dysteleology.** The science of useless and rudimentary organs. अवशेषांगिकी; अवशिष्ट-अंगविज्ञान

**Dysthymia.** Mental distress. मनस्ताप; मानसिक कष्ट

**Dystocia.** Difficult or slow labour. कष्टप्रसव; कठिनप्रसव; कठिनाई के साथ प्रसव होना

**Dystonia.** Abnormal tonicily in any of the tissues. दुस्तानता

**Dystonic.** Pertaining to dystonia. दुस्तानता सम्बन्धी

**Dystopia.** Displacement of an organ. दुःस्थानता; दुर्स्थानता; किसी अंग का सामान्य स्थिति से हट जाना

**Dystopic.** Relating to dystopia. दुःस्थानता सम्बन्धी

**Dystrophia.** See **Dystrophy.**

**Dystrophic.** Relating to dystrophy. अपविकास अथवा दुष्पोषण सम्बन्धी

**Dystrophy.** Dystrophia; imperfect or faulty nourishment. दुष्पोषण; कुपोषण; faulty development. अपविकास; दुर्विकास

**Dysuria.** Pain and difficulty in urination. मूत्रकृच्छ्र; मूत्रकृच्छ्रता

**Dysuriac.** Relating to dysuria. मूत्रकृच्छ्रता सम्बन्धी; one affected with dysuria. मूत्रकृच्छ्रग्रस्त (रोगी)

# E

**Ear.** The organ of hearing, composed of the external ear, the middle ear (tympanic cavity) and internal ear or labyrinth. कान; श्रोत्र; कर्णेन्द्रिय;

    **Inflammation of e.,** otitis. कर्णशोथ; कर्णप्रदाह; कान का प्रदाह;

    **Middle E.,** the tympanic cavity; an irregular airfilled space in the temporal bone. मध्यकर्ण;

    **E.-ache,** otalgia; pain in the ear; otodynia. कर्णशूल; कर्णपीड़ा; कान का दर्द;

    **E.-bones,** the ossicles of the tympanic cavity; malleus. कर्णास्थियाँ; कान की हड्डियाँ

    **E.-drum,** the tympanic membrane; the cavity in the middle ear; membrana tympani. कर्णपटह;

    **E.-wax,** cerumen. कर्णगूथ; कर्णमल; कान का मैल

**Earth.** Clay. मृदा; मिट्टी

**Ebullition.** The motion of a liquid by which it gives off bubbles of vapor, as in boiling. क्वथन; उत्क्वथन; उबाल; उबलने की दशा

**Eburnation.** A morbid change in bone by which it becomes hard and ivory-like. कठिनीभवन; किसी हड्डी का कठोर होकर हाथी-दान्त जैसे रूप में बदल जाना

**Ecbolic.** Producing abortion or promoting parturition. गर्भोत्सारक; गर्भस्रावी; गर्भस्रावक; गर्भपातक; गर्भपाती

**Eccentric.** Away from the centre. उत्केंद्री; केन्द्र से दूर; irregular. अनियमित; odd. विषम; erratic. चलायमान; peripheral. परिसरीय

    **E. Hypertrophy,** hypertrophy of the heart with dilatation. उत्केन्द्री अतिबृद्धि; उत्केन्द्री हृद्बृद्धि; हृदय का बढ़ना और फैल जाना

**Ecchondroma.** A benign tumour composed of the cartilage which protrudes from the surface of the bone in which it arises; ecchondrosis. बहिरुपास्थ्यर्बुद; उपास्थि-ऊतक का बाहर की ओर बढ़ना

**Ecchondromata.** Plural of **Ecchondroma.**

**Ecchondrosis.** See **Ecchondroma.**

**Ecchondrotome.** Knife for excision of cartilage. उपास्थि-उच्छेदक

**Ecchymoma.** A skin tumour caused by extravasation of blood. रक्तार्बुद; खूनी अर्बुद; खून की रसौली

**Ecchymosed.** Characterized by or affected with ecchymoma. रक्तार्बुदग्रस्त

**Ecchymoses.** Plural of **Ecchymosis.**

**Ecchymosis.** Extravasation of blood; livid spots on the skin of a bruise-like character. नीललांछन; नीलांछन; चमड़ी पर नीले-नीले धब्बे उभर आना

**Ecchymotic.** Relating to ecchymosis. नीललांछन सम्बन्धी

**Eccoprotic.** A laxative; a mild purgative. सारक; विरेचक; विसर्जन को बढ़ावा देने वाला; दस्तावर (दवा)

**Eccrine.** Pertaining to secretion. बाह्यस्रावी; उत्सर्गी

**Eccritic.** A medicine promoting excretion. सारक; विरेचक; विसर्जन को बढ़ावा देने वाला; दस्तावर

**Ecdemomania.** Wanderlust; abnormal desire to wander. भ्रमणोन्माद

**Ecderon.** Epidermis or outer portion of skin. अधस्त्वक; बहि:त्वचा; बहित्र्वचा

**Ecdysis.** Moulting of the skin; desquamation. निर्मोकोत्सर्जन; विशल्कन; प्रपतन; पपड़ी उतरना

**E.C.G.** Electrocardiography; the making and study of graphic records produced by electric currents originating in the heart. विद्युतृहृद्लेख; विद्युत्यंत्र द्वारा हृदय की गति का रेखाचित्रण

**Echinococcosis.** Infection with **Echinococcus.** फीताकृमिरोग

**Echinococcus.** A genus of tapeworms. स्फीतकृमि; पट्टकृमि; फीताकृमि

**Echo.** A reverbrated sound. प्रतिध्वनि; गूंज; अनुनाद

**Echoaortography.** Application of ultrasound techniques to the diagnosis and study of the aorta, particularly the abdominal aorta. महाधमनीप्रतिध्वनिलेखन; प्रतिध्वनिमहाधमनीलेखन

**Echocardiography.** Use of ultrasound in the diagnosis of cardiovascular lesion and recording of the size, motion and composition of various cardiac structures. प्रतिध्वनिहृद्लेख; पराध्वनिहृद्लेख

**Echoencephalography.** Passage of penetrating sound waves across the head. प्रतिध्वनिमस्तिष्कलेखन

**Echogenic.** Containing internal interfaces that reflect high frequency sound waves. प्रतिध्वनिजनक

**Echography.** The use of ultrasonic technique to produce a photograph of the echo produced when sound waves are reflected from tissues of different density; ultrasonography. प्रतिध्वनिलेखन

**Echokinesia.** See **Echopraxia.**

**Echokinesis.** See **Echopraxia.**

**Echolalia.** Aphasic repetition of another's words; echophrasia. शब्दानुकरण; अन्य व्यक्तियों द्वारा कहे गये शब्दों को पुन: बोलना

**Echopathy.** A mental disorder in which the words or actions of another are imitated and repeated by the patient. प्रतिध्वनि-रुग्णता

**Echophrasia.** See **Echolalia.**

**Echopraxia.** Spasmodic imitation of another's gesture; echokinesia; cchokincsis; echopraxis. क्रियानुकरण, नकल उतारना

**Echopraxis.** See **Echopraxia.**

**Echovirus.** A virus related to influenza which causes obscure types of infection. श्लेष्मज्वराणु; श्लैष्मिक ज्वराणु

**Eclabium.** Eversion of a lip. उद्वर्ती ओष्ठ; ओष्ठबहिर्वर्तन

**Eclampsia.** Puerperal convulsions; eclampsis. गर्भाक्षेप; प्रसवाक्षेप

**Eclampsis.** See **Eclampsia.**

**Eclamptic.** Affected with eclampsia. गर्भाक्षेपग्रस्त; प्रसवाक्षेपग्रस्त

**Eclectic.** Choosing. सर्वग्राही; सारग्राही; a certain class of physicians. चिकित्सकों की एक श्रेणी

**Eclecticism.** A system of treatment composed of various tried and selected medicines. सर्वसंग्राहक चिकित्सा प्रणाली

**Ecmnesia.** A momentary loss of memory. क्षणिकस्मरणशक्तिलोप; वर्तमान घटनाओं को कुछ क्षणों के लिये भूल जाने की अवस्था

**E. Coli.** Escherichia coli; the colon bacillus. एशेरिशिया कोलाइ; बृहदान्त्र-दण्डाणु

**Ecological.** Pertaining to ecology. पारिस्थितिक; परिस्थितिविज्ञान सम्बन्धी

**Ecology.** The modifying influence of enviroment on the physiology and behaviour of organisms. पारिस्थितिकी; परिस्थितिविज्ञान

**Economic.** Financial. आर्थिक

**Economy.** The whole animal organism. शरीर; सम्पूर्ण देह

**Ecostate.** Without ribs. अपर्शुक; पर्शुकाहीन; पसलियों से हीन

**Ecstasiá.** Dilatation; distension. विस्फार; विस्फारण; फैलाव

**Ecstasy.** A trance-like exalted state. अत्यानन्द; आह्लाद; हर्षोन्माद; हर्षातिरेक

**Ectal.** External. बाह्य; बाहरी

**Ectasia.** See **Ectasis.**

   **E. Cordis,** dilatation of the heart. हृत्विस्फार

**Ectasis.** An abnormal distension of a part; ectasia. विस्फार; किसी अंग-विशेष का असाधारण रूप से फैल जाना

**Ecthyma.** An eruption of large, round pustules, quite distinct from each other. पूयस्फोटिका; पीबभरी फुंसियों से युक्त उद्भेद

**Ectiris.** The external portion of the iris. बहिर्परितारिका; उपतारा का बाहरी भाग

**Ecto-.** Prefix meaning outside or external. 'बाह्य' तथा 'बहि:' के रूप में प्रयुक्त उपसर्ग

**Ectoantigen.** Any toxin or other excitor of antibody formation, separate or separable from its source; exoantigen. बाह्यप्रतिजन

**Ectoblast.** The outer cell-layer or ectoderm. बहि:प्रसू; बाह्यस्तर

**Ectocardia.** A displacement of the heart; ectopia cordis; exocardia. बहिर्हृदयता; हृदय की स्थानच्युति

**Ectocervix.** The portion of the canal of the uterine cervix. बहिर्जरायुग्रीवा

**Ectoderm.** The external primitive layer of the embryo; ectoblast. बहिर्जनस्तर; बहिश्चर्म

**Ectodermal.** Pertaining to the ectoderm; ectodermic. बहिर्जनस्तरीय; बहिर्जनस्तर या बहिश्चर्म सम्बन्धी

**Ectodermatosis.** See **Ectodermosis.**

**Ectodermic.** See **Ectodermal.**

**Ectodermosis.** Disease of any organ or tissue derived from the ectoderm; ectodermatosis. बहिर्जनस्तर-रुग्णता

**Ectogenous.** Originating outside the organism. बहिर्विकासी; बाहर की ओर विकसित होने वाला

**Ectomorph.** Emaciated; a constitutional body type or build in which tissues that originate from the ectoderm prevail. कृश; कृशकाय; दुर्बल; कमजोर

**Ectomorphic.** Relating to ectomorph. कृशता सम्बन्धी

**Ectoparasite.** An external parasite. बहि:परजीवी; बाह्यपरजीवी

**Ectoparasiticide.** An agent destroying the external parasites. बहि:परजीवीनाशक; बाह्यपरजीवीनाशक; बाह्यपरजीवियों को नष्ट करने वाला

**Ectopia.** An abnormality of position, usually congenital; ectopy.

अस्थानता; सहज अस्थानता; स्थानच्युति; स्थानभ्रंश;
**E. Cordis,** see **Ectocardia.**
**E. Lentis,** dislocation of the crystalline lens of the eye. लेंस-अस्थानता; नेत्र के स्फटिक लेंस की स्थानच्युति;
**E. Renis,** displacement of the kidney. वृक्कच्युति; वृक्क-अस्थानता; गुर्दे का अपने स्थान से हट जाना;
**E. Testis,** displacement of the testes. अण्ड-अस्थानता; वृषणों की स्थानच्युति;
**E. Vesicae,** protrusion of the bladder through the abdominal wall. अस्थानी विवृत मूत्राशय; अस्थानी मूत्राशय विवर्तन

**Ectopic.** Relating to ectopia. अस्थानिक; अस्थानी; स्थानच्युत; स्थानच्युति सम्बन्धी;

**E. Beat,** electrical stimulation of cardiac contraction beginning at a point than the sinoatrial node. अस्थानिक स्पन्द;
**E. Pregnancy,** extra-uterine gestation. अस्थानिक सगर्भता; बहिगर्भाशयिक सगर्भता;
**E. Rhythm,** any cardiac rhythm that is abnormal or irregular. अस्थानिक ताल;
**E. Secretion,** the secretion of hormones by tumours arising from tissues that do not normally secrete the hormone or hormones. अस्थानिक स्राव

**Ectoplasm.** The exterior protoplasm of a cell; exoplasm. बहि:प्रद्रव्य; बाह्यद्रव्य; बाह्यसत्व; बहि:परासरण

**Ectoplast.** Cell-membrane. कोशिकाकला

**Ectopy.** See **Ectopia.**

**Ectozoa.** External parasites. यूका अर्थात् जूं, आदि बहि:परजीवी

**Ectozoon.** Singular of **Ectozoa.**

**Ectrodactylia.** See **Ectrodactyly.**

**Ectrodactylism.** See **Ectrodactyly.**

**Ectrodactyly.** Congenital shortness or absence of one or more fingers or toes; ectrodactylia; ectrodactylism. सहज लघ्वंगुलिता; सहज अल्पांगुलिता; सहज अंगुल्यभाव; एक या अधिक उँगलियों का जन्मजात अभाव

**Ectrogenic.** Relating to ectrogeny. सहज अनंगता सम्बन्धी

**Ectrogeny.** A congenital absence of one or more of limbs. सहज अनंगता; किसी अंग का जन्मजात अभाव

**Ectromelia.** Hypoplasia of the long bones of the limbs. दीर्घास्थिलोप

**Ectropic.** Turned out or everted. अस्थानी; बहिरवर्त; बाहर को मुड़ा हुआ

**Ectropion.** Diversion of the eyelids; ectropium. बहिर्वर्तन; बहिर्वर्तमता; पलकों का बाहर की ओर मुड़ना

**Ectropium.** See **Ectropion.**

**Ectropody.** Total or partial absence of a foot. अपादता; पादहीनता

**Eczema.** A chronic skin condition of allergic origin. छाजन; अकौता; दाद; पामा; एक्जीमा

**Eczematoid.** Resembling eczema. छाजनाभ; छाजनवत्; छाजन से मिलता-जुलता

**Eczematous.** Affected with or like eczema. छाजनग्रस्त या छाजन जैसा

**E. D.** Effective dose. प्रभावी मात्रा

**E.D.D.** Expected date of delivery. अनुमानित प्रसव तिथि

**Edea.** The genital organs. जननांग; प्रजननांग

**Edeitis.** Inflammation of the genital organs. जननांगशोथ; प्रजननांगों का प्रदाह

**Edema.** Tissue swelling due to retained fluid, commonly called dropsy; oedema. शोफ; पानी वाली सूजन

**Edematogenic.** Causing edema; oedematogenic. शोफजनक

**Edematous.** Relating to, or marked by edema; oedematous. शोफज; शोफमय; शोफयुक्त

**Edentate.** Toothless; without teeth; edentulous. अदन्ती; दन्तहीन

**Edentia.** An absence of teeth. दन्तहीनता; दन्ताभाव; अदन्तता

**Edentulous.** Without teeth. दन्तहीन; बिना दान्तों वाला; अदन्ती

**Edeology.** A treatise on the genital organs. जननांगविज्ञान; जननांगप्रकरण

**Edible.** Suitable for food; fit to eat; non-poisonous. खाद्य; आहार योग्य

**E.E.G.** Electroencephalography. विद्युत् मस्तिष्कलेख; विद्युत् यंत्र द्वारा मस्तिष्क के कार्य-कलापों का चित्रण

**Effect.** The result or consequence of an action. प्रभाव; परिणाम

**Effective.** Powerful in effect. प्रभावी

**Effectiveness.** The ability to cause the expected or intended effect or result. प्रभाविता

**Effector.** A motor or secretory nerve-ending in a muscle, gland or organ. प्रेरक; सम्पादी; निष्पादी

**Efferent.** Conveying from a centre. अपवाही; बहिर्गामी; केन्द्र से बाहर की ओर ले जाने वाला (वाली)

**E. Nerves,** nerves that carry impulses to various parts of the body; motor nerves. अपवाही तंत्रिकायें; बहिर्गामी तंत्रिकायें; प्रेरक तंत्रिकायें

**Effervescence.** The escape of gas from a fluid, as in the so-called 'soda water'. बुद्बुदन; उबाल; जोश

**Effervescent.** Bubbling over. बुद्बुदकारी; फेनिल; आलोड़ित; उत्तेजित

**Efficiency.** Capability; skilfulness. क्षमता; सामर्थ्य; निपुणता

**Efflorescence.** An eruption on the skin resembling a blush. उत्फुल्लन; प्रस्फुटन; विस्फोट

**Efflorescent.** Drying from loss of the water of crystallization, as certain salts. उत्फुल्लनशील; प्रस्फुटित

**Effluent.** A flowing out. बहि:प्रवाह

**Effluvia.** Plural of **Effluvium.**

**Effluvium.** Exhalation. दुर्गन्ध-प्रसर्ग; vapour. वाष्प; odour. गन्ध; a shedding, especially of hair. पात; गिरना, खास तौर से बालों का गिरना

**Effluxion.** Early abortion, during the first three months. गर्भस्राव; गर्भपात

**Effusion.** An escape of the blood or any other fluid of the body from their natural position into the tissues or cavities of the body. नि:सरण; बहाव; रिसाव

**Egesta.** The excrement of the body. मल; स्राव; उत्सर्ग

**Egg.** The female sexual cell or gamete. अण्ड; अण्डा

**Eglandular.** Without glands; eglandulous. ग्रन्थिविहीन; ग्रन्थिहीन

**Eglandulous.** See **Eglandular.**

**Ego.** Refers to the unconsciousness "self"; the 'I', the part of personality that deals with the reality and is influenced by social forces. अहम्

**Egocentric.** Marked by extreme concentration of attention upon oneself; egotropic; self-centered. अहम्केन्द्रिक

**Egotropic.** See **Egocentric.**

**Eighth Cranial Nerve.** The acoustic nerve. ध्वनिकतंत्रिका

**Ejaculate.** To expel suddenly, as semen. वीर्यपात होना

**Ejaculatio Praecox.** Premature orgasm of the males. कालपूर्वस्खलन; पुरुषों का समय से पहले ही वीर्यपात हो जाना

**Ejaculation.** A sudden emission of semen from the male urethra. वीर्यस्खलन; वीर्यस्खलनता; वीर्यपात

**Ejaculator.** Muscle that ejects semen. वीर्यस्खलनकारी; वीर्यपाती (पेशी)

**Ejaculatory.** Seminiferous; relating to ejaculation. वीर्यस्खलनीय; वीर्यपाती; वीर्यपात सम्बन्धी

**Ejecta.** That which is cast away; excretion. उत्सर्ग; शरीर से बाहर निकाला हुआ द्रव्य

**Ejection.** The process of casting away. उत्सर्जन; उत्सरण

**Elaboration.** Converting crude food into high tissue-products. विस्तार; खाद्य-विस्तार; कच्चे भोजन का उच्च ऊतक-उत्पादों में बदलना

**Elastic.** Endowed with elasticity. प्रत्यास्थ; लचीला; लोचदार;

 **E. Bandage,** a rubber bandage for constant pressure. प्रत्यास्थ पट्टी; लगातार दबाव देने के लिये प्रयुक्त एक रबड़ की पट्टी;

 **E. Cartilage,** yellow cartilage, such as found in the epiglottis, pharynx, external ears and auditory tube. प्रत्यास्थ उपास्थि;

 **E. Fibres,** fibres capable of returning to their original form after being stretched or compressed. प्रत्यास्थ तंतु; लचीले तन्तु;

 **E. Tissue,** a variety of connective tissue composed of yellow elastic fibres. प्रत्यास्थ ऊतक; लचीला ऊतक

**Elasticity.** The quality or condition of being elastic. प्रत्यास्थता; लोच; लचीलापन

**Elastometer.** Device for measuring elasticity. प्रत्यास्थतामापी

**Elastometry.** The measurement of elasticity of tissues. प्रत्यास्थतामिति

**Elastosis.** Any disease of elastic tissue. प्रत्यास्थ-ऊतकविकृति

**Elation.** Joyful emotion. उल्लास

**Elbow.** The joint below the arm and forearm. कूर्पर; कोहनी; कफोणि

**Elcosis.** Foetid ulceration. दुर्गन्धित व्रण; बदबूदार घाव

**Electe.** Alongwith the milk. दूध के साथ

**Electric.** See **Electrical.**

**Electrical.** Having the nature of electricity; electric. वैद्युत्; विद्युतीय; विद्युत्-लक्षणों से युक्त

**Electricity.** A natural force or power generated by magnetism, chemism, friction, heat, etc. विद्युत्; बिजली

**Electro-.** Prefix denoting relation to electricity. 'विद्युत्' के रूप में प्रयुक्त उपसर्ग

**Electroanaesthesia.** Anaesthesia produced by the electricity; eletroanesthesia. विद्युत्-संज्ञाहरण; विद्युत्-संवेदनाहरण

**Electroanalysis.** Use of electricity in making a chemical analysis. विद्युत्विश्लेषण

**Electroanesthesia.** See **Electroanaesthesia.**

**Electrobiology.** Study of the electric properties of the living beings. विद्युत्-जैविकी; विद्युत्जीवविज्ञान

**Electrobioscopy.** Electric test to determine if life is present. विद्युत्जीवदर्शन

**Electrocardiogram.** A tracing of electromotive variations taking place in the heart during its action. विद्युत्हृद्लेख; विद्युत्यंत्र द्वारा हृदय की धड़कनों का रेखाचित्रण

**Electrocardiograph.** An instrument containing a string galvanometer through which passes the electrical current produced by the heart's contraction. विद्युत्हृद्लेखयंत्र; विद्युत्हृद्लेखी (यंत्र)

**Electrocardiographic.** Relating to electrocardiograph. विद्युत्हृद्लेखी (यंत्र) सम्बन्धी

**Electrocardiography.** See **E.C.G.**

**Electrocauterization.** Cauterization by an electric cautery. विद्युद्दहनकर्म

**Electrocautery.** A metal or platinum wire heated by electricity; an instrument for directing a high frequency current through a local area of tissue. विद्युद्दहनकर्म (उपकरण)

**Electrochemical.** Pertaining to electrochemistry. विद्युत्रासायनिक

**Electrochemistry.** The study of chemic changes produced by electricity. विद्युत्-रासायनिकी; विद्युत् द्वारा उत्पादित रासायनिक परिवर्तनों का अध्ययन

**Electrocoagulation.** Coagulation produced by an electro-cautery. विद्युतातंचन

**Electroconvulsive.** Denoting a convulsive response to an electrical stimulus. विद्युत्-आक्षेपी;

**E. Therapy,** the use of electric shock to produce convulsions; electroshock therapy. विद्युत्-आक्षेपी चिकित्सा

**Electrocorticogram.** The record obtained by electrocorticography. विद्युत्प्रान्तस्थालेख

**Electrocorticography.** The technique of surveying the electrical

**Electrocorticography**

activity of the cerebral cortex. विद्युत्मस्तिष्कप्रान्तस्थालेखन

**Electrocution.** The destruction of life by means of electric current; electrothanasia. विद्युत्मारण

**Electrode.** That part of any electric apparatus designed to be applied to the body. विद्युदग्र; विद्युत्चालक

**Electrodesiccation.** A technique of electric diathermy. विद्युत्शुष्कन

**Electrodiagnosis.** The use of graphic recording of electrical irritability of the tissues in diagnosis. विद्युत्-निदान

**Electrodiagnostic.** Pertaining to electrodiagnosis. विद्युत्-नैदानिक; विद्युत्-निदान सम्बन्धी

**Electroencephalogram.** Graphs of electric impulses that accompany brain activity. विद्युत्मस्तिष्कलेख

**Electroencephalograph.** An instrument by which electrical impulses derived from the brain can be amplified and recorded on paper. विद्युत्मस्तिष्कलेखी; विद्युत्मस्तिष्कलेखयंत्र

**Electroencephalography.** See E.E.G.

**Electrogenesis.** Production by electricity. विद्युत्जनन; बिजली द्वारा उत्पादित

**Electrograph.** A record usually graphically displayed or recorded of the electrical activity produced by biological tissue. विद्युत्लेख

**Electrolysis.** Dissolution of a compound-body by electricity. विद्युत्-अपघटन; विद्युत्पघटन; विद्युत्लयन

**Electrolyte.** A compound capable of resolution by electrolysis. विद्युत्-अपघट्य; विद्युत्पघट्य

**Electromagnetism.** The science which treats of the mutual action of electricity and magnetism. विद्युत्चुम्बकत्व

**Electromassage.** Electric treatment combined with massage. विद्युत्मर्दन

**Electrometer.** An instrument for determining electric intensity. विद्युत्मापी; विद्युत् की तीव्रता को मापने वाला यंत्र

**Electromyogram.** The graphic representation produced by an electromyograph. विद्युत्पेशीलेख

**Electromyograph.** An instrument used in electromyograph. विद्युत्पेशीलेखयंत्र

**Electromyography.** Graphic recording of electrical currents generated in active muscle. विद्युत्पेशीलेखन

**Electron.** Any one of the particles of the cathode ray. विद्युदणु

**Electronegative.** Relating to the electric condition at the negative pole of a battery. विद्युत्ऋण; विद्युत्-ऋणात्मक

**Electro-occulogram.** Graphic record of eye position and movement. विद्युत्-नेत्रलेख

**Electro-oculography.** Oculography using elecrodes placed on the skin adjacent to the lateral canthi to measure a standing potential difference between the front and the back of the eyeball. विद्युत्नेत्रलेखन

**Electrophobia.** A morbid fear of electricity. विद्युत्भीति; विद्युतातंक

**Electrophoresis.** The movement of particles in an electric field toward one or other electric pole, node, or cathode. वैद्युत्कणसंचलन

**Electrophysiology.** The study of electric phenomena in living tissues. विद्युत्शरीरक्रियाविज्ञान

**Electroplexy.** See **Electrotherapy.**

**Electropositive.** The condition of being subject to repulsion by bodies positively electrified and to attraction by bodies negatively electrified. विद्युत्-धनात्मक; विद्युत्-धन

**Electroprognosis.** The use of electricity in prognosis. विद्युत्निदान

**Electroretinogram (ERG).** Graphic record of electrical current generated in active retina. विद्युत्दृष्टिपटललेख

**Electroretinography.** The recording and study of the retinal action currents. विद्युत्दृष्टिपटललेखन

**Electroscope.** An instrument that detects intensity of radiation. विद्युत्दर्शी

**Electroshock.** See **Electrotherapy.**

**Electroshock Therapy.** See **Electroconvulsive Therapy.**

**Electrosurgery.** The use of electricity in surgery. विद्युत्शल्यकर्म; विद्युत्शल्यचिकित्सा

**Electrothanasia.** See **Electrocution.**

**Electrotherapy.** Treatment by electricity; electroplexy. विद्युत्-चिकित्सा; विद्युत्-प्रघात

**Electrotonus.** A change of condition in nerves transversed by an electric current. विद्युत्-तान; विद्युत्तान; नाड़ियों में विद्युत्-धारा से उत्पन्न परिवर्तन

**Electuary.** A confection. अवलेह

**Element.** A fundamental part or principle. तत्व; an indivisible structure or entity. घटक; अवयव

**Elephant Leg.** See **Elephantiasis.**

**Elephantiasis.** A chronic disease characterised by inflammation and obstruction of lymphatics and hypertrophy of the skin and sebaceous tissues; elephant leg. श्लीपद; हाथी-पाँव

**Elevator.** A muscle lifting a part or a surgical instrument for raising a depressed bone. उत्थापक; ऊर्ध्वकर्षक; एलिवेटर

**Elimination.** Discharged from the body. विलोपन; निःसरण; संशोधन; विसर्जन; बहिष्करण

**Elinquid.** Mute. मूक; गूंगा

**Elixation.** A decoction. क्वाथ; काढ़ा; digestion. पाचन

**Elixir.** A sweetened, aromatic solution of a drug, often containing an appreciable amount of alcohol. जल-अक्सीर; सुरस

**Elliptic.** See **Elliptical.**

**Elliptical.** Oval in shape; round; elliptic. अण्डाकार; गोल; दीर्घवृत्तीय

**Elliptocyte.** An elliptical round blood corpuscle found normally in lower vertebrates and in camels; ovalocyte. दीर्घवृत्तकोशिका

**Elliptocytosis.** Anaemia in which the red blood cells are oval. दीर्घवृत्तकोशिकता; अरक्तता का वह रूप जिसमें लाल रक्त कोशिकायें अण्डाकार रहती हैं

**Elongated.** Increased in size. विसृत; दीर्घीभूत; आकार में बढ़ा हुआ

**Elongation.** The condition of being extended, or the process of extending. दीर्घीभवन

**Elution.** Separation by washing or removal by suitable solvent. प्रोद्धावन; क्षालन

**Elutriation.** Process of separating by washing. निक्षालन; धावन; शोधन; धोकर अलग करने की क्रिया

**Elytritis.** Inflammation of vagina. योनिशोथ; योनि का प्रदाह

**Elytroptosis.** Prolapse of the vagina. योनिभ्रंश; योनि की स्थानच्युति

**Emaciate.** To cause to become excessively lean. कृशकाय अर्थात् दुबला-पतला होना

**Emaciated.** Exremely lean. कृश; कृशकाय; दुबला-पतला

**Emaciation.** Extreme loss of flesh. कृशता; मांसक्षय; दुर्बलता; शोष

**Emanation.** Exhalation. प्रसर्जन; निःसरण; निर्गम; विकिरण पदार्थों से निकलने वाला उत्पाद

**Emansio Mensium.** Delayed or suppressed menstruation. रजोलोप; अनार्तव; ऋतुस्राव अथवा मासिक धर्म का देरी से होना या लोप हो जाना

**Emasculation.** Excision of testicles or ovaries. पुंस्त्वहरण; वृषणों अथवा डिम्बग्रन्थियों को काट कर हटा देना

**Embedding.** The fixation of a tissue-specimen in a firm substance before making microscopic sections. अन्त:स्थापन; सम्पुटन

**Embole.** The same as **Embolia.**

**Embolectomy.** Removal of an embolus. अन्त:शल्यनिष्कासन; किसी अन्त:शल्य को निकाल कर हटा देना

**Embolemia.** The presence of emboli in the blood. अन्त:शल्यरक्तता; रक्त में अन्त:शल्य विद्यमान रहना

**Embolia.** See **Embolism.**

**Embolic.** Pertaining to an embolism or embolus. अन्त:शल्य सम्बन्धी; अन्त:शल्यीय

**Emboliform.** Of the form of an embolus. अन्त:शल्याभ; कीलकाभ; अन्त:शल्याकार; अन्त:शल्यरूप; resembling a nucleus. केन्द्रकाभ

**Embolism.** The obstruction of a blood-vessel by an embolus; embolia. अन्त:शल्यता; समावरोध;

Air E., obstruction by a bubble of air. वायु अन्त:शल्यता;

Fat E., obstruction by a fat-globule. वसा अन्त:शल्यता;

Paradoxical E., plugging of an artery by an embolus. अपसामान्यगतिक अन्त:शल्यता;

Pulmonary E., embolism of pulmonary arteries, most frequently by detached fragments of thrombus from a leg or pelvic vein. फुप्फुसधमनी अन्त:शल्यता;

Retrograde E., plugging of vein by a mass carried in a direction opposite to that of the normal blood current. पश्चगतिक अन्त:शल्यता

**Embolus.** A blood clot or other body occluding blood vessel. अन्त:शल्य; थक्का; जमा हुआ रक्त, जो रक्तसंचार में बाधा पैदा कर देता है

**Embrocation.** A fomentation or liniment. मर्दन; मर्दनलेप

**Embryectomy.** Surgical removal of the product of conception. भ्रूणोच्छेदन

**Embryo.** The early state of the foetus; embryon. भ्रूण; गर्भ में पलने वाला सातवें से लेकर नवें सप्ताह तक का शिशु

**Embryocardia.** A condition in which the heart's action resembles that of the foetus. भ्रूणहृदयता; भ्रूणहृदय से मिलती-जुलती क्रिया

**Embryogenetic.** Producing an embryo; embryogenic. भ्रूणजनक

**Embryogenic.** See **Embryogenetic.**

**Embryogeny.** The development of the embryo. भ्रूणविकास; भ्रूणवर्धन

**Embryography.** A description of the embryo. भ्रूणचित्र

**Embryologist.** One who specializes in embryology. भ्रूणविज्ञानी

**Embryology.** The science of embryonic evolution. भ्रूणविज्ञान; भ्रूणिकी; भ्रूण की रचना तथा विकास सम्बन्धी विज्ञान

**Embryoma.** A dermoid or embryonal tumour. भ्रूणार्बुद

**Embryon.** See **Embryo.**

**Embryonal.** Pertaining to the embryo; embryonic. भ्रूणी; भ्रूणीय; भ्रूण सम्बन्धी

**Embryonic.** See **Embryonal.**

**Embryonoid.** Resembling an embryo or foetus. भ्रूणाभ; भ्रूणवत्; भ्रूण से मिलता-जुलता

**Embryony.** The condition of being an embryo. भ्रूणता

**Embryopathy.** Disease or abnormality of the foetus. भ्रूणविकृति

**Embryo-sac.** The first rudiments of an organised being. भ्रूणकोष

**Embryotocia.** Abortion. गर्भपात

**Embryotome.** An instrument used in embryotomy. भ्रूणछेदक; भ्रूणछिद्रक; भ्रूण-उच्छेदक

**Embryotomy.** Mutilation of the foetus to facilitate removal from womb, when natural birth is impossible. भ्रूण-उच्छेदन; कठिनप्रसव में भ्रूण को काटकर निकालना

**Embryotroph.** The nutritive material supplied to embryo during development. भ्रूणपोष

**Embryotrophy.** The nutrition of the embryo. भ्रूणपोषण

**Emergency.** A sudden change in the patient's condition such that immediate medical or surgical intervention is required. आपातस्थिति

**Emesia.** See **Emesis.**

**Emesis.** Vomiting or the act of vomiting; emesia. वमन; वमनोद्रेकं; कै

**Emetic.** Medicine or substance that produces vomiting. वमनकारी; वामक; वमनोत्पादक औषधि अथवा पदार्थ

**Emiction.** Discharge of urine. मूत्रोत्सर्जन;

**Emictory.** A medicine promoting the flow of urine. मूत्रल (औषधि); पेशाब का बहाव बढ़ाने वाली (औषधि)

**Eminence.** A protuberance or process; eminentia. उत्सेध; उभार;
   **Arcuate E.,** see **Eminentia Arcuata.**

**Canine E.,** the ridge over the canine teeth. रदनक उत्सेध; रदनक दांत के ऊपर विद्यमान उभार;

**Collateral E.,** a projection of the lateral ventricle of the brain. समपार्श्वी उत्सेध; मस्तिष्क के पिछले निलय का उभार;

**Frontal E.,** the two eminences of the frontal bone above the superciliary ridges. ललाट उत्सेध; चेहरे की हड्डी का उभार;

**Nasal E.,** the prominence above the root of the nose. नासा उत्सेध; नासिकामूल के ऊपर स्थित उभार;

**Occipital E.,** protuberance on occipital bone. पश्चकपालोत्सेध; सिर की पिछली-हड्डी का उभार;

**Thenar E.,** eminence formed by muscles below the thumb on the palm of the hand. अंगुष्ठमूलोत्सेध; हथेली पर अंगूठे के नीचे का उभार

**Eminentia.** An eminence. उत्सेध; उभार;

**E. Arcuata,** an arched elevation on the surface of the petrous portion of the temporal bone over the superior semicircular canal; arcuate eminence. चापी उत्सेध;

**E. Capitata,** the head of the bone. अस्थि-उत्सेध;

**E. Conchae,** the posterior projection on the pinna corresponding to the concha. शुक्ति उत्सेध; कोंका उत्सेध

**Emissio.** A discharge; emission. उत्सर्जन; स्राव

**Emission.** An ejaculation or sending forth. उत्सर्जन; वीर्यपात; शुक्रमेह; स्वप्नदोष

**Emmenagog.** See **Emmenagogue**.

**Emmenagogue.** A medicine which is supposed to have the power of bringing on menstruation; emmenagog. आर्तवजनक; ऋतुस्रावी; ऋतुस्राव लाने वाली औषधि

**Emmenia.** The menses. आर्तव; ऋतुस्राव; रजोधर्म; माहवारी

**Emmenic.** Menstrual; pertaining to the menses. ऋतुस्रावी; आर्तव अथवा ऋतुस्राव सम्बन्धी

**Emmeniopathy.** A menstrual disorder. आर्तवदोष; ऋतुविकार

**Emmenology.** A treatise on menstruation. आर्तवप्रकरण; आर्तवविज्ञान; रजोधर्मविज्ञान

**Emmetrope.** One endowed with normal vision. सामान्यदृष्टि

**Emmetropia.** The condition of being without ametropia. सामान्यदृष्टिता

**Emollient.** An agent which softens tissues. मृदुकारी; ऊतकों को कोमलता प्रदान करने वाला पदार्थ

**Emotion.** The tone of feeling recognised in ourselves by certain bodily changes, and in others by tendencies to certain characteristic behaviour. आवेश; मनोद्वेग; भावावेग

**Emotional.** Characteristic of or caused by emotion. आवेशी; मनोद्वेगी; भावावेगी; relating to emotion. मनोद्वेग सम्बन्धी; मनोद्वेगी

**Empasm.** A powder to remove a bad personal odour; empasma. उबटन

**Empasma.** See **Empasm.**

**Emphysema.** A condition of dilatation and destruction of the air passages of the lungs, causing breathing difficulties. वातस्फीति; वायुस्फीति;

> **Atrophic E.,** senile emphysema with wasting of lung substance. शोषकर वातस्फीति;
>
> **Interstitial E.,** gas in the connective tissue of any part. अन्तरालीय वातस्फीति;
>
> **Surgical E.,** distension of subcutaneous tissue by air. अधस्त्वक् वातस्फीति;
>
> **Vesicular E.,** dilatation of the air vesicles. कोष्ठकी वातस्फीति

**Emphysematous.** Affected with emphysema. वातस्फीतिग्रस्त

**Empiric.** Practice based on experience alone; empirical. आनुभविक; अनुभव पर आधारित (चिकित्सा)

**Empirical.** See **Empiric.**

**Empiricism.** Quackery; dependence upon experience. दुश्चिकित्सा; अनुभूतचिकित्सा; अनुभव पर आधारित चिकित्सा

**Emplastic.** A constipating medicine. कोष्ठबद्धताकारी; मलबद्धताकारी; कब्ज पैदा करने वाली औषधि

**Emplastra.** Plural of **Emplastrum.**

**Emplastrum.** A plaster. प्लास्टर; पलस्तर

**Emplastrum Adhesivum.** The adhesive plaster. चिपक-पलस्तर

**Emprosthotonos.** Spasm or convulsion by which the body is bent forward; emprosthotonous. वातटंकार; अन्तरायाम

**Emprosthotonous.** See **Emprosthotonos.**

**Emptysis.** Expectoration of blood or blood-stained mucus; haemoptysis. रक्तनिष्ठीवन; बलगम में खून आना

**Empyema.** Accumulation of pus in a cavity or body, especially the chest. अन्तःपूयता; फुप्फुसावरण में पीब भर जाना;

**Pulsating E.,** that attended with pulsation of the chest-wall. स्पन्दी अन्तःपूयता;

**E. Necessitans,** empyema with a spontaneous escape of pus; empyema necessitatis. उद्भेदी अन्तःपूयता;

**E. Necessitatis,** see **Empyema Necessitans.**

**Empyemic.** Relating to empyema. अन्तःपूयता सम्बन्धी

**Empyesis.** Any pustular eruption. पूयस्फोट; पीबदार फुंसी; hypopyon. अग्रकक्षपूयता

**Emulgent.** Draining out; applied to the renal vessels. पायसीकर; स्त्राववर्धक; बाहर निकालने वाला; शोधक

**Emulsification.** The process of making or of becoming an emulsion. इमल्सीकरण; पायसीकरण

**Emulsifier.** An agent used to make an emulsion of a fixed oil. इमल्सीकारक; पायसीकारक

**Emulsify.** To form into an emulsion. इमल्सीकरण; पायसीकरण

**Emulsion.** A fine suspension of an oily substance in a watery medium. इमल्सन; पायस

**Emulsum.** An emulsion. इमल्सन; पायस

**Enamel.** The exterior coating of the teeth; enamelum. दन्तवल्क; दान्तों पर सफेद चमकदार पत्थर

**Enemeloma.** Development of a small nodule of enamel below the cementoenamel junction of molar teeth. दंतवल्कार्बुद

**Enamelum.** See **Enamel.**

**Enanthesis.** Skin eruption due to some internal disease. अन्तःरोगजनित विस्फोट; किसी आन्तरिक रोग के कारण होने वाला चर्म उद्भेद

**Enantiomorphic.** See **Enantiomorphous.**

**Enantiomorphous.** Similar but contracted in form; enantiomorphic. प्रतिबिम्बरूपी

**Enarthrosis.** A ball and socket-joint. उलूखलसन्धि; वह सन्धि जिसमें एक अस्थि का गोल सिरा दूसरी अस्थि के प्यालेनुमा मुख के अन्दर रहता है

**Encapsulation.** The process of surrounding with a capsule. परिसम्पुटन

**Enciente.** Pregnant. गर्भवती; सगर्भा

**Encelitis.** Inflammation of the abdominal viscera. उदरगह्वरशोथ; उदरगह्वर का प्रदाह

**Encephalalgia.** Severe and deep-seated headache. शीर्षार्ति; उग्र एवं गहन सिरदर्द

**Encephalatrophy.** Atrophy of the brain; cerebral atrophy. मस्तिष्कशोष

**Encephalic.** Pertaining to the brain. मस्तिष्क अथवा शीर्ष सम्बन्धी

**Encephalitic.** Relating to encephalitis. मस्तिष्कशोथ सम्बन्धी

**Encephalitis.** Inflammation of the brain and its membranes. मस्तिष्ककलाशोथ; मस्तिष्कशोथ;

   **E. Lethargica,** an epidemic form of encephalitis. जानपदिक मस्तिष्कशोथ;

   **E. Neonatorum,** a form of encephalitis occurring within the first several weeks of life. नवजात मस्तिष्कशोथ

**Encephalocele.** Hernia of the brain. मस्तिष्क-हर्निया

**Encephalogram.** X-ray picture of the cerebal ventricles. मस्तिष्कलेख

**Encephalography.** Radiographic examination of cerebal ventricles after injection of air by means of a lumbar or cisternal puncture. मस्तिष्कचित्रण

**Encephalogy.** The science of the brain. मस्तिष्कविज्ञान

**Encephaloid.** Resembling the substance of the brain. मस्तिष्काभ; मस्तिष्कोपम; मस्तिष्क जैसा

**Encephalolith.** A concretion in the brain. मस्तिष्काश्मरी

**Encephaloma.** A brain tumour; cerebroma. मस्तिष्कार्बुद; मस्तिष्क की रसौली

**Encephalomalacia.** A softening of the brain. मस्तिष्कमृदुता; मस्तिष्क की कोमलता

**Encephalomeningitis.** Combined inflammation of the brain and membranes. मस्तिष्कतानिकाशोथ; मस्तिष्कतानिका का प्रदाह

**Encephalomeningocele.** Hernia of the membranes and brain-substance. मस्तिष्कतानिका-हर्निया

**Encephalomeningopathy.** Any disorder affecting the meninges and the brain; meningoencephalopathy. मस्तिष्कतानिकाविकृति

**Encephalometer.** An apparatus for indicating on the skull the location of the cortical centres. मस्तिष्कप्रान्तस्थामापी

**Encephalomyelitis.** Inflammation of the brain and the spinal cord. मस्तिष्कसुषुम्नाशोथ; मस्तिष्क एवं सुषुम्ना का प्रदाह

**Encephalomyelopathy.** Any disease of the brain and spinal cord. मस्तिष्कसुषुम्नाविकृति; मस्तिष्क और सुषुम्ना का कोई रोग

**Encephalon.** The whole of the brain. मस्तिष्क

**Encephalopathy.** Any disease of the brain. मस्तिष्कविकृति; मस्तिष्क का कोई रोग

**Encephalopyosis.** Purulent inflammation of the brain. सपूयमस्तिष्कशोथ; मस्तिष्क का सपूय प्रदाह

**Encephalosclerosis.** Hardening of the brain. मस्तिष्ककाठिन्य; मस्तिष्क की कठोरता

**Encephalotome.** Instrument for incising brain tissue. मस्तिष्कछेदक

**Encephalotomy.** Dissection or incision of the brain. मस्तिष्कछेदन; मस्तिष्क-उच्छेदन

**Enchondroma.** A cartilaginous tumour; enchondrosis. अन्तरुपास्थ्यर्बुद; उपास्थि-अर्बुद

**Enchondromata.** Plural of **Enchondroma.**

**Enchondrosis.** See **Enchondroma.**

**Encolpitis.** Inflammation of the vaginal mucosa; endocolpitis. योनिश्लेष्मकलाशोथ; योनि की श्लैष्मिक झिल्ली का प्रदाह

**Encopresis.** Involuntary passage of the faeces. असंयतपुरीषता; निरंकुशपुरीषता

**Encrustation.** Incrustation. पर्पटीभवन; पपड़ी बनना

**Encrusted.** Incrusted. पर्पटीमय; पपड़ीमय; पपड़ीदार

**Encyesis.** Normal uterine pregnancy. सामान्य गर्भ

**Encysted.** Inclosed in a cyst or sac. अन्तर्पुटित; परिपुटित; गर्भित; कोषाच्छादित

**End.** A termination; an extremity. अन्त; अन्त्य; छोर;

   **E.-bulb.,** the terminal bulb of a nerve in the skin. अन्त्य कन्द;

   **E.-organ,** the special structure containing the terminal portion of a nerve fibre in peripheral tissue. अन्तांग; अंत्यांग

**Endarterectomy.** Surgical removal of an atheromatous corn from the artery. धमनीअन्त:अस्तर-उच्छेदन

**Endarteritis.** Inflammation of the intima of an artery; endoarteritis. अन्तर्धमनीशोथ; किसी धमनी की आन्तरिक कला का प्रदाह

**Endemic.** A disease which is of local and not of general occurrence. स्थानिक; स्थान-विशेष तक सीमित रोग

**Endemiology.** The science of endemic diseases. स्थानिकरोगविज्ञान; स्थानिक रोगों का वैज्ञानिक अध्ययन

**Endermatic.** See **Endermic**.

**Endermic.** Introduced through the skin by abrading surface; endermatic. त्वग्-प्रवेशी; त्वचा-प्रवेशी; त्वचा द्वारा दी जाने वाली

**Endo-.** Greek preposition, signifying within. 'अन्तः' के रूप में प्रयुक्त होने वाला उपसर्ग

**Endoaortitis.** Inflammation of the intima of the aorta. महाधमनी-अन्तःकलाशोथ; महाधमनी की आन्तरिक कला का प्रदाह

**Endoarteritis.** See **Endarteritis**.

**Endoblast.** The cell-nucleus; entoblast. अन्तःप्रसू; कोशिका-केन्द्रक

**Endobronchitis.** Inflammation of the bronchial mucosa. अन्तःश्वसनी-कलाशोथ; श्वसनी की आन्तरिक कला का प्रदाह

**Endocardia.** Plural of **Endocardium**.

**Endocardiac.** See **Endocardial**.

**Endocardial.** Situated within the heart; endocardia. अन्तर्हृद्; अन्तर्हृद्कला

**Endocarditic.** Relating to endocarditis. अन्तर्हृद्कलाशोथ अथवा अन्तर्हृद्शोथ सम्बन्धी

**Endocarditis.** Inflammation of the lining membrane of the heart, or endocardium. अन्तर्हृद्कलाशोथ; अन्तर्हृद्शोथ; हृदयावरक झिल्ली का प्रदाह;

**Bacterial E.,** one caused by direct invasion of bacteria. जीवाणुज अन्तर्हृद्शोथ;

**Infectious E.,** see **Infective Endocarditis**.

**Infective E.,** that caused due to infection by micro-organisms; infectious endocarditis. संक्रामी अन्तर्हृद्शोथ;

**Rheumatic E.,** endocarditis as a part of the acute rheumatic process with valvular involvement. आमवाती अन्तर्हृद्शोथ;

**Valvular E.,** when one or more heart-valves are affected. हृत्कपाटीय अन्तर्हृद्कलाशोथ; जब एक या अधिक हृत्कपाट प्रभावित रहते हैं

**Endocardium.** The lining membrane of the heart covering the valves. अन्तर्हृद्; अन्तर्हृद्कला; कपाटों को ढक कर रखने वाली हृदयावरक झिल्ली

**Endocervicitis.** Inflammation of the mucosa of the cervix uteri. अन्तर्गर्भाशयग्रीवाशोथ; जरायुग्रीवा की श्लैष्मिक झिल्ली का प्रदाह

**Endocervix.** The mucosa of the cervix uteri. अन्तर्गर्भाशयग्रीवा; जरायुग्रीवा

की श्लैष्मिक झिल्ली

**Endocolpitis.** See **Encolpitis.**

**Endocranitis.** Inflammation of the endorcranium. अन्त:करोटिशोथ; अन्त:कपालशोथ

**Endocranium.** The cerebral duramater. अन्त:करोटि; अन्त:कपाल

**Endocrine.** Secreting internally; ductless. अन्त:स्रावी, नलिकाहीन: नि:स्रोत;

   **E. Glands,** the ductless glands of the body. अन्त:स्रावीग्रन्थियाँ; नलिकाहीनग्रन्थियाँ

**Endocrinologist.** One specializing in endocrinology. अन्त:स्रावविज्ञानी

**Endocrinology.** Study of endocrine glands and internal secretions. अन्त:स्राविकी; अन्त:स्रावविज्ञान; अन्त:स्रावप्रकरण

**Endocrinopathy.** Abnormality of one or more of the endocrine glands or their secretions. अन्त:स्रावी विकृति; अन्त:स्रावी ग्रन्थियों या उनसे होने वाले स्रावों की दोषपूर्ण अवस्था

**Endocrinotherapy.** Treatment with endocrine preparation. अन्त:स्रावीचिकित्सा

**Endocrinous.** Pertaining to endocrine. अन्त:स्रावी; अन्त:स्राव सम्बन्धी

**Endocystitis.** Inflammation of the mucous membrane of the bladder. मूत्राशयश्लेष्मकलाशोथ; मूत्राशय की श्लैष्मिक झिल्ली का प्रदाह

**Endoderm.** See **Entoderm.**

**Endodermal.** Pertaining to the endoderm. अन्त:जनस्तर सम्बन्धी

**Endodontitis.** Inflammation of the internal membrane of the teeth. अन्त:दन्तकलाशोथ; दान्तों की भीतरी झिल्ली का प्रदाह

**Endogenic.** See **Endogenous.**

**Endogenous.** Originating within the body; endogenic. आन्तरिक; अन्तर्जात; बहि:सर

**Endolymph.** Fluid in the inner ear; endolymphaticus. अन्त:कर्णोदक; कान के अन्दर का तरल पदार्थ

**Endolymphatic.** See **Endolymphic.**

**Endolymphaticus.** See **Endolymph.**

**Endolymphic.** Relating to endolymph; endolymphatic. अन्त:कर्णोदकीय; अन्त:कर्णोदक समबन्धी

**Endometrectomy.** Excision of the uterine mucosa; curettage. अन्तर्गर्भाशयकला-उच्छेदन

**Endometria.** Plural of **Endometrium.**

**Endometrial.** Pertaining to the endometrium. अन्तर्गर्भाशयकला सम्बन्धी

**Endometrioma.** A tumour of misplaced endometrium. अन्तर्गर्भाशयकलार्बुद; गर्भाशय की अन्दरूनी झिल्ली की रसौली

**Endometriosis.** The presence of endometrium in abnormal sites. अन्तर्गर्भाशय-अस्थानता

**Endometritis.** Inflammation of the lining membrane of the uterus; blennometritis. अन्तर्गर्भाशयकलाशोथ; जरायु-आवरक झिल्ली का प्रदाह

**Endometrium.** Lining membrane of the uterus. अन्तर्गर्भाशयकला; जरायु की भीतरी झिल्ली

**Endoneurium.** Delicate connective tissue around nerve fibres. अन्तस्तंत्रिकाकला; स्नायु-तन्तुओं के चारों ओर विद्यमान एक कोमल संयोजी ऊतक

**Endoparasite.** An internal parasite. अन्त:परजीवी; पराश्रय परजीवी

**Endopathy.** Any internal disease of the body. अन्त:विकृति; दैहिक विकार; शरीर का कोई आन्तरिक रोग

**Endopericarditis.** Combined endocarditis and pericarditis. अन्तर्हृद्परिहृद्शोथ; हृदय तथा परिहृद् का मिश्र प्रदाह

**Endoperitonitis.** Inflammation of the mucous lining of the peritoneum. अन्त:पर्युदर्यशोथ; उदरावरण की श्लैष्मिक झिल्ली का प्रदाह

**Endophlebitis.** Inflammation of the inner coat of a vein. अन्त:शिराशोथ; अन्तर्शिरावरणप्रदाह; शिरा की अन्दरूनी झिल्ली का प्रदाह

**Endophthalmitis.** Internal infection of eye-globe, usually as a result of perforating injury. अन्तर्नेत्रशोथ; आँख का अन्दरूनी प्रदाह

**Endoplasm.** The inner or medullary part of the cytoplasm. अन्त:प्रद्रव्य

**Endoplasmic.** Relating to endoplasm. अन्त:प्रद्रव्य सम्बन्धी

**Endorhinitis.** Inflammation of the mucous membranes of the nose. अन्तर्नासाकलाशोथ

**Endosalpingitis.** Salpingitis restricted to the lining of the tube without affecting any other part. अन्तर्डिम्बवाहिनीशोथ; डिम्बवाहिनी की अन्दरूनी झिल्ली का प्रदाह

**Endosalpingoma.** Adenomyoma of the uterine tube. अन्तर्डिम्बवाहिनी-अर्बुद

**Endoscope.** An instrument for examining a body cavity through its natural outlet. गुहान्तदर्शी; अन्त:दर्शी

**Endoscopist.** A specialist in the use of endoscope. अन्तर्दर्शनविज्ञानी; गुहान्तदर्शनविज्ञानी

**Endoscopy.** Examination of the body cavities with the endoscope. गुहान्तदर्शन; अन्त:दर्शन

**Endosis.** Intermission of fever. ज्वरोपशम; ज्वरमुक्ति; बुखार उतरना

**Endoskeleton.** The bony frame of the body. अन्त:कंकाल; अस्थिपंजर

**Endosteal.** Relating to the endosteum. अन्तरस्थिकला सम्बन्धी

**Endosteitis.** See **Endostitis.**

**Endosteoma.** See **Endostoma.**

**Endosteum.** The vascular lining membrane of the medullary cavities of the bone. अन्तर्स्थिकला; हड्डी के अन्तस्था-विवरों की रक्तधर झिल्ली

**Endostitis.** Inflammation of the lining membrane of a bone; endosteitis. अन्त:अस्थिवेष्टप्रदाह; अस्थि-आवरक झिल्ली का प्रदाह

**Endostoma.** An osseous tumour within a bone; endosteoma. अन्त:अस्थ्यर्बुद; हड्डी के अन्दर की गिल्टी

**Endothelial.** Pertaining to, or consisting of endothelium. अन्त:अस्तर अथवा अन्तर्कला सम्बन्धी

**Endothelioid.** Resembling endothelium. अन्तर्कलाभ; अन्त:कलाभ; अन्दरूनी झिल्ली से मिलती-जुलती

**Endothelioma.** A tumour of the endothelium. अन्त:कलार्बुद; अन्दरूनी झिल्ली की रसौली

**Endotheliomyoma.** Muscular tumour with elements of endothelium. अन्त:पेशीकलार्बुद

**Endothelium.** The lining membrane of the vascular and serous cavities. अन्त:कला; अन्तर्कला; अन्तश्छद; अन्त:अस्तर

**Endothermal.** See **Endothermic.**

**Endothermic.** Denoting a chemical reaction during the progress of which there is absorption of heat; endothermal. ऊष्माशोषी

**Endotoxicosis.** Poisoning by an endotoxin. अन्तर्जीवविषण्णता

**Endotoxin.** A toxin which remains within the body of a bacterium. अन्तर्जीवविष

**Endotracheal.** Within the trachea. अन्त:श्वासनलीय; श्वासप्रणाल के अन्दर

**Endotracheitis.** Inflammation of the tracheal mucosa. अन्त:श्वासप्रणालशोथ

**Endotrachelitis.** Inflammation of the mucous membrane of the cervix uteri. अन्तर्गर्भाशयग्रीवाशोथ; जरायुग्रीवा की श्लेष्मकला का प्रदाह

**Endotracheloma.** A tumour of the inside of the cervix uteri. अन्तर्गर्भाशयग्रीवार्बुद; जरायुग्रीवा की अन्दरूनी रसौली

**Endyma.** See **Ependyma.**

**Enecia.** Continued fever. अविरामज्वर; सततज्वर

**Enema.** A clyster or injection, especially to move the bowels. गुदवस्ति; वस्तिकर्म; एनिमा

**Energetics.** The science of study of energy. ऊर्जाविज्ञान

**Energizer.** Any substance which increases energy. ऊर्जावर्धक; शक्तिवर्धक; ऊर्जा बढ़ाने वाला पदार्थ-विशेष

**Energy.** Vigour, the power of doing work. ऊर्जा; शक्ति;

   **E. Deficit,** insufficient energy for ordinary demands of living. ऊर्जाल्पता; अल्पूर्जा;

   **Chemical E.,** energy liberated by a chemical reaction. रासायनिक ऊर्जा;

   **Kinetic E.,** the energy of motion. गतिक ऊर्जा; गतिज ऊर्जा;

   **Latent E.,** energy that exists, but is not being used. अदृश्य ऊर्जा;

   **Potential E.,** energy existing in a body by virtue of its position or state of existence, which is not exerted at a time. स्थितिज ऊर्जा;

   **Radiant E.,** that form of energy which is transmitted through space without the support of a sensible medium. विकिरणी ऊर्जा

**Enervate.** To weaken. क्षीण करना; शक्तिहीन करना; अशक्त करना; दुर्बल करना

**Enervated.** Weak; weakened. क्षीण; अशक्त; दुर्बल; कमजोर

**Enervation.** A loss of nervous tone and reduction of strength; a weakening; a weakness. क्षीणता; दुर्बलता; कमजोरी; initial stage of impotency. नपुंसकता की प्रारम्भिक अवस्था

**Engagement.** In obstetrics, the mechanism by which the biparietal diameter of the foetal head enters the plane of inlet. आस्थिति

**Englandular.** Without glands. ग्रन्थिहीन; ग्रन्थिविहीन

**Engorged.** Congested. अतिपूरित; रक्तसंकुलं

**Engorgement.** Accumulation of fluids in vessels and hollow organs. अतिपूरण; अधिरक्तता; अतिरक्तता

**Engram.** Habits affect the protoplasm and leave more or less traces which may be inherited. छाप; चिन्ह; निशान

**Enomania.** Delirium of the drunkards. मद्योन्माद; मद्यात्यय; पियक्कड़ों का प्रलाप

**Enophthalmia.** See **Enophthalmos.**

**Enophthalmos.** Retraction of the eyeball from spasm of the extrinsic eye-muscle; enophthalmia. अन्तर्गताक्षि

**Enostosis.** A tumour in the medullary canal of the bone. अन्तरध्यास्थिता; हड्डी की अन्तस्था-नलिका की रसौली

**Ensiform.** Sword-shaped; xiphoid. खड्गाकार; खड्गवत्

**Enstrophe.** See **Entropion.**

**E.N.T.** Ear, nose and throat. कर्णनासाकण्ठ; कान, नाक और गला

**Ental.** Relating to the interior. आन्तरिक; अन्दरूनी; inside. अन्दर

**Entameba.** See **Entamoeba.**

**Entamoeba.** A genus of parasitic amoeba found in the caecum and large bowel of the human beings; entameba. एण्टअमीबा; मनुष्य की आंतों में पाया जाने वाला एक परजीवी जो पेचिश अथवा आमातिसार के लिये उत्तरदायी होता है

**Entasia.** Tonic spasm; entasis. तानिक-उद्वेष्ट

**Entasis.** See **Entasia.**

**Enteradenitis.** Inflammation of the intestinal glands. आंत्रग्रन्थिशोथ; आंतों की गिल्टियों का प्रदाह

**Enteralgia.** Neuralgia of the bowels. आंत्रशूल; आंत्रार्ति; आंतों का दर्द

**Enteramphalos.** Umbilical hernia. आंत्रबृद्धि; नाभि-हर्निया

**Enterectasia.** Dilatation of the bowels; enterectasis. आंत्रविस्फार

**Enterectasis.** See **Enterectasia.**

**Enterectomy.** Excision of a part of the intestine. आंत्रोच्छेदन; आन्त्र के किसी भाग को काट कर निकाल देना

**Enteralcosis.** Ulceration of the bowel. आंत्रव्रणता

**Enteric.** Intestinal. आंत्रिक; आंत्र सम्बन्धी;

**E. Fever,** typhoid fever. आंत्र-ज्वर; आंत्रिक-ज्वर; मोतीझीरा; टायफाइड; मियादी बुखार

**Enteritis.** A catarrhal inflammation of the intestines. आंत्रशोथ; आन्तों का प्रदाह

**Enteroanastomosis.** See **Enteroenterostomy.**

**Enterobiasis.** Infestation with threadworms. सूत्रकृमिरुग्णता; सूत्रकृमियों के कारण होने वाली बीमारी

**Enterocele.** Hernia in which a portion of intestine is protruded. आंत्र-हर्निया; आंत्र-विस्फार

**Enterocinesia.** Intestinal movement; enterocinesis; enterokinesia; enterokinesis; peristalsis. आंत्रगति

**Enterocinesis.** See **Enterocinesia.**

**Enteroclysis.** The administration of an enema. बृहदांत्रधावन; एनिमा-प्रयोग करना

**Enterocolith.** See **Enterolith**.

**Enterocolithiasis.** See **Enterolithiasis**.

**Enterocolitis.** Inflammation of the small intestines and colon. आंत्रांत्रशोथ; लघ्वांत्रबृहदांत्रशोथ; छोटी तथा बड़ी दोनों आंतों का प्रदाह

**Enterocolonopathy.** Any disease of the intestines and colon. लघ्वांत्रबृहदांत्रविकृति; छोटी आन्तों तथा बड़ी आंत का कोई रोग

**Enterocolostomy.** An operation for joining the intestines and the colon. लघ्वांत्रबृहदांत्रसम्मिलन; छोटी आंतों तथा बड़ी आंत को जोड़ने के लिये किया जाने वाला आपरेशन

**Enterocyst.** See **Enterocystoma**.

**Enterocystoma.** A cystic tumour of the intestines; enterocyst. आंत्रपुटी-अर्बुद; आन्तों का पुटी-अर्बुद

**Enterocystoplasty.** A plastic surgical procedure involving the use of a portion of intestine to enlarge the bladder. आंत्रमूत्राशयसंधान

**Enterodynia.** Pain in the intestine. आंत्रपीड़ा; आंत्रशूल; आंत्रवेदना

**Enteroenterostomy.** The formation of a fistula between two intestinal loops; enteroanastomosis. आन्त्रांत्रसम्मिलन

**Enteroepiplocele.** Hernia of the omentum and the intestine. आंत्रवपाहर्निया; आंत्रवपाविस्फार

**Enterogastric.** Pertaining to the intestines and the stomach. आंत्र एवं जठर सम्बन्धी

**Enterogastritis.** Inflammation of the stomach and intestines. जठरांत्रशोथ; आमाशय तथा आन्तों का प्रदाह

**Enterogenous.** Of intestinal origin. आंत्रमूलक; आंत्रज

**Enterogram.** Tracing or graph of intestinal movement. आंत्र गतिलेख

**Enterokinesia.** See **Enterocinesia**.

**Enterokinesis.** See **Enterocinesia**.

**Enterolite.** See **Enterolith**.

**Enterolith.** A stone in the intestines; enterolite; enterocolith. आंत्राश्मरी; मलाश्मरी; आन्तों की पथरी

**Enterolithiasis.** The formation of intestinal concretions; enterocolithiasis. आंत्राश्मरता; मलाश्मरता; आन्तों के अन्दर पथरियाँ बनना

**Enterology.** The branch of medical science concerned with the intestinal tract. आंत्रविज्ञान

**Enterolysis.** Division of the intestinal adhesions. आंत्रलयन

**Enteromegalia.** See **Enteromegaly.**

**Enteromegaly.** Abnormal enlargement of the intestine; enteromegalia. आंत्रबृद्धि

**Enteromerocele.** Crural hernia. वंक्षणांत्रविस्फार; वंक्षण की आन्त का फैलना या बढ़ना; वंक्षण-हर्निया

**Enteromycosis.** An intestinal disease of the fungal origin. आंत्रकवकता

**Enteron.** The alimentary canal. अन्ननली; भोजननली

**Enteroneuritis.** Inflammation of the intestinal nerves. आंत्रतंत्रिकाशोथ; आंतों की नाड़ियों का प्रदाह

**Enteropathy.** Any disease of the intestines. आंत्रविकृति; आन्तों की कोई बीमारी

**Enteroplasty.** Plastic operation of the intestines. आंत्रसन्धान

**Enteroptosia.** See **Enteroptosis.**

**Enteroptosis.** Prolapse of the intestines; enteroptosia. आंत्रभ्रंश; आन्तों की स्थानच्युति

**Enterorrhaphy.** Suture of the intestines. आंत्रसीवन

**Enteroscheocele.** Scrotal hernia. वृषणकोषविस्फार; अण्डकोष का हर्निया

**Enteroscope.** A device for visually examining the inside of the intestine. आंत्रदर्शी

**Enterospasm.** Increased, irregular and painful peristalsis. आंत्र-उद्वेष्ट; आंतों की ऐंठन

**Enterostenosis.** Stricture of intestines. आंत्रसंकुचन; आन्तों की अस्वाभाविक सिकुड़न

**Enterostomy.** Formation of an intestinal fistula. आंत्रछिद्रीकरण

**Enterotome.** An instrument for opening intestines. आंत्रसंधर; आंत्रछिद्रक; आंत्रछेदक

**Enterotomy.** An intestinal incision. आंत्रछेदन

**Enterotoxin.** A toxin produced in or originating in the intestinal contents. आंत्रजीवविष

**Enterovirus.** The intestinal virus. आंत्रविषाणु

**Enterozoa.** Plural of **Enterozoon.**

**Enterozoon.** An intestinal parasite; entozoon. आंत्रपरजीवी; आंतों के अन्दर रहने वाला परजीवी

**Enthelmintha.** Intestinal worm. आंत्रकृमि; कृमि

**Entheomania.** Religious insanity. धर्मोन्माद; धार्मिक विक्षिप्ति; धार्मिक उन्माद

**Entity.** That which performs a complete whole. परिपूर्णता

**Entoblast.** See **Endoblast.**

**Entoderm.** The simple cell-layer lining the cavity of the primitive intestine; endoderm. अन्त:जनस्तर; अन्तश्चर्म

**Entomology.** The branch of natural history which treats of insects. कीटविज्ञान; कीटविद्या

**Entoptic.** Pertaining to the internal parts of the eye. अन्तर्नेत्रीय; आँखों के आन्तरिक भागों से सम्बन्धित; within the eyeball. अन्तर्नेत्रगोलकीय; नेत्रगोलकों के अन्दर

**Entozoa.** A general name for worms of a variety of kinds; enterozoa. कृमि; आंत्रकृमि

**Entozoon.** Plural of **Entozoa.**

**Entrail.** The intestine; the bowel. आंत्र; आन्त्र; अन्तड़ी

**Entrolith.** A stone of the intestines. आंत्राश्मरी; आंतों की पथरी

**Entropion.** The inversion or turning inward of the eyelashes; enstrophe. अन्तर्वर्त्मता; पलकों का अन्तर्वलन होना अथवा अन्दर की ओर मुड़ना

**Entropium.** The same as **Entropion.**

**Enucleation.** A shelling out, as of a tumour. समूल-निष्कासन

**Enuresis.** Wetting of the bed during sleep; involuntary discharge of urine. असंयतमूत्रता; निरंकुशमूत्रता; शय्यामूत्रण; नींद में पेशाब कर देना;

  **Diurnal E.,** urinary incontinence during the day. दिवा-शय्यामूत्रण; दिन के समय नींद में पेशाब कर देना;

  **Nocturnal E.,** urinary incontinence during the night. निशा-शय्यामूत्रण; रात के समय नींद में पेशाब कर देना

**Envelope.** Anatomically, a structure that encloses or covers. आवरण

**Environment.** External surrounding. पर्यावरण; वातावरण; परिस्थिति

**Enzymatic.** Relating to an enzyme. पाचकरस सम्बन्धी

**Enzyme.** Substance created by living cells whose presence aids no other process within the body or speeds it to completion. प्रकिण्व; पाचकरस; एन्जाइम

**Enzymology.** Science dealing with the structure and function of enzymes. प्रकिण्वविज्ञान; पाचकरसविज्ञान; एन्जाइमिकी

**Enzymolysis.** Chemical change or disintegration due to an enzyme. पाचकरसलयन; प्रकिण्वलयन

**Enzymopenia.** Deficiency of enzyme. प्रकिण्वाल्पता; पाचकरसाल्पता

**Enzynuria.** Presence of enzyme in the urine. प्रकिण्वमेह; पाचकरसमेह

**Eosin.** A rose coloured stain or dye used in histology. इयोसिन; ऊतकविज्ञान अथवा आकारिकी में प्रयुक्त की जाने वाली एक गुलाबी रंग की छान

**Eosinophil.** Cell having an affinity for eosin; eosinophile. इयोसिनरागी; इयोसिनप्रेमी

**Eosinophile.** See **Eosinophil**.

**Eosinophilia.** Increased eosinophils in the blood. इयोसिनरागीकोशिकाबहुलता

**Eosinophilic.** See **Eosinophilous**.

**Eosinophilous.** Staining readily with eosin; eosinophilic. इयोसिनफिली

**Ep-.** Prefix meaning upon. 'अधि' के रूप में प्रयुक्त उपसर्ग

**Eparterial.** Located over or above an artery. अधिधमनीय

**Epaxial.** Above or behind any axis. अध्यक्षीय

**Ependyma.** The lining membrane of the cerebral ventricles, and the spinal cord; endyma. अन्तरीयक; आन्तरीयकला; मस्तिष्क एवं मेरुदण्ड की झिल्ली

**Ependymal.** Pertaining to ependyma. अन्तरीयक अथवा आन्तरीयकला सम्बन्धी

**Ependymitis.** Inflammation of the ependyma. आंतरीयकलाशोथ; अन्तरीयकशोथ; अन्तरीयक-प्रदाह

**Ependymoblast.** An embryonic ependymal cell. आंतरीयकलाप्रसू

**Ependymocyte.** An ependymal cell. आंतरीयकलाकोशिका

**Ependymoma.** Neoplasm arising from the lining of the cerebral ventricles of central canal of the spinal cord. आन्तरीयकार्बुद; आन्तरीयकलार्बुद

**Ephebic.** Pertaining to adolescence. यौवनकाल सम्बन्धी; यौवनकालीन

**Ephebology.** The study of puberty and its changes. यौवनविज्ञान

**Ephelides.** Plural of **Ephelis**.

**Ephelis.** Freckle. चकत्ता; मेचक

**Ephelis ab lgne.** A dermatitis induced by exposure to heat, as toasting, x-rays or other rays. ऊष्मावर्णकता; विकिरणीत्वक्शोथ

**Ephemeral.** Of short duration; lasting but a day, or briefly. अल्पकालिक; एकदिवसीय, अथवा एक दिन का, किन्तु क्षणिक

**Ephidrosis.** Abnormal or excessive sweating. अतिस्वेदलता; स्वेदाधिक्य; अत्यधिक पसीना होना

**Epi-.** Prefix meaning upon. 'अधि', 'अपि', 'उपरि', के रूप में प्रयुक्त उपसर्ग

**Epiblast.** The ectoderm; outer layer of blastoderm. आद्यबहिर्जनस्तर; आद्यकोशिकाप्रसूस्तर; अधिकोरक

**Epiblastic.** Relating to the epiblast. आद्यबहिर्जनस्तरीय

**Epibulbar.** Upon the eyeball. अधिनेत्रगोलक; अधिनेत्रगोलकीय

**Epicanthus.** The mangolian fold of skin from nose to eyebrow. अधिनेत्रकोण

**Epicardia.** The portion of the oesophagus from where it passes diaphragm to the stomach. अधिहृद्

**Epicardium.** Visceral layer of the pericardium. अधिहृद्स्तर; हृदयावरण का अन्तरांगी अस्तर

**Epicolic.** The surface of the abdomen above the colon. अधिबृहदांत्र; बड़ी आंत के ऊपर स्थित उदर-तल

**Epicondyle.** The external condyle of the humerus; epicondylus. अधिस्थूलक; अधिअस्थिकंद

**Epicondyli.** Plural of **Epicondyle**.

**Epicondylitis.** Inflammation of the epicondyle. अधिस्थूलकशोथ; अधिस्थूलक-प्रदाह

**Epicondylus.** See **Epicondyle**.

**Epicranium.** Structures covering the cranium. अधिकपाल; उपकपाल; खोपड़ी को ढक कर रखने वाली बनावटें

**Epicrisis.** The disease-phenomena succeeding crisis. सूक्ष्मसंवेदन

**Epicritic.** Pertaining to the return of a normal condition. सूक्ष्मसंवेदी; सामान्य अवस्था लौटने सम्बन्धी

**Epidemic.** Disease prevalent in a district or country, not necessarily but usually dependent on local causes. जानपदिक; महामारी के रूप में फैलनेवाला; बहुव्यापक; मारक;

    **E. Encephalitis,** sleeping sickness. निद्रारोग

**Epidemiologic.** Pertaining to the study of epidemics. जानपदिक-रोगविज्ञान सम्बन्धी

**Epidemiologist.** A specialist in epidemiology. जानपदिक-रोगविज्ञानी; बहुव्यापकरोगविज्ञानी

**Epidemiology.** The science of epidemic diseases and of epidemics. जानपदिकरोगविज्ञान; बहुव्यापकरोगविज्ञान

**Epiderma.** An outgrowth from the epidermis. बहिर्जनस्तर

**Epidermal.** Pertaining to the epidermis; epidermic. बाह्य त्वचा सम्बन्धी; अधिचर्म सम्बन्धी

**Epidermic.** See **Epidermal**.

**Epidermides.** Plural of **Epidermis**.

**Epidermis.** The outer layer of the skin. बाह्यत्वचा; अधिचर्म; उपत्वक्; बहिश्चर्म

**Epidermitis.** Inflammation of the epidermis or the superficial layer of the skin. अधिचर्मशोथ; बाहरी त्वचा का प्रदाह

**Epidermoid.** Pertaining to or resembling the cuticle. अधिचर्म सम्बन्धी; बाह्यत्वचाभ; अधिचर्माभ; बहिश्चर्म जैसा

**Epidermolysis.** A loosening of the epidermis. बाह्यत्वचालयन; बाहरी त्वचा का ढीला पड़ना

**Epidermoma.** An excrescence on the skin. अधिचर्मार्बुद

**Epididymal.** Relating to the epididymis. अधिवृषण सम्बन्धी

**Epididymectomy.** Operative removal of the epididymis. अधिवृषण-उच्छेदन

**Epididymides.** Plural of **Epididymis**.

**Epididymis.** A small oblong body attached to the posterior surface of the testes. अधिवृषण; उपकोष; उपाण्ड

**Epididymitis.** Inflammation of the epididymis. अधिवृषणशोथ; उपाण्ड-प्रदाह

**Epididymo-orchitis.** Inflammation of the epididymis and the testes. अधिवृषण-वृषणशोथ

**Epididymoplasty.** Surgical repair of the epididymis. अधिवृषणसंधान

**Epididymotomy.** Incision into the epididymis. अधिवृषणछेदन

**Epidosis.** Abnormal growth of any portion of the body. गुल्मता; बृद्धि

**Epidural.** Upon or over the dura. अधिदृढ़तानिक; दृढ़तानिका के ऊपर

**Epifolliculitis.** Inflammation of hair follicles of the scalp. अधिलोमकूपशोथ; अधिरोमकूपशोथ

**Epigastralgia.** Pain in the epigastrium. अधिजठरशूल; अधिजठरार्ति; अधिजठर वेदना

**Epigastric.** Pertaining to the region of the stomach or upper part of the body. अधिजठरीय; अधिजठर प्रदेश सम्बन्धी;

> **E. Relflex,** contraction of the upper portion of the rectus abdominis muscle when skin of the epigastric region is scratched. अधिजठर-प्रतिवर्त;

**Epigastric**

**E. Region,** epigastrium. अधिजठर प्रदेश

**Epigastrium.** The region of the upper and front part of the body. अधिजठर; उदरोर्ध्व प्रदेश

**Epigenesis.** Generation by new and successive formations. पश्चजनन

**Epigenetic.** Relating to epigenesis. पश्चजनन सम्बन्धी

**Epiglottic.** Relating to the epiglottis; epiglottidean. कण्ठच्छद सम्बन्धी

**Epiglottidean.** See **Epiglottic.**

**Epiglottidectomy.** Excision of the epiglottis. कण्ठच्छद-उच्छेदन; कण्ठच्छद को काट कर हटा देना

**Epiglottiditis.** See **Epiglottitis.**

**Epiglottis.** A thin flap-like stucture that lies over the opening to the larynx and aids in keeping fluid and other foreign matter out of air passages. कण्ठच्छद; उपकण्ठ

**Epiglottitis.** Inflammation of the epiglottis; epiglottiditis. कण्ठच्छदशोथ; उपकण्ठप्रदाह

**Epilating.** Removing hair. केशलुंचक; रोमोच्छेदक; केशोन्मूलक

**Epilation.** Eradication of hair. केशलुंचन; केशोन्मूलन; रोमोच्छेदन

**Epilatory.** Depilatory; having the property of removing hair. केशलुंचक; relating to epilation. केशलुंचन सम्बन्धी

**Epilepsia.** Disease of the brain characterized by unconsciousness, convulsive fits, etc.; epilepsy. अपस्मार; मिर्गी; मिरगी

**Epilepsy.** See **Epilepsia.**

**Cortical E.,** see **Focal Epilepsy.**

**Focal E.,** spasmodic contraction of certain groups of muscles due to disease of the cortex; cortical epilepsy. विकारस्थानी अपस्मार;

**Grand-mal E.,** major epilepsy. गुरु अपस्मार;

**Idiopathic E.,** a typical epilepsy. अज्ञातहेतुक अपस्मार;

**Myoclonic E.,** the occurrence of myoclonus and epilepsy in the same patient, the so-called association-disease; myoclonus epilepsy. पेशी-अवमोटनी अपस्मार;

**Myoclonus E.,** see **Myoclonic Epilepsy.**

**Petit-mal E.,** minor epilepsy. लघु अपस्मार; पेटीमाल अपस्मार;

**Psychomotor E.,** attacks characterized by impairment of consciousness and amnesia, often associated with semipurposeful movements of the arms or legs and sometimes with psychic disturbances, such as hallucinations. मनःप्रेरक अपस्मार;

**Reflex E.**, due to some reflex neurosis. प्रतिवर्त अपस्मार

**Epileptic.** Pertaining to epilepsy. अपस्मारक; अपस्मार सम्बन्धी; affected with epilepsy. अपस्मारग्रस्त (रोगी); मिर्गी से पीड़ित व्यक्ति; मिर्गीग्रस्त

**Epileptiform.** Of the form of epilepsy. अपस्माररूपी; मिर्गीरूप

**Epileptogenic.** Producing epilepsy; epileptogenous. अपस्मारजनक; मिर्गी उत्पन्न करने वाला

**Epileptogenous.** See **Epileptogenic.**

**Epileptoid.** Resembling epilepsy. अपस्माराभ; मिर्गी जैसा

**Epileptology.** Study of epilepsy. अपस्मारविज्ञान

**Epilose.** Without hair; bald. खल्वाट; गंजा; केशहीन

**Epimenorrhagia.** See **Epimenorrhoea.**

**Epimenorrhea.** See **Epimenorrhoea.**

**Epimenorrhoea.** Reduction of the length of the menstrual cycle. लघुचक्रीआर्तव; लघुचक्री-बहुऋतुस्राव

**Epimysiotomy.** Incision or section of a muscle within its sheath. परिपेशिकाछेदन; परिपेशिका-उच्छेदन

**Epimysium.** The sheath of areolar tissue surrounding a muscle. परिपेशिका

**Epinephritis.** Inflammation of an adrenal gland. अधिवृक्कग्रन्थिशोथ

**Epinephroma.** A lipomatoid tumour of the kidney. अधिवृक्कार्बुद

**Epinephros.** The suprarenal gland. अधिवृक्कग्रन्थि

**Epineurial.** Relating to the epineurium. परितंत्रिकाकला सम्बन्धी

**Epineurium.** The nerve-sheath. परितंत्रिकाकला

**Epiotic.** Situated above or on the cartilage of the ear. अधिकर्णिक: कर्ण-उपास्थि के ऊपर स्थित

**Epiphora.** Watery eyes; an overflow of tears. अश्रुप्रवाह; अश्रुपात

**Epiphyseal.** Pertaining to an epiphysis. अधिवर्धी; अधिवर्ध सम्बन्धी

**Epiphysis.** A process of bone attached to another by cartilage, which later ossifies. अधिवर्ध

**Epiphysitis.** Inflammation of an epiphysis. अधिवर्धशोथ

**Epiphyte.** A plant growing upon another plant. अधिपादप

**Epiplocele.** Hernia of the omentum. वपा-हर्निया; आंत्रावरणार्बुद

**Epiploenterocele.** Hernia of the omentum and intestine. वपा-आंत्रहर्निया

**Epiploic.** Relating to omentum. वपा सम्बन्धी; आंत्रावरण सम्बन्धी

**Epiploitis.** Inflammation of the omentum or the epiploon. वपाशोथ; आंत्रावरणशोथ

**Epiploon.** Omentum. वपा; आंत्रावरण

**Epiplopexy.** The suturing of the omentum of the inner surface of the abdominal wall. वपापर्युदर्यासीवन; वपास्थिरीकरण

**Episclera.** Loose connective tissue between the sclera and the conjunctiva. अधिश्वेतपटल

**Episcleral.** Upon the sclera of the eye. अधिश्वेतपटलीय; relating to the sclera of the eye. अधिश्वेतपटल सम्बन्धी

**Episcleritis.** Inflammation of the subconjunctival tissues. अधिश्वेतपटलशोथ

**Episioitis.** Inflammation of the vulva. भंगशोथ

**Episioperineoplasty.** Plastic surgery of the perineum and the vulva. मूलाधारभगसंधान

**Episioplasty.** Plastic surgery of the vulva. भगसंधान

**Episiostenosis.** Narrowing of the vulval orifice. भगद्वारसंकीर्णता

**Episiotomy.** Incision of the labia to protect the perineum in labour. भगछेदन

**Epispadial.** Relating to an epispadias. अधिमूत्रमार्ग सम्बन्धी

**Epispadias.** A urethral opening on the dorsum of the penis. अधिमूत्रमार्ग

**Epispastic.** A blistering agent. स्फोटक; स्फोटकर; फफोले अथवा छाले पैदा करने वाला

**Episplenitis.** Inflammation of the capsule of the spleen. प्लीहासम्पुटशोथ

**Epistaxis.** Bleeding from the nose; nosebleed; rhinorrhagia. नासारक्तस्रवण; नकसीर फूटना; नाक से खून आना

**Episternum.** The upper segment of the sternum. अधिउरोस्थिखण्ड

**Episthotonos.** A clonic spasm bending the body forward. वातटंकार

**Epistropheus.** Axis. अक्ष

**Epithalamus.** A small dorsomedial area of the thalamus. अधिचेतक

**Epithelia.** Plural of **Epithelium.**

**Epithelial.** Concerned with epithelium, the layer lining the cavities of the body, alimentary canal, etc. उपकलापरक; उपकला सम्बन्धी

**Epitheliochorial.** Pertaining to the epithelium and the uterus.

उपकलाजरायुज; उपकला एवं जरायु सम्बन्धी

**Epithelising.** Formation of an epithelium. उपकलानिर्माण

**Epithelitis.** Overgrowth and inflammation of the mucosal epithelium. उपकलाशोथ; अधिच्छदशोथ

**Epithelioblastoma.** Epithelial cell tumour. उपकलाप्रसूअर्बुद

**Epitheliogenetic.** See **Epitheliogenic.**

**Epitheliogenic.** Caused by epithelial proliferation; epitheliogenetic. उपकलाजनक

**Epithelioid.** Resembling epithelium. उपकलाभ; अधिच्छदाभ

**Epitheliolysis.** Death of epithelial tissue. उपकलालयन

**Epithelioma.** Cancerous growth of the skin. epithelial cancer; squamous carcinoma. कर्कट-गुल्म ;दिमउपकलार्बुद; चर्मकर्कटता; चमड़ी का कैंसर

**Epithelium.** The cells covering all cutaneous and mucous surfaces together with the secreting cells of glands developed from ectoderm. उपकला; अधिच्छद;

  **Ciliated E.,** a form in which the cells bear cilia. रोमक उपकला;

  **Columnar E.,** that composed of cylindric cells. स्तम्भाकार उपकला;

  **Cubical E.,** see **Cuboidal Epithelioma.**

  **Cuboidal E.,** simple epithelium with cells appearing as cubes in a vertical section; cubical epithelioma. घनीय उपकला;

  **Pavement E.,** a kind composed of cubic cells; simple squamous epithelium. एकस्तरीशल्की उपकला;

  **Simple Squamous E.,** see **Pavement Epithelioma.**

  **Squamous E.,** the cells have been reduced to scaly plates. शल्की उपकला;

  **Stratified E.,** the cells arranged in distinct layers. अस्तरित उपकला;

  **Transitional E.,** intermediate between simple and stratified. परिवर्ती उपकला

**Epitrichium.** Superficial layer of the foetal epidermis. अधिरोमस्तर

**Epizoa.** Plural of **Epizoon.**

**Epizoon.** An animal parasite living on the external surface of the body. पशुपरजीवी; बाह्यत्वचा पर रहने वाले क्षुद्रकीट

**Epizootic.** Widespread disease among animals. पशुपदिक; पशुओं को होने वाला एक महामारी रोग

**Eponychium.** The thickened epitrichium covering the nail-area. अधिनरव

**Epoophorectomy.** Removal of the epoophoron. अधिडिम्बग्रंथि-उच्छेदन

**Epoophori.** Plural of **Epoophoron**.

**Epoophoron.** The parovarium. अधिडिम्बग्रन्थि

**Epulis.** A small elastic tumour of the gums. पुष्पुट; मसूड़ों का एक छोटा-सा लचीला अर्बुद

**Epuloid.** A nodule or mass in the gingival tissue that resembles an epulis. पुष्पुटाभ; पुष्पुटवत्

**Epulosis.** The process of scar formation; cicatrization. पुष्पुटन; क्षतांकन

**Equation.** A collection of chemic symbols so arranged as to indicate the reaction that will take place if the bodies represented by the symbols be brought together. समीकरण

**Equator.** Line encircling a round body and equidistant from both poles. मध्यरेखा

**Equilibration.** The maintenance of equilibrium. साम्यीकरण

**Equilibrium.** A state of balance. साम्य; साम्यावस्था; सन्तुलन;

   **Dynamic E.,** in chemistry, a state of apparent repose created by two reactions proceeding in opposite direction at equal speed. गत्यात्मक साम्यावस्था;

   **Nutritive E.,** a condition in which there is a perfect balance between intake and excretion of nutritive material. आहारिक साम्यावस्था; पोषणज सन्तुलन

**Equivalent.** An equal quality or quantity. तुल्य; तुल्यांक; समान; बराबर

**Eradicate.** To entirely remove, as to eradicate a disease. उन्मूलन करना; नष्ट करना

**Erect.** Upright. उच्छ्रत; ऊर्ध्वशीर्ष; तना हुआ; खड़ा

**Erectile.** Capable of being elevated. उच्छ्रायी; तनने योग्य

**Erection.** The state achieved when erectile tissue is hyperaemic. उच्छ्रता; उत्थान; हर्षण

**Eremophobia.** Fear of being alone. एकान्तभीति

**Erethism.** Morbid energetic action or irritability. अतिक्षोभ्यता; स्नायविक उत्तेजना

**E.R.G.** Abbreviated form of **Electroretinogram**.

**Ergasiomania.** An abnormal desire to be busy at work. कार्योन्माद;

कार्य करते रहने की उत्कट इच्छा

**Ergasophobia.** Abnormal dislike for work or assuming responsibility; ergophobia. कार्यभीति

**Ergastic.** Possessing potential energy. शक्तिसम्पन्न; शक्तिशाली

**Ergophobia.** See **Ergasophobia.**

**Ergot.** A fungus-rye parasite. गदाकरस; अर्गट; अरगट

**Ergotism.** Ill-effects produced by ergot; ergot poisoning. गदाकरसात्यय; अर्गटात्यय; अर्गटविषण्णता

**Erosion.** Eating away; corrosion. अपरदन; क्षरण; कटाव; काट

**Erotic.** Pertaining to love or sexual passion. कामोत्तेजक; कामोद्दीपक; कामुक; प्रेम या रति सम्बन्धी

**Eroticism.** Morbid exaggeration of love; erotism. कामुकता; प्रेमासक्ति

**Erotism.** See **Eroticism.**

**Erotogenic.** Causing sexual excitement. कामोत्तेजक; कामोद्रेकी

**Erotology.** The study of love and its manifestations. प्रेमविज्ञान

**Erotomania.** Insanely uncontrollable sexual passion. कामोन्माद; प्रेमोन्मत्तता

**Erratic.** Irregular. अनियमित; wandering; changing. भ्रमणकारी; चलायमान; परिवर्तनशील

**Errhine.** An agent increasing nasal discharge. नस्य; नाक के स्राव को बढ़ावा देने वाला पदार्थ

**Error.** A defect. दोष; त्रुटि; गलती

**Eructation.** Ejection of wind from the stomach through the mouth; belching. उद्गिरण; डकार

**Eruption.** A discolouration or breaking out of pimples on the skin. विस्फोट; दाना; फुन्सी; उद्भेद

**Eruptive.** Attended by rash, pustules, spots or small blisters. विस्फोटक; फुन्सीदार;

    **E. Fever,** fever attended by rash, pustules, etc., such as measles, scarlatina, small-pox, nettle-rash, herpes, etc. विस्फोटक ज्वर

**Erysipelas.** Inflammatory cutaneous disease characterized by extreme redness. विसर्प

**Erysipelatous.** Having the character of erysipelas. विसर्पी; विसर्पीय

**Erysipeloid.** A non-contagious disease resembling erysipelas. विसर्पाभ; विसर्पवत्

**Erythema.** Abnormal redness of the skin due to local congestion. त्वक्रक्तिमा; त्वग्ररक्तिमा; अरुणिका; चमड़ी पर लाल-लाल दाने;

**E. ab Igne,** see **Erythema Caloricum.**

**E. Caloricum,** a reticulated, pigmented, macular eruption that occurs mostly on skin, from exposure to radiant heat; erythema ab igne. एब-इग्नी त्वग्ररक्तिमा; तापन त्वग्ररक्तिमा;

**E. Induratum,** recurrent hard nodules that frequently break down and form necrotic ulcers. दृढ़ीभूत त्वग्ररक्तिमा;

**E. Infectiosum,** a mild infection characterized by an erythematous mucopapular eruption. संक्रामी त्वग्ररक्तिमा;

**E. Nodosum,** inflammation marked by elevated nodules. पर्विल अरुणिका; पर्विल त्वग्ररक्तिमा;

**E. Toxicum,** flushing of the skin due to allergic reaction to some toxic substance. विषण्ण त्वग्ररक्तिमा

**Erythremia.** Increase of red blood corpuscles. लोहितकोशिकाबहुलता; अतिलोहितकोशिकारक्तता; लाल रक्त कणों का बढ़ना

**Erythroblast.** A rudimentary erythrocyte; hemonormoblast. लोहितकोशिकाप्रसू; लाल रक्तकणों को जन्म देने वाली कोशिका

**Erythroblastosis Foetalis.** A pathological condition in the newborn child due to a difference of child's blood and the mother's blood. गर्भलोहितकोशिकाप्रसूमयता

**Erythrochloropia.** Partial colour blindness with ability to see red and green, but not blue and yellow. नीलपीतवर्णांधता

**Erythrocyanosis.** A condition especially seen in young girls and women in which exposure of the limbs to cold causes them to become swollen and dusky red. लोहितश्यावता

**Erythrocyanosis Frigida.** Vasospastic disease with hypertrophy of arteriolar muscular coat. शीतललोहितश्यावता

**Erythrocytes.** The normal non-nucleated red cells of the circulating blood. लोहितकोशिका; लालरक्तकण; रक्ताणु;

**E. Sedimentation Rate,** see **E.S.R.**

**Erythrocythaemia.** See **Erythrocytosis.**

**Erythrocytolysis.** The alteration, dissolution or destruction of red blood cells; erythrolysis. लोहितकोशिकालयन

**Erythrocytometer.** An instrument for counting erythrocytes. लोहितकोशिकामापी; लोहितकोशिकागणनयंत्र

**Erythrocytopenia.** Deficiency in the number of red blood cells.

लोहितकोशिकाह्रास

**Erythrocytopoiesis.** See **Erythropoiesis.**

**Erythrocytosis.** Overproduction of red cells; erythrocythaemia. लोहितकोशिकाबहुलता; लोहितकोशिकाओं का अत्यधिक बढ़ना

**Erythroderma.** Excessive redness of the skin; erythrodermia. त्वग्लालिमा; रक्तिमत्वक्; त्वचा की अत्यधिक लाली

**Erythrodermia.** See **Erythroderma.**

**Erythrogenesis.** The production of red blood cells. लोहितकोशिकाजनन; लाल रक्त कोशिकाओं की उत्पत्ति होना

**Erythrogenic.** Producing red blood cells. लोहितकोशिकाजनक; लाल रक्त कोशिकाओं की उत्पत्ति करने वाला; pertaining to blood cells. रक्तकोशिकाओं सम्बन्धी

**Erythroid.** Of a reddish colour. रक्तवर्ण; concerning red blood cells. लाल रक्त कोशिकाओं सम्बन्धी

**Erythrolysis.** See **Erythrocytolysis.**

**Erythromelalgia.** A painful affection of the extremities with purplish discolouration of the parts; acromelalgia. रक्तिमशाखार्ति; बाह्यांगों का एक दर्दनाक रोग जिसमें रोगग्रस्त भाग बैंगनी रंग के हो जाते हैं

**Erythrophage.** A phagocyte absorbing haemoglobin. लोहितकोशिकाभक्षक; लाल रक्त कणों का शोषण करने वाला

**Erythropathy.** Disease of the red blood cells. लोहितकोशिकाविकृति

**Erythropenia.** Deficiency in the number of red blood cells. लोहितकोशिकाल्पता

**Erythropia.** See **Erythropsia.**

**Erythropoiesis.** The production of red blood cells; erythrocytopoiesis. लोहितकोशिकाजनन; लाल रक्त कोशिकाओं की उत्पत्ति होना

**Erythropoietic.** Producing red blood cells. लोहितकोशिकाजनक; लाल रक्त कोशिकायें उत्पन्न करने वाला

**Erythropsia.** A disordered state or vision in which everything appears red; erythropia. लोहितदृष्टि; एक रोग-विशेष, जिसमें प्रत्येक वस्तु लाल दिखाई देती है

**Erythrostasis.** Accumulation of red blood cells in vessels due to blood flow having ceased. लोहितकोशिकास्थिरता

**Erythruria.** Passage of red coloured urine. लोहितमेह

**Escape.** To escape from confinement; leak or seep out. निकास; पलायन

**Eschar.** A dry crust, scab, or slough of dead tissue. खुरण्ड; निर्मोक

**Escharotic.** A caustic substances;like potash, that causes death of the part on which it is applied. संक्षारक; दाहक

**Escherichia Coli.** See E. Coli.

**Esculent.** Good for food. भक्ष्य; खाने योग्य

**Esophageal.** Pertaining to the esophagus; oesophageal. ग्रासनली सम्बन्धी

**Esophagi.** Plural of **Esophagus.**

**Esophagismus.** Esophageal spasm; oesophagismus. ग्रासनली-उद्वेष्ट; ग्रासनली की ऐंठन

**Esophagitis.** Inflammation of the oesophagus. ग्रासनलीशोथ; ग्रासनली का प्रदाह

**Esophagocardioplasty.** A reconstructive operation on the oesophagus and cardiac end of the stomach; oesophagocardioplasty. ग्रासनलीहृद्संधान

**Esophagoenterostomy.** Operative formation of a direct communication between the esophagus and the intestine; oesophagoenterostomy. ग्रासनलीआंत्रसम्मिलन

**Esophagomalacia.** Softening of the walls of the esophagus; oesophagomalacia. ग्रासनलीमृदुता

**Esophagoplasty.** Surgical repair of a defect in the wall of the esophagus; oesophagoplasty. ग्रासनलीसंधान

**Esophagoscope.** An instrument for examining the esophagus. ग्रासनलीवीक्षकयंत्र; ग्रासनलीदर्शी

**Esophagoscopy.** An examination of the esophagus with esophagoscope. ग्रासनलीदर्शन

**Esophagostenosis.** Stricture or narrowing of the esophagus; oesophagostenosis. ग्रासनलीसंकीर्णता

**Esophagotomy.** The operation or cutting into the oesophagus. ग्रासनली-उच्छेदन

**Esophagus.** Musculo-membranous canal about nine inches (25 cm.) long extending from the pharynx to the stomach; oesophagus. ग्रासनली; भोजननली का ग्रसनी से आमाशय तक का भाग

**Esophoria.** The tending of the visual lines inward. नेत्रअभिमध्यविचलनप्रवृत्ति

**Esotropia.** An internal deviation of the eyes. नेत्रअभिमध्यविचलन

**E.S.R.** Erythrocytes sedimentation rate. लोहितकोशिका अवसादन दर; रक्त अवसादन दर

**Essence.** The inherent quality of a drug. सत्त्; सार; अर्क; आसव

**Essential.** Necessary; indispensable. आवश्यक; idiopathic. अज्ञातहेतुक

**Ester.** In organic chemistry, a compound formed by the combination of an organic acid with alcohol. ऐस्टर; जैवीअम्ल एवं सुरासार का एक योगिक

**Estervation.** Sexual excitement. कामोत्तेजना; कामोद्रेक

**Esthesia.** Sensation. सम्वेदना

**Esthesiogenesis.** Production of sensation. सम्वेदनाजनन

**Esthesiogenic.** Producing a sensation. सम्वेदनाजनक

**Esthesiology.** Science of the sense organs and functions. सम्वेदनाविज्ञान

**Esthesiometer.** An instrument for determining the state of tactile and other forms of sensibility. सम्वेदनामापी

**Esthesiometry.** Measurement of the degree of tactile and other forms of sensibility. सम्वेदनामिति

**Esthetics.** The branch of philosophy dealing with beauty; aesthetics. सौंदर्यकलाविज्ञान; सौंदर्यविज्ञान

**Esthiomene.** Lupus of the vulva. सत्रणभगशोथ

**Estrus.** Sexual desire; the orgasm. कामोन्माद; कामोद्रेक; मदचक्र

**Ethambutol.** Synthetic tubercular drug. इठाम्बुटोल; ऐलोपैथिक चिकित्सा में प्रयुक्त की जाने वाली एक जीवन-रक्षक औषधि

**Ether.** A liquid anaesthetic which evaporates readily and is inhaled. ईथर; एक निश्चेतनाकारी पदार्थ

**Ethical.** Relating to ethics. नीतिशास्त्र सम्बन्धी

**Ethics.** A code of moral principles derived from a system of values and beliefs. नीतिशास्त्र; आचारसंहिता;

Medical E., a system of principles governing medical conduct, comprising the relationship of a physician to the patient, the patient's family, fellow physicians and society at large. मेडिकल आचारसंहिता; वैद्यक आचार संहिता; वैद्यक नीतिशास्त्र; उपचार संहिता;

Nursing E., a system of principle governing conduct of a nurse. परिचारिका नीतिशास्त्र

**Ethmoid.** A bone in the base of the skull and the sinuses it contains, the latter located between the eyes. झर्झरिका; बहुछिद्रास्थि; कपाल की एक जालीदार हडडी;

**E. Bone,** sievelike spongy bone forming a roof for the nasal fossae. झर्झरिकास्थि

**Ethmoidal.** Relating to the ethmoid bone. झर्झरिका अथवा बहुछिद्रास्थि सम्बन्धी

**Ethmoidectomy.** Surgical removal of part of the ethmoid bone, usually that forming the nasal walls. झर्झरिका-उच्छेदन

**Ethnography.** A description of the races of men. संजातिवृत्त; जातिविज्ञान

**Etiolation.** Paleness; pallor. पाण्डुरता; पीतता; पीलापन; धुँधलापन

**Etiologic.** Pertaining to the etiology; aetiologic. रोगहेतु सम्बन्धी; रोग के कार्य-कारण सम्बन्धी

**Etiologist.** A specialist in etiology; aetiologist. रोगहेतुविज्ञानी

**Etiology.** The history of the causes of a disease; aetiology. रोगहेतु; हेतुकी; हेतु; रोग के कारणों का इतिहास

**Eucrasia.** A sound state of health. स्वस्थ

**Eudiometer.** Apparatus used in analysis of gases. गैसआयतनमापी

**Eugenics.** Race improvement by careful mating to avoid parental taints, peculiarities or abnormalities in offspring. सुजननिकी; सुजननविज्ञान

**Eugonic.** Denoting rapid and relatively luxuriant growth of a bacterial culture. बहुवर्धी

**Eunuch.** A castrated male. नपुंसक; षंढ; हीजड़ा; नामर्द

**Eunuchism.** Sterility in male. नपुंसकता; षंढता; पुरुषबंध्यता; नामर्दी

**Eupatorium Perfoliatum.** Boneset; it is diaphoretic. जलविजया; एक स्वेदल औषधि

**Eupepsia.** Normal digestion. सुपाचन; सामान्य पाचन

**Euphonia.** Having a normal clear voice. सुवाक्; सामान्य एवं स्पष्ट वाणी

**Euphorbium.** A vesicant extract from certain species of **Euphorbia.** यूफोर्बियम; विषैले पदार्थों से प्राप्त गोंद

**Euphoria.** A sense of health; a sense of well-being. सुखाभास; स्वास्थ्यचिंतन

**Eupnea.** See **Eupnoea.**

**Eupnoea.** Normal easy respiration; eupnea. मुक्तश्वसन; सुश्वसन; सामान्य तथा सरल श्वसन

**Eurhythmia.** Harmonious body relationships of the separate organs. सुतालता

**Eustachian Tube.** A partially collapsed canal which admits air from the throat into the middle ear and equalizes pressure on the ear drum. कम्बुकर्णीनली

**Eustachitis.** Inflammation of the eustachian tube. कम्बुकर्णीनलीशोथ; कम्बुकर्णीनली का प्रदाह

**Eutelegenesis.** Artificial insemination. कृत्रिम शुक्रसेचन

**Euthanasia.** An easy painless death. सदय अन्त; सुखद मृत्यु

**Euthenics.** Race betterment through improved hygienic or living conditions. सुजीवनिकी; मानव सुपरिस्थितिकी

**Eutocia.** Easy natural delivery. सहज प्रसव; सुख प्रसव

**Evacuant.** Anything increasing evacuation. रेचक; मलोत्सारक; उत्सारक

**Evacuation.** Movement of the bowels, or passage of urine from the bladder, etc. रेचन; मलोत्सरण; उत्सरण

**Evacuator.** A bladder-irrigating instrument. उत्सारक; मूत्रोत्सारक

**Evagination.** The protrusion of some part or organ from its normal position. बहिर्वलन

**Evaluation.** The judgement of anything. मूल्यांकन

**Evanescent.** Of short duration. क्षणस्थायी; क्षणजीवी

**Evaporating.** Passing off in a vapour. वाष्पन; भाप बन जाना

**Evaporation.** A turning into vapour. वाष्पन; वाष्पीभवन; वाष्पीकरण

**Eventration.** Extrusion of the abdominal viscera उदराशय-निस्सरण; उदरांगों का बाहर निकलना

**Eversion.** A turning out. उद्वर्ती; बाहर की ओर मुड़ना

**Evil.** Disease or illness. रुग्णता; रोग; बीमारी; मरज

**Evisceration.** Removal of the viscera or the internal organs. आशयनिष्कासन; निरसन

**Evolution.** The developing from a simple to a complex, specialized, perfect form. विकास

**Evulsion.** A forcible pulling out or extraction. उत्पाटन; उन्मूलन

**Ex-.** Prefix meaning 'out of' or 'away from'. 'बहि:', के रूप में प्रयुक्त उपसर्ग

**Exacerbation.** Increase in the severity of a disease. प्रकोपन; प्रचण्डता; तीव्रता

**Examination.** Any investigation or inspection made for the purpose of diagnosis. परीक्षा; परीक्षण; जांच

**Exangia.** Any dilatation of a blood vessel. वाहिकाविस्फार

**Exanimation.** Death. मृत्यु; मौत

**Exanthem.** See **Exanthema**.

**Exanthema.** An eruptive disease with fever, as small-pox, measles, etc.; exanthem; exanthum. विस्फोट; उद्भेद; दाना; स्फोटक ज्वर

**Exanthemata.** Plural of **Exanthema**.

**Exanthematous.** Pertaining to, or of the nature of exanthema. विस्फोटक; उद्भेदविषयक

**Exanthum.** See **Exanthema**.

**Exanthum Subitum.** A non-infectious exanthema. असंक्रामी विस्फोट

**Ex. Aq.** See **Ex. Aqua**.

**Ex. Aqua.** Alongwith water; ex. aq. जल के साथ; पानी के साथ

**Excavatio.** See **Excavation**.

**Excavation.** Hollowing out, as of the optic disc; excavatio. खात; गर्त; कोष्ठ

**Excess.** More than the usual. अत्यधिक

**Excessive.** Beyond the ordinary degree, measure or limit. अत्यधिक; बहुत ज्यादा

**Excipient.** A vehicle for administration of the drugs. अनुद्रव्य; अनुपान

**Excision.** The cutting of a part; exsection. उच्छेदन; विच्छेद; काट-छांट; कर्तन

**Excitability.** The capability of responding to stimuli. उत्तेज्यता; उद्दीप्यता

**Excitable.** See **Excitant**.

**Excitant.** An agent stimulating an organ; excitable; exciting. उत्तेजक; उद्दीपक

**Excitation.** Stimulation. उत्तेजन; उद्दीपन

**Excitement.** The state of being excited. उत्तेजना; उद्वेग; उद्दीपन

**Exciting.** See **Excitant**.

**Excitomotor.** Arousing muscular action. उत्तेजनप्रेरक; पेशीउत्तेजनप्रेरक

**Excitomuscular.** Causing muscular activity. पेशीउत्तेजक

**Excitor.** That which incites to greater activity; stimulant. उत्तेजक; उद्दीपक

**Exclusion.** A shunting out. अपवर्जन; बहिष्करण; बहिष्कार

**Excoriate.** To abrade; to strip off the skin in shreds. चर्मविदारण होना या करना; चमड़ी छिल जाना

**Excoriated.** Abraded. निस्त्वचीकृत; निस्त्वचीभूत; छिला हुआ

**Excoriating.** Scraping off of some skin. निस्त्वचनीय; त्वचा छील देने वाला

**Excoriation.** Abrasion of the skin. निस्त्वचन; चर्मविदारण

**Excrement.** Effete matter cast out from the body. उत्सर्ग; मलमूत्र

**Exerescence.** An abnormal or unnatural growth of a part, as a wart or tumour. उद्वर्ध; अपबृद्धि; गुल्म

**Excreta.** Excreted material, the natural discharge of the body. उत्सर्ग; मल-मूत्र

**Excrete.** To cast out useless material. उत्सर्जन करना; मलोत्सर्ग करना

**Excretion.** The waste product of life to be thrown off from the system. विसर्जन; उत्सर्जन; मलोत्सर्ग; मलत्याग

**Excretory.** Pertaining to the excretion. उत्सर्गी; मलोत्सर्गी

**Excruciating.** Extremely painful. यंत्रणादायक; पीड़ाप्रद; अत्यन्त दर्दनाक

**Excyclophoria.** The tendency toward outward rotation of the upper pole of the cornea. नेत्रबहिश्चक्रीविचलन-प्रवृत्ति

**Excyclotropia.** The vertical median superior pole of the eye is constantly inclined outward; a squint. नेत्रबहिश्चक्रीविचलन; तिर्यक्दृष्टिता

**Exemphalos.** Umbilical hernia. नाभि-हर्निया; नाभि-विस्फार

**Exenteration.** Removal of the viscera. निरसन; अन्तरांगों को निकालना

**Exercise.** Bodily exertion for the sake of restoring the organs and function to a healthy state, or keeping them healthy. व्यायाम; कसरत

**Exerosis.** Excision, or surgical removal of any part or organ. अंगोच्छेदन

**Exflagellation.** The act of extruding actively motile chromatin threads from the body of a male malarial parasite. कशाभोत्पत्ति

**Exfoliation.** Separating or scaling or peeling off in thin layers, as of dead bones and tissues. अपशल्कन; अपपत्रण; पपड़ियाँ उतरना

**Exhalation.** Emission of vapour, air, gas, etc. अपश्वसन; उच्छ्वसन; भाप, हवा, गैस आदि का निकलना

**Exhaustion.** Great loss of vital power. क्लान्ति; श्रान्ति; निर्वातन; थकान

**Exhibit.** To show. प्रदर्शन करना; collection of objects for public inspection. जनता को दिखाने के लिये चीजें जमा करना

**Exhibitionism.** Insanity with exposure of the genitals. प्रदर्शनीयता; पागलपन की वह अवस्था जिसमें रोगी गुप्तांगों का प्रदर्शन करता है

**Exhilarant.** An agent enlivening the mind. उल्लासक; प्रफुल्लित करने वाला

**Exhilaration.** A condition of cheerful spirits. प्रसन्नता; प्रफुल्लता

**Exhumation.** Disinterment of the body. शवोत्खनन; गड़े हुए मुर्दे को निकालना

**Exitus.** Death. मृत्यु

**Exo-.** Prefix meaning 'away from', 'out', 'out of'. 'बाह्य' अथवा 'बहि:' के रूप में प्रयुक्त उपसर्ग

**Exoantigen.** See **Ectoantigen**.

**Exocardia.** See **Ectocardia**.

**Exocardial.** Without, or external to the heart. हृद्बाह्य; बहिर्हृदयी

**Exocrine.** Glands from which the secretion passes **via** a duct; secreting externally. बहि:स्रावी; बाह्यस्रावी

**Exodeviation.** See **Exotropia**.

**Exodic.** Efferent. अपवाही; centrifugal. केन्द्रापसारी

**Exodontist.** One who extracts teeth. दन्तनिष्कासक; दान्त निकालने वाला

**Exodontology.** Branch of dentistry concerned with extraction of teeth. दन्तनिष्कासनविज्ञान

**Exogenetic.** Due to an external cause; exogenous. बहिर्जन्य; बहिर्जात

**Exogenous.** See **Exogenetic**.

**Exomphalos.** See **Exumbilication**.

**Exopathic.** See **Exoteric**.

**Exophoria.** Diverging visual lines; outward squinting. नेत्रबहिर्विचलनप्रवृत्ति; बहिर्तिर्यक्-दृष्टिता

**Exophthalmia.** Protrusion of the eyeball from its orbit. नेत्रोत्सेध; नेत्रगोलकों का अपने कोटर से बाहर की ओर फैलना

**Exophthalmic.** Pertaining to exophthalmos. नेत्रोत्सेधी;
  E. Goitre, Basedow's disease; any of the various forms of hyperthyroidism in which the thyroid gland is enlarged and exophthalmos is present. नेत्रोत्सेधी गलगण्ड; बेसडोव रोग

**Exophthalmometer.** Device for measuring the degree of protrusion of the eyeballs. नेत्रोत्सेधमापी

**Exophthalmos.** Abnormal protrusion of eyeball; exophthalmus.

नेत्रोत्सेध; बहिर्गताक्षि

**Exophthalmus.** See **Exophthalmos.**

**Exoplasm.** The peripheral portion of fluids through membranes; ectoplasm. बहि:परासरण; बाह्यप्रसरण; बहि:प्रदव्य

**Exorbitism.** The same as **Exophthalmus.**

**Exosmosis.** The outward diffusion of fluids through membranes. बहिपरासरण; बाह्यप्रसारण

**Exostoses.** Plural of **Exostosis.**

**Exostosis.** An unnatural growth from a bone. अध्यस्थिता; बाह्य-अध्यस्थि; अस्थ्यर्बुद

**Exoteric.** Of external origin; exopathic. बाह्यमूलीय

**Exothermal.** See **Exothermic.**

**Exothermic.** Concerning the external warmth; exothermal. ऊष्माक्षेपी

**Exotic.** Foreign, as exotic disease. विदेशागत

**Exotoxin.** A toxic product of bacteria which is passed into the environment of the cell during growth. बहिर्जीविविष

**Exotropia.** Outward deviation of the eyes; exodeviation. नेत्रबहिर्विचलन

**Expansion.** An increase in size, or the spreading of any structure. विस्तार

**Expectant.** Pregnant; waiting. गर्भवती; गर्भिणी; सगर्भा

**Expected Date of Dilivery.** See **E.D.D.**

**Expectorant.** Promoting ejection of mucus or other fluids from the lungs. कफोत्सारक; कफनिस्सारक; बलगम निकालने वाली

**Expectoration.** Discharge of mucus with coughing. कफ; बलगम

**Expel.** To wipe out; to drive out. निष्कासन करना; निकालना

**Experience.** The feelings of emotions and sensations as opposed to thinking. अनुभव; तजुर्बा

**Experiment.** A trial. परीक्षण; प्रयोग

**Experimental.** Concerning experiments. परीक्षणात्मक; प्रयोगात्मक; प्रायोगिक

**Expert.** One skilled in science or art. विशेषज्ञ; विज्ञानी; वेत्ता

**Expiration.** Expelling of breath from the lungs. नि:श्वसन; श्वास छोड़ना; death. मृत्यु; अवसान

**Expiratory.** Pertaining to the expiration or death. नि:श्वसन अथवा मृत्यु सम्बन्धी

**Expire.** To breath out or exhale. श्वास छोड़ना; to die. मरना; मृत्यु हो जाना

**Expired.** Breath expelled from the lungs. निःश्वसित; फेफड़ों से छोड़ा हुआ श्वास; died. मृत

**Expirium.** The same as **Expiration.**

**Exploration.** An investigation, as in physical diagnosis. अन्वेषण; जांच-पड़ताल

**Exploratory.** Pertaining to exploration. अन्वेषी; अन्वेषण सम्बन्धी

**Expression.** Facial disclosure of feelings, moods, etc. अभिव्यंजना; अभिव्यक्ति; भावाकृति

**Expulsion.** Act of expelling. निष्कासन

**Expulsive.** Tending to expel. निष्कासी; निस्सारक; उत्सर्जनात्मक; बहिष्कारक; रेचक

**Exsanguination.** The act of making bloodless. रक्तापनयन; रक्तहीन करने की क्रिया

**Exsanguinity.** Bloodlessness; anemia. रक्तापनयनता; रक्ताल्पता; अरक्तता

**Exsect.** To excise; to cut out. काट कर हटा देना

**Exsection.** See **Excision.**

**Exsiccant.** Desiccant; an agent that absorbs moisture. उच्छोषक; शुष्ककारी

**Exsiccate.** Desiccate. सुखाना

**Exsiccation.** The process of drying by heat. उच्छोषण; गर्माई देकर सुखाने की प्रक्रिया

**Extension.** Straitening, as an arm, leg or back. प्रसार; फैलाव; विस्तार

**Extensor.** A muscle called **Extensor muscle,** which causes extension of a part. प्रसारक (पेशी)

**Exterior.** Situated on the outer layer. बाह्य; बाहरी

**Externa.** See **External.**

**External.** Outer; externa; exterior. बाह्य; बहिः; बाहरी;

   E. Respiration, breathing, i.e. the visible act of inhaling and expelling breath. बहिःश्वसन; बाह्यश्वसन;

   E. Skeleton, a body framework carried on the outside of the body. बाह्यकंकाल

**Externalia.** Outer genitalia. बाह्य-जननांग

**Exteroceptor.** One of the peripheral organs of the afferent nerves in the skin or the mucous membrane, which responds to stimulation by external agents. बहिःसम्वेदी; बहिर्ग्राही

**Extirpation.** Complete removal or destruction of a part. उन्मूलन

**Extra-articular.** Outside a joint. बहिसंधिज; जोड़ के बाहर

**Extracapsular.** Outside the capsule. बहिसंम्पुटीय; सम्पुट के बाहर

**Extracardiac.** Outside the heart. हृद्बाह्य; हृदय के बाहर

**Extracellular.** Occurring outside the cell. कोशिकाबाह्य; बहिकोंशिकीय

**Extracerebellar.** Outside the cerebellum. अनुमस्तिष्कबाह्य; अनुमस्तिष्क के बाहर

**Extracerebral.** Outside the cerebrum. बहि:प्रमस्तिष्कीय; प्रमस्तिष्क के बाहर

**Extract.** The condensed active principle of a drug; extractum. सार; सत्व; निष्कर्ष;

  **Aqueous E.,** one in which the water is the solvent. जलीय सत्व;

  **Soft E.,** an extract evaporated to the consistence of honey. मृदु सत्व;

  **Solid E.,** one made solid by evaporation. घन सत्व

**Extraction.** A removal. निष्कर्षण; निकालना;

  **Extracapsular E.,** the capsule is ruptured prior to delivery of the lens. बहिसंम्पुट निष्कर्षण;

  **Intracapsular E.,** the lens is removed within its capsule. अन्त:सम्पुट निष्कर्षण

**Extractive.** An extract. सारतत्व; निष्कर्ष; सत्व

**Extractor.** A device for extracting foreign bodies. निष्कर्षक

**Extractum.** An extract. शुष्क सत्व

**Extradural.** Outside the dura-mater. बहिर्दृढ़तानिकी; दृढ़तानिका के बाहर

**Extragenital.** On areas of the body apart from genital organs. जननांगेतर

**Extrahepatic.** Outside the liver. बहिर्यकृती; यकृत् के बाहर

**Extramedullary.** Outside the medulla oblongata. बहिसुषुम्निक; बहिर्मेरुशीर्षी; बहिर्मज्जीय; सुषुम्ना के बाहर

**Extraperitoneal.** Outside the peritoneum. पर्युदर्या के बाहर; उदरावरण के बाहर

**Extrarenal.** Outside the kidney. बहिर्वृक्की; गुर्दे के बाहर

**Extrasystole.** Premature beats in the pulse rhythm. अतिरिक्तप्रकुंचन

**Extrauterine.** Outside the uterus. बहिर्गर्भाशयी; बहिर्गर्भाशयिक; गर्भाशय के बाहर;

**Extrauterine**

    **E. Gestation,** extrauterine pregnancy. अस्थानिक सगर्भता

**Extravasation.** Escape of the fluids of the body from their natural canals and diffusion in the surrounding tissues, as in the bruised conditions. परिस्राव; परिस्रवण; रिसाव

**Extremitas.** See **Extremity.**

**Extremities.** Plural of **Extremity.**

**Extremity.** The outer part of the body, as hand, foot, etc.; extremitas. बाह्यांग; प्रान्त; शाखा

**Extrinsic.** External. बहिरस्थ; बाह्य; बाहरी

**Extroversion.** The condition of being turned inside out. बाह्यावर्तन; बहिर्मुखता

**Extrovert.** Thinking of outward things. बहिर्मुखी; बहिर्चिंतन

**Extrusion.** A pushing or forcing out of a normal position. उत्सरण; बहि:सरण

**Extubation.** The removal of laryngeal tube. नलिकानिष्कासन

**Exuberant.** Excessively proliferating. अतिप्रफलनशील; समृद्ध; growth, as of a tissue or granulation. अधिमांस

**Exudate.** The product of exudation. निःस्राव; पीब; सीरम

**Exudation.** Perspiration; sweat; moisture on the skin; flow of fluid from the blood into a sore. निःस्राव; निर्यास; रिसाव

**Exudative.** Of the nature of an exudate. निःस्रावी

**Exumbilication.** Protrusion of navel; exomphalos. नाभिविस्फार

**Exuviae.** The slough; the cast-off parts. निर्मोक; केंचुली; अवशेष

**Eye.** The organ of vision. नेत्र; चक्षु; अक्षि; आँख;

    **E.-ball,** the globe, ball or apple of the eye. नेत्रगोलक;

    **E.-brow,** the hair, skin and tissues above the eye. भ्रू; भौंह;

    **E.-lash,** the hair of eyelids. अक्षिरोम; पक्ष्म; बरौनी;

    **E.-lid,** palpebra. नेत्रच्छद; वर्त्म; पलक;

    **E.-sight,** vision. दृष्टि; नजर;

    **E. Specialist,** a physician having vast knowledge of the diseases of the eyes and their treatment. नेत्ररोगविज्ञानी; नेत्ररोग विशेषज्ञ;

    **E.-teeth,** the canine teeth in the upper jaw. ऊर्ध्व चर्वणक दन्त

**Eye Bank.** A place where corneas of eyes removed immediately after death are preserved for subsequent keratoplasty. नेत्र बैंक

# F

**F.** Symbol used for **Fahrenheit.**

**Fabella.** A small sesamoid fibrocartilage or bone that sometimes develops in the head of gastrocnemius muscle. माषिका; शिम्बिका; एक तन्तु-उपास्थि अथवा तन्त्वस्थि

**Fabism.** See **Favism.**

**Fabrication.** A deliberately false statement told as if it were true. कपट-रचना; कूट-रचना

**Face.** The front part of the human head, from the head to chin. आनन; चेहरा; मुखमण्डल; ललाट;

   **F. Presentation,** the face of baby coming first in labor. आनन प्रस्तुति;

   **Hippocratic F.,** a pinched expression of the face, with sunken eyes, hollow cheeks and temples, relaxed lips and leaden complexion, observed in one dying after an exhausting illness. हिप्पोक्रैटी चेहरा;

   **Hutchinson's F.,** the peculiar facial expression produced by the drooping eyelids and motionless eyes in ophthalmoplegia. हचिंसनी चेहरा; चांद जैसा चेहरा

   **Moon F.,** full round face seen in Cushing's syndrome. चन्द्र-मुख

**Facet.** A small circumscribed articulating surface of the bone; facette. फलक; फलिका; फेसेट;

   **F. Syndrome,** dislocation of some of the gliding joints between vertebrae causing pain and muscle spasm. चलसन्धिच्युति संलक्षण

**Facetectomy.** Excision of a facet, as of a vertebra. फलकोच्छेदन

**Facette.** See **Facet.**

**Facial.** Pertaining to the face. चेहरे का; आननी; चेहरे सम्बन्धी;

   **F. Angle,** the angle between a line drawn from the upper jaw tangent to the forehead and one from the same point to the external anditory meatus. आनन कोण;

   **F. Centre,** brain centre, causing facial movements. आनन केन्द्र;

   **F. Hemiplegia,** paralysis of one side of the face. अर्ध आननघात; चेहरे के एक ओर का पक्षाघात;

## Facial

**F. Palsy,** see **Facial Paralysis.**

**F. Paralysis,** paralysis of muscles supplied by facial nerves; facial palsy; facioplegia; prosopalgia. आननघात; चेहरे का पक्षाघात;

**F. Reflex,** contraction of facial muscles following pressure on eyeball. आनन प्रतिवर्त;

**F. Spasm,** an involuntary contraction of muscles supplied by the facial nerve, involving one side of the face or the region around the eye. आनन उद्वेष्ट; चेहरे की ऐंठन अथवा अकड़न

**Facies.** The face or the surface of any structure; the expression or appearance of the face; the countenance. मुखाकृति; मुख; चेहरा;

**F. Abdominalis,** pinched, anxious, shrunken, and drawn expression seen in abdominal problems. उदर-मुख;

**F. Cadaverica,** See **Facies Hippocractica.**

**F. Hepatica,** facies seen in liver disease. यकृत् मुख;

**F. Hippocratica,** facies seen in those dying from long-continued illness or from cholera; facies cadaverica. हिप्पोक्रेटी चेहरा; मृत मुखाकृति;

**F. Leontina,** lion-like face seen in certain forms of leprosy. सिंह मुखाकृति;

**F. Ovariana,** the emaciated countenance seen in patients with large ovarian cysts. कृश मुखाकृति;

**Adenoid F.,** open mouthed; vacant expression due to the deafness from enlarged adenoids. ग्रन्थिल मुखाकृति;

**Parkinsonian F.,** a mask-like appearance with infrequent blinking of the eye. पार्किन्सनी मुखाकृति

**Facing.** A tooth-coloured material used to hide the buccal or labial surface of a gold crown to give the outward appearance of a natural tooth. लेपन; दन्ताभलेप

**Facio-.** Prefix denoting firm relation to face. 'मुख' अथवा 'आनन' के रूप में प्रयुक्त उपसर्ग

**Faciobrachial.** Pertaining to the face and arm. आननप्रगण्डपरक; चेहरे व बाजू सम्बन्धी

**Faciocephalgia.** Neuralgia of the face and head. आननशीर्षार्ति

**Faciocervical.** Pertaining to the face and neck. आननग्रैव; चेहरे व गर्दन सम्बन्धी

**Faciolingual.** Relating to the face and the tongue. आननजिह्वापरक; चेहरे व जीभ सम्बन्धी

**Facioplasty.** A plastic operation on the face. आननसंधान

**Facioplegia.** See **Facial Paralysis.**

**Facioscapulohumeral.** Pertaining to the face, shoulder and the arm. आननस्कन्धप्रगण्डीय; चेहरे, कंधे व बाजू सम्बन्धी

**Factitial.** Artificially produced; not natural. कृत्रिम; नकली; बनावटी

**Factitious.** Artificial; unnatural; self-induced. कृत्रिम; नकली; बनावटी;

**F. Disorders,** disorders that are not real, genuine or natural. कृत्रिम विकार; नकली अथवा बनावटी बीमारियां

**Factor.** An agent that is necessary to bring about a given result; one of the contributing causes in any action. कारक; कारण; one of the components which by multiplication makes a number or expression. घटक; gene. जीन; vitamin or other essential element. विटामिन अथवा अन्य आवश्यक तत्व

**Rh. F.,** an antigen present on the surface of erythrocytes. 'रे' फैक्टर; रीसस घटक

**Facultative.** Having the power of living under different conditions; conditional. अनाग्रही; विकल्पी; विकल्पजीवी;

**F. Hyperopia,** a division of manifest hyperopia. विकल्पी दूरदृष्टिता

**Faculty.** Any specific power or function, especially a mental one. गुण; क्षमता; ज्ञान; योग्यता; शक्ति; संकाय

**Faecal.** Pertaining to the faeces; fecal. मल-विषयक; बिष्ठा सम्बन्धी

**Faecalith.** See **Faecolith.**

**Faecolith.** Enterolith, stercolith; fecolith; faecalith; a concretion formed in the bowel from faecal matter. मलाश्मरी; मलपथरी

**Faecaloid.** See **Fecaloid.**

**Faeces.** The stool; the alvine evacuation; feces. बिष्ठा; मल

**Faeniculum Vulgar.** See **Fennel.**

**Faetor.** See **Fetor.**

**F. Oris,** four breathing. दुर्गन्धित श्वास

**Fahrenheit.** The thermometric scale; the freezing point of water is $32°$ F and its boiling point $212°$ F. फारेनहाइट

**Failure.** Inability to function or perform satisfactorily. पात; असफलता;

**Cardiac F.,** See **Heart Failure.**

**Coronary F.,** acute coronary insufficiency; cardiac failure. हृद्पात;

**Respiratory F.,** condition in which the lungs are unable to perform adequately their function of moving air into and carbon–dioxide out of the lungs. श्वासपात; श्वासरोध

**Faint.** Syncope; swooning; a condition of languor. मूर्च्छा; बेहोशी

**Fainting.** See **Faint**.

**Faintness.** A sensation of impending loss of consciousness. निश्चेतनाभाव; बेहोशी; a sensation due to lack of food. खालीपन; खोखलापन

**Falcate.** See **Falciform**.

**Falces.** Plural of **Falx**.

**Falciform.** Sickle-shaped; falcate; falcular. दात्राकार; हंसियाकार;

**F. Ligament,** the triangular ligament attached to sides of the sacrum and coccyx by its base. दात्राकार बन्धन;

**F. Process,** the falx cerebri; the portion of the falciform ligament along the inner margin of the ramus of the ischium. दात्राकार प्रवर्ध; दात्राकार प्रक्रम; प्रमस्तिष्क दात्र

**Falcula.** See **Falx Cerebelli**.

**Falcular.** Falciform. दात्राकार; हंसियाकार; relating to the falx cerebelli. अनुमस्तिष्क दात्र सम्बन्धी

**Fallectomy.** Cutting away the part of the Fallopian tube. डिम्बवाहीनली-उच्छेदन

**Falling of womb.** Displacement or prolapse of uterus; prolapsus uteri. जरायुभ्रंश; गर्भाशयच्युति

**Falling Sickness.** Epilepsy. अपस्मार; मिर्गी

**Fallopian.** Described by or attributed to Fallopius. फेलोपी;

**F. Acqueduct,** see **Fallopian Canal**.

**F. Canal,** the canal in the petrous bone, through which the facial nerve passes; Fallopian acqueduct. फेलोपी नलिका; डिम्बवाही नलिका

**F. Gestation,** tubal gestation. डिम्बवाही गर्भ; डिम्बाशयिक सगर्भता;

**F. Ligament,** long ligament of the uterus. जरायु-बन्ध;

**F. Tube,** one of the two tubes opening out the uppear part of the uterus; the oviduct. डिम्बवाही नली; डिम्बवाही नलिका; फेलोपी नलिका

**Fallotomy.** Division of the Fallopian tube. डिम्बवाहीनली-विभाजन

**False.** Not true; spurium. कूट; मिथ्या; कृत्रिम; अयथार्थ; बनावटी

   **F. Aneurysm,** one due to rupture of the coats of an artery, the effused blood being retained in the tissues. कूट धमनीविस्फार;

   **F. Ankylosis,** adhesive, not bony, union of a part or joint. कूट अस्थिसमेकन;

   **F. Image,** the image formed by the deviating eye in diplopia. कूट प्रतिबिम्ब;

   **F. Membrane,** a morbid product resembling a membrane. कूट कला; अयथार्थ झिल्ली

   **F. Pains,** pains like or resembling labor pains. कूट प्रसववेदनायें; अयथार्थ प्रसव पीड़ायें

   **F. Passage,** a laceration of the urethra by the forcible introduction of an instrument. कूट पथ; कूट द्वार;

   **F. Pelvis,** that portion of the pelvis above the iliopectinal line. कूट गोणिका; कूट वस्ति;

   **F. Ribs,** the five inferior ribs. कूट पर्शुकायें; नीचे की पांच पसलियाँ

**Falx.** Any sickle-shaped structure. दात्र; हंसिया;

   **F. Cerebelli,** a sickle-like process between the cerebellar lobes; falcula. अनुमस्तिष्क दात्र;

   **F. Cerebri,** the portion of the duramater separating the two cerebral hamispheres; falciform process. प्रमस्तिष्क दात्र;

   **F. Ligamentosa,** the broad ligament of the liver. यकृत् दात्र

**Fames.** Hunger. क्षुधा; भूख

**Familial.** Pertaining to the family, as of a disease affecting several members of the same family. पारिवारिक; परिवार सम्बन्धी

**Family.** A group of blood relatives, strictly, the parents and the children. परिवार

**Family Planning.** The planning and spacing of conception of children according to the wishes of the couple rather than to chance. परिवार कल्याण

**Family Practice.** Comprehensive medical care with particular emphasis on the family unit, in which the physician's continuing responsibility for health care is not limited by the patient's age or sex, nor by particular organ, system or disease entity. पारिवारिक चिकित्सा

**Famine.** Severe continued hunger. दुर्भिक्ष; अकाल;

**Famine**

**F. Fever,** relapsing, or typhus fever. दुर्भिक्ष ज्वर

**Fang.** The root or a socketed part of a tooth. दंतमूल; विषदंत

**Fantasy.** A peculiar imagination, where images or chains of images are directed by the desire or pleasure of the thinker, normally accompanied by a feeling of unreality. विलक्षण कल्पना; अद्भुत कल्पना

**Far.** At a distance. दूर;

**F. Point,** the farthest point at which an object can be distinctly seen with the eye in repose. दूरबिन्दु;

**F.-sightedness,** a colloquial term for hypermetropia. दूरदृष्टि

**Farad.** The unit of electric capacity. विद्युत्धारा

**Faradic.** Pertaining to induced electric currents. विद्युत्धारा सम्बन्धी

**Faradisation.** The use of the induced electric current; faradization. विद्युत्प्रेरण;

**Faradism.** The form of electricity furnished by a faradic machine. विद्युत्-रूप; application of induced currents to the treatment of disease. विद्युत्-चिकित्सा

**Faradization.** See **Faradisation.**

**Faradotherapy.** Treatment of disease by faradic current. विद्युत्-चिकित्सा

**Farcinoma.** Glanders. ग्लैण्डर्स

**Farcy.** A chronic form of glanders. चिरकारी ग्लैण्डर्स;

**Farina.** The powdered fecula of grain. तलछट

**Farinaceous.** Containing starch; starchy, i.e. made of flour or grain. मण्डात्मक; मण्डयुक्त; मण्डमय; मण्डीय; pertaining to cerebral substances. प्रमस्तिष्कीय पदार्थों सम्बन्धी

**Farpoint.** The farthest point of vision at which objects can be seen distinctly with eyes in complete relaxation. दूर बिन्दु

**Farsighted.** Pertaining to farsightedness. दूरदृष्टिता सम्बन्धी

**Farsightedness.** Hyperopia; an irror of refraction in which, with accommodation completely relaxed, parallel rays come to a focus behind the retina. दूरदृष्टिता

**Fascia.** A connective tissue sheath consisting of fibrous tissue and fat which unite the skin to the underlying tissues. प्रावरणी; बन्धन; डोरी; पिधानक;

**F. Dentata,** the grey substance of dentate convolution of the cerebrum; dentate fascila. दन्तुर प्रावरणी;

**F. Lata,** the dense fibrous aponeurosis surrounding the thigh. ऊरु प्रावरणी;

**F. Transversalis,** see **Transverse Fascia.**

**Anal F.,** fascia of connective tissue covering levator ani muscle from the perineal aspect. गुदा प्रावरणी

**Aponeurotic F.,** thick fascia that provides attachment for a muscle. कण्डराकला प्रावरणी;

**Cervical F.,** see **Deep Cervical Fascia.**

**Cremasteric F.,** a thin covering of the stretched fibres of the cremaster muscle over the spermatic cord. वृषण-उत्कर्षिका प्रावरणी;

**Cribriform F.,** the sieve-like covering of the sphenous opening. चालनीरूप प्रावरणी;

**Deep Cervical F.,** invests the muscles of the neck and incloses the vessels and nerves. गभीर ग्रैव प्रावरणी;

**Dentate F.,** see **Fascia Dentata.**

**Infundibuliform f.,** the funnel-shaped membrane inclosing the spermatic cord and tastis in a distinct pouch. कीपाकार प्रावरणी;

**Renal F.,** the condensation of the fibroareolar tissue and fat surrounding the kidney to form a sheath for the organ. वृक्क प्रावरणी;

**Superficial F.,** that just beneath the skin. उपरिस्थ प्रावरणी;

**Transverse F.,** the inner surface of the abdominal musculature and the peritoneum; fascia transversalis. अनुप्रस्थिका प्रावरणी

**Fasciae.** Plural of **Fascia.**

**Fascial.** Pertaining to the fascia. प्रावरणीय; प्रावरणी सम्बन्धी;

**F. Reflex,** muscular contraction resulting from percussing facial fascia. प्रावरणीय प्रतिवर्त

**Fascicle.** A small bundle of fires; fasciculus; fasicle. पूलिका; गुच्छा;

**Cuneate F.,** the continuation of the posteromedian column of the spinal cord. कीलाकार पूलिका;

**Fundamental F.,** a portion of the anterior column extending into the oblongata. आधारिक पूलिका;

**Pyramidal F.,** a portion of the anterior column of the cord extending to the pyramid. पिरामिदी पूलिका;

**Solitary F.,** fibres connecting the internal capsule and lenticular nucleus with parts below. एकाकी गुच्छा

# Fascicular

**Fascicular.** Pertaining to a fasciculus; fasciculate; fasciculated. पूलिका सम्बन्धी

**Fasciculate.** See **Fascicular.**

**Fasciculated.** See **Fascicular.**

**Fasciculation.** A visible flickering of muscle. स्फुरण; formation of fascicles. पूलिकाभवन; spontaneous contractions of muscle fibres without causing movement at a joint. पेशीसंकीर्णन

**Fasciculi.** Plural of **Fasciculus.**

**Fasciculus.** A little bundle of fibres, muscles or nerves; fascicle. गुच्छा; पूलिका;

F. Cuneatus, see **Cuneate Fasciculus.**

F. **Fronto-occipitalis,** a bundle of fibres extending from the cortex of the frontal lobe to the cortex of the occipital lobe; fronto-occipital fasciculus. ललाटपश्च-मस्तिष्क पूलिका;

F. **Perpendicularis,** a vertical bundle of fibres from the inferior parietal and superior occipital gyri to the inferior temporal and occipital and the fusiform gyri; fasciluculus rectus. लम्ब-पूलिका;

F. Rectus, see **Fasciculus Perpendicularis.**

F. **Subcallosus,** a tract of fibres passing under the callosum and connecting the frontal, parietal and occipital lobes. अर्धोमहासंयोजक पूलिका;

F. **Unciformis,** fibres connecting the frontal and temporosphenoidal lobes; fasciculus uncinatus; uncinate fasciculus. अंकुश पूलिका;

F. Uncinatus, see **Fasciculus Unciformis.**

**Cuneate F.,** the continuation of the posteromedian column of spinal cord; fasciculus cuneatus. कीलक पूलिका

**Uncinate F.,** see **Fasciculus Unciformis.**

**Fronto-occipital F.,** see **Fasciculus Fronto-occipitalis.**

**Fasciectomy.** Excision of strips of fascia; fasciotomy. प्रावरणी-उच्छेदन; प्रावरणीछेदन

**Fasciitis.** See **Fascitis.**

**Fascioplasty.** A plastic operation on the fascia. प्रावरणीसंधान

**Fasciorrhaphy.** Suture of a fascia or aponeurosis; aponeurorrhaphy. प्रावरणीसीवन

**Fasciotomy.** See **Fasciectomy.**

**Fascitis.** Inflammation of a fascia; fasciitis. प्रावरणीशोथ

**Fasicle.** See **Fascicle.**

**Fast.** To abstain from a food. उपवास; व्रत; resistant to change. स्थाई;
  **Acid-f.,** term applied to bacteria, especially the **Mycobacteria,** that after staining, are not decolourized when treated with acid. अम्लस्थाई

**Fastigii.** Plural of **Fastigium.**

**Fastigium.** (1) The acme; the highest point of a fever or the period of full development of a disease. चरमति; चरमसीमा

**Fasting.** Going without food. उपवास करना; भूखा रहना

**Fastness.** Ability of bacteria to resist stains or destructive agents.

**Fat.** Adipose tissue. वसा ऊतक; वसोतक; an oily substance found in meats, fish, cheese, milk and some vegetables. वसा; स्नेह; भेद; चर्बी; स्निग्ध; corpulent. स्थूलकाय; मोटा
  **F.-cell,** a connective tissue-cell containing oil. वसा-कोशिका;
  **F.-column,** columnar-shaped adipose tissue found in the thicker parts of cutis vera. वसा-खण्ड;
  **F.-necrosis,** necrosis of the fatty tissue occurring in small white areas. वसा-परिगलन;
  **F. Soluble,** capable of being dissolved in body fat. वसा विलेय; चर्बी के साथ घुल जाने वाला

**Fatal.** Pertaining to, or causing death. घातक; मारक;
  **F. Dose,** the dose that kills; lethel dose. घातक मात्रा

**Father.** The male parent. पिता; जनक

**Fatiguability.** Condition in which fatigue is easily induced. क्लान्तिशीलता

**Fatigue.** Weariness, usually from overexertion. थकान; थकावट; श्रान्ति; क्लान्ति
  **F. Diseases,** diseases caused by the constant repetition of certain muscular movements; fatigue fever. क्लान्ति रोग; क्लान्ति ज्वर;
  **F. Fever,** see **Fatigue Diseases.**

**Fatty.** Pertaining to, or combined with fat; oily or greasy. वसीय; वसामय; वसायुक्त; मेदमय;
  **F. Acid,** any acid derived from fats. वसाम्ल;

**Fatty**

> **F. Casts,** that seen in the urine. वसीय निर्मोक; वसा-निर्मोक;
>
> **F. Degeneration,** degeneration of tissues which results in appearance of fatty droplets in cytoplasm, found especially in the diseases of the liver. वसापजनन
>
> **F. Heart,** see Under **Heart.**
>
> **F. Liver,** one marked with fatty degeneration and inflammation. वसा-यकृत्; दसीय यकृत्; मेदमय यकृत्

**Fauces.** The cavity between the mouth and throat bounded by the tongue, the uvula and tonsils and the pharynx, or at the commencement of the throat. गलतोरणिका

**Faucial.** Pertaining to the fauces. गलतोरणिकापरक; गलतोरणिका सम्बन्धी;

> **F. Reflex,** gagging or vomiting resulting from irritation of fauces. गलतोरणिका-प्रतिवर्त

**Faucitis.** Inflammation of fauces. गलतोरणिकाशोथ; गलतोरणिका का प्रदाह

**Faveoli.** Plural of **Faveolus.**

**Faveolus.** A small pit or depression, especially of the skin. गर्त; खात

**Favism.** Fabism, a condition caused in some by eating certain beans, or inhalation of pollen or its flowers, characterized by fever, headache, abdominal pain, severe anaemia, prostration and coma. अदारुणता; दाद का एक रूप जो कुछ फलियां खाने से प्रकट होता है

**Favosus.** A severe type of chronic rengworm, characterized by development of yellow cup-shaped crusts, especially on the scalp. अदारुण; दाद; चमड़ी का एक पपड़ीदार रोग; मण्डलकुष्ठ का एक रूप

**Favus.** Fungal skin disease characterized by pinhead to peasized, saucer-shaped, yellowish crusts over hair follicles and accompanied by musty odour and itching. फेवस; कवकचर्मरोग

**F.D.** Abbreviation for **Fatal Dose.**

**Fear.** Apprehension; dread; alarm; fright; the emotional reaction to an environmental threat. भय; डर

**Feature.** Any single part of the face. मुखाकृति; रूप

**Febricide.** Destructive to fever. ज्वरनाशक; ज्वरहारी

**Febricula.** A mild fever of short duration. ज्वरांश; हरारत; मन्द ज्वर; हल्का-हल्का बुखार

**Febrifacient.** Causing fever; febrifarous; febrific. ज्वरोत्पादक; ज्वरकारी; ज्वरकारक; बुखार पैदा करने वाला

**Febrifarous.** See **Febrifacient.**

**Febrific.** See **Febrifacient.**

**Febrifugal.** See **Febrifuge.**

**Febrifuge.** An agent that lessens fever; febrifugal; antipyretic. ज्वरशामक; ज्वरनाशक

**Febrile.** Pertaining to, or accompanied by fever; feverish; pyretic. ज्वरीय; सज्वर; ज्वर सम्बन्धी

**Febriphobia.** Anxiety or fear induced by a rise in body temperature. ज्वरभीति; ज्वरातंक

**Febris.** Fever. ज्वर; बुखार;

    **F. Amatoria,** chlorosis. रक्ताल्पता; अरक्तता; हरित्पाण्डुता;

    **F. Enterica,** enteric or typhoid fever. आंत्रिक ज्वर;

    **F. Flava,** yellow fever. पीत ज्वर;

    **F. Nervosa,** nervous fever. स्नायविक ज्वर; typhus. मोह ज्वर

**Fecal.** See **Faecal.**

    **F. Vomit,** faeces in vomitus. मल वमन

**Fecalith.** Coproma; coprolith; मलाश्मरी; मलपथरी

**Fecaloid.** Resembling feces; faecaloid. मलाभ; बिष्ठाभ

**Fecaloma.** Coproma; a large mass of accumulated feces in the rectum resembling a tumour; scatoma; stercoroma. मलार्बुद; मलपथरी

**Fecaluria.** Secretion of fecal matter in the urine. मलमेह; बिष्ठामेह

**Feces.** See **Faeces.**

**Fecula.** The starchy part of a seed. हरितरस; हरी वनस्पतियों से निकला माण्ड; sediment. तलछट; अवसाद

**Feculent.** Having sediment, तलछटयुक्त; foul, दुर्गन्धित; excrementitious; fecal. मलाभ; बिष्ठाभ

**Fecund.** Fruitful; capable of conceiving and bearing young; fertile. उर्वर; उपजाऊ

**Fecundate.** To impregnate, fertilize or render fertile. गर्भाधान करना; उर्वर करना; निषेचन करना; संफलन करना

**Fecundated.** Impregnated. उर्वरित; संफलित; निषेचित

**Fecundation.** Fertilization; impregnation; the act of rendering fertile. गर्भाधान; संफलन; निषेचन; निषेक; उर्वर;

    **Artificial F.,** impregnation by injecting the seminal fluid into the uterus by mechanical means; artificial insemination. कृत्रिम गर्भाधान

**Fecundity.** The power of reproduction; ability to produce offspring; fertility. उर्वरता; बहुप्रजता; प्रजननशक्ति; प्रजननता; सुजननता; जननशक्ति

**Feeble.** Weak. दुर्बल; कमजोर; क्षीण; मन्द;

**F.-minded,** of low perception; moron. मन्द-बुद्धि

**Feeding.** Taking or giving nourishment. आहार; भोजन; संभरण;

**Artificial F.,** feeding of a baby with food other than the mother's milk; providing liquid food preparation through a tube passed into the stomach or the rectum. कृत्रिम आहार; कृत्रिम भोजन;

**Breast F.,** feeding of an infant at the breast. स्तनपान

**Feeling.** The conscious phase of nervous activity. अनुभूति

**Feet.** The pedal extremities of the legs. पाद; पैर; पांव

**Fehling's Solution.** An alkaline, copper solution used for the detection and estimation of the amount of the sugar. फाहलिंग घोल

**Fehling's Test.** A glucose test carried out for detecting diabetes. फाहलिंग जांच

**Fel.** Bile. पित्त

**Fellatio.** Coitus per mouth; the sexual act of taking a penis into the mouth. मुखमैथुन; मुखीमैथुन

**Fellifluous.** Flowing with gall. पित्त के साथ बहने वाला

**Felon.** Very painful tumour found on the fingers or toes; whitlow. चिप्प; अंगुलबेढ़ा

**Felty's Syndrome.** Enlargement of liver, spleen and lymph nodes as a complication of rheumatoid arthritis. फेल्टी संलक्षण; यकृत्-बृद्धि

**Female.** In zoology, denoting the sex that bears the young, or the sexual cell which develops into a new organism. स्त्री; महिला; मादा; नारी; त्रिया; औरत;

**F. Catheter,** a short urethral catheter. लघु-मूत्रशलाका

**Feminine.** Concerning or being of the female sex. स्त्री सम्बन्धी; नारीपरक

**Feminization.** The acquisition of female characteristics by the male. स्त्रीभवन; स्त्रीकरण; पुरुष द्वारा स्त्री जैसे लक्षणों का उपार्जन

**Femora.** See **Femur.**

**Femoral.** Relating to the femur or the thigh-bone. और्विक; जघनास्थिक; जांघ की हड्डी से सम्बन्धित;

**F. Artery,** artery that begins at the external iliac artery and terminates behind the knee as the popliteal artery on the inner side of the femur. ऊरु-धमनी;

**F. Canal,** inner compartment of the femoral sheath. ऊरु-नलिका;

**F. Ligament,** the falciform process of the fascia lata. ऊरु-बन्धन;

**F. Reflex,** extension of knee and flexion of foot resulting from irritation of skin over upper anterior third of thigh. ऊरु-प्रतिवर्त;

**F. Ring,** the abdominal end of femoral canal. ऊरु-मुद्रिका;

**F. Sheath,** the fascia covering the femoral vessels. ऊरु-पिधान;

**F. Vein,** continuation of the popliteal vein upward toward the external iliac vein. और्विक शिरा; ऊरु-शिरा

**Femoris.** See **Femur.**

**Os F.,** the thigh bone. जघनास्थि; ऊर्विकास्थि

**Femorocele.** Femoral hernia. ऊरु-हर्निया; और्विक हर्निया; ऊरुस्रंस

**Femoropopliteal.** Usually referring to the femoral and popliteal vessels. ऊरुजानुपृष्ठीय; ऊर्विकाजानुपृष्ठीय

**Femorotibial.** Relating to the femur and the tibia. ऊर्विकान्तर्जंविकी; ऊर्विका तथा अन्तर्जंघा सम्बन्धी

**Femur.** The thigh-bone; the longest and strongest bone in the body; femora; femoris. ऊर्विका; ऊरु-अस्थि; ऊर्वस्थि; नितम्बास्थि; जांघ की हड्डी

**Fenestra.** A windowlike opening. गवाक्ष; द्वार; an aperture frequently closed by a membrane. छिद्र; रंध्र;

**F. Cochleae,** the opening leading into the cochlea. कर्णावर्त्ती गवाक्ष;

**F. Vestibuli,** an oval opening on the inner wall of the middle ear to tympanum leading to the vestibule into which the base of the stapes fits. प्रघाण गवाक्ष

**Fenestrae.** Plural of **Fenestra.**

**Fenestrated.** Having apertures or windowlike openings. गवाक्षित

**Fenestration.** The condition of being perforated. गवाक्षीकरण

**Fennel.** The herb of **Faeniculum vulgar;** the seeds are aromatic and carminative. सौंफ

**Feral.** Deadly. घातक; मारक

**Ferment.** Yeast; a substance which, in small quantities, is capable of setting up changes in another substance without itself undergoing much change. किण्व; खमीर

**Fermentation.** The chemical changes brought about by the action of ferments, usually accompanied by liberation of heat and gas. किण्वन; खमीरण

**Fermentative.** Causing or having the ability to cause fermentation. किण्वनशील; खमीरणशील

**Fermented.** Excited fermentation in. किण्वित; खमीरीकृत; खमीरयुक्त; उफना हुआ

**Fermentemia.** The presence of a ferment in the blood. किण्वरक्तता

**Fermentometer.** An instrument for measuring the fermentation. किण्वनमापी

**Fermentum.** Yeast; a ferment. किण्व; खमीर

**Fern.** A flowerless plant. पर्ण; पर्णांग; फर्न; एक प्रकार का पौधा जिसमें कभी फूल नहीं लगता

**-ferous.** Suffix meaning producing. 'जनक' तथा 'उत्पादक' का अर्थ देने वाला प्रत्यय

**Ferrated.** Combined with, or containing, iron. लौहयुक्त; लौहमिश्रित

**Ferri-, Ferro-.** Prefix used to indicate presence of iron. 'लौह' अथवा 'अयस' का अर्थ देने वाले उपसर्ग

**Ferric.** Pertaining to, or containing iron; ferrous; लोहे सम्बन्धी अथवा लौहयुक्त; denoting a compound containing iron in its trivalent form. लौहयुक्त; लोहस; लौहमिश्रित; अयसी

**Ferrin.** An iron-containing compound isolated from liver tissue. फेरिन

**Ferrokinetics.** The study of iron metabolism using radioactive iron. लोहगतिविज्ञान; लौहचयापचय सम्बन्धी अध्ययन

**Ferrometer.** An apparatus for determining the amount of iron present in the blood. लौहरक्तमापी

**Ferropexia.** Iron fixation. लौहस्थिरीकरण

**Ferrotherapy.** Use of iron in treating anaemia. लौहचिकित्सा; अयसोपचार

**Ferrous.** See **Ferric.**

**Ferruginous.** Associated with or containing iron, लोहमय; लौहयुक्त; लोहस; अयसमय; अयसयुक्त; colour of iron-rust. अयसजंगवर्ण; लोहे पर लगे जंग के रंग जैसा

**Ferrule.** A band or ring of metal applied to the end of the root or crown of a tooth in order to strengthen it. फेरूल; पट्टी या छल्ला

**Ferrum.** The iron. लौह; लोहा; अयस

**Fertile.** Profile; fruitful; fecund, अबन्ध्य; जननक्षम; उर्वर; fertilized; impregnated. संसेचित; निषेचित

**Fertilisation.** The impregnation of an ovum by a spermatozoon; fertilization. संसेचन; निषेचन; उर्वरीकरण; गर्भाधान

**Fertility.** The ability to become a parent; the state of being fertile; fecundity. प्रजननशक्ति; जननक्षमता; जनने की शक्ति; उर्वरता; माता-पिता बनने की योग्यता

**Fertilization.** See **Fertilisation.**

**Fertilizers.** The union of sperm and ovum in conception. संसेचक; निषेचक; उर्वरक

**Fervescence.** Increase of fever. ज्वरबृद्धि; अतिज्वरता

**Fester.** To become inflamed. प्रदाहित होना; to suppurate. पूतिस्राव होना; पीब बनना; an ulcer. व्रण; घाव

**Festers.** Ulcers. व्रण; घाव

**Festinant.** Rapid; quick, द्रुत; तेज; hastening; accelerating त्वरक; त्वरित्र

**Festinating Gait.** See **Festination.**

**Festination.** An involuntary hastening in gait as seen in paralysis agitans; festinating gait. क्षिप्रता; द्रुतगामिता; उछल-उछल कर चलना

**Fetal.** Pertaining to a foetus; foetal. भ्रूण सम्बन्धी;

**F. Membranes,** the membranous structures that serve to protect and support the embryo or foetus and provide its nutrition. भ्रूण कलायें

**Fetation.** See **Foetation.**

**Fetid.** Having a stench or offensive odour; foetid. दुर्गन्धित; बदबूदार

**Fetishism.** A condition in which a particular object is regarded with a strong emotional attachment. वस्तुकामुकता

**Fetochorionic.** Pertaining to the foetus and the chorion or chorionic membrane of the placenta. भ्रूण तथा गर्भाशय सम्बन्धी अथवा अपरा की गर्भाशयिक झिल्ली सम्बन्धी

**Fetography.** Radiography of the foetus in utero; foetography. भ्रूणचित्रण

**Fetology.** The branch of medicine concerned with the study, diagnosis and treatment of the foetus in utero; foetology. भ्रूणविज्ञान

**Fetometry.** Estimation of the size of the foetus, especially of its head, prior to delivery; foetometry. भ्रूणमिति

**Fetopathy.** Disease in a foetus after the third month of pregnancy; Foetopathy; embryopathy. भ्रूणरोग

**Fetoplacental.** Relating to the foetus and its placenta; foetoplacental. भ्रूण तथा अपरा सम्बन्धी

**Fetor.** An offensive odour; stench; faetor; foeter; foetor. दुर्गन्ध; बदबू;

    **F. Exore,** see **Fetor Oris.**

    **F. Oris,** bad breath; halitosis; fetor exore. दुर्गन्धित श्वास; बदबूदार श्वास

**Fetoscope.** A fiberoptic endoscope used in fetoscopy; foetoscope. भ्रूणदर्शन

**Fetoscopy.** Use of a fiberoptic endoscope to view the foetus and placenta, and for collection of foetal blood; foetoscopy. भ्रूणदर्शी

**Fetotoxic.** Anything that is toxic to the foetus. भ्रूणविषण्ण

**Fetus.** See **Foetus.**

    **Papyraceous F.,** see under **Foetus.**

**Fetuses.** Plural of **Fetus.**

**Fever.** Elevation of body temperature above the normal, i.e. $98.4^0$ F or $37^0$ C, though it is still considered normal if it is $1^0$ above or $2^0$ below of this value; pyrexia. ज्वर; बुखार; शरीर का तापमान $98.4^0$ F या $37^0$ C से अधिक होना;

    **Asthenic F.,** one marked by weak circulation, clammy skin and nervous depression. दुर्बलकारी ज्वर; जीर्ण ज्वर;

    **Bilious F.,** with vomiting of bile. पित्त ज्वर;

    **Blackwater F.,** a fatal contagious disease of tropics, with fever, chills, vomiting and dyspnoea. कालामेह ज्वर;

    **Brain F.,** meningitis. मस्तिष्कावरणशोथ; मस्तिष्क ज्वर; दिमागी बुखार;

    **Breakbone F.,** dengue. अस्थिभंजक ज्वर; डेंगू (ज्वर);

    **Camp F.,** typhus. मोह ज्वर; कैम्प ज्वर; सन्निपात ज्वर;

    **Catheter F.,** fever due to the use of the catheter. मूत्रशलाका ज्वर; कैथेटर ज्वर;

    **Cerebrospinal F.,** malignant epidemic fever, with lesions of the cerebral and spinal membranes. प्रमस्तिष्कमेरु ज्वर;

    **Chagres F.,** malignant malarial fever. दुर्दम मलेरिया; सांघातिक मलेरिया;

    **Childbed F.,** puerperal fever. सूतिका ज्वर; प्रसूति ज्वर;

    **Continued F.,** one with an uninterrupted course. सतत ज्वर;

    **Dandy F.,** dengue. डेंगू (ज्वर);

**Dum-dum F.,** kala-azar. काला-आजार; दम-दम ज्वर;
**Enteric F.,** typhoid fever. आंत्रिक ज्वर;
**Eruptive F.,** when accompanied by an eruption; exanthematous fever. विस्फोटक ज्वर;
**Exanthematous F.,** see **Eruptive Fever.**
**Famine F.,** a severe form of relapsing fever. दुर्भिक्ष ज्वर;
**Fracture F.,** one following bone fracture. अस्थिभंग ज्वर;
**Gastric F.,** fever with gastric disturbances. जठरविकृति ज्वर;
**Glandular F.,** epidemic fever of children, with marked swelling of the carotid lymph-glands. ग्रंथि ज्वर; ग्लैंडुलर ज्वर;
**Hay F.,** seasonal disease of nasal mucous membranes, with coryga, catarrhal inflammation and lacrimation. परागज ज्वर;
**Hectic F.,** a type of intermittent fever, with sweats and chills, associated with tuberculosis and septic poisoning. यक्ष्मज ज्वर;
**Intermittent F.,** a fever with periods of apyrexia. विरामी ज्वर; सविराम ज्वर;
**Jungle F.,** malaria. मलेरिया; जंगल ज्वर;
**Low F.,** an asthenic type of fever. जीर्ण ज्वर; दुर्बलतांकारी ज्वर;
**Lung F.,** lobar pneumonia. फुप्फुस-ज्वर; खण्ड-फुप्फुसपाक; खण्डकीय निमोनिया;
**Malarial F.,** malaria; jungle fever. मलेरिया ज्वर;
**Marsh F.,** see **Helodes.**
**Miliary F.,** miliaria. कंगु-विस्फोट; an infectious disease characterized by fever, profuse sweating and the production of sudamina, occurring in severe epidemics. कंगु ज्वर;
**Milk F.,** slight puerperal septicaemia. स्तन्य ज्वर;
**Paratyphoid F.,** an acute infectious disease with symptoms and lesions resembling those of typhoid fever, though milder in character. परांत्रिक ज्वर; आंत्रिक ज्वर का एक मृदु रूप;
**Puerperal F.,** a contagious febrile affection of women in childbed, due to septic poisoning. सूतिका ज्वर; प्रसूति ज्वर;
**Recurrent F.,** see **Relapsing Fever.**
**Relapsing F.,** a contagious fever often associated with famine and poverty; recurrent fever. पुनरावर्ती ज्वर;
**Remittent F.,** one with remision, but no complete apyrexia. अल्पविरामी ज्वर; अल्पविसर्गी ज्वर;

**Fever**

> **Rheumatic F.**, acute rehematism. आमवाती ज्वर; उग्र आमवात;
> **Scarlet F.**, scarlatina. आरक्त ज्वर;
> **Septic F.**, one due to septic poison in the blood septicaemia. पूति ज्वर;
> **Splenic F.**, true anthrax. प्लीहा-ज्वर;
> **Sthenic F.**, one marked by rapid pulse, high temperature and delirium. प्रबल ज्वर;
> **Typhoid F.**, enteric fever. आंत्रिक ज्वर; टाइफाइड ज्वर;
> **Typhus F.**, an epidemic, contagious fever, with eruption and great depression, but no lesion. मोह ज्वर; सन्निपात ज्वर;
> **Yellow F.**, an epidemic disease, with high fever, jaundice, black vomit, etc.; Kandal's fever. पीत ज्वर

**Feverish.** Affected by, indicating, or resembling, a fever. ज्वरमय; ज्वर्वत्; pertaining to fever. ज्वर सम्बन्धी

**Fiat.** Latin term used in recipes which means let there be made; fiant. बनाइये; बनाओ;

> **F. Haustus (Ft. haust.)**, make a draught. एक घूंट बनाओ

**Fiant.** See **Fiat**.

**Fiber.** A filament; threadlike structure; fibre. तन्तु; सूत्र; रेशा;

> **Arciform F.'s**, see **Arcuate Fibers**.
> **Arcuate F.'s**, bow-shaped fibers on the anterior aspect of the oblongata; arciform fibers. चापाकार तन्तु;
> **Association F.**, fiber joining neighbouring or distant areas of the cortex of the same hemisphere. संयोजन तन्तु;
> **Axial F.**, the axial band of a nerve-fiber. अक्षाकार तन्तु;
> **Commissural F.**, fiber joining an area of the cortex of one hemisphere to a similar area of the other hemisphere. परियोजी तन्तु;
> **Projecting F.**, fiber joining the cerebral cortex to lower centres and vice versa; projection fiber. प्रक्षेप तन्तु;
> **Projection F.**, see **Projecting Fiber**.

**Fiberoptic.** Pertaining to fiberoptics. अक्षितन्तुतन्त्र सम्बन्धी

**Fiberoptics.** An optical system whereby light or an image is conveyed by compact, coherent bundle of fine flexible glass or plastic fibers. अक्षितन्तुतन्त्र

**Fiberscope.** An optical instrument that transmits images by fiberoptics. अक्षितन्तुदर्शी

**Fibra.** Fiber. तन्तु

**Fibrae.** Plural of **Fibra.**

**Fibre.** See **Fiber.**

**Fibril.** See **Fibrilla.**

**Fibrilla.** A minute fiber or filament; fibril. सूक्ष्मतन्तु; तन्तुकी

**Fibrillage.** Plural of **Fibrilla.**

**Fibrillar.** Fibrillary; relating to a fibril or fibrilla. सूक्ष्मतन्तु सम्बन्धी

**Fibrillary.** See **Fibrillar.**

**Fibrillate.** To make or to become fibrillar. तन्तुकृत; fibrillated. तन्तुमय

**Fibrillated.** Composed of fibrils; fibrillate. तन्तुमय; सूत्रमय

**Fibrillation.** The formation of fibrils. तन्तुर्विकसन; तन्तुरचना; an irregular, usually rapid rate of excitation of the heart muscles. विकम्पन;

> **Atrial F.,** see **Auricular Fibrillation.**
>
> **Auricular F.,** fibrillation in which the normal rhythmical contractions of the cardiac atria are replaced by rapid irregular twitchings of the muscular wall; atrial fibrillation. अलिन्द विकम्पन;
>
> **Ventricular F.,** fine, rapid, fibrillary movements of the ventricular muscle that raplace the normal contraction. निलय विकम्पन

**Fibrillogenesis.** The development of fine fibrils normally present in collagenous fibers of connective tissue. तन्तुजनन

**Fibrin.** A whitish portion from the body and the serous fluid of the body. फाइब्रिन; आतंच; रक्त जमाने वाला एक वर्णहीन तरल पदार्थ; तांत्विन;

> **F.-ferment,** the ferment turning fibrinogen into fibrin. आतंच-किण्व; फाइब्रिनी खमीर;
>
> **F.-foam,** a white, dry, spongy material made from fibrinogen. आतंच-फेन; फाइब्रिनी झाग

**Fibrination.** Increasing the blood fibrin. फाइब्रिनीभवन; रक्त में फाइब्रिन पदार्थ बढ़ना

**Fibrinocellular.** Composed of fibrin and cells. फाइब्रिनकोशिकी

**Fibrinogen.** A soluble protein of the blood from which is produced the insoluble protein called fibrin and is essential to blood coagulation; fibrogen. फाइब्रिनोजन; फाइब्रोजन

**Fibrinogenesis.** The formation or production of fibrin. फाइब्रिनजनन

**Fibrinogenic.** Pertaining to fibrinogen. फाइब्रिन सम्बन्धी; producing fibrin. फाइब्रिनजनक

**Fibrinogenolysis.** The inactivation or dissolution of fibrinogen in the blood. फाइब्रिनोजनलयन

**Fibrinogenopenia.** Lack of normal concentration of fibrinogen in the blood. अल्पफाइब्रिनरक्तता

**Fibrinogenous.** See **Fibrinogenic**.

**Fibrinoid.** Resembling fibrin. फाइब्रिनवत्; फाइब्रिन से मिलता-जुलता

**Fibrinolysin.** Blood stream enzyme thought to dissolve fibrin occurring after minor injuries; plasmin. फाइब्रिनोलाइसिन; प्लासमिन

**Fibrinolysis.** The hydrolysis or dissolution of fibrin. फाइब्रिनोलयन

**Fibrinopurulent.** Pertaining to pus or suppurative exudate that contains a relatively large amount of fibrin. फाइब्रिनपूतिता सम्बन्धी

**Fibrinosis.** A condition characterized by excess of fibrin. फाइब्रिनता

**Fibrinosus.** See **Fibrinous**.

**Fibrinous.** Composed of fibrin; fibrinosus. फाइब्रिनयुक्त; तान्तुक

**Fibrinuria.** The presence of fibrin in the urine. फाइब्रिनमेह

**Fibroadenoma.** A benign tumour containing fibrous and glandular tissue. तन्त्वर्बुद

**Fibroadipose.** Relating to, or containing both fibrous and fatty structures. तन्तुवसीय

**Fibroareolar.** Composed of fibrous and areolar tissue. तन्तुवृन्तमय

**Fibroblast.** A cell which gives rise to connective tissue; fibrocyte. तन्तुप्रसू

**Fibroblastic.** Relating to fibroblast. तन्तुप्रसू सम्बन्धी

**Fibroblastoma.** Tumour of the connective tissue or fibroplastic (fibre-forming) cells. तन्तुप्रसू-अर्बुद

**Fibrocarcinoma.** Scirrhous carcinoma; a hard, indurated form of cancer. तन्तुकर्कट; तन्तुकैंसर; सिर्सी कैंसर

**Fibrocartilage.** Cartilage containing fibrous tissue. तन्तूपास्थि; तन्तु-उपास्थि

**Fibrocartilaginous.** Relating to, or composed of fibrocartilage. तन्तूपास्थिक

**Fibrocaseous.** A soft, cheesy mass infiltrated by fibrous tissue, formed by fibroblast. तन्तुकिलाटी

**Fibrocellular.** Both fibrous and cellular. तन्तुकोशिकी; तन्तुकी

**Fibrochondritis.** Inflammation of fibrocartilage. तन्तूपास्थिशोथ;

तन्तु-उपास्थि का प्रदाह

**Fibrochondroma.** A benign neoplasm of cartilaginous tissue. तन्तूपास्थ्यर्बुद

**Fibrocyst.** A cystic fibroma; a fibroma which has undergone cystic degeneration. तन्तुपुटी; पुटी-अर्बुद

**Fibrocystic.** Containing fibrous and cystic matter, or pertaining to fibrocyst. तन्तुपुटीय; तन्तुप्रत्यास्थ

**Fibrocystoma.** Fibroma with cystoma. तन्तुपुटी-अर्बुद

**Fibrocyte.** See **Fibroblast.**

**Fibrodysplasia.** Abnormal development of fibrous connective tissue. तन्तुदुर्विकसन

**Fibroelastic.** Composed of collagen and elastic fibers. तन्तुप्रत्यास्थऊतिमय

**Fibroelastosis.** Excessive proliferation of collagenous and elastic fibrous tissue. तन्तुप्रत्यास्थऊतिता

**Fibroenchondroma.** An enchondroma in which neoplastic cartilage cells are situated within an abundant fibrous stoma. तन्तूपास्थि-अर्बुद; तन्तूपास्थ्यर्बुद

**Fibroepithelioma.** A skin tumour composed of fibrous tissue intersected by thin anastomosing bands of basal cells of the epidermis. तन्तूपकलार्बुद

**Fibrogen.** See **Fibrinogen.**

**Fibroglioma.** A fibroid glioma. तन्तुतंत्रिकाबंधार्बुद

**Fibroid.** Having a fibrous structure. तन्तुरूप; तान्तव; तन्त्वाभ; सूत्रोपम; a fibromuscular tumour usually found in the uterus. तन्तुपेशी-अर्बुद; गर्भाशयतन्तुपेशी-अर्बुद; जरायुतन्तुपेशी-अर्बुद;

   **F. Degeneration,** transformation of membraneous tissue into fiberlike material. तन्तुपेशी-अर्बुदापजनन;

   **F. Heart,** a heart affected with fibroid degeneration. तन्तु-हृद्;

   **F. Induration,** see **Fibroid Substitution.**

   **F. Substitution,** cirrhosis; fibroid induration. सिरोसिस; अधितन्तुरुजा; सूत्रण रोग;

   **F. Tumour,** a fibroma. तन्त्वर्बुद

**Fibroidectomy.** Surgical removal of a fibroid tumour. तन्त्वर्बुद-उच्छेदन

**Fibrolipoma.** A fibrous and fatty tumour. तन्तुवसार्बुद

**Fibroma.** A benign tumour composed of fibrous tissue. तन्तु-अर्बुद; तन्त्वर्बुद; सूत्रार्बुद;

**Telangiectatic F.**, angiofibroma. वहिकातंत्वर्बुद

**Fibromatoid.** A focus, nodule or mass that resembles a fibroma, but is not regarded as neoplastic. तन्त्वर्बुदाभ; तन्तु-अर्बुद से मिलता-जुलता

**Fibromatosis.** The occurrence of multiple fibromas, with a relatively large distribution; abnormal hyperplasia of fibrous tissue. तन्तु-अर्बुदता; तन्त्वर्बुदता;

**Palmar F.**, nodular fibroblastic proliferation in the palmar fascia of one or both hands. करतल तन्त्वर्बुदता

**Plantar F.**, nodular fibroblastic proliferation in plantar fascia of one or both feet. पदतल तन्त्वर्बुदता

**Fibromatous.** Pertaining to, or of the nature of, a fibroma. तन्त्वर्बुदीय

**Fibromuscular.** Pertaining to fibrous and muscular tissue. तन्तुपेशीय; तन्तुपेशी-ऊतक सम्बन्धी

**Fibromyectomy.** Excision of a fibromyoma. तन्तुपेश्यर्बुद-उच्छेदन

**Fibromyitis.** Inflammation of a muscle. तन्तुपेशीशोथ

**Fibromyoma.** A muscular and fibrous tumour. तन्तुपेश्यर्बुद; तन्तुपेशी-अर्बुद

**Fibromyositis.** Chronic inflammation of a muscle with an overgrowth, or hyperplasia, of the connective tissue; myogelosis. तन्तुपेशीशोथ

**Fibromyxoma.** A mucous and fibrous tissue. श्लेष्मतन्तूतक

**Fibroneuroma.** A neuroma with fibroid tissue; neurofibroma. तन्तुतंत्रिकार्बुद

**Fibropapilloma.** A papilloma characterized by conspicuous amount of fibrous connective tissue at the base and forming the cores upon which the neoplastic epithelial cells are massed. तन्तु-अंकुरार्बुद; तन्त्वंकुरार्बुद

**Fibroplasia.** Production of fibrous tissue, usually implying an abnormal increase of non-neoplastic fibrous tissue. तन्तुविकसन

**Fibroplastic.** Fiber-forming; producing fibrous tissue. तन्तुजन; तन्तु-निर्माणक;

**F. Tumour**, a small spindle-celled sarcoma. तन्तुजनार्बुद

**Fibroreticulate(d).** Consisting of a network of fibrous tissue. तन्तुजालमय; तन्तुजालाकार

**Fibrosarcoma.** A sarcomatous fibroid tumour. तन्तु-सार्कोमा; सार्कोमी-तन्त्वर्बुद

**Fibrosarcomata.** Plural of **Fibrosarcoma.**

**Fibroserous.** Composed of fibrous tissue in a structure, as a reparative or reactive process. तन्तुसीरमी

**Fibrosis.** The formation of fibrous tissue in a structure, as a reparative or reactive process. तन्तुमयता; तन्तुरुजा

**Fibrositis.** Inflammation of any fibrous tissue. तन्तुशोथ; किसी तन्तु-ऊतक का प्रदाह; muscular rheumatism. पेशी-वात

**Fibrotic.** Pertaining to, or characterized by fibrosis. तन्तुमय; तान्तव

**Fibrous.** Composed of, or containing fibroblasts. तान्तव; तन्तुमय;

    **F. Tissue,** the connective tissue of the body. तन्तु-ऊतक; तन्तूतक

**Fibula.** One of the longest and thinnest bones of the body, situated on the outer side of the leg. बहिर्जंघिका; पिण्डली की बाहरी लम्बी हड्डी

**Fibular.** Pertaining to the fibula. बहिर्जंघिकी; बहिर्जंघिका सम्बन्धी

**Fibulocalcaneal.** Relating to the fibula and the calcaneus. बहिर्जंघिका तथा पार्ष्णिका सम्बन्धी

**Fidgety.** Troublesome uneasiness of the nerves and muscles of the legs, or arms, and an irresistible desire to change their position; uneasy; restless. अशान्त; अधीर; बेचैन

**Field.** A definite area of plane surface. क्षेत्र;

    **F. of vision,** the area in which objects can be seen by the fixed eye; visual field. दृष्टि क्षेत्र;

    **Auditory F.,** the space included within the limits of hearing of a definite sound, as of tuning fork. श्रवण क्षेत्र;

    **Visual F.,** see **Field of Vision.**

**Fifth Nerve.** The trigeminal nerve. पंचम तंत्रिका; त्रिधारा तंत्रिका

**Fig-wart.** Fig-like appearance of a wart. अंजीरी-मस्सा; गूमड़ी

**Filament.** A thread-like structure or membrane. सूत्र; तन्तु

**Filaria.** Parasitic thread-like worm found mainly in the tropics and subtropics. फाइलेरिया; सूत्रवत् कृमि

**Filariasis.** Infestation with filaria, or disease due to filaria in the blood. फाइलेरिया रोग; नारू-रोग; नारू-ज्वर

**Filter-paper.** A coarse paper used for filtration. फिल्टर-पेपर

**Filtration.** The process of staining a liquid through a filter. निस्यंदन

**Filum.** A thread or filament. सूत्र; तन्तु

**Fimbria.** Any structure resembling fringe or border. झल्लरी; झालर

**Finger-print.** An impression of the inked bulb of the distal phalanx of a finger, used as a means of identification. अंगुलि चिन्ह

**Finger-stall.** A rubber cap for a finger. अंगुलि-धानी

**Fins.** Membranous organs of fishes. मीनपंख; मत्स्यपंख; मछलियों के झिल्लीदार अंग

**First-Aid.** Primary help or immediate assistance given in the case of injury or sudden illness. प्राथमिक चिकित्सा; प्रथम सहायता

**First Cranial Nerve.** The olfactory nerve; nerve supplying the nasal olfactory mucosa. घ्राण तंत्रिका

**Fisher's brain-murmur.** A systolic murmur heard ot the anterior fontanelle or in the temporal region in rachitic infants. प्रकुंचन-मर्मर; फिशर-ब्रेन-मर्मर

**Fisher's sign.** A presystolic murmur heard in cases of adherent pericardium without valvular disease. प्रकुंचनपूर्व-मर्मर; फिशर-चिन्ह

**Fish-skin Disease.** See **Ichthyosis**.

**Fission.** A method of reproduction by splitting the bacteria and protozoa in two equal parts; splitting of the nucleus of an atom. विभंजन; विखण्डन;

> **Binary F.,** simple fission in which the two new cells are approximately equal in size. द्वियंगी विखण्डन;
>
> **Simple F.,** division of the nucleus and then the cell body into two parts. सामान्य विभंजन

**Fissiparity.** Origin by fission; schizogenesis. विखण्डनशीलता

**Fissiparous.** Propagating or reproducing by fission. विखण्डनशील

**Fissura.** A groove, cleft, or narrow opening; a fissure. विदर; दरार; दरण; फटन;

> **F. Oris,** the oral fissure. मुख विदर;
>
> **F. Prima,** the main fissure. प्रमुख विदर;
>
> **F. Secunda,** the secondary fissure. गौण विदर

**Fissurae.** Plural of **Fissura.**

**Fissure.** A deep furrow, cleft or slit. विदर; दरार; दरण; फटन; a developmental break or fault in the enamel of a tooth. दंतवल्क-दरण;

> **Anal F.,** a linear ulcer at the margin of the anus. गुदा विदर;
>
> **Auricular F.,** one in petrous bone. बहिकर्ण विदर;
>
> **Dental F.,** see **Dentate Fissure.**

Dentate F., the dental fissure. दन्त विदर;

Occipital F., a deep fissure between the occipital and parietal lobes of the brain. पश्चकपाल विदर;

Oral F., see **Fissura Oris**.

Palpebral F., the opening between the eyelids. नेत्रच्छद विदर; वर्त्म विदर;

Sphenoid F., see **Sphenoidal Fissure**.

Sphenoidal F., a cleft between the great and small wings of the sphenoid bone. जतूक विदर;

Transverse F., one crossing the lower surface of the right lobe of the liver. अनुप्रस्थ विदर;

Umbilical F., the anterior portion of the longitudinal fissure of the liver. नाभिविदर

**Fistula.** An abnormal communication between two body surfaces or cavities. नालव्रण; नासूर;

F. Auris Congenita, congenital fistula of the externla ear. सहज बहिर्कर्ण-नालव्रण; बाहरी कान का जन्मजात नासूर;

F.-in-ano, anal or rectal fistula. गुदा नालव्रण; गुदाव्रण; भगंदर;

F. Lachrymalis, fistula of the lachrymal sac; fistula lacrimalis. अश्रुनालव्रण; अश्रुनली का नासूर;

Anal F., one near the anus, may or may not communicate with the bowel. गुदा-नालव्रण;

Arteriovenous F., an abnormal communication between an artery and a vein. धमनीशिरा-नालव्रण;

Blind F., a fistula opening at one end only; incomplete fistula. अन्ध-नालव्रण; अपूर्ण नालव्रण;

Complete F., one having an internal and external opening. पूर्ण नालव्रण;

External F., a fistula between a hollow viscus and the skin. बहिर्नालव्रण;

Faecal F., one communicating with the intestine; fecal fistula; stercoral fistula; intestinal fistula. बिष्ठा नालव्रण;

Fecal F., see **Faecal Fistula**.

Gastric F., a fistulous tract from the stomach to the abdominal wall. जठर नालव्रण;

Incomplete F., see **Blind Fistula**.

**Fistula**

**Internal F.,** a fistula between hollow visceras. अन्तरांगी नालव्रण; अन्त: नालव्रण;

**Intestinal F.,** see **Faecal Fistula.**

**Parietal F.,** a fistula, either blind or complete, opening on the wall of the thorax or abdomen. भित्तिक नालव्रण; पार्श्विक नालव्रण;

**Salivary F.,** an opening between a salivary duct or gland and the cutaneous surface, or into the oral cavity through other than the normal anatomical pathway. लाला नालव्रण;

**Stercoral F.,** see **Faecal Fistula.**

**Vesico-vaginal F.,** one opening from the bladder into the vagina. मूत्राशय-योनि नालव्रण

**Fistulae.** Plural of **Fistula.**

**Fistulation.** Formation of a fistula in a part; becoming fistulous; fistulization. नालव्रणता

**Fistulatome.** An instrument for cutting a fistula. नालव्रण-उच्छेदक

**Fistulectomy.** Excision of a fistula; syringectomy. नालव्रण-उच्छेदन.

**Fistulization.** See **Fistulation.**

**Fistulotomy.** Incision or surgical enlargement of a fistula; syringotomy. नालव्रणछेदन

**Fistulous.** Of the nature of fistula. नालव्रणाभ; नालव्रण जैसा

**Fit.** A convulsion; a sudden paroxysm. दौरा; आक्षेप; मूर्च्छा; आवेश

**Fixation.** A making firm or rigid. स्थिरीकरण; बन्धन; दृढ़ीकरण;

**F.-forceps,** forceps for holding a part during operation. स्थिरीकरण संदंशिका;

**F.-point,** the point for which accommodation of the eye is adjusted. स्थिरीकरण बिन्दु;

**Complement F.,** when antigen and homologous antibody unite to form a complex. पूरक बन्धन; पूरक स्थिरीकरण;

**External F.,** fixation of the fractured bones by splints, plastic dressinags or transfixion pins. बहिर्बन्धन; बाह्य स्थिरीकरण;

**Internal F.,** stabilization of fractured bony parts by direct fixation to one another with surgical wires, screws, pins, plates, etc. अन्तर्बन्धन; अन्त:स्थिरीकरण;

**Fixative.** Serving to fix, bind, or make firm or stable. बन्धक; स्थिरकारी; दृढ़कारी

**Fixing.** Preserving the natural form of tissue in microscopy.

स्थिरीकरण

**Flaccid.** Soft; flabby; yielding to touch; not firm; without tone; relaxed. शिथिल; श्लथ; कोमल

**Fiaccidity.** Softness; flabbiness. शिथिलता; श्लथता; कोमलता

**Flagella.** Plural of **Flagellum.**

**Flagellar.** Relating to a flagellum, or to the extremity of a protozoa. कशाभी; कशाभ

**Flagellate (s).** Furnished with flagella. कशाभी

**Flagellated.** Possessing one or more flagella. कशाभित

**Flagellation.** Flogging or stroking, recommended as a means of checking post-partem haemorrhage. कशाभोत्पत्ति

**Flagellosis.** Infection with flagellated protozoa in the intestinal or genital tract. कशाभता; कशाभ-रुग्णता

**Flagellum.** A whip; fine; hair-like appendage, capable of lashing movement. कशाभ; कशाभिका

**Flail-chest.** Unstable thoracic cage due to fracture. शिथिल-वक्ष

**Flail-foot.** A congenital or acquired deformity, marked by depression of the arches of the feet. शिथिल पाद

**Flail-joint.** An abnormally mobile joint. शिथिल सन्धि; चल-सन्धि

**Flake.** A crust. शल्क; निर्मोक; पपड़ी

**Flaking.** Desquamation. शल्कन; शल्कीभवन; निर्मोकन; पपड़ियाना

**Flammable.** Likely to burn. ज्वलनशील; दाहक

**Flank.** Latus; the side of the body between the pelvis and the ribs. पार्श्व; बगल

**Flap.** A loose, partly detached portion of skin and tissues. प्रालम्ब; आस्फाल; उत्क्षेप; पल्ला;

   **F.-amputation,** amputation with flap-formation. प्रालम्ब-उच्छेदन;

   **F.-extraction,** the extraction of a cataract by cutting a flap of cornea. प्रालम्ब निष्कर्षण;

   **Arterial F.,** includes a direct cutaneous artery within its longitudinal axis. धमनी-प्रालम्ब;

   **Composite F.,** see **Compound Flap.**

   **Compound F.,** a skin flap incorporating underlying muscle, bone or cartilage; composite flap. विवृत प्रालम्ब; यौगिक प्रालम्ब;

   **Cross F.,** a skin flap transferred from one arm, breast, eyelid, finger, foot, lip, leg, etc, to the other. व्यत्यस्त प्रालम्ब;

**Direct F.**, one raised completely and transferred at the same stage; immediate flap. प्रत्यक्ष प्रालम्ब;

**Distant F.**, a flap in which donor site is distant form the receipient area. दूरस्थ प्रालम्ब;

**Flat F.**, a flap in which, during transfer, the pedicle is left flat or open; open flap. सपाट प्रालम्ब;

**Hinged F.**, a turnover flap transferred by lifting it over on its pedicle as though the pedicle was hinge. अवलम्बी प्रालम्ब;

**Immediate F.**, see **Direct Flap.**

**Local F.**, one transferred to an adjacent area. स्थानिक प्रालम्ब;

**Open F.**, see **Flat Flap.**

**Pedicle F.**, a flap sustained by a blood-carrying stem from the donor site during transfer. वृन्त प्रालम्ब;

**Rotation F.**, a pedicle flap rotated from the donor site to an adjacent receipient area, usually as a direct flap. घूर्णी प्रालम्ब;

**Subcutaneous F.**, a pedicle flap in which the pedicle is denuded of epithelium and buried in the subcutaneous tissue of the receipient area. अधस्त्वक् प्रालम्ब;

**Tubed F.**, a flap in which the sides of the pedicle are sutured together to create a tube, with the entire surface covered by the skin. नलकित प्रालम्ब

**Flare.** A diffuse redness of the skin extending beyond the local reaction to the application of an irritant. फ्लेयर; त्वग्लालिमा

**Flat-foot.** A congenital or acquired deformity marked by depression of the arches of the feet; talipes planus. सपाट-पाद; चपटा-पाद

**Flatness.** The percussion note produced by airless bodies. ठोस ध्वनि

**Flat Pelvis.** A pelvis in which the anteroposterior diameter of the brim is reduced, causing pelvic contraction. सपाट-श्रोणि

**Flattened.** Made flat. चपटा; बिल्कुल सीधा या समतल

**Flatulence.** Accumulation of wind or gas in the stomach. आध्मान; अफारा; अधोवायु; उदरवायु

**Flatulent.** Affected with wind or gas generated in the stomach and bowels, through imperfect digestion and other causes. साध्मान; आध्मानयुक्त; अधोवायुमय

**Flatus.** Gas or air in the alimentary canal, which may be expelled through the anus. अधोवायु; आंत्रवायु

**Flavism.** Paleness of hair; having a yellow tinge. पीतलोमता; बालों का पीलापन

**Flay.** To remove skin or outerlayer. निस्त्वचन करना; छीलना; खाल उतारना

**Flea.** An insect of the genus **Pulex,** marked by lateral compression, sucking mouth parts and extraordinary jumping power. पिस्सू

**Fleam.** A lancet used in phlebotomy. फ्लीम; शिराकर्तक; शिराकर्तनी

**Flesh.** A soft tissue of the body; the meat of animals used for food. मांस; गोश्त; आभिष; muscular tissue. पेशी-ऊतक;

   **Proud F.,** exuberant granulation in the granulation tissue on the surface of a wound. मांसांकुर

**Flex.** To bend; to move a joint in such a direction as to approximate the two parts which it connects. झुकाना; मोड़ना

**Flexibilitas.** Flexibility. नम्यता; लोच; लचक; लचीलापन;

   **F. Cerea,** a cataleptic condition in which the limbs remain fixed as they are placed. मोमी नम्यता; मोमी लोच

**Flexibility.** The act of bending. नम्यता; लोच; लचक; लचीलापन

**Flexible.** That which may be bent; flexile. नम्य; लचीला; लोचदार

**Flexile.** See **Flexible.**

**Flexion.** The process of flexing or bending; the condition of being bent or flexed. कुंचन; आकुंचन; नमन; मोड़

**Flexner's bacillus.** A pathogenic, gram-negative rod becterium, which is the most common cause of bacillary dysentery epidemics, and sometimes infantile gastroenteritis. ग्राम-ऋण दण्डाणु; फ्लेक्सनर बेसिलस

**Flexor.** A muscle, which on contraction flexes or bends a part or joint. आकुंचक; आकुंचिका; आकुंचिनी; आकोचक

**Flexur.** See **Flexure.**

**Flexura.** See **Flexure.**

**Flaxurae.** Plural of **Flexura.**

**Flexural.** Relating to a flexure. वंक सम्बन्धी

**Flexure.** A bending; flexur; flexura. वंक; आनमन; मोड़;

   **Caudal F.,** the bend at the lower portion of the embryo. पुच्छ-वंक;

   **Cephalic F.,** the arch at the cephalic end of the embryo; cranial flexure. मस्तिष्क-वंक;

   **Cervical F.,** the ventrally concave bend at the juncture of the brain-stem and spinal cord in the embryo. ग्रीवा-वंक;

**Flexure**

>Cranial F., see **Cephalic Flexure.**
>
>Dorsal F., one in the mid-dorsal region in the embryo. पृष्ठ-वंक;
>
>Hepatic F., the bend between the ascending and transverse colon beneath the liver; right colic flexure. यकृत् वंक;
>
>Left Colic F., see **Splenic Flexure.**
>
>Lumbar F., the normal ventral curve of the vertebral column in the lumbar region. कटि-वंक;
>
>Right Colic F., see **Hepatic Flexure.**
>
>Sigmoid F., the S-shaped bend at the lower end of the descending colon. अवग्रहान्त्र वंक;
>
>Splenic F., is situated at the junction of the transverse and the descending parts of the colon; left colic flexure. प्लीहा-वंक;
>
>Telecephalic F., a flexure appearing in the region of embryonic forebrain. दूरमस्तिष्क-वंक

**Floaters.** Floating bodies in the vitreous humor (of the eye) which are visible to the person. प्लवमान-पिण्ड; नजर के सामने तैरती चीजें

**Floating.** Free to move about; wandering. प्लवमान; स्वच्छन्दगतिक; चल;

>F. Bodies, see **Floaters.**
>
>F. Kidney, an abnormally mobile kidney. प्लवमान वृक्क; स्वच्छन्दगतिक गुर्दा; चल वृक्क;
>
>F. Ribs, the free ribs - the two lower pairs. प्लवमान पर्शुकायें; चल पर्शुकायें

**Floccilation.** An aimless plucking at the bedclothes, as if one were picking off the threads or tufts of cotton, occurring in the delirium of a fever. वस्त्र-लुंचन

**Flocci Volitantes.** Specks floating before the eyes. दृष्टिचित्तिता; आँखों की आगे उड़ती चिनगारियां

**Floccular.** Relating to a flocculus of any sort. ऊर्णपिण्डिकी; ऊर्णपिण्डिका सम्बन्धी

**Flocculate.** To become flocculent. गुफ्फेदार होना

**Flocculation.** The coalescence of colloidal particles in the suspension resulting in their aggregation into larger discrete masses which are often visible to the naked eye; flocculence. ऊर्णन

**Flocculence.** See **Flocculation.**

**Flocculent.** In the form of flocks; containing shreds; flaky. ऊर्णी; गुफ्फेदार; ऊनी; रोमिल

**Flocculi.** Plural of **Flocculus.**

**Flocculus.** A small lobule of the cerebellum. मस्तिष्क-खण्ड; a tuft or shred of cotton or wool or anything resembling it. ऊर्णपिण्डिका; गुम्फिका; गुच्छा

**Flood.** To bleed profusely from the uterus, as after childbirth or in cases of menorrhagia. जरायु से प्रचुर रक्तस्राव होना

**Flooding.** Profuse flow of blood, especially from the uterus. प्रचुर रक्तस्राव, प्रमुखतया जरायु से

**Flora.** Plant life, usually of a certain locality. वनस्पतिजीवन; the various bacterial and other microscopic forms of life inhibiting an individual. सूक्ष्माणु; सूक्ष्मजीवाणु

**Florid.** Flushed. रक्तिम; high coloured. गहरे रंग का; of a bright red colour. चमकते हुए लाल रंग का

**Flow.** The movement of a fluid or gas passing a given point per unit of time. प्रवाह; बहाव

**Flowers.** A mineral substance in a powdery state after sublimation. अवपेषण; चूर्ण

**Flowmeter.** A measuring instrument for flowing gas or liquid. प्रवाहमापी

**Fluctuate.** To vary, to change from time to time, as in referring to any quantity or quality. उतार-चढ़ाव होना; घटना-बढ़ना

**Fluctuation.** The undulatory movement of a fluid collected in a natural or artificial cavity of the body which is left by pressure, स्पर्शतरंग; a sudden rise or fall in the temperature. तापमान में आकस्मिक उतार-चढ़ाव होना

**Fluent.** Flowing. प्रवाही; बहता हुआ

**Fluid.** A substance whose molecules move freely upon one another. द्रव्य; द्रव; तरल;

    **Allantoic F.,** the fluid contents of the allantois or the allantoic cavity. अपरापोषकीय द्रव्य; अपरापोषिक द्रव्य;

    **Amniotic F.,** a serous liquor filling the cavity of the amnion. उल्व द्रव्य;

    **Cerebrospinal F.,** the fluid between the arachnoid membrane and the pia-mater; subarachnoid fluid. मस्तिष्कमेरु द्रव्य;

**Pleural F.,** the thin film of fluid between the viscerae and parietal pleurae. फुप्फुस द्रव्य;

**Prostatic F.,** a whitish secretion that is one of the constituents of the semen. पुरःस्थ द्रव्य;

**Seminal F.,** semen. वीर्य; शुक्र;

**Subarachnoid F.,** see **Cerebrospinal Fluid.**

**Fluidity.** Liquidity. द्रवता; तरलता

**Fluidization.** Liquidation. द्रवण; तरलीकरण; तरलीभवन

**Fluidounce.** A liquid measure, eight fluidrams. द्रव-औंस; आठ द्रव ड्राम

**Fluidrachm.** See **Fluidram.**

**Fluidram.** A liquid measure equalling 56.96 grains of distilled water or 1/8 of a fluidounce; fluidrachm; a teaspoonful. द्रवड्राम; १ चाय के चम्मच के बराबर का माप

**Fluke.** A broad flat parasite, or worm, infesting the liver of the sheep, goat, etc. पर्णकृमि; पट्टकृमि

**Fluor.** A secretion or discharge. स्राव;

**F. Albus,** leucorrhoea, white discharge. प्रदरस्राव; श्वेतप्रदर

**Fluorescence.** Power of body to change wave-rate of light passing through it. प्रतिदीप्ति

**Fluorescent.** Possessing the quality of fluorescence. प्रतिदीप्त

**Fluoride.** A salt sometimes present in water, which prevents caries, but in gross excess causes mottling of the teeth. फ्लोराइड; फ्लूओरिड; जल में पाया जाने वाला नमक

**Fluorometer.** A device for adjusting the shadow of the skiagram. प्रतिदीप्तिमापी

**Fluoroscope.** An instrument for holding the fluorescent screen in x-ray examination. प्रतिदीप्तिदर्शी

**Fluoroscopic.** Concerning fluoroscopy. प्रतिदीप्तिदर्शी (यंत्र) सम्बन्धी

**Fluoroscopy.** The process of examining the tissues by a fluoroscope. प्रतिदीप्तिदर्शन

**Flush.** A suffusion of the face with blood from fear, modesty or shame, or more excitement, passion, joy, etc. तमतमाहट; लालिमा; to wash out with a full stream of fluid. भलीभांति पानी से धो कर साफ करना

**Flutter.** Agitation or tremulousness, especially of heart; twitching. स्फुरण; फड़फड़ाहट

**Flutter-fibrillation.** An electro-cardiographic pattern of atrial activity with features of both fibrillation and flutter. आस्फालनीय विकम्पन

**Flux.** An excessive flow of any of the body excretion. प्रवाह; अत्यधिक; स्राव होने की अवस्था;

    **Alvine F.,** diarrhoea. अतिसार; प्रवाहिका; दस्त;

    **Bloody F.,** dysentery. रक्तातिसार; खूनी पेचिश

**Fluxion.** The gathering of fluid in any part of the body. द्रवसंचय

**Flying.** Rapidly wandering. भ्रमणकारी; चलायमान; उड़ान भरता;

    **F. Blister,** a blister rapidly moving from place to place. तेजी से स्थान बदलता हुआ छाला

**Focal.** Pertaining to a focus. विकारस्थानिक;

    **F. Depth,** that capacity of an objective to define objects out of focus. विकारस्थानिक घनता;

    **F. Distance,** the distance from the centre of a lens or mirror to its focus. विकारस्थानिक दूरी;

    **F. Lesion,** a lesion of the spinal cord or brain limited in extent. विकारस्थानिक विक्षति

**Foci.** Plural of **Focus**.

**Focus.** The principle seat of a disease. विकारस्थान; the meeting point of rays made convergent by a convex lens or a concave mirror. प्रेरणस्थान; केन्द्रबिन्दु; फोकस;

    **Ghon's F.,** the pulmonary lesion of primary tuberculosis; Ghon's tubercle or primary lesion. घोन फोकस; प्रारम्भिक यक्ष्मा; फुप्फुस विक्षति

**Foeniculum.** See **Fennel**.

**Foetal.** Pertaining to a foetus; fetal. भ्रूणज; भ्रूण अथवा गर्भ सम्बन्धी

**Foetation.** Pregnancy; gestation; fetation. गर्भ; सगर्भता

**Foeter.** See **Fetor**.

**Foeticide.** Destructive of foetus in the uterus; feticide. भ्रूणनाशक; गर्भनाशक; गर्भपातक

**Foetid.** Bad-smelling; fetid. दुर्गन्धित; बदबूदार

**Foetography.** See **Fetography**.

**Foetology.** See **Fetology**.

**Foetometry.** See **Fetometry.**
**Foetopathy.** See **Fetopathy.**
**Foetoplacental.** See **Fetoplacental.**
**Foetor.** See **Fetor.**
**Foetoscope.** See **Fetoscope.**
**Foetoscopy.** See **Fetoscopy.**
**Foetus.** The product of conception; the embryo when in womb; unborn child; fetus. भ्रूण; गर्भ;

    **Dead F.,** see **Papyraceous Foetus.**

    **Papyraceous F.,** a dead foetus flattened by the living twin, which has become flattened and mummified. कागजी भ्रूण; मृत भ्रूण; मृत गर्भ; पत्रवत् गर्भ

**Foetuses.** Plural of **Foetus.**

**Fogging.** A method of refraction in which accommodation is relaxed by over-correction with a convex spherical lens. फोगिंग

**Fold.** A thin, recurved margin, or doubling; plica. पुटक; बलि; वलय; तह; सिलवट; शिकन

    **Amniotic F.,** a fold of amniotic membrane enclosing the vitelline duct and extending from the point of insertion of the umbilical cord to the yolk sac. उल्व पुटक;

    **Nail F.,** a groove in the cutis in which lie the margins and proximal edge of the nail; plica unguis. नख पुटक;

    **Neural F.,** the elevated margin of the neural groove; plica neuralis. तंत्रिका पुटक;

    **Tail F.,** the ventral folding of the caudal extremity of the embryonic disk; plica caudalis. पुच्छ पुटक

**Folia.** Plural of **Folium.**

**Folium.** A leaf. पर्ण; पत्ता; पत्ती; one of the many folds of the cerebellum. पुटक

**Follicle.** A very minute excretory or secretory sac or gland; folliculus. कूप; पुटक; गर्त; कोषक;

    **Graafian F.,** one of the minute vesicles contained in the stoma of an ovary. डिम्ब कूप;

    **Hair F.,** the depression containing the root of the hair; follicula pilorum. लोम कूप; रोम कूप;

    **Lymph F.,** collections of a denoid tissue in mucous membranes. लसीका पुटक;

**Sebaceous F.,** one of the sacs beneath the skin, secreting the oily fluid that softens the skin. वसा कूप;

**Solitary F.,** one of the small, discrete, lymph-follicles found in the intestinal mucous membrane. एकल पुटक

**Folliclis.** A skin disease of the tubercular subjects characterized by a macular eruption which later becomes nodular and then pustular. कूपविकृति

**Follicula Pilorum.** See **Hair Follicle.**

**Follicular.** Relating to, or containing follicles. कूपिक; पुटकीय;

**F. Tumour,** the sebaceous cyst. पुटकार्बुद;

**F. Hormone,** the female sex hormone. पुटक-हार्मोन

**Folliculi.** Plural of **Folliculus.**

**Folliculitis.** Inflammation of one or more follicles. कूपशोथ; पुटकशोथ;

**F. Barbae,** inflammation of the hair follicles of the beard; sycosis. दाढ़ी के लोम कूपों का प्रदाह;

**F. Decalvans,** inflammatory disease of the hair follicles resulting in patches of baldness. लोम कूपों के प्रदाह के कारण होने वाला रोग, जिसके फलस्वरूप बाल चकत्तों के रूप में उड़ते हैं

**Folliculoma.** A tumour of a follicle. पुटकार्बुद

**Folliculose.** Full of follicles. पुटकपूर्ण; पुटकों से परिपूर्ण

**Folliculosis.** Hypertrophy of follicles. पुटकबृद्धि;

**Conjunctival F.,** overgrowth of conjunctival follicles. नेत्रश्लेष्मला-पुटकबृद्धि

**Folliculus.** See **Follicle.**

**Foment.** A warm application or bath with hot water. सेंकना; गर्म जल से सिकाई करना

**Fomentation.** External application of hot, moist flannel. सिकाई; सिंकाई; a warm application; a poultice. सेंक; सेक; पुल्टिस

**Fomes.** A porous substance absorbing and transmitting the contagium of disease. संक्रामक पदार्थ; संक्रमणी पदार्थ; छूत की बीमारी के कीटाणु फैलाने वाले पदार्थ

**Fomites.** Plural of **Fomes.**

**Fontanel.** See **Fontanelle.**

**Fontanelle.** Aperture in the infant skull at the junction of the suture; fontanel; fonticulus. ब्रह्मरन्ध्र; रन्ध्र; कलान्तराल; करोटि-अन्तराल

**Fonticuli**

**Fonticuli.** Plural of **Fonticulus.**

**Fonticulus.** See **Fontanelle.**

**Food.** Any substance taken for the growth of the body. खाद्य; आहार; भोजन; अन्न; पोषण; पदार्थ खाना;

**F.-poisoning,** poisoning by tainted food or some substance naturally poisonous; ptomaine poisoning. खाद्य-विषण्णता

**Foot.** The organ at the extremity of leg; pedis. पाद; पद; पैर; पांव; चरण;

**F.-drop,** inability to dorsiflex foot, as in severe sciatica and nervous disease affecting lower lumbar regions of the cord; drop foot. पादपात;

**Athlete's F.,** ringworm of the foot; tinea pedis. पाद-दडु; पैरों का दाद;

**Claw F.,** a condition characterized by hyperextension at the metatarsophalangeal joints as a fixed contracture. नखर पाद;

**Drop F.,** see **Foot-drop.**

**Flat F.,** a deformity in which the arch of the foot is broken down, the entire sole touching the ground; talipes planus; pes planus; splay foot. सपाट पाद; चपटा पाद;

**Fungus F.,** see **Madura Foot.**

**Immersion F.,** the same as **Trench Foot.**

**Madura F.,** a fungus infection, occurring in tropical and subtropical regions; mycetoma; fungus foot. मदुरा पाद; कवक पाद;

**Splay F.,** see **Flat Foot.**

**Trench F.,** occurs in frost-bite or other conditions of exposure where there is local deprivation of blood supply. खाई पाद

**Football-knee.** Periostitis from overuse of the extensors of the thigh. जानुशोथ; जानुकलाशोथ; घुटने की हड्डी की झिल्ली का प्रदाह

**Footling-presentation.** Labor in which the foetal feet present. भ्रूणपाददर्शन

**Foramen.** A hole or opening through a bone or membranous structure. रन्ध्र; विवर; छिद्र;

**F. Magnum,** a large hole in the occipital bone through which the oblongata becomes continuous with the spinal cord; great foramen. महारन्ध्र;

**F. Ovale,** an oval opening situated in the partition which separates the right and left auricles in the foetus. अण्डाकार रन्ध्र;

**F. Rotundum,** a round aperture in great wing of sphenoid bone for the superior maxillary nerve. वर्तुल रन्ध्र;

**F. Spinosum,** passage in great wing of the sphenoid bone for the middle meningeal artery. कण्टक रन्ध्र;

**Aortic F.,** an opening in the diaphragm transmitting the aorta. महाधमनी रन्ध्र;

**Apical F.,** the passage at the end of the root of the tooth for the neural supply to the dental pulp. शिखर रन्ध्र;

**Arachnoid F.,** an opening in the roof of the fourth ventricle. जालतानिका रन्ध्र;

**Conjugate F.,** a foramen formed by the notches of two bones in apposition. संयुग्मी रन्ध्र;

**Epiploic F.,** the passage below and behind the portal fissure of the liver, connecting the two sacs of the peritoneum. वपा रन्ध्र;

**Esophageal F.,** passage for the oesophagus through the diaphragm; oesophageal foramen. ग्रासनलीय रन्ध्र;

**Frontal F.,** the supraorbital notch. लालाट रन्ध्र;

**Great F.,** see **Foramen Magnum.**

**Incisor F.,** aperture of the incisor canal in the alveolar margin. कृन्तक रन्ध्र;

**Infraorbital F.,** passage for the infraorbital nerve and artery. अवनेत्र रन्ध्र;

**Intervertebral F.,** passage for the spinal nerves between the pedicles of adjacent vertebras. अन्तर्कीशेरुका रन्ध्र;

**Mastoid F.,** small aperture behind the mastoid process. कर्णमूल रन्ध्र;

**Medullary F.,** the canal conveying the nutrient vessels to the medullary cavity of a bone. अन्तस्था रन्ध्र;

**Mental F.,** opening in the lower jaw for mental nerves and vessels. चिबुक रन्ध्र;

**Obturator F.,** the large aperture between the ischium and pubis. गवाक्ष रन्ध्र;

**Occipital F.,** a large hole in the occipital bone through which the oblongata is continuous with the spinal cord. पश्चकपाल रन्ध्र;

**Oesophageal F.,** see **Esophageal Foramen.**

**Olfactory F.,** one of many foramens in the cribriform plate of the ethmoid. घ्राण रन्ध्र;

**Foramen**

**Optic F.,** passage at apex of orbit for the optic nerve and ophthalmic artery. नेत्रगुहा रन्ध्र;

**Parietal F.,** one near the posterior angle of the parietal bone. पार्श्विका रन्ध्र;

**Suprorbital F.,** a groove, sometimes converted into a foramen, in the superior margin of the orbit transmitting the supraorbital vessels and nerves. ऊर्ध्वाक्षि रन्ध्र;

**Thyroid F.,** one in the ala of the thyroid cartilage. अवटूपास्थि रन्ध्र;

**Vertebral F.,** the space between the body and arch of a vertebra. कशेरुका रन्ध्र

**Foramina.** Plural of **Foramen.**

**Force.** Power; strength; that which produces or arrests motion. बल; शक्ति; ताकत; जोर;

**Electromotive F.,** the force producing an electric current. विद्युत्प्रेरक बल;

**Masticatory F.,** the motive force created by the dynamic action of the muscles during the physiological act of mastication. चर्वण बल;

**Occlusal F.,** the result of muscular force applied on opposing teeth. अधिधारण बल;

**Reciprocal F.,** the force whereby the resistance of teeth is utilized to move one or more opposing teeth. अन्योन्य बल;

**Reserve F.,** the energy residing in an organ or any of its parts above that required for its normal functioning. आरक्षित बल; संचित बल

**Forced Feeding.** Compulsory feeding, as of the insane. सबल भोजन कराना

**Forceps.** Pincers, a two-bladed instrument for extracting, संदंश; संदंशिका; चिमटी; फारसेप्स; the curved bundles of fibres passing from the callosum to the hemisphere. पूलिका;

**F. Major,** a curved band of fibres passing from splenium to the occipital lobe; posterior forceps. बृहत् संदंशपूलिका;

**F. Minor,** a curved band of fibres passing from the genu of the callosum to the frontal lobe; anterior forceps. लघु संदंशपूलिका;

**Alligator F.,** long forceps with a small hinged jaw on the end. एलीगेटर संदंश;

**Alveolar F.**, forceps used in removing portions of the alveolar process. वायुकोशीय संदंश;

**Anterior F.**, the **Forceps Minor**.

**Arterial F.**, a forceps with sloping blades for grasping the end of a blood vessel in order to perform ligation. धमनी संदंश;

**Axis-traction F.**, an obstetrical forceps specially constructed to enable pulling in the direction of the pelvic axis. अक्षकर्षक संदंश;

**Bone F.**, a forceps for cutting bone. अस्थि संदंश;

**Bulldog F.**, forceps for occluding a blood vessel. बुल्लडाग संदंश;

**Bullet F.**, forceps within curved blades with serrated grasping surfaces, for extracting a bullet from tissues. बुल्लेट संदंश;

**Capsule F.**, fine, strong forceps used for removing the capsule of the lens in cataract. सम्पुट संदंश;

**Clip F.**, a small forceps with spring to catch hold a bleeding vessel. क्लिप संदंश;

**Dental F.**, forceps used for the extraction of teeth; extracting forceps. दन्त संदंश; दन्तनिष्कर्षक;

**Dressing F.**, forceps used for handling surgical dressings. ड्रेसिंग संदंश;

**Epilating F.**, forceps for pulling out hairs. लोम संदंश;

**Extracting F.**, see **Dental Forceps**.

**Fixation F.**, forceps for holding structures in a fixed position during an operation. स्थिरक संदंश;

**Hemostatic F.**, forceps used in compressing bleeding vessels. रक्तवाहिका संदंश;

**Obstetric F.**, forceps used for extracting the foetus; obstetrical forceps. प्रसूति संदंश

**Obstetrical F.**, see **Obstetric Forceps**.

**Posterior F.**, see **Forceps Major**.

**Speculum F.**, a slender forceps for use through a speculum; a form of tubular forceps. वीक्षक संदंश;

**Thumb F.**, forceps used by compression with thumb and forefinger. अंगुष्ठ संदंश;

**Torsion F.**, one used for making torsion on an artery to arrest haemorrhage. मरोड़ संदंश;

**Tubular F.,** a long slender forceps intended for use through a cannula or other tubular instruments. नलिकी संदंश;

**Vulsella F.,** forceps with hooks at the tip of each blade; vulsellum forceps. वुलसेला संदंश

**Vulsellum F.,** see **Vulsella Forceps.**

**Forcipate.** Shaped like forceps. संदंशाकार; पूलिकाकार

**Forcipressure.** The arrest of minor haemorrhage by compressing a blood vessel with forceps. संदंश दाब

**Forearm.** The part of the arm between the elbow and the wrist; antibrachium. प्रकोष्ठ; बांह; भुजा; बाजू का कोहनी से कलाई तक का भाग

**Forebrain.** The anterior part of the brain; prosencephalon. अग्रमस्तिष्क; मस्तिष्क का अगला भाग

**Forefinger.** Index finger. तर्जनी; अंगूठे के पास वाली उँगली

**Foregut.** A cavity raised at the cephalic end of the embryo. अग्रान्त्र

**Forehead.** The front part of the head; frons. ललाट; माथा

**Foreign Body.** Any substance which is left in wound and keeps up irritation to the deteriment of its cure, such as splinter, nail, bullet, a piece of broken glass, etc. आगन्तुक शल्य; बाह्य शल्य

**Forensic.** Pertaining to a court of law or the legal proceedings. विधिविषयक; न्याय सम्बन्धी;

**F. Medicine,** the application of medical knowledge to questions of law; legal medicine. न्याय-वैद्यक; विधि-वैद्यक

**Foreplay.** Stimulative sexual play preceding sexual intercourse. क्रीड़ा; कामोत्तेजक क्रीड़ा; कामोद्रेकी क्रीड़ा

**Foreskin.** The prepuce or skin covering the glans penis; preputium. अग्रच्छद; शिश्नमुण्डच्छद; लिंगमुण्डच्छद

**Form.** Shape. आकार; रूप; प्ररूप

**Formatio.** A formation; a structure of definite shape or cellular arrangement. रचना; विरचना; निर्माण; जनन;

**F. Reticularis,** an intermingling of oblique and longitudinal fibres resembling a network in certain parts of the spinal cord, mid-brain and pons. जाल रचना

**Formation.** See **Formatio.**

**Formationes.** Plural of **Formatio.**

**Forme Fruste.** Incomplete or atypical form of a disease. अपूर्ण रूप

**Formes Frustes.** Plural of **Forme Fruste.**

**Formication.** A creeping sensation felt on the body as though ants were crawling over it. पिपीलिका सरणानुभूति; रेंगन

**Formula.** A prescribed method; a prescription; a recipe; a series of symbols denoting the chemical composition of a substance; a concise statement of the composition of a body. सूत्र; फार्मूला;

    **Empirical F.,** indicating the kind and number of atoms in the molecules of a substance or its composition, but not the relation of the atoms to each other or the intimate structure of the molecule; molecular formula. अनुभूत फार्मूला; आनुभविक सूत्र; अनुभव पर आधारित फार्मूला;

    **Molecular F.,** see **Empirical Formula.**

    **Official F.,** a formula contained in the pharmacopoeia or the National Formulary. आधिकारिक सूत्र; अधिकृत फार्मूला; शासकीय सूत्र;

    **Rational F.,** a formula that indicates the constitution as well as the composition of a substance. तर्कसंगत सूत्र

    **Structural F.,** a formula in which the connections of the atoms and groups of atoms, as well as their kind and number, are indicated. रचना-सूत्र

**Formulae.** Plural of **Formula.**

**Formulary.** A collection of formulas for compounding the medicinal preparation. सूत्रसंहिता

**Formulas.** Plural of **Formula.**

**Fornicate.** To commit fornication to have sexual intercourse with an unmarried partner. कौमार्यसंगम करना

**Fornicate Convolution.** A long convolution on the median surface of the brain above the corpus callosum. मस्तिष्क संवलन

**Fornication.** The sexual intercourse between unmarried persons. कौमार्यसंगम; अविवाहितों के मध्य लैंगिक सम्भोग

**Fornices.** Plural of **Fornix.**

**Fornicolumn.** Anterior pillar of the fornix. तोरणिकाग्रस्तम्भ

**Fornix.** An arched portion of the brain; a medullary body beneath the corpus callosum. तोरणिका; चापिका;

    **Conjunctival F.,** the line of reflection of the conjunctiva from the eyelids on to the eyeball. नेत्रश्लेष्मला-तोरणिका

**Fortification Spectrum.** Temporary amblyopia with subjective images, often an accompaniment of migraine; teichopsia. प्रदीप्त रेखाभास

**Fossa**. A depression, furrow or sinus. खात; विवर; कोटर; झुर्री;

**F. Acetabuli**, see **Acetabular Fossa**.

**F. Mandibularis**, see **Mandibular Fossa**.

**F. Navicularis**, navicular fossa; the dilation of the urethra at the glans penis; a hollow between the vaginal aperture and the fourchette. नौकाभ खात; नौकाभ विवर;

**F. Ovalis**, one in the right auricle of the heart; the remains of the oval foramen of the foetus. अण्डाकार खात;

**F. Pararectalis**, see **Pararectal Fossa**.

**F. Paravesicalis**, see **Paravesical Fossa**.

**F. Patellaris**, see **Hyaloid Fossa**.

**Acetabular F.**, a depressed area in the floor of the acetabulum above the acetabular notch; fossa acetabuli. उलूखल खात;

**Axillary F.**, armpit; axilla. कक्षा खात;

**Canine F.**, a depression on the external surface of the superior maxilla. रदनक खात;

**Coronoid F.**, a depression in the humerus receiving the coronoid process of the ulna. चंचु-खात;

**Epigastric F.**, the pit of the stomach. अधिजठर खात;

**Glenoid F.**, see **Mandibular Fossa**.

**Hyaloid F.**, a hollow for the lens in the anterior substance of the vitreous body; fossa patellaris. काचाभ खात;

**Lacrimal F.**, one in the orbit plate of the frontal bone receiving the lacrimal gland; lachrymal fossa. अश्रु खात;

**Lacrymal F.**, see **Lacrimal Fossa**.

**Mandibular F.**, the depression in the temporal bone; fossa mandibularis; glenoid fossa. अधोहनु खात;

**Navicular F.**, see **Fossa Navicularis**.

**Ovarian F.**, a depression in the parietal peritoneum of the pelvis that lodges the ovary. डिम्बग्रन्थि खात;

**Pararectal F.**, a depression in the peritoneum on the side of the rectum; fossa pararectalis. परामलाशय खात;

**Paravesical F.**, one on the either side of the bladder; fossa paravesicalis. परावस्ति खात;

**Pituitary F.**, a hollow in the sphenoid bone lodging the pituitary body. पीयूषिका खात;

**Sublingual F.,** a hollow on the inside of the lower jaw-bone containing the sublingual gland. अवजिह्वा खात;

**Submaxillary F.,** the hollow on the inside of the lower jaw-bone containing submaxillary gland. अवहनु खात;

**Temporal F.,** the space on the side of the cranium bounded by the temporal lines and terminating below at the level of the zygomatic arch. शंरवास्थि खात;

**Zygomatic F.,** a cavity below and on the inner side of the zygoma. गण्डास्थि खात

**Fossae.** Plural of **Fossa.**

**Fosset.** See **Fossula.**

**Fossette.** A small fossa. खातिका; a deep corneal ulcer of small diameter. कनीनिका का एक छोटा-सा किन्तु गहरा व्रण

**Fossil.** Putrified remains of animals under the earth. जीवाश्म; जीवावशेष

**Fossula.** A small fossa; fosset. खातिका; सूक्ष्मविवर

**Fossulae.** Plural of **Fossula.**

**Foul.** Putrid; bad-smelling. दुर्गन्धित; बदबूदार

**Foulage.** Kneading and pressure of the muscles, consisting a form of message. पेशीसम्पीडन

**Foundation.** A base; a supporting structure. नींव; आधार

**Fourchet.** See **Fourchette.**

**Fourchette.** The fold of mucous membrane at the posterior junction of the labia minora; fourchet. भगांजलि; फूर्शे

**Fourth Disease.** Any disease resembling measles or scarlet fever. विस्फोटक रोग; रोमान्तिका अथवा आरक्त ज्वर से मिलती-जुलती कोई बीमारी

**Fourth Nerve.** The trochlear nerve. चक्रक तंत्रिका

**Fourth Ventricle.** A space between the cerebellum and pons and medulla. चतुर्थ निलय

**Fovea.** A small cup-shaped pit, depression or fossa. गर्तिका; खातिका; क्षुद्र विवर; लघु कोटर;

**F. Centralis Retinae,** a depression in the centre of the macula retinae, where only cones are present and blood vessels are lacking; central fovea. अक्षिपट केन्द्र गर्तिका;

**F. Sublingualis,** a shallow depression on either side of the mental spine on the inner surface of the body of the mandible; sublingual fovea. अवजिह्वा गर्तिका;

**F. Sublingualis,** a shallow depression on either side of the mental spine on the inner surface of the body of the mandible; sublingual fovea. अवजिह्वा गर्तिका;

**F. Submandibularis,** the depression on the medial surface of the body of the mandible; submandibular fovea. अवअधोहनु गर्तिका;

**Central F.,** see **Fovea Centralis Retinae.**

**Sublingual F.,** see **Fovea Sublingualis.**

**Submandibular F.,** see **Fovea Submandibularis.**

**Foveae.** Plural of **Fovea.**

**Foveate.** Pitted. विवरित

**Foveas.** Plural of **Fovea.**

**Foveation.** Pitted scar formation, as in small-pox, chicken-pox, or vaccina. गर्तिकाभवन

**Foveola.** A minute fovea or pit. सूक्ष्मगर्तिका; सूक्ष्मखातिका

**Foveolae.** Plural of **Foveola.**

**Foveolar.** Pertaining to a foveola. सूक्ष्मगर्तिका सम्बन्धी

**Foveolate.** Having minute pits or small depressions on the surface. सूक्ष्मगर्तिकामय; सूक्ष्मगर्तिकायुक्त

**Fraction.** Quotient of two quantities. प्रभाज

**Fracture.** A broken bone or cartilage. अस्थिभंग; विभंग; हड्डी का टूट-फूट जाना;

**Bending F.,** bending of a long bone due to multiple micro-fractures. नत अस्थिभंग;

**Closed F.,** see **Simple Fracture.**

**Colles F.,** a fracture of the radius with displacement of the distal fragment dorsally. कॉलीस अस्थिभंग;

**Comminuted F.,** a fracture in which the bone is broken into pieces. विखण्डित अस्थिभंग;

**Complete F.,** one with injury of the adjacent parts. पूर्णअस्थिभंग;

**Complicated F.,** one with injury of adjacent parts. जटिल अस्थिभंग;

**Compound F.,** one with a communicating wound of the skin; open fracture. विवृत अस्थिभंग;

**Compression F.,** usually of lumbar or dorsal region due to hyperflexion of the spine. सम्पीडन अस्थिभंग;

**Depressed F.,** one with the fractured part depressed below the normal level. अवनत अस्थिभंग;

**Depressed Skull F.,** a fracture with inward displacement of a part of the calvarium. अवनत करोटिभंग;

**Dislocation F.,** a fracture of a bone near an articulation with its concomitant dislocation from that joint. च्युत अस्थिभंग;

**Double F.,** a fracture in two parts of the same bone. द्विगुण अस्थिभंग;

**Fatigue F.,** a fine hairline fracture that appears without evidence of soft tissue injury; stress fracture. श्रान्ति अस्थिभंग; आयास अस्थिभंग;

**Fissured F.,** see **Linear Fracture.**

**Greenstick F.,** that in which one side of the bone is broken, the other bent; incomplete fracture; interperiosteal fracture. अपूर्ण अस्थिभंग;

**Hairline F.,** a minor fracture in which all the portions of the bones are in perfect alignment. लोमाकार; अस्थिभंग; सूक्ष्मरेखी अस्थिभंग;

**Impacted F.,** in which one end of the broken bone is driven into the other. अन्तर्घट्टित अस्थिभंग;

**Incomplete F.,** see **Greenstick Fracture.**

**Indirect F.,** a fracture, especially of the skull, that occurs at a point not at the site of impact. अप्रत्यक्ष अस्थिभंग; परोक्ष अस्थिभंग;

**Interperiosteal F.,** see **Greestick Fracture.**

**Intrauterine F.,** a fracture of one or more bones of a foetus occurring before birth. अन्तर्गर्भाशय अस्थिभंग;

**Linear F.,** a fracture running parallel with the long axis of the bone; fissured fracture. रेखित अस्थिभंग;

**Longitudinal F.,** one involving the bone in the line of its axis. लम्ब-अस्थिभंग;

**March F.,** a fatigue fracture of one of the metatarsals. प्रगम अस्थिभंग;

**Multiple F.,** a fracture of several bones occurring simultaneously. बहु-अस्थिभंग;

**Oblique F.,** a fracture the line of which runs obliquely to the axis of the bone. तिर्यक अस्थिभंग; बक्र अस्थिभंग;

**Open F.,** see **Compound Fracture.**

**Pathologic F.,** one caused by local disease of bone; pathological fracture. वैकृत अस्थिभंग;

**Pathological F.,** see **Pathologic Fracture.**

**Pott's F.,** occurs at the lower end of the fibula. पॉट अस्थिभंग;

**Simple F.,** one without rupture of the underlying skin; closed fracture. सरल अस्थिभंग;

**Spiral F.**, one produced by twisting of long bone. सर्पिल अस्थिभंग;

**Spontaneous F.**, one due to slight force, as and when there is a disease of the skin. स्वत: अस्थिभंग;

**Stellate F.**, one in which the lines of break radiate from a central point. ताराकार अस्थिभंग;

**Stress F.**, see **Fatigue Fracture.**

**Torsion F.**, a fracture resulting from twisting of the limbs. मरोड़-अस्थिभंग;

**Transverse F.**, a fracture the line of which forms a right angle with the axis of the bone. अनुप्रस्थ अस्थिभंग;

**Trophic F.**, one caused by trophic disturbances. पोषणज अस्थिभंग;

**Ununited F.**, one in which bony union has failed. असंयोजी अस्थिभंग

**Fracture Fever.** Fever due to fracture of a bone. अस्थिभंग ज्वर; हड्डी टूट जाने के कारण होने वाला बुखार

**Fraenotomy.** See **Frenotomy.**

**Fraenum.** A fold of membrane which checks or limits movement of an organ; frenum. फ्रीनम; बन्ध;

**Fragilitas.** Brittleness; fragility. भंगुरता;

**F. Crinium**, brittleness of the hair. लोम-भंगुरता;

**F. Ossium**, brittleness of the bones; osteogenesis imperfecta. अस्थि-भंगुरता;

**F. Unguium**, brittleness of the nails. नख-भंगुरता

**Fragility.** See **Fragilitas.**

**Fragment.** A small part broken from a larger entity. टुकड़ा; खण्ड; to break into small parts. टुकड़े-टुकड़े कर देना

**Fragmentation.** A subdivision into fragments. खण्डात्मकता; विखण्डन; छोटे-छोटे टुकड़ों में बांट देना

**Frambesia.** See **Framboesia.**

**Framboesia.** Yaws; a contagious cutaneous disease with raspberry-like tubercles; frambesia. याज

**Frame.** A structure made of parts fitted together. ढांचा; आकृति; आकार

**Framework.** The skeleton. पंजर; हड्डियों का ढांचा

**Frank.** Unmistakable; manifest; clinically evident. सही

**F.R.C.P.** Abbreviation for Fellow of Royal College of Physicians. एफ० आर० सी० पी०

**F.R.C.S.** Abbreviation for Fellow of Royal College of Surgeons. एफ० आर० सी० एस०

**Freckle.** Lentigo; circumscribed spots on the skin; ephelis. मेचक; चकत्ता; लेन्टीगो

**Freezing.** Congealing, stiffening, or hardening by exposure to cold. हिमीकरण; हिमीभवन; फ्रीजिंग

**Freezing-point.** The temperature at which the water freezes. हिमांक बिन्दु; फ्रीजिंग पाइन्ट

**Freiberg's disease.** Osteochondritis of the second metatarsal head. फ्रीबर्ग रोग; अस्थ्युपास्थिशोथ

**Fremitus.** Palpable vibration, as of a chest–wall. स्पृश्यकम्प;

**Friction F.,** see under **Friction.**

**Hydatid F.,** vibration felt in the palpation over a hydatid cyst. जलस्फोटी स्पृश्यकम्प;

**Pleural F.,** vibration in the chest-wall produced by the rubbing together of the roughned opposing surfaces of the pleura. फुप्फुस-स्पृश्यकम्प;

**Rhonchal F.,** vibration caused by the passage of air through a large bronchial tube containing mucus. घर्घर-स्पृश्यकम्प;

**Tactile F.,** thrill felt by the hand applied to the chest of a person speaking. स्पर्श-स्पृश्यकम्प;

**Tussive F.,** thrill felt by the hand applied to the chest of one coughing. कास-स्पृश्यकम्प;

**Vocal F.,** thrill caused by speaking and heard through the chest-walls. वाक्-स्पृश्यकम्प

**Frena.** Plural of **Frenum.**

**Frenal.** Relating to any frenum. बन्धविषयक; फ्रीनम सम्बन्धी

**Frenectomy.** See **Frenotomy.**

**Frenkel's exercises.** Exercises for tabes dorsalis to teach muscle and joint sense. फ्रेंकल व्यायाम

**Frenkel's sign.** Hypotonia of the muscles of the lower extremities in tabes dorsalis. फ्रेंकल चिन्ह

**Frenoplasty.** Surfical correction of an abnormally attached fraenum. बन्धसंधान; फ्रीनमसंधान

**Frenotomy.** Surgicial severance of a frenum; fraenotomy; frenectomy. बन्ध-उच्छेदन; फ्रीनम-उच्छेदन

**Frenotomy.** Surgical severance of a frenum; fraenotomy; frenectomy. बन्ध-उच्छेदन; फ्रीनम-उच्छेदन

**Frenula.** See **Frenulum**.

**Frenulum.** A small fraenum; frenula. बन्ध; क्षुद्रबन्ध;
   **F. Clitoridis,** the line of union of the inner portions of the labia minora on the undersurface of the glans clitoridis. भगशिश्निका बन्ध;
   **F. Linguae,** a fold of mucous membrane extending from the floor of the mouth to the midline of the undersurface of the tongue. जिह्वा बन्ध;
   **F. Preputii,** fraenum uniting the prepuce to the glans penis. शिश्नमुण्ड-बन्ध

**Frenum.** See **Fraenum**.

**Frenums.** Plural of **Frenum**.

**Frenzy.** Violent mania; furor. क्रोधोन्मत्त; गुस्से से भरा हुआ; क्रोधी

**Frequency.** The number of repetition of a phenomenon in a certain period of time. आवृत्ति; बारम्बारता

**Fret.** An abrasion; chafing. खरोंच; रगड़न; herpes. हर्पीज; दाद

**Fretum.** A constriction. संकुचन; सिकुड़न

**Freyer's operation.** Suprapubic transversial type of prostatectomy. फ्रीयर ऑपरेशन

**Friable.** Easily crumbled, pulverized, broken, or reduced to powder. अवपेषणीय

**Friction.** The act of rubbing of one surface against another. घर्षण; रगड़
   **F. Fremitus,** a thrill of the chest-wall produced by the rubbing together of two dry roughened surfaces such as the parietal and visceral pleuras. घर्षण स्पृश्यकम्प;
   **F. Murmur,** the sound heard through the stethoscope when two rough or dry surfaces rub together, as in pleurisy and pericarditis. घर्षण मर्मर;
   **F. Rub,** the distinct two dry surfaces are rubbed together. घर्षण ध्वनि

**Fright.** Fear. भय; डर; उद्वेग

**Frigid.** Cold; temperamentally, especially sexually, cold or irresponsive. अनुत्तेजक; निर्मद; ठण्डा; शीतल; विरक्त

**Frigidity.** Literally coldness, especially lack of normal sexual desire. शैत्य; अनुत्तेजन; विरक्ति; वैराग्य; उदासी; निर्मदता; मंदकामुकता

**Frigolabile.** Subject to destruction by cold. शीतनाशी; ठण्ड से नष्ट

होने वाला

**Frigorific.** Cold producing agent. शीतजन्य; शीतलतादायक; ठण्डा करने वाला;

    **F. Nerve,** the vasoconstrictor nerve. वाहिकासंकीर्णक तंत्रिका

**Frigostabile.** See **Frigostable.**

**Frigostable.** Not subject to destruction by a low temperature. शीतस्थिरकारी

**Frog-belly.** Tympany of a child's belly. दादुर-पेट; बच्चों का पेट अफरा जाना

**Frog-face.** A distortion of the face from a swelling or tumour. दादुराननन

**Frog-in-throat.** A collection of mucus in the larynx causing hoarseness and an inclination to hawk. दादुर-कण्ठ

**Frog-plaster.** Conservative treatment of a congenital dislocation of the hip, whereby the dislocation is reduced by gentle manipulation and both hips are immobilized in plaster of Paris, both limbs abducted to 80 degress. फ़ॉग-प्लास्टर; दादुर पलस्तर

**Frolement.** Light friction or massage with the palm of the hand. मर्दन; हथेली से हल्की-हल्की मालिश करना

**Frons.** Forehead; brow; the part of the face between the eyebrows and the hairy scalp; frontis. माथा; ललाट; पेशानी

**Front.** The anterior. अग्र; the forehead. माथा; ललाट; पेशानी

**Frontal.** Relating to the anterior part of a body; in front. ललाटीय; ललाट सम्बन्धी;

    **F. Bone,** the bone of the forehead. ललाटास्थि; माथे की हड्डी;

    **F. Section,** a transverse vertical section. ललाट-खण्ड;

    **F. Sinuses,** air-spaces in the frontal bone. ललाट-विवर; ललाट-गह्वर

**Frontalis.** Frontal, referring to the frontal coronal plane, or to the frontal bone or forehead. ललाटीय; ललाट अथवा माथे सम्बन्धी

**Frontis.** See **Frons.**

**Frontomalar.** Relating to the frontal and malar bones; frontozygomatic. ललाटगण्डास्थिक

**Frontomaxillary.** Relating to the frontal bone and the upper jaw bone. ललाट-हन्वस्थिक; ललाट एवं ऊर्ध्व हन्वस्थि सम्बन्धी

**Frontonasal.** Relating to the frontal and the nasal bones. ललाटनासास्थिक; ललाट व नाक की हड्डियों सम्बन्धी

**Fronto-occipital.** Relating to the frontal and the occipital bones, or to the forehead and the occiput. ललाटपश्चकपालास्थिक; ललाट एवं पश्चकपालास्थियों सम्बन्धी

**Frontoparietal.** Relating to the frontal and parietal bones. ललाटपार्श्विकास्थिक; ललाट एवं पार्श्विकास्थियों सम्बन्धी

**Frontotemporal.** Relating to the frontal and the temporal bones. ललाटशंखास्थिक

**Frontozygomatic.** See **Frontomalar.**

**Frost.** A deposit resembling that of frozen vapour or dew. तुषार; हिमसिक्त ओस;

**F.-bite,** devitalized skin or deeper areas due to exposure to cold; chilblains. शीतदंश; हिमदाह; हिमोपहति; तुषारदंश; शीतक्षत

**Froth.** The saliva. लाला; लार; थूक; foam. झाग; फेन

**Frothy.** Full of foam or froth. फेनिल; झागदार

**Frottage.** The rubbing movement in massage; production of sexual excitement by rubbing against someone. गर्दन

**F.R.S.** Abbreviation for Fellow of the Royal Society. एफ० आर० एस०

**Fructose.** The fruit-sugar; a monosaccharide found with glucose in plants; laevulose. फलशर्करा; फलों से निर्मित चीनी

**Fructosuria.** Fruit-sugar in the urine. फलशर्करामेह

**Fruit.** The developed ovary of a plant. डिम्बफल; the offspring of an animal. संतति

**Frustration.** Inability to achieve personal goals, gratify a desire or to satisfy an urge or need. हताशा; विफलता; नैराश्य; निराशा

**FSH.** Follicle stimulating hormone, secreted by the anterior lobe of the hypophysis. पुटक-उद्दीपक हॉर्मोन

**Fugacity.** The tendency of a fluid, as a result of all forces acting on it, to leave a given site in the body. पलायनशीलता

**Fugitive.** Wandering; erratic. पलायनशील; भ्रमणकारी; चलायमान

**Fugue.** An attempt to escape from reality. पलायन; सच्चाई से भागने की कोशिश; a period of loss of memory. स्मृतिलोपकाल; चेतनाविकार

**Fulcrum.** The fixed point against which a lever operates. टेकन; सहारा

**Fulgurant.** Severe and terrific; sharp and piercing; fulgurating. तीखा; विदीर्णकारी

**Fulgurating.** Fulgurant. विदीर्णकारी; relating to fulguration. विद्युत्दहन अथवा विदीर्णता सम्बन्धी;

**F. Pain,** pain in momentary exacerbations. विदीर्णकारी पीड़ा

**Fulguration.** Lightning stroke. विद्युत्दहन; lancinating pain. विदीर्णकारी पीड़ा; destruction of tissue by diathermy. ऊतकलयन

**Full-term.** Mature when pregnancy has lasted 40 weeks. पूर्णकालीन; पूर्णकालिक; परिपक्व

**Fulminant.** Occurring with sudden severity; fulminating. स्फूर्जक; उग्र

**Fulminating.** See **Fulminant**.

**Fulmination.** In chemistry, the explosion or detonation of certain preparation by heat or friction. स्फूर्जन

**Fumigant.** Any vapourous substance used as a disinfectant or pesticide. धूमद; धूमनकारी (पदार्थ)

**Fumigate.** To expose to the action of smoke or of fumes of any kind as a means of disinfection. धूमन करना; धुँआरना; धूनी देना

**Fumigation.** Exposure to disinfectant vapours. धूमन; the use of a fumigant. धूमद अथवा धूमनकारी पदार्थ का उपयोग करना

**Fuming.** Smoking; emitting a visible vapour. सधूम; धूमायमान; धुँआ छोड़ने वाला

**Function.** The active condition or object of an organ. कार्य

**Functional.** Pertaining to functions. क्रियात्मक; कार्य अथवा क्रिया सम्बन्धी; non-organic, not caused by a structural defect. अजैवी; अनांगिक;

**F. Disease,** a disease disturbing the function of a part, but without bringing the structural changes in the body. क्रियात्मक रोग

**Fundal.** Pertaining to the fundus; fundic. बुघ्नपरक; बुघ्नविषयक; बुघ्न सम्बन्धी;

**F. Placenta,** a placenta normally attached near the uterine fundus. बुघ्न अपरा

**Fundament.** The base. आधार; भित्ति; the anus. गुदा; गुद; मलद्वार

**Fundectomy.** See **Fundusectomy**.

**Fundi.** Plural of **Fundus**.

**Fundic.** See **Fundal**.

**Fundiform.** Looped; sling-shaped; of the form of a fundus. बुघ्नरूप; बुघ्नाकार

**Fundus.** The bottom or the lowest part of a sac or hollow organ, as the womb. बुघ्न; तलदेश; पेंदी; अंगमूल; आधार; तल;

**Fundus**

    **F. Glands,** microscopic tubular glands in the cardiac portion of the gastric mucous membrane. बुघ्न ग्रन्थियाँ;

    **F. Oculi,** posterior inner part of the eye. नेत्रबुघ्न; आँख का पिछला अन्दरूनी भाग;

    **F. Uteri,** that portion of the womb cephalad from the line joining the entrances of the oviducts. गर्भाशय बुघ्न;

    **F. Ventriculi,** fundus of the stomach that lies above the cardiac notch. आमाशय बुघ्न

**Funduscopic.** Relating to the visualization of the eyegrounds with the ophthalmoscope. बुघ्नदर्शन सम्बन्धी

**Fundusectomy.** Excision of the fundus of an organ; fundectomy. बुघ्न-उच्छेदन

**Fungal.** See **Fungous.**

**Fungi.** Plural of **Fungus.**

**Fungicidal.** Denoting a fungicide. कवकनाशी; कवकनाशक

**Fungicide.** An agent which is lethal to fungi. कवकनाशक; कवकनाशी

**Fungiform.** Resembling or of the form of a mushroom or fungus. कवकरूप; कवकवत्; छत्रक से मिलता-जुलता;

    **F. Papillas,** reddish papillas of the tongue, larger than the cervical papillas. कवकरूप अंकुरक

**Fungistat.** See **Fungistatic.**

**Fungistatic.** An agent which inhibits the growth of fungi; fungistat. कवकस्तम्भक; कवकरोधक

**Fungoid.** Having the form of a mushroom. कवकाभ; कवकरूप; छत्रक जैसा;

    **F. Growth,** see **Fungosity.**

**Fungosity.** A soft, spongy fungus-like growth or a fungoid growth. कवक-गुल्मता; मृदुगुल्म

**Fungous.** Relating to a fungus; fungal. कवकविषयक; कवक सम्बन्धी

**Fungus.** A spongelike morbid growth on the body that resembles fungi; a vegetable cellular organism that subsists on organic matter. कवक; छत्रक; छत्ता; फफूंद; फंगस;

    **F.-foot,** madura foot. कवक-पाद; मदुरा-पाद;

    **F. Haematoides,** a bleeding and ulcerated vascular tumour. रक्तस्रावी कवक कर्कटता; रक्तस्रावी तथा सव्रण अर्बुद

**Funic.** See **Funicular.**

**Funicle.** A little cord of aggregated fibres; funiculus. बीजांड-वृन्त

**Funicular.** Pertaining to the funiculus; funic. वृषणरज्जु सम्बन्धी;

    **F. Hernia,** hernia into the spermatic or umbilical cord. वृषणरज्जु-हर्निया;

    **F. Process,** the peritoneal prolongation descending with the testicles. वृषणरज्जु-जाल

**Funiculi.** Plural or **Funiculus.**

**Funiculitis.** Inflammation of funiculus, especially of the spermatic or umbilical cord. वृषणरज्जुशोथ; नाभिरज्जुशोथ; नाभिरज्जु-प्रदाह; inflammation of that portion of a spinal nerve that lies within the intervertebral canal. मेरुतंत्रिकाशोथ

**Funiculopexy.** Suturing of the spermatic cord to the surrounding tissue in the correction of an undescended testicle. वृषणरज्जुबन्धन; नाभिरज्जुबन्धन

**Funiculum.** See **Funiculus.**

**Funiculus.** A cordlike structure, as the spermatic cord or umbilical cord; a small bundle; funicle; funiculum. वृषणरज्जु; रज्जु;

    **F. Cuneatus,** the continuation into the oblongata of the posterolateral column of the cord. कीलाकार रज्जु; नोकदार रज्जु;

    **F. Gracilis,** the continuation into the oblongata or the posteromedian column of the cord. तनु-रज्जु;

    **F. Solitarius,** a bundle of nerve fibres in the medulla made up of the descending fibres of the glossopharyngeal and vagus nerve. एकल रज्जु;

    **F. Teres,** a column on each side of the median furrow on the floor of the fourth ventricle. गोलाकार रज्जु;

    **F. Umbilicalis,** the definitive connective stalk between the embryo or foetus and the placenta; umbilical cord. नाभि-रज्जु

**Funiform.** Ropelike; cordlike. रज्जुवत्; रस्सी जैसा

**Funis.** The spermatic or umbilical cord. वृषणरज्जु अथवा नाभिरज्जु; a cordlike structure. रज्जुवत्

**Funnel Breast.** A depression in the lower part of the sternum; funnel chest. कीपवक्ष

**Funnel Chest.** See **Funnel Breast.**

**Fur.** A coating of morbid matter on the tongue. परत

**Furcal.** Forked. विशाखित

**Furcation.** A forking, or a forklike part or branch; the region of a multirooted tooth at which the roots divide. विशाखन

**Furcula.** Furculum; a forked elevation in the floor of the embryonic pharynx. द्विशल; भ्रूण की ग्रसनी का उभार

**Furculum.** See **Furcula.**

**Furfuraceous.** Resembling bran; branny, or composed of small scales; denoting a form of desquamation. भूसीवत्; भूसी जैसा

**Furor.** Madness; insanity; frenzy. उन्मत्तता; विक्षिप्ति; पागलपन; rage. क्रोध; गुस्सा;

   **F. Epilepticus,** attacks of anger to which epileptics are occasionally subject. अपस्मारी क्रोध;

   **F. Uterinus,** nymphomania. कामोन्माद (स्त्रियों में)

**Furrow.** A groove, crease, fold or sulcus. खातिका; खांच; वलि; तह;

   **Digital F.,** one of the grooves on the palmar surface of a finger, at the level of an interphalangeal joint. अंगुलि खातिका;

   **Genital F.,** a groove on the genital tubercle in the embryo, appearing toward the end of the second month. जननांगी खातिका;

   **Gluteal F.,** the space between the surface of the tooth and the free gingiva; sulcus gluteus. नितम्ब खातिका;

   **Primitive F.,** the groove in the primitive streak. आद्य खातिका

**Furuncle.** A circumscribed abscess, commonly called boil. पनसिका; फोड़ा; फुंसी

**Furuncular.** Pertaining to a furuncle; furunculous. पनसिका सम्बन्धी;

   **F. Diathesis,** furunculosis. पनसिका रोग; फुन्सी रोग

**Furunculi.** Plural of **Furunculus.**

**Furunculoid.** Resembling a furuncle. पनसिकाभ; पनसिकावत्; पनसिका जैसा

**Furunculosis.** The systemic condition favouring boil-formation; furuncular diathesis. पनसिका रोग; फुन्सी रोग;

   **F. Malignans,** carbuncle; furunculus malignans. दुर्दम पनसिका; सांघातिक फोड़ा; नासूर; छिद्रार्बुद

**Furunculous.** See **Furuncular.**

**Furunculus.** A furuncle. पनसिका; फोड़ा; फुन्सी;

   **F. Malignans,** See **Furunculosis Malignans.**

**Fusible.** That which is easily fused or melt. द्रवशील; गलनीय; पिघलने या पिघलाने योग्य

**Fusiform.** Spindle-shaped; tapering at both ends. तर्कुरूप; तर्क्वाकार;

**F. Lobule,** the inferior temporo-occipital convolution. तर्कुरूप खण्ड

**Fusion.** Reduction of a solid body, by exposure to the action of heat, to the liquid form. संलयन; पिघलाव; विलय; union, as by joining together. संयुक्ति; संयोजन;

**Spinal F.,** see **Vertebral Fusion.**

**Vertebral F.,** an operative procedure to accomplish bony ankylosis between two or more vertebrae; spinal fusion. कशेरुकासंयोजन

# G

**Gadus Callarias.** Cod-fish; gadus morrhua. कॉड-मत्स्य; कॉड-मीन; कॉड-मछली

**Gadus Morrhua.** See **Gadus Callarias.**

**Gaertnerian cyst.** A cystic tumour developed from Gaertner's duct. गेर्टनर पुटक

**Gaertner's duct.** A tube extending from the broad ligament to the walls of the uterus and vagina during intrauterine life. गेर्टनर नली

**Gag.** A device for placing between the teeth to prevent closure of the jaws during surgery. गैग; मुखबन्धनी; मुखरोधनी; मुँह खुला रखने के लिये दांतों के बीच रखा जाने वाला उपकरण; to retch or to cause to retch. उबकाई आना; to prevent from talking. बातचीत करने से रोकना

**Gain.** Increase. बृद्धि; profit. लाभ; to increase something, such as weight, strength or health. बृद्धि करना; किसी चीज को बढ़ाना;

**Primary G.,** alleviation of anxiety derived from conversion of emotional concerns into demonstrably organic illness. प्राथमिक बृद्धि;

**Secondary G.,** in psychiatry, interpersonal or social advantages gained indirectly from organic illness. गौण बृद्धि

**Gait.** The mode or manner of walking. चाल; गति; चलने का ढंग;

**Antalgic G.,** a staggering or unsteady gait resulting from pain. आर्तिहर चाल;

**Ataxic G.**, an incoordinate or abnormal gait. भंग गति; असामंजस्यपूर्ण अथवा असाधारण चाल;

**Cerebellar G.**, one with rolling, staggering, lurching movements, seen in cerebellar diseases. अनुमस्तिष्कीय चाल; लड़खड़ाती चाल;

**Cow G.**, a swaying movement due to knock-knee. गो-चाल;

**Equine G.**, that of peroneal paralysis in which the foot is raised high by flexing the thigh on the abdomen. अश्व-चाल;

**Frog G.**, the hopping gait of infantile paralysis. मेंढक चाल; दादुर चाल;

**Hemiplegic G.**, the gait of hemiplegics characterized by swinging the affected leg in a half circle. अर्धांगघाती चाल;

**Scissors G.**, one in whihc the legs cross each other in walking. कैंची चाल;

**Spastic G.**, that in which the legs are held together and move stiffly, the toes seeming to drag and catch. संस्तम्भी चाल;

**Steppage G.**, that in which the foot and toes are lifted high and the heel brought down first. पद चाल; उछलती चाल;

**Waddling G.**, like a duck's gait in which feet are wide apart during a walk. डगमगाती चाल; बत्तख चाल; बत्तख जैसी चाल

**Galactacrasia.** See **Galactacrasis**.

**Galactacrasis.** Abnormal composition of breast milk; galactacrasia. अतिस्तन्यता; स्तनों में अस्वाभाविक रूप से दूध बनना

**Galactagog.** See **Galactagogue**.

**Galactagogue.** Substances that induce or promote the flow of milk; galactagog; galactophora. स्तन्यवर्धक; दूध की मात्रा बढ़ाने वाले पदार्थ

**Galactemia.** Milk in the blood, or a milky condition of the body. दुग्धरक्तता; रक्तदुग्धता; रक्त में दूध विद्यमान रहना अथवा शरीर की दुग्ध-धवल अवस्था

**Galactia.** Defective or abnormal secretion of milk. सदोष दुग्धस्राव

**Galactic.** Pertaining to milk. दुग्ध सम्बन्धी; promoting the flow of milk. स्तन्यवर्धक; दुग्धस्राववर्धक

**Galactidrosis.** The sweating of milk-like fluid. दुग्धस्वेदनता; दुग्धस्वेदता

**Galactocele.** A milk tumour or cyst. दुग्धार्बुद; स्तन्यार्बुद; स्तन्यपुटी; hydrocele containing milk, or fluid resembling milk. दुग्धजलवृषण

**Galactoid.** Resembling milk. दुग्धवत्; दूध जैसा

**Galactometer.** Lactometer; device for measuring the specific gravity of milk. दुग्धमापी; लैक्टोमीटर

**Galactophagous.** Subsisting on milk. or feeding upon milk. दुग्धाहारी; दूध पर निर्भर रहने वाला या पलने वाला

**Galactophora.** See **Galactagogue.**

**Galactophore.** A milk-duct. दुग्धनली

**Galactophoritis.** Inflammation of the milk-ducts. दुग्धनलीशोथ

**Galactophorous.** Lactigerous; milk-bearing; giving or conveying milk. दुग्धोत्पादक; दुग्धजनक

**Galactophthisis.** Consumption caused by long lactation. स्तन्यक्षय; स्तन्य-यक्ष्मा

**Galactophygous.** Retarding milk-secretion; arresting flow of milk. दुग्धरोधी

**Galactopoiesis.** Milk-production. दुग्धोत्पादन; दुग्धजनन

**Galactopoietic.** Pertaining to galactopoeisis. दुग्धोत्पादन सम्बन्धी; a substance that promotes the secretion of milk. दुग्धोत्पादक

**Galactoposia.** The milk-cure. दुग्धोपचार; milk-diet. दुग्धाहार

**Galactopara.** See **Galactopyretus.**

**Galactopyretus.** Milk-fever; galactopara. स्तन्यज्वर; दुग्धज्वर

**Galactorrhea.** See **Galactorrhoea.**

**Galactorrhoea.** An excessive flow of milk; incontinence of milk; galactorrhea; lactorrhoea. अतिस्तन्यस्रवण; स्तनों से अधिक मात्रा में दुग्धस्राव होना

**Galactosaemia.** See **Galactosemia.**

**Galactose.** A crystalline sugar obtained by the action of dilute acids on lactose. गैलेक्टोज; दुग्धशर्करा; क्षीरशर्करा

**Galactosemia.** Excess of galactose in the milk; galactosaemia. अतिदुग्धशर्करा; दूध में शर्करा की अत्यधिक बढ़ी हुई मात्रा

**Galactosis.** The secretion of milk. दुग्धक्षरण; दुग्धस्राव; दुग्धस्रवण; क्षीरस्राव

**Galactostasis.** Suppression of the milk-secretion. दुग्धस्थैर्य; दुग्धदमन; a stasis of milk in a breast. स्तन्यस्थैर्य

**Galactosuria.** Excretion of glactose in the urine. दुग्धशर्करामेह; पेशाब में दुग्धशर्करा जाना; गैलेक्टोजमेह

**Galactotherapy.** The treatment of infants at the breast by administering medicine to the nursing mother; the milk-cure. स्तन्योपचार; दुग्धोपचार; दुग्धचिकित्सा

**Galacturia.** Passage of turbid, milky urine. दुग्धमेह; पेशाब में दूध जाना; chyluria. वसालसीकामेह

**Galaxia.** The thoracic duct. वक्ष-नली; वक्ष-प्रणाली

**Galea.** A bandage for the head. शिरोबन्ध; शीर्षपट्टी; the amnion or canal. उल्व अथवा नलिका; a structure shaped like a helmet. शिरस्त्राण;

   **G. Aponeurotica,** the aponeurosis containing the occipital and frontal muscles. शिरस्त्राणीय कण्डराकला

**Gall.** The bile. पित्त; an excoriation. निस्त्वचन; रगड़न;

   **G. Bladder,** the pear-shaped reservoir for the bile on the undersurface of the liver. पित्ताशय; पित्तकोश;

   **G. Cyst,** the gall-bladder. पित्ताशय; पित्तपुटी;

   **G.-ducts,** the ducts conveying the bile. पित्तनलियां; पित्तवाहिनियां;

   **G.-stones,** stones formed in the gall-bladder and its ducts. पित्ताश्मरियां; पित्तपथरियां

**Gallie's operation.** The use of fascial strips from the thigh for radical cure after reduction of a hernia. गैली ऑपरेशन

**Gallipot.** A small vessel for lotions. गैलीपाट

**Gallon.** A standard liquid measure; four quarts. गैलन; चार क्वार्ट्स

**Galloping Consumption.** A rapid form of the tuberculosis of the lungs. तीव्र फुप्फुसक्षय

**Galvanic.** Pertaining to galvanism. विद्युत्धारा सम्बन्धी;

   **G. Battery,** series of cells producing electricity by chemic reaction and so arranged as to secure the combined effect of the units. विद्युत् बैटरी;

   **G. Electricity,** see **Galvanism.**

**Galvanism.** Voltaic electricity which is generated by the action of a chemical liquid on two plates of metal, as copper or zinc, contained in a cell; galvanic electricity; voltasm. गैलवनीधारा; विद्युत्धारा; विद्युत्शक्तिविज्ञान

**Galvanization.** The transmission of a galvanic current through a part of the body. गैलवनीकरण; विद्युत्संचरण

**Galvanocauterization.** The use of wire heated by galvanic current to destroy tissue. विद्युत्दहन

**Galvanocautery.** A cautery heated by a galvanic current. विद्युत्दहनयंत्र

**Galvanocontractility.** Contractility on galvanic stimulation. विद्युताकुंचनशीलता

**Galvanometer.** An instrument for measuring an electric current. विद्युत्धारामापी; विद्युत्शक्तिमापी (यंत्र)

**Galvanoscope.** Instrument for revealing a galvanic current. विद्युत्धारादर्शी

**Galvanotherapeutics.** See **Galvanotherapy.**

**Galvanotherapy.** Treatment by means of galvanism; galvanotherapeutics. विद्युत्-चिकित्सा; विद्युत्धारा द्वारा की जाने वाली चिकित्सा

**Galvanothermy.** The galvanic production of heat. विद्युत्तापन

**Galvanotonus.** A tonic contraction from galvanism. विद्युत्तानसंकीर्णन

**Galvanotropism.** The turning movements of growing organs under the influence of electric current. विद्युत्प्रतिक्रिया

**Gameta.** See **Gamete.**

**Gamete.** A sexual reproductive cell, e.g. sperm, ovum; gameta. युग्मक; गैमीट; निषेकाणु; जन्यु

**Gametocidal.** See **Gametocide.**

**Gametocide.** An agent destructive to gamete, especially the malarial gametocyte; gametocidal. युग्मकनाशी; जन्युनाशी

**Gametocyte.** A cell different from the ordinary individuals of the species from which the gamete is derived. युग्मककोशिका

**Gametogenesis.** Formation and development of gametes. युग्मकजनन

**Gamma Globulin.** A protein substance in blood serum concerned with immunity against infections. गामारक्तगोलिका; रक्तसीरम में एक पौष्टिक पदार्थ जिसका सम्बन्ध रोगक्षमता से होता है

**Gamma Rays.** Non-charged hard x-rays. गामा रश्मियां; गामा किरणें; अपरिवर्तित कठोर एक्स-रे चित्र

**Gamogenesis.** Sexual reproduction. कामोद्रेक

**Ganglia.** Plural of **Ganglion.**

**Ganglial.** See **Ganglionic.**

**Gangliasthenia.** Asthenia from disease of the ganglia. गण्डिकावसाद

**Gangliate.** See **Gangliated.**

**Gangliated.** Provided with ganglia; having ganglia; gangliate; ganglionated. गण्डिकामय

**Gangliectomy.** See **Ganglionectomy.**

**Gangliform.** Of the form of a ganglion; ganglioform. गण्डिकारूप; गण्डिकाकार;

**Gangliitis.** See **Ganglionitis.**

**Ganglioblast.** An embryonic cell giving rise to ganglionic cells. गण्डिकाप्रसू

**Gangliocyte.** Ganglion cell; a neuron of the cell body which is located outside the limits of the brain and the spinal cord. गण्डिकाकोशिका

**Gangliocytoma.** See **Ganglioma.**

**Ganglioform.** See **Gangliform.**

**Gangliolum.** A little ganglion. क्षुद्रगण्डिका

**Gangliolysis.** Dissolution or breaking up of a ganglion. गण्डिकालयन

**Ganglioma.** A swelling of a lymphatic gland; gangliocytoma; ganglioneuroma. लसीकाग्रन्थ्यर्बुद; लसीका ग्रंथि की सूजन; ganglioneuroma. गण्डिकातन्त्रिकार्बुद

**Ganglion.** A collection of nerves and fibres forming a subsidiary nerve centre within the main nerve system. गण्डिका; कण्डरापुटी; गुच्छिका; तंत्रिका-उपकेन्द्र;

**G. Cell,** see **Gangliocyte.**

**Auricular G.,** see **Otic Ganglion.**

**Carotid G.,** one in the lower part of the cavernous sinus. मन्या-गण्डिका; केरोटिड गण्डिका;

**Ciliary G.,** that in the posterior part of the orbit; lenticular ganglion; ophthalmic ganglion; orbital ganglion. रोमकगण्डिका;

**Coccygeal G.,** that on the anterior surface of the tip of the occyx. अनुत्रिक-गण्डिका;

**Gasserian G.,** see **Semilunar Ganglion.**

**Geniculate G.,** a gangliform enlargement of the seventh nerve in the Fallopian canal. बक्र-गण्डिका;

**Hepatic G.,** one around the hepatic artery. यकृत्-गण्डिका;

**Jugular G.,** one in the upper part of the jugular foramen. मन्या-गण्डिका;

**Lenticular G.,** see **Ciliary Ganglion.**

**Lingual G.,** see **Submaxillary Ganglion.**

**Lumbar G.'s,** four or five, on each side and behind the

abdominal aorta. कटि-गण्डिकायें;

**Lymphatic G.,** any lymphatic gland. लसीका-गण्डिका;

**Nodose G.,** the ganglion on the trunk of the vas just before the jugular foramen. पर्विल गण्डिका;

**Ophthalmic G.,** see **Ciliary Ganglion.**

**Orbital G.,** see **Ciliary Ganglion.**

**Otic G.,** one below the foramen ovale; auricular ganglion. कर्ण-गण्डिका;

**Petrous G.,** one on the lower border of the petrous bone. अश्म-गण्डिका;

**Pharyngeal G.,** one near the ascending pharyngeal artery. ग्रसनी-गण्डिका;

**Phrenic G.,** one under the diaphragm. मध्यच्छद-गण्डिका;

**Renal G.,** one around the renal artery. वृक्क-गण्डिका;

**Sacral G.'s,** four or five, on the ventral surface of the sacrum. त्रिक-गण्डिकायें;

**Semilunar G.,** deeply situated within the skull, on the sensory root of the fifth cranial nerve; gasserian ganglion. अर्धचन्द्र-गण्डिका; नवचन्द्र-गण्डिका;

**Spinal G.'s,** those on the spinal nerves. मेरुरज्जु-गण्डिकायें; सुषुम्ना गण्डिकायें;

**Subaxilalry G.,** one above the submaxillary gland; lingual ganglion. अवहनु-गण्डिका;

**Thoracic G.'s,** twelve pairs on the thoracic sympathetic cord between the transverse process of the vertebras and the heads of the ribs. वक्ष-गण्डिकायें;

**Tympanic G.,** that in the canal between the lower surface of the petrous bone and the tympanum. मध्यकर्ण-गण्डिका;

**Vestibular G.,** that in the aqueduct of Fallopius (Fallopian canal). प्रघाण-गण्डिका

**Ganglionar.** Pertaining to, or having the characteristics of, a ganglion. गण्डिकी

**Ganglionated.** See **Gangliated.**

**Ganglionectomy.** Surgical excision of a ganglion; gangliectomy. गण्डिकोच्छेदन; गण्डिका-उच्छेदन

**Ganglioneure.** A cell of a nervous ganglion. गण्डिकातंत्रिका

**Ganglioneuroma.** A tumour of the nerve of a ganglion; ganglioma; gangliocytoma; neurocytoma. गण्डिकातंत्रिकार्बुद

**Ganglionic.** Pertaining to a ganglion; ganglial. गण्डिका सम्बन्धी; कण्डरापुटीय

**Ganglions.** Plural of **Ganglion.**

**Ganglionitis.** Inflammation of a ganglion; gangliitis. गण्डिकाशोथ; कण्डरापुटीशोथ; गण्डिका अथवा कण्डरापुटी का प्रदाह

**Ganglionostomy.** Making an opening into a ganglion. गण्डिकासम्मिलन

**Ganglioplegia.** Paralysis of a ganglion. गण्डिकाघात; कण्डरापुटीघात

**Ganglioplegic.** An agent which paralysis a ganglion. गण्डिकाघाती; गण्डिकाघातक

**Gangosa.** A tropical disease characterized by a destructive ulceration of the nasopharynx and adjacent structures. नासाग्रसनीव्रण; कण्ठनासाव्रण

**Gangraena Oris.** Cancrum oris; gangrenous stomatitis of mouth in debilitated children. मुख-कोथ

**Gangrene.** Mortification or death of a part of the tissues of the body. कोथ; गलन; विगलन;

**Diabetic G.,** a complication of diabetes. मधुमेही कोथ; मधुमेहज कोथ;

**Dry G.,** occurs when the drainage of blood from the affected part is inadequate. शुष्क कोथ;

**Embolic G.,** due to an embolus cutting off the blood-supply. घनास्री कोथ;

**Hospital G.,** a contagious gangrene arising in crowded conditions where there is absence of antisepsis. अस्पताली कोथ;

**Moist G.,** with abundance of serous exudation. आर्द्र कोथ;

**Primary G.,** without preceding inflammation of a part. प्राथमिक कोथ;

**Secondary G.,** a form with preceding inflammation. गौण कोथ;

**Senile G.,** a gangrene of the extremities in the aged. जराजन्य कोथ;

**Symmetric G.,** that attacking corresponding parts on opposite sides. सममित कोथ;

**White G.,** a moist gangrene due to anemia and lymphatic obstruction. श्वेत कोथ

**Gangrenopois.** Putrid sore-throat. सपूय कण्ठदाह; पूतित कण्ठदाह; गलित मुखक्षत

**Gangrenous.** Mortified. कोथयुक्त; कोथमय; relating to gangrene. कोथ सम्बन्धी; affected with gangrene. कोथग्रस्त

**Ganserstate.** A hysterical condition, stimulating dementia. वातोन्माद

**Gap.** A fissure. दरार; विदर; a hiatus or opening in a structure; an interval or discontinuity in any series or sequence. अन्तराल; at empty space. रिक्तस्थान; खाली जगह;

    **Cranial G.,** congenital fissure of the skull. कपाल विदर

**Gape.** Yawning. जम्भाई; जम्हाई; जंभ

**Gargarism.** A gargle; gargarisma. गरारा, गण्डूष

**Gargarisma.** See **Gargarism.**

**Gargarismata.** Plural of **Gargarisma.**

**Gargle.** A medicated fluid used for gargling; a wash for the throat गरारा; गण्डूष; to wash or rinse the fauces with fluid in the mouth through which expired breath is forced to produce a bubbling effect while the head is held far back. गरारा करना

**Garlic.** The plant **Allium Sativum;** it is a tonic. लहसुन

**Garrot.** A compressing bandage used in haemorrhages. गैरेट; एक रक्तस्त्रावरोधक पट्टी

**Gas.** A thin, fluid, like air, capable of indefinite expansion but convertible by compression and cold into a liquid and, eventually, solid. गैस; to subject to the action of a gas. गैस बनना; वायुग्रस्त होना

    **Anaesthetic G.,** a compound above its boiling point at room temperature, capable of producing general anaesthesia upon inhalation. चेतनाहारी गैस;

    **Tear G.,** a gas that causes irritation of the conjunctiva and profuse lachrymation. अश्रु गैस

**Gaseous.** Of the nature of gas. गैसीय; वायवी;

    **G. Pulse,** a very full, soft pulse. वायवी नाड़ी

**Gasometric.** Relating to gasometry. गैसमापी अथवा गैसमिति सम्बन्धी

**Gasometry.** Determination of the relative proportion of gases in a mixture. गैसमिति

**Gasp.** Opening the mouth to catch breath. हाँफना; हवा के लिये छटपटाना

**Gasserectomy.** Surgical excision of the gasserian ganglion. अर्धचन्द्रगण्डिका-उच्छेदन

**Gassing**

**Gassing.** Poisoning by irrespirable or otherwise noxious gases. गैसविषण्णता

**Gaster.** The stomach. आमाशय; जठर; पाकाशय; पेट

**Gasterasthenia.** Debility of the stomach. आमाशयदौर्बल्य; पाचनदौर्बल्य

**Gasterhysterotomy.** An abdominal incision of the uterus. छेदन; औदरिक गर्भाशयछेदन

**Gastr-.** See **Gastro-.**

**Gastradenitis.** Inflammation of the glands of the stomach. आमाशयग्रंथिशोथ; आमाशयग्रंथि का प्रदाह

**Gastral.** Pertaining to the stomach. आमाशयिक; आमाशय अथवा पेट सम्बन्धी

**Gastralgia.** Neuralgia of the stomach. जठरार्ति; जठरशूल; आमाशयशूल; पेटदर्द

**Gastrectasia.** See **Gastrectasis.**

**Gastrectasis.** Dilatation of the stomach; gastrectasia. जठरविस्फार; आमाशयविस्फार; पेट फैलना

**Gastrectomy.** Removal of a part or the whole of the stomach. जठरोच्छेदन; आमाशय-उच्छेदन; जठरनिर्गम को काट कर हटा देना

**Gastrelcosis.** Ulceration of the stomach. जठरव्रणता; पेट के अन्दर फोड़ा बनना

**Gastric.** Relating to the stomach. जठरीय; आमाशयिक; आमाशयी; पाचक; पेट सम्बन्धी;

   **G. Calculus,** See **Gastrolith.**

   **G. Crises,** paroxysms of pain in the epigastrium in locomotor ataxia. जठरशूल;

   **G. Digestion,** digestion in the stomach. आमाशयिक पाचन;

   **G. Fever,** fever with gastric derangements. जठर ज्वर;

   **G. Influenza,** a term used when gastrointestinal symptoms predominate. जठर प्रतिश्याय;

   **G. Juice,** the acid digestion fluid secreted by the glands of the stomach. पाचक रस; जठर रस;

   **G. Suction,** may be intermittent or continuous to keep the stomach empty after some abdominal operation. आमाशय चूषण;

   **G. Ulcer,** occurs in the stomach. उदर-व्रण; जठर-व्रण

**Gastricism.** Dyspepsia. अग्निमांद्य; मंदाग्नि; अपच; अजीर्ण

**Gastrin.** A hormone secreted by the gastric mucosa on entry of food, which causes a further flow of gastric juice. गैस्ट्रिन; पाचक रस पैदा करने वाला एक हॉर्मोन

**Gastrins.** Plural of **Gastrin.**

**Gastritis.** Inflammation of the mucous membranes of the stomach. जठरशोथ; पाकाशयशोथ;

  **G.Polyposa,** see **Polypous Gastritis.**

  **Atrophic G.,** a chronic form with atrophy of the mucous membrane. शोषी जठरशोथ;

  **Catarrhal G.,** gas with excessive secretion of mucus. अभिष्यंदी जठरशोथ;

  **Exfoliative G.,** gastritis with excessive shedding of mucosal epithelial cells. अपशल्की जठरशोथ;

  **Hypertrophic G.,** gastritis with hyperplasia of the mucous membrane. अतिबृद्ध जठरशोथ;

  **Interstitial G.,** inflammation of the stomach involving the submucosa and muscle coats. अन्तरालीय जठरशोथ;

  **Phlegmonous G.,** a form with abscesses in the stomach walls. श्लेष्मल जठरशोथ;

  **Polypous G.,** gastritis polyposa; chronic gastritis in which there is irregular atrophy of the mucous membrane with cystic glands. पॉलिपी जठरशोथ;

  **Pseudomembranous G.,** a kind in which patches of false membrane occur within the stomach. कूटकला-जठरशोथ

**Gastro–, Gastr-.** Prefixes signifying relation to the stomach. 'जठर' के रूप में प्रयुक्त उपसर्ग

**Gastroanastomosis.** The formation of a communication between the two pouches of the stomach; gastrogastrostomy. जठरशाखामिलन

**Gastroblenorrhoea.** Excessive mucus discharge from the stomach. जठरअतिश्लेष्मस्राव; पेट से प्रचुर श्लैष्मिक स्राव होना

**Gastrobrosis.** Perforation of the stomach. जठरछिद्रण; जठरछिद्रता

**Gastrocardiac.** Relating to both stomach and the heart. जठर एवं हृदय सम्बन्धी

**Gastrocele.** Hernia of a portion of the stomach. जठर-हर्निया; जठरभ्रंश; जठरखंस; पाकाशयभ्रंश

**Gastrocnemius.** The large two-headed muscle of the calf. उपरिस्थपिण्डिका (पेशी)

**Gastrocolic.** Pertaining to the stomach and the colon. जठर तथा बृहदांत्र सम्बन्धी;

**G. Omentum,** the great omentum. महावपाजाल;

**G. Reflex,** sensory stimulus arising on entry of food into stomach, resulting in strong peristaltic waves in the colon. जठरबृहदांत्र-प्रतिवर्त

**Gastrocolitis.** Inflammation of the stomach and the colon. जठरबृहदांत्रशोथ; आमाशय तथा बड़ी आंत का प्रदाह

**Gastrocoloptosis.** Prolapse of the stomach and colon. जठरबृहदांत्रच्युति; जठरबृहदांत्रभ्रंश; आमाशय तथा बड़ी आंत का अपने स्थान से हट जाना

**Gastrocolostomy.** The formation of a fistula between the stomach and the colon. जठरबृहदांत्रसम्मिलन

**Gastrocolotomy.** Incision of the stomach and the colon. जठरबृहदांत्रछेदन

**Gastrocolpotomy.** An abdominal incision through the vagina. योनिमार्गी उदरछेन

**Gastroduodenal.** Relating to the stomach and the duodenum. जठर तथा ग्रहणी सम्बन्धी

**Gastroduodenitis.** Inflammation of the stomach and the duodenum. जठरग्रहणीशोथ

**Gastroduodenoscopy.** Visualization of the interior of the stomach and duodenum by a gastroscope. आमाशयजठरदर्शन

**Gastroduodenostomy.** A surgical anastomosis between the stomach and the duodenum. जठरग्रहणीसम्मिलन; शल्यकर्म द्वारा आमाशय तथा ग्रहणी को एक दूसरे से जोड़ देना

**Gastrodynia.** Pain in the stomach. जठरवेदना; जठरार्ति; जठरशूल; जठरपीड़ा; आमाशय-वेदना; पेटदर्द

**Gastroenteralgia.** Pain in the stomach and the intestine. जठरांत्रशूल; जठरांत्रवेदना

**Gastoenteric.** See **Gastrointestinal.**

**Gastroenteritis.** Inflammation of the mucous membranes of the stomach and small intestine. जठरांत्रशोथ; आमाशय तथा आंतों का प्रदाह

**Gastroenterocolitis.** Inflammation of the stomach, intestines and the colon. जठरांत्रबृहदांत्रशोथ; आमाशय, आंतों तथा बड़ी आंत का प्रदाह

**Gastroenterologist.** A specialist in the diseases of the stomach and intestines. जठरांत्ररोगविज्ञानी; जठरांत्रविज्ञानी; जठररोग-विशेषज्ञ

**Gastroenterology.** Study of the stomach and intestines and their diseases. जठरांत्ररोगविज्ञान; जठरांत्रविज्ञान; आमाशय एवं आंतों का वैज्ञानिक अध्ययन

**Gastroenteropathy.** Any disease of the stomach and intestines. जठरांत्रविकृति; आमाशय तथा आंतों का कोई रोग

**Gastroenteroplasty.** Operative repair of the defects in the stomach and the intestine. जठरांत्रसंधान

**Gastroenteroptosis.** Prolapse of the stomach and intestines. जठरांत्रभ्रंश; आमाशय तथा आंतों की स्थानच्युति

**Gastroenterostomy.** Surgical anastomosis between the stomach and small intestine. जठरांत्रसम्मिलन

**Gastroenterotomy.** An intestinal incision through the abdominal wall. जठरांत्रछेदन

**Gastroepiploic.** Pertaining to both the stomach and the omentum. जठरवपात्मक; जठरवपाविषयक; जठरवपा अथवा आमाशय तथा चिबुक सम्बन्धी

**Gastroesophageal.** Relating to both stomach and oesophagus; gastro-oesophageal. जठरग्रासनलीपरक; आमाशय तथा ग्रासनली सम्बन्धी

**Gastroesophagitis.** Inflammation of the stomach and oesophagus; gastro-oesophagitis. जठरग्रासनलीशोथ; आमाशय तथा ग्रासनली का प्रदाह

**Gastroesophagostomy.** Establishment of a new opening between the oesophaus and stomach; gastro-oesophagostomy. जठरग्रासनलीसम्मिलन

**Gastrogastrostomy.** See **Gastroanastomosis**.

**Gastrogenic.** Deriving from or caused by the stomach. आमाशयजनक

**Gastrograph.** A device for learning the mechanical action of the stomach. जठरलेख

**Gastrohelcosis.** Ulceration of the stomach. जठरव्रणता

**Gastrohepatic.** Relating to the stomach and the liver. जठरयकृत्विषयक; आमाशय तथा जिगर सम्बन्धी

**Gastrohepatitis.** Inflammation of the stomach and the liver. जठरयकृत्शोथ; आमाशय तथा जिगर का प्रदाह

**Gastrohysterectomy.** Uterine excision through the abdomen. औदरिकगर्भाशय-उच्छेदन; उदरमार्गीगर्भाशय-उच्छेदन

**Gastrohysterotomy.** Caesarean section. जठरगर्भाशय-उच्छेदन; शल्यजनन

**Gastroileitis.** Inflammation of the alimentary canal in which the stomach and ileum are preponderantly involved. जठरशेषान्त्रशोथ

**Gastroileostomy.** A surgical joining of stomach to ileum. जठरशेषान्त्रसम्मिलन

**Gastrointestinal.** Referring to the stomach and intestines; gastroenteric. जठरांत्रपरक, आमाशय तथा आंतों सम्बन्धी

**Gastrojejunocolic.** Referring to the stomach, jejunum and colon. जठरमध्यांत्रबृहदांत्रपरक; आमाशय मध्यान्त्र तथा बृहदांत्र सम्बन्धी

**Gastrojejunostomy.** The formation of a fistula between the stomach and the jejunum. जठरमध्यांत्रसम्मिलन; आमाशय तथा मध्यांत्र को एक-दूसरे से मिला देना

**Gastrolienal.** Pertaining to the stomach and the spleen; gastrosplenic. जठर एवं प्लीहा सम्बन्धी; आमाशय तथा तिल्ली सम्बन्धी

**Gastrolith.** A calcareous formation in the stomach; gastric calculus. जठराश्मरी; पेट में पथरी बनना

**Gastrolithiasis.** The presence or formation of gastroliths जठराश्मरीयता

**Gastrologist.** One varsed in gastric disorders. जठरविज्ञानी; जठररोगविज्ञानी; जठररोग-विशेषज्ञ

**Gastrology.** A treatise on the stomach. जठरविज्ञान; जठररोगविज्ञान; जठरप्रकरण

**Gastrolysis.** The loosening of adhesions between the stomach and adjacent organs; surgical division of epigastric adhesions. जठरलयन

**Gastromalacia.** Morbid softening of the walls of the stomach. जठरमृदुता; आमाशय की विकारक कोमलता

**Gastromegaly.** Enlargement of the abdomen or the stomach. जठरवृद्धि; उदर अथवा आमाशय का बढ़ जाना

**Gastromenia.** Gastric vicarious menstruation. जठरानुकल्परज:

**Gastromyxorrhea.** See **Gastromyxorrhoea.**

**Gastromyxorrhoea.** Excessive secretion of mucus in the stomach; gastromyxorrhea. अतिश्लेष्मजठरता

**Gastro-oesophageal.** See **Gastroesophageal.**

**Gastro-oesophggitis.** See **Gastroesophagitis.**

**Gastro-oesophagostomy.** See **Gastroesophagostomy.**

**Gastropancreatic.** Pertaining to the stomach and the pancreas. जठराग्न्याशयिक; आमाशय तथा अग्न्याशय सम्बन्धी

**Gastroparalysis.** Paralysis of the muscular coat of the stomach. जठरपात; जठरघात; आमाशयिक पेशी-अस्तर का पक्षाघात

**Gastroparesis.** A slight degree of gastroparalysis. आंशिक-जठरपात

**Gastropathic.** Relating to the diseases of the stomach. जठरविकृति सम्बन्धी; आमाशयिक रोगों सम्बन्धी

**Gastropathy.** Any disease of the stomach. जठरविकृति; आमाशयिक रुग्णता; आमाशय-विकार; पेट का कोई रोग

**Gastroperiodynia.** Intense periodic pain in the stomach. जठरार्ति; जठरवेदना; पेटदर्द

**Gastropexy.** Surgical fixation of a displaced stomach. जठरस्थिरीकरण

**Gastrophrenic.** Pertaining to both stomach and the diaphragm. आमाशय तथा मध्यच्छद सम्बन्धी

**Gastroplasty.** Any plastic operation on the stomach or the lower oesophagus to remove its defect. जठरसंघान

**Gastroplegia.** Paralysis of the stomach. जठरघात; आमाशयिक पक्षाघात; पेट का फालिज

**Gastroplication.** An operation for the cure of dilated stomach by stitching the walls. जठरसंघान

**Gastroptosis.** Downward displacement of the stomach. जठरभ्रंश; आमाशयभ्रंश; आमाशय की स्थानच्युति

**Gastroptyxis.** In gastric dilatation, an operation to reduce the size of the stomach; gastroptyxy. जठरसंकुचन

**Gastroptyxy.** See **Gastroptyxis.**

**Gastropulmonary.** Relating to the stomach and the lungs; pneumogastric. जठरफुफ्फुसी; आमाशय तथा फेफड़ों सम्बन्धी

**Gastropylorectomy.** Excision of the pyloric end of stomach. जठरनिर्गमोच्छेदन; जठरनिर्गम को काट कर हटा देना

**Gastropyloric.** Relating to the stomach and the pylorus. आमाशय तथा जठरनिर्गम सम्बन्धी

**Gastrorrhagia.** Haemorrhage from the stomach. जठररक्तस्राव

**Gastrorrhaphy.** Suture of a wound of the stomach. जठरसीवन

**Gastrorrhea.** See **Gastrorrhoea.**

**Gastrorrhoea.** Secretion of an excessive quantity of mucus from the lining membrane of the stomach; gastrorrhea. अतिजठरस्राव; आमाशयिक अस्तर-कला से प्रचुर श्लैष्मिक स्राव होना

**Gastroschisis.** Fissure of the abdominal wall; celoschisis. उदरप्राचीर-विदर

**Gastroscope.** An instrument for inspecting the interior of the stomach; endoscope. जठरदर्शी; जठरदर्शकयंत्र; आमाशय के अन्दरूनी भाग की जांच में प्रयुक्त यंत्र

**Gastroscopic.** Relating to gastroscopy. जठरदर्शन सम्बन्धी

**Gastroscopy.** Inspection of the stomach-cavity through gastroscope or endoscope. जठरदर्शन; आमाशय के अन्दरूनी भाग की जांच करना

**Gastrosis.** Any disease of the stomach. जठर-रोग; आमाशयिक रोग; पेट की कोई बीमारी

**Gastrospasm.** Spasmodic contraction of the walls of the stomach. जठर-उद्वेष्ट

**Gastrosplenic.** See **Gastrolienal.**

**Gastrostaxis.** Oozing of blood from the mucous membrane of the stomach. जठररक्तच्यवन

**Gastrostenosis.** Contraction of the cavity of the stomach. जठरसंकीर्णन

**Gastrostomy.** A surgically established fistula between the stomach and the exterior abdominal wall, usually for artificial feeding. जठरछिद्रीकरण

**Gastrosuccorrhea.** Hypersecretion of gastric juices; gastrosuccorrhoea. अतिजठररसस्राव

**Gastrosuccorrhoea.** See **Gastrosuccorrhea.**

**Gastrotome.** An instrument to perform gastrotomy. जठरछेदक; उदरछेदक; आमाशयछेदक

**Gastrotomy.** Incision into the stomach or abdomen. जठरछेदन; उदरछेदन; आमाशयछेदन

**Gastrotonometry.** Measurement of intragastric pressure. जठरतानमिति

**Gastrotubotomy.** Oviduct incision through the abdomen. जठरनलीछेदन

**Gastrotympanites.** Gaseous distention of the stomach. जठराध्मान; प्रत्याध्मान

**Gastroxia.** An abnormal acidity of the stomach-contents; gastroxynsis. जठराम्लता

**Gastroxynsis.** See **Gastroxia.**

**Gastrula.** An early embryonic stage in which, by blastular invagination, there is formed a hollow, double-coated vesicle with an aperture. गैस्ट्रूला; द्वि-अस्तरभ्रूण

**Gastrulation.** The formation of the gastrula. गैस्ट्रूलाभवन; द्वि-अस्तरभ्रूण-भवन

**Gauge.** A thin, light cloth used in surgical dressing; gauze. गॉज; जाली; घावों की मरहम पट्टी करने के लिये प्रयुक्त किया जाने वाला एक पतला, महीन जालीदार कपड़ा

**Gauss.** A unit of magnetic field intensity. गौस; चुम्बक-क्षेत्र की तीव्रता की एक इकाई

**Gaussian.** Relating to, or described by Johann K.F. Gauss. जॉन के० एफ० गौस सम्बन्धी अथवा जॉन के० एफ० गौस द्वारा वर्णित

**Gauze.** See **Gauge.**

**Gavage.** Forced or tube-feeding, as of infants. नलिका-पोषण; नली द्वारा पेट के अन्दर भोजन पहुँचाना; therapeutic use of high-potency diet. चिकित्सा के निमित्त उच्च-शक्ति वाला आहार

**Gaze.** The act of looking steadily in one direction for a period of time. प्रेक्षण; अनिमेष अथवा एकटक देखते रहना

**Geiger-Muller Counter.** A device for detecting and registering radioactivity. गीजर म्यूलर यंत्र (उपकरण); रेडियोसक्रियता प्रदर्शित करने वाला यंत्र

**Gel.** Jelly, or the solid or semi-solid phase of a colloidal solution. लप्सी; जेली; कलिल घोल; to form a gel or jelly; to convert a solid into a jelly. जेली बनाना; किसी ठोस पदार्थ को लप्सी में बदल देना

**Gelatification.** A conversion into gelatine. जेलेटिनभवन; जेलेटिनकरण

**Gelatin.** See **Gelatine.**

**Gelatine.** A protein-containing gluelike substance obtained by boiling bones, skin and other animal tissues; gelatin. श्लेष; शिलिष; सरेस; जिलेटिन

**Gelatiniferous.** Producing gelatine. सरेस जैसा; जिलेटिनरूप; श्लेषाकार

**Gelatiniform.** Resembling gelatine. सरेस जैसा; जिलेटिनरूप; श्लेषाकार

**Gelatinise.** See **Gelatinize.**

**Gelatinize.** Gelatinise; to convert into gelatine. जेलेटिनकरण; to become gelatinous. जेलेटिनभवन

**Gelatinous.** Having the character or nature of gelatine or jelly; jelly-like. लेसदार; चिपचिपा; लप्सी जैसा; relating to gelatine. सरेस सम्बन्धी; जिलेटिनी;

   **G. Tissue,** mucous tissue. श्लेष्म-ऊतक

**Gemellipara.** A woman who has given birth to twins. युगलप्रसवा; यमलप्रसूता

**Gemellus.** Double; in pairs. यमला; युगल; जोड़ों में

**Geminate.** Occurring in pairs; geminous. युग्म

**Gemination.** Embryologic partial division of a primordium. युग्मीकरण

**Geminous.** See **Geminate.**

**Gemmation.** Reproduction by budding. नेमोद्भवन; कलिकोत्पादन; जनन

**Gemmule.** A small bud that projects from the parent cell, and finally becomes detached, forming a cell of a new generation. दायकण; जेम्यूल

**Gen.** See **Gene.**

**Gena.** Cheek. कपोल; गाल

**Genal.** Pertaining to gena or the cheek. कपोल सम्बन्धी;

    **G. Line,** a furrow on the cheek produced by abdominal disease. कपोल-वलि

**Gender.** Anatomical sex of an individual. लिंग

**Gene.** A factor in the chromosome responsible for transmission of hereditary characteristics; gen. जीन; पित्रैक; परम्पराकरण; गुणसूत्र के अन्तर्गत विद्यमान वंश परम्परा को निर्धारित करने वाली इकाई

**Genealogy.** History of the descent of a person or family. जीनविज्ञान

**Genera.** Plural of **Genus.**

**General.** Pertaining to the whole body. सार्वदैहिक; सर्वांगीण; not special. सामान्य; साधारण;

    **G. Paralysis of Insane (GPI),** involvement of the brain by syphilitic infection with consequent dementia; general paresis. पागल का व्यापक अंगघात;

    **G. Paresis,** see **General Paralysis of Insane (GPI).**

**Generalist.** A general or family physician. who takes care of the majority of non-surgical diseases. पारिवारिक चिकित्सक; कायचिकित्सक

**Generalize.** To make general, as a disease. सर्वव्यापक बनाना, जैसे किसी रोग को

**Generate.** To produce; to beget. उत्पन्न करना; जनन करना

**Generation.** The begetting of offspring. जनन; प्रजनन; gene. वंश; पीढ़ी;

    **Asexual G.,** reproduction by fission or gemmation. अलिंगी जनन;

**Sexual G.,** reproduction by union of a male and female element. लिंगी जनन;

**Spontaneous, G.,** generation of living from non-living matter. स्वत:स्फूर्त जनन

**Generative.** Having the power of reproduction. जनक; प्रजनक; जननक्षम; उत्पादक; relating to generation. प्रजनन अथवा वंश सम्बन्धी

**Generator.** An apparatus for conversion of chemical, mechanical, atomic, or other forms of energy into electricity. जनित्र; जनरेटर

**Generic.** Pertaining to, or denoting the same genus. समजीनी; general. सामान्य अथवा व्यापक; characteristic or distinctive. चारित्रिक अथवा विशिष्ट

**Genesial.** Pertaining to generation or genes; genesic; genetic. जीनी; आनुवंशिक; औत्पत्तिक; वंश-परम्परा सम्बन्धी

**Genesic.** See **Genesial.**

**Genesiology.** The science of reproduction. पुनर्जननविज्ञान

**Genesis.** The act of begetting an origin or beginning process. जनन; प्रजनन; उत्पत्ति; सर्जन

**Genetic.** See **Genesial.**

**Geneticist.** A specialist in genetics. आनुवंशिकीविज्ञ

**Genetics.** Study of the part played by nuclear and extranuclear cellular structures in human heredity. आनुवंशिकी;

**Clinical G.,** the means of diagnosis, management, and prevention of genetic disease. नैदानिक आनुवंशिकी;

**Medical G.,** the study of the aetiology, pathogenesis and natural history of diseases that are least partially genetic in origin. चिकित्सा-आनुवंशिकी

**Genetous.** Congenital. सहज; आजन्म; जन्मजात

**Genial.** Pertaining to the chin; genian. चिबुक अथवा ठोढ़ी सम्बन्धी;

**G. Tubercles,** the four tubercles on the internal surface of lower maxilla. चिबुकान्तर्गुलिकायें; ठोढ़ी के अन्दरूनी तल पर चार गुलिकायें (गांठें)

**Genian.** See **Genial.**

**Genicula.** Plural of **Geniculum.**

**Genicular.** Commonly used to mean genual, i.e. relating to knee. जानु सम्बन्धी; घुटने सम्बन्धी

**Geniculate.** Geniculated; bent like a knee. जानुवत्; घुटने जैसा; बक्र

**Geniculatum.** See **Geniculum.**

**Geniculum.** One of the knee-like bodies; geniculatum. बक्र; जानुवत्; घुटने जैसा

**Genion.** Point at the apex of the lower genial tubercle; the tip of the mental spine, a point in craniometry. चिबुक-बिन्दु

**Genioplasty.** The operation for restoring the chin; mentoplasty. चिबुक-संधान

**Genital.** Relating to reproduction, or generation, or the organs of reproduction. जननांगी; जननांग; गुप्तांगी; प्रजनन अथवा जनन सम्बन्धी;

    **G. Organs,** the organs of generation. जननांग; प्रजननांग; गुप्तांग

**Genitalia.** See **Genitals**.

    **External G.,** the vulva in the female, and the penis and scrotum in the male. बाह्य जननांग

**Genitals.** Plural of **Genital;** genitalia. जननांग; प्रजननांग; गुप्तांग

**Genitocrural.** Pertaining to the genital area and the thighs. जननांगों तथा ऊरुओं सम्बन्धी

**Genitofemoral.** See **Genitocrural**.

**Genitourinary.** Pertaining to the reproductive and urinary organs; urogenital. जननमूत्रांगी; जननांगों तथा मूत्रांगों सम्बन्धी

**Genotype.** The inherent endowment of the individual. जीनप्ररूप; समजीनी; व्यक्ति की परम्परागत अथवा आनुवंशिक बनावट

**Genotypical.** Relating to the genotype. जीनप्ररूपी; जीनप्ररूप सम्बन्धी

**Genu.** The knee. जानु; घुटना; any structure of angular shape resembling a flexed knee. घुटने से मिलती-जुलती कोई कोणाकार आकृति (बनावट);

    **G. Extrorsum,** see **Genu Varum**.

    **G. Introrsum,** see **Genu Valgum**.

    **G. Recurvatum,** backward curvature of knee-joint. पश्च-बक्र; घुटने के जोड़ का पिछला मोड़;

    **G. Valgum,** leg distorted outward throwing knee inside of normal line; knock-knee; genu introrsum; tibia valga. बहिर्नत जानु; संघट्ट जानु;

    **G. Varum,** leg distorted inward throwing the knee outside of normal line; bow-leg; genu extrorsum; tibia vara. अन्तर्नत जानु; धनुर्जंघा

**Genua.** Plural of **Genu**.

**Genual.** Genicular; relating to the knee. जानुपरक; घुटने सम्बन्धी

**Genuflex.** Bent at the knee. जानुनत; घुटने पर झुका हुआ

**Genupectoral.** The knee-chest posture, the patient resting upon the knees and chest. जानुवक्षस्थिति; घुटनों को छाती से सटा कर रखने की स्थिति

**Genus.** A species with characteristics which differentiate them from the species. वंश; जीनस

**Genus Epidemicus.** The prevailing type of a disease. महामारी; व्यापकरोग; महामारी के रूप में फैलने वाला रोग

**Genyantritis.** Inflammation of the mucous membrane of the maxillary antrum. कपोलकोटरशोथ

**Genyplasty.** An operation for restoring the cheek. कपोलसंघान

**Geo-.** Prefix denoting relation to the earth, or to soil. 'मृदा' अथवा 'मिट्टी' के रूप में प्रयुक्त किया जाने वाला उपसर्ग

**Geographic Tongue.** A rare disease of the tongue in which there are irregular areas of denudation. चित्रित जिह्वा

**Geophagia.** See **Geophagism.**

**Geophagism.** The practice of clay-eating; geophagia; geophagy. मृदाभक्षण

**Geophagy.** See **Geophagism.**

**Geriatician.** One who specializes in gariatrics. जराचिकित्सक

**Geriatric.** Relating to old age or to geriatrics. बृद्धावस्था अथवा जराचिकित्सा विज्ञान सम्बन्धी

**Geriatrics.** The branch of the medical science dealing with old age and its diseases. जराचिकित्साविज्ञान

**Germ.** A microbe or bacterium; a unicellular micro-organism. बीजांकुर; बीजाणु; बीज; जीवाणु; रोगाणु; an ovum; a spore; an undeveloped embryo. डिम्ब; अविकसित भ्रूण;

G.-cell, a cell resulting from a fecundated germinal vesicle. बीज-कोशिका; जनन-कोशिका;

G.-disease, any disease of microbic origin. बीजाणु-रोग;

G. Epithelium, the cylindric cell on the median plate of the mesoblast; germ-ridge. बीज-उपकला;

G.-force, plastic or constructive force. जननशक्ति;

G.-plasm, germinal protoplasm transmitting inherited peculiarities. बीज-द्रव्य;

G.-ridge, see **Germ Epithelium.**

**G. Theory,** the theory of the bacterial origin of disease; the doctorine of the origin of every organism from a germ. जीवाणु सिद्धान्त;

**Enamel G.,** the enamel organ of a developing tooth. दन्तवल्क बीज;

**Tooth G.,** the enamel organ and dentin papilla, constituting the developing tooth. बीज-दन्त

**German Measles.** See **Rubella.**

**Germicidal.** See **Germicide.**

**Germicide.** An agent which kills the germs; germicidal. रोगाणुनाशक; रोगाणुनाशी; जीवाणुनाशक; जीवाणुनाशी

**Germinal.** Pertaining to a germ or germination; germinative. बीजाणु; जीवाणुक; जननिक; रोगाणुक; बीजांकुरक; बीजाणु, रोगाणु अथवा जीवाणु सम्बन्धी;

**G. Area,** the white spot on one side of the vitelline membrane; germinal disc. बीजाणु क्षेत्र;

**G. Disc,** see **Germinal Area.**

**G. Membrane,** the blastoderm. बीजकला; बीज-अस्तर;

**G. Vesicle,** the nucleus of the ovule. बीज-पुटिका

**Germination.** The development of a seed or germ. अंकुरण; बीज अथवा जीव का विकास

**Germinative.** See **Germinal.**

**Germinoma.** A neoplasm of germinal tissue that normally differentiates to form sperm cells or ova. बीजार्बुद

**Geroderma.** The atrophic skin of the aged; any condition in which the skin is thinned and wrinkled, resembling the integument of old age. वलीयत्वक्; झुर्रीदार त्वचा

**Gerodontics.** Dentistry concerned with the problems of the elderly; gerodontology. जरादन्तविज्ञान

**Gerodontology.** See **Gerodontics.**

**Geromorphism.** Appearance of old age in the young; a condition of premature senility. अकालजरावस्था

**Gerontal.** Relating to old age; gerontic. बृद्धावस्था सम्बन्धी

**Gerontic.** See **Gerontal.**

**Gerontological.** Pertaining to gerontology. जराविज्ञान सम्बन्धी

**Gerontologist.** A specialist in gerontology. जराविज्ञानी

**Gerontology.** Scientific study of the process and problems of aging. जराविज्ञान; जराप्रकरण

**Gestation.** Pregnancy. गर्भ; सगर्भता

**G.F.R.** Glomerular filtration rate. केशिकास्तवक निस्यंदन दर

**Ghon's Focus.** Primary complex. प्रारम्भिक फुप्फुसक्षय

**Ghost.** A phantom. भूत-प्रेत; प्रेतात्मा; छाया

**Giantism.** the same as **Gigantism.**

**Gibbon's Hydrocele.** Hydrocele with hernia. सजलवृषणहर्निया; हर्निया के साथ जलवृषण

**Gibbous.** Bunched or bulged out. कुबड़ा; उभरा हुआ

**Giddiness.** Vertigo; a sensation of whirling; giddy. शिरोघूर्णन; भ्रमि; सिर चकराना; चक्कर

**Gigantism.** An abnormal overgrowth, especially in height. महाकायता; बृहत्-कायता

**Gills.** The respiratory organs of fishes and frogs. गलश्वसनिकायें; मछलियों तथा मेंढकों के श्वासांग

**Ginger.** An aromatic root with carminative properties. अदरक; सोंठ

**Gingiva.** The gum; the dense fibrous tissue, covered by mucous membrane, that envelopes the alveolar process of the upper and lower jaws that surround the neck of the teeth. मसूड़ा;
  **Alveolar G.,** gingival tissue supplied to the alveolar bone. दन्तउलूखल मसूड़ा; कोष्ठिक मसूड़ा;
  **Attached G.,** that part of the oral mucosa firmly bound to the tooth and alveolar process. अभिलग्न मसूड़ा;
  **Free G.,** that portion of the gingiva that surrounds the tooth and is not directly attached to the tooth surface. उन्मुक्त मसूड़ा

**Gingivae.** Plural of **Gingiva.**

**Gingival.** Pertaining to the gums. मसूड़ों सम्बन्धी;
  **G. Index,** an index of the periodontal disease based upon the severity and location of the lesion. मसूड़ा-सूचकांक;
  **G. Line,** the dark line on the gums produced by certain metallic poisons. मसूड़ा-रेखा;
  **G.-periodontal Index,** an index of the gingivitis, gingival irritation and advanced periodontal disease. मसूड़ापरिदन्त-सूचकांक

**Gingivalgia.** Neuralgia of the gums. मसूड़ार्ति; मसूड़ाशूल; मसूड़ों का दर्द

**Gingivectomy.** Excision of a portion of the gums, usually for pyrrhoea; gum resection. मसूड़ा-उच्छेदन; दन्तमांसोच्छेदन

**Gingivitis.** Inflammation of the gums. मसूड़ाशोथ; मसूड़ों का प्रदाह;
  **Pregnancy G.,** occurs due to hormonal changes. सगर्भ मसूड़ाशोथ

**Gingivoglossitis.** Inflammation of the gums and the tongue. दन्तमांसजिह्वाशोथ; मसूड़ों तथा जीभ का प्रदाह

**Gingivoplasty.** Surgical reshaping and recontouring of the gingival tissue to attain aesthetic, physiologic and functional form. मसूड़ासंधान; दन्तमांससंधान

**Gingivus.** The gum. मसूड़ा; मसूढ़ा

**Ginglyform.** See **Ginglymoid.**

**Ginglymoid.** Resembling, or of the form of a hinge-joint;

ginglyform. कोर-संध्याभ; कोर-संधिरूप

**Ginglymus.** A hinge-joint, or ginglymoid joint. कोर-संधि

**Girdle.** A band or belt to go around a body. मेखला; वलय; कटिबन्ध;
  **G. Anesthesia,** an anesthetic ring around the body. मेखला असंवेदनता;
  **G. Pain,** a constricting pain round the waist region; girdle sensation. कटिवेदना; कमरदर्द; मेखलार्ति
  **G. Sensation,** see **Girdle Pain.**
  **Pelvic G.,** comprising the two innominate bones, sacrum and coccyx. श्रोणि मेखला; श्रोणि वलय;
  **Shoulder G.,** comprising the two clavicles and scapulae. स्कन्ध-मेखला; अंसवलय

**Glabella.** The small space between the eyebrows; a point midway between the two supraorbital ridges; glabellum. स्थपनी; भ्रूमध्य; भ्रूमध्य बिन्दु; दोनों भौंहो के बीच वाला स्थान

**Glabellum.** See **Glabella.**

**Glabrate.** See **Glabrous.**

**Glabrification.** The process of becoming smooth; glistening and hairless. अलोमीकरण; अलोमीभवन; चमचमाता तथा केशहीन

**Glabrous.** Hairless, smooth, without projections; glabrate. रोमहीन; लोमहीन; केशहीन; अलोम

**Glacial.** Assuming a crystalline form. काचाभ; काचमय

**Gladiolus.** The middle piece of the sternum. उरोस्थिकाय; उरोस्थि का मध्य भाग

**Glairy.** Viscous; slimy; albuminous. स्निग्ध; चमकीला; अन्नसारिक; चिपचिपा

**Gland.** A soft body, the function of which is to secrete some fluid. ग्रन्थि; गिल्टी;
  **Absorbent G.,** a lymphatic gland. अवशोषक ग्रन्थि;
  **Acinous G.,** a gland in which the secretory unit has a saclike shape and a very small lumen; alveolar gland. कोष्ठक ग्रन्थि;
  **Adrenal G.,** a flattened, roughly triangular body upon upper end of each kidney; suprarenal gland. अधिवृक्क ग्रन्थि;
  **Aggregate G.'s,** see **Cowper's Glands.**
  **Alveolar G.,** see **Acinous Gland.**
  **Apocrine G.,** a coiled tubular gland the cells of which were believed to contribute part of their protoplasmic substance to their secretion. शिखरस्रावी ग्रन्थि;
  **Areolar G.'s,** a number of cutaneous glands forming small,

rounded projections from the surface of the areola of the mamma. मण्डल ग्रन्थियां;

**Axillary G.'s,** the lymph-gland in the axilla; axillary lymphnodes. कक्षा ग्रन्थियां;

**Bartholin's G.,** the vulvovaginal gland; one of the two mucoid-secreting tubuloalveolar glands on either side of the lower part of the vagina. बार्थोलिन ग्रन्थि; योनिकपाट ग्रन्थि; महाप्रघाण ग्रन्थि;

**Cardiac G.,** a coiled tubular gland located in the cardiac region of the stomach. हृद्-ग्रन्थि;

**Carotid G.,** a ductless gland at the bifurcation of the common carotid artery. मन्या ग्रन्थि;

**Ceruminous G.'s,** glands secreting the cerumen of the ears. कर्णगूथ ग्रन्थियां; कर्णमल छोड़ने. वाली ग्रन्थियां;

**Cervical G.'s,** the lymph-glands of the neck. ग्रीवा ग्रन्थियां;

**Coccygeal G.,** a small vascular body at the tip of the coccyx (tail-bone). अनुत्रिक ग्रन्थि;

**Compound G.,** a gland whose larger excretory ducts branch repeatedly into smaller ducts which ultimately drain secretory units. विवृत ग्रन्थि; योगिक ग्रन्थि; मिश्र ग्रन्थि;

**Cowper's G.'s,** the two small compound racemose glands, which produce a mucoid secretion; aggregate glands. कूपर ग्रन्थियां; शिश्नमूल ग्रन्थियां;

**Ductless G.'s,** glands that have no ducts, their secretions being observed directly into the blood; endocrine glands. निःस्रोत ग्रन्थियां; अन्तःस्रावी ग्रन्थियां; नलिकाहीन ग्रन्थियां; वाहिकाहीन ग्रन्थियां;

**Duodenal G.'s,** small, branched, coiled tubular glands that occur mostly in the submucosa of the first part of the duodenum. ग्रहणी ग्रन्थियां;

**Endocrine G.'s,** see **Ductless Glands.**

**Excretory G.,** a gland separating waste material from the blood. उत्सर्गी ग्रन्थि;

**Exocrine G.,** a gland from which secretions reach a free surface of the body by ducts. बाह्यस्रावी ग्रन्थि; बहिःस्रावी ग्रन्थि;

**Hematopoietic G.'s,** glands that take part in the blood-formation, as the spleen, thymus, etc. रक्तोत्पादक ग्रन्थियां;

**Intestinal G.,** one of the isolated lymph-glands distributed through the intestinal mucous membrane; solitary gland. आंत्र ग्रन्थि;

**Lacrimal G.,** a compound racemose gland in the upper and outer part of the orbit that secrets tears. अश्रु-ग्रन्थि;

**Lymph G.,** see **Lymphatic Gland.**

**Lymphatic G.,** does not secret, but is connected with filtration

# Gland

of the lymph; lymph nodes; lymph gland. लसीका ग्रन्थि; लसीकापर्व ग्रन्थि;

**Mammary G.,** the milk-secreting organ. स्तन ग्रन्थि;

**Maxillary G.,** one of two salivary glands in the neck; submandibular gland. ऊर्ध्वहनु ग्रन्थि;

**Muciparous G.,** see **Mucous Gland.**

**Mucous G.,** one that secrets mucus; muciparous gland. श्लेष्म-ग्रन्थि;

**Parotid G.,** the largest of the salivary glands in front of the ear. कर्णमूल-ग्रन्थि; कर्णपूर्व-ग्रन्थि;

**Pineal G.,** the pineal body. पिनियल ग्रन्थि;

**Pituitary G.,** a term for the hypophysis of the brain. पीयूषिका ग्रन्थि;

**Prostate G.,** a glandular body situated around the neck of the bladder in the male. पुरःस्थ ग्रन्थि;

**Pyloric G.'s,** glands of the stomach near the pylorus secreting pepsin. जठरनिर्गम-ग्रन्थियां;

**Racemose G.,** a compound gland resembling a bunch of grapes. गुच्छितग्रन्थि;

**Salivary G.,** any one secreting saliva. लार ग्रन्थि;

**Sebaceous G.'s,** the glands in the epidermis which secrete the fat. वसा ग्रन्थियां;

**Serous G.'s,** glands secreting a thin watery fluid. सीरमी ग्रन्थियां;

**Simple G.,** a gland having but one secreting sac and a single tube. सरल ग्रन्थि;

**Solitary G.,** see **Intestinal Gland.**

**Sublingual G.,** a salivary gland on each side beneath the tongue. अवजिह्वा-ग्रन्थि;

**Submandibular G.,** see **Maxillary Gland.**

**Submaxillary G.,** a salivary gland below the angle of the jaw. अवहनु-ग्रन्थि;

**Sudoriparous G.'s,** see **Sweat Glands.**

**Suprarenal G.,** see **Adrenal Gland.**

**Sweat G.'s,** the convoluted glands in the skin secreting sweat; sudoriparous glands. स्वेद ग्रन्थियां;

**Thymus G.,** a glandular organ in the anterior superior

mediastinum, usually disappearing in adult life. बाल्यग्रन्थि; थाइमस ग्लैण्ड;

**Thyroid G.,** a ductless glandular body at the upper part of the trachea consisting of two lateral lobes connected centrally by an isthmus. अवटु-ग्रन्थि;

**Vaginal G.,** one of the glands of the vaginal mucous membrane. योनि-ग्रन्थि;

**Vulvovaginal G.,** see **Bartholin's Gland.**

**Glanders.** A contagious febrile, ulcerative disease communicable from horses, mules and asses to man. ग्लैण्डर रोग; घोड़ों तथा खच्चरों को होने वाला एक संकामक रोग

**Glandes.** Plural of **Glans.**

**Glandilemma.** The capsule of a gland. ग्रन्थिसम्पुट

**Glandula.** A small gland or glandule. सूक्ष्मग्रन्थि; क्षुद्रग्रन्थि; लघुग्रन्थि

**Glandulae.** Plural of **Glandula.**

**Glandular.** Of the nature of, or pertaining to a gland; glandulous. ग्रन्थिल; ग्रन्थि वाला; ग्रन्थि सम्बन्धी

**Glandule.** See **Glandula.**

**Glandulin.** An extract from gland-tissue. ग्रन्थिरस; ग्लैण्डुलिन

**Glandulosity.** A collection of, or full of glands. ग्रन्थिलता

**Glandulous.** See **Glandular.**

**Glans.** The bulbous extremity of the penis and clitoris, मुण्ड (जैसे शिश्नमुण्ड तथा भगशिश्निकामुण्ड); a gland. ग्रन्थि; गिल्टी;

**G. Clitoridis,** a small mass of the erectile tissue capping the body of the clitoris. भगशिश्निकामुण्ड;

**G. Penis,** the conical expansion of the body of the penis. शिश्नमुण्ड

**Glaserian.** Relating to, or described by Johann H. Glaser. ग्लैसरी; जॉन एच० ग्लैसर सम्बन्धी अथवा उनके द्वारा वर्णित

**Glaserian Artery.** The tympanic artery. मध्यकर्ण धमनी; ग्लैसरी धमनी

**Glaserian Fissure.** The glenoid or petrotympanic fissure which divides transversely the glenoid fossa of the temporal bone. अंसगर्त विदर; ग्लैसरी विदर

**Glasses.** Spectacles; lens for correcting refractive errors in the eyes. ऐनक; चश्मा

**Glassy.** Resembling glasses. ऐनक जैसा; कांच जैसा; कांचाभ; bright. चमकदार; चमकता हुआ

**Glaucina.** The natural form of cow-pox. गो-मसूरिका

**Glaucoma.** A hardening of the eyeball due to interference with normal circulation of the eye-fluids; glaucosis. अधिमंथ; सबलवायु; आंखों का एक रोग जिसमें दृष्टि धुंधली पड़ जाती है

**Glaucomatous.** Affected with or like glaucoma. अधिमंथग्रस्त; अधिमंथवत्; अधिमंथ जैसा

**Glaucosis.** See **Glaucoma**.

**Gleet.** A chronic stage of gonorrhoea with mucopurulent discharge. जीर्ण प्रमेह; चिरकारी प्रमेह; सूजाक रोग; ग्लीट

**Gleety.** Resembling or affected with gleet. सूजाक रोग जैसा या सूजाक-ग्रस्त

**Glenohumeral.** Pertaining to the glenoid cavity and the humerus. अंसगर्तप्रगण्डिकी; अंसगर्त तथा प्रगण्डिका सम्बन्धी;

    **G. Ligaments,** three ligaments of the capsule of the shoulder-joint. अंसगर्तप्रगण्डिका-बन्ध

**Glenoid.** Pitlike; shallow; resembling a socket. अंसगर्त; गर्तवत्; गर्ताभ; कूपाभ;

    **G. Cavity,** a fossa in the head of the scapula for the humerus. अंसगर्त गह्वर;

    **G. Fossa,** a depression in the temporal bone receiving the condyle of the lower jaw. अंसगर्त खात

**Glia.** Neuroglia; non-neuronal cellular elements of the central and peripheral nervous system. तंत्रिकाबन्ध

**Gliacyte.** A neurolglial cell. तंत्रिकाबन्ध-कोशिका

**Glial.** Pertaining to glia or neuroglia. तंत्रिकाबन्ध सम्बन्धी

**Glioblastoma.** A neuroglial cell tumour, or a glioma, occurring most frequently in the cerebrum of adults. तंत्रिकाबन्धप्रसू-अर्बुद; मस्तिष्क का एक सांघातिक अर्बुद;

    **G. Multiforme,** a highly malignant brain tumour. बहुरूपी तंत्रिकाबन्धप्रसू-अर्बुद

**Glioma.** A tumour composed of neuroglia; a malignant growth which does not give rise to secondary deposits. तंत्रिकाबन्धार्बुद

**Gliomatosis.** The formation of a glioma; neurogliomatosis. तंत्रिकाबन्धार्बुदता;

    **G. Cerebri,** the cerebral glioma. प्रमस्तिष्क तंत्रिकाबन्धार्बुदता

**Gliomatous.** Pertaining to, or characterized by a glioma.

तंत्रिकाबन्धार्बुदीय

**Gliomyoma.** A tumour of nerve and muscle tissue; glioma mixed with myoma. तंत्रिकापेश्यर्बुद; तंत्रिकाबन्धार्बुद तथा पेश्यर्बुद दोनों साथ मिले हुए

**Gliomyxoma.** A glioma with a mucoid degeneration. तंत्रिकाबन्धश्लेष्मार्बुद

**Glioneuroma.** A combined glioma and neuroma. तंत्रिकाबन्धतंत्रिकार्बुद

**Gliosarcoma.** A sarcomatous glioma. तंत्रिकाबन्धकर्कटार्बुद

**Gliosis.** A diffuse proliferation of the neuroglial cells. तंत्रिकाबन्धवृद्धि

**Global.** Complete, generalized, overall, or total aspect. पूर्ण; सम्पूर्ण

**Globate.** Sphenoid; shaped like a globe. गोलाकार

**Globe.** A ball, as of the eye. गोलक;

   **G. of the eye,** the eyeball. नेत्र-गोलक; अक्षि-गोलक

**Globi.** Plural of **Globus.**

**Globin.** A protein which combines with haematin to form haemoglobin. ग्लोबिन; रक्तगोलिका; हेमोग्लोबिन का एक प्रोटीन

**Globular.** Shaped like a globe. गोलकाकार; गोलाकार

**Globule.** A small round particle, or body. पिण्ड; ग्लोब्यूल; a fat droplet in milk. दूध में एक वसा बिन्दुक

**Globulicidal.** Destroying blood-corpuscles. रक्तकोशिकानाशी

**Globulins.** A group of porteins found in animal tissues which differs from the albumins in the heat. रक्तगोलिकायें; ग्लोब्यूलिन्स

**Globulinuria.** The presence of globulins in the urine. रक्तगोलिकामेह

**Globulous.** Shaped like a globe. गोलकाकार; गोलाकार

**Globus.** A ball or globe; a round body. गोलक; गोला; पिण्ड;

   **G. Hystericus,** the sensation of a ball in the throat in hysteria. वायुगोला;

   **G. Major,** the head of the epididymis. बृहत् वायुगोला; बृहत् पिण्ड;

   **G. Minor,** the lower end of the epididymis. लघु वायुगोला; क्षुद्र पिण्ड;

   **G. Pallidus,** the light-coloured inner portion of the lenticular nucleus. पीत-पिण्ड; पाण्डुर पिण्ड

**Glomal.** Relating to, or involving a glomus. कोशिकागुच्छ अथवा वाहिकागुच्छ सम्बन्धी

**Glomangioma.** A painful neoplasm composed of specialized pericytes and neurites, usually in single encapsulated nodular masses that occur almost exclusively in the skin; angiomyoneuroma; angioneuromyoma; glomus tumour. केशिकागुच्छार्बुद; वाहिकागुच्छार्बुद

**Glomangiosis.** The occurrence of multiple complexes of small vascular channels, each resembling a glomus. केशिकागुच्छार्बुदता; वाहिकागुच्छार्बुदता

**Glomectomy.** Excision of a glomus tumour. केशिकागुच्छार्बुद-उच्छेदन; वाहिकागुच्छार्बुद-उच्छेदन

**Glomerate.** Clustered. गुच्छित; grouped. समूहीकृत

**Glomerular.** Relating to, or affecting a glomerulus or the glomerule; glomerulose. केशिकास्तवकीय; केशिकागुच्छीय; केशिकाजाल सम्बन्धी

**Glomerule.** The important functioning unit of the kidney; glomerulus. केशिकास्तवक; केशिकागुच्छ; केशिकाजाल; गुर्दे की महत्वपूर्ण क्रियात्मक इकाई

**Glomeruli.** Plural of **Glomerulus.**

**Glomerulitis.** Acute suppurative inflammation of the glomeruli of the kidney. केशिकास्तवकशोथ

**Glomerulonephritis.** Disease affecting the glomerules which perform the principal kidney functions. स्तवकवृक्कशोथ

**Glomerulopathy.** Glomerular disease of any type. केशिकास्तवकरोग; केशिकागुच्छरोग

**Glomerulosclerosis.** Fibrosis of the kidney, the result of renal inflammation, arteriosclerosis or diabetes. स्तवकवृक्ककाठिन्य

**Glomerulose.** See **Glomerular.**

**Glomerulus.** See **Glomerule.**

**Glomus.** A glomerule. केशिकास्तवक; केशिकागुच्छ; केशिकाजाल; a ball of the blood vessels. वाहिकागुच्छ;

G. **Aorticum,** the aortic body. धमनी-वाहिकागुच्छ;

G. **Caroticum,** the carotid or intercarotid body. मन्या-केशिकागुच्छ; मन्या-वाहिकागुच्छ;

G. **Choroideum,** an elongated balllike mass in the choroid plexus at the junction of the central part and descending horn of the lateral ventricle. रंजितपटल वाहिकागुच्छ;

G. **Tumour,** see **Glomangioma.**

**Glossa.** The tongue; lingua. जिह्वा; जीभ

**Glossagra.** See **Glossalgia**.

**Glossal.** Pertaining to the tongue; lingual. जिह्वापरक; जीभ सम्बन्धी

**Glossalgia.** Pain in the tongue; glossagra; glossodynia. जिह्वार्ति; जिह्वाशूल; जीभ का दर्द

**Glossectomy.** The amputation or excision of the tongue; glossotomy; lingulectomy. जिह्वा-उच्छेदन; जीभ को काट कर निकाल देना

**Glossitis.** Inflammation of the tongue. जिह्वाशोथ; जीभ का प्रदाह

**Glossocele.** A swollen or an oedematous tongue. जिह्वाविस्फार; जिह्वात्रंस; शोफज जिह्वा; सूजी हुई जीभ

**Glossodynia.** See **Glossalgia**.

**Glossoepiglottic.** Relating to the tongue and the epiglottis; glossoepiglottidean. जिह्वाकण्ठच्छदीय

**Glossoepiglottidean.** See **Glossoepiglottic**.

**Glossograph.** An instrument for showing the movements of the tongue in speaking. जिह्वालेख

**Glossography.** A description of the tongue. जिह्वाचित्रण; जिह्वालेखन

**Glossohyal.** Pertaining to the tongue and the hyoid bone; hyoglossal. जिह्वाकण्ठिकास्थिज; जीभ तथा कण्ठिकास्थि सम्बन्धी

**Glossoid.** Resembling the tongue. जिह्वाभ; जीभ जैसा

**Glossolalia.** Unintelligible jargon. वाग्दोष; दोषपूर्ण उच्चारण

**Glossology.** The science of the tongue; glottology. जिह्वाविज्ञान; जिह्वाप्रकरण

**Glossolysis.** Paralysis of the tongue; glossoplegia. जिह्वाघात; जिह्वालयन; जीभ का पक्षाघात (लकवा)

**Glossopathy.** Any disease of the tongue. जिह्वारोग; जीभ की कोई बीमारी

**Glossopharyngeal.** Pertaining to the tongue and the pharynx. जिह्वा तथा ग्रसनी सम्बन्धी;

    **G. Nerve,** the ninth cranial nerve. जिह्वाग्रसनी तंत्रिका

**Glossophygia.** Parasitic glossitis. परजीवी जिह्वाशोथ

**Glossophytia.** A dark discolouration of the tongue from an epithelial accumulation. श्यामजिह्वा

**Glossoplasty.** Plastic surgery of the tongue. जिह्वासंधान

**Glossoplegia.** See **Glossolysis**.

**Glossorrhaphy.** Suture of a wound of the tongue. जिह्वासीवन

**Glossospasm.** A spasm of the muscles of the tongue. जिह्वाकर्ष

**Glossotomy.** See **Glossectomy.**

**Glossotrichia.** Hair tongue. लोमजिह्वा

**Glossy.** Shining and smooth. चमचमाती; चमकती हुई; स्निग्ध;

   **G. Skin,** neurosis of the skin marked by shining smoothness, attended with intense pain. स्निग्ध चर्म

**Glottic.** Relating to the tongue, or to the glottis. जिह्वा अथवा कण्ठद्वार सम्बन्धी

**Glottides.** Plural of **Glottis.**

**Glottis.** The opening into the windpipe at the larynx; aperture between the arytenoid cartilages of the larynx. कण्ठद्वार; घांटी; श्वासनली का मुख

**Glottitis.** Inflammation of the glottis or glottic portion of the larynx. कण्ठद्वारशोथ; घांटी का प्रदाह

**Glottology.** See **Glossology.**

**Glover's suture.** A form of continuous suture. ग्लोबर बन्ध

**Glucides.** Carbohydrates. श्वेतसार; कार्बोहाड्रेट्स

**Glucocid.** A body containing glucose and an organic principle; glucocide; glucosid; glucoside. शर्करा; मधुमेय; ग्लूकोसाइड; ग्लूकोसिड

**Glucocide.** See **Glucocid.**

**Glucogenesis.** See **Glycogenesis.**

**Glucogenic.** A saccharine state of blood; glycohemia. शर्करारक्तता

**Glucose.** Grape sugar, blood sugar or dextrose. (The form in which carbohydrates are absorbed through the intestinal tract and circulated in the blood). ग्लूकोज; शर्करा

**Glucosid.** See **Glucocid.**

**Glucoside.** See **Glucocid.**

**Glucosuria.** See **Glycosuria.**

**Glue.** A hard brittle substance obtained by boiling to a jelly, the skin, hoops, etc, of animals. गोंद; सरेस;

   **G.-like Tumour,** a glioma. तंत्रिकाबन्धार्बुद

**Gluside.** A coal-tar derivation. ग्लूसिड

**Glutaeus.** See **Gluteus.**

**Glutaeusmaximus.** A giant muscle of the hip. महानितम्बिकापेशी; कूल्हे की बड़ी पेशी

**Glutamine.** A vegetable compound. ग्लूटामिन; एक शाक्-मिश्रण

**Gluteal.** Pertaining to the buttocks. नितम्बों अर्थात् कूल्हों सम्बन्धी;
   **G. Bursas,** three bursas below the glutei muscle. नितम्ब श्लेषपुटी;
   **G. Reflex,** contraction of the glutei on stimulation of the skin over them. नितम्ब प्रतिवर्त

**Glutei.** The muscles of the buttocks. नितम्बपेशियां; कूल्हों की पेशियां

**Gluten.** The insoluble protein constituent of wheat and other grains. आश्लेष; चिपचिपी वस्तु

**Gluteofemoral.** Relating to the buttocks and the thigh. कूल्हों तथा जांघ सम्बन्धी

**Gluteoinguinal.** Relating to the buttocks and the groin. कूल्हों तथा ऊरु सम्बन्धी

**Gluteus.** One of the three muscles of the hip; glutaeus. नितम्बपेशी; नितम्बिका; कूल्हे की पेशी

**Glutin.** The viscid constituent of the wheat-gluten. निशास्ता; अन्नसार

**Glutinous.** Viscid; adhesive; tenacious; sticky. चिपचिपा; लसदार; निशास्तेदार; like glue or gluten. गोंद अथवा आश्लेष जैसा

**Glutitis.** Inflammation of the glutei muscles. नितम्बपेशीशोथ; कूल्हे की पेशियों का प्रदाह

**Glycaemia.** Presence of glucose in the blood; glycemia. शर्करारक्तता; रक्त में शर्करा विद्यमान रहना

**Glycemia.** See **Glycaemia.**

**Glycerin.** The chemical of the alcohol group; the sweetish principle of oils and fats; glycerine. ग्लिसरिन;
   **G.-jelly,** a mixture of glycerin and jelly. ग्लिसरिन-जेली

**Glycerine.** See **Glycerin.**

**Glycerol.** A medicine for outward application prepared with mixture of glycerine; glycerole. मधुरव; ग्लिसरॉल

**Glycerole.** See **Glycerol.**

**Glyco-.** Prefix denoting relationship to sugars in general. 'मधु' अथवा 'शर्करा' का अर्थ देने वाला उपसर्ग

**Glycogen.** See **Glycogene.**

**Glycogenase.** An enzyme necessary for the conversion of glucogene into glucose. ग्लाइकोजिनेस; ग्लिकोजिनेस

**Glycogene.** Starch stored in the body to be converted as needed, into sugar; glycogen. मधुजन; ग्लाइकोजन

**Glycogenesis.** Glycogen formation from glucose; glucogenesis. शर्कराजनन

**Glycogenetic.** Relating to glycogenesis; glycogenic; glycogenous. शर्कराजनन सम्बन्धी

**Glycogenic.** See **Glycogenetic.**

**Glycogenolysis.** The hydrolysis of glycogen to glucose. शर्कराजनापघटन

**Glycogenous.** See **Glycogenetic.**

**Glycohemia.** See **Glucohemia.**

**Glycolysis.** The hydrolysis of sugar in the body. शर्करालयन; शर्करापघटन

**Glycolytic.** Relating to glycolysis. शर्करालायी;

  **G. Ferment,** a glucose decomposing ferment. शर्करालायी खमीर

**Glycopenia.** Dificiency of sugar in the blood. रक्तशर्कराल्पता; रक्त में शर्करा की कमी

**Glycophilia.** A condition in which there is a distinct tendency to develop hyperglycemia. शर्करारागिता

**Glycoptyalism.** See **Glycosialia.**

**Glycorrhachia.** Presence of sugar in the cerebrospinal fluid. शर्कराप्रमस्तिष्कमेरुद्रवता

**Glycorrhea.** A discharge of saccharine fluid from the body; glycorrhoea. शर्करास्राव

**Glycorrhoea.** See **Glycorrhea.**

**Glycosecretory.** Causing or involved in the secretion of glycogen. शर्करास्रावी

**Glycosemia.** The presence of glucose in the blood. शर्कराक्तता; खून में शर्करा विद्यमान रहना

**Glycosialia.** Presence of sugar in the saliva; glycoptyalism. शर्करालारता

**Glycosialorrhea.** An excessive secretion of saliva that contains sugar; glycosialorrhoea. शर्करालालास्राव

**Glycosialorrhoea.** See **Glycosialorrhea.**

**Glycoside.** Natural substance composed of a sugar with another compound. ग्लाइकोसिड

**Glycostatic.** Denoting the property of certain extracts of the anterior hypophysis that permit the body to maintain its glycogen stores in muscle, liver and other tissues. शर्करास्थिर

**Glycosuria.** The excretion of carbohydrates or sugar in the urine; glucosuria; glycouresis. शर्करामेह; पेशाब में शर्करा जाना;

   **Alimentary G.,** developing after the ingestion of a moderate amount of sugar or starch. पोषणज शर्करामेह;

   **Renal G.,** recurring or persistent excretion of glucose in the urine. वृक्क-शर्करामेह

**Glycouresis.** See **Glycosuria.**

**Glycouretics.** Agents which increase sugar in the urine. शर्करामेहज तत्व

**Glycyrrhiza.** Liquorice root; demulcent, slightly luxative, expectorant and used as a flavouring agent. मधुयष्टिमूल

**Glycyrrhiza Glabra.** A genus of plants including its demulcent root; also called **Glycyrrhiza Glandulifera** and **Glycyrrhiza Violacea.** मधुयष्टिपादप; अतिमधुरपादप; मुलहटी पादप; मुलेठी का पेड़

**Gm.** Abbreviation for **Gram.** 'ग्राम' का संक्षिप्त रूप

**Gnat.** A two-winged fly; a midge. मच्छर; मच्छड़; डाँस

**Gnath-.** See **Gnatho-.**

**Gnathalgia.** Pain in the jaw. हनुवेदना; हन्वार्ति; जबड़े में दर्द

**Gnathic.** Pertaining to the jaw, or alveolar process. हनु सम्बन्धी; हनुप्रसर;

   **G. Index,** a number expressing the amount of projection of the jaw. हनुप्रसर सूचकांक

**Gnathion.** The lowest median point of the inferior maxilla. चिबुकाग्र-बिन्दु

**Gnathitis.** Inflammation of the jaw. हनुशोथ; जबड़े का प्रदाह

**Gnatho-,Gnath-.** Prefixes denoting relation to the jaw. 'हनु' का अर्थ देने वाले उपसर्ग

**Gnathocephalus.** A foetus without a head, but with large jaw. हनुशीर्ष

**Gnathodynamics.** The study of the relationship of the magnitude and direction of the forces developed by and upon the components of the masticatory system during function; gnathology. हनुविज्ञान; चर्वणविज्ञान

**Gnathodynamometer.** A device for measuring biting pressure. हनुदाबमापी

**Gnathological.** Pertaining to gnathodynamics or gnathology. चर्वणविज्ञान सम्बन्धी

**Gnathology.** See **Gnathodynamics.**

**Gnathometer.** An instrument for measuring the jaw. हनुमापी; हनुमापक यंत्र

**Gnathoplasty.** A plastic operation on the jaw. हनुसंधान

**Goblet Cells.** Cuplike cells in the intestinal epithelium. चषक कोशिकायें

**Goggle-eye.** The eye of the exophthalmic goitre. नेत्रोत्सेधीगलगण्ड-नेत्र; गॉग्गल-नेत्र

**Goiter.** See **Goitre.**

**Goitre.** A chronic enlargement of the thyroid gland; goiter. गलगण्ड; घेंघा;

>    **Aberrant G.,** enlargement of supernumerary thyroid gland. विपथ गलगण्ड;
>
>    **Adenomatous G.,** goitre due to one or more encapsulated adenomas or multiple nonencapsulated colloid nodules within its substance. ग्रन्थ्यर्बुदीय गलगण्ड;
>
>    **Colloid G.,** goitre in which the contents of the follicles increase greatly and cause pressure atrophy of the epithelium. कलिल गलगण्ड; कोलाइड गलगण्ड;
>
>    **Cystic G.,** one due to the presence of one or more cysts within the gland. पुटीय गलगण्ड;
>
>    **Diving G.,** a freely movable goitre that is sometimes above and sometimes below the sternal notch; wandering goitre. चल गलगण्ड; भ्रमणकारी गलगण्ड;
>
>    **Exophthalmic G.,** goitre with exophthalmos and cardiac palpitation; Basedow's disease; Grave's disease. नेत्रोत्सेधी गलगण्ड;
>
>    **Fibrous G.,** a firm hyperplasia of the thyroid and its capsule. तान्तव गलगण्ड;
>
>    **Follicular G.,** See **Parenchymatous Goitre.**
>
>    **Lingual G.,** a tumour of thyroid tissue involving the embryonic rudiment at the base of the tongue. जिह्वा-गलगण्ड;
>
>    **Non-toxic G.,** goitre not accompanied by hyperthyroidism. अविषण्ण गलगण्ड;

**Parenchymatous G.**, goitre in which there is a great increase in the follicles with proliferation of the epithelium; follicular goitre. सारऊतकीय गलगण्ड; कूपिक गलगण्ड;

**Simple G.**, a condition in which the patient does not show any signs of excessive thyroid activity. सरल गलगण्ड;

**Suffocative G.**, a goitre that by pressure causes extreme dyspnoea. श्वासरोधी गलगण्ड;

**Toxic G.**, a condition in which the enlarged gland secretes an excess of thyroid hormone. विषण्ण गलगण्ड;

**Wandering G.**, see **Diving Goitre.**

**Goitrogen.** An agent causing goitre. गलगण्डजनन

**Goitrogenic.** Goitre-producing; causing goitre. गलगण्डजनक

**Goitrous.** Denoting or characteristic of a goitre. गलगण्डी; गलगण्डिक

**Gold.** Aurum; aurum metallicum; a yellow metallic element. स्वर्ण; सोना

**Gomphiasis.** Looseness of the teeth. दन्तश्लथता; दान्तों का ढीलापन

**Gomphosis.** A form of synarthrosis; peg-and-socket joint. दंतमूलसन्धि

**Gonad.** A male or female sex gland; an organ that produces sex cells, the testis or ovary. जननग्रन्थि; जननपिण्ड; जननद

**Gonadal.** Relating to a gonad. जननग्रन्थि सम्बन्धी

**Gonadectomy.** Removal of the testis or an ovary. जननग्रन्थि-उच्छेदन; वृषण-उच्छेदन; डिम्बग्रन्थि-उच्छेदन

**Gonadopathy.** Disease affecting the gonads. जननग्रन्थिरोग

**Gonadotroph.** A cell of the adenohypophysis that affects certain cells of the ovary or testis. जननग्रन्थि; पीयूषिका ग्रन्थि की एक कोशिका

**Gonadotrophic.** Having an affinity for, or influence on the gonads, gonadotropic. जननग्रन्थिपोषक; जननग्रन्थिप्रेरक

**Gonadotrophin.** Any gonad-stimulating hormone; gonadotropin. जननग्रन्थिपोषी

**Gonadotropic.** See **Gonadotrophic.**

**Gonadotropin.** See **Gonadotrophin.**

**Gonaduct.** Seminal duct. शुक्रनली; uterine tube. जरायुनली

**Gonagra.** Gout in the knee or knee-joint. जानुसन्धिवात; जानुवात; घुटने या घुटने के जोड़ का गठिया

**Gonalgia.** Pain in the knee. जानुशूल; घुटने में दर्द

**Gonangiectomy.** Vasectomy. शुक्रवाहिकोच्छेदन

**Gonarthritis.** Inflammation of the knee-joint. जानुसन्धिशोथ; जानुशोथ; घुटने या घुटने के जोड़ का प्रदाह

**Gonarthrocace.** White swelling of the knee. जानुश्वेतस्फीति; घुटने की सफेद सूजन

**Gonarthrotomy.** Knee-joint incision. जानुसन्धिछेदन

**Gonecyst.** Seminal vesicle; gonecystis. शुक्रपुटी; वीर्यपुटी

**Gonecystic.** Pertaining to the seminal vesicles. शुक्रपुटी अथवा वीर्यपुटी सम्बन्धी

**Gonecystis.** See **Gonecyst.**

**Gonecystitis.** Inflammation of a seminal vesicle. शुक्रपुटीशोथ; वीर्यपुटीशोथ

**Gonecystolith.** A concretion or calculus in a seminal vesicle. शुक्राश्मरी; वीर्यपुटी की पथरी

**Goneitis.** See **Gonitis.**

**Gonepoiesis.** A secretion of semen. शुक्रस्राव; वीर्यस्राव

**Gonepoietic.** Pertaining to the secretion of the semen. शुक्रस्राव सम्बन्धी अथवा शुक्रस्रावी

**Gonia.** Plural of **Gonion.**

**Gonio-.** Combining form meaning angle. 'कोण' का अर्थ देने वाला उपसर्ग

**Goniometer.** An instrument for measuring angles. कोणमापी

**Gonion.** The angle of the lower jaw. बाह्यकोणिका; निचले जबड़े का कोण

**Goniopuncture.** An operation for congenital glaucoma in which a puncture is made in the filtration angle of the anterior chamber. नेत्रकोणवेधन

**Gonioscope.** An apparatus used in noting the varying angles made by the optic axis with the lines of muscle action. नेत्रकोणदर्शी

**Gonioscopy.** Measuring angle of the anterior chamber of eye with a gonioscope. नेत्रकोणदर्शन

**Goniosynechia.** Adhesion of the iris to the posterior surface of the cornea in the angle of the anterior chamber; peripheral anterior synechia. नेत्रकोणसंसक्ति

**Goniotomy.** Operation for glaucoma. नेत्रकोणछेदन; अधिमन्थ के उपचारार्थ किया जाने वाला आँख का आपरेशन

**Gonitis.** Inflammation of the knee; goneitis. जानुशोथ; घुटने का प्रदाह

**Gonocele.** A cystic lesion of the epididymis rete testis resulting from obstruction and containing secretions from the testis. अधिवृषणस्रंस; अधिवृषण-हर्निया

**Gonocide.** Destructive to gonococci; gonococcicide. प्रमेहाणुनाशक

**Gonococcaemia.** See **Gonococcemia.**

**Gonococcal.** Relating to the gonococcus or the gonococci; gonococcic. प्रमेहाणु सम्बन्धी

**Gonococcemia.** Presence of gonococci in the blood; gonococcaemia; gonohemia. प्रमेहाणुरक्तता

**Gonococci.** Plural of **Gonococcus.**

**Gonococcic.** See **Gonococcal.**

**Gonococcicide.** See **Gonocide.**

**Gonococcus.** The specific germ of gonorrhoea. प्रमेहाणु; सूजाक पैदा करने वाला विशिष्ट विषाणु

**Gonohemia.** See **Gonococcemia.**

**Gonorrhea.** See **Gonorrhoea.**

**Gonorrhoea.** Contagious inflammation caused due to impure sexual intercourse and characterized by a purulent discharge from the genitals; gonorrhea. प्रमेह; सूजाक

**Gonorrhoeal.** Resulting from, or pertaining to gonorrhoea. प्रमेहज; प्रमेहजनित; प्रमेह अथवा सूजाक सम्बन्धी;

G. **Arthritis,** a metastatic manifestation of gonorrhoea. प्रमेहज सन्धिशोथ;

G. **Ophthalmia,** a form of ophthalmia neonatorum. प्रमेहज नेत्राभिष्यन्द;

G. **Rheumatism,** a rheumatic affection of the joints following gonorrhoea. प्रमेहज आमवात

**Gonotoxin.** The poison of gonococcus. प्रमेहाणुविष

**Gonyalgia.** Pain in the knee. जानुशूल; घुटने में दर्द

**Gonycampsis.** Ankylosis or any abnormal curvature of the knee. जानुसन्धिग्रह

**Gonyocele.** White swelling of the knee. जानुस्फीति; घुटने की सफेद सूजन

**Gonyoncus.** A tumour or swelling of the knee. जानु-यर्बुद अथवा जानुस्फीति

**Goose-flesh.** See **Goose-skin.**

**Goose-skin.** Prominence of the skin about the hair follicles; goose-

**Gorget**

flesh. झुर्रीदार त्वचा; वलयी त्वचा; वलयी त्वक्; लोम-पुटकों के आस-पास उभरी हुई चमड़ी

**Gorget.** A grooved instrument used in lithotomy. गॉर्जेट; मूत्राशयिक पथरी को निकालने के लिये प्रयुक्त किया जाने वाला यंत्र

**Gossypium.** The genus of plants furnishing cotton. कपास का पौधा;

   **G. Barbadense,** gossypium. कपास का पौधा;

   **G. Harbaceum,** the cotton. कपास;

   **G. Hirsutum,** gossypium. कपास का पौधा;

   **G. Peruvianum,** gossypium. कपास का पौधा;

   **G. Purificatum,** purified cotton. रुई

**Gouge.** An instrument with a grooved blade for cutting away a bone or hard tissue. गूज; हड्डी या किसी कठोर ऊतक को काटने के लिये प्रयुक्त किया जाने वाला यंत्र

**Gout.** A disease associated with inflammation of joints, swelling, uric acid in the blood, etc. गठिया; गाउट;

   **Latent G.,** a state ascribed to a gouty habit but without the typical symptoms of gout; masked gout. गुप्त गठिया;

   **Masked G.,** see **Latent Gout.**

   **Misplaced G.,** a form with severe internal manifestations without arthritic symptoms; retrocedent gout. अस्थानस्थ गठिया;

   **Retrocedent G.,** see **Misplaced Gout.**

   **Secondary G.,** gout resulting from increased nucleoprotein metabolism and uric acid production in patients suffering from the diseases of the blood and bone-marrow. गौण गठिया

**Gouty.** Pertaining to, or of the nature of gout. गठिया सम्बन्धी; गठियारूप; गठियावाती;

   **G. Diathesis,** the peculiar state of the body predisposing to gout; gouty habit. गठिया-प्रवण;

   **G. Habit,** see **Gouty Diathesis.**

   **G. Kidney,** a chronically contracted kidney due to gout. गठिया-वृक्क

**GPI.** General paralysis of insane. पागल का व्यापक अंगघात

**Gr.** Abbreviation for **Grain.** 'ग्रेन' का संक्षिप्त रूप

**Graafian Follicles.** Minute vesicles contained in the stoma of an ovary, each containing a single ovum. ग्राफी पुटक; क्षुद्र कोश

**Gracile.** Slender. तनु; लम्बा-तड़ंगा

**Gracilis.** The rectus internus femoris muscle. तनुपेशी

**Gradient.** Rate of change of temperature, pressure, or other variables as a function of disease. प्रवणता; क्रमिकता

**Graduate.** A glass vessel marked with liquid measurement. अंशांकित कांचपात्र; one who has a college degree. स्नातक

**Graduated.** Divided into degrees, or marked to denote capacity, percentage, etc. अंशांकित; अंशों में विभाजित

**Graefe's Knife.** Finely-pointed knife with narrow blade, used for making incisions across anterior chamber of eye prior to removal of cataract. ग्रैफी छुरिका

**Graft.** Anything inserted into something else so as to become an integral part of the latter. निरोप; उपरोप; संधान;

**Accordion G.,** a skin graft in which multiple slits have been made so that it can be stretched to cover a large area. वलयी निरोप;

**Allogeneic G.,** allograft or homograft. समनिरोप;

**Chip G.,** a graft utilizing small pieces of cartilage or bone packed into a bone defect. चिप-अस्थिनिरोप;

**Composite G.,** a graft composed of several structures. सम्मिश्र निरोप;

**Corneal G.,** keratoplasty. स्वच्छपटल-संधान;

**Free G.,** a graft transplanted without its normal attachments. मुक्त निरोप;

**Periosteal G.,** a graft of the periosteum. पर्यस्थिकला निरोप

**Grafting.** Implantation of skin or tissue from a healthy side to an injured side. निरोपण

**Grain.** A small pill; the 60th part of a drachm. ग्रेन; कण; आधारत्ती; एक ड्राम का साठवां भाग; a seed of cereals. दाना; the smallest division of a pound. एक पौण्ड का क्षुद्रतम भाग; a minute hard particle of any substance. सूक्ष्मकण

**Gram.** The unit of weight in the metric system, equivalent of 15.432 grains; gramme. ग्राम; समतुल्य १५.४३२ ग्रेन;

**G.-meter,** a unit of energy equal to 100 gram-centimeters. ग्राम-मीटर;

**G.-method,** a method of staining bacteria. ग्राम-पद्धति;

**G.-molecule,** the amount of a substance with a mass of the number of grams of its molecular weight. ग्राम-अणु;

**G.-negative,** said of bacteria which do not retain the stain when acted upon by Gram's solution. ग्राम-ऋण; ग्रामवर्ण-अग्राही;

**G.-positive,** retains the stain despite Gram's solution. ग्राम-धन; ग्राम वर्णग्राही

**Gram's solution.** A solution of iodine, potassium iodide and water, used as a stain for bacteria. ग्राम घोल

**Gram's stain.** A bacteriological stain for differentiation of germs. ग्राम-छान

**Gramme.** See **Gram.**

**Grand-mal.** Major or generalized epilepsy. दुर्दम अपस्मार; महामिर्गी

**Granula.** The granules or microsomes of protoplasm. कण; कणिकायें

**Granular.** Composed of, or resembling granules or granulations. कणीय; कणिकीय; दानेदार;

**G. Conjunctivitis,** trachoma; granular lids. कणिकीय नेत्रश्लेष्मलाशोथ;

**G. Lids,** See **Granular Conjunctivitis.**

**Granulatio.** Granulation. कणांकुरण

**Granulation.** The healing of a wound or ulcer by the formation of grainlike fleshy masses. कणांकुरण; formation into grains or granules. कणीकरण; कणीभवन;

**G. Tissue,** the young soft tissue so formed. कणांकुरण ऊतक

**Granulationes.** Plural of **Granulatio.**

**Granule.** A small rounded grain. कण; दाना; a granulation. कणांकुरण; a spore. बीजाणु; a very small pill. कणिका;

**G. Layer,** one of the retinal layers; also the subcortical layer of the cerebellum. कणिका अस्तर

**Granulocyte.** A cell containing granules in its cytoplasm. कणिकाकोशिका; a mature granular leukocyte, including neutrophils, eosinophils and basophils. कणिका-श्वेतकोशिका

**Granulocytopenia.** An aplastic anaemia with an acute febrile course and high mortality; granulopenia. कणिकाकोशिकाल्पता

**Granulocytopoiesis.** See **Granulopoiesis.**

**Granulocytopoietic.** See **Granulopoietic.**

**Granulocytosis.** A condition characterized by more than the normal number of granulocytes in the circulating blood or in the tissues. कणिकाकोशिकता

**Granuloma.** A tumour formed of granulation tissues. कणिकागुल्म;

   **G. Inguinale,** ulcerating granuloma of the pudenda; granuloma venereum. वंक्षण कणिकागुल्म;

   **G. Tropium,** yaws. न्युपदंश; याज;

   **G. Venereum,** see **Granuloma Inguinale.**

**Granulomatosis.** Any condition characterized by multiple granulomas. कणिकागुल्मता

**Granulomatous.** Having the characteristics of a granuloma. कणिकागुल्मीय

**Granulopenia.** See **Granulocytopenia.**

**Granuloplastic.** Forming granules. कणिकासंधानक;

**Granulopoiesis.** Formation of the granulocytes; granulocytopoiesis. कणिकाकोशिका-उत्पत्ति

**Granulopoietic.** Pertaining to granulopoiesis; granulocytopoietic. कणिकाकोशिका-उत्पत्ति सम्बन्धी

**Granulosis.** A mass of minute granules of any character. कणांकुरण

**Granulosum.** Granular. कणीय; कणिकीय

**Granum.** A grain. ग्रेन

**Grape-cure.** The treatment of pulmonary tuberculosis by ingestion of quantities of grapes. द्राक्षोपचार

**Grape-sugar.** Glucose. द्राक्षाशर्करा; ग्लूकोज

**Graphanaesthesia.** Inability to recognize figures written on the skin; graphanesthesia. लेख-असंवेदनता

**Graphanesthesia.** See **Graphanaesthesia.**

**Graphite.** Black lead, a native form of carbon. काला-सीसा; ग्रैफाइट

**Graphology.** The study of the handwriting for the purpose of diagnosing nerve-disease. हस्तलेखविज्ञान; हस्तलेखप्रकरण

**Graphospasm.** Writers' cramp. मुष्टिका-उद्वेष्ट; लेखन-उद्वेष्ट; मुट्ठी की ऐंठन; लेखकों के बाँयटे

**Grating.** The sound produced by the friction of rough surfaces. किसना; करकराना; रगड़न से होने वाली कर्कश ध्वनि

**Grattage.** Scraping, curetting, or brushing to stimulate the healing process. आखुरण; खुरचना; कुतरना

**Grave.** Serious; dangerous. गम्भीर; अरिष्ट; relating to or described by Dr. Robert J. Grave. ग्रैव सम्बन्धी अथवा डा० राबर्ट जे० ग्रैव द्वारा वर्णित

   **G.'s Disease,** thyrotoxicosis; Basedow's disease; exophthalmic

# Grave

goitre. ग्रैव रोग; अवटुविषण्णता; नेत्रोत्सेधी गलगण्ड;

**G.'s Sign,** increase of the systolic impulse often noted in the beginning of pericarditis. ग्रैव चिन्ह;

**G.-wax,** adipocere. वसासिक्थ

**Gravedo.** Coryza; catarrh of upper air passages. ऊर्ध्ववायुमार्गी प्रतिश्याय

**Gravel.** A calculus or stone formed in the kidney and passed through the ureter, bladder and urethra. अश्मरी; पथरी

**Gravid.** Pregnant; being with child; gravida. गर्भिणी; गर्भवती; सगर्भा

**Gravida.** See **Gravid.**

**Gravidic.** Relating to pregnancy or a pregnant woman. गर्भ अथवा गर्भवती स्त्री के सम्बन्धित

**Gravidity.** Number of pregnancies. गर्भसंख्या

**Gravidocardiac.** Relating to an affection of the heart during pregnancy. गर्भहृद्रुग्णता सम्बन्धी

**Gravimetric.** Relating to, or determined by weight. भारमितिक

**Gravireceptors.** Highly specialized receptor organs and nerve endings in the inner ear, joints, tendons and muscles, that give the brain information about body position. तीव्रसंज्ञाग्राही

**Gravitation.** The force by which bodies are drawn to the earth's centre. गुरुत्वाकर्षण; मध्याकर्षण;

**Gravitational.** Being attracted by force of gravity. गुरुत्वाकर्षक;

**G. Ulcer,** vericose ulcer. गुरुत्वाकर्षक व्रण; शिरानाल व्रण

**Gravity.** Property of possessing weight. गुरुत्व;

**Specific G.,** the weight of a substance compared with that of an equal volume of water. विशिष्ट गुरुत्व

**Gray.** A colour between white and black; grey; griseum; grisia. धूसर; भूरा;

**G. Matter,** the substance forming the outer part of the brain and the inner part of the cord containing the specialized cells of these parts; gray substance. धूसर पदार्थ; भूरा पदार्थ;

**G. Softening,** an inflammatory softening of the brain or cord with a gray discolouration. धूसर मृदुता;

**G. Substance,** see **Gray Matter.**

**Grazing.** The sound of rubbing or touching lightly. मंदघर्षणध्वनि; मंदस्पर्शध्वनि

**Green.** Of the colour of grass or sea-water. हरित; हरा; हरी;
  **G. Blindness,** an inability to distinguish the green colour. हरितान्धता; हरित-वर्णान्धता; हरा रंग पहचानने की अयोग्यता;
  **G. House,** a glass house in which tender plants are kept. हरित गृह; ग्रीन हाउस;
  **G. Sickness,** chlorosis. हरित्पाण्डुरोग;
  **G. Softening,** purulent softening of nervous matter. हरित मृदुता
**Greffotome.** An instrument for making tissue-grafts. ऊतकनिरोपयंत्र; ग्रेफ्फोटोम
**Gregarious.** Showing preference for living in a group; liking to mix. यूथचर; यूथचारी
**Grey.** See **Gray.**
**Grief.** A normal emotional response to an external loss. शोक; संताप; विषाद
**Grimaces.** An affected expression of the face. मुँह बनाना; नकल उतारना
**Grinders.** The molars or double teeth; grinding teeth. चर्वणक; चबाने वाले; चर्वण दन्त; दाढ़ें
**Grinding-in.** Correcting occlusal disharmonies by grinding the natural or artificial teeth. अवघर्षण
**Grinding Pain.** Pain prevailing in the first stage of labour. प्रसवपूर्व-पीड़ा; प्रसवपूर्व-वेदना
**Grinding Teeth.** See **Grinders.**
**Grip.** Influenza. इन्फ्लुएंजा; शीतज्वर; श्लैष्मिक ज्वर; grasp or clasp. जकड़न
**Gripe.** Colic. शूल; उदरशूल; पेददर्द
**Griping.** Colicky. शूल प्रकृति का;
  **G. Pain,** colicky pain. उदरशूल; पेटदर्द;
  **Intestinal G.,** colicky pain in the bowels. आंत्रशूल; आंतों में दर्द
**Grippal.** Pertaining to influenza. इन्फ्लुएंजा सम्बन्धी
**Grippe.** Influenza; cold in the head; catarrh. इन्फ्लुएंजा; शीतज्वर; श्लैष्मिक ज्वर
**Grippotoxin.** The specific poison of influenza. इन्फ्लुएंजाविष; ग्रिप्पोटॉक्सिन
**Griseum.** See **Gray.**

**Grisia.** See **Gray.**

**Gristle.** Cartilage. उपास्थि

**Groan.** A low moaning sound. कराहना

**Grocer's itch.** Inveterate eczema; contact dermatitis, especially from flour or sugar; a peculiar psoriasis or eczema of the hands. चिरस्थायी छाजन

**Groin.** The depressed part in the body between the belly and the thigh. वंक्षण; ऊरुसन्धि; ऊरुमूल

**Groove.** A furrow, channel, crease or fold. खातिका; खात; खांचा; परिखा; लीक

**Gross.** Coarse. खुरदरा; great. महान; घोर; total. सकल; पूर्ण

**Group.** A class scientifically connected. वर्ग; समूह; गण; समुच्चय;

**G. Reaction.** a reaction with an antibody which is characteristic of a whole group of bacteria. वर्ग प्रतिक्रिया

**Growing-pains.** Neuralgic pains in the limbs during youth. वर्धिष्णु दर्द; यौवनकालिक अंगपीड़ा

**Growth.** An excrescence. गुल्म; गांठ; development. विकास; an increase. बृद्धि;

**Appositional G.,** growth by the addition of new layers on those previously formed. सन्निधानक बृद्धि;

**Interstitial G.,** growth from a number of different centres within an area. अन्तरालीय बृद्धि;

**New G.,** neoplasm. नवोत्पत्ति

**Grub.** An affection of the skin follicles; a comedo. सूंडी; मस्सा; एक चर्मपुटक रोग; चमड़ी पर निकलने वाला काला दाना

**Gruel.** A decoction of cereal in water. कंजी; विलेपी

**Grumose.** Viscid. चिपचिपा; thick. गाढ़ा; clotted. थक्केदार

**Grumous.** The same as **Grumose.**

**Grunting.** Uttering a short sound. बुड़बुड़ाना; बड़बड़ाना

**Gryposis.** An abnormal inward curvature of the nails. नखबक्रता; नाखुनों का अन्तर्मुखी टेढ़ापन

**Gtt.** Symbol fot Latin word **Gutta.**

**Gubernaculum.** A fibrous cord connecting two structures. रज्जु; बन्ध; a structure that guides. निदेशक; निर्देशक; पथप्रदर्शक;

**G. Dentis,** a connective tissue band uniting the tooth sac with the gum. दंतसंयोजी रज्जु;

**G. Testis,** a foetal cord directing the descent of the testes. वृषणनिदेशक रज्जु

**Guide.** Any device or instrument by which another is led into its proper course. गाइड; निर्देशक; पथप्रदर्शक

**Guinea-pig.** A small rodent used in laboratory research. शूकर-शावक; गिनी-पिग

**Guinea-worm.** Nematode parasite of tropics responsible for drancontiasis; dracunculus medinensis. नहरुआ; नहरवा; गिनीकृमि

**Gullet.** The passage from the mouth to the stomach for the food; oesophagus. ग्रासनली; अन्ननली

**Gum.** The root of a tooth. गसूड़ा; the concrete juice of certain plants. गोंद;

   **G. Acacia,** gum from Acacia senegal; gum Arabica. बबूल-गोंद; बबूल का गोंद; अरबी गोंद;

   **G. Arabica,** see **Gum Acacia.**

   **G.-boil,** an affection at the root of a tooth which drains through gum. मसूड़ा फोड़ा; मसूड़े का फोड़ा;

   **G.-resin,** a concrete vegetable juice. रेजिन-गोंद

**Gumma.** A localized area of vascular granulation tissue which develops in the later stages of syphilis; a syphilitic tumour. गम्मा; गम्माबुंद

**Gummas.** Plural of **Gumma.**

**Gummata.** Plural of **Gumma.**

**Gummatous.** Pertaining to, or characterized by the features of a gumma. गम्माबुंदाभ; गम्माबुंद जैसा; गम्माबुंदीय

**Gummy.** Gummatous. गम्माबुंदाभ; resembling gum. गोंद जैसा

**Gums.** Gingiva. मसूड़े;

**Gurgling.** The sound of air passing through the fluid in a cavity. गड़गड़ाहट

**Gustation.** The act of tasting. रसास्वादन; स्वाद लेना; the sense of taste. स्वादानुभूति

**Gustative.** See **Gustatory.**

**Gustatory.** Pertaining to the sense of taste; gustative. स्वाद सम्बन्धी

**Gut.** The intestine. आंत्र; आंत; embryonic digestive tube. आहार नली; catgut. आंत्रतन्ति

**Gutta.** A Drop. बूंद;

   **G.-opaca,** cataract. मोतिया; मोतियाबिन्द;

**Gutta**

**G.-rosacea,** red or purple spots upon the face and nose; acne rosacea. गुलाबी मुहासे;

**G.-serena,** amaurosis. अन्धता

**Guttate.** Of the shape of, or resembling a drop, characterizing certain cutaneous lesion. बूंदाकार

**Guttatim.** Drop by drop; guttatin. बूंद-बूंद करके

**Guttatin.** See **Guttatim.**

**Guttur.** The throat, with reference to the trachea. कण्ठ; गला

**Guttural.** Relating to the throat; throaty. कण्ठ्य; कण्ठ सम्बन्धी

**Gutturotetany.** Pharyngeal spasm with stammering. ग्रसनी-आकर्ष; ग्रसनी-उद्वेष्ट

**Gymnasium.** A place for systematic muscular exercise. व्यायामशाला; अखाड़ा

**Gymnastic.** Pertaining to gymnastics. व्यायामविद्या सम्बन्धी

**Gymnastics.** The science of a systematic bodily exercise. व्यायामविद्या

**Gymnocyte.** A cell without a limiting membrane. अभिभित्तिककोशिका

**Gynaecic.** Pertaining to, or associated with women; gynecic. स्त्रीविषयक; स्त्रीपरक

**Gynaecography.** Radiological visualization of internal female genitalia after pneumoperitoneum; gynecography. स्त्रीजननेन्द्रियचित्रण

**Gynaecoid.** Resembling a woman in form and structure; gynecoid. स्त्रीरूप

**Gynaecologic.** Pertaining to gynaecology; gynecologic. स्त्रीरोगविज्ञानविषयक; स्त्रीरोगविज्ञान सम्बन्धी

**Gynaecologist.** A surgeon who specializes in gynaecology; gynecologist. स्त्रीरोगविज्ञ

**Gynaecology.** The medical speciality concerned with the diseases of the women; gynecology. स्त्रीरोगविज्ञान

**Gynaecomastia.** An abnormal development of the male mammary glands; gynecomastia. पुंस्तनबृद्धि; पुरुषों में असाधारण स्तनबृद्धि

**Gynaephobia.** Morbid aversion to women; gynephobia. स्त्रीभीति; औरतों से डर अथवा अरुचि

**Gynandria.** See **Gynandrism.**

**Gynandrism.** A developmental abnormality characterized by hypertrophy of the clitoris and union of the labia majora;

**gynandria.** उभयलिंगता

**Gynandroid.** Exhibiting gynandrism. उभयलिंगताभ

**Gynandromorph.** An individual exhibiting gynandromorphism. स्त्रीपुंरूप; पुरुष तथा स्त्री दोनों के लक्षणों से युक्त

**Gynandromorphism.** A combination of male and female characteristics. स्त्रीपुंरूपता

**Gynandromorphous.** Having both male and female characteristics. स्त्रीपुंरूपी

**Gynatresia.** Imperforation of vagina. योनि-अभेद्यता

**Gynecography.** See **Gynaecography.**

**Gynecic.** See **Gynaecic.**

**Gynecoid.** See **Gynaecoid.**

**Gynecologic.** See **Gynaecologic.**

**Gynecologist.** See **Gynaecologist.**

**Gynecology.** See **Gynaecology.**

**Gynecomastia.** See **Gynaecomastia.**

**Gynephobia.** See **Gynaephobia.**

**Gyniatrics.** The treatment of diseases of women. स्त्रीरोगचिकित्सा

**Gynogenesis.** Egg-development activated by a spermatozoon, but to which the male gamete contributes no genetic material. स्त्रीजननता

**Gynoplastics.** Reparative or reconstructive surgery of the female genital organs. स्त्रीजननांगसंधान

**Gynoplasty.** See **Gynoplastics.**

**Gypsum.** Plaster of Paris; native calcium sulphate. चिरोड़ी; कुलनार; जिप्सम

**Gyrate.** Of convoluted or ring shape. कर्णकित

**Gyration.** Revolving in a circle. घूर्णन; वलय; चक्कर

**Gyre.** A cerebral convolution. कर्णक

**Gyrectomy.** Surgical removal of a gyrus, a convoluted portion of cerebral cortex. कर्णक-उच्छेदन

**Gyrencephalic.** Pertaining to a brain having numerous convolutions. बहुकर्णकी

**Gyrencephalus.** Having a brain with numerous convolutions. बहुकर्णक

# Gyri

**Gyri.** Plural of **Gyrus.**

   **G. Brevis Insulae,** short gyri of insula. लघुद्वीपिका कर्णक;

   **G. Insulae,** short and long gyri of insulae. द्वीपिका कर्णक;

   **G. Orbitales,** see **Orbital Gyri.**

   **G. Temporales Transversi,** see **Transverse Temporal Gyri.**

   **Heschl's Gyri,** see **Transverse Temporal Gyri.**

   **Orbital G.,** a number of small irregular convolutions occupying the concave inferior surface of each frontal lobe of the cerebrum; gyri orbitales. नेत्रगुहा-कर्णक;

   **Transverse Temporal G.,** three convolutions running transversely on the upper surface of the temporal lobe; gyri temporales transversi. अनुप्रस्थ शंख-कर्णक.

**Gyroma.** A tumour of the ovary. डिम्बाशयार्बुद; डिम्बाशय की रसौली

**Gyrometer.** An instrument for measuring the gyri indirectly. कर्णकमापी

**Gyrosa.** Vertigo due to stomach trouble. भ्रमि; चक्कर; घुमरी

**Gyrospasm.** A rotatory spasm of the head. घूर्णीशिरोद्वेष्ट

**Gyrus.** A convolution of the brain. कर्णक; घुमेड़;

   **Angular G.,** the posterior part of that one between the intraparietal fissure in front and above and the horizontal limb of the Sylvian fissure. कोण-कर्णक; कोणीय कर्णक;

   **Annectent G.,** four small convolutions connecting the occipital with temporosphenoid and parietal lobes; transitional gyrus. संयोजी कर्णक;

   **Callosal G.,** the convolution immediately above the callosum. महासंयोजिका कर्णक;

   **Dentate G.,** in man, a rudimentary one in the hippocampal fissure. दन्तुर कर्णक;

   **Frontal G.,** the convolution of the frontal lobe. ललाट कर्णक;

   **Hippocampal G.,** that part of the fornicate convolution that winds around the splenium of the corpus callosum. हिपोकैम्पी कर्णक;

   **Marginal G.,** the median surface of the first frontal convolution. उपान्त-कर्णक;

   **Medifrontal G.,** the convolution between the superfrontal and subfrontal fissures; middle frontal gyrus. मध्यललाट कर्णक;

   **Meditemporal G.,** the convolution between the supertemporal and meditemporal fissures; middle temporal gyrus. मध्यशंख कर्णक;

**Mesorbital G.**, the convolution between the intercerebral and olfactory fissures. मध्यनेत्रगुहा-कर्णक;

**Middle Frontal G.**, see **Medifrontal Gyrus.**

**Middle Temporal G.**, see **Meditemporal Gyrus.**

**Occipital G.**, the convolution making the occipital lobe. पश्चकपाल कर्णक;

**Olfactory G.**, the roots of the olfactory tract; striae olfactoriae. घ्राण कर्णक;

**Paracentral G.**, one on the mesial surface of the brain representing the junction of the upper ends of the ascending frontal and ascending parietal convolutions. पराकेन्द्रिक कर्णक; पराकेन्द्रीय कर्णक;

**Parietal G.**, those of the parietal lobe. पार्श्विका कर्णक

**Postparietal G.**, the convolution between the posterior limb of the meditemporal fissure and the paroccipital fissure. पश्चपार्श्विका कर्णक;

**Subfrontal G.**, the convolution between the meditemporal and the subtemporal fissures. अवललाट कर्णक;

**Superfrontal G.**, the convolution between the Sylvian and the supertemporal fissures. अधिललाट कर्णक;

**Supertemporal G.**, the anterior part of one between the intraparietal fissure in front and above the horizontal limb of the Sylvian fissure. अधिशंख कर्णक;

**Temporal G.**, those of the temporal lobe. शंख कर्णक;

**Transitional G.**, see **Annectent Gyrus.**

**Transtemporal G.**, one of a number of small gyri on the opercular surface of the temporal lobe. पारशंख कर्णक

# H

**H.** Symbol for **Hydrogen.** 'हाइड्रोजन' के लिये प्रयुक्त संकेत चिन्ह

**Habena.** A bandage. पट्टी; पट्टिका; a frenum or restricting fibrous band. फ्रीनम अथवा बंध

**Habenae.** Plural of **Habena.**

**Habenal.** Relating to a habena; habenar. पट्टी, पट्टिका, फ्रीनम अथवा बंध सम्बन्धी

**Habenar.** See **Habenal.**

**Habenula.** A peduncle or stalk attached to the pineal body of the brain. वृन्तक; a narrow bandlike structure; a frenum or whiplike structure. पट्टिका

**Habenulae.** Plural of **Habenula.**

**Habenular.** Relating to a habenula, especially the stalk of the pineal body. वृन्तक अथवा पट्टिका सम्बन्धी

**Habit.** A particular state of body and mind. स्वभाव; प्रकृति; आदत; अभ्यास; addiction to the use of drugs or alcoholic beverages. अभ्यस्तता; व्यसन

**Habitat.** The natural locality of an animal or plant. आवास; मूलस्थान

**Habitspasm.** Habitual spasmodic action of the voluntary muscles. अभ्यासाकर्ष

**Habituation.** Dependence. निर्भरता; addiction. व्यसन; अभ्यस्तता; Drug H., a state arising from repeated administration of a drug on a pariodic or continuous basis. औषध-व्यसन; औषध-अभ्यस्तता

**Habitus.** Physical characteristics of a person. किसी व्यक्ति-विशेष का शारीरिक गठन

**Habromania.** A gay form of insanity. आनन्दोन्माद; पागलपन का एक प्रफुल्लित रूप

**Hacking.** Short and interrupted. खुसखुसी; हुकहुकी;
  H. Cough, a short, dry, frequent cough. खुसखुसी खांसी; हुकहुकी के साथ होने वाली खांसी

**Haem-, Haema-, Haemo-, Hem-, Hemat-, Hemo-.** Prefixes meaning blood. 'रक्त', 'लोहित', अथवा 'रुधिर' के अर्थ देने वाले उपसर्ग

**Haema-.** See **Haem-.**

**Haemacyte.** A blood cell; hemacyte; haematocyte; hematocyte. रक्तकोशिका; रुधिरकोशिका; लोहितकोशिका

**Haemadsorption.** See **Hemadsorption.**

**Haemagglutination.** See **Hemagglutination.**

**Haemagglutinin.** See **Hemagglutinin.**

**Haemagog.** See **Haemagogue.**

**Haemagogic.** Promoting the flow of blood; hemagogic. रक्तप्रवाही

**Haemagogue.** Medicine that promotes the catamenial and haemorrhoidal discharges; haemagog; hemagog; hemagogue. रक्तस्रावी (औषधि)

**Haemal.** Pertaining to the blood; hemal. रक्त सम्बन्धी; रुधिर सम्बन्धी;

**H.-arch,** the ribs, breastbone and that part of the vertebrae that enclose the heart and viscera. रुधिर-चाप

**Haemalopia.** An effusion of the blood into the globe of the eye; bloodshot eye; hemalopia. रक्तिमनेत्र

**Haemameba.** See **Hemameba.**

**Haemamebiasis.** See **Hemamebiasis.**

**Haemamoeba.** See **Hemameba.**

**Haemamoebiasis.** See **Hemamebiasis.**

**Haemanalysis.** Analysis of the blood; hemanalysis. रक्तविश्लेषण

**Haemangiectasis.** Dilatation of a blood vessel; hemangiectasis. रक्तवाहिकाविस्फार; रक्तवाहिनी का फैल जाना

**Haemangio-, Hemangio-.** Prefixes meaning blood vessel. 'रक्तवाहिका' का अर्थ देने वाले उपसर्ग

**Haemangioblast.** A primitive embryonic cell of mesodermal origin that produces cells giving rise to vascular endothelium, reticuloendothelial elements and blood-forming cells; hemangioblast. रक्तवाहिकाप्रसू

**Haemangioblastoma.** A benign, slowly growing, cerebellar neoplasm composed of capillary vessel-forming endothelial cells; hemangioblastoma. रक्तवाहिकाप्रसू-अर्बुद

**Haemangioendothelioblastoma.** A neoplasm of the epithelial cells lining the blood vessels; hemangioendothelioblastoma. रक्तवाहिकांतर्कलाप्रसू-अर्बुद

**Haemangioendothelioma.** An overgrowth of the endothelium of the minute capillary vessels; hemangioendothelioma. रक्तवाहिकांतर्कलार्बुद

**Haemangiofibroma.** A fibrous haemangioma; hemangiofibroma. रक्तवाहिकातन्त्वर्बुद; रक्तवाहिकासूत्रार्बुद

**Haemangioma.** A malformation of blood vessels; hemangioma. रक्तवाहिकार्बुद

**Haemangiomatosis.** Presence of numerous haemangiomas; hemangiomatosis. रक्तवाहिकार्बुदता

**Haemangiopericytoma.** A tumour arising in capillaries, which is presumably derived from the pericytes; hemangiopericytoma. रक्तवाहिका-परिकोशिकार्बुद

**Haemangiosarcoma.** A malignant neoplasm characterized by rapidly proliferating and, extensively infiltrating anaplastic cells derived from blood vessels and lining blood-filled spaces; hemangiosarcoma. रक्तवाहिकासार्कार्बुद

**Haemapoiesis.** Blood formation; hemapoeisis. रक्तनिर्माण; खून बनना

**Haemarthrosis.** The presence of blood in a joint cavity; hemarthrosis. रक्तसन्धि

**Haemat-, Hemat-.** Prefixes meaning blood. 'रक्त' अथवा 'रुधिर' का अर्थ देने वाले उपसर्ग

**Haematachometer.** An instrument for measuring the rapidity of the circulation of blood; hematachometer. रक्तगतिमापकयंत्र; रक्तगतिमापी

**Haematemesis.** Vomiting of blood; hematemesis. रक्तवमन; खून की उल्टी; खूनी कै होना

**Haematencephalon.** Cerebral haemorrhage; hematencephalon. प्रमस्तिष्क-रक्तस्राव

**Haemathorax.** An effusion of blood into the pleural cavities; hemathorax. रक्तवक्ष; वक्षरक्तता

**Haematic.** Hematic; hemic; relating to blood. रक्त सम्बन्धी; bloody. रक्तिम; रक्तमिश्रित; खून मिला

**Haematica.** Agents affecting the blood; hematica. रक्तविकारी; खून गंदा करने वाले तत्व

**Haematidrosis.** Excretion of blood or blood pigment in the sweat; hematidrosis; haemidrosis. रक्तस्वेदन; रक्तमिश्रित पसीना होना

**Haematin.** An iron-containing constituent of haemoglobin; hematin. रक्तरंजक; रक्तकणरंजक; रक्तकणों को लाल रंग देने वाला पदार्थ; हेमाटिन

**Haematinaemia.** Presence of heme in the circulating blood; haematinemia; hematinaemia; hematinemia. हेमाटिनरक्तता

**Haematinemia.** See **Haematinaemia.**

**Haematinic.** An agent improving blood-quality; hematinic. रक्तगुणवर्धक; रक्त की गुणवत्ता में वृद्धि करने वाला पदार्थ

**Haematinuria.** The presence of haematin in the urine; hematinuria. रक्तकणरंजकमेह; रक्तरंजकमेह; पेशाब में रक्तकणरंजक द्रव्य जाना

**Haematite.** A kind of silicosis. रक्ताम्बु

**Haemato-, Hemato-.** Prefixes meaning blood. 'रक्त' अथवा 'रुधिर' का अर्थ देने वाले उपसर्ग

**Haematocele.** Swelling of the scrotum or the spermatic cord containing blood; a blood tumour; hematocele. रक्तार्बुद; रक्तगुल्म; खून की गिल्टी

**Haematochezia.** Passage of bloody stools; hematochezia. रक्तातिसार; खूनी पाखाना होना

**Haematochyluria.** Presence of blood and chyle in the urine; hematochyluria. वसालसीकारक्तमेह

**Haematocolpometra.** Accumulation of blood in the uterus and in the vagina; hematocolpometra. रक्तपूरितयोनिगर्भाशय; योनि तथा गर्भाशय के अन्दर रक्तसंचय हो जाना

**Haematocolpos.** Retention of the menstrual blood due to the congenital obstruction of vagina; hematocolpos. रक्तपूरितयोनि; योनि की जन्मजात अवरुद्धता के कारण ऋतुस्राव न होना

**Haematocyst.** A blood cyst; hematocyst. रक्तपुटी

**Haematocystitis.** An effusion of blood into the bladder; hematocystitis. रक्तपूरितमूत्राशयशोथ

**Haematocyte.** See **Haemacyte.**

**Haematocytometer.** A device for counting the corpuscles in a given volume of blood; hematocytometer. रक्तकणिकामापी; लोहितकणिकामापी; रक्तकणिकागणित्र; लोहितकोशिकागणित्र

**Haematogenesis.** The development of the blood; hematogenesis. रुधिरजनन; रक्तोत्पादन

**Haematogenic.** Hematogenic; haematogenous; hematogenous; haemopoietic; pertaining to anything produced, derived from, or transported by the blood. रुधिरजनन अथवा रक्तोत्पादन सम्बन्धी

**Haematogenous.** See **Haematogenic.**

**Haematography.** A description of the blood; hematography. रक्तचित्रण

**Haematohidrosis.** Bloody sweat; hematohidrosis. रक्तस्वेदन; खूनी पसीना

**Haematoid.** Bloodlike; having the nature or appearance of blood; hematoid. रक्ताभ; रक्तवत्; खून जैसा

**Haematologist.** A physician specializing in haematology; hematologist. रुधिरविज्ञानी; रक्तविशेषज्ञ

**Haematology.** The medical speciality concerned with the anatomy, physiology, pathology, symptomatology and therapeutics related to the blood and blood-forming tissues; haemology; hematology; hemology. रुधिरविज्ञान; रक्तविज्ञान

**Haematolymphangioma.** A congenital anomaly consisting of numerous lymphatic vessels of varying sizes; hematolymphangioma. रक्तलसीकावाहिकार्बुद

**Haematolysis.** See **Haemolysis.**

**Haematolytic.** See **Haemolytic.**

**Haematoma.** The blood tumour; a circumscribed collection of blood in the tissues; hematoma. रक्तार्बुद; रक्तगुल्म;

  **H. Auris,** the blood tumour of the external ear. बहिर्कर्ण-रक्तार्बुद; बाह्यकर्ण-रक्तगुल्म

**Haematometra.** An accumulation of blood or menstrual flow in the uterus; hematometra; haemometra; hemometra. रक्तगर्भाशय; रक्तजरायु

**Haematomphalocele.** An umbilical hernia into which an effusion of blood has taken place; hematomphalocele. रक्तपूरितनाभिस्रंस; रक्तपूरितनाभि-हर्निया

**Haematomyelia.** Haemorrhage into the substance of the spinal cord; hematomyelia. मेरुरक्तस्राव

**Haematopathology.** The subdivision of pathology concerned with diseases of the blood and of haemopoietic and lymphoid tissues; hematopathology; haemopathology; hemopathology. रुधिरविकृतिविज्ञान

**Haematophobia.** A morbid fear of blood; hematophobia. रुधिरभीति; रक्तभीति

**Haematoplastic.** Blood-forming; hematoplastic. रक्तनिर्माणक

**Haematopoiesis.** See **Haemopoiesis.**

**Haematopoietic.** See **Haemopoietic.**

**Haematopsia.** Haemorrhage into the eye; hematopsia. नेत्ररक्तता

**Haematorrhachis.** A spinal haemorrhage; hematorrhachis; hemorrhachis. कशेरुकानाल-रक्तस्राव;

**H. Externa,** haemorrhage into the spinal canal external to the cord. बहि:कशेरुकानाल-रक्तस्राव;

**H. Interna,** haematomyelia. अन्त:कशेरुकानाल-रक्तस्राव; मेरुरक्तस्राव;

**Haematosalpinx.** A collection of blood in the Fallopian tube; haemosalpinx; hematosalpinx; hemosalpinx. रक्तपूरितडिम्बवाहिनी; डिम्बवाही नली में खून जमा हो जाना

**Haematoscheocele.** Accumulation of blood in the scrotal cavity; hematoscheocele. रक्तपूरितवृषणकोष

**Haematosis.** The formation of blood; hematosis. रक्तोत्पादन; रक्तनिर्माण; रक्तजनन; खून बनना

**Haematospermatocele.** A spermatocele that contains blood; hematospermatocele. रक्तपूरितशुक्रपुटी

**Haematospermia.** The discharge of blood-stained semen; hematospermia; haemospermia; hemospermia. रक्तशुक्रता; वीर्य में खून जाना

**Haematostatic.** Hematostatic; haemostatic; stagnation or arrest of blood in the vessels of a part. रक्तस्तम्भक

**Haematostaxis.** Spontaneous bleeding due to a disease of blood; hematostaxis. स्वत:रक्तस्राव

**Haematotoxic.** See **Haemotoxic.**

**Haematotoxin.** See **Haemotoxin.**

**Haematotrachelos.** Distention of the cervix uteri with accumulated blood; hematotrachelos. रक्तपूरितजरायुग्रीवा; रक्तपूरितगर्भाशयग्रीवा

**Haematotympanum.** See **Haemotympanum.**

**Haematozoa.** Parasites living in the blood; hematozoa. रक्तकीट; रक्तपरजीवी; खून में पलने वाले परजीवी

**Haematozoon.** Singular of **Haematozoa.**

**Haematuresis.** See **Haematuria.**

**Haematuria.** Blood in the urine; haematuresis; hematuresis; hematuria. रक्तमेह; पेशाब में खून जाना;
  **Renal H.,** haematuria resulting from extravasation of blood into the glomerular spaces, or tubules, or pelvis of the kidneys. वृक्क-रक्तमेह;
  **Urethral H.,** haematuria in which the site of bleeding is in the urethra. मूत्रमार्गी रक्तमेह;
  **Vesical H.,** haematuria in which the site of bleeding is in the urinary bladder. मूत्राशयिक रक्तमेह

**Haemaxis.** Blood-letting; hemaxis. रक्तमोषण; रक्तमोचन; खून निकालना

**Haeme.** Reduced haematin; the prosthetic, oxygen-carrying, colour-furnishing constituent of haemoglobin; heme. अल्परक्तकणरंजक

**Haemic.** Pertaining to, or containing blood; hematic; hemic. रक्तज; रक्तक; रक्त सम्बन्धी या रक्तमिश्रित

**Haemidrosis.** See **Haematidrosis.**

**Haemin.** A crystallized substance obtained from the dry blood; hemin. हीमिन; रक्तपर्पटी

**Haemo-.** See **Haem-.**

**Haemochromatosis.** A congenital error in iron-metabolism with increased iron deposition in tissues; hemochromatosis. रक्तवर्णकता; रुधिरलौहवर्णकता

**Haemoconcentration.** Relative increase of volume of red blood cells to volume of plasma; hemoconcentration. रक्तसान्द्रण

**Haemocytometer.** An instrument for measuring the number of blood corpuscles; hemocytometer; hemacytometer; hemocytometer. रुधिरकोशिकामापी; लोहितकोशिकामापी; रक्तकोशिकामापी

**Haemocytometry.** The counting of red blood cells; hemocytometry. रुधिरकोशिकामिति; लोहितकोशिकामिति; रक्तकोशिकामिति

**Haemodialysis.** A process of removing waste products from, and replacing essential constituents in the blood by a process of dialysis; hemodialysis. रक्त-अपोहन

**Haemogenesis.** The formation of blood; hemogenesis. रक्तजनन; रक्तोत्पादन

**Haemogenic.** Producing blood; hemogenic. रक्तजनक; रक्तोत्पादक

**Haemoglobin (Hb).** The colouring matter of red blood corpuscles, which has a strong affinity for oxygen and used to carry it to the body tissues; hemoglobin. रक्तकणरंजकद्रव्य; हीमोग्लोबिन; रक्तकणों को लाल रंग देने वाला पदार्थ-विशेष

**Haemoglobinometer.** An instrument for estimating the haemoglobin in the blood; hemoglobinometer. रक्तकणरंजकद्रव्यमापी; रक्तकणरंजकद्रव्यमापक (यंत्र); हीमोग्लोबिनमापी

**Haemoglobinometry.** Measuring of haemoglobin in the blood; hemoglobinometry. रक्तकणरंजकद्रव्यमिति; रक्तकणरंजकद्रव्यमापन; हीमोग्लोबिनमिति

**Haemoglobinopathy.** Abnormality of the haemoglobin; hemoglobinopathy. रक्तकणरंजकद्रव्यरोग; हीमोग्लोबिनरुग्णता

**Haemoglobinophilic.** Relating to certain micro-organisms that cannot be cultured except in the presence of haemoglobin; hemoglobinophilic. हीमोग्लोबिन सम्बन्धी

**Haemoglobinuria.** Presence of blood in the urine; hemoglobinuria. रक्तकणरंजकद्रव्यमेह; हीमोग्लोबिनमेह

**Haemoglobinuric.** Relating to, or marked by haemoglobinuria; hemoglobinuric. हीमोग्लोबिनमेह सम्बन्धी; रक्तकणरंजकद्रव्यमेह सम्बन्धी; रक्तकणरंजकमेहग्रस्त

**Haemogram.** A microphotograph of the blood; hemogram. रक्ताणुवीक्षण; रक्ताणुचित्र

**Haemoid.** Resembling blood; hemoid. रक्ताभ; रुधिराभ; खून जैसा

**Haemolith.** A blood calculus; hemolith. रक्ताश्मरी; रुधिराश्मरी; रक्तपथरी

**Haemology.** See **Haematology.**

**Haemolymph.** Bloody lymph or the blood and lymph; hemolymph. रुधिरलसीका

**Haemolysis.** Disintegration of red blood cells, with liberation of contained haemoglobin; hemolysis; haematolysis; hematolysis. रुधिरलयन; रक्तलयन; रक्त-अपघटन; रक्तापघटन

**Haemolytic.** Destructive to blood cells, resulting in liberation of haemoglobin; haematolytic; hemolytic; hematolytic. रुधिरलायी; रक्तलायी

**Haemometra.** See **Haematometra.**

**Haemopathology.** See **Haematopathology.**

**Haemopathy.** An abnormal condition or disease of the blood or haemopoietic tissues; hemopathy. रक्तविकार; रक्तरोग

**Haemopericardium.** Blood in the cavity of the pericardium; hemopericardium. रक्तपरिहृद्; रक्तहृदयावरण

**Haemoperitoneum.** Blood in the peritoneal cavity; hemoperitoneum. रक्तपर्युदर्या; रक्त-उदरावरण

**Haemophagocyte.** A white blood corpuscle; hemophagocyte. श्वेतरक्तकोशिका

**Haemophilia.** Hemophilia; bleeder's disease; an hereditary blood disease characterized by greatly prolonged coagulation time. अधिरक्तस्राव; abnormal tendency to haemorrhage. रक्तस्राव की असाधारण प्रवृत्ति

**Haemophiliac.** Affected with haemophilia; hemophiliac. हीमोफीलियाग्रस्त (रोगी)

**Haemophilic.** Relating to haemophilia; hemophilic. हीमोफीलिया सम्बन्धी; अधिरक्तस्रावी

**Haemophilus.** A genus of parasitic bacteria containing minute, gram-negative rod-shaped cells; hemophilus. हीमोफिलस

**Haemophthalmia.** Bleeding into the eyeball; hemophthalmia. रक्तनेत्र; नेत्रगोलकों के अन्दर खून उतरना

**Haemoplastic.** See **Haemopoietic.**

**Haemopneumothorax.** The presence of blood and air in the pleural cavity causing compression of lung tissues; hemopneumothorax रक्तवातवक्ष; फुप्फुस-गह्वर में खून तथा हवा भरना

**Haemopoiesis.** The formation of blood; haematogenesis; haematopoiesis; hematopoiesis; hemopoiesis. रक्तजनक; रक्तोत्पादक; रक्तनिर्माणक; खून बनाने वाला

**Haemopoietic.** That which produces blood; haematopoietic; hematopoietic; haemoplastic; hemoplastic; hemopoietic. रक्तजनक; रक्तनिर्माणक; खून बनाने वाला

**Haemoptoe.** See **Haemoptysis.**

**Haemoptysis.** The spitting or expectoration of blood; haemoptoe; hemoptoe; hemoptysis. रक्तनिष्ठीवन; बलगम में खून आना

**Haemorrhage.** The escape of blood from a vassel; bleeding; hemorrhage. रक्तस्राव; रक्तप्रवाह; खून बहना;
    **Postpartum H.,** one following labor. प्रसवोत्तर रक्तस्राव

**Haemorrhagenic.** Causing or producing haemorrhage; hemorrhagenic. रक्तस्रावजनक

**Haemorrhagic.** Pertaining to haemorrhage or bleeding; hemorrhagic. रक्तस्रावी; रक्तप्रवाही; रक्तस्राव सम्बन्धी

**Haemorrhoidal.** Hemorrhoidal; relating to haemorrhoids. अर्श अथवा बवासीर सम्बन्धी

**Haemorrhoidectomy.** Surgical removal of the haemorrhoids; hemorrhoidectomy. अर्शोच्छेदन; बवासीर के मस्सों को काट कर हटा देना

**Haemorrhoids.** Varicosity of the veins around the anus, commonly called piles; hemorrhoids. अर्श; बवासीर

**Haemosalpinx.** See **Haematosalpinx.**

**Haemospermia.** See **Haematospermia.**

**Haemostasis.** Arrest of bleeding; stagnation of blood within its vessels; hemostasis. रक्तस्तम्भन; वाहिनियों के अन्दर खून रुक जाना

**Haemostatic.** Hemostatic; an agent arresting the flow of blood within the vessels. रक्तस्तम्भक; रक्तस्तम्भी; रक्तसंचार रोकने वाला पदार्थ

**Haemothermal.** Warm-blooded; hemothermal. गर्ममिजाज; जोशीला

**Haemothorax.** Effusion of blood into the chest; hemothorax. रक्तवक्ष; छाती के अन्दर खून का रिसाव होना

**Haemotoxic.** Causing blood poisoning; haematotoxic; haemolytic; hematotoxic; hemotoxic. रक्तविषण्णकारी

**Haemotoxin.** Any substance that causes destruction of red blood cells; haematotoxin; hematotoxin; hemotoxin. लालरक्तकोशिकानाशक

**Haemotympanum.** Presence of blood in the middle ear; haematotympanum; hemotympanum. मध्यकर्णरक्तता

**Hahnemann.** Doctor Christian Friedrich Samuel Hahnemann; the German physician known as founder of the Homoeopathic System of Medicine. हैनीमैन; होम्योपैथिक चिकित्सा के जनक जर्मनी के डाक्टर का नाम

**Hahnemannian.** Enunciated by Hahnemann or relating to his doctrine. हैनीमैनप्रणीत; हैनीमैन द्वारा निर्दिष्ट सिद्धान्तों पर आधारित

**Hair.** Threadlike appedages present on all parts of human skin, except palms, soles, glans penis and that surrounding the terminal phalanges. केश; बाल; रोम; लोम;

**H. Bulb,** expanded portion at the lower end of a hair root. लोमकन्द; रोमकन्द;

**H. Cast,** a small nodular accretion of epithelial cells and keratinous debris. लोम-निर्मोक;

**H. Follicle,** a recess lodging the root of a hair. रोमकूप; लोपकूप; रोमपुटक; लोमपुटक; केशपुटक;

**Club H.,** a hair in resting state, prior to shedding, in which the bulb has become a club-shaped mass. मुद्गर लोम;

**Stellate H.,** hair split into several stands at free end. अन्तःशलाका-लोम

**Halation.** Blurring of the visual image by irradiation of light. प्रभावविकिरण

**Halisteresis.** A deficiency of lime salts in the bones. कैल्सियम-अपनयन

**Halisteretic.** Relating to, or marked by halisteresis. कैल्सियम-अपनयनी

**Halitosis.** Unpleasant or foul breath; fetor exore. दुर्गन्धित श्वास; दुर्गन्धित प्रश्वसन; श्वास में बदबू होना

**Halitus.** Any exhalation, as of a vapour or breath. उच्छ्वास, जैसे वाष्प, भाप अथवा निःश्वास अर्थात् छोड़ा हुआ श्वास

**Hallucal.** Relating to the hallux. पादांगुष्ठविषयक; पादांगुष्ठ सम्बन्धी

**Halluces.** Plural of **Hallux**.

**Hallucination.** A false perception or image about sight, sound, smell, taste or touch. विभ्रम; दृष्टिभ्रम; तहम

**Hallucinogenic.** Relating to a hallucinogen. भ्रामक; भ्रम पैदा करने वाला

**Hallucinogens.** Chemicals capable of producing hallucination. विभ्रमजनक औषधियां; भ्रामक औषधियां; भ्रम पैदा करने वाले रसायन

**Hallucinosis.** A psychosis in which the patient is grossly hallucinated; a syndrome, of organic origin, characterized by more or persistent hallucination. विभ्रमता; विभ्रम; भ्रम; वहम

**Hallus.** See **Hallux**.

**Hallux.** The great toe, the first digit of the foot; hallus. पादांगुष्ठ; पैर का अंगूठा;

   **H. Dolorosus,** a condition in which walking causes severe pain in the metatarsophalangeal joint of the great toe. पादांगुष्ठवेदना; पादांगुष्ठार्ति; पैर के अंगूठे में दर्द होना;

   **H. Flexus,** hammer toe, involving the first toe; hallux malleus. मुद्गर पादांगुष्ठ;

   **H. Malleus,** see **Hallux Flexus.**

   **H. Rigidus,** ankylosis of the metatarsophalangeal articulation. पादांगुष्ठस्तम्भ;

   **H. Valgus,** an outward bending of the great toe. पादांगुष्ठ-बहिर्नति; बहिर्नत पादांगुष्ठ;

   **H. Varus,** an inward bending of the great toe. पादांगुष्ठ अन्तर्नति; अन्तर्नत पादांगुष्ठ

**Halo.** A brownish circle around the female nipple; areola. परिवेश; an annular flare of light surrounding a luminous body. प्रभामण्डल; ज्योतिमण्डल;

   **Anaemic H.,** pale, relatively a vascular area in the skin seen sometimes in acute macular eruptions. रक्ताल्प प्रभामण्डल;

**Glaucomatous H.**, a yellowish white ring surrounding the optic disc, indicating atrophy of the choroid in glaucoma. अधिमंथज प्रभामण्डल

**Halometer.** An instrument for measuring the diffraction halo of a red blood cell or ocular halos. लोहितकोशिका-व्यासमापी

**Halophil.** See **Halophile**.

**Halophile.** A micro-organism whose growth is enhanced by or dependent on a high salt concentration; halophil; halophilic. लवणरागी

**Halophilic.** See **Halophile**.

**Ham.** The buttock and back part of the thigh. ऊरु; पुट्ठा; रान का पिछला हिस्सा

**Hammer.** Malleus. हथौड़ी; हथौड़ा; मुद्गर; मूसली

**Hamstrings.** Tendons at the back of the knee bounding the popliteal space on either side. मंदिराशिरा; घुटने के भीतर की नाड़ी; रान की नाड़ी

**Hamular.** Shaped like a hook; unciform. अंकुशवत्; अंकुशाभ

**Hamuli.** Plural of **Hamulus**.

**Hamulus.** The hook or hooklike process of a bone. अंकुश अथवा अंकुशाभ प्रवर्धन

**Hand.** Manus; the distal portion of the superior limb, comprising of carpus, metacarpus and digits. हस्त; हाथ

**Handicap.** A physical, mental or emotional condition that interferes with one's functioning. विकलांगता

**Handicapped.** The term applied to a person with a defect that interferes with the normal activity and achievement. विकलांग; अपंग; अंगहीन

**Hangnail.** A narrow strip of skin partly detached from the nail fold. छिलौरी; नाखुन की जड़ में उखड़ा मांस

**Hangover.** A non-technical term for describing the malaise that may be present following the ingestion of a considerable amount of alcoholic beverages, tobacco-smoking or other central nervous system depressant. नशेड़ियों में पाई जाने वाली घबराहट, बेचैनी, आदि

**Hansen's Disease.** Leprosy. कुष्ठ; कोढ़

**Haphalgesia.** Pain by touching any object; haphalgia. वस्तुस्पर्शार्ति; किसी चीज को छूने से दर्द होना

**Haphalgia.** See **Haphalgesia**.

**Haphephobia.** A morbid fear of touching the things. वस्तुस्पर्शभीति; वस्तुस्पर्शातंक; चीजों को छूने का डर

**Haploid.** Denoting the number of chromosomes in sperm or ova. अगुणित

**Haploscope.** An instrument used in testing the visnal axes. त्रिविमदर्शी; दृष्टि-जांच में प्रयुक्त किया जाने वाला यंत्र विशेष

**Hapten.** Incomplete or partial antigen. अपूर्णप्रतिजन; हैप्टेन

**Haptics.** The science concerned with the tactile sense. स्पर्शज्ञानप्रकरण

**Hard.** Rigid. कठोर; कठिन; ठोस;

    **H. Chancre,** the true Hunterian chancre of syphilitic origin. कठिन-क्षत;

    **H. Palate,** the osseous framework of the palate. कठोर-तालु

**Hardness.** Rigidness; rigidity. कठोरता; ठोसपन

**Harelip.** The congenital cleft of one or both the lips but usually of the upper lip; cleft lip. स्त्रण्टोष्ठ; दोनों होंठों, प्रगुखतया ऊपर वाले होंठ का जन्म से ही खण्डित (कटा-फटा) रहना

**Harmony.** Coordination. समन्वय; सामंजस्य; समंजन; संगति; सुमेल

**Haschisch.** See **Hashish.**

**Hashish.** Hashisch; a form of **Cannabis** that consists largely of resin from the flowering tops and sprouts of cultivated female plants; Cannabis Indica; the Indian hemp. हशीश; पोश्त; भांग

**Haunches.** Hips and buttocks. नितम्ब और कूल्हे

**Haust.** Abbreviated form of **Haustus.**

**Haustra.** Plural of **Haustrum.**

**Haustral.** Relating to a haustrum. आवलीविषयक; आवलीपरक; आवली सम्बन्धी

**Haustration.** The formation of a haustrum; an increase in prominence of the haustra. आवलन

**Haustrum.** One of a series of saccules or pouches, such as sacculations of the colon caused by longitudinal bands that are slightly shorter than the gut. आवली

**Haustus.** A draft of medicine; haust. घूंट

**Haver's canal.** One of the mintute canals found in the compact substance of the bone containing blood vessels and medullary matter. हैवर-नलिका; हड्डियों के अन्दर की रक्तवहानली

**Haversian.** Relating to the various osseous structures described by Clopton Havers. हैवरप्रणीत; हैवर के सिद्धान्तों पर आधारित

**Hawking.** Making constant efforts to clear the throat. खखारना

**Hay-fever.** One form of allergy affecting the nose and the eyes and prevalent in the falls. परागज-ज्वर, जो अगस्त-सितम्बर में घास-फूस सड़ने से होता है

**Hb.** Abbreviation used for **Haemoglobin.**

**HCN.** Symbol for **Hydrocyanic Acid.** हाइड्रोस्यानिक एसिड के लिये प्रयुक्त संकेत चिन्ह

**H.D.** Hora decubitus; at the bed-time. सोते समय

**Head.** The upper part of the body containing brain; caput. सिर; शीर्ष; शिर; मुण्ड; सर

**Headache.** Pain in the head; cephalalgia. सिरदर्द; शिरोवेदना; सिर में दर्द या पीड़ा;
  **Sick H.,** migraine; hemicrania. अर्धकपाली; आधासीसी का दर्द; अर्धशिरोवेदना;
  **Spinal H.,** headache associated with nervous tension, anxiety, etc. तनावी शिरोवेदना

**Head-louse.** Pediculus capitis. यूका; जूं

**Heal.** The natural process of cure or repair of the tissues; healing. विरोहण; स्वस्थ होने या घाव भरने की प्रक्रिया; to cure. रोगमुक्त करना; आरोग्य करना

**Healing.** See **Heal.**

**Health.** The normal condition of mind and body. स्वास्थ्य; आरोग्यता;
  **Mental H.,** the absence of mental or behavioural disorder. मानसिक स्वास्थ्य;
  **Public H.,** the art and science of community health, concerned with statistics, epidemiology, hygiene and prevention and eradication of epidemic disease. जन-स्वास्थ्य

**Healthy.** Conducive to health; well; in a state of normal functioning; free from disease. स्वस्थ; आरोग्य; नीरोग; नीरुज;
  **H. Ulcer,** an ulcer showing tendency to heal. स्वस्थ घाव; नीरुज व्रण

**Hearing.** Special sense by which sounds are appreciated. श्रवण; ज्ञानेन्द्रिय-विशेष, जिसके कारण सुनाई देता है;
  **H. Aid,** an electronic amplifying device designed to bring sound more effectively into the ear; consists of a microphone, amplifier, and receiver. श्रवण यंत्र; हियरिंग एड

**Heart.** An organ keeping up the circulation of blood; cor. हृद्; हृदय; हृत्पिण्ड; दिल;
  **H.-beat,** pulsation of the heart. हृत्स्पन्द; हृदय की धड़कन;
  **H.-block,** disassociation of the auricular and ventricular rhythms due to interference with the contraction process. हृद्रोध; हृदय के निलय तथा अलिन्द का सम्पर्क टूट जाने से दोनों का अलग-अलग ताल देना
  **H.-burn,** see **Pyrosis.**
  **H. Disease,** any disease of the heart. हृद्रोग; हृदय की बीमारी;
  **H. Failure,** complete arrest of the activity of the heart. हृद्पात; हृदय की गति रुक जाना;
  **Athletic H.,** hypertrophy of the heart supposedly due to

overindulgence in athletics. एथलेटी हृद्; मल्लहृदय;
**Fatty H.,** fatty degeneration of the myocardium. वसा-हृद्; वसा-हृदय;
**Tobacco H.,** cardiac irritability marked by irregular action, palpitation, and sometimes pain, occurring as a result of the excessive use of tobacco. तम्बाकू हृद्; तम्बाकू हृदय

**Heat.** The sensation of warmth produced by proximity to fire, etc. ताप; उत्ताप; गर्मी; ऊष्मा; आतप;
**H. Apoplexy,** sun-stroke. लू लगना; तापाघात; आतपरक्ताघात; लू लगने से अपसन्यास प्रकट होना;
**H. Exhaustion,** collapse due to excessive exposure to heat. आतपश्रांति; गर्मी के कारण भारी कमजोरी आ जाना;
**H.-labile.** destroyed by heat; thermolabile. ताप-अस्थिर;
**H.-stable,** thermostable. तापस्थिर;
**H.-stroke,** final stage in heat-exhaustion. तापाघात; ऊष्माघात;
**Prickly H.,** an eruption of papules and vesicles at the mouths of the sweat follicles, accompanied by redness and inflammatory reaction of the skin; miliaria rubra. घमौरी

**Hebetic.** Pertaining to the period of puberty. यौवनारम्भकालीन; यौवनारम्भकालिक

**Heberden's Disease.** Angina pectoris. हेबर्डेन रोग; हृच्छूल; हृदयशूल

**Hectic.** A condition pertaining to a slowly wasting disease, as consumption. प्रलेपक; क्षय अथवा यक्ष्मा सम्बन्धी;
**H. Fever,** habitual fever of phthisis. प्रलेपक ज्वर; यक्ष्मा ज्वर; क्षय ज्वर

**Hecto-.** Prefix used in the metric system to signify one hundred. मीटरिक प्रणाली में 'शत' अर्थात् 'सौ' का अर्थ देने वाला उपसर्ग

**Hectocele.** Prolapse of the intestine through the anus. गुदांत्रभ्रंस; गुदांत्रच्युति

**Heel.** The hinder most part of the foot; calx. पार्ष्णि; पार्ष्णिका; एड़ी;
**H-bone,** the os calcis. पार्ष्णिकास्थि; एड़ी की हड्डी

**Hegar's Sign.** Marked softening of the cervix in early pregnancy. हीगर चिन्ह; जरायुग्रीवा (गर्भाशयग्रीवा) की मृदुता

**Height.** Vertical measurement. ऊंचाई

**Helcoid.** Resembling an ulcer. व्रणाभ; क्षताभ; घाव जैसा

**Helcology.** The science of ulcers. व्रणविज्ञान; क्षतविज्ञान; फोड़ाविज्ञान

**Helcosis.** The formation of ulcers. व्रणोद्भव; व्रणोद्भवन; फोड़ा बनना

**Helical.** Helicine. सर्पिल; relating to a helix. कर्णकुण्डलिनी सम्बन्धी; helicoid. कर्णकुण्डलिनीवत्

**Helicine.** Spiral; coiled; helical. सर्पिल; चक्करदार

**Helicoid.** Resembling a helix; helical. कर्णकुण्डलिनीवत्

**Helicopod Gait.** See **Helicopodia.**

**Helicopodia.** A gait seen in some conversion reactions or hysterical disorders, in which the feet discribe half circles; helicopod gait. अर्धवृत्त चाल

**Heliencephalitis.** Inflammation of the brain following sunstroke. सूर्यतापमस्तिष्कशोथ; लू लगने के कारण होने वाला मस्तिष्क-प्रदाह

**Heliophobia.** A morbid fear of sunlight. सूर्यरश्मिभीति; सूरज की किरणों का डर

**Heliotherapy.** Treatment of diseases by exposure to sunlight. सूर्यरश्मिचिकित्सा; सूरज की किरणों द्वारा की जाने वाली चिकित्सा

**Helium.** A gaseous element, used as a diluent of medicinal gases. हेलियम

**Helix.** The margin of the external ear or the auricle. कर्णकुण्डलिनी; बाहरी कान का किनारा

**Helminth.** An intestinal vermiform parasite. कृमि; आंत्रकृमि

**Helminthagog.** See **Helminthagogue.**

**Helminthagogue.** Any remedy used for expelling worms; helminthagog; anthelmintic. कृमिनिस्सारक (औषधि); पेट के कीड़े निकालने वाली औषधि

**Helminthemesis.** Vomiting of worms. कृमिवमन; कै या उल्टी में कीड़े निकलना

**Helminthiasis.** A morbid condition due to infection with worms; helminthogenesis. कृमिरोग; कृमिरुग्णता; कृमिरोगप्रवणता

**Helminthic.** Anthelmintic. कृमिनिस्सारक

**Helminthogenesis.** See **Helminthiasis.**

**Helminthoid.** Wormlike. कृम्याभ; कृमिवत्; पेट के कीड़ों जैसा

**Helminthology.** A treatise on worms. कृमिविज्ञान; कृमिप्रकरण

**Helminthoma.** A discrete nodule of granulomatous inflammation caused by Helminth or its products. कृमि-अर्बुद; कृम्यर्बुद

**Helminthous.** Wormy. कृम्याभ; कृमिवत्

**Helodes.** Marsh fever. दलदल ज्वर; मलेरिया

**Heloma.** A corn; a callosity; clavus. किण; घट्टा; गुल्म; ठेंठ;

   **H. Durum,** hard corn. कठिन किण; कठोर घट्टा;

   **H. Molle,** soft corn. मृदु किण; कोमल घट्टा

**Helosis.** Eversion of the eyelids. बहिर्वर्त्मता; पलकों का बाहर की ओर मुड़ जाना

**Helotomy.** The surgical treatment of corns. किण-उच्छेदन; घट्टा काट

कर हटा देना
**Hem-.** See **Haem-**.
**Hema-.** See **Haem-**.
**Hemacyte.** See **Haemacyte**.
**Hemacytometer.** See **Haemocytometer**.
**Hemadsorption.** A phenomenon manifested by an agent or substance adhering to, or being absorbed on the surface of a red blood cell; haemadsorption. रक्त-अधिशोषण
**Hemagglutination.** Agglutination of red blood cells; haemagglutination. लोहितकोशिका-समूहन
**Hemagglutinin.** An antibody or other substance that causes hemagglutination; haemagglutinin. रक्त-ऐग्लूटिनिन; लाल रक्त कणों को एकत्र करने वाला प्रतिपिण्ड
**Hemagog.** See **Haemagogue**.
**Hemagogic.** See **Haemagogic**.
**Hemagogue.** See **Haemagouge**.
**Hemal.** See **Haemal**.
**Hemalopia.** See **Haemalopia**.
**Hemameba.** Haemameba; haemamoeba; a parasitic ameboid micro-organism of the blood. रक्तअमीबाणु
**Hemamebiasis.** Any infection with ameboid forms of parasite in red blood cells, as in malaria; haemamebiasis; haemamoebiasis. रक्तअमीबाणुता
**Hemanalysis.** See **Haemanalysis**.
**Hemangiectasis.** See **Haemangiectasis**.
**Hemangio-.** See **Haemangio-**.
**Hemangioblast.** See **Haemangioblast**.
**Hemamngioblastoma.** See **Haemangioblastoma**.
**Hemangioendothelioblastoma.** See **Haemangioendothelioblastoma**.
**Hemangioendothelioma.** See **Haemangioendothelioma**.
**Hemangiofibroma.** See **Haemangiofibroma**.
**Hemangioma.** See **Haemangioma**.
**Hemangiomatosis.** See **Haemangiomatosis**.
**Hemangiopericytoma.** See **Haemangiopericytoma**.
**Hemangiosarcoma.** See **Haemangiosarcoma**.
**Hemapoiesis.** See **Haemopoiesis**.
**Hemarthrosis.** See **Haemarthrosis**.
**Hemat-.** See **Haemat-**.
**Hematachometer.** See **Haematachometer**.
**Hematemesis.** See **Haematemesis**.
**Hematencephalon.** See **Haematencephalon**.

Hemathorax. See Haemathorax.
Hematic. See Haematic.
Hematica. See Haematica.
Hematidrosis. See Haematidrosis.
Hematin. See Haematin.
Hemetinaemia. See Haematinaemia.
Hematinemia. See Haematinaemia.
Hematinic. See Haematinic.
Hematinuria. See Haematinuria.
Hemato-. See Haemato-.
Hematocele. See Haematocele.
Hematochezia. See Haematochezia.
Hematochyluria. See Haematochyluria.
Hematocolpometra. See Haematocolpometra.
Hematocolpos. See Haematocolpos.
Hematocyst. See Haematocyst.
Hematocystitis. See Haematocystitis.
Hematocyte. See Haemacyte.
Hematocytometer. See Haematocytometer
Hematogenesis. See Haematogenesis.
Hematogenic. See Haematogenic.
Hematogenous. See Haematogenic.
Hematography. See Haematography.
Hematohidrosis. See Haematohidrosis.
Hematoid. See Haematoid.
Hematologist. See Haematologist.
Hematology. See Haematology.
Hematolymphangioma. See Haematolymphangioma.
Hematolysis. See Haemolysis.
Hematolytic. See Haemolytic.
Hematoma. See Haematoma.
Hematometra. See Haematometra.
Hematomphalocele. See Haematomphalocele.
Hematomyelia. See Haematomyelia.
Hematopathology. See Haematopathology.
Hematophobia. See Haematophobia.
Hematoplastic. See Haematoplastic.
Hematopoiesis. See Haemopoiesis.
Hematopoietic. See Haemopoietic.
Hematopsia. See Haematopsia.
Hematorrhachis. See Haematorrhachis.
Hematosalpinx. See Haematosalpinx.

**Hematoscheocele.** See **Haematoscheocele.**
**Hematosis.** See **Haematosis.**
**Hematospermatocele.** See **Haematospermatocele.**
**Hematospermia.** See **Haematospermia.**
**Hematostatic.** See **Haematostatic.**
**Hematostaxis.** See **Haematostaxis.**
**Hematothermal.** Warm-blooded. गर्ममिजाज; जोशीला; क्रोधी; गुसैल
**Hematotoxic.** See **Haemotoxic.**
**Hematotoxin.** See **Haemotoxin.**
**Hematotrachelos.** See **Haematotrachelos.**
**Hematotympanum.** See **Haemotympanum.**
**Hematozoa.** See **Haematozoa.**
**Hematozoon.** The Same as **Haematozoon.**
**Hematuresis.** See **Haematuria.**
**Hematuria.** See **Haematuria.**
**Hemaxis.** See **Haemaxis.**
**Heme.** See **Haeme.**
**Hemeralope.** One affected with day-blindness. दिवान्ध; दिनान्ध; ऐसा व्यक्ति जिसे दिन में दिखाई नहीं देता
**Hemeralopia.** Day-blindness; inability to see as distinctly in a bright light as in a dim one; night-sight. दिवान्धता; दिनौंधी; दिन में दिखाई न देने की बीमारी
**Hemi-.** Prefix meaning half. 'अर्ध' तथा 'पक्ष' का अर्थ देने वाला उपसर्ग
**Hemiachromatopsia.** Absent colour-perception in one half of the field of vision; colour hemianopia. अर्धवर्णान्धता; पक्षवर्णान्धता
**Hemianaesthesia.** A loss of sensibility on one side of the body; hemianesthesia. पक्ष-असंवेदनता; एक-पार्श्वी सम्वेदना का अभाव
**Hemianalgesia.** A loss of sense of pain on one side of the body. पक्षनिर्वेदना; एक पार्श्व में पीड़ा-ज्ञान का अभाव
**Hemianencephaly.** Anencephaly on one side only, or involving one side much more extensively than the other. अर्ध-अमस्तिष्कता; पक्ष-अमस्तिष्कता
**Hemianesthesia.** See **Hemianaesthesia.**
**Hemianopia.** Blindness of one-half of the visual field; hemianopsia; hemiopia. अर्धदृष्टिता; दृष्टिदोष-विशेष, जिसमें आधा ही दिखाई देता है;
  **Absolute H.,** hemianopia in which the affected field is totally insensitive to all visual stimuli. शुद्ध अर्धदृष्टिता;
  **Binasal H.,** blindness in the nasal field of vision of both eyes. नासा-अर्धदृष्टिता;

**Bitemporal H.,** blindness in the temporal field of vision of both eyes. द्विशंखी अर्धदृष्टिता;
**Colour H.,** see **Hemiachromatopsia.**
**Complete H.,** hemianopia involving full half of the visual field. पूर्ण अर्धदृष्टिता;
**Unilateral H.,** loss of sight in half the visual field of one eye; uniocular hemianopia. एकपार्श्वी अर्धदृष्टिता;
**Uniocular H.,** see **Unilateral Hemianopia.**

**Hemianopic.** Affected with hemianopia; hemiopic. अर्धदृष्टि; अर्धदृष्टिक

**Hemianopsia.** See **Hemianopia.**

**Hemianoptic.** Pertaining to hemianopia. अर्धदृष्टि सम्बन्धी

**Hemianosmia.** Loss of the sense of smell on one side. अर्ध-अघ्राणता; पक्ष-अघ्राणता

**Hemiapraxis.** Apraxia affecting one side of the body. अर्ध-चेष्टाक्षमता

**Hemiataxia.** An inability to coordinate on one side of the body. पक्षगतिविभ्रम; एक-पार्श्वी समंजन की अयोग्यता

**Hemiathetosis.** Athetosis affecting one hand, or one hand and foot, only. अर्ध-अस्थिरता

**Hemiatrophy.** Impaired nutrition on one side of the body. अर्धांगशोष; शरीर की एक-पार्श्वी अपुष्टि

**Hemiballism.** See **Hemiballismus.**

**Hemiballismus.** Violent writing and choreic movements involving one side of the body; hemiballism. अर्धांग-उद्वेष्टलास्य

**Hemiblock.** Arrest of the impulse in one of the two main divisions of the left branches of the conducting bundle, in heart-block. अर्धरोध; पक्षरोध

**Hemic.** See **Haemic.**

**Hemicanities.** Greyness of hair on one side only. अर्धपार्श्विक-केशधूसरता

**Hemicardia.** Half of a four-chambered heart. अर्धहृद्; पक्षहृद्

**Hemicephalalgia.** See **Hemicrania.**

**Hemicephalia.** See **Hemicephaly.**

**Hemicephaly.** An absence of a lateral half of the skull; hemicephalia. अर्धमस्तिष्कता; सिर का एक हिस्सा गायब रहना

**Hemichorea.** Chorea confined to one side of the body. अर्धांगलास्य

**Hemicolectomy.** Removal of approximate half of the colon. अर्धबृहदांत्र-उच्छेदन; बड़ी आंत का आधा भाग काट कर हटा देना

**Hemicrania.** Neuralgia of half of the head; migraine; hemicephalalgia. अर्धकपाली; आधासीसी, अथवा आधे सिर का दर्द

**Hemicranial.** Relating to one side of the head. अर्धकपालीय;

अर्धकपालिक; आधीसीसी का; आधे सिर का; अर्धकपाली सम्बन्धी

**Hemicraniosis.** Enlargement of one side of the cranium. अर्धकपालबृद्धि

**Hemidiaphoresis.** Unilateral sweating of the body; hemihidrosis; hemidrosis. एकपार्श्वीस्वेदन; एकपार्श्विकस्वेदन

**Hemidrosis.** See **Hemidiaphoresis**.

**Hemidystrophy.** Undevelopment of one lateral half of the body. अर्धपार्श्विक-अपविकास; पक्ष-अपविकास

**Hemiectromelia.** Defective development of the limbs on one side of the body. एकपार्श्विक-अंगदोष; पक्षांगदोष

**Hemiepilepsy.** Epilepsy in which the convulsive movements are confined to one side of the body. एकपार्श्विक-अपस्मार

**Hemifacial.** Pertaining to one side of the face. अर्धआननीय; आधे चेहरे से सम्बन्धित

**Hemigastrectomy.** Excision of the distal half of the stomach. अर्धामाशय-उच्छेदन

**Hemiglossectomy.** Removal of approximately half of the tongue. अर्धजिह्वा-उच्छेदन; आधी जीभ काट कर निकाल देना

**Hemiglossitis.** A vesicular eruption on one side of the tongue and the corresponding inner surface of the cheek. अर्धजिह्वाशोथ

**Hemignathia.** Defective development of one side of the mandible. अर्धचिबुकता; आधी ठोढ़ी गायब रहना

**Hemihidrosis.** See **Hemidiaphoresis**.

**Hemihypalgesia.** Partial loss of sensibility to pain affecting one lateral half of the body. पक्षांगअल्पसम्वेदिता; एकपार्श्विकअल्पसम्वेदिता

**Hemiparaesthesia.** Increased tactile and painful sensibility affecting one side of the body. पक्षांगअपसम्वेदना

**Hemihyperidrosis.** Excessive sweating confined to one side of the body. पक्षांगअतिस्वेदनता; एकपार्श्विकअतिस्वेदनता; एकपार्श्वीस्वेदाधिक्य

**Hemihypertrophy.** Muscular hypertrophy of one side of the face or body. एकपार्श्विकअतिबृद्धि

**Hemihypotonia.** Partial loss of muscular tonicity on one side of the body. एकपार्श्विक अल्पतानता

**Hemilaminectomy.** Removal of a portion of a vertebral lamina. अर्धकशेरुकाफलक-उच्छेदन

**Hemilaryngectomy.** Excision of a lateral half of the larynx. अर्धस्वरयंत्र-उच्छेदन

**Hemilateral.** Relating to one lateral half. एकपार्श्विक; एकपार्श्व सम्बन्धी

**Hemimelia.** A condition marked by defects in the limbs. अर्धांगदोष

**Hemin.** See **Haemin.**

**Hemineurasthenia.** One-sided neurasthenia. पक्षतंत्रिकावसाद; तंत्रिकाओं (नाड़ियों) का एकपार्श्वी. अवसाद

**Hemiopia.** See **Hemianopia.**

**Hemiopic.** See **Hemianopic.**

**Hemiparaesthesia.** Paraesthesia of one side of the body. पक्षांगअपसंवेदनता; एकपार्श्वीअपसंवेदना; एकपार्श्विकअपसंवेदना

**Hemiparaplegia.** Paralysis of the lower limb on one side. अर्धनिम्नांगघात; पक्षनिम्नांगघात; निम्नांगों का एकपार्श्वी अथवा एकपार्श्विक पक्षाघात

**Hemiparesia.** See **Hemiparesis.**

**Hemiparesis.** Paresis of one lateral half of the body; hemiparesia. अर्धपार्श्विकघात; शरीर के एक पार्श्व का आंशिक पक्षाघात

**Hemipexia.** The same as **Hemiplegia.**

**Hemiphonia.** Half-voice; half-whisper. अर्धध्वनि; अर्धवाक्; आधी आवाज

**Hemiplegia.** Paralysis of one side of the body; hemiplexia. अर्धांगघात; अर्धांगवात; शरीर के एक पार्श्व का पक्षाघात;

**Crossed H.**, that affecting one side of the face and the trunk and the extremities of the other; alternating hemiplegia; stauroplegia. विपरीतांगघात; विपरीतांगी पक्षाघात;

**Facial H.**, paralysis of one side of the face. अर्धाननघात; आधे चेहरे का पक्षाघात;

**Spastic H.**, a hemiplegia with increased tone in the antigravity muscles of the affected side. संस्तम्भी अर्धांगघात

**Hemiplegic.** Relating to hemiplegia. अर्धांगघाती; अर्धांगघात सम्बन्धी; affected with hemiplegia. अर्धांगघातग्रस्त

**Hemiplexia.** See **Hemiplegia.**

**Hemisection.** Division of one-half of a part. अर्धपरिच्छेद; समविखण्डन; किसी अंश को दो समान भागों में बांट देना

**Hemispasm.** A spasm affecting but one side of the body. अर्धांगाकर्ष; पक्षाकर्ष; शरीर की एकपार्श्वी अकड़न

**Hemisphere.** Half a sphere, or half of a spherical structure or organ. गोलार्ध

**Hemisystole.** Contraction of left ventricle following every second atrial contraction only, so that there is but one pulse beat to every two heart beats. अर्धप्रकुंचन

**Hemithorax.** One side of the thorax. अर्धवक्ष

**Hemivertebra.** A congenital defect on the spine in which one side of a vertebra fails to develop completely. अर्धकशेरुक

**Hemizygosity.** Possessing only one of the gene pair that determines a particular genetic trait. अर्धयुग्मनजता

**Hemo-.** See **Haem-**.

**Hemoblast.** See **Hemocytoblast**.

**Hemoblastosis.** A proliferative condition of the hematopoietic tissues in general. रक्तकणिकाप्रसू-अर्बुद

**Hemocatheresis.** See **Hemocytocatheresis**.

**Hemocatheretic.** Pertaining to, or characterized by hemocatheresis; hemocytocatheretic. रक्तकणिकानाशी

**Hemocholecyst.** A cyst containing blood and bile. रक्तपित्तपुटी; रक्तपित्तपुटक; nontraumatic haemorrhage or old blood accumulated in the gall-bladder. पित्ताशयरक्तपुटी

**Hemocholecystitis.** Haemorrhagic cholecystitis. रक्तस्रावीपित्ताशयशोथ; पित्ताशयरक्तपुटीशोथ

**Hemochromatosis.** See **Haemochromatosis**.

**Hemoclasia.** See **Hemoclasis**.

**Hemoclasis.** Rupture, dissolution, or other type of destruction of red blood cells; haemolysis; hemoclasia. रक्तलयन; रक्तापघटन; रुधिरलयन; लाल रक्तकणों का टूटना

**Hemoclastic.** Pertaining to hemoclasis. रुधिरलायी; रक्तलायी; रक्तलायक

**Hemoconcentration.** See **Haemoconcentration**.

**Hemocyte.** A blood-corpuscle; any cell or formed element of the blood. रक्तकणिका

**Hemocytoblast.** A primitive blood cell found in bone marrow from which all cells normally present in blood are thought to arise; hemoblast. रक्तकणिकाप्रसू

**Hemocytocatheresis.** Hemolysis, or other type of destruction of red blood cells; hemocatheresis. रक्तकणिकानाशन

**Hemocytocatheretic.** See **Hemocatheretic**.

**Hemocytolysis.** The dissolution of blood cells, including hemolysis. रक्तकणिकापघटन

**Hemocytometer.** See **Haemocytometer**.

**Hemocytometry.** See **Haemocytometry**.

**Hemodiagnosis.** Diagnosis by means of examination of the blood. रक्तरोगनिदान

**Hemodialysis.** See **Haemodialysis**.

**Hemodialyzer.** A machine for hemodialysis in acute or chronic renal failure; artificial kidney. रक्त-अपोहनयंत्र; कृत्रिम वृक्क

**Hemodilution.** Increase in the volume of plasma in relation to red blood cells. रक्ततनूकरण

**Hemodynamics.** The study of the dynamics of the blood circulation. रक्तसंचारप्रकरण; रक्तसंचारविज्ञान
**Hemogenesis.** See **Haemogenesis.**
**Hemogenic.** See **Haemogenic.**
**Hemoglobin.** See **Haemoglobin.**
**Hemoglobinonemia.** Presence of free haemoglobin in the blood plasma. रक्तप्लाविकाहीमोग्लोबिनता
**Hemoglobinolysis.** Destruction or chemical splitting of haemoglobin. हीमोग्लोबिनापघटन
**Hemoglobinometer.** See **Haemoglobinometer.**
**Hemoglobinometry.** See **Haemoglobinometry.**
**Hemoglobinopathy.** See **Haemoglobinopathy.**
**Hemoglobinophilic.** See **Haemoglobinophilic.**
**Hemoglobinuria.** See **Haemoglobinuria.**
**Hemoglobinuric.** See **Haemoglobinuric.**
**Hemogram.** See **Haemogram.**
**Hemoid.** See **Haemoid.**
**Hemolith.** See **Haemolith.**
**Hemology.** See **Haematology.**
**Hemolymph.** See **Haemolymph.**
**Hemolysis.** See **Haemolysis.**
**Hemolytic.** See **Haemolytic.**
**Hemometra.** See **Haematometra.**
**Hemomediastinum.** Blood in the mediastinum. मध्यस्थानिकारक्तता
**Hemonephrosis.** Blood in the pelvis of the kidney. वृक्कगोणिकारुधिरता; वृक्कगोणिकारक्तता
**Hemonormoblast.** See **Erythroblast.**
**Hemopathology.** See **Haematopathology.**
**Hemopathy.** See **Haemopathy.**
**Hemopericardium.** See **Haemopericardium.**
**Hemoperitoneum.** See **Haemoperitoneum.**
**Hemophagocyte.** See **Haemophagocyte.**
**Hemophil.** Applied to micro-organisms growing preferably in media containing blood; hemophile. रक्तग्राही; रुधिरग्राही
**Hemophile.** See **Hemophil.**
**Hemophilia.** See **Haemophilia.**
**Hemophiliac.** See **Haemophiliac.**
**Hemophilic.** See **Haemophilic.**
**Hemophilus.** See **Haemophilus.**
**Hemophthalmia.** See **Haemophthalmia.**
**Hemoplastic.** See **Haemopoietic.**

**Hemopneumothorax.** See **Haemopneumothorax.**
**Hemopoiesis.** See **Haemopoiesis.**
**Hemopoietic.** See **Haemopoietic.**
**Hemoptoe.** See **Haemoptysis.**
**Hemoptysis.** See **Haemoptysis.**
**Hemorrhachis.** See **Haematorrhachis.**
**Hemorrhage.** See **Haemorrhage.**
**Hemorrhagenic.** See **Haemorrhagenic.**
**Hemorrhagic.** See **Haemorrhagic.**
**Hemorrhagins.** A group of toxins, found in certain venoms and poisonous material from some plants, that causes degeneration and lysis of endothelial cells in capillaries and small vessels, thereby resulting in numerous small haemorrhages in tissues. रक्तस्रावक (तत्व); रक्तस्रावी (तत्व)
**Hemorrhea.** See **Hemorrhoea.**
**Hemorrhoea.** Haemorrhage; hemorrhea. रक्तस्राव
**Hemorrhoidal.** See **Haemorrhoidal.**
**Hemorrhoidectomy.** See **Haemorrhoidectomy.**
**Hemorrhoids.** See **Haemorrhoids.**
**Hemosalpinx.** See **Haematosalpinx.**
**Hemospermia.** See **Haematospermia.**
**Hemostasis.** See **Haemostasis.**
**Hemostat.** An antihaemorrhagic agent. रक्तस्तम्भक (पदार्थ); an instrument for arresting haemorrhage by compression of the bleeding vessel. रक्तस्तम्भक (यंत्र/उपकरण)
**Hemostatic.** See **Haemostatic.**
**Hemotherapy.** Treatment of disease by the use of blood or blood derivatives, such as transfusion. रक्तोपचार; रक्त द्वारा की जाने वाली चिकित्सा
**Hemothermal.** See **Haemothermal.**
**Hemothorax.** See **Haemothorax.**
**Hemotoxic.** See **Haemotoxic.**
**Hemotoxin.** See **Haemotoxin.**
**Hemotympanum.** See **Haemotympanum.**
**Hemp.** Cannabis Indica; the Indian hemp. गांजा; भांग
**Hepaptosis.** See **Hepatoptosis.**
**Hepar.** The liver or liverlike structures; hepatis. यकृत् अथवा यकृताकार;
  **H. Lobatum,** a liver having numerous lobes. यकृत् बहुखण्डकता; असंख्य खण्डों वाला जिगर अथवा यकृत् पिण्ड;

**Hepatr**

 H. Siccatum, dried liver. शुष्क यकृत्; सूखा जिगर

**Hepat-, Hepatico-, Hepato-.** Prefixes denoting the liver. 'यकृत्' का अर्थ देने वाले उपसर्ग

**Hepatalgia.** Painful affection of the liver; hepatic colic; hepatodynia. यकृत्शूल; यकृतार्ति; यकृत् (जिगर) का दर्दनाक रोग

**Hepatatrophia.** See **Hepatatrophy**.

**Hepatatrophy.** Atrophy of the liver; hepatatrophia. यकृत्शोष

**Hepatectomised.** The excised liver. उच्छिन्न-यकृत्

**Hepatectomy.** Excision of a part of the liver. यकृतुच्छेदन; यकृत् के किसी अंश को काट कर हटा देना

**Hepatic.** Pertaining to the liver. यकृती; यकृत् सम्बन्धी;

 H. Colic, see **Hepatalgia**.

 H. Duct, the duct conveying the bile from liver towards the duodenum. यकृत्-नली; पित्त-नली

**Hepatico-.** See **Hepat-**.

**Hepaticodochotomy.** Combined choledochotomy and hepaticotomy. पिताशययकृत्नलीछेदन

**Hepaticoduodenostomy.** Establishment of a communication between the hepatic duct and the duodenum. यकृत्ग्रहणीसम्मिलन

**Hepaticoenterostomy.** Establishment of a communication between the hepatic duct and the intestine. यकृतांत्रसम्मिलन

**Hepaticogastrostomy.** Establishment of a communication between the hepatic duct and the stomach. यकृतामाशयसम्मिलन

**Hepaticolithotomy.** Removal of the calculus from a hepatic duct. पित्तनली-अश्मरीहरण; पित्तनली की पथरी निकाल देना

**Hepaticolithotripsy.** Crushing a biliary calculus in the hepatic duct. यकृत्पित्ताश्मरीहरण

**Hepaticostomy.** Establishment of an opening into the hepatic duct. यकृत्नली-सम्मिलन

**Hepaticotomy.** Incision into the hepatic duct. पित्तनलीछेदन

**Hepatis.** The liver. यकृत्; जिगर

**Hepatitic.** Relating to hepatitis. यकृत्शोथज; यकृत्शोथ सम्बन्धी

**Hepatitis.** Inflammation of the liver, formerly called infectious jaundice. यकृत्शोथ; जिगर का प्रदाह

**Hepatization.** Conversion of a loose tissue into a liverlike substance. यकृतीभवन;

 Grey H., the second stage of hepatitis in pneumonia, when the yellowish-grey exudate is beginning to degenerate prior to breaking down. धूसर यकृतीभवन;

**Red H.,** the first stage of hepatitis in which the exudate is blood-stained. लोहित यकृतीभवन;

**Yellow H.,** the final stage of hepatitis in which the exudate is becoming purulent. पीत यकृतीभवन

**Hepato-.** See **Hepat-.**

**Hepatobiliary.** Pertaining to the liver and bile. यकृत्-पित्तज; यकृत् तथा पित्त सम्बन्धी

**Hepatoblastoma.** A malignant neoplasm of the liver, occurring in children. यकृत्प्रसू-अर्बुद

**Hepatocarcinoma.** See **Malignant Hepatoma.**

**Hepatocele.** Hernia of the liver. यकृत्-हर्निया; यकृत्स्रंस

**Hepatocellular.** Pertaining to, or affecting the liver cells. यकृत्कोशिकीय; यकृत्-कोशिकाओं सम्बन्धी अथवा उन्हें रुग्ण करने वाला;

**H. Carcinoma,** see **Malignant Hepatoma.**

**Hepatocholangiojejunostomy.** Union of the hepatic duct to the jejunum. यकृत्नलीमध्यान्त्रसम्मिलन

**Hepatocholangiostomy.** Creation of an opening into the common bile duct to establish drainage. यकृत्पित्तनलीसम्मिलन

**Hepatocholangitis.** Inflammation of the liver and biliary tract. यकृत्पित्तनलीशोथ

**Hepatocystic.** Relating to the gall-bladder, or to both liver and gall-bladder. पित्ताशय अथवा यकृत् तथा पित्ताशय दोनों से सम्बन्धित

**Hepatocyte.** A parenchymal liver cell. यकृत्कोशिका

**Hepatodynia.** See **Hepatalgia.**

**Hepatoenteric.** Relating to the liver and the intestine. यकृतांत्रज; यकृत् तथा आंत्र सम्बन्धी

**Hepatogastric.** Relating to the liver and the stomach. यकृतामाशयिक; यकृत् तथा आमाशय सम्बन्धी

**Hepatogenic.** See **Hepatogenous.**

**Hepatogenous.** Produced by the liver; formed in the liver; of hepatic origin; hepatogenic. यकृत्जन्य; यकृत्जनित

**Hepatography.** A description of the liver. यकृत्चित्रण

**Hepatoid.** Resembling the liver. यकृताभ; यकृत् जैसा

**Hepatolith.** A concretion or stone in the liver; a biliary calculus. यकृताश्मरी; पित्ताश्मरी; जिगर की पथरी

**Hepatolithectomy.** Removal of a calculus from the liver. यकृताश्मरी-उच्छेदन; यकृताश्मरीहरण; जिगर की पथरी निकाल देना

**Hepatolithiasis.** Formation or presence of stone in the liver. यकृताश्मरता; पित्ताश्मरता; पित्तपथरी बनना

**Hepatology.** The science of the nature, structure, diseases, etc. of the liver. यकृत्विज्ञान; यकृत् की प्रकृति, बनावट, रोगावस्थाओं, आदि का वैज्ञानिक अध्ययन

**Hepatoma.** Primary carcinoma of the liver. यकृतार्बुद; यकृत् का प्राथमिक कैंसर;

**Malignant H.**, a carcinoma derived from parenchymal cells of the liver; hepatocellular carcinoma; hepatocarcinoma. दुर्दम यकृतार्बुद

**Hepatomalacia.** Softening of the liver. यकृत्मृदुता; मृदुयकृत्; यकृत् की कोमलता

**Hepatomegaly.** Hypertrophy or enlargement of the liver; megalohepatica. यकृत्बृद्धि;· यकृत्-विवर्धन; जिगर बढ़ना

**Hepatomelanosis.** Deep pigmentation of the liver. यकृत्मेलेनिनमयता

**Hepatomphalocele.** Umbilical hernia with involvement of the liver. यकृत्नाभिहर्निया; यकृत्नाभिस्रंस

**Hepatonephric.** Relating to the liver and the kidney; hepatorenal. यकृत् तथा वृक्क सम्बन्धी

**Hepatopathic.** Damaging the liver. यकृत्पिण्डनाशक

**Hepatopathy.** Any disease of the liver. यकृत्रोग; जिगर की कोई बीमारी

**Hepatopexy.** Fixation of the wandering liver. यकृत्स्थिरीकरण

**Hepatopneumonic.** Relating to the liver and the lungs; hepatopulmonary. यकृत् तथा फुप्फुसों सम्बन्धी

**Hepatoportal.** Relating to the portal system of the liver. यकृत्प्रतिहारी

**Hepatoptosis.** The movable liver; hepaptosis. यकृत्भ्रंश; चलयकृत्; यकृत्पात

**Hepatopulmonary.** See **Hepatopneumonic**.

**Hepatorenal.** See **Hepatonephric**.

**Hepatorrhaphy.** Suture of a wound of the liver. यकृत्सीवन

**Hepatorrhea.** See **Hepatorrhoea**.

**Hepatorrhexis.** Rupture of the liver. यकृत्विदर; यकृत्-हर्निया

**Hepatorrhoea.** Bilious diarrhoea; hepatorrhea. पित्तातिसार; पैत्तिक दस्त होना

**Hepatoscopy.** Examination of the liver. यकृत्दर्शन

**Hepatosplenitis.** Inflammation of the liver and the spleen. यकृत्प्लीहाशोथ; जिगर तथा तिल्ली का प्रदाह

**Hepatosplenography.** Use of contrast dyes to depict the liver and spleen radiographically. यकृत्प्लीहाचित्रण

**Hepatosplenomegaly.** Hypertrophy of the liver and the spleen. यकृत्प्लीहातिबृद्धि; जिगर तथा तिल्ली बढ़ जाना

**Hepatosplenopathy.** Disease of the liver and the spleen. यकृत्प्लीहाविकृति; जिगर तथा तिल्ली की बीमारी

**Hepatotomy.** Incision into the liver. यकृत्छेदन

**Hepatotoxic.** Having an injurious effect on the liver cells. यकृत्विषकारी; यकृत्-कोशिकाओं को हानि पहुँचाने वाला

**Hepatotoxin.** A toxin that is destructive to parenchymal cells of the liver. यकृत्विष

**Hepatotoxaemia.** Autointoxication originating in the liver; hepatotoxemia. यकृत्विषण्णता

**Hepatotoxemia.** See **Hepatotoxaemia.**

**Hepta-.** Prefix denoting seven. 'सप्त' अथवा 'सात' का अर्थ देने वाला उपसर्ग

**Herb.** Any plant, having a soft stem. शाक्; वनस्पति; पौधा; झाड़ी; क्षुप

**Herbivora.** Eating vegetation; herbivorous. शाक्भक्षी; वनस्पतियों को खाने वाला

**Herbivorous.** See **Herbivora.**

**Hereditary.** Parental; relating to heredity. पैत्रिक; वंशगत; आनुवंशिक

**Heredity.** That factor responsible for the persistence of characteristics in successive generations. पैत्रिकता; वंशगतता; आनुवंशिकता; वंश-परम्परा

**Heredo-.** Prefix denoting heredity. 'पैत्रिकता', 'अनुवंश', 'वंशगतता' अथवा 'आनुवंशिकता' का अर्थ देने वाला उपसर्ग

**Heredofamilial.** Denoting an inherited constitution present in more than one member of a family. अनुवंशपरिवारगत

**Hermaphrodism.** See **Hermaphroditism.**

**Hermaphrodite.** One whose generative organs combine those of both sexes. उभयलिंगी

**Hermaphroditism.** The condition of hermaphrodite; hermaphrodism. उभयलिंगिता

**Hermetic.** Denoting a container closed or sealed in such a way that it is airtight. वातरक्षित

**Hernia.** Rupture; the abnormal protrusion of a part or structure through the tissues containing it. हर्निया; बहि:सरण; वर्ध्म; स्रंस;
   **H. Cerebri,** see **Cerebral Hernia.**
   **H. Testis,** see **Scrotal Hernia.**
   **Abdominal H.,** a protrusion of a part of the viscera through the abdominal wall. उदर हर्निया;
   **Cerebral H.,** protrusion of brain substance through a defect in the skull; hernia cerebri. मस्तिष्कस्रंस; मस्तिष्क-हर्निया;

**Hernia**

**Congenital H.,** a hernia existing at birth into the vaginal process of the peritoneum. सहज हर्निया; जन्मजात हर्निया;

**Crural H.,** see **Femoral Hernia.**

**Diaphragmatic H.,** hernia of the abdominal viscera into the thorax. मध्यच्छद-हर्निया; मध्यच्छदीय हर्निया;

**Epigastric H.,** hernia through the linea alba above the navel. अधिजठर-हर्निया;

**Femoral H.,** one alongside the femoral blood vessels as they pass into the thigh; crural hernia; enteromerocele; femorocele. और्विक हर्निया; ऊरु-हर्निया

**Gastro-oesophageal H.,** a hiatal hernia into the thorax. जठर-ग्रासनलीय हर्निया;

**Hiatal H.,** see **Hiatus Hernia.**

**Hiatus H.,** hernia of a part of the stomach through the oesophageal hiatus of the diaphragm; hiatal hernia. विदरित हर्निया;

**Incarcerated H.,** an old occluded hernia causing obstruction of the bowels. आंत्ररोधज हर्निया;

**Incisional H.,** hernia occurring through a surgical incision or scar. छेदनोत्तर हर्निया;

**Inguinal H.,** one at the inguinal region. वंक्षण हर्निया;

**Interstitial H.,** a hernia in which the protrusion is between any two of the layers of the abdominal wall. अन्तरालीय हर्निया;

**Irreducible H.,** a hernia that cannot be reduced without an operation. पुनरस्थाप्य हर्निया;

**Ischiatic H.,** a hernia through the sacrosciatic foramen. आसनास्थिक हर्निया;

**Labial H.,** one into the labium majus; cremnocele. भगोष्ठ-हर्निया;

**Parietal H.,** hernia in which only a portion of the wall of the intestine is engaged. भित्तिक हर्निया;

**Perineal H.,** hernia protruding through the pelvic diaphragm; perineocele. मूलाधारी हर्निया;

**Reducible H.,** a hernia in which the contents of the hernial sac can be returned to their normal location by manipulation. पुनःस्थाप्य हर्निया;

**Retrograde H.,** a double loop hernia, the central loop of which lies in the abdominal cavity. पश्चगतिक हर्निया;

**Sciatic H.,** protrusion of intestine through the great sacrosciatic foramen; ischiocele. आसनास्थिक हर्निया; आसनास्थिभ्रंस;

**Scrotal H.,** inguinal hernia in which the protrusion has entered the scrotum; hernia testis; oscheocele. वृषणकोष-हर्निया; अण्डग्रन्थि-हर्निया;

**Strangulated H.,** one so tightly constricted as to interfere with its return with the circulation of blood and with the passage of faeces. विपाशित हर्निया;

**Umbilical H.,** one in which the bowel protrudes through the abdominal wall under the skin at the umbilicus; exomphalos. नाभि-हर्निया;

**Vesicle H.,** protrusion of a segment of the bladder through the abdominal wall or into the inguinal canal and into the scrotum. पुटिका हर्निया;

**Vitreous H.,** internal prolapse of the vitreous into the anterior chamber. विट्रियस हर्निया

**Hernial.** Relating to hernia. हर्नियाविषयक; हर्निया सम्बन्धी

**Herniated.** Denoting any structure protruded through a hernial opening. संस्त्रित; बहिसरणित

**Herniation.** Formation of a hernia. बहि:सरण

**Hernio-.** Prefix indicative of hernia. 'हर्नियासूचक' उपसर्ग

**Hernioid.** Resembling hernia. हर्नियाभ; हर्निया जैसा

**Herniology.** The science of hernia. हर्नियाविज्ञान; बहि:सरणविज्ञान

**Hernioplasty.** An operation for hernia, in which an attempt is made to prevent recurrence. हर्नियासंधानकर्म

**Herniorrhaphy.** An operation for hernia, in which the weak area is reinforced by some of the patients, own tissues, or by some other material. हर्नियासीवन

**Herniotome.** A special knife with a blunt tip, used for the operation of hernia. हर्निया-उच्छेदक

**Herniotomy.** Surgical correction of a hernia by cutting; celotomy; kelotomy. हर्निया-उच्छेदन

**Heroic.** Denoting an aggressive and daring procedure. पराक्रमशील; वीरोचित

**Herpangina.** Minute vesicles and ulcers at the back of the mouth. मुखीपरिसर्प; मुख के पिछले भाग में छोटे-छोटे स्फोट तथा व्रण उत्पन्न होना

**Herpes.** A skin disease with patches of distinct vesicles. परिसर्प; विसर्प; विसर्पिका; छाजन; दाद; हर्पीज;

**H. Circinatus,** ringworm. मण्डलकुष्ठ; दद्रु; दाद;

**H. Genitalis,** see Herpes Preputialis.

**H. Preputialis,** herpes of the genitals, i.e. penis of males, or the cervix, perineum, vagina, or vulva of females; herpes genitalis. जननांगी विसर्प;

**H. Simplex**, fever blister; cold sore. सरल हर्पीज;

**H. Zoster**, zoster; zona; shingles. वर्तुलाकार छाजन; परिसर्पीय छाजन; भैंसिया छाजन (दाद)

**Herpetic.** Pertaining to, or characterized by herpes. हर्पीज सम्बन्धी.अथवा हर्पीज जैसा; परिसर्पी; विसर्पी

**Herpetiform.** Having the appearance of herpes. हर्पीजसम; हर्पीजरूप; परिसर्पसम; विसर्पसम; परिसर्प से मिलता-जुलता

**Hertz (Hz).** A unit of frequency equivalent to 1 cycle per second. हर्ट्ज

**Hesitancy.** An involuntary delay or inability in starting the urinary stream. उत्संग; झिझक

**Heter-.** See **Hetero-**.

**Heterecious.** Having more than one host. विषमपोषी; असमपोषी

**Hetero-, Heter-.** Prefixes meaning unlikeness, dissimilarity, different or other. 'असम' या 'विषम' का अर्थ देने वाले उपसर्ग

**Heteroantibody.** Antibody that is heterologous with respect to antigen. असमप्रतिपिण्ड; विषमप्रतिपिण्ड

**Heteroblastic.** Developing from more than a single type of tissue. असमप्रसू; विषमप्रसू

**Heterocellular.** Formed of cells of different kinds. असमकोशिकीय; विषमकोशिकीय

**Heterochromia.** A condition of diversity of colour. असमवर्णकता; विषमवर्णकता

**Heterochromic.** A diversity of colour; heterochromous. असमवर्णी; विषमवर्णी

**Heterochromous.** See **Heterochromic**.

**Heterochronia.** The origin or development of tissues or organs at an unusual time or out of the regular sequence. विषममूल; असममूल

**Heterochronic.** See **Heterochronous**.

**Heterochronous.** Relating to heterochronia; heterochronic. विषममूलक; असममूलक

**Heterocrine.** Denoting the secretion of two or more kinds of material. विषमस्रावी

**Heterodromous.** Moving in opposite direction. विषमदिक्; असमदिक्

**Heterogametic.** Pertaining to an individual having both dominant and recessive germ cells; heterogametous. विषमयुग्मकी

**Heterogametous.** See **Heterogametic**.

**Heterogamous.** Relating to heterogamy. विषमयुग्मकता अथवा विषमवंश सम्बन्धी

**Heterogamy.** Conjugation of unlike gametes. विषमयुग्मकता; विषमजन्युता; alteration of generations in which two kinds of sexual generations alternate. विषमवंशगतता; विषमआनुवंशिकता

**Heterogeneic.** Pertaining to different gene constitutions, especially with respect to different species; heterogenic. विषमजीनी; असमजीनी

**Heterogeneity.** The state of being heterogeneous. विषमांगता; असमांगता

**Heterogeneous.** Composed of parts having various and dissimilar characteristics or properties. विषमांगी; असमांगी

**Heterogenesis.** Production of offspring unlike the parents. असम-उत्पत्तिक; विषम-उत्पत्तिक

**Heterogenetic.** Relating to heterogenesis. विषम-उत्पत्ति सम्बन्धी

**Heterogenic.** See **Heterogeneic.**

**Heterogenous.** Of different kinds; of unlike origin. असमांग; विषमांग; विजातीय

**Heterograft.** A graft transferred from an animal of one species to one of another species; heterotransplant; heterologous, heteroplastic, heterospecific or interspecific graft. विषमनिरोप; असमनिरोप

**Heterolalia.** A form of aphasia characterized by habitual substitution of meaningless or inappropriate words for those intended; heterophasia; heterophemia. विषमवाक्; असमवाक्

**Heterolateral.** Contralateral. विषमपार्श्विक; असमपार्श्विक

**Heterologous.** Differing from the normal in structure or form; derived from different species. असमधर्मी; विषमधर्मी

**Heterolysis.** Dissolution or digestion of cells or protein components from one species by a lytic agent from a different species. विषमलयन

**Heterolytic.** Pertaining to heterolysis. विषमलायी

**Heterometaplasia.** Tissue transformation resulting in the production of a tissue foreign to the part where produced. विषमइतरविकसन; विषमइतरविकास

**Heterometropia.** A condition in which the degree of refraction is unlike in the two eyes. विषमापवर्तन

**Heteromorphosis.** Development of one tissue from a tissue of another kind or type; embryonic development of tissue or an organ inappropriate to its site. विषमोत्पत्ति; विषमरूप; विषमविकास

**Heteromorphous.** Of abnormal form; differing from the normal type. असमरूप; विषमरूप; विषमाकृतिक

**Heteronomous.** Abnormal; different from the type; subject to direction or law of another; not self-governing. असमनियमी; विषमनियमी; भिन्ननियमी

**Heteronomy.** The condition or state of being heteronomous. असमनियमता; विषमनियमता

**Heteronymous.** Crossed; in opposite relation. विषमखण्डी; असमखण्डी

**Heteropathy.** Allopathy. ऐलोपैथी; ऐलोपैथिक चिकित्सा; abnormal sensitivity to stimuli. अतिसम्वेदिता

**Heterophasia.** See **Heterolalia.**

**Heterophemia.** See **Heterolalia.**

**Heterophil.** See **Heterophile.**

**Heterophile.** Activity of a product of one species against that of another; heterophil. विषमरागी; इतररागी

**Heterophonia.** A change of voice, especially at puberty; any abnormality in the voice sounds. विषमवाक्; इतरवाक्; वाग्दोष; आवाज बदल जाना

**Heterophoralgia.** Painful heterophoria. सपीडनेत्रविचलनप्रवृत्ति

**Heterophoria.** The tending of the visual lines away from parallelism. नेत्रविचलनप्रवृत्ति

**Heterophthalmus.** A difference in the appearance of the two eyes. विषमनेत्री

**Heteroplasia.** Development of cytologic and histologic elements that are normal for the organ or part in question. विषमतन्तुजता; इतरविकास; malposition of tissue or a part that is otherwise normal. विस्थिति

**Heteroplastic.** Pertaining to, or manifesting heteroplasia. इतरविकास सम्बन्धी; relating to tissue transplantation from one species to another. विषमतन्तुजता सम्बन्धी

**Heteropyknosis.** Any state of variable density. इतरघनता; विषमघनता

**Heterosexual.** Attracted towards the opposite sex. इतरलैंगिक; इतरलिंग-कामुक; विपरीत लिंग की ओर आकर्षित होने वाला/वाली

**Heterosexuality.** Erotic attraction, predisposition, or sexual behaviour between persons of the opposite sex. इतरलिंगी-कामुकता

**Heterosuggestion.** Suggestion received from another person. इतरसंसूचन

**Heterotaxia.** Abnormal arrangement of organs or parts of the body in relation to each other. विषमांगता; असमांगता

**Heterotaxic.** Abnormally placed or arranged. विषमांगी; असमांगी

**Heterotonia.** Abnormality or variation in tension or tonus. विषमतानता

**Heterotopia.** See **Heterotopy.**

**Heterotopic.** Relating to heterotopia. विस्थिति अथवा विस्थापन सम्बन्धी; ectopic. अस्थानी; अस्थानिक

**Heterotopy.** Heterotopia; an abnormal position of a part; ectopia. विस्थिति; विस्थापन; किसी अंश-विशेष की असाधारण स्थिति

**Heterotransplant.** See **Heterograft.**

**Heterotransplantation.** Transfer of a heterograft. इतरप्रतिरोपण

**Heterotroph.** A micro-organism that obtains its carbon, as well as its energy, from organic compounds. परपोषी

**Heterotrophic.** Relating to a heterotroph. परपोषित

**Heterotropia.** Deviation of the eyes from the normal position; strabismus. नेत्रविचलन; आँखों की सामान्य स्थिति न होना

**Heterotypic.** See **Heterotypical.**

**Heterotypical.** Differing from type or form; heterotypic. विषमप्ररूपी; भिन्नप्ररूपी

**Heteroaxial.** Having mutually perpendicular axes of unequal length. विषमाक्षीय; असमाक्षीय

**Hex-, Hexa-.** Prefixes meaning six. 'षट्' अथवा 'छ:' का अर्थ देने वाले उपसर्ग

**Hexadactylism.** See **Hexadactyly.**

**Hexadactyly.** Presence of six digits on one or both hands or feet; hexadactylism. षटंगुलिता

**Hexaploidy.** The state of a cell nucleus containing three or a higher multiple of the haploid number of chromosomes; polyploidy. षट्गुणसूत्री

**Hg.** Abbreviation for **Hydrargyrum** (mercury). पारद के लिये प्रयुक्त किया जाने वाला संक्षिप्त चिन्ह

**Hiatal.** Relating to a hiatus. द्वार, छिद्र अथवा विदर सम्बन्धी

**Hiatus.** An aperture or fissure; a space, gap, opening or foramen. द्वार; छिद्र; छेद; मुख; विदर; vulva. भग;

    **H. Hernia,** see under **Hernia.**

**Hibernation.** A sleeping throughout the winter. शीतनिष्क्रियता; सर्दियों में काम-काज से पूर्णतया अलग रहना

**Hiccough.** A diaphragmatic spasm causing a sudden inhalation which is interrupted by a spasmodic closure of the glottis; hiccup. हिचकी; हिक्का

**Hiccup.** See **Hiccough.**

**Hidr-.** See **Hidro-.**

**Hidradenitis.** Inflammation of one or more sweat glands. स्वेदग्रंथिशोथ; स्वेदग्रंथियों का प्रदाह

**Hidradenoma.** A tumour of the sweat gland. स्वेदग्रन्थ्यर्बुद; स्वेदग्रन्थि की रसौली

**Hidro-, Hidr-.** Prefixes meaning sweat or sweat gland. 'स्वेद', अथवा 'स्वेदग्रन्थि' का अर्थ देने वाले उपसर्ग

**Hidrocystoma.** A cystic form of hydradenoma. स्वेदपुटी-अर्बुद

**Hidropedesis.** Excessive sweating. अतिस्वेदनता; अत्यधिक पसीना होना

**Hidropoiesis.** Formation of sweat. स्वेदनोत्पत्ति; स्वेदोत्पत्ति

**Hidropoietic.** Relating to hidropoiesis. स्वेदोत्पत्ति सम्बन्धी

**Hidroschesis.** Suppression of sweating. स्वेददमन

**Hidrose.** Full of sweat. स्वेदावृत्त; पसीने से तर

**Hidrosis.** Production and excretion of sweat. स्वेदोत्पादन; स्वेदनोत्पादन; पसीना आना या बनना

**Hidrotic.** Relating to, or causing hidrosis. स्वेदोत्पादन सम्बन्धी अथवा स्वेदोत्पादक

**Hila.** Plural of **Hilum.**

**Hilar.** Pertaining to hilus. विदर, नाभि अथवा बीज सम्बन्धी

**Hilitis.** Inflammation of the lining membrane of any hilus. विदरशोथ

**Hillock.** In anatomy, any small elevation or prominence. क्षुद्रोत्थापन

**Hilum.** A depression on the surface of an organ where vessels, ducts, etc. enter and leave; hilus. विदर; दरार; नाभि; बीज; हाइलम

**Hilus.** See **Hilum.**

**Hind.** Relating to the rear extremity. पश्च; पीछे का; पिछला;

   **H.-brain,** the encephalon. पश्चकपाल;

   **H.-gut,** the posterior intestine, i.e. the large intestine, rectum and anal canal; the caudal or terminal part of the embryonic gut. पश्चान्त्र; आहार नली का पिछला भाग;

   **H. Water,** hydrorrhoea gravidarum; liquor amnii. गर्भोदक; उल्वोदक

**Hinge-joint.** The synovial joint; diarthrosis. चलसन्धि

**Hip.** The upper part of the thigh. नितम्ब; कूल्हा; श्रोणि; पुट्ठा;

   **H.-bath,** term for a half-bath or the hips only. नितम्ब-स्नान; कटि-स्नान;

   **H. Disease,** a scrofulous affection, otherwise styled morbus coxarum. नितम्ब रोग;

   **H.-joint,** the joint of the upper part of the thigh. नितम्ब-सन्धि;

   **H.-joint Disease,** a tuberculous lesion of the hip-joint. नितम्ब-सन्धि रोग

**Hipnotic.** Sleep-producing. स्वापक

**Hippocrates.** Famous Greek physician and philospher who started the old school of medicine, called Allopathy. हिप्पोक्रैट्स; ऐलोपैथिक चिकित्सा प्रणाली के जनक

**Hippocratic.** Relating to, described by, or attributed to Hippocrates. हिप्पोक्रैटी; हिप्पोक्रैट्स के सिद्धान्तों पर आधारित व सिद्धान्तों सम्बन्धी

**Hippus.** Spasmodic, rhythmical pupillary dilatation and constriction, independent of illumination, convergence or psychic stimuli. ताराकम्पन

**Hirci.** Plural of **Hircus.**

**Hircus.** One of the hair of the axilla. कक्षारोम; कांख के बाल; the odour of the axillae. कक्षागंध; कांखों की गंध; the tragus. तुंगिका

**Hirsute.** Hairy. रोमिल; रोमयुक्त; केशयुक्त; बालयुक्त

**Hirsuties.** See **Hirsutism.**

**Hirsutism.** Presence of excessive bodily and facial hair, especially in women; hirsuties. अतिरोमता; अत्यधिक बाल उगना

**Hirudo.** The leech. जलौंक; जोंक;
H. Medicinalis, those commonly used in medicine. उपचारक जलौंक;
H. Quen Que Striata, the same as **Hirudo.**

**Histamine.** A naturally occurring chemical substance in the body tissue which is a powerful stimulant of gastric secretion, constrictor of bronchial smooth muscle and vasodilator (capillaries and arterioles). हिस्टामिन; शरीर के ऊतकों में स्वत: प्रकट होने वाला रासायनिक पदार्थ;
H.-fast, indicating the absence of the normal response to histamine, especially in speaking of true gastric anacidity. हिस्टामिन-स्थाई; हिस्टामिनसह

**Histaminemia.** Presence of histamine in the circulating blood. हिस्टामिनरक्तता

**Histaminuria.** Excretion of histamine in the urine. हिस्टामिनमेह

**Histio-.** Prefix meaning. 'ऊतक' का अर्थ देने वाला उपसर्ग

**Histioblast.** A tissue-forming cell; histoblast. ऊतकप्रसू

**Histiocyte.** A macrophage present in connective tissue; histocyte. ऊतककोशिका

**Histiocytoma.** A tumour composed of histiocytes. ऊतककोशिकार्बुद

**Histiocytosis.** A generalised multiplication of histiocytes; histocytosis. ऊतककोशिकता

**Histiogenic.** See **Histogenous.**

**Histioma.** See **Histoma.**

**Histo-.** Prefix meaning tissue. 'ऊतक' का अर्थ देने वाला उपसर्ग

**Histoblast.** See **Histioblast.**

**Histochemistry.** Chemistry of organic tissue; cytochemistry. ऊतकरसायनविज्ञान; ऊतकरसायनशास्त्र

**Histocompatibility.** A state of immunologic similarity or identity of tissue sufficient to permit successful transplantation. ऊतकसंयोज्यता

**Histocyte.** See **Histiocyte.**

**Histocytosis.** See **Histiocytosis.**

**Histodifferentiation.** The morphologic appearance of tissue characteristics during development. ऊतकविभेदन

**Histogenesis.** Development of organic tissue. ऊतकविकास; ऊतकजनन; ऊतिजनन; ऊतकों का निर्माण और विकास

**Histogenetic.** Relating to the histogenesis. ऊतकजनन अथवा ऊतकविकास सम्बन्धी

**Histogenous.** Formed by tissues; histiogenic. ऊतकजनित; ऊतकनिर्मित

**Histological.** Producing tissue. ऊतकजनक; ऊतिजनक; relating to histology. ऊतकविज्ञान सम्बन्धी

**Histologist.** One who specializes in histology; microanatomist. ऊतकविज्ञानी; ऊतिविज्ञानी; ऊतिविज्ञानवेता

**Histology.** Microscopic study of the minute structures of cells, tissues and organs in relation to their functions; microanatomy. ऊतकविज्ञान; ऊतकों की बनावट का वैज्ञानिक अथवा सूक्ष्म अध्ययन

**Histolysis.** Disintegration of tissue. ऊतकलयन; ऊतिलयन

**Histoma.** A tissue tumour; histioma. ऊतकार्बुद

**Histometaplastic.** Stimulating the metaplasia of tissue. ऊतकइतरविकासी

**Histone.** One of a number of simple proteins that contains a high proportion of basic amino-acids. हिस्टोन

**Histonuria.** Excretion of histone in the urine. हिस्टोनमेह

**Histopathogenesis.** Abnormal embryonic development or growth of tissue. ऊतकविकृतिजनक

**Histopathology.** The science concerned with the cytologic and histologic structures of abnormal or diseased tissue. ऊतकविकृतिविज्ञान

**Histophysiology.** Microscopic study of tissues in relation to their functions. ऊतकभौतिकी; ऊतकों का सूक्ष्मदर्शी अध्ययन

**Histotome.** An instrument for making sections of tissues for examination under the microscope; microtome. ऊति-उच्छेदक; ऊत्युच्छेदक

**Histotomy.** The making of thin sections of tissues for examination under the microscope; microtomy. ऊति-उच्छेदन; ऊत्युच्छेदन

**Histotoxic.** Relating to poisoning of the respiratory enzyme system of the tissues. ऊतकविषी

**Histotrophic.** Nourishing or favouring the formation of tissue. ऊतकपोषक

**Histotropic.** Attracted toward tissues; denoting certain parasites, stains and chemical compounds. ऊतकप्रेरक

**Hives.** Nettle-rash; urticaria; an allergic reaction of the body with itching. शीतपित्त; जुलपित्ती; छपाकी; पित्ती

**Hoarse.** Having a rough, harsh quality of voice. कर्कश; खराशयुक्त

**Hoarseness.** Roughness of voice. कर्कशता; खराश; स्वररूक्षता; कण्ठ की कर्कशता; गले की खराश

**Hobnail Liver.** Nutmeg liver; firm nodular liver. गुरखुल यकृत्; ठोस व गठीला जिगर

**Hobnailed.** Set with hobnails. गुरखुलदार

**Hodgkin's Disease.** Pseudoleukemia; progressive hyperplasia of the lymphatic glands associated with anemia; lymphadenoma. हॉज्किन रोग; कूटश्वेतरक्तता; कैंसर

**Hodgkin's Granuloma.** Lyphadenoma; a variety of cancer. हाज्किनकणिकागुल्म; कैंसर का एक रूप

**Holagog.** See **Holagogue**.

**Holagogue.** A radical remedy; holagog. सम्यगौषधि

**Holism.** In psychology, the approach to the study of a psychological phenomenon through the analysis of the phenomena as a complete entity in itself. पूर्णता; परिपूर्णता

**Holistic.** Pertaining to the characteristic of holism or holistic psychologies. परिपूर्ण

**Hollow.** Containing an empty space. खोखला; खाली; रिक्त

**Holo-.** Prefix denoting entirely or relationship to a whole. 'पूर्ण' का अर्थ देने वाला उपसर्ग

**Holoacardius.** Complete absence of heart. पूर्ण-अहृदयता; हृत्पिण्ड का पूर्ण अभाव

**Holoblastic.** Denoting the involvement of the entire ovum in cleavage. पूर्णभंजी

**Holocrine.** A cell or gland, all of which forms and yields a secretion and then disappears. पूर्णस्रावी

**Holodiastolic.** Relating to, or occupying the entire diastole. पूर्णहृत्प्रसारी

**Holoendemic.** Endemic in the entire population. पूर्णस्थानिक

**Holoenzyme.** The complete enzyme. पूर्णप्रकिण्व

**Holophytic.** Having a plantlike mode of obtaining nourishment. पूर्णपादप; पूर्णपादपीय

**Holoprosencephaly.** Failure of the forebrain to devide into hemispheres or lobes. पूर्णअग्रमस्तिष्कता; पूर्णग्रशीर्षता

**Holorachischisis.** Spinal bifida of the entire spinal column. पूर्णमेरुनलिकाविदर

**Holosystolic.** Lasting throughout systole, extending from first to second heart sound; pansystolic. पूर्णप्रकुंचनीय

**Holozoic.** Animal-like in mode of obtaining nourishment. जन्त्वाभभोजी

**Homaxial.** Having all the axes alike, as a sphere. समाक्षिक

**Homeo-,Homoeo-,Homo-.** Prefixes meaning similar, alike, or the same. 'सम' अथवा 'सदृश' का अर्थ देने वाले उपसर्ग

**Homeomorphous.** Of similar shape, but not necessarily of the same composition. समाकृतिक

**Homeopath.** A physician practising homoeopathy; homeopathist; homoeopath; homoeopathist. होम्योपैथ; होम्योचिकित्सक

**Homeopathic.** Homoeopathic; relating to homoeopathy; homeotherapeutic. होम्योपैथी अथवा होम्योपैथिक चिकित्सा सम्बन्धी

**Homeopathist.** See **Homeopath.**

**Homeopathy.** A method of treating diseases by the **Law of Similars,** enunciated by Dr. Samuel Hahnemann; homoeopathy. होम्योपैथिक चिकित्सा; होम्योपैथी; सदृश विधान पर आधारित वह चिकित्सा प्रणाली जिसका आविष्कार डा० सैमुइल हैनीमैन ने किया था

**Homeoplasia.** Formation of new tissue of the same character as are already existing in the part. समविकसन; समविकास

**Homeoplastic.** Relating to, or characterized by homeoplasia. समविकासी

**Homeostasis.** The state of equilibrium in the body. समस्थिति

**Homeotherapeutic.** Homoeopathic; relating to homoeopathy or homoeotherapy. होम्योपैथिक चिकित्सा सम्बन्धी

**Homeotherapy.** See **Homoeotherapy.**

**Home-sickness.** Longing for home; nostalgia; a variety of melancholy; an overpowering desire to return to one's country, attended by wasting and hectic fever. गृहातुरता; घर जाने की आतुरता अथवा उत्सुकता

**Homicide.** Killing of a man or woman; murder. मानववध; हत्या; परहत्या; किसी मनुष्य की हत्या करना

**Homo-.** See **Homeo-.**

**Homoeo-.** See **Homeo-.**

**Homoeopath.** See **Homeopath.**

**Homoeopathic.** See **Homeopathic.**

**Homoeopathy.** See **Homeopathy.**

**Homoeotherapy.** Treatment or prevention of a disease by means of a product similar to, but not identical with the active causal agent; homeotherapy. होम्योपैथिक चिकित्सा

**Homogametic.** Producing only one type of gamete with respect to sex chromosomes. समयुग्मकी

**Homogamy.** Similarity of husband and wife in a specific trait. सगोत्रपरिणय

**Homogeneity.** Sameness of kind or nature. समजातता; समांगता

**Homogeneous.** Of uniform structure or composition throughout; of a similar nature with like offspring; homogenous. सजातीय; समांग

**Homogenesis.** The generation of a progeny showing the same cycle of developmental changes as the parent; homogeny. समजनन

**Homogenous.** See **Homogeneous.**

**Homogeny.** See **Homogenesis.**

**Homograft.** A tissue or organ which is transplanted from one individual to another of the same species. समनिरोप

**Homoiothermal.** Maintaining a uniform temperature; homoiothermic. नियततापी; समतापी; मिततापी; स्थिरतापी

**Homoiothermic.** See **Homoiothermal.**

**Homolateral.** Pertaining to objects situated on the same side; ipsilateral. समपार्श्वी

**Homologous.** Corresponding in origin and structure; having the same form or function; homologus. समजात; समधर्मी; समरूप

**Homologus.** See **Homologous.**

**Homology.** The doctorine of similarity of structures. सदृशता; सजातीयता; समरूपता

**Homolysin.** A sensitizing, hemolytic antibody formed as the result of stimulation by an antigen derived from an animal of the same species. समनाशी; समनाशक; समापघट्य; होमोलाइसिन

**Homolysis.** Lysis of red blood cells by a homolysin and complement. समलयन; समापघटन

**Homomorphic.** Denoting two or more structures of similar size and shape. समाकृतिक

**Homononomous.** Governed by the same law. समनियमी; denoting parts, having similar form and structure, arranged in a series, as the digits. समाकार

**Homonymous.** Having the same name or position. समदिक्; समस्थितिक

**Homophil.** Denoting an antibody that reacts only with the specific antigen that induced its formation. समरागी

**Homoplastic.** Similar in form and structure, but not in origin. समसंधानक

**Homoplasty.** Repair of a defect by a homograft. समसंधान

**Homorganic.** Produced by the same organs, or by homologous organs. समांगजनित

**Homosexual.** Of same sex; denoting or characteristic of homosexuality. समलैंगिक; समलिंगी; one who practices homosexuality. समलिंगकामी

**Homosexuality.** Erotic attraction, predisposition or sexual behaviour of persons of the same sex. समलिंगिकामुकता

**Homothermal.** Warm-blooded. गरममिजाज; जोशीला; क्रोधी; उष्णरक्तक

**Homotonic.** Of uniform tension or tonus. समतानिक

**Homotopic.** Pertaining to, or occurring at the same place or part of the body. समस्थानिक अथवा समांगिक

**Homotransplant.** Tissues or organs transplanted from non-identical members of the same species. समप्रतिरोप; समनिरोप

**Homotype.** A corresponding part or organ of the same structure on the opposite side of the body. समप्रतिरूपी; समरूपी

**Homotypic.** See **Homotypical.**

**Homotypical.** Of the same type or form; homotypic. समप्रतिरूपीय; समरूपीय

**Homozygosity.** The state of having identical genes at one or more paired foci in homologous chromosomes. समयुग्मजता

**Homozygote.** A homogygous individual. समयुग्मज

**Homozygous.** Having identical genes in the same locus on one of the chromosome pairs. समयुग्मजी

**Honorarium.** A physician's fee. मानदेय; चिकित्सक की फीस

**Hookworm.** Common name for blood sucking nematodes of the members of **Ankylastoma, Necator** and **Uncinaria.** अंकुशकृमि

**Hooping Cough.** Whooping cough; pertussis. कूकर-कास; काली खांसी

**Hora.** Hour. घण्टा;

  **H. Decubitus,** on lying down. Abbreviation : **H.D.** लेटते समय;

  **H. Somni,** at the bedtime. Abbreviation : **H.S.** सोते समय;

  **H. Somni Sumendum,** to be taken at the bedtime. Abbreviation: **H.S.S.** सोते समय सेवनीय

**Hordeolum.** A stye on the eyelid. गुहेरी; गुहाञ्जनी; अञ्जनी; बिलौनी

**Hordeum.** Barley. यव; जौ

**Horis.** Hour. घण्टा

**Hormion.** The anteromedian point of the spheno-occipital bone.

जतूक-सीरिकाबिन्दु

**Hormonal.** Pertaining to hormones. हॉर्मोन सम्बन्धी

**Hormone.** The secretion from a ductless gland, which passes in the blood stream to excite activity in other tissues. हॉर्मोन; किसी नलिकाहीन ग्रन्थि से होने वाला स्राव, जो रक्त में मिलकर अन्य ऊतकों की क्रिया को उत्तेजित करता है

**Hormonogenesis.** The formation of hormones; hormonopoiesis. हॉर्मोनजनन

**Hormonogenic.** Pertaining to the formation of hormones; hormonopoietic. हॉर्मोनजनक; हार्मोनजनन सम्बन्धी

**Hormonology.** The science of hormones. हॉर्मोनविज्ञान

**Hormonopoiesis.** See **Hormonogenesis.**

**Hormonopoietic.** See **Hormonogenic.**

**Hormonotherapy.** Therapeutic use of hormones. हॉर्मोनोपचार; हॉर्मोन-चिकित्सा

**Horn.** A cutaneous outgrowth composed chiefly of keratin or a hornlike projection. शृंगी उभार; शृंगी गुल्म; cornu. शृंग; सींग

**Horny.** Of the nature or structure of horn; corneous; keratic; keratinous; keratoid. शृंगी; शृंगवत्

**Horopter.** The sum of all the points seen singly by the two retinas while the fixation point remains stationary. दृष्टिपरिधि

**Horripilation.** A sense of creeping in the hair; a bristling of the hair. रोमांच; लोमहर्षण

**Horrors.** Delirium tremens. कम्पोन्माद

**Hospice.** An institution that provides a centralized programme of palliative and supportive services to dying persons and their families. आश्रम; शरणस्थल

**Hospital.** An institution for the treatment, care and cure of the sick and wounded persons. चिकित्सालय; अस्पताल

**Hospitalisation.** Indoor treatment of the sick in a hospital; hospitalization. चिकित्सालय-आश्रयण; चिकित्सालयीयन; अन्तरंग रोगी-चिकित्सा

**Hospitalization.** See **Hospitalisation.**

**Host.** The organic structure upon which perasites thrive. पोषद; परपोषी; सत्कारी

**Hot Flash.** A vasomotor symptom of the climacterium; hot flush. तमतमाहट; गर्म चौंध

**Hot Flush.** See **Hot Flash.**

**Hour Glass Contraction.** An irregular contraction of the uterus.

डमरूवत् जरायु-संकोच; जरायु की अनियमित सिकुड़न

**Housemaid's knee.** Bursitis; an inflammation of the patellar bursa. श्लेषपुटीशोथ; स्नेहपुटीशोथ; जानुसन्धिशोथ; जान्वस्थि तथा स्नेहपुटी का प्रदाह

**H.S.** Abbreviated form of **Hora Somni.**

**H.S.G.** Hysterosalpingography. गर्भाशय-डिम्बवाहिनीचित्रण

**H.S.S.** Abbreviated form of **Hora Somni Sumendum.**

**Hub.** Umbilicus. नाभि

**Hue.** Colour. वर्ण; वर्णाभा; रंग

**Hum.** A low continuous murmur. क्ष्वेड; लगातार धीमी-धीमी मर्मर-ध्वनि होते रहना

**Humectant.** A preparation intended to preserve moisture in the body. आर्द्रकारी; आर्द्रतास्थायी; नमीदार

**Humeral.** Pertaining to the humerus. प्रगण्डकीय; प्रगण्डीय; प्रगण्डिका सम्बन्धी

**Humeri.** Plural of **Humerus.**

**Humeroradial.** Pertaining to the humerus and the radius. प्रगण्डबहि:-प्रकोष्ठक

**Humeroscapular.** Relating to both humerus and scapula. प्रगण्डस्कन्धफलकीय

**Humeroulnar.** Relating to both humerus and ulna. प्रगण्ड-अन्त:प्रकोष्ठक

**Humerus.** The large bone of the upper arm, articulating with the scapula above and the radius and ulna below. प्रगण्डिका; कन्धे से कोहनी तक की हड्डी

**Humid.** Moist. आर्द्र; नम

**Humidification.** To render moist; humification. आर्द्रीकरण; नम करना

**Humidity.** The amount of moisture or dampness in the atmosphere. आर्द्रता; नमी

**Humification.** see **Humidification.**

**Humor.** Any fluid of the body; humoris; humour. देहद्रव; शारीरिक रसादि;

    **Aqueous H.,** the fluid filling the anterior and posterior chambers in front of the optical lens; humoris aquosus. नेत्रोद;

    **Vitreous H.,** the gelatinous mass filling the interior of the eyeball from the lens to the retina; humoris vitreus. नेत्रकाचाभद्रव

**Humoral.** Pertaining to the natural fluids of the body or the humour; humoural. देहद्रवी; शारीरिक रसादि

**Humoris.** See **Humor.**

    **H. Aquosus,** see **Aqueous Humor.**

    **H. Vitreus,** see **Vitreous Humor.**

**Humour.** See **Humor.**

**Humoural.** See **Humoral.**
**Humpback.** Hunchback; kyphosis. कुब्ज; कुबड़ा
**Humpfoot.** The same as **Talipes Cavus.**
**Hunchback.** See **Humpback.**
**Hungarian Disease.** Typhus fever. सन्निपात ज्वर; मोह ज्वर
**Hunger.** A longing, strong desire, or craving, usually for food. क्षुधा; भूख; बुभुक्षा;
**Air H.,** inspiratory distress characterized by sighing and gasping. वायु-क्षुधा; वायु-बुभुक्षा;
**H. Cure,** treatment by restricted diet. अस्याशन चिकित्सा; प्रमिताशन चिकित्सा;
**H. Pain,** epigastric pain which is relieved by taking food. क्षुधा-पीड़ा; बुभुक्षा-वेदना
**Hunterian Chancre.** A hard chancre; the initial lesion of syphilis. कठिनक्षत; उपदंशक्षत
**Hutchinson's teeth.** Defect of the upper incisors. विषमदन्तता; ऊपर वाले भेदक दांतों की दोषपूर्ण अवस्था
**Hyal-.** See **Hyalo-.**
**Hyalin.** A clear, eosinophilic, homogeneous substance occurring in degeneration. स्फटिककला
**Hyaline.** Like glass; glassy; crystalline; hyaloid. काचाभ; शीशे जैसा; स्फटिकाभ
**Hyalinization.** Formation of hyaline. काचाभीकरणा; काचाभीभवन
**Hyalinosis.** Hyaline degeneration, especially that of relatively extensive degree. स्फटिककलामयता
**Hyalinuria.** Excretion of hyaline or casts of hyaline material in the urine. स्फटिककलामेह
**Hyalitis.** Inflammation of the hyaloid membrane or the vitreous humour; hyaloiditis. स्फटिककलाशोथ; स्फटिक झिल्ली का प्रदाह
**Hyalo-, Hyal-.** Prefixes meaning glassy. 'काचाभ' अथवा 'स्फटिकाभ' का अर्थ देने वाले उपसर्ग
**Hyaloid.** Transparent; resembling a glass; hyaline. काचाभ; स्फटिकाभ; शीशे जैसा; काचोपम; पारदर्शी
**Hyaloiditis.** See **Hyalitis.**
**Hyalophagia.** Eating or chewing of glass. काचभक्षण
**Hyaloplasm.** A clear, transparent protoplasm. काचीद्रव्य; काचद्रव; एक स्वच्छ, पारदर्शी जीवद्रव्य
**Hyaloserositis.** Inflammation of a serous membrane with fibrinous exudate undergoing hyaline transformation. काचाभसीरमीकलाशोथ

**Hybrid.** The product of two distinct species. संकर; वर्णसंकर; दोगला

**Hybridoma.** A tumour of hybrid cells. संकरकोशिकार्बुद

**Hydatid.** The cyst formed by larvae of tapeworm. हाइडेटिड; फ़ीताकृमियों के अण्डों से निर्मित पुटी; a vesicular structure. जलस्फोट

**Hydatidiform.** Pertaining to, or resembling a hydatid. जलस्फोटरूप; हाइडेटिड अथवा जलस्फोट सम्बन्धी या हाइडेटिड अथवा जलस्फोट से मिलता-जुलता

**Hydatidocele.** A cystic mass composed of one or more hydatids formed in the scrotum. जलस्फोटस्त्रंस; जलस्फोट-हर्निया

**Hydatidoma.** A benign neoplasm in which there is prominent formation of hydatid. जलस्फोटार्बुद

**Hydatidosis.** The diseased state caused by the presence of hydatid cysts. जलस्फोटीरुग्णता

**Hydatidostomy.** Surgical evacuation of a hydatid cyst. जलस्फोटीपुटकरिक्तीकरण

**Hydr-.** See **Hydro-**.

**Hydraemia.** A relative excess of plasma volume as compared with cell volume of the blood; hydremia. जलरक्तता

**Hydragog.** See **Hydragogue**.

**Hydragogue.** Purgative; causing watery discharges; hydragog. रेचक; विरेचक; जलनिस्सारक

**Hydramnion.** See **Hydramnios**.

**Hydramnios.** Presence of an excessive amount of amniotic fluid; hydramnion. अति-उल्वोदकता; अत्युल्वोदकता; उल्वोदक की प्रचुर मात्रा विद्यमान रहना

**Hydranencephaly.** Congenital absence of the cerebral hemisphere. सहज-अमस्तिष्कता

**Hydrargism.** The same as **Hydrargyrism**.

**Hydrargyria.** See **Hydrargyrism**.

**Hydrargyrism.** Mercurial disease; mercury poisoning; hydrargyria. पारदविकृति; पारदविषण्णता; पारदरोग

**Hydrargyrum.** Mercury or quick-silver. पारद; पारा

**Hydrarthrodial.** Relating to hydrarthrosis. जलसन्धिपरक; जोड़ों में पानी भर जाने सम्बन्धी

**Hydrarthrosis.** Effusion of a serous fluid into a joint cavity. जलसन्धि; जोड़ों में पानी भर जाना

**Hydrarthrus.** White swelling. श्वेत सूजन; dropsy of the knee-joint. जानुसन्धिशोफ; घुटने के जोड़ की पनीली सूजन

**Hydrate.** See **Hydrated**.

**Hydrated.** Combined chemically with water; hydrate. उदकित; जलयोजित

**Hydration.** Impregnation with water. जलयोजन

**Hydremia.** See **Hydraemia.**

**Hydrencephalocele.** Protrusion through a defect in the skull of brain substance expanded into a sac containing fluid; hydrocephalocele; hydroencephalocele. जलमस्तिष्कपुटी; जलशीर्षस्रंस

**Hydrencephalomeningocele.** A protrusion through a defect in the skull of a sac containing meninges, brain substance and spinal fluid. जलशीर्षमस्तिष्कावरणपुटी

**Hydrencephalus.** See **Hydrocephalus.**

**Hydric.** Relating to hydrogen in chemical combination. जलयोजन सम्बन्धी

**Hydro-, Hydr-.** Prefixes meaning water or association with water. 'जल' का अर्थ देने वाले उपसर्ग

**Hydroa.** Certain vesicular eruptions with erythematous lesions. जलस्फोटी-त्वग्रोग;

   **H. Aestivale,** a vesicular or bullous disease occurring in children. आतप जलस्फोटी-त्वग्रोग; आतपस्फोट;

   **H. Vacciniforme,** a more severe hereditary form in which scarring ensues. गोशीतला; जलस्फोटी त्वग्रोग

**Hydroadenitis.** Inflammation of the sweat glands. स्वेदग्रन्थिशोथ; स्वेद ग्रन्थियों का प्रदाह

**Hydroblepharon.** Oedematous swelling of the eyelids. वर्त्मशोफ; पलकों की पानी वाली सूजन

**Hydrocalycosis.** A rare symptomless anomaly of the renal calix, which is dilated from obstruction of the infundibulum. जलालवाल

**Hydrocarbon.** A compound containing only hydrogen and carbon. जलकार्बन; हाइड्रोकार्बन

**Hydrocele.** Dropsy of the scrotum or testicles. जलवृषण; जलसंग्रह; वृषणकोष अथवा वृषणों में पानी भर जाना;

   **Gibbon's H.,** hydrocele with hernia. गिब्बनी जलवृषण; जलवृषण के साथ हर्निया

**Hydrocelectomy.** Excision of a hydrocele. जलवृषण-उच्छेदन

**Hydrocephalic.** Relating to hydrocephalus. जलशीर्ष सम्बन्धी

**Hydrocephalocele.** See **Hydrencephalocele.**

**Hydrocephaloid.** Resembling hydrocephalus. जलशीर्षाभ; जलशीर्ष जैसा

**Hydrocephalus.** Collection of fluid in the head; hydrencephalus; hydrocephaly. जलशीर्ष; सिर में पानी जमा हो जाना

**Hydrocephaly.** See **Hydrocephalus.**

**Hydrochloric Acid.** The acid of gastric juice. हाइड्रोक्लोरिक अम्ल

**Hydrochloride.** A compound by the addition of a hydrochloric acid molecule to related substance. हाइड्रोक्लोराइड

**Hydrocholecystis.** Effusion of serous fluid into the gall-bladder. जलपित्ताशयता

**Hydrocholeresis.** Increased output of a watery bile of low specific gravity, viscosity and solid contents. जलपित्तता

**Hydrocholeretic.** Pertaining to hydrocholeresis. जलपित्तता सम्बन्धी

**Hydrocirsocele.** Hydrocele complicated with varicocele. जलवृषण–शिरापस्फीति

**Hydrocolpocele.** Accumulation of mucus or other non-sanguineous fluid in the vagina; hydrocolpos. जलयोनिपुटी

**Hydrocolpos.** See **Hydrocolpocele.**

**Hydrocyanic Acid.** A colourless liquid poison with the odour of bitter almonds; prussic acid; hydrogen cyanide. Symbol: **HCN.** हाइड्रोस्यानिक अम्ल

**Hydrocyst.** A cyst with clear, watery contents. जलपुटी; जलस्फोट

**Hydroderma.** Dropsy of the skin. त्वक्शोफ; त्वचा की पानी वाली सूजन

**Hydroencephalocele.** See **Hydrencephalocele.**

**Hydrogen.** A colourless, combustible gaseous element. Symbol: **H.** उद्जन; हाइड्रोजन;

**H. Chloride,** a very soluble gas which, in solution, forms hydrochloric acid. हाइड्रोजन क्लोराइड;

**H. Cyanide,** see **Hydrocyanic Acid.**

**Hydrogenation.** Addition of hydrogen to a compound, especially of an unsaturated fat or fatty acid. उद्जनीकरण; उद्जनीभवन

**Hydrogenoid.** Of the nature of hydrogen. उद्जनाभ; उद्जनात्मक

**Hydrokinetic.** Pertaining to the motion of fluids and the force giving rise to such motion. जलगतिक

**Hydrology.** The science of hydrogen. उद्जनविज्ञान; जलविज्ञान

**Hydrolysate.** A solution containing the products of a hydrolysis. जलापघटितघोल

**Hydrolysis.** The splitting into more simple substance by the addition of water. जलापघटन; जललयन

**Hydrolytic.** Relating to, or causing hydrolysis. जलापघटनीय; जललायी

**Hydroma.** A cyst filled with serous fluid; hygroma. जलार्बुद; पानी से भरी रसौली

**Hydromel.** Honey and water. मधुजल; शहद और पानी

**Hydromeningitis.** Meningitis with watery effusion. सजलमस्तिष्कावरणशोथ; पश्चकपालशोथ

**Hydromeningocele.** Protrusion of the meninges of brain or spinal cord through defect in the bony wall. जलमस्तिष्कावरणस्रंस

**Hydrometer.** An instrument for measuring the amount of moisture in the air; gravimeter. उत्प्लव-घनत्वमापी; हवा में नमी की मात्रा को मापने का यंत्र

**Hydrometra.** A collection of fluid in the womb. जरायुशोफ; जलगर्भाशयता; गर्भाशय के अन्दर तरल द्रव जमा होना

**Hydrometric.** Relating to, or concerned with the measurement of the degree of moisture. उत्प्लव-घनत्वमितिक; द्रवमितिक; आर्द्रतामापन सम्बन्धी

**Hydrometrocolpos.** Distention of uterus and vagina by fluid other than blood or pus. जलपूरितयोनि

**Hydrometry.** Determination of the specific gravity of a fluid by means of a hydrometer. उत्प्लव-घनत्वमिति

**Hydromicrocephaly.** Microcephaly associated with an increased amount of cerebrospinal fluid. जललघुशिरस्कता

**Hydromphalus.** A cystic tumour at the umbilicus. नाभिपुटी

**Hydromyelia.** A condition in children in which cystic cavities form in the spinal cord. जलमेरुरज्जु

**Hydromyelocele.** The protrusion of a sac with cerebrospinal fluid through a spinal bifida. जलसुषुम्नापुटी

**Hydromyoma.** Cystic fibroid, usually uterine, filled with fluid. जलपेश्यर्बुद

**Hydroncus.** A watery tumour. जलार्बुद; पानी की रसौली

**Hydronephrosis.** Dilatation of the pelvis and calices of one or both kidneys resulting from obstruction to the flow of urine; uronephrosis; renal dropsy. जलवृक्कता; वृक्कशोफ; गुर्दे में पानी भरना

**Hydronephrotic.** Relating to hydronephrosis. वृक्कशोफ सम्बन्धी

**Hydropathy.** Treatment of diseases by the use of water. जलचिकित्सा; जलोपचार; पानी द्वारा रोगों का इलाज करना

**Hydropericarditis.** Pericarditis with a large serous effusion. जलपरिहृद्शोथ; जल-हृदयावरणशोथ; सद्रव-हृदयावरणशोथ

**Hydropericardium.** A serous non-inflammatory effusion within the pericardium resembling ascites or hydrothorax. जलहृदयावरण; जलपरिहृद्

**Hydroperitoneum.** Ascites. जलपर्युदर्या; पर्युदर्याशोफ; उदरावरणशोफ

**Hydrophilia.** A tendency of the blood and tissues to absorb fluid. जलरागिता; हाइड्रोफीलिया

**Hydrophilic.** Denoting the property of attracting or associated with water molecules, possessed by polar radicals or ions, as opposed to hydrophobic. जलरागी

**Hydrophilous.** Absorbing of water; taking up moisture. जलशोषक

**Hydrophobia.** Dog madness; rabies in man. जलभीति; जलसंत्रास; जलातंक; अलर्क रोग; पानी से डर लगने की बीमारी

**Hydrophobic.** Relating to, or suffering from hydrophobia. जलातंक सम्बन्धी अथवा जलातंकग्रस्त

**Hydrophthalmia.** Dropsy of the eyeballs; hydrophthalmus. नेत्रगोलकशोफ; नेत्रगोलकों में पानी जमा होने की बीमारी

**Hydrophthalmus.** See **Hydrophthalmia.**

**Hydrophysometra.** A collection of water and gas in the womb. वायुजलगर्भाशयता; जलवातगर्भाशयविस्फार; जलजरायुविस्फार; गर्भाशय का पानी और हवा से फूल जाना

**Hydropic.** Having the property of absorbing moisture from air. जलसंचयी

**Hydropneumatosis.** Combined emphysema and oedema. जलवातवक्ष

**Hydropneumopericardium.** Presence of a serous effusion and of gas in the pericardial sac; pneumohydropericardium. जलफुप्फुसपरिहृद्; जलफुप्फुसहृदयावरण

**Hydropneumoperitoneum.** Presence of gas and serous fluid in the peritoneal cavity; pneumohydroperitoneum. जलफुप्फुसपर्युदर्या; जलफुप्फुस-उदरावरण

**Hydropneumothorax.** A collection of both gas and liquids in the pleural cavity; pneumohydrothorax. जलवातवक्ष; फुप्फुसावरक नली में गैस और द्रव जमा होना

**Hydrops.** Dropsy; accumulation of clear, watery fluid in any of the tissues or cavities of the body as in ascites, anasarca, oedema, etc. जलशोफ; पानी वाली सूजन

**Hydropyonephrosis.** Presence of purulent urine in the pelvis and calices of the kidney following obstruction of the ureter. जलवृक्कता

**Hydrorrhea.** A copious watery discharge; hydrorrhoea. अतिजलस्राव; जलस्राव; प्रचुर परिमाण में पानी बहना;
  **H. Gravidarum,** discharge of a watery fluid from the vagina during pregnancy; hindwater. सगर्भ जलस्राव

**Hydrorrhoea.** See **Hydrorrhea.**

**Hydrosalpinx.** Accumulation of serous fluid in the Fallopian tube. जलडिम्बवाहिनी; डिम्बवाही नली में पानी भरना

**Hydrosarcocele.** A chronic swelling of the testis complicated with hydrocele. जलवृषणमांसार्बुद

**Hydrosis.** The formation and excretion of sweat. जलस्वेदन; पसीना बनना और आना

**Hydrosol.** A water-soluble colloid. जलविलेय; पानी में घुल जाने वाला

**Hydrostatic.** Relating to the science of liquids in a state of rest. द्रवस्थैतिक

**Hydrosyringomyelia.** Syringomyelia; distention of the central canal of the spinal cord with effusion of fluid and formation of cavities. जलमेरुरज्जुता

**Hydrotaxis.** Movement of cells or organisms in relation to water. जलगतिकता

**Hydrotherapy.** The use of water as a therapeutic agent. जलचिकित्सा; जलोपचार; पानी द्वारा रोगों का इलाज करना

**Hydrothorax.** Dropsy of the pleura; a non-inflammatory serous effusion into the pleural cavity. जलवक्ष; फुप्फुसगह्वर का शोफ

**Hydrotis.** Dropsy of the ear. कर्णशोफ; जलकर्ण; कानों की शोफज अवस्था

**Hydrotropism.** The property in growing organisms of turning toward or away from moisture. जलानुवर्तिता

**Hydrotubation.** Injection of liquid medication or saline solution through the cervix into the uterine cavity and Fallopian tubes for dilatation and medication of the tubes. जलनलीकरण

**Hydroureter.** Abnormal distension of the ureter with urine; uroureter. जलगवीनी; मूत्रनली का असाधारण रूप से फूल जाना

**Hydrovarium.** A collection of fluid in the ovary. जलडिम्बाशयता

**Hydruria.** An excessive flow of watery urine; polyuria. उदकमेह; अतिजलमूत्रता; पानी जैसा प्रचुर पेशाब होना; बहुमूत्रता

**Hydruric.** Relating to hydruria or polyuria. अतिजलमूत्रता अथवा बहुमूत्रता सम्बन्धी

**Hygiene.** The means of preventing health; the science of health. स्वास्थ्यविज्ञान; स्वास्थ्यवृत्त; स्वास्थ्य;

    **Mental H.,** the science and practice of maintaining and restoring mental health. मानसिक स्वास्थ्यवृत्त; मनोस्वास्थ्य;

    **Oral H.,** cleaning of oral structures by means of brushing, irrigating, massaging or the use of other devices. मुखी स्वास्थ्यवृत्त

**Hygienic.** Pertaining to hygiene; healthful. स्वास्थ्यकर; स्वास्थ्य सम्बन्धी

**Hygienist.** One skilled in the science of health. स्वास्थ्यविज्ञानवेत्ता

**Hygr-, Hygro-.** Prefixes meaning moist, moisture or humidity. 'आर्द्र' अथवा '**नम**' का अर्थ देने वाले उपसर्ग

**Hygroma.** A cystic swelling containing a serous fluid; hydroma. लसपुटी; पानी की रसौली; **सीरमीपुटी**

**Hygrometer.** An instrument used to determine the degree of moisture of the atmosphere. आर्द्रतामापी (यंत्र); जलवायु की आर्द्रता को मापने का यंत्र

**Hygrometry.** The discipline pertaining to psychological and mental testing; psychometrics; psychometry. आर्द्रतामिति; आर्द्रतामापन

**Hygroscopic.** Capable of readily absorbing and retaining moisture from the air. आर्द्रताग्राही; indicative of moisture. आर्द्रतासूचक

**Hygrostomia.** Chronic salivation. जीर्णलालास्राव; जीर्णलारस्राव

**Hymen.** A membranous perforated structure stretching across the vaginal entrance; vaginal membrane. योनिच्छद; सतीच्छद; योनिद्वार की झिल्ली

**Hymenal.** Relating to hymen. योनिच्छद सम्बन्धी

**Hymenectomy.** Surgical excision of the hymen. योनिच्छद-उच्छेदन

**Hymenitis.** Inflammation of the hymen. योनिच्छदशोथ; योनिच्छद का प्रदाह

**Hymenotomy.** Surgical incision of a hymen. योनिच्छदछेदन

**Hymenology.** The branch of anatomy and physiology with the membranes of the body. योनिच्छदविज्ञान; योनिच्छदप्रकरण

**Hyoepiglottic.** Pertaining to the epiglottis and hyoid bone; hypoepiglottidean. कण्ठिकाकण्ठच्छदीय; कण्ठिका तथा कण्ठच्छद सम्बन्धी

**Hyoepiglottidean.** See **Hyoepiglottic.**

**Hyoglossal.** Pertaining to the tongue and hyoid bone; glossohyal. जिह्वा तथा कण्ठिकास्थि सम्बन्धी

**Hyoid.** Shaped like U or V. कण्ठिका;
   H. Bone, the U-shaped bone at the root of the tongue. कण्ठिकास्थि; जिह्वामूलास्थि

**Hyomandibular.** Pertaining to both the hyoid bone and the mandible. कण्ठिका-अधोहनुज

**Hyoscyamus.** Hen-bane leaves and flowers. पारसीक यवानी; खुरासानी अजवायन

**Hyp-.** See **Hypo-.**

**Hypacusis.** Hearing impairment attributable to deficiency in the peripheral organs of hearing; hypoacusis. अल्पश्रवणता; मंदश्रवणता; श्रवणाल्पसंवेदिता

**Hypalbunemia.** See **Hypoalbuminaemia.**

**Hypalgesia.** Decreased sensibility to pain; hypoalgesia; hypalgia. अल्पसंवेदिता

**Hypalgesic.** Relating to hypalgia; hypalgetic. अल्पसंवेदिता सम्बन्धी

**Hypalgetic.** See **Hypalgesic.**

**Hypalgia.** See **Hypalgesia.**

**Hypamnios.** Presence of an abnormally small amount of amniotic fluid. अल्पउल्वोदकता

**Hypanakinesis.** Diminution in the normal gastric or intestinal movements. जठराल्पगतिकता

**Hypaxial.** Beneath the body-axis. निम्नाक्षीय

**Hypemia.** Anaemia. रक्ताल्पता; अल्परक्तता; रक्तस्वल्पता; खून की कमी

**Hyper-.** Prefix meaning excessive or above the normal. 'अति' का अर्थ देने वाला उपसर्ग

**Hyperacid.** Excessive acid. अत्यम्ल; अत्यधिक अम्ल

**Hyperacidity.** An excessive degree of acidity. अत्यम्लता; अत्यधिक अम्लता

**Hyperactivity.** Excessive activity or general restlessness. अतिसक्रियता; अत्यधिक सक्रियता; सर्वांगीण बेचैनी

**Hyperacusis.** Morbid acuteness of the sense of hearing; hyperakusis; hypercusis. श्रवण-अतिसम्वेदिता; सुनने की भारी सम्वेदनशीलता

**Hyperadenosis.** Enlargement of glands, especially of the lymphatic glands. अतिग्रन्थिलता; ग्रन्थियों का बढ़ जाना, वह भी खास तौर से लसीका ग्रन्थियों का

**Hyperadiposis.** Excessive fat in any part of the body. अतिमेदता; अतिवसामयता

**Hyperaemia.** Excessive blood in any part; hyperemia. अतिरक्तता; किसी भाग में रक्त की मात्रा बढ़ जाना;

   **Active H.,** that due to an excessive flow of blood; arterial hyperaemia; fluxionary hyperaemia. सक्रिय अतिरक्तता;

   **Arterial H.,** see **Active Hyperaemia.**

   **Fluxionary H.,** see **Active Hyperaemia.**

   **Passive H.,** that due to retardation of the outflow and consequent accumulation of blood; venous hyperaemia. निष्क्रिय अतिरक्तता; शैरिक अतिरक्तता;

   **Venous H.,** see **Passive Hyperaemia.**

**Hyperaemic.** Denoting hyperaemia; hyperemic. अतिरक्तक

**Hyperaesthesia.** Excessive sensibility; hyperesthesia. अतिसम्वेदिता; अत्यधिक संवेदनशीलता;

   **H. Acoustica,** morbid acuteness of the sense of hearing. श्रवण-अतिसम्वेदिता;

   **Tactile H.,** see **Hyperaphia.**

**Hyperakusis.** See **Hyperacusis.**

**Hyperalgesia.** Excessive sensitiveness to painful stimuli;

hyperalgia. अत्यार्ति; अत्यधिक पीड़ा; अतिशय वेदना
**Hyperalgesic.** Relating to hyperalgesia; hyperalgetic. अत्यार्ति सम्बन्धी
**Hyperalgetic.** See **Hyperalgesic.**
**Hyperalgia.** See **Hyperalgesia.**
**Hyperalimentation.** Administration or consumption of nutrients beyond normal requirements; superalimentation. अतिपोषणता
**Hyperamylasemia.** Elevated serum amylase, seen as one of the features of acute pancreatitis. अतिएमिलेजता
**Hyperanakinesis.** Excessive gastric or intestinal movements; hyperanakinezia. जठरातिगतिकता
**Hyperanakinezia.** See **Hyperanakinesis.**
**Hyperaphia.** Extreme sensitiveness to touch; tactile hyperaesthesia. स्पर्श-अतिसम्वेदिता; अतिस्पर्शसम्वेदिता
**Hyperaphic.** Marked by hyperaphia. स्पर्श-अतिसम्वेदी; अतिस्पर्शसम्वेदी
**Hyperasthenia.** Extreme weakness. अतिदौर्बल्य; अत्यधिक कमजोरी
**Hyperbaric.** At greater pressure, specific gravity or weight, than normal, with respect to solutions, more dense than the diluent or medium. अतिघनीय
**Hyperbarism.** Disturbance in the body resulting from the pressure of ambient gases. अतिघनीयता
**Hyperbilirubinemia.** An abnormally large amount of bilirubin in the circulating blood. अतिबिलिरूबिनता
**Hypercalcaemia.** Excessive calcium in the blood; hypercalcemia. अतिकैल्सियमरक्तता
**Hypercalcemia.** See **Hypercalcaemia.**
**Hypercalciuria.** Greatly increased calcium excretion in the urine. अतिकैल्सियममेह; पेशाब में अत्यधिक कैल्सियम जाना
**Hypercapnia.** Presence of an abnormally large amount of carbondioxide in the circulating blood; hypercarbia. अतिकैप्निया; रक्त में कार्बनडाइआक्साइड की बढ़ी हुई मात्रा
**Hypercarbia.** See **Hypercapnia.**
**Hypercatharsis.** Excessive purging. मलाधिक्य; अतिमलोत्सर्ग; अतिमलोत्सर्जन
**Hypercellularity.** Increased number of cells in any location, but especially in the bone-marrow. अतिकोशिकता
**Hypercementosis.** An overgrowth of cementum on the root of a tooth which may be caused by localized trauma or inflammation, metabolic dysfunction, or developmental defect. अतिदन्तवल्कता
**Hyperchloremia.** An abnormally large amount of chloride ions in the circulating blood; chloremia. अतिक्लोराइडता

**Hyperchlorhydria.** The presence of an excess amount of hydrochloric acid in the stomach; chlorhydria. अतिहाइड्रोक्लोरिकाम्लता; अतिजठराम्लता

**Hypercholia.** Condition in which an abnormally large amount of bile is formed in the liver. अतिपित्तता; पित्ताधिक्य

**Hyperchromasia.** See **Hyperchromatism**.

**Hyperchromatic.** Abnormally highly coloured, excessively stained, or overpigmented; hyperchromic. अतिरंजक; अतिरंज्य; अतिक्रोमी

**Hyperchromatism.** Hyperchromasia; hyperchromia; excessive pigmentation; increased staining capacity; increased chromatin in cell-nuclei. अतिरंजकता; अतिरंज्यता

**Hyperchromemia.** Abnormally high colour index of the blood. अतिरक्तरंजकता; अतिरक्तरंज्यता

**Hyperchromia.** See **Hyperchromatism**.

**Hyperchromic.** See **Hyperchromatic**.

**Hypercoagulability.** Increased ability to coagulate, especially the blood. अतिस्कन्दनता

**Hyperchylia.** Excessive secretion of gastric juice. अतिजठरस्राव

**Hypercryalgesia.** See **Hypercryesthesia**.

**Hypercryesthesia.** Extreme sensibility to cold; hypercryalgesia. अतिशीतसंवेदनता

**Hypercupremia.** An abnormally high level of plasma copper. अतिताम्रता

**Hypercupruria.** Discharge of excessive coppery substance in the urine. अतिताम्रमेह; पेशाब में प्रचुर ताम्र पदार्थ जाना

**Hypercusis.** See **Hyperacusis**.

**Hypercyanotic.** Marked by excessive cyanosis. अतिश्याव; अत्यधिक नीला

**Hypercythemia.** Presence of an abnormally high number of red blood cells in the circulating blood; hypererythrocythemia. अतिलोहितकोशिकता

**Hypercytosis.** An abnormal increase in the number of cells in the circulating blood or the tissues. अतिकोशिकता

**Hyperdactyly.** Presence of more than five digits on either foot or hand; polydactyly. बहु-अंगुलिता; पांच से अधिक उँगलियां होना

**Hyperdicrotic.** Pronouncedly dicrotic. अतिद्विस्पन्दी

**Hyperdiuresis.** An excessive secretion of urine. अतिमूत्रता; मूत्राधिक्य; अत्यधिक मूत्रस्राव होना

**Hyperechema.** Auditory magnification or exaggeration. अतिश्राव्यता

# Hyperelastosis

**Hyperelastosis.** Excessive elasticity. अतिप्रत्यास्थता; अत्यधिक लचीलापन

**Hyperelectrolytaemia.** Dehydration associated with high serum sodium and chloride levels. अतिविद्युतपघट्यरक्तता

**Hyperemesis.** Excessive vomiting. अतिवमन; अत्यधिक वमन होना

**Hyperemetic.** Marked by excessive vomiting. अतिवामक; अतिवमनकारी

**Hyperemia.** See **Hyperaemia**.

**Hyperemic.** See **Hyperaemic**.

**Hypereosinophilia.** A greater degree of abnormal increase in the number of eosinophilic granulocytes in the circulating blood or the tissues. अतिइयोसिनरागिता

**Hyperergasia.** Increased or excessive functional activity; hyperergia; hyperergy. अतिक्रियात्मकता; बढ़ी हुई क्रियात्मक शक्ति

**Hyperergia.** Hyperergasia; hyperergy; hypergia. अतिक्रियात्मकता; abnormal sensitivity to allergens. अतिप्रत्यूर्जता

**Hyperergic.** Relating to hyperergia; hypergic. अतिक्रियात्मकता अथवा अतिप्रत्यूर्जिता सम्बन्धी

**Hyperergy.** See **Hyperergia**.

**Hypererythrocythemia.** See **Hypercythemia**.

**Hyperesophoria.** A tendency of one eye to deviate upward and inward. अतिनेत्राभिमध्यविचलनप्रवृत्ति

**Hyperesthesia.** See **Hyperaesthesia**.

**Hyperesthetic.** Marked by hyperesthesia. अतिसम्वेदनशील

**Hyperexcitability.** Excessive excitability. अति-उत्तेज्यता; अति-उत्तेजनशीलता; अत्यधिक उत्तेजना

**Hyperexophoria.** A tendency of one eye to deviate upward and outward. अतिनेत्रबहिर्विचलनप्रवृत्ति

**Hyperextension.** Excessive extension; overextension. अतिविस्तार; अतिप्रसार; अत्यधिक फैलाव

**Hyperferraemia.** Excess of iron in the blood; hyperferremia. अतिअयसरक्तता; अतिअयसता; खून में लोहे की बढ़ी हुई मात्रा

**Hyperferremia.** See **Hyperferraemia**.

**Hyperfibrinogenemia.** Increased level of fibrinogen in the blood; fibrinogenemia. अतिफाइब्रिनजनकता

**Hyperfibrinolysis.** Markedly increased fibrinolysis. अतिफाइब्रिनलयन; अतिफाइब्रिनापघटन

**Hyperflexion.** Flexion of a limb or part beyond the normal limit. अतिकुंचन; किसी अंग या अंश का अत्यधिक सिकुड़ जाना

**Hyperfunction.** Overactivity. अतिकार्यता; अतिक्रियता

**Hypergalactia.** Excessive secretion of milk; hypergalactosis. अतिस्तन्यता; स्तनों से अत्यधिक दुग्धस्राव होना

**Hypergalactosis.** See **Hypergalactia.**

**Hypergenesis.** Excessive development or over-production of parts or organs of the body. अतिजननता

**Hypergenetic.** Relating to hypergenesis. अतिजननीय

**Hypergeusia.** Abnormal acuteness of the sense of taste; gustatory hyperaesthesia; oxygeusia. स्वादाधिक्य

**Hypergia.** See **Hyperergia.**

**Hypergic.** See **Hyperergic.**

**Hyperglandular.** Characterized by overactivity or increased size of a gland. अतिग्रन्थिल

**Hyperglobulia.** An increase above the normal in the number of red cells in the blood; erythrocythaemia; polycythaemia. अतिलोहितकोशिकता

**Hyperglobulinemia.** Abnormally large amount of globulins in the circulating blood plasma. अतिग्लोब्यूलिनरक्तता

**Hyperglycaemia.** Excessive glucose in the circulating blood; hyperglycemia. अतिग्लूकोजरक्तता; अतिशर्करारक्तता; रक्त में अत्यधिक शर्करा विद्यमान रहना

**Hyperglycemia.** See **Hyperglycaemia.**

**Hyperglycogenolysis.** Excessive glycogenolysis. अतिग्लाइकोजनापघटन; अतिमधुजनलयन

**Hyperglycorrhachia.** Excessive amount of sugar in the cerebrospinal fluid. मस्तिष्कमेरुद्रव्यशर्कराधिक्य

**Hyperglycosuria.** Persistent excretion of unusually large amounts of glucose in the urine. अतिशर्करामेह; पेशाब में अत्यधिक शर्करा जाना

**Hyperhidrosis.** Excessive or profuse sweating; hyperidrosis; hyperhydrosis; polyhidrosis. अतिस्वेदलता; अतिस्वेदन; अत्यधिक पसीना होना

**Hyperhydration.** Excesive water content of the body; overhydration. अति-उदकता; अत्युदकता; अतिजलमयता

**Hyperhydrosis.** See **Hyperhidrosis.**

**Hyperidrosis.** See **Hyperhidrosis.**

**Hyperinsulinism.** Morbid condition through excess of insulin. अतिइन्सुलिनता; इन्सुलिन की अधिकता के कारण होने वाली दुरावस्था

**Hyperinvolution.** An abnormal inside turning of the uterus; superinvolution. अतिप्रत्यावर्तन; जरायु का अस्वाभाविक रूप से अन्दर की ओर मुड़ जाना

**Hyperirritability.** Excessive irritability. अतिक्षोभ्यता; अत्यधिक उत्तेजना या चिड़चिड़ापन

**Hyperkeratosis.** Hypertrophy of the horny layer of the epidermis. अतिशृंगीयता; अतिकिरेटिनता

**Hyperketonemia.** Accumulation of excess of ketone bodies in the blood. अतिकीटोनता

**Hyperketonuria.** Increased quantity of ketones in the urine. अतिकीटोनमेह

**Hyperkinemia.** Increased volume flow through the circulation. अतिप्रवाहिता

**Hyperkinesia.** An exaggerated motor function or activity; hyperkinesis. अतिगतिकता; अतिगतिक्रम

**Hyperkinesis.** See **Hyperkinesia.**

**Hyperkinetic.** Pertaining to, or characterized by hyperkinesia. अतिगतिक अथवा बढ़ी हुई गति सम्बन्धी

**Hyperlactation.** Continuance of lactation beyond the normal period. अतिस्तन्यता

**Hyperleukocytosis.** An unusually great incease in the number and proportion of leukocytes in the circulating blood or the tissues. अतिश्वेतकोशिकता

**Hyperlipaemia.** Excessive fat in the blood; hyperlipemia. अतिवसारक्तता; रक्त में अत्यधिक चर्बी होना

**Hyperlipaemic.** Affected with or pertaining to hyperlipaemia; hyperlipemic. अतिवसारक्ती; अतिवसारक्तक; अतिवसारक्तता सम्बन्धी

**Hyperlipemia.** See **Hyperlipaemia.**

**Hyperlipemic.** See **Hyperlipaemic.**

**Hyperliposis.** Excessive adipostiy. अतिवसामयता; an extreme degree of fatty degeneration. अतिवसापजनन

**Hypermastia.** Excessively large mammary glands. बृहद्स्तनता; polymastia; a condition in which, in the human, more than two breasts are present. बहुस्तनता

**Hypermenorrhea.** See **Hypermenorrhoea.**

**Hypermenorrhoea.** Excessively prolonged or profuse menses; hypermenorrhea; menorrhagia; menostaxis. अत्यार्तव; दीर्घकालीन अथवा प्रचुर ऋतुस्राव होना

**Hypermetabolism.** Abnormal heat production by the body. अतिचयापचय

**Hypermetria.** A manifestation of ataxia characterized by overreaching a desired object or goal. अतिगतिकता

**Hypermetrope.** Affected with hypermetropia. दूरदृष्टिक

**Hypermetropia.** Farsightedness; hyperopia. दूरदृष्टिता;
    **Absolute H.,** that which cannot be corrected by accommodation. अवशिष्ट दूरदृष्टिता;
    **Facultative H.,** manifest hyperopia which can be corrected by accomodation. विकल्पी दूरदृष्टिता;
    **Latent H.,** the difference between total and manifest hypermetropia. गुप्त दूरदृष्टिता;
    **Manifest H.,** the amount of hypermetropia represented by the strongest convex lens which a person will accept without paralysis of the accommodation. स्पष्ट दूरदृष्टिता;
    **Total H.,** the entire hyperopia, both latent and manifest. समग्र दूरदृष्टिता

**Hypermnesia.** An abnormal power of memory; hypermnesis. अतिस्मृति; असाधारण स्मरण-शक्ति

**Hypermnesis.** See **Hypermnesia.**

**Hypermotility.** Increased movement, as peristalsis. अतिचरता; अतिगतिकता

**Hypermyotonia.** Excessive muscular tonus. अतिपेशीतानता

**Hypermyotrophy.** Muscular hypertrophy. पेशी-अतिबृद्धि; पेशी-विबृद्धि

**Hyperonychia.** Excessive growth or hypertrophy of the nails. अतिनखता; नाखुनों का अत्यधिक बढ़ना

**Hyperope.** One who is farsighted. दूरदृष्टिक

**Hyperopia.** See **Hypermetropia.**

**Hyperorchidism.** Increased size or functioning of the testes. वृषणातिक्रियता; वृषण-अतिक्रियता

**Hyperorexia.** Excessive or morbid hunger; bulimia. अतिक्षुधा; अतिबुभुक्षा; अत्यधिक भूख लगना

**Hyperosmia.** A morbidly acute sense of smell. घ्राण-अतिसम्वेदिता; अतिघ्राणसम्वेदिता; सूंघने की अत्यधिक सम्वेदनशीलता

**Hyperostosis.** A hypertrophy of bone tissue. अतिअध्यास्थिता; अस्थि-ऊतक का अत्यधिक बढ़ना; exostosis. अस्थ्यर्बुद

**Hyperparasitism.** A condition in which a secondary parasite develops within a previously existing parasite. अतिपरजीविता

**Hyperparathyroidism.** Overaction of the parathyroid glands with an increase in serum calcium level. अतिपरावटुता; परावटु ग्रंथियों की अत्यधिक बढ़ी हुई अवस्था

**Hyperperistalsis.** Excessive rapidity of the passage of food through the stomach and intestine. अतिपुरःसरण; अतिक्रमाकुंचन

**Hyperphagia.** Excessive, morbid hunger. अतिभक्षण; भस्मक रोग; अत्यधिक भूख लगने की बीमारी

**Hyperphonesis.** Increase in the percussion sound, or of the voice sound, in auscultation. अतिपरिताड़नता

**Hyperphoria.** A tendency of the visual axis of one eye to deviate upward. नेत्रऊर्ध्वविचलनप्रवृत्ति

**Hyperpiesia.** High pressure, especially of blood; hyperpiesis; essential hypertension. अज्ञातहेतुक-अतिरक्तदाब;

**Hyperpiesis.** See **Hyperpiesia.**

**Hyperpigmentation.** Increased or excessive pigmentation. अतिवर्णकता

**Hyperpituitarism.** Abnormal activity of pituitary gland. अतिपीयूषिकता; पीयूषिका-अतिक्रियता; पीयूषिका ग्रन्थि की असाधारण क्रिया

**Hyperplasia.** Overgrowth of a part due to a multiplication of its elements. अतिविकसन; अतिविकास

**Hyperplastic.** Relating to hyperplasia. अतिविकास सम्बन्धी

**Hyperpnea.** See **Hyperpnoea.**

**Hyperpnoea.** Panting; excessive respiration; hyperpnea. अतिश्वसन; हांफना

**Hyperpolarization.** An increase in polarization of membranes or nerves or muscle cells. अतिध्रुवीकरण

**Hyperponesis.** Exaggerated activity within the motor portion of the nervous system. अतिसक्रियता; अतिक्रियता

**Hyperpraxia.** Excessive activity. अतिक्रियता; restlessness. व्यग्रता; बेचैनी

**Hyperproteinemia.** An abnormally large concentration of protein in plasm. अतिप्रोटीनता

**Hyperproteosis.** A condition due to an excessive amount of protein in the diet. अतिप्रोटीनमयता

**Hyperpyretic.** Relating to hyperpyrexia; hyperpyrexial. ज्वराधिक्य सम्बन्धी

**Hyperpyrexia.** Too high rise in temperature; extremely high fever. अतिज्वर; ज्वराधिक्य

**Hyperpyrexial.** See **Hyperpyretic.**

**Hyper-reflexia.** A condition in which the deep tendon reflexes are exaggerated. अतिप्रतिवर्त्तता

**Hyper-resonance.** Resonance increased above the normal, and often of lower pitch, on percussion of the body. अति-अनुनाद; अत्यनुनाद

**Hyper-resonant.** Over-resonant. अति-अनुनादी; अत्यनुनादी

**Hypersalivation.** Excessive salivation; sialism. अतिलालास्राव; अतिलारता

**Hypersecretion.** Excessive secretion. अतिस्रवण; अतिस्राव
**Hypersensibility.** See **Hypersensitivity.**
**Hypersensitisation.** See **Hypersensitization.**
**Hypersensitive.** Oversensitive. अतिसुग्राही; अतिग्राही; अतिसम्वेदी; अतिसम्वेदनशील
**Hypersensitiveness.** See **Hypersensitivity.**
**Hypersensitivity.** Abnormal sensitiveness; oversusceptibility; oversensitiveness; oversensitivity; hypersensibility; hypersensitiveness; a condition in which the response to a stimulus is excessive in degree. अतिसुग्राहिता; अतिग्राहिता; अतिसम्वेदिता; अतिसम्वेदनशीलता
**Hypersensitization.** The immunological process by which hypersensitiveness is induced; hypersensitisation. अतिसुग्राहीकरण
**Hypersexuality.** Excessive lasciviousness. अतिकामुकता; अत्यधिक बढ़ी हुई वासना
**Hypersomnia.** Excessive sleep. अतिनिद्रा; अत्यधिक नींद आना
**Hypersplenism.** Term used to describe depression of erythrocyte, granulocyte and platelet counts by enlarged spleen in the presence of active bone-marrow. प्लीहा-अतिक्रियता; प्लीहातिक्रियता; तिल्ली की अत्यधिक बढ़ी हुई क्रिया
**Hypersthenia.** Excessive tension or strength; hypersthesia. अतिबल; अत्यधिक तनाव अथवा शक्ति
**Hypersthenic.** Pertaining to, or marked by hypersthenia. अतिबल सम्बन्धी अथवा अतिशक्तिसम्पन्न
**Hypersthesia.** See **Hypersthenia.**
**Hypertelorism.** Genetically determined cranial anomaly (low forehead and pronounced vertex) associated with mental subnormality. दीर्घ-अंगान्तरता; दीर्घांगान्तरता
**Hypertension.** High blood pressure. अतिरक्तदाब; उच्चरक्तदाब; उच्चरक्तचाप; बढ़ा हुआ रक्त का दबाव;
  **Benign H.,** essential hypertension that runs a relatively long and symptomless course. सुदम अतिरक्तदाब;
  **Essential H.,** hypertension without pre-existing renal disease or known cause; primary hypertension. अज्ञातहेतुक अतिरक्तदाब;
  **Malignant H.,** severe hypertension that runs a rapid course, causing necrosis of arteriolar walls, haemorrhagic lesions, and a poor prognosis. दुर्दम अतिरक्तदाब;
  **Portal H.,** increased pressure in the portal veins caused by obstruction of flow of blood through the liver. प्रतिहारी अतिरक्तदाब;

**Primary H.,** see **Essential Hypertension.**

**Pulmonary H.,** hypertension in the pulmonary circulation due to pulmonary or cardiac disease. फुप्फुसी अतिरक्तदाब;

**Renal H.,** hypertension accompanied by renal disease. वृक्कज अतिरक्तदाब

**Hypertensive.** Belonging to, or marked by hypertension. अतिरक्तदाबी; उच्चरक्तदाबी; उच्चरक्तदाब सम्बन्धी

**Hypertensor.** Producing increased blood pressure; pressor. अतिरक्तदाबजनक

**Hyperthelia.** The presence of more than two nipples. बहुचूचुकता

**Hyperthermalgesia.** Unusual or extreme sensitiveness to heat. अतितापार्ति

**Hyperthermia.** Very high body temperature. अतिताप; शरीर का अत्यधिक बढ़ा हुआ तापमान;

**Malignant H.,** hyperpyrexia; rapid onset of extremely high fever with muscular rigidity. दुर्दम अतिताप

**Hyperthrombinemia.** An abnormal amount of thrombin in the blood. अतिथ्रोम्बिनरक्तता

**Hyperthymic.** Pertaining to hyperthymism. अतिबाल्यग्रन्थिता सम्बन्धी

**Hyperthymism.** Excessive activity of the thymus gland. अतिबाल्यग्रन्थिता; बाल्यग्रन्थि की बढ़ी हुई क्रिया

**Hyperthyroidism.** The exophthalmic goitre of the older writers; Grave's disease; Basedow's disease; disease of the thyroid gland in which its secretion is usually increased and is no longer under regulatory control of hypothalamic-pituitary centres. अवटु-अतिक्रियता; अवटुग्रन्थि की अत्यधिक बढ़ी हुई क्रिया

**Hypertonia.** Overtension; great tonicity; hypertonicity; extreme tension of the muscles or arteries. अतितानता; अतितनावता; अतिपरासारिता

**Hypertonic.** Pertaining to hypertonia; spastic; having a greater degree of tension. अतितनावी; अतिपरासारी

**Hypertonicity.** Excessive tonicity; hypertonia. अतितानता; अतितनावता; अतिपरासारिता

**Hypertrichiasis.** Extreme hairiness; hypertrichosis. अतिलोमता; अतिरोमता; लोमातिबृद्धि; रोमातिबृद्धि

**Hypertrichosis.** See **Hypertrichiasis.**

**Hypertrophic.** Affected with hypertrophy. विबृद्धिग्रस्त

**Hypertrophy.** Unnatural enlargement of a part or organ of the body. अतिबृद्धि; विबृद्धि; शरीर का अस्वाभाविक रूप से बढ़ना;

**Compensatory H.,** that due to overactivity of an organ to make up deficiency in a paired organ or in itself. क्षतिपूरक अतिबृद्धि;

**Complementary H.,** increase in size or expansion of an organ or tissue to fill the space left by the destruction of another portion of the same organ or tissue. सम्पूरक अतिबृद्धि; पूरक अतिबृद्धि;

**Concentric H.,** increased thickness of the walls of the heart, without enlargement, but with diminished capacity. संकेन्द्री अतिबृद्धि;

**Eccentric H.,** hypertrophy of an organ with dilatation. उत्केन्द्री अतिबृद्धि;

**False H.,** increase in someone constituent tissue of an organ. कूट अतिबृद्धि; अयथार्थ अतिबृद्धि;

**Functional H.,** temporary increase in size of an organ or part due to natural rather than pathological factors; physiologic (al) hypertension. क्रियात्मक अतिबृद्धि;

**Physiologic (al) H.,** see **Functional Hypertrophy.**

**True H.,** increase of all component tissues of an organ. यथार्थ अतिबृद्धि;

**Vicarious H.,** hypertrophy of an organ or part to provide for a natural increase of function such as occurs in the walls of the uterus and in the mammae during pregnancy. अपथप्रवृत्तार्तवबृद्धि

**Hypertropia.** The deviation of one visual line above the other. नेत्रऊर्ध्वविचलन

**Hyperuricemia.** Enhanced blood concentrations of uric acid. अतिमिहेयाम्लता

**Hyperuricemic.** Relating to, or characterized by hyperuricemia. अतिमिहेयाम्लिक

**Hypervascular.** Abnormally vascular; containing an excessive number of blood vessels. अतिरक्तधर; अतिवाहिकामय

**Hyperventilation.** Increased alveolar ventilation relative to metabolic carbondioxide production. अतिवातायनता

**Hypervitaminosis.** Any condition arising from an excess of vitamins, especially vitamin D. अतिविटामिनता

**Hypervolemia.** Abnormally increased volume of blood; plethora. रक्तायतनबृद्धि; रक्तबहुलता

**Hypervolemic.** Pertaining to, or characterized by hypervolemia. रक्तबहुल; रक्तायतनबृद्धि सम्बन्धी

**Hypesthesia.** Diminished sensitivity to stimulation; hypoaesthesia; hypoesthesia. अल्पसम्वेदिता

**Hypha.** A branching tubular cell characteristic of the growth of filament fungi. कवकतन्तु

**Hyphae.** Plural of **Hypha**.

**Hyphedonia.** A habitually lessened or attenuated degree of pleasure. निरानन्दानुभूति

**Hyphema.** Haemorrhage into the anterior chamber of eye. अग्रकक्षरक्तता

**Hyphemia.** A deficiency in the normal amount of blood in the body; hypovolaemia; oligaemia. रक्तायतनह्रास; रक्तस्वल्पता

**Hyphidrosis.** See **Hypohidrosis**.

**Hypn-.** See **Hypno-**.

**Hypnagog.** See **Hypnagogue**.

**Hypnagogue.** An agent producing sleep; hypnagog. निद्रावर्धी; निद्राकारक; स्वापक

**Hypno-, Hypn-.** Prefixes denoting relation to sleep or hypnosis. 'निद्रा' अथवा 'नींद' का अर्थ देने वाले उपसर्ग

**Hypnogenesis.** Induction of sleep or of the hypnotic state. निद्राजनन

**Hypnogenetic.** Sleep-producing. निद्रापक; निद्राकर; निद्राजनक

**Hypnogenic.** Relating to hypnogenesis. निद्राजनन सम्बन्धी

**Hypnoidal.** Resembling hypnosis. सम्मोहनवत्

**Hypnolepsy.** Morbid sleepiness; narcolepsy. निद्राधिक्य; अतिनिद्रारुग्णता

**Hypnology.** A treatise upon sleep. निद्राविज्ञान; नींदविज्ञान

**Hypnosis.** A state of suspended consciousness; a condition of abnormal sleep. निद्रापकता; सम्मोहन

**Hypnotherapy.** Treatment of diseases by means of hypnotism or inducing prolonged sleep. सम्मोहनोपचार; सम्मोहन-चिकित्सा

**Hypnotic.** Something, usually a drug, that induces sleep. निद्रापक; निद्राकारी; निद्राकर; निद्राजनक; नींद लाने वाली; relating to hipnotism. सम्मोहन सम्बन्धी

**Hypnotism.** Mesmerism; the process or act of inducing hypnosis; the practice or study of hypnosis. सम्मोहनविद्या; वशीकरण; सम्मोहन

**Hypnotist.** One who practices hypnotism. सम्मोहनविज्ञ

**Hypnotize.** To induct one into hypnosis. सम्मोहित करना; वश में करना

**Hypo-, Hyp-.** Prefixes denoting a location beneath something else. 'अधः' तथा 'अल्प' का अर्थ देने वाले उपसर्ग

**Hypoacidity.** Insufficient acidity. अल्पाम्लता

**Hypoacusis.** See **Hypacusis**.

**Hypoadenia.** Decreased activity of glands. ग्रन्थि-अल्पक्रियता

**Hypoadrenalism.** Reduced adrenocortical function. अल्पअधिवृक्कता

**Hypoaesthesia.** See **Hypesthesia.**

**Hypoalbuminaemia.** Decreased albumin in the blood; hypalbuminemia. अल्पान्नसाररक्तता; रक्त में अन्नसार की घटी हुई मात्रा

**Hypoalgesia.** See **Hypalgesia.**

**Hypoalimentation.** A condition of insufficient nourishment. अल्पपोषणता; अल्पपोषण

**Hypoazoturia.** Excretion of abnormally small quantities of urea in the urine. अल्पमूत्राम्लमेह

**Hypoblast.** The inner cell layer or entoderm, which develops during gastrulation. अल्पप्रसू

**Hypoblastic.** Relating to, or derived from the hypoblast. अल्पप्रसू सम्बन्धी अथवा अल्पप्रसूजनित

**Hypocalcaemia.** Decreased calcium in the blood; hypocalcemia. अल्पकैल्सियमरक्तता; खून में कैल्सियम की घटी हुई मात्रा

**Hypocalcemia.** See **Hypocalcaemia.**

**Hypocalcification.** Deficient calcification of bone or teeth. अल्पकैल्सीभवन

**Hypocapnia.** Abnormally low tension of carbondioxide in the circulating blood; hypocarbia. अल्पकैप्नियता; रक्त में कार्बनडाइऑक्साइड का अत्यल्प तनाव

**Hypocarbia.** See **Hypocapnia.**

**Hypochloremia.** An abnormally low level of chloride ions in the circulating blood. अल्पक्लोराइडता

**Hypochlorhydria.** A deficiency of the gastric hydrochloric acid. अल्पजठराम्लता

**Hypochloruria.** Excretion of abnormally small quantities of chloride ions in the urine. अल्पक्लोराइडमेह

**Hypocholesterolemia.** Abnormally small amount of cholestrol in the circulating blood. अल्परक्तवसामयता; अल्पकोलेस्ट्रालरक्तता

**Hypochondria.** Below the ribs. अधःपर्शुकीय; पसलियों के नीचे; hypochondriasis. रोगभ्रम; plural of **Hypochondrium.**

**Hypochondriac.** Hypochondriacal; a victim of hypochondriasis. रोगभ्रमी; beneath the ribs. अधःपर्शुकीय; relating to the hypochondrium. अधःपर्शुकप्रदेश सम्बन्धी

**Hypochondriacal.** Relating to, or suffering from hypochondriasis; hypochondriac. अधःपर्शुक प्रदेश सम्बन्धी अथवा रोगभ्रमाक्रान्त

**Hypochondriasis.** Depression of spirits, with languor, listlessness and despair of recovery, as a result of morbid fear of being sick; hypochondria. रोगभ्रम; चित्तोन्माद

**Hypochondrium.** The two superior regions of the abdomen just below the short ribs. अध:पर्शुकप्रदेश; कोख

**Hypochromasia.** Lack of haemoglobin in the red blood cells. अल्पक्रोमिता; अल्पवर्णता

**Hypochromatic.** Hypochromic; containing a small amount of pigment, or less than the normal amount for the individual tissue. अल्पक्रोमी; अल्पवर्णी

**Hypochromatism.** The condition of being hypochromatic; hypochromia. अल्पक्रोमिता; अल्पवर्णता

**Hypochromia.** Condition of the blood in which the red blood cells have a reduced haemoglobin content; hypochromatism. अल्पक्रोमिता; अल्पवर्णता

**Hypochromic.** Hypochromatic; deficiency in colouring of pigmentation. अल्पक्रोमी; अल्पवर्णी; pertaining to hypochromia. अल्पवर्णता सम्बन्धी

**Hypochylia.** Deficiency of gastric juice. जठररसाल्पता

**Hypocorticalism.** Addison's disease; a disease marked by a peculiar bronzed pigmentation of the skin with severe prostration and progressive anaemia. अल्पलोहितरक्तता; एडीसन रोग; विनाशक अरक्तता; सांघातिक रक्ताल्पता

**Hypocratic.** Sunken; corpselike; Hippocratic. मृतवत्; मृतक जैसा मुरझाया हुआ; हिप्पोक्रैटी

**Hypocupraemia.** Decreased quantity of copper in the blood; hypocupremia. अल्पताम्ररक्तता; रक्त में ताम्बे की घटी हुई मात्रा

**Hypocupremia.** See **Hypocupraemia**.

**Hypocythemia.** Decreased blood cells, especially red blood cells. अल्परक्तकोशिकता

**Hypodactyly.** Less than the normal number of digits. अल्पांगुलिता

**Hypodermic.** Used of medication inserted beneath the skin with a hollow needle and syringe; subcutaneous. अधस्त्वचीय; अन्तर्वचीय; अधस्त्वक्

**Hypodermoclysis.** Subcutaneous injection of a saline or other solution. अधस्त्वक्द्रवाधान

**Hypodontia.** Diminished development or absence of teeth; oligodontia. अल्पदन्तता

**Hypodynamic.** Possessing or exhibiting subnormal power or force. अल्पशक्ति; अशक्त; दुर्बल; कमजोर

**Hypodynia.** A mild type of pain. अल्पवेदना; हल्की पीड़ा

**Hypoergia.** See **Hyposensitiveness**.

**Hypoergy.** See **Hyposensitiveness**.

**Hypoesophoria.** Combined downward and inward deviation of the eyeball. अल्पनेत्राभिमध्यविचलनप्रवृत्ति

**Hypoesthesia.** See **Hypesthesia.**

**Hypoexophoria.** Combined outward and downward deviation of the eyeball. अल्पनेत्रबहिर्विचलनप्रवृत्ति

**Hypoferraemia.** Decreased quantity of iron in the blood. अल्पलौहरक्तता; रक्त में लोहे की घटी हुई मात्रा

**Hypofunction.** Diminished, reduced, low or inadequate function or performance. अल्पक्रिया; कार्याल्पता; अल्पकार्यशीलता

**Hypogalactia.** Diminised secretion of milk. अल्पस्तन्यता

**Hypogalactous.** Producing or secreting diminished amount of milk. अल्पदुग्धस्रावी; अल्पदुग्धोत्पादक

**Hypoganglionosis.** A reduction in the number of ganglionic nerve cells. अधोगण्डिकता

**Hypogastric.** Pertaining to hypogastrium or the lower part of the abdomen. अधोजठरीय; अधोजठरप्रदेशीय; उदर के निचले भाग से सम्बन्धित

**Hypogastrium.** The lower interior part of the abdomen; pubic region. अधोजठरप्रदेश; उदर का निचला अन्दरूनी भाग

**Hypogastrocele.** Hernia in the hypogastrium. अधोजठरहर्निया; जधोजठरस्रंस

**Hypogastroschisis.** Congenital fissure in the hypogastric region. अधोजठरविदरता

**Hypogenesis.** General underdevelopment of parts or organs of the body. अल्पविकसन; अल्पविकास

**Hypogenetic.** Relating to hypogenesis. अल्पविकास सम्बन्धी

**Hypogenitalism.** Partial or complete failure of maturation of genitalia. अल्पजनननांगता

**Hypogeusia.** A blunting of, or subnormal sense of taste. अल्पस्वादसम्वेदना

**Hypoglossal.** Under the tongue; subglossal. अवजिह्वी; अवजिह्वक; जीभ के नीचे

**Hypoglottis.** The undersurface of the tongue; ranula. अधोजिह्वा; अधोकण्ठ; जीभ का निचला भाग

**Hypoglycaemia.** Deficiency of sugar in the blood; hypoglycemia. अल्पग्लूकोजरक्तता; अल्पशर्करारक्तता; रक्त में शर्करा की घटी हुई मात्रा

**Hypoglycaemic.** Pertaining to, or characterized by hypoglycaemia; hypoglycemic. अल्पग्लूकोजरक्तता सम्बन्धी अथवा अल्पग्लूकोजरक्तताग्रस्त

**Hypoglycemia.** See **Hypoglycaemia.**

**Hypoglycemic.** See **Hypoglycaemic.**

**Hypognathus.** Having a congenitally defectively developed lower jaw. अल्पहनु

**Hypogonadism.** Inadequate gonadal function. अल्पजननग्रन्थिता

**Hypogonadotropic.** Concerning or caused by deficiency of gonadotrophins. अधोजननग्रन्थिपोषी

**Hypohidrosis.** A deficiency in the water of the tissues; hyphidrosis. अल्पस्वेदनता; पसीने की कमी

**Hypohidrotic.** Characterized by diminished sweating. अल्पस्वेदनताग्रस्त

**Hypoinsulinism.** Insulin deficiency. अल्पइन्सुलिनता; इन्सुलिनाल्पता; इन्सुलिन की कमी

**Hypokinesia.** A weak and imperfect response of a muscle to stimuli; hypokinesis; hypomotality. अल्पगतिकता

**Hypokinesis.** See **Hypokinesia.**

**Hypomania.** A moderate degree of maniacal exaltation. अल्पोन्माद

**Hypomastia.** Atrophy or congenital smallness of the breasts. अल्पस्तनता

**Hypomenorrhea.** See **Hypomenorrhoea.**

**Hypomenorrhoea.** A diminution of the flow or a shortening of the duration of menstruation; hypomenorrhea. अल्पार्तव; ऋतुस्राव की घटी हुई मात्रा

**Hypometabolism.** Decreased production of body heat; low metabolic rate. अल्पचयापचयदर

**Hypomnesia.** Impaired memory. अल्पस्मरणशक्ति

**Hypomotality.** See **Hypokinesia.**

**Hypomyotonia.** Diminished muscular tone. अल्पपेशीतानता

**Hypomyxia.** Diminished secretion of mucus. अल्पश्लेष्मस्राव

**Hyponeuria.** Weakness of nerve power. स्नायुदौर्बल्य; तंत्रिकावसाद

**Hyponychial.** Subungual. अवनखी; relating to the hyponychium. अवनख सम्बन्धी

**Hyponychium.** The epithelium of the nail-bed, particularly its posterior part in the region of the lunula (semilunar area). अवनख

**Hyponychon.** An ecchymosis beneath a finger or toe nail. अवनखीनीलांछन

**Hypopancreatism.** A condition of diminished activity of the pancreas. अल्पाग्न्याशयता; अल्पक्लोमग्रन्थिता

**Hypoparathyroidism.** A pathologial state due to partial loss or insufficient parathyroid tissue. अल्पपरावटुता

**Hypophalangism.** Congenital absence of one or more of the phalanges of a digit. अल्पांगुलिपर्वता

**Hypopharynx.** That portion of the pharynx lying below and behind the larynx, correctly called the laryngopharynx. अधोग्रसनी; अधोकण्ठ

**Hypophonesis.** In percussion or auscultation, a sound that is diminished or fainter than usual. मन्दध्वनि

**Hypophoria.** A tendency of visual axis of one eye to be below than that of the other. नेत्रअधोविचलनप्रवृत्ति

**Hypophosphatemia.** Abnormally low concentration of phosphates in the circulating blood. अल्पफास्फेटरक्तता; अल्पस्फुर-अम्लरक्तता

**Hypophosphaturia.** Reduced urinary excretion of phosphates. अल्पफास्फेटमेह; अल्पस्फुर-अम्लमेह

**Hypophyseal.** Relating to hypophysis; hypophysial. पीयूषिकां सम्बन्धी

**Hypophysectomy.** Surgical removal of pituitary gland. पीयूषिका-उच्छेदन; पीयूषिका-ग्रन्थि को काट कर हटा देना

**Hypophysial.** See **Hypophyseal.**

**Hypophysis.** The pituitary or master gland. पीयूषिका; पीयूषिका-ग्रन्थि

**Hypopiesis.** See **Hypotension.**

**Hypopion.** Effusion of pus in the anterior chamber of the eyes; hypopyon. अग्रकक्षपूयता; अग्रकक्षपूतिता

**Hypopituitarism.** Pituitary gland insufficiency, especially of the anterior lobe. पीयूषिकाल्पक्रियता; पीयूषिका-ग्रन्थि की मंद क्रिया

**Hypoplasia.** Defective development of tissue. अल्पविकसन; अल्पविकास; ऊनवृद्धि; अल्पवृद्धि; सदोष रचना

**Hypoplastic.** Pertaining to, or characterized by hypoplasia. अल्पविकास सम्बन्धी अथवा अल्पविकसित

**Hypoploid.** Characterized by hypoploidy. अल्पगुणसूत्री

**Hypoploidy.** State of having fewer chromosomes than the normal number. अल्पगुणसूत्रता

**Hypopnea.** Deficient respiration; hypopnoea. अल्पश्वसन; श्वासाल्पता

**Hypopnoea.** See **Hypopnea.**

**Hypoposia.** Decreased intake of fluids. अल्पद्रवग्रहणता

**Hypopraxia.** Deficient activity. अल्पक्रियाशीलता

**Hypoptyalism.** Deficient secretion of saliva; hyposalivation. अल्पलालास्राव; अल्पलालास्रवण

**Hypopyon.** See **Hypopion.**

**Hyporeflexia.** Deminished or weakened reflexes. अल्पप्रतिवर्तता; मंदप्रतिवर्तता

**Hyposalivation.** See **Hypoptyalism.**

**Hyposecretion.** Diminished secretion, as by a gland. अल्पस्रवण; अल्पस्राव; स्रावाल्पता

**Hyposensitiveness.** Hypoergia; hypoergy; subnormal sensitiveness or sensitivity. अल्पसम्वेदनशीलता; अल्पसम्वेदिता

**Hyposmia.** Decrease in the normal sensitivity to smell; diminished sense of smell. अल्पघ्राणता; गंध के प्रति घटी हुई सम्वेदनशीलता

**Hyposomnia.** Deficient sleep. अल्पनिद्रा

**Hypospadia.** See **Hypospadias**.

**Hypospadiac.** Relating to hypospadia. अधोमूत्रमार्गता सम्बन्धी

**Hypospadias.** A congenital fissure in the undersurface of the penis; hypospadia. अधोमूत्रमार्गता

**Hypostasis.** A standing asunder. अध:स्थिति; formation of a sediment or deposit at the bottom of the liquid. तलछट; परत

**Hypostatic.** Pertaining to hypostasis. अध:स्थितिक; sedimentary. परतदार अथवा तलछट सम्बन्धी

**Hyposthenia.** A want of strength; debility; weakness. अल्पबल; अल्पशक्ति; दुर्बलता; कमजोरी

**Hyposthenic.** Of subnormal power; debilitating; weak. अल्पबलकारी; दुर्बलताकारी; कमजोर करने वाला

**Hypostomia.** Congenital defect in which the mouth is small. अल्पमुखता

**Hypotension.** Hypopiesis; low blood pressure (systolic below 110 mm mercury, diastolic 70 mm). अल्परक्तदाब; निम्नरक्तदाब; निम्नरक्तचाप; reduced pressure or tension of any kind. अल्पदाब; अल्पतनाव

**Hypotensive.** Characterized by low blood pressure or causing a reduction in the blood pressure. अल्परक्तदाबी; अल्पतनावी

**Hypotensor.** Depressor; an agent producing decreased blood pressure. अल्परक्तदाबी

**Hypothalamic.** Belonging to hypothalamus. अध:श्चेतकी; अध:श्चेतक सम्बन्धी

**Hypothalamus.** Name given to the structures of the forebrain under the thalamus. अध:श्चेतक

**Hypothenar.** An eminence on the ulnar side of the palm; antithenar. कनिष्ठामूल

**Hypothermal.** Tepid; lukewarm; denoting hypothermia. अल्पोष्ण; अल्पतप्त; कोसा; हल्का गर्म

**Hypothermia.** A state of lowered temperature of the body (i.e. below 98.4° F or 37°C); hypothermy. अल्पोष्णता; अल्पतप्तंता; अल्पताप

**Hypothermy.** See **Hypothermia**.

**Hypothesis.** Imagination; speculation. परिकल्पना; अनुमान

**Hypothymia.** Depression of spirits. आत्मावसाद; आत्मग्लानि; आत्मविषाद

**Hypothymism.** Inadequate function of the thymus. बाल्यग्रन्थि-अल्पक्रियता

**Hypothyroid.** Marked by reduced thyroid function. अवटु-अल्पता

**Hypothyroidism.** Imperfect or complete loss of the function of the thyroid gland; myxedema; myxoedema. अवटु-अल्पक्रियता; अवटु ग्रन्थि की अपूर्ण क्रिया अथवा पूर्ण निष्क्रियता

**Hypotonia.** Lower tension than normal, as of the blood; hypotonicity; hypotonus; hypotony. अल्पतनाव; अल्पपरासारिता

**Hypotonic.** Having a lower osmotic pressure. अल्पतनावी; अल्पपरासारी

**Hypotonicity.** Hypotonia; a decreased osmotic pressure. अल्पपरासारिता; अल्पतनाव

**Hypotonus.** See **Hypotonia**.

**Hypotony.** See **Hypotonia**.

**Hypotoxicity.** A reduced or lessened toxicity. अल्पविषण्णता

**Hypotrichosis.** A less than normal amount of hair on the head and/or body. अल्परोमता

**Hypotropia.** Downward deviation of the visual axis of one eye. नेत्रअधोविचलन

**Hypotympanotomy.** Complete surgical extirpation of small tumours confined to the lower tympanic cavity. मध्यकर्णसंधान

**Hypotympanum.** The middle ear; the lower part of the tympanic cavity. मध्यकर्ण; कर्ण-गह्वर का निचला भाग

**Hypoventilation.** Diminished breathing or underventilation. अल्पसंवातन; अल्पश्वसन

**Hypovitaminaemia.** Deficiency of vitamin in the blood. अल्पविटामिनरक्तता; रक्त में विटामिनों की कमी

**Hypovitaminosis.** Any condition due to lack of vitamins. अल्पविटामिनरुग्णता; विटामिनों की कमी के कारण होने वाली रुग्णता

**Hypovolaemia.** Diminished total quantity of blood; hyphemia; hypovolemia; oligaemia. अल्पायतनरक्तता; रक्त की पूर्ण घटी हुई मात्रा

**Hypovolemia.** See **Hypovolaemia**.

**Hypovolia.** Diminished water content or volume of a given compartment. उदकाल्पता; जलाल्पता

**Hypoxemia.** Subnormal oxygenation of arterial blood. अल्प-ऑक्सीमियता

**Hypoxia.** Diminished amount of oxygen in air, blood, or tissue; short of anoxia. अल्प-ऑक्सीयता

**Hypsophobia.** A morbid fear of height. उत्तुंगभीति; ऊँचाई का डर

**Hyster-.** See **Hystero-**.

**Hystera.** The uterus; the womb. गर्भाशय; जरायु; बच्चेदानी

**Hysteralgia.** Uterine neuralgia; hysterodynia; pain in the womb. जरायुशूल; गर्भाशयशूल; जरायुवेदना; जरायुपीड़ा; गर्भाशयार्ति

**Hysteratresia.** Atresia of the uterine cavity. जरायु-अविवरता

**Hysterectomy.** Excision of the womb. गर्भाशयोच्छेदन; जरायूच्छेदन; जरायु-उच्छेदन; गर्भाशय-उच्छेदन;
   **Abdominal H.,** removal of the uterus through an incision in the abdominal wall; abdominohysterectomy. उदरमार्गी गर्भाशयोच्छेदन;
   **Cesarean H.,** cesarean section followed by hysterectomy. सीजेरियन गर्भाशयोच्छेदन;
   **Vaginal H.,** removal of the uterus through the vagina without incising the abdominal wall. योनिमार्गी गर्भाशयोच्छेदन

**Hystereurysis.** Dilatation of the lower segment and cervical canal of the uterus. अधःजरायुखण्डविस्फार

**Hysteria.** A disordered state of nervous system characterized by the acute attacks of functional spasm and paralysis resulting from irritating impressions. वातोन्माद; गुल्मवायु; हिस्टीरिया

**Hysteriac.** A hysterical person. वातोन्मादी; वातोन्मादग्रस्त (रोगी); गुल्मवायु रोगी

**Hysteric.** See **Hysterical.**

**Hysterical.** Relating to, or suffering from hysteria; hysteric. वातोन्माद सम्बन्धी अथवा वातोन्मादग्रस्त

**Hysterics.** An expression of emotion accompanied by crying, laughing and screaming. वातोन्मादीभावभंगिमा

**Hysteritis.** Inflammation of the womb. जरायुशोथ; गर्भाशयशोथ; गर्भाशय-प्रदाह; जरायु-प्रदाह

**Hystero-, Hyster-.** Prefixes denoting the uterus. 'गर्भाशय' अथवा 'जरायु' का अर्थ देने वाले उपसर्ग

**Hysterocatalepsy.** Hysteria with cataleptic manifestations. जरायुपेशीप्रतिष्टम्भ

**Hysterocele.** Falling off of the womb; prolapsus uteri, especially when gravid. जरायु-हर्निया; जरायुभ्रंश; गर्भाशयच्युति

**Hysterocleisis.** Operative occlusion of the uterus. जरायुसंरोध

**Hysterodynia.** See **Hysteralgia.**

**Hysteroepilepsy.** Hysteria with epileptiform convulsions. वातोन्मादी आक्षेप; वाताक्षेप; वातोन्माद के साथ मिर्गीरूप अकड़न

**Hysterogenic.** Causing hysterical symptoms or reactions. वातोन्मादी

**Hysterogram.** A radiograph of the uterus; a record of the strength of the uterine contraction. जरायुलेख; गर्भाशयलेख

**Hysterograph.** An apparatus for recording the strength of uterine contraction. जरायुचित्र; गर्भाशयचित्र

**Hysterography.** X-ray examination of the uterus; the procedure of recording uterine contractions. जरायुचित्रण; गर्भाशयचित्रण

**Hysteroid.** Resembling hystera. जरायुवत्; गर्भाशयाभ; resembling hysteria. वातोन्माद जैसा

**Hysterolith.** Uterine calculus. जरायु-अश्मरी; गर्भाशयाश्मरी; बच्चेदानी की पथरी

**Hysterology.** The science of uterus. जरायुविज्ञान; गर्भाशयविज्ञान

**Hysterolysis.** Breaking up of adhesions between the uterus and the neighbouring parts. जरायुलयन; गर्भाशयापघटन

**Hysteromania.** Lascivious madness of females. कामोन्माद; स्त्रीकामोन्माद; स्त्रियों में बढ़ी हुई सम्भोग की इच्छा

**Hysterometer.** A graduated sound for measuring the depth of the uterine cavity; uterometer. जरायुमापी; गर्भाशयमापी

**Hysteromyoma.** A myoma of the uterus. जरायुपेश्यर्बुद

**Hysteromyomectomy.** Operative removal of a uterine myoma. जरायुपेश्यर्बुदोच्छेदन

**Hysteromyotomy.** Incision into the uterine muscles. जरायुपेशीछेदन

**Hystero-oophorectomy.** Surgical removal of the uterus and the ovaries. जरायुडिम्बग्रन्थि-उच्छेदन; गर्भाशय तथा डिम्बग्रन्थियों को काट कर हटा देना

**Hysteroparalysis.** Paralysis of the uterine walls. जरायुघात; गर्भाशयघात; जरायु-प्राचीरों का पक्षाघात

**Hysteropathy.** Any disease of the uterus. जरायुरोग

**Hysteropexy.** Surgical fixation of a misplaced or abnormally movable uterus; uteropexy; uterofixation. जरायुस्थिरीकरण

**Hysteroplasty.** A plastic operation on the uterus; uteroplasty. जरायुसंधान; गर्भाशयसंधान

**Hysterorrhaphy.** Sutural repair of a lacerated uterus. जरायुसीवन

**Hysterorrhexis.** Rupture of the uterus. जरायुविदर

**Hysterosalpingectomy.** Excision of the womb and usually both uterine tubes. गर्भाशयडिम्बवाहिनी-उच्छेदन; गर्भाशय तथा डिम्बवाही नलियों को काट देना

**Hysterosalpingography.** X-ray examination of the uterus and tubes after injection of a contrast medium; hysterotubography. गर्भाशयडिम्बवाहिनीचित्रण

**Hysterosalpingo-oophorectomy.** Excision of the uterus, oviducts and ovaries. गर्भाशयडिम्बवाहिनीडिम्बाशयोच्छेदन

**Hysterosalpingostomy.** Anastomosis between an oviduct and the uterus. गर्भाशयडिम्बवाहिनीसम्मिलन

**Hysteroscope.** A uterine speculum with reflector for the visual examination of the womb; uteroscope. जरायुदर्शी; गर्भाशयदर्शी

**Hysteroscopy.** Inspection of the uterus with the hysteroscope; uteroscopy. जरायुदर्शन; गर्भाशयदर्शन

**Hysterospasm.** Spasm of the uterus. जरायु-आकर्ष; गर्भाशयाकर्ष

**Hysterostomatomy.** Excision of the cervix uteri. गर्भाशयग्रीवा-उच्छेदन

**Hysterotomy.** The dissection of the uterus; uterotomy. गर्भाशय-उच्छेदन; गर्भाशयोच्छेदन; जरायूच्छेदन;

  **Abdominal H.,** transabdominal incision into the uterus; abdominohysterotomy. उदरमार्गी गर्भाशयछेदन;

  **Vaginal H.,** incision into the uterus via the vagina. योनिमार्गी गर्भाशयछेदन

**Hysterotrachelectomy.** Surgical removal of the cervix uteri. जरायुग्रीवा-उच्छेदन; गर्भाशयग्रीवा-उच्छेदन

**Hysterotracheloplasty.** Plastic repair of the cervix uteri. जरायुग्रीवासंधान; गर्भाशयग्रीवासंधान

**Hysterotrachelorrhaphy.** Sutural repair of a lacerated cervix uteri. जरायुग्रीवासीवन

**Hysterotrachelotomy.** Incision of the cervix uteri. जरायुग्रीवाछेदन

**Hysterotubography.** See **Hysterosalpingography.**

**Hysterovaginectomy.** Excision of both uterus and vagina. गर्भाशययोनि-उच्छेदन

**Hystriciasis.** A hair disease in which they stand erect; hystricism. केशोनुत्तानता; बालों का एक रोग जिसमें वे सीधे खड़े रहते हैं

**Hystricism.** See **Hystriciasis.**

**Hz.** Abbreviation for **Hertz.**

# I

**Iamatology.** The science of remedies. औषधिविज्ञान; औषधियों का वैज्ञानिक अध्ययन

**Iatria.** Therapeutics. चिकित्साविधान; चिकित्साशास्त्र

**Iatric.** Relating to medicine or to a physician. चिकित्साशास्त्र अथवा

चिकित्सक सम्बन्धी

**Itro-.** Prefix denoting relation to physicians, medicine, treatment. 'चिकित्सक', 'चिकित्साशास्त्र', अथवा 'चिकित्सा' सम्बन्धी अर्थ देने वाला उपसर्ग

**Iatrogenic.** A secondary condition arising from treatment of a primary condition. चिकित्साजन्य; चिकित्साजनित; चिकित्सकजनित; चिकित्सकप्रेरित

**Iatrology.** The science of medicine. औषधविज्ञान; चिकित्साविज्ञान

**Iatros.** A physician. चिकित्सक; वैद्य; हकीम

**Iatrotechnic.** The art of healing. विरोहणकला; आरोग्यकला

**Ichor.** A foetid watery discharge flowing from ulcers, wounds, etc. तीखाव्रणस्राव

**Ichoroid.** Denoting a thin, purulent discharge. दुर्गन्धित

**Ichorous.** Of the nature of, or relating to ichor. तीखा; पूतिरक्तमय; पूयरक्तयुक्त; तीखेव्रणस्राव सम्बन्धी

**Ichthyism.** Poisoning by fish; ichthyotoxism. मत्स्यविषण्णता; मीनविषण्णता

**Ichthyo-.** Prefix meaning fish. 'मत्स्य' अथवा 'मीन' का अर्थ देने वाला उपसर्ग

**Ichthyoid.** Fish-shaped; resembling a fish. मत्स्याकार; मीनाकार; मत्स्यरूप; मत्स्यवत्; मीनरूप; मीनसदृश; मछली से मिलता-जुलता

**Ichthyology.** The science of fishes. मत्स्यविज्ञान

**Ichthyosarcotoxism.** Alcoholism. मद्यात्यय; मद्यविषण्णता; मद्यविषाक्तता; शराब पीने से होने वाली रोगावस्था

**Ichthyosis.** Fishlike dry, scaly and horny skin; fish-skin disease. शल्कचर्मता; शल्कीत्वचा; मीनकुष्ठ; मीनचर्मता; मत्स्यचर्मता; मछली की खाल जैसी सूखी, पपड़ीदार तथा शृंगी चमड़ी

**Ichthyotic.** Relating to ichthyosis. शल्कचर्मता अथवा मीनचर्मता सम्बन्धी

**Ichthyotoxism.** See **Ichthyism.**

**Icing Liver.** Chronic perihepatitis. जीर्ण परियकृत्शोथ; जीर्ण यकृतावरणशोथ; यकृतावरण का जीर्ण प्रदाह

**Ictal.** Relating to, or caused by a stroke or seizure. आघात सम्बन्धी अथवा आघातजन्य या आघातजनित

**Icter.** Jaundice; icterus. कामला; पीलिया; कँवलवायु; कमल; पाण्डु;

**I. Hepatitis,** hepatitis with jaundice. कामलजयकृत्शोथ; पाण्डुयकृत्शोथ

**Icteric.** Affected with, marked by, or relating to jaundice (icterus). कामलाग्रस्त; कामलारोगी अथवा कामला सम्बन्धी

**Icterine.** Pallid; yellow. पाण्डुर; पीत; पीला

**Icteritious.** Resembling jaundice; icteroid. कामलाभ; कामला रोग से मिलता-जुलता; पीलिया जैसा

**Ictero-.** Prefix denoting relationship to icterus. 'कामला' का अर्थ देने वाला उपसर्ग

**Icterode.** Having or affected with jaundice. कामलाग्रस्त; पीलियाग्रस्त; कामलारोगी

**Icterogenic.** Causing or producing jaundice. कामलाजनक

**Icterohepatitis.** Inflammation of the liver with jaundice as a prominent symptom. कामलजयकृत्शोथ

**Icteroid.** See **Icteritious.**

**Icterus.** See **Icter.**

   **I. Albus,** chlorosis. हरित्पाण्डु रोग;

   **I. Gravis,** acute yellow atrophy of the liver. उग्र कामला; गंभीर कामला; गम्भीर कामला;

   **I. Index,** measurement of concentration of bilirubin in the plasma. कामला सूचकांक;

   **I. Neonatorum,** the jaundice of the newborn. शिशु-कामला; नवजात-कामला

**Ictus.** A stroke or attack. आघात; प्रहार;

   **I. Solis,** sun-stroke. तापाघात; लू लगना

**I.C.U.** Intensive Care Unit. गहन चिकित्सा केन्द्र

**Idea.** A mental image, concept or picture. विचार; मत; धारणा; प्रतिकृति; अनुमान;

   **Compulsive I.,** a fixed and inappropriate idea. दुराग्रही विचार;

   **Dominant I.,** an idea that governs all the actions and thoughts of the individual. प्रबल धारणा; प्रभावी विचार;

   **Fixed I.,** an exaggerated motion, belief or delusion that persists and controls the mind. स्थिर धारणा; निश्चित धारणा; तर्कसंगत विचार

**Ideal.** Pertaining to an idea. विचार अथवा प्रतिकृति सम्बन्धी; a standard of perception. आदर्श

**Ideation.** The capacity of the mind to form ideas. प्रत्ययन; चिन्तन; कल्पना

**Ideational.** Relating to ideation. प्रत्ययन, चिन्तन अथवा कल्पना सम्बन्धी

**Identification.** Recognition. पहचान; in behavioural sciences, an imitation, sense of oneness, or psychic continuity with another person or group. समीकरण; तद्रूपण

**Identity.** The social role of the person and his perception of it. अभिज्ञान; अन्योन्यता; तद्रूपता; पहिचान

**Ideology.** The philosophy of mind, i.e. the composite system of ideas, beliefs, and attitudes that constitutes an individual's or group's organized view of others. मनोविज्ञान; वैचारिकी; विचारधारा

**Idiocy.** A condition of extreme mental deficiency. मूर्खता; जड़बुद्धिता; मूढ़ता; जड़ता

**Idioglossia.** Disorder of speech marked by substituting one consonant for another. असम्बद्धोच्चारण; असम्बद्ध-उच्चारण

**Idiomuscular.** Peculiar to muscle tissue. पेशीविशिष्ट

**Idioneurosis.** Any disease having its origin in the nerves. तंत्रिकामूलक; तंत्रिकाजनित; तंत्रिकाजन्य

**Idiopathic.** Without apparent cause; agnogenic; spontaneous; denoting a primary disease. अज्ञातहेतुक; प्रारम्भिक; स्वत:; relating to the original disease. मूलरोग सम्बन्धी

**Idiopathy.** A pathologic state of unknown or spontaneous origin; a primary disease. प्रत्यात्मविकृति; मूलरोग; अज्ञेय अथवा स्वमूल (स्वत:मूल) की कोई रोगावस्था

**Idiophrenic.** Relating to, or originating in the mind or brain alone; not reflex or secondary. स्वमनोजात

**Idiosyncrasy.** Peculiarity of temperament of an individual. प्रकृतिप्रत्यात्मता; प्रकृतिवैशिष्ट्य; संवेदनवैशिष्ट्य; स्वभावगत 'विलक्षणता

**Idiot.** A person with defective mental faculties. जड़बुद्धि; मूर्ख; बेवकूफ; निर्बुद्धि; मूढ़

**Idiotism.** Weakness of intellect from the birth. जड़बुद्धिता; मूर्खता; मूढ़ता; बेवकूफी

**Idioventricular.** Pertaining to the cardiac ventricles. हृद्निलयी; हृद्निलय सम्बन्धी

**Idrosis.** Morbid increase of perspiration; hidrosis. अतिस्वेदलता; स्वेदनाधिक्य; स्वेदाधिक्य; पसीने की अधिकता

**Igneus.** Pertaining to, or containing fire. अग्नि सम्बन्धी अथवा अग्नियुक्त

**Ignipuncture.** The original procedure of closing a retinal break in retinal separation by transfixation of the break with cautery. अग्निछिद्रीकरण

**Ignis.** A fire. अग्नि; आग

**Ileac.** Pertaining to the ileum or to ileus; ileal. शेषान्त्र अथवा आन्त्रावरोध सम्बन्धी

**Ileal.** See **Ileac.**

**Ileectomy.** Excision of the ileum. शेषान्त्रोच्छेदन; शेषान्त्र-उच्छेदन; लघ्वान्त्रोच्छेदन

**Ileitis.** Inflammation of the ileum. शेषान्त्रशोथ; शेषान्त्र-प्रदाह; लघ्वान्त्रशोथ

**Ileo-.** Prefix denoting relationship to the ileum. 'शेषान्त्र' अथवा 'लघ्वान्त्र' का अर्थ देने वाला उपसर्ग

**Ileocaecal.** Pertaining to both ileum and caecum; ileocecal. शेषान्त्रोण्डुकीय; शेषान्त्र-उण्डुकीय; शेषान्त्र तथा अन्धान्त्र सम्बन्धी

**Ileocaecostomy.** Anastomosis of ileum to caecum; ileocecostomy. शेषान्त्र-अन्धान्त्रसम्मिलन

**Ileocecal.** See **Ileocaecal.**

**Ileocecostomy.** See **Ileocaecostomy.**

**Ileocolic.** Pertaining to the ileum and the colon. शेषान्त्रबृहदान्त्रीय; शेषान्त्र तथा बृहदान्त्र सम्बन्धी

**Ileocolitis.** Inflammation of the ileum and the colon. शेषान्त्रबृहदान्त्रशोथ; शेषान्त्र तथा बृहदान्त्र का प्रदाह

**Ileocolostomy.** The formation of a fistula between the ileum and the colon. शेषान्त्रबृहदान्त्र-सम्मिलन

**Ileocystoplasty.** Surgical reconstruction of the bladder. शेषान्त्रमूत्राशयसंधान

**Ileoileostomy.** Surgical establishment of a passage through the abdominal wall into the ileum. शेषान्त्र-उदरसम्मिलन

**Ileopexy.** Surgical fixation of ileum. शेषान्त्रस्थिरीकरण

**Ileoproctostomy.** Surgical establishment of a communication between the ileum and the rectum. शेषान्त्रमलान्त्रसम्मिलन

**Ileorrhaphy.** Suturing the ileum. शेषान्त्रसीवन

**Ileosigmoidostomy.** Surgical establishment of a communication between the ileum and the sigmoid colon. शेषान्त्रावग्रहान्त्रसम्मिलन

**Ileostomy.** The surgical establishment of a passage through the abdominal wall into the ileum. शेषांत्रछिद्रीकरण

**Ileotomy.** Incision into the ileum. शेषान्त्रछेदन

**Ileum.** The lower third portion of the small intestine. शेषान्त्र; लघ्वान्त्र; आंत का निचला आधा भाग

**Ileus.** Intestinal obstruction attended with severe colicky pain, vomiting and often fever and dehydration. आन्त्रावरोध; आन्त्रान्त्रप्रवेश;

    **Adynamic I.,** see **Paralytic Ileus.**

    **Dynamic I.,** obstruction due to spastic contraction of a segment of the bowel; spastic ileus. संस्तम्भी आंत्रावरोध;

    **Mechanical I.,** obstruction of the bowel due to some mechanical cause. भौतिक आन्त्रावरोध;

    **Meconium I.,** intestinal obstruction in the newborn following inspissation of meconium. जातबिष्ठा आन्त्रावरोध;

    **Occlusive I.,** complete mechanical blocking of the intestinal lumen. अन्तर्रोधी आन्त्रावरोध;

    **Paralytic I.,** non-mechanical obstruction of bowel wall; adynamic ileus. घाती आन्त्रावरोध;

**Spastic I.,** see **Dynamic Ileus.**

**Ilia.** Plural of **Ilium.**

**Iliac.** Belonging to the ilium or flanks. श्रोणिफलकीय; श्रोणि अथवा श्रोणिफलक सम्बन्धी;

   **I. Passion,** deep-seated, acute, obstinate pain in the bowels. आन्त्रशूल;

   **I. Region,** the side of the abdomen between ribs and hips. श्रोणि-प्रदेश

**Ilio-.** Prefix denoting relationship to the ilium. 'श्रोणि' अथवा 'श्रोणिफलक' का अर्थ देने वाला उपसर्ग

**Iliococcygeal.** Pertaining to the ilium and the coccyx. श्रोणिपुच्छास्थिक; श्रोणिअनुत्रिकीय; श्रोणिफलक तथा अनुत्रिक (पुच्छास्थि) सम्बन्धी

**Iliofemoral.** Relating to the ilium and the femur. श्रोणिफलक तथा ऊर्विका सम्बन्धी

**Ilioinguinal.** Pertaining to the iliac region and the groin. श्रोणिफलक तथा वंक्षण सम्बन्धी

**Iliolumbar.** Relating to the iliac and the lumbar regions. श्रोणिफलक तथा कटि (कमर) सम्बन्धी

**Iliopectineal.** Pertaining to the ilium and the pectineus muscle (pubis). श्रोणिफलक तथा कंकत पेशी (जघन) सम्बन्धी

**Iliopsoas.** Pertaining to the ilium and the loin. श्रोणिफलक तथा कटिलम्बिका सम्बन्धी;

   **I. Muscles,** the combined iliac and psoas muscles. श्रोणिफलक-कटिलम्बिकायें

**Iliotibial.** Pertaining to the ilium and the tibia. श्रोणिफलक तथा जंघिका सम्बन्धी

**Ilium.** The upper part of the innominate bone, as ilium. श्रोणिफलक; नितम्बास्थि; कूल्हे की हड्डी

**Ill.** Sick; unwell. रुग्ण; अस्वस्थ; बीमार; व्याधिग्रस्त

**Illness.** Sickness; a diseased condition. रुग्णता; अस्वस्थता; व्याधि; बीमारी; स्वास्थ्य की बिगड़ी हुई अवस्था;

   **Compression I.,** decompression sickness. विसम्पीडन रुग्णता

**Illumination.** The act of directing light upon an object. प्रदीप्ति; प्रकाश; रोशनी; ज्योति;

   **Oblique I.,** illumination from one side. तिर्यक् प्रदीप्ति

**Illusion.** A false perception of an object. भ्रम; भ्रांति

**Illusional.** Relating to, or of the nature of an illusion. भ्रामक; भ्रांतिमय

**Illutation.** The act of besmearing any part of the body with mud. कीचालेपन

**Image.** A picture of an object to the eyes or mind. प्रतिबिम्ब; परछाईं;
  **False I.,** the image in the deviating eye in strabismus. कूट प्रतिबिम्ब;
  **Optical I.,** an image formed by the refraction or reflection of light. दृष्टिज-प्रतिबिम्ब;
  **Sensory I.,** an image based on one or more types of sensation. सम्वेदी प्रतिबिम्ब;
  **Tactile I.,** an image of an object as perceived by the sense of touch. स्पर्श-प्रतिबिम्ब;
  **Virtual I.,** the image produced by the imaginary focus of the rays. आभासी प्रतिबिम्ब

**Imagination.** The power of forming mental images. कल्पना

**Imaginary.** Not real; unreal. काल्पनिक; कल्पित

**Imago.** The insect after the completion of its metamorphosis. पूर्णकीट

**Imbalance.** Out of balance; the term refers commonly to the upset of acid-base relationship and the electrolytes in body fluids. असंतुलन; अतुल्यता; असमतोलन

**Imbecile.** Feeble in mind. जड़बुद्धि; मूर्ख; मूढ़; बेवकूफ; अल्पबुद्धि; अल्पमति; जड़मति; मंदबुद्धि

**Imbecility.** Mental defect, or weakness. जड़बुद्धिता; मूढ़ता; मानसिक दुर्बलता

**Imbibition.** The absorption of fluids by solid bodies without chemical changes. अन्तःशोषण; निपान

**Imbricate.** See **Imbricated.**

**Imbricated.** Overlapped, as scales in skin diseases, e.g. shingles; imbricate. कोरछादित

**Immersion.** The plunging of a body into a liquid. निमज्जन; गोता लगाना; डूबना

**Immiscible.** Not capable of being mixed. अमिश्र्य; मिश्रण के अयोग्य

**Immobility.** Stiffness; incapable of motion. अकड़न; जकड़न; ऐंठन

**Immobilization.** The act of rendering a part immobile. अचलीकरण; गतिहीनता

**Immobilize.** To render fixed or incapable of moving. अचल करना; गतिहीन करना

**Immune.** Not susceptible to an infection. रोगक्षम; प्रतिरक्षित

**Immunifacient.** Making immune; producing immunity. रोगक्षमकारी; प्रतिरक्षाकारी; प्रतिरक्षणकारी

**Immunisation.** The process of increasing specific antibody in the tissues; immunization. रोगक्षमीकरण; प्रतिरक्षीकरण; प्रतिरक्षण

**Immunity.** The capacity of the body to resist infection. रोगक्षमता; प्रतिरक्षा;

    **Acquired I.,** that conveyed by recovery from the infectious disease; active immunity. उपार्जित रोगक्षमता; सक्रिय रोगक्षमता;

    **Active I.,** see **Acquired Immunity.**

    **Congenital I.,** that with which the individual is born; natural immunity; genetic immunity; inherent immunity; innate immunity. सहज रोगक्षमता; नैसर्गिक रोगक्षमता; प्राकृतिक रोगक्षमता;

    **General I.,** that associated with widely diffused mechanisms that tend to protect the body as a whole. सार्वदैहिक रोगक्षमता;

    **Genetic I.,** see **Congenital Immunity.**

    **Inherent I.,** see **Congenital Immunity.**

    **Innate I.,** see **Congenital Immunity.**

    **Natural I.,** see **Congenital Immunity.**

    **Passive I.,** that conferred by the introduction of antibodies or vaccines. निष्क्रिय रोगक्षमता; कृत्रिम रोगक्षमता

**Immunization.** See **Immunisation.**

**Immunize.** To render immune. रोगक्षम करना

**Immuno-.** Prefix meaning immune, or relating to immunity. 'रोगक्षम' का अर्थ देने वाला उपसर्ग

**Immunoblast.** An antigenetically stimulated lymphocyte. रोगक्षमप्रसू

**Immunocyte.** A leukocyte capable, actively or potentially, of producing antibodies. रोगक्षमकोशिका

**Immunodeficiency.** Immunological immunity, or immune deficiency. रोगक्षम-अपर्याप्तता

**Immunogen.** Antigen; allergen. रोगक्षमजन; प्रतिरक्षाजन; प्रतिजन

**Immunogenic.** Producing immunity; antigenic. प्रतिजनक; रोगक्षमताजनक; प्रतिरक्षाजनक

**Immunogenicity.** The ability to produce immunity; antigenicity. प्रतिजनकता; रोगक्षमजनकता; प्रतिरक्षाजनकता

**Immunologist.** One versed in the science of immunity. रोगक्षमताविज्ञानी; प्रतिरक्षाविज्ञानी

**Immunology.** The special study of immunity. रोगक्षमताविज्ञान; प्रतिरक्षाविज्ञान

**Immunosuppressant.** Denoting an agent that effects immunosuppression; immunosuppressive. प्रतिरक्षादमनकारी

**Immunosuppression.** Preventing the occurrence of an immune reaction. प्रतिरक्षादमन

**Immunosuppressive.** See **Immunosuppressant.**

**Immunotherapy.** Any treatment used to produce immunity. रोगक्षमताचिकित्सा; रोगक्षमचिकित्सा; प्रतिरक्षाचिकित्सा

**Immunotransfusion.** Transfusion of blood from a donor previously rendered immune by repeated inoculations with given agent from the receipient. प्रतिरक्षीरक्ताधान

**Impacted.** Used in obstetrics, with reference to the head of a child, when fixed in the pelvic cavity. अन्तर्घट्टित

**Impaction.** The blocking of a passage by accumulation of some of its contents. अन्तर्घट्टन; कस कर भरना

**Impalpable.** Not capable of being felt or palpated. अपरिस्पर्शनीय; स्पर्शातीत

**Impar.** Odd or unequal. असम; विषम; अयुग्मी; एकल

**Impatient.** Anxious. अधीर; अशांत

**Impedance.** Obstruction. अवरोध; प्रतिबाधा

**Imperfect.** Incomplete. अपूर्ण; अधूरा; अधूरी

**Imperforate.** Without opening; not open or pervious; natural closure of an opening, as the anus, hymen, etc.; atresic. अछिद्री; छिद्रहीन; अभेद्य; अप्रवेश्य

**Imperforation.** The condition of being imperforate, atretic, occluded, or closed. अछिद्रता; अभेद्यता

**Impermeable.** See **Impervious.**

**Impervious.** Not permitting a passage; impermeable. अछिद्री; छिद्रहीन; अभेद्य; अप्रवेश्य

**Impetiginous.** Relating to impetigo. सपूयचर्मस्फोटीय; सपूयचर्मस्फोटक

**Impetigo.** A superficial highly contagious skin infection. सपूयचर्मस्फोट; पीब वाली फुंसियों से युक्त चर्म रोग;

   **I. Contagiosa,** a contagious form of impetigo. सांसर्गिक सपूयचर्मस्फोट;

   **I. Herpetiformis,** a grave form affecting pregnant women and resembling herpes. परिसर्पी सपूयचर्मस्फोट;

   **I. Neonatorum,** bullous impetigo of the newborn. नवजात सपूयचर्मस्फोट;

   **I. Syphilitica,** a specific form resembling syphilis. उपदंशज सपूयचर्मस्फोट

**Implacental.** Having no placenta. अपराहीन; अपराविहीन

**Implant.** To graft or insert. रोपना; material inserted or grafted into tissues. रोपणशील पदार्थ

**Implantation.** The insertion of living cells or solid materials into the tissues. रोपण; आरोपण

**Imponderables.** Agents having no sensible weights, as light, heat, electricity, magnetism, etc. भारहीन-तत्त्व

**Impotence.** See **Impotency.**

**Impotency.** Absence or failure of sexual function in the males; impotence. नपुंसत्व; नपुंसकता; षण्ढता; नामर्दगी; नामर्दी

**Impotent.** One who lacks the sexual power. नपुंसक; षण्ढ; नामर्द

**Impregnate.** To render pregnant; to fecundate; to cause to conceive. गर्भाधान करना; संसेचन करना

**Impregnation.** Fecundation of ova. गर्भाधान; संसेचन; saturation. संतृप्तीकरण

**Impressio.** See **Impression.**

**Impression.** Impressio; a hollow depression or indentation made by the pressure of one organ on the surface of another. गर्त; खात; an effect produced upon the mind by some external object acting through the organs of sense. प्रभाव; छाप

**Imprint.** A particular kind of learning characterized by its occurrence in the first few hours of life, and which determines species-recongnition behaviour; imprinting. मुद्रा; छाप; चिन्ह; निशान

**Imprinting.** See **Imprint.**

**Impuber.** Not arrived at the adult age. नाबालिग

**Impulse.** The tendency to act without deliberation; a sudden pushing or driving force; the action potential of a nerve fibre. आवेग; धड़कन; झटका; जोर; प्रेरणा; अन्तःप्रेरणा; मनोवेग; धक्का

**Impulsion.** An abnormal urge to perform certain activity, often unpleased. प्रणोदन; संवेग; मनःप्रेरणा

**Impulsive.** Relating to, or actuated by an impulse, rather than controlled by reason. आवेगी; आवेगशील; संवेगशील

**Impurity.** Want of purity; want of clearness. अशुद्धता; अशुचिता; मलिनता; अपद्रव्य; अशुद्धि

**Inactivate.** To destroy the activity or the effects of an agent or substance. निष्क्रिय कर देना

**Inactivation.** The destruction of activity of a body fluid. निष्क्रियण; निष्क्रिय हो जाना

**Inactivity.** Indisposition to action or exertion. निष्क्रियता; क्रियाहीनता

**Inadequacy.** Insufficiency. अपर्याप्तता; अल्पता; कमी

**Inanimate.** Lifeless; dead; not alive. निर्जीव; निष्प्राण

**Inanition.** Exhaustion from want of nourishment. निर्जलान्नता; पोषण-तत्त्व के अभाव में दुर्बल हो जाना

**Inappetence.** Loss or want of appetite; lack of desire or craving. क्षुधाभाव; भूख का अभाव; खान-पान से अरुचि हो जाना

**Inarticulate.** Not articulate in the form of intelligible speech; unable to satisfactorily express oneself in words. अस्पष्ट; अव्यक्त (उच्चारण)

**Inassimilable.** Incapable of assimilation; not assimilable. अस्वांगीकर; अपच्य; स्वांगीकरण के अयोग्य

**Inborn.** Innate; inherited; implanted during development in utero. अंतर्जात

**Inbreeding.** Mating of individuals that are closely related or have very similar genetic constitutions. अन्त:प्रजनन

**Incarcerated.** Imprisoned; confined; strangulated; constricted; trapped; incapable of reduction. बंधित; बाधित

**Incarceration.** Imprisonment of a part. बन्धीकरण; legal confinement. वैध-प्रसव

**Incarnatio.** Becoming flesh; granulation. मांसांकुरण; अंकुरण

**Incest.** Sexual intercourse between blood relations. संगोत्रगमन; खूनी रिश्तों से लैंगिक सम्भोग करना

**Incestuous.** Pertaining to incest. संगोत्रगमन सम्बन्धी

**Incidence.** The number of new cases of a disease in a population over a period of time. आघटन; आंकड़ा

**Incineration.** Cremation; reduction to ashes; destruction by fire. भस्मीकरण; जला कर राख कर देना

**Incipient.** Commencing; beginning. आरभमाण; प्रारम्भिक

**Incisal.** Cutting; relating to the cutting edges of the incisor and cuspid teeth. कृन्तक

**Incise.** To cut with a knife. छिन्न करना; छुरी से काट देना

**Incised.** Applied to wound made with a sharp-edged instrument; cut. छिन्न; उत्कीर्ण;

 I. Wound, the wound made with a sharp-edged instrument. उत्कीर्ण घाव; छिन्न क्षत

**Incision.** Separation of surfaces by a sharp knife; a surgical wound; a cut. छेदन; उत्कीर्णन; कर्तन; भेदन;

 Diagnostic I., see **Exploratory Incision.**

 Exploratory I., section for diagnostic purposes; diagnostic incision. अन्वेषी छेदन

**Incisiva.** Incisor. कृन्तक; अगला दांत

**Incisive.** Cutting; having the power to cut. कृन्तकी; pertaining to incisor teeth. कृन्तक (अगले दांतों) सम्बन्धी

**Incisor.** One of the cutting teeth, or incisor teeth, four in number in each jaw at the apex of the dental arch; incisiva. कृन्तक;

**I. Teeth,** incisors. कृन्तक; अगले आठ दांत

**Incisors.** Plural of **Incisor.**

**Incisura.** An incision, a slit or notch; incisure. भंगिका;
  **I. Cardiaca,** a notch in the anterior border of the left lung. हृद्मुख-भंगिका

**Incisure.** See **Incisura.**

**Inclination.** A leaning or sloping, as of the pelvis. नति; झुकाव

**Inclusion.** The state of being inclosed or included. अन्तर्वेशन; अन्तर्विष्ट; अन्तस्थ

**Incoherent.** Not connected or coherent. असंगत; असम्बद्ध; अनमेल

**Incombustible.** Incapable of being burnt. अदह्य; अदहनीय; दुर्दह्य

**Incompatibility.** Inability to unite. असंगति; असंयोज्यता; जुड़ने की अयोग्यता

**Incompatible.** Not capable of being united in solution. असंयोज्य; denoting persons who cannot freely associate together without resulting anxiety and conflict. असंगत; बेमेल; बेजोड़

**Incompetence.** Inability to perform a natural function; incompetency. अक्षमता; असमर्थता; अयोग्यता

**Incompetency.** See **Incompetence.**

**Inconcocted.** Not fully digested. अपचित; अनपचा

**Incongruity.** Incoordination. असामंजस्य; असंगति

**Inconsistence.** Variable; irregular. अनियमित

**Incontinence.** Incontinentia; inability to retain discharges, as incontinence of urine; involuntary evacuation. असंयति; असंयतता; असंयम

**Incontinentia.** See **Incontinence.**

**Incoordination.** Inability to produce smooth, harmonious muscular movements. असमंजन; असमन्वय; विषमता; समंजन अथवा समन्वय का अभाव

**Incorporation.** The making into a homogenous mass. समावेश; समावेशन; संयोजन

**Incrassation.** Thickness. स्थूलता; मोटापा; मोटाई

**Increment.** A change in the value of a variable, usually an increase. बृद्धि

**Incrustation.** The formation of a crust; a coating of some adventitious material or an exudate; a scab. निर्मोकन; पर्पटीभवन; खुरण्ड बनना; पपड़ियाना; परत चढ़ना; तह जमना

**Incubation.** The period that elapses between the introduction of a morbific principle into the system and the development of disease. उद्भवन; रोगोद्भवन; संक्रमण से लेकर रोग-लक्षण प्रकट होने तक की अवधि; maintenance of controlled environmental conditions for the purpose of favouring growth or development of microbial or tissue cultures of an artificial environment, usually for a premature infant. ऊष्मायन

**Incubator.** A device for rearing prematurely born children, or for the cultivation of bacteria. ऊष्मायित्र

**Incubus.** Nightmare. दुःस्वप्न; an evil spirit which lays upon and oppresses sleeping persons. दुरात्मा

**Incudal.** Relating to the incus. स्थूणक सम्बन्धी

**Incudectomy.** Removal of the incus of the tympanum. स्थूणक-उच्छेदन

**Incudes.** Plural of **Incus**.

**Incudis.** See **Incus**.

**Incurable.** That which is not amenable to any mode of treatment. असाध्य; ठीक न होने वाला

**Incurvation.** An inward curvature; a bending inward. अन्तर्बक्रता; अन्तर्नति

**Incus.** Incudis; the name of one of the three ossicles of the middle ear. स्थूणक; निधात्यस्थिका; मध्यकर्ण की तीन में से एक कोमल हड्डी

**Incyclotropia.** A form of squint in which the vertical median superior pole is constantly inclined inward. अंतश्चक्रीनेत्रविचलन

**Indentation.** A notch, or depression. खांचा

**Indes.** Daily. Abbreviation : **In dies.** हर रोज

**Index.** The ratio of one part to another taken as a standard, guide, indicator, symbol or number. सूचकांक; अंक; सूचक; सूची; forefinger; index finger, i.e. the second finger (the first being the thumb). देशिनी; तर्जनी; अंगूठे के साथ वाली पहली उँगली;

**Alveolar I.,** the degree of prominence of the jaws measured by the basialveolar length multiplied by 100 and divided by the basinasal length. उलूखल सूचकांक;

**Cardiac I.,** the amount of blood ejected by the heart in a unit of time divided by the body surface area. हृद्-सूचकांक;

**Cephalic I.,** the breadth of the skull multiplied by 100 and devided by its length. शीर्ष सूचकांक;

**Cerebral I.,** the ratio of the greatest transverse to the greatest anteroposterior diameter of the cranial cavity. मस्तिष्क सूचकांक;

**Colour I.,** the ratio between the amount of haemoglobin and the number of red blood cells. वर्णांक; रंगांक;

**Gnathic I.,** the ratio of the distance between the basion and the alveolar point to the distance between the basion and nasal point. हनुप्रसर सूचकांक;

**Icterus I.**, the value that indicates the relative level of bilirubin in serum or plasma. कामला सूचकांक;
**Refractive I.**, the coefficient of refraction. अपवर्तक सूचकांक; अपवर्तनी सूचकांक; अपवर्तनांक;
**Saturation I.**, an indication of the relative concentration of haemoglobin in the red blood cells. संतृप्ति सूचकांक; संतृप्तीकरणांक;
**Thoracic I.**, the ratio of anteroposterior diameter to the transverse. वक्ष सूचकांक;
**Vital I.**, the ratio of births to death within a population during a given time. जन्म-मृत्यु सूचकांक
**Indexes.** Plural of **Index**.
**Indian Hemp.** Cannabis indica; hashish. भांग; गांजा
**Indication.** The pointing out of a proper remedy; a sign. संकेत; निर्देश
**Indicator.** A substance that indicates chemic reaction by a colour change. निर्देशक; सूचक; संकेतक (पदार्थ)
**Indices.** Alternative plural of **Index**.
**In dies.** Daily. प्रतिदिन; हर रोज
**Indifferent.** Of no interest. विरक्त; उदासीन; उदास; neutral. निष्पक्ष
**Indiffusible.** Incapable of being diffused. अविसरणीय
**Indigenous.** Native to a certain locality or country. देसी; देशी; स्वदेशी
**Indigestible.** Not digestible. अपच्य; न पचने वाला
**Indigestion.** Digestive distress or upset due to many different causes; dyspepsia. अपच; अजीर्ण; मंदाग्नि; अग्निमांद्य
**Indignation.** Anger excited by meanness. आक्रोश; रोष; क्रोध
**Indigo.** A blue dye-stuff from various species of **Indigo era**. नील; जम्बुकी
**Indirect.** Not direct. अप्रत्यक्ष; परोक्ष
**Indisposition.** Slight disorder of the healthy functions of the body. अस्पृहा; अरुचि; विरक्ति
**Indium.** A metallic element. इण्डियम; एक धातु
**Indol.** See **Indole**.
**Indole.** A product of intestinal putrefaction, basis of many biologically active substances. इण्डोल; आंतों की पीब का एक उत्पाद
**Indolence.** Sluggishness; tiredness. अकर्मण्यता; आलस
**Indolent.** Inactive; sluggish; slow of action; painless or nearly so. अकर्मण्य; आलसी; मन्दरोही
**Induction.** The act of bringing on or causing to occur. प्रेरण; प्रेरणा; production or causation. उत्पादन या कारण

**Inductor.** An agent bringing about induction. प्रेरक; an organizer. संचालक

**Indurated.** Hardened, usually used with reference to soft tissues becoming extremely firm but not as hard as bone. कठोर; दृढ़

**Induration.** Hardness. कठोरता; दृढ़ता; process or state of becoming extremely hard or firm. दृढ़ीभवन;
   **Black I.,** the hard, pigmented condition of the lungs in anthracosis. श्याम दृढ़ता;
   **Brown I.,** a hardening of the lung-tissue with deposition of pigmented matter. बभ्रु दृढ़ता;
   **Cyanotic I.,** induration related to persistent, chronic venous congestion in an organ or tissue. श्याव दृढ़ता;
   **Grey I.,** a condition occurring in lungs during and after pneumonic process. धूसर दृढ़ता;
   **Red I.,** a condition observed in lungs in which there is an advanced degree of acute passive congestion, acute pneumonitis, or a similar pathologic process. लोहित दृढ़ता

**Indurative.** Pertaining to induration. दृढ़ता अथवा कठोरता सम्बन्धी; causing, or characterized by induration. दृढ़ीभूत

**Inebriants.** Intoxicating substances. मादक पदार्थ; नशीली चीजें

**Inebriates.** Alcoholics; drunkards. पियक्कड़; शराबी

**Inebriation.** Intoxication, as by alcohol; inebriety. मदहोशी; मतवालापन

**Inebriety.** See **Inebriation.**

**Inelastic.** Not elastic. अप्रत्यास्थ; लोचहीन

**Inert.** Having no action; slow in action; sluggish; devoid of active chemical properties; having no pharmacologic or therapeutic action. निष्क्रिय; जड़; गतिहीन; निश्चल

**Inertia.** Inactivity or lack of force; lack of mental or physical vigour. जड़ता; जड़त्व; निश्चेष्टता; निष्क्रियता; निश्चलता; क्रियाहीनता; गतिहीनता

**Inertness.** Inactivity. जड़ता; निष्क्रियता; निश्चेष्टता; निश्चलता; गतिहीनता

**In extremis.** At the point of death. आसन्नमृत्यु; मरणासन्न; मृत्यु के कगार पर

**Infancy.** Early childhood; generally covering the age from birth to seventh month. शैशव; बचपन

**Infant.** A baby or young child under the age of one year. शिशु; बच्चा;
   **Liveborn I.,** the product of a livebirth. सप्राणजात शिशु;
   **Stillborn I.,** an infant who shows no evidence of life after birth. निष्प्राणजात शिशु; मृतजात शिशु

**Infanticide.** The murder of an infant. शिशुहत्या; शिशुवध

**Infantile.** Relating to infancy. शैशवकालीन; शैशव अथवा शिशु सम्बन्धी; बच्चों का;

   **I. Convulsions,** general clonic, epileptiform acute spasms occurring during infancy and childhood. शिशु-आक्षेप;

   **I. Paralysis,** acute anterior poliomyelitis. शिशु-अंगघात; पोलियो;

   **I. Skull,** an undeveloped skull. शिशुकरोटि; अविकसित खोपड़ी;

   **I. Uterus,** an undeveloped womb. शिशु-गर्भाशय; शिशु-जरायु; अविकसित जरायु

**Infantilism.** The persistence of infantile characteristics into the adult life. शिशुता; शैशव;

   **Sexual I.,** failure to develop secondary sexual characteristics after the normal time of puberty. संगम-शिशुता

**Infarct.** An area of the tissue-death due to blocking of its blood supply, usually referred to the heart. रोधगलितांश

**Infarction.** The production of an infarct. रोधगलन; रोधगलितांशोत्पत्ति;

   **Cardiac I.,** infarction of an area of the heart muscle; myocardial infarction. हृद्रोधगलन; हृत्पेशीरोधगलन;

   **Myocardial I.,** see **Cardiac Infarction.**

**Infect.** To communicate germs of a disease. संक्रमण होना या करना

**Infection.** Invasion of the body by germs, viruses or parasites. संक्रमण; संसर्ग; उपसर्ग; छूत की बीमारी;

   **Cross I.,** infection spread from one source to another. पारसंक्रमण;

   **Droplet I.,** infection acquired through the inhalation of droplets or sputum containing micro-organisms expelled by another person. बिन्दुक संक्रमण;

   **Focal I.,** an old term that distinguishes local infections from generalized infections. विकारस्थानिक संक्रमण

**Infectious.** Capable of being communicated by contact or otherwise infective. संक्रामक; संक्रामी; सांसर्गिक; औपसर्गिक

**Infective.** Disease transmissible from one host to another. संक्रमी; संक्रामी; सांसर्गी; औपसर्गी;

   **I. Hepatitis,** catarrhal jaundice. संक्रामी यकृत्शोथ; प्रतिश्यायी कामला

**Infectsiosa.** An infectious disease. संक्रामक रोग; छूत से फैलने वाला रोग

**Infecundity.** Sterility; barrenness. बंध्यता; बांझपन

**Inferior.** Lower; beneath; situated below or directed downward; situated nearer the soles of the feet in relation to a specific reference point. अधः; निम्न; घटिया; निचला;

   **I. Organs,** lower parts of the body. अधोअंग; निम्नांग

**Inferiority.** The condition or state of being or feeling inadequate or inferior. हीनता; हीनभावना

**Infertile.** Sterile; unable to become a parent. बंध्य; बांझ; अनुर्वर

**Infertility.** Inability to become a parent; relative sterility; diminished or absent fertility. बंध्यता; बांझपन; प्रसवन-अशक्ति; अनुर्वरता

**Infest.** To infect. रोगसंक्रमण करना; बीमारी फैलाना

**Infestation.** The presence of animal parasites in or on the human body; the act or process of infesting. पर्याक्रमण; जन्तुबाधा

**Infiltrate.** To ooze into interstitial spaces of a tissue. अन्त:संचरण करना या होना; to percolate; to enter or cause to enter the pores of a substance, denoting a liquid. परिस्राव होना; रिसाव होना

**Infiltration.** The entering of fluid into a serous part of the body; the act of passing into or interpenetrating a substance, cell, or tissue; the gas fluid, or dissolved matter that has entered any substance, cell or tissue. अन्त:संचरण; अन्त:स्यन्दन; परिस्राव; रिसाव;
**Adipose I.,** growth of normal adult fat cells in sites where they are not usually present. मेदुर अन्त:संचरण;
**Fatty I.,** a deposit of fat in the tissues or the presence of oil in the interior of a cell. वसीय अन्त:संचरण

**Infinite.** Immeasurable. सूक्ष्म; अमाप्य

**Infinitesimal.** The lowest quantity. सूक्ष्मातिसूक्ष्म

**Infirm.** Weak; feeble. दुर्बल; कमजोर; शिथिल

**Infirmar.** See **Infirmary.**

**Infirmary.** A small hospital, especially in an institution for the care of chronic patients; infirmar. जीर्णरोगीशाला

**Infirmity.** A weakness; an abnormal, more or less disabling, condition of mind or body. दुर्बलता; कमजोरी; शैथिल्य; शिथिलता

**Inflame.** To undergo inflammation. शोथमय अथवा शोथग्रस्त होना

**Inflammation.** A redness or swelling of any part of the body, usually attended with heat, pain and fever. शोथ; प्रदाह; शरीर के किसी भाग की लाली या सूजन, जिसके साथ प्राय: उत्ताप, दर्द और ज्वर विद्यमान रहता है;
**Acute I.,** any inflammation that has a fairly rapid onset and then relatively soon comes to a crisis, with clear and distinct termination. तरुण शोथ; उग्र प्रदाह;
**Catarrhal I.,** inflammation occurring on a mucous surface and causing the shedding of its epithelium. श्लेष्मस्रावी शोथ; प्रतिश्यायीशोथ
**Chronic I.,** that in which there is a formation of new connective tissue. चिरकारी शोथ; चिरशोथ; चिर प्रदाह; जीर्ण प्रदाह;

**Exudative I.,** inflammation in which the conspicuous or distinguishing feature is an exudate, which may be chiefly serous, serofibrinous, fibrinous, or mucous. निःस्रावी शोथ;

**Fibrinous I.,** an exudative inflammation in which there is a disproportionately large amount of fibrin. फाइब्रिनी शोथ;

**Purulent I.,** see **Suppurative Inflammation.**

**Serous I.,** an exudative inflammation in which the exudate is predominantly fluid. सीरमी शोथ; सीरमी प्रदाह;

**Subacute I.,** an inflammation intermediate in duration between an acute inflammation and a chronic inflammation. अनुतीव्र शोथ; अर्धजीर्ण शोथ;

**Suppurative I.,** that attended by formation of pus; purulent inflammation. सपूय शोथ;

**Toxic I.,** that due to poison. विषण्ण शोथ; किसी विषाक्त अवस्था के कारण होने वाला प्रदाह

**Inflammatory.** Affected with, or pertaining to inflammation. शोथयुक्त; शोथज; प्रदाहक

**Inflation.** Swelling up or distention, especially by air or any gaseous body; vesiculation. वातस्फीति; वातप्रधमन; वायुसंचय; स्फीति; हवा भर जाना; फुलाव

**Inflection.** A bending inward; inflexion. अन्तर्नति; अन्दर की ओर मुड़ा हुआ या घूमा हुआ

**Inflexion.** See **Inflection.**

**Influenza.** A group of various respiratory infections, commonly called flu; la grippe. इन्फ्लुएंजा; श्लैष्मिक ज्वर

**Influenzal.** Relating to, or marked by, or resulting from, influenza. इन्फ्लुएंजा सम्बन्धी; इन्फ्लुएंजापरक; इन्फ्लुएंजाजनित

**Influx.** An inflow. अन्तर्वाह; रेल-पेल

**Infra-.** Prefix denoting a position below the part denoted by the word to which it is joined. 'अव', 'नीचे', 'निचला' का अर्थ देने वाला उपसर्ग

**Infra-axillary.** Situated below the axilla. अवकक्षी; कांख के नीचे स्थित

**Infracardiac.** Below the heart. अवहृदयी

**Infraclavicular.** Relating to the clavicle. अवजत्रुकी; जत्रुक सम्बन्धी

**Infraclusion.** See **Infraocclusion.**

**Infracostal.** Under the ribs. अवपर्शुकी; पसलियों के नीचे

**Infraction.** Incomplete fracture of a bone. अपूर्णास्थिभंग

**Infrahyoid.** Below the hyoid bone. अवकंठिकी; कण्ठास्थि के नीचे

**Inframarginal.** Below any margin or edge. अवसीमांतक

**Inframaxillary.** Below the jaw. अवहनुज; जबड़े के नीचे
**Infraocclusion.** Failure of apposition of one or more teeth when the jaws are closed; infraclusion; infraversion. अवअधिधारण
**Infraorbital.** Below the orbital cavity. अवनेत्रगुही; नेत्रगुहा अथवा चक्षुगह्वर के नीचे
**Infrapatellar.** Pertaining to parts below the patella. अवजानुफलकीय; जानुफलक के निचले भागों सम्बन्धी
**Infrapsychic.** Denoting ideas or actions originating below the level of consciousness. अवमनोजात
**Infrared.** Beyond the red end of the spectrum. अवरक्तीय
**Infrasonic.** Pertaining to sounds with frequencies below the human range of hearing. अवध्वनिक
**Infraspinous.** Below the scapular spine. अवकण्टकी; कंधे की रीढ़ की हड्डी के नीचे
**Infratrochlear.** Below the trochlea. अवचक्रकी
**Infraversion.** A turning downward; rotation of both eyes downward; infraocclusion. अववर्तन
**Infricetur.** Rub it. इसे मलिये
**Infundibula.** Plural of **Infundibulum.**
**Infundibular.** Pertaining to the infundibulum. कीपविषयक; कीप सम्बन्धी; infundibuliform. कीपाकार
**Infundibulectomy.** Excision of the infundibulum. कीपोच्छेदन
**Infundibuliform.** Funnel-shaped; choanoid. कीपाकार
**Infundibuloma.** A tumour of the infundibulum. कीपार्बुद
**Infundibulum.** A funnel or funnel-shaped passage. कीप; कीपमार्ग
**Infused.** Steeped. भीगा हुआ; तर; extracted. निस्सारित
**Infusible.** Incapable of being fused. अद्राव्य; अघुलनशील; घुलने के अयोग्य
**Infusion.** Fluid flowing by gravity into the body. फांट; आधान; अर्क
**Infusor.** An instrument for slow injection of liquid into a vein. आधानक
**Infusum.** An aqueous preparation made by steeping a vegetable substance in water without boiling. आधान; फांट; अर्क
**Ingesta.** Substances taken into the body, as food and drink. अन्नपान; भोजन; खाद्य अथवा पेय पदार्थ
**Ingestion.** The act of taking food or medicine into the stomach; the taking in of particles by phagocyte cells. अशन; अन्तर्ग्रहण
**Ingestive.** Relating to ingestion. अन्तर्ग्रहण सम्बन्धी
**Ingravescent.** Increasing in severity. दु:साध्य

**Ingredient.** Any part of a compound. अवयव; घटकांग

**Ingrowing Toenail.** Spreading of the nail into the lateral tissue, causing inflammation. अन्तर्वर्धी-नख; नखान्त:बृद्धि

**Inguen.** The groin. वंक्षण; ऊरु

**Inguinal.** Belonging to the groin. वंक्षणीय; वंक्षणपरक; वंक्षण सम्बन्धी;
   **I. Hernia,** hernia through an abdominal ring. वंक्षण हर्निया

**Inguinodynia.** Pain in the groin. वंक्षणार्ति

**Inhalant.** That which is inhaling; insufflation; finely powdered or liquid drugs that are carried to the respiratory passages by the use of special devices. नि:श्वसनी; सूंघने की दवा

**Inhalation.** The act of inhaling or breathing in; inspiration. अभिश्वसन; अन्त:श्वसन; श्वास लेना

**Inhale.** Inspire; to draw in breath. श्वास लेना

**Inhaler.** The apparatus for inhalation; respirator. श्वासित्र; श्वास लेने का यंत्र

**Inherent.** Natural; ancestoral; innate; inborn. प्राकृतिक; वंशगत; वंशागत; वंशानुगत; आनुवंशिक; विरासती

**Inheritance.** Characters or qualities that are transmitted from parents to offspring; that which is so transmitted. वंशागति

**Inherited.** Derived from an ancestor; transmitted by inheritance; inborn. वंशागत; वंशगत; आनुवंशिक; विरासती

**Inhibit.** To curb or restrain. संदमन करना; रोकना

**Inhibition.** Loss or partial loss of function either mental or physical as a result of mental influence. संदमन; निरोध; निषेध

**Inhibitor.** An agent that restricts or retards physiologic, chemical or enzymatic action; a nerve, stimulation of which represses activity. संदमी; संदमक; निरोधक; निषेधक

**Inhibitory.** Having the power to retain; restraining; tending to inhibit. संदमी; संदमक; निरोधक; निषेधक

**Inion.** The external protuberance of the occiput. पश्चकपालबिन्दु; मन्यासन्धिबिन्दु

**Initial.** Beginning. प्रारम्भिक; आरभमाण

**Initis.** Inflammation of fibrous tissue. तन्तुऊतिशोथ; myositis. पेशीशोथ

**Inject.** To introduce into the body. इंजेक्शन लगाना; अन्त:क्षेपण करना; सुई लगाना

**Injected.** Congested; having the blood-vessels visibly distended with blood. रक्तिम; denoting a fluid introduced into the body. इंजेक्शन लगाना

**Injection.** The act of throwing a liquid into the part. अन्त:क्षेपण;

इंजेक्शन्; सूचिकाभरण; congestion in hyperaemia. रक्तसंलयन

**Injury.** A wound or hurt or any damage to body. क्षति; क्षतिग्रस्तता; अभिघात; चोट; घाव

**Inlet.** Enterance; a passage leading into a cavity. अन्तर्गम

**Innate.** Inborn; dependent on genetic constitution. प्राकृतिक; स्वाभाविक; नैसर्गिक; वंशगत; वंशानुगत; अन्तर्जात; पैत्रिक; कुदरती

**Innervation.** The nervous influence necessary for the maintenance of life and the functions of various organs. तंत्रिकाप्रेरण; तंत्रिकावितरण; तंत्रिकाविन्यास

**Innidiation.** The growth and multiplication of abnormal cells in another location to which they have been transported by means of lymph or the blood stream, or both. विस्थानी-कोशिकता

**Innocent.** Benign; not malignant; not apparently harmful. सुदम; सौम्य; free from moral wrong. अनभिज्ञ; निर्दोष

**Innocuous.** Harmless. अहानिकर; अनपकारी

**Innominate.** Nameless; applied to several anatomical structures. अनामी; बेनाम;
  **I. Bone**, the hip-bone including the pubis, ilium and ischium. नितम्बास्थि; श्रोणिफलक

**Innominatus.** Having no name. अनामी; बेनाम

**Innutrition.** A want of nutrition. पोषणाभाव; अपुष्टि; पोषाहार का अभाव

**Inoculability.** The quality of being inoculable. टीकाग्राहिता; टीकाव्याधिक्षमता

**Inoculable.** Susceptible to a disease transmissible by inoculation. टीकाग्राही; टीकाव्याधिक्षम

**Inoculate.** To introduce the agent of a disease or other antigenic material into the subcutaneous tissue or a blood vessel or through an abraded or absorbing surface for preventive, curative, or experimental purposes. टीका लगाना; to implant micro-organisms or infectious material into or upon culture media. रोपण करना; to communicate a disease by transferring its virus. संरोपण करना

**Inoculation.** The introduction of specific virus into the system. टीका; टीकाकरण; संरोपण; टीका लगाना

**Inoculum.** The micro-organism or other material introduced by inoculation. संरोप

**Inocuous.** Harmless. अहानिकर; लाभदायक

**Inodorous.** Having no smell. निर्गन्ध; गन्धहीन

**Inoma.** Fibrous tumour. तन्त्वबुंद; तान्तवार्बुद

**Inoperable.** Denoting that which cannot be operated upon, or cannot be corrected or removed by an operation. शस्त्रकर्म-अयोग्य;

शस्त्रकर्म-असाध्य

**Inorganic.** Not formed by living organism; not organic. अकार्बनिक; अजैवी

**Inoscopy.** A method for the detection of the tubercle bacilli in any exudate. यक्ष्माणुदर्शन

**Inosculation.** The union of the extremities of blood vessels. योजन; योग; आपस में मिल जाना अथवा जुड़ जाना

**Inotropic.** Pertaining to influences which modify the contractility of the heart. पेशीप्रेरक; पेश्याकुंचप्रभावी; बलप्रभावी

**In phiala.** In a phial or bottle. बोतल में; शीशी में

**Inquest.** The legal inquiry held by a coroner into the cause of sudden or unexpected death. अपमृत्युसमीक्षा; अपमृत्युमीमांसा; मृत्युसमीक्षा; मृत्युविचारण

**Inquisition.** The systemic legal investigation. अन्वेषण; छान-बीन; तहकीकात; समीक्षा; खोज

**Insalivation.** A mixture of food with saliva during mastication. लालामिश्रण; लारमिश्रण

**Insane.** Diseased in mind; crazy; mad. विक्षिप्त; उन्मत्त; पागल;
  **General Paralysis of I.,** involvement of the brain by syphilitic infection with consequent dementia. पागल का व्यापक अंगघात

**Insanitary.** Not sanitary or healthful. अस्वास्थ्यकर; स्वास्थ्य के अयोग्य

**Insanity.** Madness; unsoundness of mind. विक्षिप्ति; उन्मत्तता; पागलपन; मानसरोग;
  **Acquired I.,** that arising after a long period of mental integrity. उपार्जित उन्मत्तता;
  **Circular I.,** a form recurring in cycles, melancholy following mania and that followed by a lucid interval; cyclic insanity. चक्री उन्मत्तता;
  **Communicated I.,** that transmitted by association with an insane person. साहचर्य मानसरोग;
  **Cyclic I.,** see **Circular Insanity.**
  **Impulsive I.,** that marked by uncontrollable desire to commit violence. संवेगी मानसरोग;
  **Moral I.,** a form marked by depravity. नैतिक मानसरोग

**Insatiable.** Not to be satisfied. अतृप्त; अतृप्य; अतोषणीय

**Inscription.** The ingredient part of a prescription. अन्त:निर्देश; अन्तर्निर्देश; औषधि-निर्देश

**Insect.** Articulated animals that have six legs, never more than four wings. कीट; कीटाणु;

**I. Repellent,** a preparation to be applied to skin for the purpose of discouraging biting insects. कीटनिवारक पदार्थ; कीटाणुनाशक पदार्थ

**Insecticide.** An gent destructive to insects. कीटनाशी; कीटनाशक; कीटाणुनाशक

**Insecurity.** A feeling of unprotectedness and helplessness. असुरक्षा

**Insemination.** Introduction of semen into the vagina, normally by sexual intercourse; semination. शुक्रसेचन; वीर्यरोपण;

**Artificial I.,** the introduction of semen of the husband or of another into the vagina otherwise than through the act of coitus. कृत्रिम शुक्रसेचन

**Insensibility.** Loss or absence of sensations. संज्ञाहीनता; सम्वेदनाभाव

**Insensible.** Devoid of sensibility; unconscious. संज्ञाहीन; सम्वेदनाहीन; बेहोश

**Insertion.** The act of setting or placing in. निवेश; अन्तर्न्यास

**Insidious.** Coming on stealthily and imperceptibly; hidden; latent; treacherous. प्रच्छन्न; अदृश; अलक्ष्य; गुप्त

**Insight.** Ability to accept one's limitations but at the same time to develop one's potentialities. अन्तर्दृष्टि; सूक्ष्मदृष्टि; तीक्ष्णदृष्टि

**In situ.** In a given or natural position; confined to site or origin. स्वस्थानी; यथावत्; अपने स्थान पर

**Insolation.** Sun-stroke. सूर्याभिताप; सूर्याघात; सूर्यातप; लू लगना

**Insoluble.** Not capable of being dissolved. अविलेय; अघुलनशील; घुलने के अयोग्य

**Insomnia.** An unnatural deficiency or loss of sleep; wakefulness; sleeplessness. निद्रालोप; अनिद्रा; नींद न आने की बीमारी

**Insomniac.** One who has insomnia. अनिद्राग्रस्त

**Inspection.** Examination by naked eyes. परिदर्शन; जांच; निरीक्षण

**Inspersion.** Sprinkling with a fluid or a powder. छिड़काव

**Inspiration.** Intake of breath; inhalation. अन्तःश्वसन; प्रश्वसन; श्वास लेना

**Inspiratory.** Pertaining to inspiration. प्रश्वसनीय; श्वास लेने अथवा प्रश्वसन सम्बन्धी

**Inspire.** To take breath; inhale. प्रश्वसन करना; श्वास लेना; सांस लेना

**Inspissated.** Thickened; rendered thicker by evaporation. शुष्कीकृत; शुष्कित; सांद्रित; सघन; घनीभूत; गाढ़ा

**Inspissation.** The act of thickening by evaporation or by the absorption of fluid. शुष्कीकरण; सान्द्रण

**Instep.** The arch of foot on the dorsal surface. पादकमान; पैर का ऊपरी

भाग टखने और उँगलियों के बीच होना

**Instill.** To insert by drops. बिन्दुपात करना; बूंद-बूंद करके डालना

**Instillandus.** Put a drop. एक बूंद डालिये

**Instillation.** Insertion of drops into a cavity. बिन्दुपातन; टपकाना; किसी गह्वर के अन्दर बूंद-बूंद करके टपकाना

**Instinct.** An inborn tendency to act in certain way in a given situation. मूलप्रवृत्ति; सहजवृत्ति; प्रवृत्ति;
  **Death I.,** the instinct of all living creatures toward self-destruction, death, or a return to the inorganic lifelessness from which they arose; instinctia. मृत्यु सहजवृत्ति;
  **Life I.,** the instinct of self-preservation and sexual procreation. जीवन प्रवृत्ति

**Instinctia.** See **Instinct.**

**Instinctive.** Prompted by natural impulse. सहजवृत्तिक; सहजज्ञानमूलक; relating to instinct. प्रवृत्ति अथवा सहजवृत्ति सम्बन्धी

**Instinctual.** The same as **Instinctive.**

**Instrument.** A mechanical tool used in surgery. यंत्र; उपकरण

**Instrumental.** Pertaining to an instrument. यांत्रिक; यंत्र अथवा उपकरण सम्बन्धी

**Instrumentarium.** A collection of instruments and other equipments for an operation or for a medical procedure. उपकरणसंग्रह; उपकरणसमूह

**Instrumentation.** The care and use of instruments. उपकरण-प्रयोग

**Insudate.** Oedematous swelling within an arterial wall. धमनीप्राचीरशोफ

**Insufficiency.** Incapacity of normal action; lack of completeness of function or of power; incompetence. अपर्याप्तता; कमी;
  **Adrenocortical I.,** loss of adrenocortical function. अधिवृक्कप्रान्तस्था अपर्याप्तता;
  **Aortic I.,** see **Valvular Insufficiency.**
  **Cardiac I.,** myocardial insufficiency; inability of heart muscles to function normally. हृद्-अपर्याप्तता; हृत्पेशी-अपर्याप्तता;
  **Coronary I.,** inadequate coronary circulation leading to anginal pain. हृद्धमनी अपर्याप्तता;
  **Mitral I.,** see **Valvular Insufficiency.**
  **Myocardial I.,** see **Cardiac Insufficiency.**
  **Pulmonary I.,** see **Valvular Insufficiency.**
  **Tricuspid I.,** see **Valvular Insufficiency.**
  **Valvular I.,** failure of the cardiac valves to close perfectly; aortic insufficiency; mitral insufficiency; pulmonary insufficiency;

**Insufflate** 580

tricuspid insufficiency. हृत्कपाटीय अपर्याप्तता;

**Venous I.**, inadequate drainage of venous blood from a part. शैरिक अपर्याप्तता

**Insufflate.** To blow into. प्रधमन करना; नाक आदि में फूंक मार कर दवा पहुँचाना

**Insufflation.** Blowing powder into a cavity. प्रधमन; inhalant. निःश्वसनी; सूंघने की दवा; the act or process of insufflating. प्रश्वसन; श्वास खींचना

**Insufflator.** An instrument used for insufflation. प्रधमनित्र; श्वास लेने का यंत्र

**Insula.** The oval-shaped region of the cerebral cortex. द्वीपिका

**Insular.** Pertaining to any insula. द्वीपिकी; denoting an islandlike structure. द्वीपिकाकार; isolated in condition. पृथक्कृत

**Insulation.** Cutting off of the communication with other bodies. रोधन; पृथक्करण; विसंवाहन

**Insulator.** A non-conductor. रोधी; पृथक्कारी

**Insuli.** Plural of **Insula.**

**Insulin.** The internal secretion of the islets of Langerhans, situated within the pancreas; its deficiency causes diabetes mellitus. इन्सुलिन; अग्न्याशय का एक द्रव्य जिसकी कमी से मधुमेह रोग हो जाता है

**Insulinaemia.** See **Insulinemia.**

**Insulinemia.** Abnormally large concentrations of insulin in the circulating blood; insulinaemia. अतिइन्सुलिनरक्तता; रक्त में इन्सुलिन की अधिकता

**Insulogenesis.** Production of insulin by the islets of Langerhans. इन्सुलिनजनन; इन्सुलिनोत्पादन

**Insulinogenic.** Relating to insulinogenesis; insulogenic. इन्सुलिनजनक अथवा इन्सुलिनजनन सम्बन्धी

**Insulinoma.** Adenoma of the islets of Langerhans in the pancreas; insuloma. द्वीपिका-कोशिकार्बुद

**Insulogenic.** See **Insulinogenic.**

**Insulitis.** A histologic change in which the islets of Langerhans are oedematous and contain small numbers of leukocytes. द्वीपिकाकोशिकाशोथ

**Insuloma.** See **Insulinoma.**

**Insult.** An injury, attack or trauma. क्षति, आक्रमण अथवा चोट

**Insusceptibility.** Immunity. रोगक्षमता; अग्राहकता

**Integration.** The state of being combined, or the process of combining, into a complete and harmonious whole. समाकलन

**Integrity.** Soundness or completeness of structure; a sound or unimpaired condition. सम्पूर्णता; पूर्णता; अखण्डता

**Integument.** A covering, especially the skin. अध्यावरण; त्वचा; आवरण; शरीर को ढकने वाला प्राकृतिक आवरण (चर्म)

**Integumentary.** Relating to, or composed of integuments. अध्यावरणी; त्वचा सम्बन्धी

**Intellect.** Reasoning power; thinking faculty. प्रज्ञा; बुद्धि; सहजज्ञान

**Intellectualization.** An unconscious defence mechanism. बौद्धिकरण; मनीषीकरण

**Intelligence.** Inborn mental ability. प्रज्ञा; बुद्धि; सहजज्ञान

**Intemperence.** Immoderate indulgence to appetite, especially to alcoholic drinks. मद्यात्यय

**Intensity.** A high tension, energy or activity. तीव्रता; उच्च तनाव, ऊर्जा अथवा कार्य; extension. विस्तार; प्रसार; फैलाव

**Intensive Care Unit.** See **I.C.U.**

**Intention.** An objective. चेष्टा; a process or operation, in surgery. शल्यकर्म

**Inter-.** Prefix signifying between, and or denoting intervals. 'अन्तरा' का अर्थ देने वाला उपसर्ग

**Interatrial.** Between two atrias of the heart; interauricular. अन्तरा-अलिन्दी

**Interauricular.** See **Interatrial.**

**Interbody.** Between the bodies of two adjacent vertebrae. अन्तरापिण्ड

**Intercadence.** The occurrence of an extra beat between the two regular pulse beats; extreme dicrotism; interpolated extrasystole. अन्तरास्पन्द

**Intercadent.** Irregular in rhythm; characterized by intercadence. अन्तरास्पन्दी

**Intercalary.** Occurring between two others, as in pulse tracing. अन्तरानिविष्ट; बीचों-बीच

**Intercalated.** Inserted between two others; intercalatus. अन्तरानिहित; अन्तर्विष्ट

**Intercalatus.** See **Intercalated.**

**Intercellular.** Situated between the cells. अन्तराकोशिकी; कोशिकाओं के बीचों-बीच

**Interchondral.** Between cartilages. अन्तरोपास्थिक; उपस्थियों के बीचों-बीच

**Interclavicular.** Between the clavicles. अन्तराजत्रुकी; जत्रुकों के बीचों-बीच

**Intercondylar.** See **Intercondyloid.**

**Intercondyloid.** Between the condyles; intercondylar. अन्तरास्थाणुक

**Intercostal.** Between the ribs. अन्तरापर्शुकी; पसलियों के बीच

**Intercourse.** Communication or dealings between two or among more people. संगम; सम्पर्क; रति; भोग; interchange of ideas. परस्पर व्यवहार;

**Sexual I.,** coitus; coition. सम्भोग; रतिक्रिया; मैथुन

**Intercristal.** Between the surmounting ridges of a bone, an organ, or a process. अन्तराशिखी

**Intercurrent.** Occurring between; intervening. मध्यवर्ती; अन्त:प्रवाही; अन्तर्वर्ती

**Interdental.** Between the teeth; denoting the relationship between the proximal surfaces of the teeth of the same arch. अन्तरादन्ती

**Interdigit.** That part of the sloping extremity of the hand or foot lying between any two adjacent fingers or toe. अन्तरांगुलि

**Interdigital.** Between the fingers. अन्तरांगुलिक; उँगलियों के बीच

**Interdigitation.** The mutual interlocking of toothed or tonguelike processes. अन्तरांगुलन

**Interface.** A surface that forms a common boundary of bodies. अन्तरापृष्ठ

**Interictal.** Denoting the interval between convulsions. अन्तराक्षेपी

**Interlobar.** Between the lobes. अन्तराखण्डी; खण्डों के बीच

**Interlobitis.** Inflammation of the pleura, separating two pulmonary lobes. अन्तराखण्डशोथ

**Interlobular.** Between the lobules. अन्तराखण्डकी; खण्डकों के बीच

**Intermaxillary.** Between the maxillary bones. अन्तराहनुज; अन्तराहनुक; जबड़े की हड्डियों के बीच

**Intermediate.** Between two extremes; intermedius; interposed. माध्यमिक; मध्य; मध्यवर्ती

**Intermedius.** See **Intermediate.**

**Intermission.** An interval. मध्यान्तर; intermittency. सविरामता

**Intermittency.** See **Intermission.**

**Intermittent.** Ceasing at intervals, as an intermittent fever. सविराम; सविरामी; विरामी;

**I. Fever,** a fever with periods of apyrexia. सविराम ज्वर; विरामी ज्वर

**Intermitting.** Ceasing for a time. विरामी; सविरामी; कुछ समय के लिये रुक जाने वाला

**Intern.** A young physician, graduated from medical school who is gaining experience in a hospital; interne. अन्त:शिशु; रेजीडेण्ट डाक्टर; गृह चिकित्सक; निवासी चिकित्सक

**Internal.** Inward; interior. आन्तरिक; आभ्यन्तर; आन्तर;
   **I. Medicine,** the speciality concerned with illnesses of non-surgical nature, mainly in adults. आन्तर-चिकित्सा;
   **I. Piles,** the blind haemorrhoids. वातार्श;
   **I. Respiration,** that portion of the respiration process which takes place inside the organism. अन्त:श्वसन;
   **I. Skeleton,** bony frame-work inside of the body which grows with the body, as in man. अन्त:पंजर; आन्तरकंकाल

**Interne.** See **Intern.**

**Interneuronal.** Lying between neurons. अन्तरातंत्रिकाणुक; तंत्रिकाणुओं के बीच स्थित

**Interneurons.** Combinations or groups of neurons between sensory and motor neurons which govern coordinated activity. अन्तरातंत्रिकाणु

**Intermist.** A physician trained in intenal medicine. आन्तरचिकित्सक

**Internoctem.** During night. रात में

**Internode.** The space between adjacent nodes. अन्तरापर्व

**Internuclear.** Between nerve cell groups in the brain or retina. अन्तराकेन्द्रकी

**Internus.** Internal. आभ्यन्तर; आन्तरिक

**Interoceptive.** Relating to the sensory nerve cells innervating the viscera, their sensory end-organs, or the information they convey to the spinal cord and the brain. अन्त:सम्वेदी; अन्तरासम्वेदी

**Interoceptor.** One of the various forms of small sensory end-organs situated within the walls of the respiratory and gastrointestinal tracts or in other viscera. अन्त:सम्वेदक; अन्तर्ग्राही

**Interosseous.** Between bones. अन्तरास्थिक; हड्डियों के बीच

**Interparoxysmal.** Occurring between successive paroxysms of a disease. अन्तराप्रवेगी

**Interphase.** The stage between two successive divisions of a cell nucleus; interkinesis. अन्तराप्रावस्था; अन्तरावस्था

**Interposed.** See **Intermediate.**

**Interpretation.** The characteristic therapeutic intervention, or drawing inteferences and formulating the meaning in terms of the psychological dynamics inherent in an individual's responses to psychological tests. व्याख्या; विवरण

**Interpubic.** Between the pubes. अन्तराजघनक; जांघ की हड्डियों के बीच

**Interrupted.** Broken. विच्छिन्न; खण्डित; भग्न; टूटा हुआ; टूटी हुई

**Interscapular.** That which is between the shoulders. अन्तरांसीय; अंसफलकांतरीय; कंधों के बीच स्थित

**Intersexuality.** The possession of both male and female characteristics. उभयलिंगता; मिश्रलिंगता

**Interspinous.** Between spinous processes, especially those of the vertebrae. अन्तराकण्टकी

**Interstice.** A small area, space, or hole in the substance of an organ or tissue; interstitium. अन्तराल

**Interstices.** Plural of **Interstice.**

**Interstitial.** Lying or placed between; relating to spaces or interstices in any structure. अन्तरालीय

**Interstitium.** See **Interstice.**

**Intertrigo.** Erythema from friction or rubbing. त्वग्वलिशोथ; घर्षण अथवा खरोंच से होने वाली ग्वरक्तिमा

**Intertrochanteric.** Between the trochanters, e.g. a femoral line. अन्तरागण्डकी

**Intertubular.** Between the tubules. अन्तरानलिकी

**Interval.** A lapse or space either of time or distance. अन्तराल; समयान्तराल; मध्यान्तर; समयावकाश; अन्तर

**Intervening.** See **Intercurrent.**

**Intervenous.** Between the veins. शिरान्तरीय; अन्तराशिरीय; अन्तराशैरिक; शिराओं के बीच

**Intervention.** Interference, so as to modify a process or situation. हस्तक्षेप

**Interventrical.** See **Interventricular.**

**Interventricular.** Between the ventricles; interventrical. अन्तरानिलयी; निलयों के बीच

**Intervertebral.** Between the vertebrae or bones of the spine. अन्तराकशेरुक; कशेरुकाओं के बीच

**Intestinal.** Pertaining to intestines. आंत्रिक; आंत्र अथवा आंतों सम्बन्धी

**Intestine.** The bowel; the digestive tract passing from the stomach to the anus. आंत्र; आंत;

   **Large I.,** the portion of the digestive tract extending from the ileocaecal valve to the anus. बृहदांत्र; बड़ी आंत;

   **Small I.,** the portion of the digestive tract between the stomach and the caecum or beginning of the large intestine. लघ्वांत्र; छोटी आंत

**Intestinum Crassum.** The large intestine; colon. बृहदांत्र; बड़ी आंत

**Intima.** The internal coat; tunica intima. अन्त:अस्तर

**Intimal.** Relating to the intima or inner coat of a vessel. अन्त:अस्तरीय; अन्त:अस्तर सम्बन्धी

**Intimitis.** Inflammation of an intima. अन्त:अस्तरशोथ

**Intolerance.** Inability to bear pain or a discomfort. असह्यता; असहनशीलता

**Intoxicant.** Having the power to intoxicate; an intoxicating agent, such as alcohol. मादक; नशीला; नशीली

**Intoxication.** Poisoning. विषण्णता; acute alcoholism. मद्यात्यय; मद्यविषण्णता; the state of being intoxicated. मादकता; मद; नशा

**Intra-.** Prefix meaning within. 'अन्त:' के रूप में प्रयुक्त होने वाला उपसर्ग

**Intra-abdominal.** Within the belly; inside the abdomen. अन्तरुदरीय; उदर के अन्दर

**Intra-amniotic.** Within or into the amniotic fluid. अन्त:उल्वज

**Intra-arterial.** Within the artery. अन्त:धमनिक; धमनी के अन्दर

**Intra-articular.** Within a joint. अन्त:सन्धिज; सन्धि (जोड़) के अन्दर

**Intracanalicular.** Within a canaliculus. अन्त:नलिकी; अन्तर्नलिकी; किसी नलिका के अन्दर

**Intracapsular.** Within the capsule of a joint. अन्त:सम्पुटी; अन्तर्सम्पुटी; किसी जोड़ या सन्धि के सम्पुट के अन्दर

**Intracardiac.** Within the heart; intracardial. अन्त:हृदी; अन्तर्हृदी; हृदय के अन्दर

**Intracardial.** See **Intracardiac.**

**Intracartilagenous.** Within a cartilage. अन्तरुपास्थिक; किसी उपास्थि के अन्दर

**Intracatheter.** A plastic tube, usually attached to the puncturing needle, inserted into a blood vessel for infusion, injection or pressure monitoring. अन्त:कैथेटर; अन्तर्कैथेटर; अन्त:मूत्रनिस्सारकनली

**Intracellular.** Within a cell. अन्त:कोशिक; किसी कोशिका के अन्दर

**Intracerebellar.** Within the cerebellum. अन्त:अनुमस्तिष्कीय; अनुमस्तिष्क के अन्दर

**Intracerebral.** Within the cerebrum. अन्त:प्रमस्तिष्कीय; प्रमस्तिष्क के अन्दर

**Intracorporeal.** Within the body. अन्त:शारीरी; शरीर के अन्दर

**Intracranial.** Within the skull. अन्त:कपालिक; अन्त:कपालीय; खोपड़ी के अन्दर

**Intractable.** Incurable or resistant to therapy; obstinate. दु:साध्य; असाध्य

**Intracutaneous.** Within the skin tissue. अन्तस्त्वगूतकीय; त्वचा के ऊतकों के अन्दर

**Intrad.** Toward the inner part. अन्तरांगी; अन्दरूनी अंगों की ओर

**Intradermal.** Within the epidermis; intradermic. अन्त:त्वचीय; अन्तर्वचीय; त्वचा के अन्दर

**Intradermic. See Intradermal.**
**Intraductal.** Within a duct. अन्तर्वाहिनिक; किसी वाहिका या नली के अन्दर
**Intradural.** Inside the dura mater. अन्त:मेरुनालिक; मेरुनाल के अन्दर
**Intraepithelial.** Within the epithelium. अन्तरुपकलायी; उपकला के अन्दर
**Intrahepatic.** Within the liver. अन्तर्यकृती; यकृत् के अन्दर
**Intralobar.** Within a lobe. अन्तर्खण्डी; किसी खण्ड के अन्दर
**Intralobular.** Within a lobule. अन्तर्खण्डकी; अन्त:खण्डकी; किसी खण्डक के अन्दर
**Intramedullary.** Within the bone-marrow, the spinal cord or the medulla oblongata. अन्तरस्थिक; अन्त:मज्जीय; अन्तर्मज्जीय; अस्थिमज्जा के अन्दर
**Intramembranous.** Within a membrane. अन्त:कलाभ; किसी कला या झिल्ली के अन्दर
**Intramural.** In the substance of the walls of an organ. अन्तर्भित्तिक
**Intramuscular.** Within a muscle. अन्त:पेशीय; अन्तर्पेशीय; किसी पेशी के अन्दर
**Intranasal.** Within the nasal cavity. अन्तर्नासिकीय; अन्तर्नासी; अन्त:नासिक; नासा-गह्वर के अन्दर
**Intranatal.** At the time of birth; intrapartum. प्रसवकालीन; प्रसव के दौरान
**Intraoral.** Within the mouth, as an intraoral appliance. अन्तर्मुखी; मुँह के अन्दर
**Intraparietal.** Within the parietes. अन्त:पार्श्विक; अन्तर्भित्तिक
**Intrapartum. See Intranatal.**
**Intraperitoneal.** Within the peritoneum. अन्त:पर्युदर्यीय; उदरावरण के अन्दर
**Intrapulmonary.** Within the lungs. अन्त:फुफ्फुसी; फेफड़ों के अन्दर
**Intraserous.** Within a serous membrane. अन्त:सीरमी; सीरमी कला के अन्दर
**Intraspinal.** Within the spinal canal. अन्त:मेरुनालीय; मेरुनाल के अन्दर
**Intrathecal.** Within the meninges. अन्त:मस्तिष्कावरणीय; मस्तिष्कावरण के अन्दर
**Intrathoracic.** Within the thorax. अन्तर्वक्षीय; वक्ष अथवा छाती के अन्दर
**Intratracheal.** Within or through the trachea. अन्त:श्वासप्रणालीय; श्वासप्रणाल के अन्दर या रास्ते
**Intrauterine.** Within the womb. अन्तर्गर्भाशयी; अन्तर्गर्भाशयिक; गर्भाशय के अन्दर
**Intravascular.** Within the blood vessels. अन्तर्वाहिकी; रक्तवाहिनियों के अन्दर

**Intravenous.** Within a vein. शिराभ्यन्तर; अन्त:शिराभ; किसी शिरा के अन्दर; **I. Pylography,** radiographic visualization within the veins of the renal pelvis and the ureter. अन्त:गोणिकाचित्रण

**Intraventricular.** Within a ventricle. अन्तर्निलयी; किसी निलय के अन्दर

**Intravital.** During the period of life. अन्तर्जीवी

**Intrinsic.** Inherent or inside; belonging entirely to a part. अन्त:स्थ; आभ्यन्तरिक

**Intro-.** Prefix meaning in or into. 'अन्त:' के रूप में प्रयुक्त उपसर्ग

**Introducer.** An instrument or style for the introduction of a flexible instrument, such as catheter, endotracheal tube, etc. अन्त:प्रवेशक

**Introflection.** See **Introflexion.**

**Introflexion.** A bending inward; introflection. अन्तर्बक्रता

**Introitus.** The entrance into a body, canal or hollow organ, as the vagina. द्वार, जैसे योनिद्वार

**Introjection.** A psychological defence mechanism involving appropriation of external happening and its assimilation by the personality, making it a part of the self. अन्तर्निदेशन; अन्तर्निर्देश

**Intromission.** The insertion or introduction of one part into another. अन्तर्निवेश; अन्तरोंपण; अन्तर्निवेशन

**Intromittent.** Conveying or sending into a body or cavity. अन्तर्निवेशक

**Introspect.** To examine one's own mind. स्वानुशीलन करना; आत्मनिरीक्षण करना

**Introspection.** Study by a person of his own mental processes; looking within. स्वानुशीलन; आत्मनिरीक्षण; अन्तर्निरीक्षण; अपने ही ज्ञान द्वारा स्वयं का चिंतन करना

**Introspective.** Relating to introspection. स्वानुशीलन अथवा आत्मनिरीक्षण सम्बन्धी

**Introsusception.** The same as **Intussusception.**

**Introversion.** The turning of a structure into itself. अन्तर्मुखीकरण; a trait of preoccupation with oneself, in contrast to extraversion. अन्तर्मुखता

**Introvert.** One who tends to be introspective and self-centered and who takes small interest in the affairs of the others. अन्तर्मुखी; to turn a structure into itself. अन्तर्मुखीकरण

**Intubate.** To perform intubation. नलिकाप्रवेश करना

**Intubation.** Insertion of a tube into any canal (as larynx) and other part. नलिकाप्रवेशन; स्वरयंत्र के अन्दर कोई नली डालना

**Intuition.** Awareness of facts or occurrences not ordinarily perceptible to the senses; cryptesthesia. अन्त:प्रज्ञा; सहजप्रज्ञा; अन्तर्बोध

**Intumesce.** To swell up; to enlarge. सूज जाना; फूल जाना; बढ़ जाना

**Intumescence.** The swelling of a part or in the whole of the body. उत्फुल्लन; the process of enlarging or swelling. बढ़ने या फूलने की प्रक्रिया

**Intumescent.** Enlarging. बृद्धि; swelling. फुलाव; सूजन; becoming enlarged or swollen. बढ़ा हुआ या सूजा हुआ

**Inturnus.** Internal; an eye-muscle. अन्तःस्थ; आभ्यन्तरिक; आँख की एक पेशी

**Intussusception.** A portion of the intestine falling into the adjoining part and choking up the opening and producing strangulation. आन्त्ररोध; आंत्रावरोध; invagination. अन्तर्वेशन; अन्तर्वलन

**Intussusceptive.** Relating to, or characterized by intussusception. आन्त्रान्त्रप्रवेशी

**Intussusceptum.** In an intussusception, that part of the bowel which is received within the other part. आन्त्रविष्टांश

**Intussuscipiens.** The intestine receiving the intussusceptum. आन्त्रान्त्रवेष्टक

**Inunction.** The act of rubbing in an ointment; anointing. मर्दन; किसी मलहम में रगड़ने की क्रिया

**In utero.** Inside the uterus. गर्भाशयान्तर्गत; गर्भाशय (जरायु) के अन्दर

**Invagination.** Intussusception; the receiving of one part into another, as in a sheath; the state of being invaginated. अन्तर्वेशन; अन्तर्वलन

**Invalid.** One who is not well; a sickly person suffering from a disabling, but not necessarily completely incapacitating disease; weak. अपंग; अशक्त; दुर्बल; कमजोर

**Invalidism.** Chronic ill-health. अशक्तता; चिरकारी रुग्णता; चिर रुग्णता; जीर्ण रुग्णता

**Invasion.** The beginning of a disease; an attack. आक्रमण; हमला; extension. प्रसार; फैलाव

**Invermination.** Becoming affected by worms. कृमिरुग्णता

**Inversion.** A turning inward, upside down, or in any direction contrary to the existing one. प्रतीपता; अन्तर्वलन; व्युत्क्रमण

**Invertebral.** Having no vertebral or back-bone. अकशेरुक; कशेरुकाहीन

**Invertebrate.** Not possessed of a spinal or vertebral column. अपृष्ठवंशी; रीढ़ रहित; रीढ़हीन; अकशेरुक

**Invertin.** A ferment from yeast and intestinal juice. किण्व; ख़मीर

**Invertor.** A muscle that inverts or causes inversion or turns a part, such as a foot inward. अपवर्तनी (पेशी)

**Inveterate.** Resisting treatment; chronic; deep-seated; firmly established; said of a disease or of confined habit. दु:साध्य; असाध्य; चिरस्थाई; लाइलाज

**In vitro.** In the glass. अन्त:काचपत्री; कांच के अन्दर; in an artificial environment. कृत्रिम वातावरण में

**In vivo.** In the living body or tissue. अन्तर्जीवी; जीवित ऊतक के अन्दर

**Involucra.** Plural of **Involucrum**.

**Involucrum.** An enveloping membrane; an envelope. विविक्तच्छद; आवरण

**Involuntary.** Independent of the will; not volitional; unknowingly; contrary to the will. अनैच्छिक; निरंकुश; असंयत;
   **I. Muscle,** unstriated muscle tissue which acts independently of the will to govern automatic physical function. निरंकुश पेशी;
   **I. Urination,** enuresis. निरंकुशमूत्रता; असंयतमूत्रता

**Involution.** Catagenesis; the return of an enlarged organ to normal size. प्रत्यावर्तन; किसी बढ़े हुए अंश का सामान्य आकार में बदल जाना; the turning inward of the edges of a part. अन्तर्वलयन

**Involutional.** Relating to involution. प्रत्यावर्तन अथवा अन्तर्वलयन सम्बन्धी

**Iodate.** A salt of Iodic acid. जम्बिक लवण; आयोडीन का नमक; आयोडेट

**Iodide.** Compound of Iodine and a base. जम्बेय; आयोडाइड; अन्य तत्वों से आयोडीन का मिश्रण

**Iodinate.** To treat or combine with Iodine. आयोडीनीकृत

**Iodine.** A poisonous, nonmetallic element with a metallic cluster, used in medicine as an alternative; Iodum. आयोडीन

**Iodinophil.** Staining readily with Iodine; iodinophile; iodinophilous. आयोडीनरागी

**Iodinophile.** See **Iodinophil**.

**Iodinophilous.** See **Iodinophil**.

**Iodism.** A poisonous effect from continued use of Iodine. आयोडात्यय; आयोडीनविषण्णता

**Iodize.** To treat or impregnate with Iodine. आयोडीनोपचार करना या आयोडीन के साथ संसेचन करना

**Iododerma.** An eruption of follicular papules and pustules caused by Iodine. आयोडीनचर्मता

**Iodoform.** A yellow antiseptic powder used largely in medicine. आयोडोफार्म

**Iodotherapy.** Treatment with Iodine. आयोडीनचिकित्सा; आयोडीनोपचार

**Iodum.** See **Iodine**.

**Ioduria.** Urinary excretion of Iodine. आयोडीनमेह; मूत्र में आयोडीन जाना

**Ion.** An element set free by electrolysis. आयन
**Ionic.** Relating to an ion or ions. आयनी
**Ionisation.** Treatment whereby ions of various substances, e.g. zinc, chloride, iodine, histamine, are introduced into the system by means of a constant electric current; ionization. आयनीकरण; आयनीभवन; आयनन
**Ionization.** See **Ionisation.**
**Ionize.** To separate into ions. आयनों में अलग-अलग कर देना
**Ionophore.** The compound or substance that forms a complex with an ion and transports it across a membrane. आयनवाहक
**Inophoresis.** Electrophoresis; the movement of particles in an electric field toward one or the other electric pole, node or cathode. आयनसंचलन
**Ionophoretic.** Relating to ionophoresis. आयनसंचलनीय; आयनसंचलन सम्बन्धी
**Iontophoresis.** Introduction into the tissue, by means of an electric current, of the ions of a chosen medicament. आयनप्रवेशन
**Iontophoretic.** Relating to iontophoresis. आयनप्रवेशनीय; आयनप्रवेशन सम्बन्धी
**Ipsilateral.** On the same side. समपार्श्विक; समपार्श्वी
**Irascibility.** Rage. क्रोधशीलता
**Iridal.** Relating to the iris; iridial; iridian; iridic. परितारिका अथवा उपतारा सम्बन्धी
**Iridalgia.** Neuralgia of the iris. परितारिकार्ति; परितारिकाशूल; उपताराशूल
**Iridauxesis.** Thickening of the iris following plastic iritis. परितारिकावमोटन
**Iridectomy.** Excision of a portion of the iris. परितारिका-उच्छेदन; उपतारा-उच्छेदन
**Iridectropium.** Eversion of the anterior edge of the secondary optic vesicle at the pupillary margin; ectropion uveae. परितारिकाबहिर्वर्तन
**Iridemia.** Bleeding from the iris. परितारिकारक्तस्राव
**Iridencleisis.** Incarceration of a portion of the iris in a wound of the cornea as an operative measure in glaucoma to effect filtration. परितारिकाबन्धीकरण
**Iridentropium.** Inversion of the pupillary margin; entropion uveae. परितारिकान्तर्वर्तन
**Irideremia.** An iris so rudimentary that it seems to be absent; aniridia. अपरितारकता; आँख की पुतली अथवा उपतारा का अभाव
**Irides.** Plural of **Iris.**
**Iridesis.** Ligature of a portion of the iris brought out through an

incision in the cornea; iridodesis. परितारिकाबन्ध; उपताराबन्ध

**Iridial.** See **Iridal.**

**Iridian.** See **Iridal.**

**Iridic.** See **Iridal.**

**Iridium.** A white, silvery metallic element. धनातु; इरीडियम

**Iridoavulsion.** A tearing away of the iris. परितारिकापदारण

**Iridocapsulitis.** Iritis with accompanying inflammation of the capsule of the crystalline lens. परितारिकासम्पुटशोथ

**Iridocele.** Protrusion of a portion of the iris through a corneal defect. परितारिकास्रंस; उपतारास्रंस; परितारिकीय हर्निया

**Iridochoroiditis.** Inflammation of both iris and choroid. परितारिकारंजितपटलशोथ; उपतारा तथा रंजितपटल का प्रदाह

**Iridocoloboma.** A coloboma or congenital defect of the iris. सहजपरितारिकाविदर; सहजपरितारिकादोष

**Iridoconstrictor.** Causing contraction of the pupil. परितारिकासंकीर्णक; उपतारासंकीर्णक

**Iridocyclectomy.** Removal of the iris and ciliary body for excision of a tumour. परितारिकारोमकपिण्ड-उच्छेदन

**Iridocyclitis.** Inflammation of the iris and the ciliary body. परितारिकारोमकपिण्डशोथ; उपतारा तथा रोमकपिण्ड का प्रदाह

**Iridocyclochoroiditis.** Inflammation of the iris and choroid, involving the ciliary body. परितारिकारंजितपटलरोमकपिण्डशोथ; उपतारा तथा रंजितपटल और रोमकपिण्ड का प्रदाह

**Iridocystectomy.** An operation for removal of a cyst from the iris. परितारिकापुटी-उच्छेदन

**Iridodesis.** See **Iridesis.**

**Iridodialysis.** A separation of the iris from the ciliary body. परितारिकाविगलन; अक्षिपिण्ड से उपतारा का पृथक् होना

**Iridodilator.** Causing dilatation of the pupil. नेत्रपटलविस्फारक

**Iridodonesis.** Agitated motion or trembling of the iris. ताराकम्पन; परितारिकाकम्पन; आँख की पुतली की कम्पन

**Iridokinesia.** See **Iridokinesis.**

**Iridokinesis.** The movement of the iris in contracting and dilating the pupil; iridokinesia. परितारिकागतिकता

**Iridokinetic.** Relating to the movements of the iris; iridomotor. परितारिकागतिक

**Iridomalacia.** Degenerative softening of the iris. परितारिकामृदुता

**Iridomesodialysis.** Separation of adhesions around the inner margin of the iris. उपतारा-आसंजविगलन

**Iridomotor.** See **Iridokinetic.**
**Iridoncosis.** Thickening of the iris. परितारिकावमोटन
**Iridoncus.** A tumefaction of the iris. परितारिकास्फीति
**Iridoparalysis.** See **Iridoplegia.**
**Iridopathy.** Pathologic lesions in the iris. परितारिकारोग; उपतारारोग
**Iridoplegia.** Paralysis of the iris; iridoparalysis. परितारिकाघात; आँख की पुतली अर्थात् उपतारा का लकवा
**Iridoptosis.** Prolapse of the iris. परितारिकाभ्रंश; परितारिकापात
**Iridorrhexis.** Tearing the iris from its peripheral attachment. परितारिकाविदारण; उपताराविदारण
**Iridoschisis.** Separation of the anterior layer of the iris from the posterior layer. परितारिकास्तरविलग्नता
**Iridosclerotomy.** An incision involving both sclera and iris. परितारिकाश्वेतपटलछेदन
**Iridotomy.** Transverse division of some of the fibres of the iris; corotomy; iritomy; irotomy. परितारिकाछेदन; उपताराछेदन
**Iris.** The coloured layer of the eye, surrounding the pupil. परितारिका; उपतारा; आँख की पुतली
**Irish-button.** Syphilis. उपदंश
**Iritic.** Relating to iritis. परितारिकाशोथज; परितारिकाशोथ अथवा उपताराशोथ सम्बन्धी
**Iritides.** Plural of **Iritis.**
**Iritis.** Inflammation of the iris. परितारिकाशोथ; उपताराशोथ; आँख की पुतली का प्रदाह
**Iritomy.** See **Iridotomy.**
**Iron.** Ferrum; a metallic element of bluish-grey colour. अयस; लौह; लोहा; लोह
**Irotomy.** See **Iridotomy.**
**Irradiate.** To apply radiation from a source to a structure or organism. किरणित करना
**Irradiation.** Exposure or subjection to the action of radiant energy for diagnostic or therapeutic purpose. किरणन
**Irrational.** Unreasonable or unreasoning; not rational. अपरिमेय; अयुक्त
**Irreducible.** Not reducible; incapable of being made smaller or simpler. अखण्डनीय; अलघुकरणीय; अलघुकारी
**Irregular.** Not symmetric; not regular. अनियमित; अव्यवस्थित
**Irresuscitable.** Incapable of being revived. अपुनर्जीव्य

**Irrigate.** To wash out a cavity or wound with a fluid. धावन करना; धोना

**Irrigation.** The constant application of water. धावन; संसेचन; निरन्तर जल-प्रयोग करना

**Irritability.** An excess of nervous excitement. क्षोभ्यता; क्षोभशीलता; क्षोभण; चिड़चिड़ापन

**Irritable.** Susceptible to irritation. चिड़चिड़ा

**Irritant.** Any agent causing irritation; irritating. क्षोभक

**Irritating.** See **Irritant.**

**Irritation.** Overexcitation. क्षोभ; क्षोभण; चिड़चिड़ापन

**Irritative.** Causing irritation. क्षोभक; क्षोभण पैदा करने वाला

**Irruption.** The act or process of breaking through to a surface. विभेदन

**Ischaemia.** Local and temporary deficiency of blood; ischemia. स्थानिक-अरक्तता

**Ischaemic.** Pertaining to ischaemia; ischemic. स्थानिक-अरक्तता सम्बन्धी

**Ischemia.** See **Ischaemia.**

**Ischemic.** See **Ischaemic.**

**Ischia.** Plural of **Ischium.**

**Ischiac.** Sciatic; ischiadic; ischiatic. पृथुस्नायुपरक; पृथुस्नायु सम्बन्धी

**Ischiadic.** See **Ischiac.**

**Ischiadica.** See **Ischium.**

**Ischiagra.** Pain in the hip. नितम्बशूल; कूल्हे का दर्द

**Ischial.** Pertaining to the ischium. आसनास्थिक; आसनास्थि सम्बन्धी

**Ischialgia.** Neuralgia of the hip; ischiodynia; sciatica. आसनास्थिशूल; नितम्बस्नायुशूल; गृध्रसी; सायटिका

**Ischias.** Gout or rheumatic affection of the hip-joint. नितम्बसन्धिवात

**Ischiatic.** See **Ischiac.**

**Ischidrosis.** The suppression of sweat; anhidrosis. स्वेदाल्पता; पसीना दब जाना

**Ischiocapsular.** Relating to the ischium and the capsule of hip-joint. आसनास्थि तथा सम्पुट सम्बन्धी

**Ischiocavernosus.** The erector penis muscle, or erector clitoridis. शिश्नप्रहर्षणी; शिश्न या भगशिश्निका की उत्तेजक पेशी

**Ischiocele.** Sciatic hernia. आसनास्थिस्त्रंस

**Ischiococcygeal.** Relating to the ischium and the coccyx. आसनास्थि तथा अनुत्रिक सम्बन्धी

**Ischiococcygeus.** The coccygeus muscle. आसनानुत्रिकपेशी

**Ischiodynia.** See **Ischialgia.**

**Ischiofemoral.** Pertaining to the ischium and the femur. आसनास्थि एवं ऊर्विकास्थि सम्बन्धी

**Ischiofibular.** Relating to, or connecting the ischium and the fibula. आसनास्थिबहिर्जंघिकी; आसनास्थि तथा बहिर्जंघिका सम्बन्धी

**Ischionitis.** Inflammation of the ischium. आसनास्थिशोथ; नितम्बास्थिशोथ

**Ischiopagus.** A double monster united by the ischia. बद्धासनास्थिययमलीय

**Ischiorectal.** Pertaining to the ischium and rectum. आसनास्थि एवं मलांत्र सम्बन्धी

**Ischiovertebral.** Relating to the ischium and the vertebral column. आसनास्थि तथा कशेरुका-खण्ड सम्बन्धी

**Ischium.** The inferior part of the hip bone; os ischii; ischiadica. आसनास्थि; नितम्बास्थि; कूल्हे की हड्डी

**Ischuretic.** Relating to, or relieving ischuria. मूत्ररोध सम्बन्धी अथवा मूत्रनिस्सारक

**Ischuria.** Retention or suppression of urine. मूत्ररोध; मूत्रक्षय

**Island.** In anatomy, any isolated part, separated from the surrounding tissues by a groove, or marked by difference in structure; insula. द्वीप;
   **I.'s of Langerhans,** see **Islets of Langerhans.**

**Islet.** A small island. द्वीपिका;
   **I.'s of Langerhans,** collection of special cells scattered throughout the pancreas; islands of Langerhans. लैंगरहन द्वीपिकायें

**-ismus.** Suffix customarily used to imply spasm or contraction. 'उद्वेष्ट' अथवा 'आकर्ष' के रूप में प्रयुक्त होने वाला प्रत्यय

**Iso-.** Prefix signifying equality. 'सम' अथवा 'तुल्य' के रूप में प्रयुक्त होने वाला उपसर्ग

**Isoagglutination.** Agglutination of red blood cells as a result of the reaction between an agglutinin and specific antigen in or on the cells; isohemagglutination. समलोहितकोशिकासमूहन

**Isoagglutinin.** An isoantibody that causes agglutination of cells; isohemagglutinin. समलोहितकोशिकासंश्लेषक

**Isoagglutinogen.** An isoantigen that induces agglutination of the cells to which it is attached upon exposure to its specific isoantibody. समलोहितकोशिकासंश्लेषकजन

**Isoantibody.** An antibody that occurs only in some individuals of a species, and reacts specifically with the corresponding antigen. समप्रतिपिण्ड

**Isoantigen.** An antigenic substance that occurs only in some individuals of a species. समप्रतिजन

**Isocellular.** Composed of cells of equal size or of similar character. समकोशिकी

**Isochromatic.** Of uniform colour; denoting two objects of the same colour. समवर्णक

**Isochromatophil.** Having an equal affinity for the same salt. समलवणरागी

**Isochronous.** Occurring at equal period of time, as pulsation of heart. तुल्यकम्पी; समकालिक

**Isocoria.** Equality in the size of the two pupils. समक्षिपटलता

**Isodactylism.** A condition in which each of the fingers or toes are approximately of equal length. समांगुलिता

**Isodiameteric.** Having the same diameter throughout. समव्यासमितिक

**Isodynamic.** Of equal force or strength. समगतिक; समबल

**Isoelectric.** Equally electric throughout. समविभवी; समविद्युत्विभव; समविभव

**Isoenergetic.** Exerting equal force. समशक्तिशाली; equally active. समक्रियाशील

**Isogamete.** One of two or more similar cells by the conjugation or fusion of which, with subsequent division, reproduction occurs. समयुग्मक

**Isogamy.** The sexual union of similar gametes. समजन्युता; समपिण्ड; समभोग

**Isogeneic.** See **Isogenic**.

**Isogenesis.** Identity of morphologic development. समजनन

**Isogenic.** Relating to a group of individuals or a strain of animals genetically alike with respect to specified gene pairs; isogeneic. समजीनी

**Isogenous.** Of the same origin, as in development from the same tissue or cell. सममूलक

**Isograft.** A tissue or organ transplanted between genetically identical individuals. समनिरोप; समनिरोपण

**Isohemagglutination.** See **Isoagglutination**.

**Isohemagglutinin.** Se **Isoagglutinin**.

**Isohypercytosis.** A condition in which the number of leukocytes in the circulating blood is increased. समश्वेताणुबृद्धि; समश्वेतकोशिकाबहुलता

**Isohypocytosis.** An abnormally small number of leukocytes in the circulating blood. समश्वेताणुह्रास; समश्वेताणुकोशिकाल्पता

**Isolate.** To separate from one another. पृथक् करना; वियुक्त करना; विच्छेदन करना

**Isolated.** Separated from one another; cut off from surroundings or associates. पृथक्भूत; पृथक्कृत; वियुक्त

**Isolation.** The seclusion of patients with contagious diseases. पृथक्करण; पार्थक्य; विच्छेदन; विच्छेद; अलगाव

**Isomer.** The isomeric substance. समावयवी पदार्थ

**Isomeric.** Exhibiting isomerism. समावयवी

**Isomerism.** Having an identical chemical composition. समावयविता; समावयवता

**Isomerization.** A process in which one isomer is formed from another. समावयवीभवन; समावयवीकरण

**Isometric.** Of equal measure or dimensions. सममितीय; सममितिक; धनीय; त्रिसमलंबाक्ष

**Isometropia.** Equality in kind and degree of refraction in the two eyes. समापवर्तन

**Isomorphic.** See **Isomorphous**.

**Isomorphism.** A similarity in crystalline form. समाकृतिकता

**Isomorphous.** Like-shaped; isomorphic. समाकार

**Isopathy.** The treatment of disease by means of a product of the same disease and also the treatment of a diseased organ by an extract of the same organ from a healthy animal. समोपचार; सदृशचिकित्सा

**Isophoria.** A state in which the tension of the vertical muscles of each eye is equal and the visual lines lie in the horizontal plane. नेत्रअविचलनप्रवृत्ति

**Isosexual.** Relating to the existence of characteristics or feelings of both sexes in one person. समलिंगी

**Isothermal.** Of equal temperature; isothermic. समतापी

**Isothermic.** See **Isothermal**.

**Isotonia.** See **Isotonicity**.

**Isotonic.** Having equal tension. समपरासारी; समतानी; समतानिक; समओजी

**Isotonicity.** Equality of the tension of blood; isotonia. समतनाव; समतानता

**Isotopes.** Two or more forms of the same element having identical chemicals, but differing in physical properties. समस्थानिक

**Isotropic.** Singly refractive; isotropous. समदिक्; समवृत्तिक

**Isotropous.** See **Isotropic**.

**Issue.** Pregnancy. सगर्भता; सन्तति; a discharge of pus, blood or other matter. पूतिस्त्राव अथवा रक्तस्त्राव; a suppurating or discharging sore. पूतिस्त्रावी घाव

**Isthmectomy.** Excision of the midportion of the thyroid. संकीर्णपथ-उच्छेदन; अवटुग्रन्थिपथ-उच्छेदन

**Isthmuses.** Plural of **Isthmus.**

**Isthmi.** Plural of **Isthmus.**

**Isthmitis.** Inflammation of the isthmus. संकीर्णपथशोथ

**Isthmus.** The neck or constricted part of an organ. संकीर्णपथ; संकीर्णसंयोजक

**Itch.** Scabies; pruritus. कण्डू; खुजली; खारिश; खाज;
I. Mite, a minute parasite found in, or near the pustules of the itch. खाज परजीवी

**Itching.** Pruritus. खुजली; खारिश

**Iter.** A passageway in the body. वीथि; नलिकापथ

**Iteral.** Relating to an iter. वीथि अथवा नलिकापथ सम्बन्धी

**-itis.** This termination implies inflammation. 'शोथ' अथवा 'प्रदाह' के रूप में प्रयुक्त किया जाने वाला शब्दान्त

**Ivory.** The dentinal substance of various animals, especially the elephants. गजदन्त; हाथीदांत

**I.V.P.** Abbreviation for **Intravenous Pyelography.**

**Ixodiasis.** Skin lesions caused by the bites of certain ticks. कीलनीचर्मता; कीलनियों द्वारा डंक मारे जाने के कारण होने वाले चर्म रोग

**Ixodic.** Relating to, or caused by ticks. कीलनियों सम्बन्धी

# J

**Jaborandi.** The leaves of various species of **Pilocarpus**, trees of Brazil. जैबोरेंडी; स्वेदन-पत्र

**Jacket.** A short coat. बाह्यावरण; जैकेट; बण्डी; छोटा कोट

**Jactation.** See **Jactitation.**

**Jactitation.** Tossing of the body; restlessness; jerking; jactation. तिलमिलाहट; तड़पन; व्याकुलता; बेचैनी

**Jagged.** Having notches or teeth. खुरदरा; कंटीला

**Jail Fever.** Thyphus fever. जेल ज्वर; कारा ज्वर; मोह ज्वर; सन्निपात ज्वर

**Jalapa.** The root of **Ipomoea Jalapa** of Mexico; it is actively cathartic. जलापा; एक विचेरक

**Jaundice.** Bile pigment in the blood and tissues giving them a yellow appearance; icterus. कामला; पीलिया; पाण्डुरोग; कँवल; कमल;

    **J. of the newborn,** icterus neonatorum. शिशु-कामला;

    **Acholuric J.,** one with excessive amount of unconjugated bilirubin in the circulatory blood and without bile pigment in the blood. अपित्तमेही कामला;

    **Catarrhal J.,** that due to catarrhal inflammation of bile-ducts. प्रतिश्यायी कामला; अभिष्यन्दी कामला;

    **Cholestatic J.,** jaundice produced by bile plugs in small biliary passages in the liver. पित्तरुद्ध कामला;

    **Congenital J.,** a jaundice occurring at or shortly after bith. सहज कामला; जन्मजात पीलिया (कामला);

    **Haemolytic J.,** one resulting from excessive amount of haemoglobin. रक्तसंलायी कामला;

    **Hapatic J.,** jaundice resulting from disease of liver. यकृत् कामला;

    **Malignant J.,** acute yellow atrophy of the liver; icterus gravis. दुर्दम कामला; सांघातिक कामला;

    **Obstructive J.,** jaundice resulting from obstruction to the flow of bile into the duodenum. रुद्धपथ कामला; रोधज कामला;

    **Retention J.,** that due to insufficiency of the liver in secreting bile pigment. अवधारण कामला

**Jaw.** The maxilla. हनु; जबड़ा;

    **J.-bone,** the bone of the jaw, containing the teeth. हन्वस्थि; जबड़े की हड्डी

**Jecur.** The liver. यकृत्

**Jejunal.** Pertaining to the jejunum. मध्यान्त्रीय; मध्यान्त्र सम्बन्धी

**Jejunitis.** Inflammation of the jejunum. मध्यान्त्रशोथ; मध्यान्त्र का प्रदाह

**Jejunoileitis.** Inflammation of the jejunum and the ileum. मध्यान्त्रशेषान्त्रशोथ; मध्यान्त्र तथा शेषान्त्र का प्रदाह

**Jejunum.** A portion of small intestine between duodenum and ileum. मध्यान्त्र; बीच की छोटी आन्त

**Jelly.** A soft substance which is gelatinous. लप्सी; जेल्ली; जैली; एक कोमल लसलसा पदार्थ

**Jerk.** A sudden pull. क्षेप; प्रतिक्षेप; झटका;

**Finger-j.**, a disease in which the flexion or extension of a finger is accompaniad by a jerk; jerk-finger. अंगुलि-प्रतिक्षेप;

**J.-finger**, see **Finger-jerk.**

**Jaw-j.**, movement as a result of tapping the mandible when the jaw in half open. हनु-प्रतिक्षेप;

**Knee-j.**, forward jerk of lower leg upon striking patellar tendon when knee is flexed at right angles. जानु-प्रतिक्षेप;

**Tendon-j.**, the contraction of muscle after tapping the tendon. कण्डरा-प्रतिक्षेप

**Jerking.** Making a sudden motion; moving by starts. प्रतिक्षेपण; झटका लगना

**Jigger.** Chigger; a flea, prevalent in the tropics. चिगर

**Joint.** The junction of two or more bones; articulatio; articulation. संधि; जोड़;

**Ankle-j.**, a hinge joint between the tibia and fibula above and the talus below. गुल्फ-संधि;

**Ball-and-socket J.**, a multiaxial joint in which a sphere on the head of one bone fits into a rounded cavity in the other bone as in the hipjoint; enarthrodial joint. उलूखल संधि;

**Cubital J.**, see **Elbow Joint.**

**Elbow J.**, a compound hinge joint between the humerus and the bones of the forearm; cubital joint. कूर्पर संधि; कोहनी का जोड़;

**Enarthrodial J.**, see **Ball-and-socket Joint.**

**False J.**, false joint formation subsequent to a fracture. कूट संधि;

**Fibrous J.**, one connected by fibrous tissue. तंतु संधि;

**Flail J.**, a joint with loss of function. शिथिल संधि;

**Gliding J.**, diarthrosis permitting a gliding motion. संसर्पी संधि;

**Hinge J.**, a joint in which a broad, transverse, cylindrical convexity on one bone fits into a corresponding concavity on the other. कोर संधि;

**Hip J.**, the ball-and-socket joint between the head of the femur and the acetabulum; articulatio coxae. नितम्ब संधि; कूल्हे का जोड़;

**Immovable J.**, a joint in which a cavity is lacking between the bones; synarthrodial joint. अचल संधि;

**Knee J.**, the joint between the femur, patella and tibia. जानु संधि; घुटने का जोड़;

**Midcarpal J.**, a joint separating the navicular, lunate and triangular bones from the distant row of carpal bones. मध्यमणिबंध संधि;

**Movable J.**, slightly or freely movable joint. चल संधि;

**Pivot J.**, a joint that permits rotation of a bone; rotatory joint; trachoid joint; articulatio trochoidea. धुराग्र संधि;

**Receptive J.**, see **Saddle Joint.**

**Rotatory J.**, see **Pivot Joint.**

**Saddle J.**, a joint in which the opposing surfaces are reciprocally concavoconvex; receptive joint; articulatio sellaris. पर्याण संधि;

**Shoulder J.**, a ball-and-socket joint between the head of humerus and the glenoid cavity of the scapula; articulatio humeri. स्कन्ध संधि; कंधे का जोड़;

**Simple J.**, a joint composed by two bones. सरल संधि;

**Synarthrodial J.**, see **Immovable Joint.**

**Synovial J.**, a joint separated by space containing synovial fluid. श्लेषक संधि;

**Trochoid J.**, see **Pivot Joint.**

**Wrist J.**, the joint between the distal end of the radius and its articular disk, and the proximal row of carpal bones; articulatio manus. मणिबन्ध संधि

**Jugal.** Connecting or uniting. योगिक; योजक;

   **J. Bone**, the malar bone. कपोलास्थि; गाल की हड्डी

**Jugular.** Pertaining to the throat. कण्ठ सम्बन्धी;

   **J. Veins**, the two large veins at the side of the neck. मात्रिका शिरायें; मन्या शिरायें; ग्रैव शिरायें

**Jugulum.** Throat. कण्ठ; गला

**Juice.** The fluid part of an animal or a plant. रस; यूष; सार; सुरा;

**Alimentary J.**, the digestive juice. पाचक रस;

**Digestive J.**, see **Alimentary Juice.**

**Gastric J.**, secretions of the stomach. जठर रस;

**Intestinal J.**, a clear, yellowish, viscid fluid, alkaline in reaction. आंत्र रस;

**Pancreatic J.**, a clear, viscid, alkaline digestive juice in which the pancreas poured into the duodenum. अग्न्याशय रस

**Junctio.** A joint; junction. सन्धि; जोड़; संगम

**Junction.** See **Junctio.**

    **Amelodental J.,** see **Dentinoenamel Junction.**

    **Amelodentinal J.,** see **Dentinoenamel Junction.**

    **Dentinoenamel J.,** the surface at which the enamel and the dentin of the crown of a tooth are joined; amelodental junction; amelodentinal junction. वल्कदन्त संगम; दन्तवल्क संगम;

    **Mucocutaneous J.,** the site of a transition from epidermis to the epithelium of a mucous membrane. श्लेष्मत्वक् संगम;

    **Myoneural J.,** the synaptic connection of the axon of the motor neuron with a muscle fibre. पेशीतंत्रिका संगम

**Junctura.** A junction. सन्धि; जोड़; मेल; संगम

**Jungle Fever.** A malignant remittent fever occurring in the jungles of India. विषम-ज्वर; जंगल-ज्वर; मलेरिया

**Juris.** The science which treats of the practical inter-relation of law and medicine; jurisprudence; forensic medicine. न्यायशास्त्र; व्यवहारशास्त्र; नीतिशास्त्र

**Jurisprudence.** See **Juris.**

    **Medical J.,** see under **Medical.**

**Jusculum.** Broth or soup; gruel. शोरबा

**Juxtaglomerular.** Close to, or adjoining a renal glomerulus. स्तवकासन्न

**Juxtaposition.** In close relationship. सन्निधि; सानिध्य

**Juxtavesical.** Near the bladder. मूत्राशयासन्न; मूत्राशय के पास

# K

**Kakotrophy.** Malnutrition. कुपोषण

**Kala-Azar.** An epidemic fever of Assam in India. काला-आजार; भारत के असम प्रदेश में महामारी के रूप में फैलने वाला ज्वर

**Kali.** Abbreviated form of **Kalium** which means potash; alkali. पोटाश; क्षार; अलकली

**Kalium.** Potassium. पोटाशियम; पोटैशियम; कैलियम; संक्षिप्त रूप 'काली'

**Karyocyte.** A young, immature normoblast. मूललोहितकोशिका

**Karyokinesis.** Indirect nuclear division; mitosis. सूत्रीविभाजन; विषमकोशिकाविभाजन

**Karyology.** Study of the nucleus. केन्द्रकविज्ञान

**Karyolysis.** Apparent destruction of the nucleus of a cell. केन्द्रकलयन

**Karyolytic.** Relating to karyolysis. केन्द्रकलयन सम्बन्धी

**Karyoplasm.** The nuclear substance of a cell; nucleoplasm. केन्द्रक-द्रव्य

**Karyorrhexis.** Dissolution of the chromatin of the nucleus. केन्द्रक-भंग

**Katabolism.** See **Catabolism.**

**Katatonia.** A form of insanity progressing to imbecility. विक्षिप्ति; पागलपन

**Katharol.** An antiseptic. कैथराल; एक पूतिरोधक औषधि

**Kation.** An electropositive element; cation. धनायन

**Keloid.** A new growth or tumour of the skin which is fibrous and usually occurring at the site of the scar. कीलाइड; चर्मक्षतार्बुद; चर्मगुल्म

**Kendall's Fever.** Yellow fever. पीत ज्वर

**Kenophobia.** A fear of large empty spaces. बृहद्‌रिक्तस्थानभीति; बड़े-बड़े खाली स्थानों का भय

**Kenotoxin.** A poisonous substance developed in the tissues during their activity and responsible for their fatigue. कीनोटॉक्सिन; एक विषैला पदार्थ

**Keratalgia.** Pain in the cornea. स्वच्छपटलार्ति; कनीनिकाशूल

**Keratectasia.** Bulging of the cornea; keratectasis. स्वच्छपटल-बहि:सरण; स्वच्छपटल का बाहर की ओर फैल जाना

**Keratectasis.** See **Keratectasia.**

**Keratectomy.** Removal of a portion of the cornea. कनीनिका-उच्छेदन; स्वच्छपटल-उच्छेदन

**Keratic.** Pertaining to the cornea. स्वच्छमण्डलीय; स्वच्छमण्डल सम्बन्धी

**Keratin.** A protein found in all horny tissues. केरेटिन; शृंगी ऊतकों में पाया जाने वाला एक प्रोटीन

**Keratinous.** Containing keratin. केरेटिनयुक्त; किरेटिनी; शृंगमय

**Keratitis.** Inflammation of the cornea; ceratitis. कनीनिकाशोथ; स्वच्छपटलशोथ;

K. Bullosa, see Bullous Keratitis.

K. Punctata, see Punctate Keratitis.

Bullous K., the formation of blebs upon the cornea; keratitis bullosa. स्फोटी स्वच्छपटलशोथ;

Deep K., see Interstitial Keratitis.

Dendriform K., a form of herpetic inflammation of cornea; dendritic keratitis. शाखी स्वच्छपटलशोथ;

Dendritic K., see Dendriform Keratitis.

Interstitial K., a chronic from of keratitis due to congenital syphilis; deep keratitis. अन्तरालीय स्वच्छपटलशोथ;

Mycotic K., keratitis produced by fungi. कवक स्वच्छपटलशोथ;;

Phlyctenular K., a form of keratitis marked by the presence of papules or pustules. अदलीय स्वच्छपटलशोथ;

Purulent K., a form of keratitis marked by the formation of pus. सपूय स्वच्छपटलशोथ;

Punctate K., a secondary affection of the cornea marked by the formation of opaque dots; keratitis punctata. बिन्दुकित स्वच्छपटलशोथ;

Sclerosing K., inflammation of the cornea complicating scleritis characterized by opacification of corneal stroma. काठिन्यज स्वच्छपटलशोथ;

Traumatic K., keratitis caused by a wound of cornea. चोटमूलक स्वच्छपटलशोथ

**Keratocele.** Hernia of the cornea. स्वच्छपटलस्रंस; केरेटोसील; कनीनिका-हर्निया

**Keratoconjunctivitis.** Inflammation of the cornea and conjunctiva. स्वच्छपटलश्लेष्मलाशोथ; स्वच्छपटल एवं आँखों की श्लैष्मिक झिल्ली का प्रदाह

**Keratoconus.** Conical protrusion of the centre of the cornea without inflammation. शुंकुक-स्वच्छपटल

**Keratoectasia.** Dilatation of the cornea. स्वच्छपटलविस्फार; कनीनिकाविस्फार

**Keratogenous.** Pertaining to the formation of horny growths. स्वच्छपटलजनक

**Keratoglobus.** A distension and protrusion of the cornea. स्वच्छपटलविस्फार; गोलकस्वच्छपटल

**Keratoid.** Horn-like. शृंगोपम; शृंगाभ; सींग जैसा

**Keratoiritis.** Inflammation of the cornea and the iris. स्वच्छपटपरितारिकाशोथ; कनीनिका और पुतली का प्रदाह

**Keratoid.** Resembling the cornea. स्वच्छपटलाभ; स्वच्छपटल जैसा

**Keratolysis.** A throwing off of the skin. त्वक्लयन; चर्मविशल्कन

**Keratolytics.** Having the property of breaking down keratinized epidermis. विशल्कक; चर्मविशल्कक

**Keratoma.** A tumour of the cornea. स्वच्छपटलार्बुद; callosity. घट्टा; किण

**Keratomalacia.** A softening of the cornea. स्वच्छपटलमृदुता; कनीनिका की कोमलता

**Keratome.** A knife used for incising the cornea ; keratotome. स्वच्छपटलछुरिका

**Keratometer.** An instrument for measuring curve of the cornea. स्वच्छपटलमापी; कनीनिकामापी

**Keratometry.** The use of the keratometer. स्वच्छपटलमिति; कनीनिकामिति; कनीनिकामापन

**Keratomycosis.** A fungoid growth of the cornea. स्वच्छपटलकवकता; कनीनिका का कवक गुल्म

**Keratoplasty.** A plastic operation on the cornea for removal of pain of the cornea, containing an opacity; corneal graft. स्वच्छपटलसंधान;

   **Optic K.,** transplantation of transparent corneal tissue to replace a leucoma or scar that obstructs vision. दृष्टि-स्वच्छपटलसंधान;

   **Tectonic K.,** grafting of corneal material on a part where it has been lost, without attempt to restore the transparency. रूपद स्वच्छपटलसंधान

**Keratoscope.** An instrument for examining the cornea. स्वच्छपटलदर्शी; कनीनिकादर्शी

**Keratoscopy.** The use of the keratoscope. स्वच्छपटलदर्शन; कनीनिकादर्शन

**Keratosis.** A form of skin disease with thickened epidermis. केरेटोसिस; शृंगीयता;

   **Senile K.,** a dry, harsh condition of the skin in the aged. जरा-केरेटिनता

   **K. Pilaris,** a horny formation around the hair-follicles. लोम-केरेटिनता

**Keratothelcosis.** Ulceration of the cornea. स्वच्छपटलव्रणता

**Keratotome.** See **Keratome.**

**Keratotomy.** An incision of the cornea. स्वच्छपटलछेदन

**Kernicterus.** Bile staining of the basal ganglia in the brain of the newborn. प्रमस्तिष्कीनवजातकामला

**Kernig's sign.** Contracture or flexion of the knee and hip-joint, at times also of the elbow, when the patient is made to assume the sitting posture. कर्निग चिन्ह; जानु, नितम्बसन्धि तथा कोहनी की सिकुड़न

**Ketogenesis.** Production of ketone bodies. कीटोनजनन; कीटोन-उत्पादन; कीटोनोत्पादन

**Ketogenetic.** Producing ketone bodies; ketogenic. कीटोनजनक; कीटोन-उत्पादक; कीटोनोत्पादक

**Ketogenic.** See **Ketogenetic.**
    **K. Diet,** a high fat content producing ketosis. कीटोनोत्पादक आहार

**Ketone.** Ketone bodies in ketosis. कीटोन; कीटोनपिण्ड

**Ketonuria.** The presenc of ketone bodies in the urine; ketosuria. कीटोनमेह; पेशाब में कीटोनपिण्ड जाना

**Ketose.** Sugar which is the ketone of the complex alcohol. कीटोज

**Ketosis.** Accumulation of ketone bodies in the blood. कीटोनमयता

**Ketosuria.** See **Ketonuria.**

**Kidney.** The urine secreting organ. वृक्क; गुर्दा;
    **Contracted K.,** a diffusely scattered kidney. संकुचित वृक्क;
    **Floating K.,** one loosened and displaced; movable kidey; wandering kidney. चल वृक्क;
    **Horse-shoe K.,** a congenital union of the kidneys. अश्वनाल वृक्क;
    **Movable K.,** see **Floating Kidney.**
    **Wandering K.,** see **Floating Kidey.**

**Kidney-failure.** Diminished function of the kidney. वृक्कपात

**Kidney-stone.** Presence of calculus in the pelvis of kidney. वृक्काश्म; वृक्काश्मरी; गुर्दे की पथरी

**Kinaesthesia.** See **Kinesthesis.**

**Kinaesthesis.** Muscle sense; perception of movement; kinaesthesia; kinesthesia; kinesthesis. गतिसंवेदना

**Kinaesthetic.** See **Kinesthetic.**

**Kinematics.** The study of motion. गतिविज्ञान; गतिकी

**Kinesalgia.** Pain on muscular movement. पेशीगतिशूल

**Kinesthesia.** See **Kinaesthesis.**

**Kinesthesis.** See **Kinaesthesis.**

**Kinesthetic.** Peraining to kinesthesis; kinaesthetic. गतिसंवेदी; गतिबोधक; गतिसंवेदना सम्बन्धी

**Kinetic.** Pertaining to, or producing motion. गतिज; गतिक

**Kinetics.** The study of motion, acceleration, or rate of change. बलगतिविज्ञान; बलगतिकी

**Kinetocardiogram.** Graphic recording of the vibration of the chest wall produced by cardiac activity. चलहृदलेख

**Kinetocyte.** A wandering cell. भ्रमणकोशिका; चलकोशिका

**King's evil.** Scrofula. गण्डमाला; कण्ठमाला

**Kinometer.** An instrument for measuring the amount of uterine displacement. जरायुभ्रंशमापी

**Kiss of life.** Method of artificial respiration. कृत्रिमश्वासपद्धति

**Kleptomania.** Madness with an irresistible propensity to theft. चोरणोन्माद; चोरी करने की अप्रतिहत इच्छा

**Kleptomaniac.** A person exhibiting kleptomania. चोरणोन्मादी

**Kleptophobia.** Fear of becoming thief. चोरणभीति; चोर बनने का भय

**Knee.** The articulation between the femur and the tibia, covered anteriorly by a patella; genu. जानु; घुटना;

   **House-maid's k.,** inflamed condition of bursa anterior to the patella with accumulation of fluid therein; prepatellar bursitis. गृहसेविका जानु; दासी जानु;

   **Knock-k.,** a crooked knee; genu valgum. बहिर्नत जानु; संघट्ट जानु;

   **K.-cap,** the patella; knee-pan. जानुका;

   **K.-jerk,** the contraction of the quadriceps extensor femoris muscle as a result of a light blow on the patellar tendon. जानुक्षेप; जानु-प्रक्षेप;

   **K.-jerk Reflex,** the reflex contraction of qudriceps muscle. जानुक्षेप प्रतिवर्त;

   **K.-joint,** the articulation of the femur and tibia. जानु-संधि; घुटने का जोड़;

   **K.-pan,** see **Knee-cap.**

**Knife.** An instrument for cutting. छुरिका; छुरी; चाकू;

   **Electric K.,** a knife that functions by use of a high-frequency cutting culture. विद्युत्-छुरिका

**Knob.** A knot; a protuberance. गांठ; उभार

**Knock-knee.** See under **Knee**.

**Knot.** See **Knob**.

**Knuckle.** The dorsal aspect of any of the joints between the phalanges and the metacarpal bones, or between the phalanges. अंगुलिपर्व; पोर

**Koch's bacillus.** A term used for the tubercle bacillus and named after Koch. यक्ष्माणु; क्षयरोगाणु

**Koilonychia.** Concave, or spoon-like nails. दर्वीनख्र; चम्मचाकार नाखुन

**Kolyseptic.** Preventing putrefaction. पूतिरोधक; पूतिरोधी

**Koplik's signs.** See **Koplik's spots**.

**Koplik's spots.** Minute bluish-white spots surrounded by a reddish areola. कॉपलिक धब्बे, जो रोमान्तिका के आक्रमण के पहले दिन मुख के अन्दर सफेद धब्बों के रूप दिखाई देते हैं

**Koumyss.** The whey of the mare's milk; kumiss; kumyss. कूमिस; घोड़ी का दूध

**Kreatin.** A nitrogenous constituent of the muscles. क्रिएटिन; पेशियों का एक नाइट्रोजनमय घटक

**Krukenberg Tumour.** Secondary malignant tumour of the ovary. दुर्दमडिम्बग्रन्थ्यर्बुद; डिम्बाशय का एक दुर्दम अर्बुद

**Kumiss.** See **Koumyss**.

**Kumyss.** See **Koumyss**.

**Kyllosis.** Club-foot. मुद्गरपाद; आजन्म पादबक्रता

**Kymograph.** An instrument for recording pressure, pulsations, sound waves, etc. on a revolving drum. गतिलेखी

**Kymography.** The use of kymograph. गतिलेखन; काइमोग्राफी

**Kymoscope.** An instrument for studying the blood-current. रुधिरधारादर्शीयंत्र

**Kyphoscoliosis.** Combined kyphosis and scoliosis. पृष्ठपार्श्वकुब्जता

**Kyphosis.** Hump-back; angular curvature of the spine. कुब्जता; कुबड़ापन

**Kysthitis.** Vaginitis; inflammation of the vagina. योनिशोथ; योनि का प्रदाह

# L

**Labia.** Plural of **Labium.**

    **L. Leporina,** the hare-lip. खण्डोष्ठ;

    **L. Majora,** the two large folds, constituting the external orifice of the pudendum. बृहत् भगोष्ठ;

    **L. Minora,** the two smaller folds, situated with the labia majora and frequently termed nymphae. लघु भगोष्ठ; क्षुद्र भगोष्ठ;

    **L. Oris,** the lips bounding the cavity of the mouth. ओष्ठ: होंठ; अधर;

    **L. Pudendi,** the lips of the vulva. बहिर्योनि भगोष्ठ

**Labial.** Pertaining to labia or the lips. ओष्ठ अथवा होंठों सम्बन्धी

**Labialism.** Speech marred by lip-sounds. ओष्ठोच्चार; होंठों से बोलना; अधरोच्चार

**Labii.** See **Labium.**

**Labile.** Gliding from place to place; unstable or unsteady; not fixed. चल; चंचल; अस्थिर; अस्थायी; परिवर्ती

**Lability.** Instability; the state of being labile. अस्थिरता

**Labiochorea.** A chronic spasm of the lips. ओष्ठलास्य; ओष्ठकम्प; ओष्ठाकर्ष

**Labioclination.** Inclination of a tooth more toward the lips. ओष्ठदन्तुरण

**Labiodental.** Pertaining to the lips and the teeth. अधर अथवा ओष्ठ एवं दान्तों सम्बन्धी

**Labiograph.** An instrument for recording the movements of the lips in speaking. ओष्ठलेखयंत्र; ओष्ठलेखी

**Labiomacy.** Comprehending speech by lip-movements. ओष्ठोच्चार; अधरोच्चार: होंठों से बोलना

**Labiomental.** Relating to the lips and the chin. ओष्ठचिबुक अर्थात् होंठों तथा ठोड़ी सम्बन्धी

**Labionasal.** Relating to the upper lip or both the lips and the nose. होंठों तथा नाक सम्बन्धी

**Labioplasty.** Plastic operation on a lip. ओष्ठसंधान

**Labis.** Forceps. संदंश; पूलिका; चिमटी

**Labium.** A lip; labii. ओष्ठ; अधर; भगोष्ठ;

   **L Majus,** one of the two folds of the skin of the female external genital organs, arising just below the mons veneris and surrounding the vulvar entrance. बृहत् भगोष्ठ;

   **L. Minor,** one of the two folds of the mucous membrane at the inner surfaces of the labia majora. लघु भगोष्ठ; क्षुद्र भगोष्ठ

   **L. Oris,** see **Lip.**

**Labor.** Parturition; childbirth; labour. प्रसव; वह प्रक्रिया जिसमें गर्भवती स्त्री गर्भाशय से शिशु को योनि-मार्ग से बाहर निकालती है;

   **Artificial L.,** that effected by other means than the forces of the maternal organism. कृत्रिम प्रसव; प्रेरित प्रसव;

   **Dry L.,** when there is a deficiency of the liquor amnii. शुष्क प्रसव, जिसमें गर्भाशय की सिकुड़न आरम्भ होने से पहले ही उल्वकोष फट जाता है तथा उल्व-द्रव शिशु के साथ ही बाहर निकल आता है;

   **Induced L.,** that brought on by artificial means. प्रेरित प्रसव, जिसमें प्रसव यंत्रों की सहायता के अतिरिक्त अन्य साधन भी अपनाये जाते हैं;

   **Missed L.,** retention of the dead foetus in utero beyond the period of normal gestation. लीन प्रसव, जिसमें प्रसवकाल पूर्ण होने पर भी मृत भ्रूण गर्भ में बना रहता है;

   **Precipitate L.,** that in which delivery takes place with undue rapidity. सहसा प्रसव; आकस्मिक प्रसव;

   **Premature L.,** that taking place before the normal period of gestation but when the foetus is viable. अकाल प्रसव; कालपूर्व प्रसव; नियत समय से पूर्व होने वाला प्रसव;

   **Protracted L.,** that prolonged beyond the usual limit. अतिदीर्घ प्रसव;

   **Spontaneous L.,** that requiring no artificial aid. स्वाभाविक प्रसव; स्वत: प्रसव

**Labour.** See **Labor.**

**Labra.** Plural of **Labrum.**

**Labrum.** Labium. ओष्ठ; लैब्रम; होंठ

**Labyrinth.** Part of the inner ear. आन्तरकर्ण; गहन;

   **Bony L.,** see **Osseous Labyrinth.**

   **Membranous L.,** the membranous cavity within the osseous labyrinth. कला-गहन;

   **Osseous L.,** the bony portion of the internal ear; bony labyrinth. अस्थि-गहन

**Labyrinthectomy.** Surgical removal of part or the whole of the membranous labyrinth of the internal ear. गहनोच्छेदन; आन्तरकर्ण-उच्छेदन

**Labyrinthine.** Relating to labyrinth. गहन अथवा आन्तरकर्ण सम्बन्धी

**Labyrinthitis.** Inflammation of the labyrinth. गहनशोथ; आन्तरकर्णशोथ

**Labyrinthotomy.** Incision into the labyrinth of the ear. आन्तरकर्णछेदन; गहनछेदन

**Lac.** Milk or any milk-like medicinal preparation; lacta. दुग्ध अथवा दुग्धवत् पदार्थ

**Lacerated.** Torn; rent; having a ragged edge. विदीर्ण; कटा-फटा

**Laceration.** Tearing; the act of being lacerated or torn. विदार; विदारण; विदीर्ण करना; चीर-फाड़ करना

**Lacertus Fibrosus.** An aponeurotic band from the biceps-tendon to fascia of the forearm. तान्तव लघुपूलिका

**Lacerum Foramen.** Two irregular openings between the occipital and temporal bones. पश्चकपाल तथा कर्णपटास्थियों के मध्य स्थित दो टेढ़े-मेढ़े द्वार

**Lachrima.** See **Lachryma.**

**Lachryma.** A tear; lachrima; lacrima; lacryma. अश्रु; आँसू

**Lachrymal.** Pertaining to the tears; lacrimal; lacrymal. अश्रुप्रवाही; अश्रुपाती; अश्रु सम्बन्धी;

   L. Duct, the duct of the lacrimal gland. अश्रुनली;

   L. Sac, the same as **Lachrymal Duct.**

**Lachrymation.** Discharge of water from the eyes; lacrimation. अश्रुपात; अश्रुप्रवाह; अश्रुस्राव; अश्रुस्रवण

**Lacrima.** See **Lachryma.**

**Lacrimal.** See **Lachrymal.**

**Lacrimation.** See **Lachrymation.**

**Lacryma.** See **Lachryma.**

**Lacrymal.** See **Lachrymal.**

**Lacrymation.** See **Lachrymation.**

**Lacta.** See **Lac.**

**Lactagog.** See **Lactagogue.**

**Lactagogue.** An agent inducing milk-secretion; lactagog. स्तन्यवर्धक; दुग्धवर्धक

**Lactalbumin.** A protein found in milk. दुग्धान्नसार; दूध में पाया जाने वाला एक प्रोटीन

**Lactant.** Suckling. स्तनपायी

**Lactation.** Secretion of milk while nursing; giving suck. स्तन्यस्रवण; दुग्धस्रवण; दुग्धपान; the production of milk. दुग्धोत्पादन

**Lacteal.** The commencing lymphatic duct in the intestinal villi. दुग्धवाही; pertaining to milk. दूध सम्बन्धी

**Lacteous.** See **Lacteus.**

**Lacteus.** Milky; lacteous. दुग्धाभ; दुग्धवत्; दुग्धिल; दूधिया; दूध जैसा

**Lactic.** Made of milk. दुग्धयुक्त; दुग्धनिर्मित; relating to milk. दुग्धविषयक; दुग्ध अर्थात् दूध सम्बन्धी,

    **L. Acid,** the acid that causes the souring of the milk. दुग्धाम्ल; दुग्धक्षार;

    **L. Fermentation,** the souring of milk. दुग्ध-खमीरण

**Lactiferous.** Conveying or secreting milk. दुग्धवाही; दुग्धस्रावी; दुग्धजन; दुग्धमय

**Lactifuge.** Any agent which suppresses the milk-secretion. दुग्धशोषक; दुग्धशोधक; स्तन्यहर; दुग्ध-स्राव को कम करने वाला

**Lactigenous.** Milk-producing. दुग्धोत्पादक; दुग्धवर्धक; दूध बढ़ाने वाला

**Lactigerous.** Producing milk. दुग्धोत्पादक; दुग्धजनक

**Lactin.** Sugar of milk; lactose. दुग्धशर्करा; लैक्टोज

**Lactinated.** Containing sugar of milk. दुग्धशर्करायुक्त

**Lactis.** Pertaining to milk; lactus. दुग्धविषयक; दूध सम्बन्धी

**Lactivorous.** Subsisting on milk-diet exclusively; lactivorus. दुग्धाहारी; दुग्धजीवी; मात्र दूध पर ही पलने वाला प्राणी

**Lactivorus.** See **Lactivorous.**

**Lactocele.** A collection of milk-like fluid; galactocele. स्तन्य-पुटी

**Lactogen.** An agent that stimulates milk production or secretion. दुग्धजन; लैक्टोजन

**Lactogenesis.** Milk-production. दुग्धोत्पादन

**Lactogenic.** Stimulating milk production. दुग्धजनक; दुग्धवर्धक; दूध की मात्रा बढ़ाने वाला; relating to lactogenesis. दुग्धोत्पादन सम्बन्धी

**Lactometer.** An instrument for measuring the specfic gravity of the milk. दुग्धमापी; दुग्धघनत्वमापी; लैक्टोमीटर

**Lactorrhea.** See **Lactorrhoea.**

**Loctorrhoea.** Incontinence of milk; lactorrhea. असंयतदुग्धस्राव

**Lactose.** A sugar found in the milk; sugar of milk; lactin. दुग्धशर्करा; लैक्टोज

**Lactosuria.** Sugar of milk in the urine. दुग्धशर्करामेह; लैक्टोजमेह; पेशाब में दुग्धशर्करा जाना

**Lactotherapy.** Milk-therapy; galactotherapy. दुग्धोपचार; दूध से की जाने वाली चिकित्सा

**Lactus.** See **Lactis.**

**Lacuna.** An abnormal space between the cellular elements of the epidermis. रिक्तिका; कोशिकान्तर;
    **L. Magna,** the largest of the mucous glands of the male urethra. बृहत् रिक्तिका

**Lacunae.** Plural of **Lacuna.**

**Lacunar.** Pertaining to lacunas. रिक्तिकीय

**Lacunas.** Plural of **Lacuna.**

**Lacunule.** A very small lacuna. क्षुद्ररिक्तिका

**Lacus.** A small hollow or cavity. क्षुद्र गह्वर; नली; a lake. सर;
    **L. Lachrymalis,** the lachrymal sac; lacrimal lake. अश्रुनली; अश्रुसर; आँसू की थैली;
    **L. Seminalis,** the vault of the vegina after insemination; seminal lake. शुक्रसर

**Laevus.** Left. बाम; बायाँ

**Lagophthalmos.** Unable to close the eyes; lagophthalmus. अल्पनिमेषी; आँखों को पूर्णतया बन्द करने में अक्षम

**Lagophthalmus.** See **Lagophthalmos.**

**La Grippe.** Influenza. श्लैष्मिक ज्वर; इन्फ्लुएंजा

**Lake.** A small cavity of fluid; lacus. सर;
    **Capillary L.,** the total mass of blood contained in capillary vessels. कोशिका-सर;
    **Lacrimal L.,** see **Lacus Lachrymalis.**
    **Seminal L.,** see **Lacus Seminalis.**

**Lallation.** See **Lalling.**

**Lalling.** Stammering; the imperfect pronunciation of a letter; lallation. तुतलाना; हकलाना

**Lalopathy.** Any disorder of the speech. वाणीविकार; वाग्विकार; बोलने का दोष

**Laloplegia.** Paralysis of the muscles concerned in the mechanism of speech. वाणीघात; वाचाघात

**Lamella.** A thin plate or scale. पक्षक; पत्रक; पटलिका;
> **Articular L.**, the compact layer of bone on its articular surface that is firmly attached to the overlying articular cartilage. सन्धि-पटलिका;
> **Bone L.**, thin layer of ground substance of osseous tissue. अस्थि-पटलिका

**Lamellar.** Disposed in lamellas; scaly. पत्रकी; पटलित

**Lamellae.** Plural of **lamella.**

**Lameness.** Weakness of the limbs. पंगुता; खंजता; लूलापन; लंगड़ापन्

**Lamina.** A thin layer, scale or plate, usually of bone. पटल; फलक; फलिका; अस्तर; आवरण; पत्रदल; पत्रिका; अस्तरिका;
> **L. Cribrosa,** a cribriform plate. चालनीवत् फलक; चालनीरूप फलक;
> **L. Denticulata,** a cartilaginous plate on the superior and external portion of the osseous spiral lamina; dental lamina. दन्त-फलक;
> **L. Fusca,** the internal pigmented layer of the sclera. कृष्ण-फलक;
> **L. Papyracea,** that of the ethmoid. पत्र-फलक;
> **L. Perpendicularis,** the vertical plate of the ethmoid or mesethmoid. लम्ब फलक;
> **L. Spiralis,** the spiral partition dividing the cochlear cavity. सर्पिल फलक;
> **L. Spiralis Ossea,** the bony spiral portion dividing the cochlear cavity. अस्थिमय सर्पिल फलक;
> **L. Suprachorioidea,** a thin layer of connective tissue between the sclera and the choroid. अधिरंजितपटल फलक;
> **L. Terminalis,** the thin sheet of tissue forming the anterior border of the third ventricle. अन्त्य फलक

**Laminae.** Plural of **Lamina.**

**Laminagram.** A film taken by a laminagraph. अस्तरचित्र

**Laminagraph.** An x-ray technique for producing a laminagram. अस्तर-आलेख

**Laminagraphy.** Study of body tissues by use of laminagrams. अस्तरचित्रण

**Laminar.** Ralating to any lamina. अस्तर सम्बन्धी

**Laminated.** Arranged in layers. पटलित; अस्तरित; परतदार

**Lamination.** Arrangement in plates or layers. पटलन; अस्तरण

**Laminectomy.** Excision of the vertebral lamina. फलकोच्छेदन; कशेरुकाफलकोच्छेदन

**Laminitis.** Inflammation of the laminas of horse's foot. सुमशोथ

**Lamp.** An illuminating device; a source of light and heat. लैम्प; दीपक; दीया;

   **Slit L.,** lamp constructed so that an intense light is emitted through a slit, used for examination of eyes. स्लिट लैम्प

**Lancet.** A sharp-pointed two-edged surgical knife. छुरिका; कुन्तिका; लैन्सेट; छोटा, नुकीला और दो धार वाला चाकू

**Lancinate.** To lacerate or tear. विदीर्ण करना; फाड़ना

**Lancinatig.** Piercing, as with a sharp-pointed instrument. विदीर्णकारी

**Landry's paralysis.** Acute ascending paralysis. तीव्र आरोही अंगघात; नीचे से ऊपर को बढ़ता हुआ उग्र पक्षाघात

**Landscurvy.** Purpura haemorrhagica. रक्तचित्तिता

**Languor.** Feebleness; weakness; lassitude. आलस; सुस्ती; शिथिलता

**Lanolin.** Wool fat containing 30 percent water; lanoline. ऊर्ण वसा; शुद्ध वसोपम पदार्थ, जिसका प्रयोग मलहम बनाने में किया जाता है

**Lanoline.** See **Lanolin.**

**Lanugo.** The downy hair on the foetus. गर्भलोम; गर्भरोम; भ्रूणरोम

**L.A.O.** Left anterior oblique. बाम-अग्र-तिर्यक; बामाग्रतिर्यक

**Lapactic.** Emptying; purgative. रेचक; विरेचक; रिक्तकारी

**Laparo-.** Prefix meaning abdomen. 'उदर' के रूप में प्रयुक्त उपसर्ग

**Laparocele.** Abdominal hernia. उदर-हर्निया

**Laparorrhaphy.** Suture of wound in the abdominal wall. उदरसीवन

**Laparoscope.** An instrument for examining the abdomen. अन्तरुदरदर्शी; उदर-जांच के लिये प्रयुक्त किया जाने वाला यंत्र

**Laparoscopy.** Examination of the abdomen. अन्तरुदरदर्शन; उदर के अन्दरूनी भाग की जांच

**Laparotomy.** An abdominal incision; celiotomy. उदरछेदन; पेट का आपरेशन

**Lapis.** A stone. अश्म; अश्मरी; पथरी; पत्थर; पाषाण

**Lard.** Fat. वसा; चर्बी; wax. मोम

**Lardaceous.** Fatty or waxy. वसाभ; मोमी; चर्बी या मोम जैसा

**Larva.** An embryo which is independent before it has assumed the characteristic features of its parents. लार्वा; डिम्भक; इल्ली; अर्भक; प्रौढ़ता प्राप्त करने से पूर्व भ्रूण की अवस्था

**Larvae.** Plural of **Larva.**

**Larval.** Relating to larva. लार्वा सम्बन्धी

**Larvicidal.** Destructive to larva. लार्वानाशी

**Larvicide.** Any agent which destroys larvae. लार्वानाशक; लार्वानाशी; इल्लीनाशी; अर्भकनाशी

**Laryngeal.** Pertaining to the larynx. स्वरयंत्रगरक; स्वरयंत्रज; रबरयंत्र सम्बन्धी;

    **L. Catarrh,** catarrh affecting chiefly the larynx. स्वरयंत्रज प्रतिश्याय; स्वरयंत्र को ही प्रमुख रूप से प्रभावित करने वाला सर्दी-जुकाम

**Larygectomy.** Extirpation of the larynx. स्वरयंत्र-उच्छेदन; स्वरयंत्रोच्छेदन; स्वरयंत्र को काट कर हटा देना

**Larynges.** Plural of **Larynx.**

**Laryngismus.** A spasmodic affection of the larynx. स्वरयंत्राकर्ष; स्वरयंत्र-उद्वेष्ट; स्वरयंत्र का ऐंठनयुक्त रोग;

    **L. Paralyticus,** a paralytic spasm of the larynx. पक्षाघाती स्वरयंत्राकर्ष;

    **L. Stridulus,** spasm of the larynx with hoarseness. घर्घर स्वरयंत्राकर्ष; स्वरयंत्रघर्घर; स्वरयंत्र का आक्षेप

**Laryngitic.** Relating to, or caused by laryngitis. स्वयंत्रशोथज

**Laryngitis.** Inflammation of the larynx. स्वरयंत्रशोथ; स्वरयंत्र-प्रदाह

**Larygocele.** A saccular dilatation of the larynx. स्वरयंत्रविपुटी; स्वरयंत्र का थैली जैसा फैलाव होना

**Laryngofissure.** A division of the thyroid cartilage; laryngotomy; thyrotomy. स्वरयंत्रछेदन; कण्ठछेदन; अवटूपास्थिछेदन अवटु-उपास्थि का विभाजन

**Laryngology.** The science of the larynx. स्वरयंत्रविज्ञान; स्वरयंत्र की रचना तथा बीमारियों सम्बन्धी वैज्ञानिक अध्ययन

**Laryngomalacia.** A softening of the larynx. स्वरयंत्रमृदुता; स्वरयंत्र की कोमलता

**Laryngoparalysis.** Paralysis of the laryngeal muscles;

**Laryngopathy**

laryngoplegia. स्वरयंत्रघात; स्वरयंत्रपेशीघात; स्वरयंत्र की पेशियों का पक्षाघात

**Laryngopathy.** Any disease of the larynx. स्वरयंत्ररोग

**Laryngopharyngeal.** Relating to the larynx and the pharynx. स्वरयंत्र तथा ग्रसनी सम्बन्धी

**Laryngopharyngectomy.** Excision of both larynx and pharynx. स्वरयंत्रग्रसनी-उच्छेदन

**Laryngopharyngitis.** Inflammation of both larynx and pharynx. स्वरयंत्रग्रसनीशोथ

**Laryngopharynx.** The portion of the pharynx above the larynx. स्वरयंत्रग्रसनी; ग्रसनी का स्वरयंत्र भाग

**Laryngoplasty.** Reparative surgery of the larynx. स्वरयंत्रसंधान

**Laryngoplegia.** See **Laryngoparalysis.**

**Laryngoptosis.** An abnormally low position of the larynx. स्वरयंत्रपात; स्वरयंत्रच्युति

**Laryngorhinology.** The branch of medical science concerned with the larynx and the nose. स्वरयंत्रनासाविज्ञान

**Laryngorrhea.** See **Laryngorrhoea.**

**Laryngorrhoea.** Excessive secretion from the larynx; laryngorrhea. स्वरयंत्र-अतिस्राव; स्वरयंत्र से अत्यधिक स्राव होना

**Laryngoscope.** Instrument for visualization of the larynx. स्वरयंत्रदर्शी; स्वरयंत्र की जांच में प्रयुक्त यंत्र-विशेष

**Laryngoscopy.** An inspection of the larynx. स्वरयंत्रदर्शन; स्वरयंत्र की जांच

**Laryngospasm.** Spasmodic contracture of the glottis. स्वरयंत्राकर्ष; कण्ठद्वार की उद्वेष्टकारी सिकुड़न

**Laryngostenosis.** Constriction of the larynx. स्वरयंत्रकाठिन्य; स्वरयंत्रसंकीर्णन; स्वरयंत्र की सिकुड़न

**Laryngostomy.** Establishment of a permanant opening from the neck into the larynx. स्वरयंत्रछिद्रीकरण

**Laryngotomy.** See **Laryngofissure.**

**Laryngotracheitis.** See **Laryngotrachitis.**

**Laryngotracheobronchitis.** Inflammation of the larynx, trachea and bronchi. स्वरयंत्रश्वासप्रणालश्वसनीशोथ; स्वरयंत्र, श्वासप्रणाल एवं श्वसनिकाओं का प्रदाह

**Laryngotrachitis.** Inflammation of the larynx and trachea;

laryngotracheitis. स्वरयंत्रश्वासप्रणालशोथ; स्वरयंत्र एवं श्वासप्रणाल का प्रदाह

**Laryngoxerosis.** Dryness of the larynx. स्वरयंत्रशुष्कता; स्वरयंत्र का रूखापन

**Larynx.** The organ of voice situated at the front of the neck beginning below the base of the tongue and being continuous with the wind pipe. स्वरयंत्र; कण्ठनली

**Lascivious.** Lustful; wanton; amorous. कामुक; कामासक्त; आसक्त; लम्पट

**Lasciviousness.** Lustfulness; amorousness. कामुकता; कामासक्ति; लम्पटता

**Laser.** A device that concentrates high energies into a narrow beam of visible, nonspreading, monochromatic light, used in surgery to cut and disslove tissue. लेसर; रश्मिएकीकरणयंत्र;

**L. Cane,** an experimental cane that helps a blind person detect objects ahead of, above and below his or her path. लेसर केन

**Lassitude.** A morbid sensation of languor, frequently preceding and accompanying disease. आलस; सुस्ती

**Latent.** Concealed; not manifest. गुप्त; प्रच्छन्न; अदृश; अप्रकट; अव्यक्त; अन्तर्हित;

**L. Period,** the period before the actual onset of a disease. गुप्त काल; प्रच्छन्न काल

**Latera.** Plural of **Latus.**

**Lateral.** At or pertaining to a side. पार्श्विक; पार्श्वीय; पार्श्व सम्बन्धी;

**L. Sinus,** transverse and sigmoid portion of two cranial venous sinuses. पार्श्व-शिरानाल

**Laterality.** Condition of being on one side or toward the side. पार्श्वीयता; पार्श्विकता

**Lateris.** See **Latus.**

**Lateroflexion.** A bending to one side. एकपार्श्विकनति; एकपार्श्वनति; एक ओर को झुका हुआ

**Lathyrism.** Poisoning with chickpea. कलायखंज; लेथीरस-रुग्णता

**Latus.** Flank; the side of the body between the pelvis and the ribs; lateris. पार्श्वभाग; कोख; बगल; broad. चौड़ा; विस्तृत

**Laudable.** Commendable. स्तुत्य; श्लाघ्य; प्रशंसा योग्य

**Laudanum.** The tincutre of opium. अफीम का अर्क अथवा टिंचर

**Lavage.** The washing out of a body cavity, as the stomach or bowels; lavation. धावन; प्रक्षालन; पानी से धोना

**Lavation.** See **Lavage.**

**Lavement.** Clyster; enema; an injection to move the bowels. वस्तिकर्म; एनीमा देना

**Law.** Scientifically, a statement that is found to hold true uniformly for a whole class of natural occurrences; a principle or rule. नियम; विधान; विधि; कानून; संहिता; सिद्धान्त

**Lax.** Loose; slack. ढीला-ढाला; शिथिल; rare. विरल

**Laxative.** A mild aperient. मृदुविरेचक; सारक; रेचक औषधि; दस्तावर दवा; जुलाब लाने वाली दवा

**Laxity.** Atony; a relaxed condition. अतानता; ढीलापन; ढीली-ढाली अवस्था

**Layer.** A mass of nearly uniform thickness spread over an area. अस्तर; तह; परत;

   **Horny L.,** the outer layer of the skin. शृंगी अस्तर

**Lazeretto.** Quarantine station for contagious disease. संक्रामक रुग्णालय; संक्रामक रोगियों को अलग रखने का स्थान

**Lb.** Abbreviation for **Libra.**

**L.D.** Lethal dose; a fatal dose. घातक मात्रा

**Lead.** A dangerous chemical, producing poison when swallowed. सीसा; रांग;

   **L. Colic,** an affection produced by lead. सीसज उदरशूल;

   **L. Palsy,** paralysis caused by lead-poisoning. सीसज पक्षाघात;

   **L. Pipe Contraction,** a cataleptic state in which the limbs maintain any position given to them. पेशी-प्रतिष्टम्भ;

   **L. Plaster,** an adhesive plaster containing lead-oxide. सीसा-पलस्तर;

   **L. Poisoning,** poisoning caused by lead either due to ingestion or inhalation. सीसज विषण्णता;

   **Red L.,** red oxide of lead. सिंदूर

**Leaf.** Folium. पत्ता; पत्र; पर्ण

**Lean.** Without flesh; emaciated. कृशतन; कृशकाय; दुबला

**Leaping Ague.** A species of dancing mania. लास्योन्माद; नृत्योन्माद; नाचने के पागलपन का एक रूप

**Lecithin.** A phosphorized substance occurring widely in the body and in plant-tissues. योक; डिम्बान्न; लेसीथिन; शरीर तथा पौधों में पाया जाने वाला पदार्थ

**Leech.** A cataloid worm, largely used to the local abstraction of the blood. जोंक; जलौका; जलीय तन्तु, जिसका प्रयोग रक्त को बाहर निकालने

के लिये किया जाता है;

**German L.**, speckled leech. बिन्दुकित जोंक; जर्मन जोंक;

**Hungarian L.**, green leech. हरी जोंक; हंगेरी जोंक

**Leeches.** A disease of mules and cattles. पशुकवकचर्मता; खच्चरों तथा अन्य पालतू पशुओं को होने वाली चमड़ी की एक बीमारी

**Left.** Sinistral; opposite of right. बाम; बायाँ

**Leg.** The lower extremity, especially from the knee-down. टांग; जंघा;

**Bow L.**, leg distorted inward throwing the knee outside of the normal line. धनुर्जंघा;

**Milk L.**, phlegmasia alba dolans; white leg. श्वेतजंघा; श्वेतपाद;

**White L.**, see **Milk Leg.**

**Legitimacy.** The state of being born in wedlock. धर्मजता

**Legume.** Pod; plant; edible part of a fruit; legumin. फली; दाना; शिम्ब

**Legumin.** See **Legume.**

**Leguminous.** Pertaining to, or consisting of a legume. शिंबित; शिम्बीधान्य का प्रोटीन

**Leiodermia.** Smooth, glossy skin. स्निग्धचर्मता; त्वचा अत्यधिक चिकनी व चमकदार होने की अवस्था

**Leiomyoma.** A tumour of unstripped muscular fibres. आरेखीपेशी-अर्बुद

**Leishman Donovan Bodies.** Small parasite-like bodies found in the liver and seen in the patients suffering from Kala-Azar; Leishmania Donovani. लीशमैन डोनोवन पिण्ड; लीशमैनिया; काला-आजारग्रस्त रोगियों के जिगर में पाये जाने वाले छोटे-छोटे परजीवी-पिण्ड

**Leishmania Donovani.** See **Leishman Donovan Bodies.**

**Lemnisci.** Plural of **Lemniscus.**

**Lemniscus.** A white band lying to the outer side of the superior peduncles of the cerebellum. तन्तुबन्ध

**Lens.** A transparent convex or concave disc; lentis. लेंस; ताल; वीक्ष; आँख का पर्दा;

**Achromatic L.**, one the dispersing power of which is exactly neutralized by another lens with the same curvature but a different refractive index. अवर्णिक लेंस; वर्ण-विपथन को ठीक करने वाला लेंस;

**Biconcave L.**, one concave on both surfaces; concavoconcave lens. उभयावत्तल लेंस;

**Lens**

> **Biconvex L.,** one with two convex lens; concavoconvex lens. उभयोत्तल लेंस;
>
> **Bifocal L.,** one having a double focus. द्विखण्डांशी लेंस; द्विकेन्द्री लेंस; बाइफोकल लेंस; ऐसा लेंस जिसमें दो खण्ड होते हैं, तथा जिनमें ऊपर वाले लेंस-खण्ड से दूर की वस्तु देखी जाती है और निचले लेंस-खण्ड से पास की वस्तु देखी जाती है;
>
> **Concave L.,** a dispersing lens. अवतल लेंस; नतोदर लेंस; परिक्षेपी किरणों को इधर-उधर छितरा देने वाला लेंस;
>
> **Concavoconcave L.,** see **Biconcave Lens.**
>
> **Concavoconvex L.,** see **Biconvex Lens.**
>
> **Contact L.,** a lens that fits over the cornea in direct contact with the sclera or cornea. सम्पर्क लेंस; कॉन्टैक्ट लेंस;
>
> **Convergent L.,** see **Converging Lens.**
>
> **Converging L.,** a double convex or planoconvex lens that focuses rays of light; convergent lens. उत्तल लेंस; अभिसारी लेंस;
>
> **Crystalline L.,** the lens of the eye. स्फटिक लेंस;
>
> **Dispersing L.,** see **Concave Lens.**
>
> **Photochromic L.,** a light-sensitive spectacle-lens that automatically darkens in sunlight and clears in reduced light. फोटोक्रॉमिक लेंस; प्रकाशवर्णी लेंस;
>
> **Spheric L.,** one with a curved surface; spherical lens. वर्तुलाकार लेंस; गोलाकार लेंस;
>
> **Spherical L.,** see **Spheric Lens.**

**Lensectomy.** Removal of lens, usually done by puncture incision. लेंसोच्छेदन; लेंसछेदन

**Lenticonus.** A clinical projection of the anterior or posterior surface of the lens occurring as a developmental anomaly. शंकुक लेंस

**Lenticular.** Pertaining to lens; lenticularis. लेंस सम्बन्धी

**Lenticularis.** See **Lenticular.**

**Lenticuli.** Plural of **Lenticulus.**

**Lenticulus.** An intraocular lens of inert plastic placed in the anterior chamber or behind the iris after cataract extraction. लेण्टिकुलस; अन्तराक्षिलेंस

**Lentiform.** Shaped like a lens. लेंसाकार; लेंस के आकार जैसा

**Lentigines.** Plural of **Lentigo.**

**Lentigo.** A brown macule resembling a freckle. मेचक; वर्णक; धब्बा; दाग

**Lentil.** A cheap and nutritious legumin containing a large amount of protein. मसूर; दाल

**Lentis.** See **Lens.**

**Lentitis.** Inflammation of the eye-lens. लेंसशोथ; लेंसप्रदाह

**Leontiasis.** Enlargement of face and head giving a lion-like appearance. सिंहमुखता; शेर के मुख के समान चेहरा और सिर का बढ़ जाना

**Leper.** One affected with leprosy. कुष्ठरोगी; कुष्ठग्रस्तरोगी; कोढ़ी

**Lepra.** Leprosy. कुष्ठ; कोढ़

**Leprae.** Plural of **Lepra.**

**Leprasorium.** A hospital or institute for the treatment of leprotic patients; leprosary; leprosarium. कुष्ठाश्रम; कोढ़ियों का अस्पताल

**Leprologist.** One who specializes in the study and treatment of leprosy. कुष्ठरोगविज्ञानी

**Leproma.** A leprous tumour or swelling. कुष्ठिक; कुष्ठवत् अर्बुद या सूजन

**Lepromatous.** Resembling leprosy. कुष्ठार्बुदवत्; कुष्ठार्बुद जैसा; pertaining to leprosy. कुष्ठ सम्बन्धी

**Leprosarium.** See **Leprasorium.**

**Leprosary.** See **Leprasorium.**

**Leprostatic.** Inhibiting the growth of **Mycobacterium Leprae.** कुष्ठाणुरोधक

**Leprosy.** A chronic transmissible disease caused by the **Myobacterium Leprae.** कुष्ठ; कोढ़; कुष्ठाणुओं द्वारा फैलने वाला रोग; Anaesthetic L., leprosy chiefly affecting the nerves; trophoneurotic leprosy. असम्वेदी कुष्ठ;

Lepromatous L., leprosy in which nodular cutaneous lesions are infiltrated. कुष्ठिका-कुष्ठ;

Nodular L., see **Tuberculoid Leprosy.**

Trophoneurotic L., see **Anaesthetic Leprosy.**

Tuberculoid L., a benign, stable and resistant form. यक्ष्मिकाभ कुष्ठ; गुलिकाभ कुष्ठ

**Leprotic.** Infected with leprosy. कुष्ठरोगी; कुष्ठग्रस्तरोगी; कोढ़ी; pertaining

**Leprous**

to leprosy. कुष्ठ सम्बन्धी; कुष्ठविषयक

**Leprous.** Pertaining to leprosy, which is a cutaneous scaly disease. कुष्ठविषयक; कुष्ठ सम्बन्धी; infected with leprosy. कुष्ठग्रस्त; कोढ़ी

**Lepto-.** Prefix meaning thin or soft. 'तनु' अथवा 'कृश' के रूप में प्रयुक्त उपसर्ग

**Leptocephalus.** A foetus with an abnormally small head. तनुशीर्ष; तनुशिरी; कृशकपाली; संकीर्णकपाली; बहुत छोटे सिर वाला भ्रूण

**Leptocytosis.** Thin, flattened, circulating red blood cells. कृशलोहित-कोशिकता; पतली, चपटी, संचरणशील लाल रक्त कोशिकायें

**Leptomeningitis.** Inflammation of the pia and arachnoid membranes. मृदुजालतानिकाशोथ; मिश्रमस्तिष्कावरणशोथ

**Leptoprosope.** Having a long narrow face. तनुआननता

**Leptoprosopic.** One with a long narrow face. तनुआननी

**Leptorrhin.** Having a thin nose; leptorrhine. तनुनासा

**Leptorrhine.** See **Leptorrhin.**

**Leptosome.** Emaciated; person of thin slight strature. कृश; कृशकाय; तनु; दुर्बल

**Leptospirosis.** Swine-herder's disease; infectious jaundice. संक्रामी कामला

**Lepus.** A hare. शशक; लीपस

**Lesbian.** One who practices lesbianism. स्त्रीसमलिंगकामुक;

    **L. Love,** see **Lesbianism.**

**Lesbianism.** Sexual attraction of a woman to another; lesbian love. स्त्रीसमलिंगकामुकता

**Lesion.** A structural tissue change caused by violence or disease. विक्षति; घाव;

    **Focal L.,** lesion of a small definite area. स्थानिक विक्षति

**Letal.** See **Lethal.**

**Lethal.** Deathly; fatal; letal. घातक; मारक;

    **L. Dose,** fatal dose. घातक मात्रा

**Lethargy.** A condition of drowsiness; a kind of coma. आलस; सुस्ती; तन्द्रा

**Lethum.** Death. मृत्यु; मौत

**Leucocyte.** A white blood corpuscle; leukocyte. श्वेतकोशिका; श्वेताणु

**Leucocytosis.** The presence of leucocytes in the blood; leukocytosis.

श्वेतकोशिकाबहुलता; श्वेताणुवृद्धि

**Leucoderma.** Abnormal whiteness of the skin or albinism in the blood; leukoderma. श्वित्र; श्वेतकुष्ठ; सफेद कोढ़; सफेद दाग;

   **Acquired L.,** vitiligo. अर्जित श्वित्र;

   **Syphilitic L.,** a fading of the roseola of secondary syphilis, leaving reticulated depigmented and hyperpigmented areas located chiefly on the sides of the neck. उपदंशज श्वित्र

**Leucoma.** White opaque spot on the cornea; leukoma. श्वेतफुल्ली; स्वच्छपरान्धता; स्वच्छपटल पर सफेद अपारभासी धब्बा होना

**Leuconychia.** White spots on the nails; leukonychia. श्वेतनखता; नाखुनों की श्वेतचित्तिता; नाखुनों पर सफेद धब्बे होना

**Leucopathy.** Albinism; the condition of an albino; leukopathy. पीतवर्णता; पीलिया; पीलिमा

**Leucopenia.** See **Leukopenia.**

**Leucophlegmatic.** Torpid or sluggish temperament. मन्द; शिथिल

**Leucoplacia.** See **Leucoplakia.**

**Leucoplakia.** The formation of white spots or plates on the epidernis of epithelium; also called smoker's patches; leukoplakia; leukoplasia; leukokeratosis. श्वेतशल्कता; मुँह के अन्दर सफेद धब्बे होना

**Leucoplakic.** Pertaining to, or affected with leucoplakia; laukoplakic. श्वेतशल्की

**Leucopoiesis.** The formation of white blood cells. श्वेतकोशिकाजनन; श्वेताणुजनन

**Leucopyria.** Hectic fever. यक्ष्माज्वर; प्रलेपकज्वर

**Leucorrhea.** See **Leucorrhoea.**

**Leucorrhoea.** Whites; a discharge of white, yellowish or greenish mucus from the vagina; leucorrhea; leukorrhoea. प्रदर; श्वेतप्रदर

**Leucosis.** Any disease of lymphatics; abnormal pallor of the skin; leukosis. श्वेतरक्तता

**Leukaemia.** See **Leukemia.**

**Leukaemoid.** See **Leukemoid.**

**Leukemia.** A disease in which white blood cells become too numerous in the blood stream, due to disease of bone-marrow, probably cancerous; leukaemia. श्वेतरक्तता; अधिश्वेतकोशिकारक्तता;

   **Myelogenic L.,** see **Myelogenous Leukemia.**

**Myelogenous L.**, that in which the bone-marrow is involved; myelogenic leukemia. कणिका-श्वेतरक्तता

**Leukemic.** Pertaining to, or affected with leukemia. श्वेतरक्तक; श्वेतरक्तता सम्बन्धी

**Leukemogen.** That which is known to be a causal factor in occurrence of leukemia. श्वेतकोशिकाणुजन

**Leukemogenesis.** Induction, development and progression of a leukemic disease. श्वेतकोशिकाणुजनन

**Leukemogenic.** Pertaining to leukemogenesis or leukemogen. श्वेतकोशिकाणुजनक

**Leukemoid.** Of the nature of leukemia; laukaemoid. श्वेतरक्ताभ

**Leukoblast.** The germ of leucocyte. श्वेतकोशिकाणुप्रसू

**Leukoblastosis.** Abnormal proliferation of leukocytes. श्वेतकोशिकाणुप्रसूमयता

**Leukocyte.** See **Leucocyte**.

**Leukocythaemia.** An abnormal increase in the number of white corpuscles, with glandular enlargement. अतिश्वेताणुकोशिकता; ग्रन्थियाँ बढ़ने के साथ श्वेत रक्तकणों की संख्या में अस्वाभाविक वृद्धि होना

**Leukocytogenesis.** Formation and development of leukocytes. श्वेताणुजनन

**Leukocytolysis.** Dissolution of leukocytes. श्वेताणुलयन

**Leukocytopenia.** See **Leukopenia**.

**Leukocytosis.** See **Leucocytosis**.

**Leukoderma.** See **Leucoderma**.

**Leukokeratosis.** See **Leukoplakia**.

**Leukoma.** See **Leucoma**.

**Leukonychia.** See **Leuconychia**.

**Leukopaenia.** See **Leukopenia**.

**Leukopathy.** See **Leucopathy**.

**Leukopenia.** Decrease of leucocytes; leucopenia; leukopaenia; leukocytopenia. क्षाररागीश्वेतकोशिकाल्पता; बेसरागीश्वेताणुह्रास;

**Eosinophilic L.**, a decrease in the number of eosinophilic granulocytes. इयोसिनरागी श्वेतकोशिकाल्पता

**Leukopenic.** Relating to leukopenia. श्वेताणुह्रास सम्बन्धी

**Leukoplakia.** See **Leucoplakia**.

**Leukoplakic.** See **Leucoplakic.**

**Leukoplasia.** See **Leucoplakia.**

**Leukopoiesis.** Formation and deveopment of various types of white blood cells. श्वेतकोशिकाजनन

**Leukopoietic.** Pertaining to, or characterized by leukopoiesis. श्वेतकोशिकाजनक

**Leukorrhoea.** See **Leucorrhoea.**

**Leukosis.** Abnormal pallor of the skin. पीतवर्णता; पीलिया; पीलिमा

**Laukotaxis.** Artificially produced leukocytosis. श्वेतकोशिकाकर्षण; कृत्रिम रूप से श्वेताणुओं की वृद्धि होना

**Leukotomy.** Incision into the white matter of the frontal lobe of the brain; lobotomy. मस्तिष्करवण्डच्छेदन

**Leukotoxic.** Destructive to leucocytes. श्वेताणुनाशक

**Leukotrichia.** Whiteness of the hair. श्वेतलोमता

**Levator.** A muscle that elevates a part. उत्तोलक; उत्थापिका

**Levigation.** The trituration of a substance. पिष्टीकरण; किसी पदार्थ का अवपेषण बनाना या बनना

**Levocardia.** Having the heart on the left of the body. वामहृदयता

**Libido.** A venereal desire. कामलिप्सा; कामोत्तेजना; वासना

**Libra.** Pound. Symbol : **lb.** पौंड; balance. तुला

**Lice.** Plural of **Louse.**

**Lichanus.** The index or forefinger. तर्जनी

**Lichen.** A papular inflammation of the skin; aggravated or obstinate eczema. लाइकेन; शैवाक; पिटकमय त्वक्शोथ;

    **L. Planus,** a form having broad, flat papules. समतल शैवाक

**Licheniasis.** The formation of lichen. लाइकेनोत्पत्ति; शैवाकोत्पत्ति;

**Lichenification.** Thickening of the skin, usually secondary to scratching. शैवाकीभवन

**Lid.** The eyelid. वर्त्म; पलक

**Lien.** The spleen; lienalis. प्लीहा; तिल्ली

**Lienalis.** See **Lien.**

**Lienitis.** Inflammation of the spleen. प्लीहाशोथ; तिल्ली का प्रदाह

**Lienomalacia.** A softening of the spleen. प्लीहामृदुता; तिल्ली की कोमलता

**Lienorenal.** Pertaining to the spleen and the kidney. प्लीहा (तिल्ली) एवं वृक्क (गुर्दे) सम्बन्धी

**Lienteria.** Passage of undigested food with the motion; lientery. अजीर्णातिसार; अपच के साथ दस्त होना

**Lienteric.** Pertaining to lienteria. अजीर्णातिसार सम्बन्धी

**Lientery.** See **Lienteria.**

**Life.** Vitality; the power by which an organism exists and exercises its functions. जीवन; जिन्दगी; प्राण; आयु

**Ligament.** Membrane which assists in holding the joints together; ligamentum. स्नायु; बन्ध; बन्धन;

   **Accessory L.'s,** ligaments about a joint, in addition to the articular capsule. सहायक स्नायु;

   **Annular L.,** any ring-shaped ligament. वलयी स्नायु;

   **Arcuate L.'s,** the arched ligaments that connect the body of the diaphragm to the last rib and the lumbar vertebras; ligamentum arcuata. चापाकार स्नायु;

   **Broad L.,** the peritoneal fold extending laterally from the uterus to the pelvic wall; the ligament supporting the liver. पृथुस्नायु;

   **Capsular L.,** the fibrous framework surrounding a joint. सम्पुट-स्नायु;

   **Collateral L.'s,** ligaments on either side of and acting as radius of movement of, a hinge joint, as of the elbow, knee and wrist. समपार्श्वी स्नायु;

   **Coracoclavicular L.,** that joining the coracoid process of the scapula and the clavicle; ligamentum coracoclaviculare. तुण्ड-जत्रुक स्नायु;

   **Coracohumeral L.,** that joining the coracoid process of the scapula and the upper and posterior portion of the shoulder joint and the upper part of the humerus. तुण्डप्रगण्डिका स्नायु;

   **Coronary L.,** a peritoneal fold extending from the posterior edge of the liver to the diaphragm. किरीटी स्नायु;

   **Crucial L.,** one of the two ligaments of the knee. स्वस्तिक स्नायु;

   **Cruciform L.,** that formed by the transverse ligament of the atlas and a vertical ligament running from the middle of this to the body of the axis. स्वस्तिकार स्नायु;

   **Crural L.,** see **Inguinal Ligament.**

   **Deltoid L.,** lateral internal ligament of the ankle; ligamentum deltoideum. त्रिकोणिका स्नायु;

**Falciform L.**, the broad ligament of the liver. दात्र स्नायु;

**Iliofemoral L.**, a ligament of the hip-joint; ligamentum iliofemorale. श्रोणिफलक-ऊर्विका स्नायु;

**Iliotrochanteric L.**, a portion of the iliofemoral ligament. श्रोणिफलकगण्डक स्नायु;

**Inguinal L.**, ligament extending from anterior superior spine to pubic tubercle; crural ligament; ligamentum inguinale. वंक्षण स्नायु;

**Interclavicular L.**, one joining the sternal extremities of the clavicles and the sternum. अन्तराजत्रुक स्नायु;

**Round L.**, that of the hip, of liver, of forearm and of uterus. गोल स्नायु;

**Spinoglenoid L.**, that one unites the spine of the scapula with the margins of the glenoid cavity. कंटक-अंसगर्त स्नायु;

**Suspensory L.**, the suspensory ligament of the crystalline lens. निलम्बी स्नायु;

**Sutural L.**, a delicate membrane binding the bones at the cranial suture. सीवनी स्नायु;

**Synovial L.**, one of the large synovial folds in a joint. श्लेषक स्नायु;

**Transverse L.**, that of atlas, of hip-joint and of knee. अनुप्रस्थ स्नायु;

**Triangular L.**, that of the urethra. त्रिकोण स्नायु

**Ligementa.** Plural of **Ligamentum.**

**Ligamentous.** Relating to ligament. स्नायु अथवा बन्ध सम्बन्धी; of the form or structure of a ligament. स्नायुवत् अथवा बन्धन जैसा

**Ligamentum.** A ligament. स्नायु; बन्धन; बन्ध;

**L. Arcuata,** see **Arcuate Ligament.**

**L. Coracoclaviculare,** see **Coracoclavicular Ligament.**

**L. Deltoideum,** see **Deltoid Ligement.**

**L. Denticulatum,** a notched ligament on each side of the myelon. दन्तुर स्नायु;

**L. Iliofemorale,** see **Iliofemoral Ligament.**

**L. Inguinale,** see **Inguinal Ligament.**

**L. Nuchae,** one at the nape of the neck. मन्या स्नायु;

**L. Patellae,** the ligament securing the patella to the tibia. जानुकपालिक स्नायु;

**L. Teres,** the round ligament. गोल स्नायु

**Ligate.** To tie, as of the blood vessels etc., at operation. बांधना

## Ligation

**Ligation.** The art of tying a vessel. बन्धन; आवेष्टन;
  **Tubal L.,** interruption of the continuity of the oviduct by cutting, cautery, or a device, to prevent future conception. डिम्बवाहिनी बन्धन

**Ligature.** A thread for tying blood vessels to prevent haemorrhage. बन्ध; पट्टी

**Light.** The agent, which produces vision. प्रकाश; रोशनी; बत्ती

**Lightening.** Term used to denote the relief of pressure on the diaphragm by the abdominal viscera, when the presenting part of the foetus descends into the pelvis in the last three weeks of pregnancy. हल्कापन; अपरोहण

**Lightning Pains.** Symptomatic of tabes dorsalis; paroxysmal swift cutting stabs in the lower limbs. तड़ित दर्द; चमचमाते हुए दर्द

**Ligneous.** Wood-like. काष्ठाभ; काष्ठवत्; लकड़ी जैसा

**Lignum.** Wood. काष्ठ; लकड़ी

**Ligula.** See **Ligule.**

**Ligule.** A tongue-shaped organ; ligula. जीभ जैसी बनावट

**Limb.** A leg or an arm; an extremity. अंग; अंश; शाखा; अवयव

**Limbi.** Plural of **Limbus.**

**Limbic.** Marginal. सीमांत

**Limbus.** A margin, edge, border or fringe of a part. किनारी

**Lime.** Oxide of calcium; calx. चूना; कैल्शियमऑक्साइड; fruit of the lime tree. नीम्बू;
  **L. Water,** solution of calcium hydroxide. चूने का पानी

**Limen.** Threshold; entrance; the external opening of a canal. देहली; द्वार; छिद्र

**Limes.** A boundary, limit or threshold. सीमा अथवा देहली

**Liminal.** Least; Lowest; minimal. अल्पतम; अल्पिष्ठ; कम से कम; pertaining to a threshold. देहली सम्बन्धी

**Limitans.** Limiting; bounding. सीमाकर; सीमान्त

**Limpid.** Clear; pure; transparent. स्वच्छ; शुद्ध; पारदर्शक; साफ-सुथरा; निर्मल

**Lincture.** See **Linctus.**

**Linctus.** A sweet syrupy liquid; lincture. लेह

**Line.** See **Linea.**
  **Mammary L.,** a line from one nipple to the other. स्तन रेखा;
  **Mylohyoid(ean) L.,** a ridge on the internal surface of the lower

jaw. चर्वककंठिका रेखा;

**Nuchal L.**, one on the external surface of the occiput. मन्या रेखा;

**Parasternal L.**, the imaginary vertical line midway between the margin of the sternum and the mammillary line. पराउरोस्थि-रेखा

**Linea.** A line; a long narrow mark, strip or streak. रेखा; लाइन;

   **L. Alba,** the white line in the middle of the abdomen. उदरमध्य रेखा;

   **L. Albicans,** a white cutaneous scar from linear atrophy; linea albicantis; stria gravidarum. श्वेत रेखा;

   **L. Albicantis,** see **Linea Albicans.**

   **L. Aspera,** a rough line on the posterior surface of the femur. ऊर्विका रेखा;

   **L. Splendens,** a fibrous band in the middle of the spinal piamater. दीप्तिमान रेखा;

   **L. Terminalis,** arcuate line of pelvis. अन्त्य रेखा; श्रोणिचाप रेखा;

   **L. Transversa,** one of the tendinous intersections of the rectus abdominis muscle. अनुप्रस्थ रेखा

**Lineae.** Plural of **Linea.**

**Lineament.** Feature; first trace of the embyo. रेखण

**Linear.** Of, or pertaining to a line. रेखित

**Lingua.** The tongue. जिह्वा; जीभ; जबान

**Lingual.** Pertaining to the tongue; glossal. जिह्वापरक; जीभ सम्बन्धी;

   **L. Bone,** the hyoid bone. जिह्वास्थि; कण्ठास्थि;

   **L. Gyrus,** the lobule of the tongue. जिह्वा-कर्णक; जिह्वा-खण्डक

**Lingula.** A small lobule or tongue-shaped process. जिह्विका; खण्डक;

   **L. Cerebelli,** a small lobule of the cerebellum. अनुमस्तिष्क खण्डक; सिर के पिछले भाग का एक छोटा-सा खण्डक;

   **L. Pulmonis,** the pulmonary lobule. फुप्फुस-जिह्वा; फुप्फुस-खण्डक

**Lingulectomy.** Excision in the lingular portion of the left upper lobe of the lung. फुप्फुसखण्डक-उच्छेदन; glossectomy. जिह्वाखण्डक-उच्छेदन

**Liniment.** A liquid to be applied to the skin by gentle friction; linimentum. लेप; विलेपन; मर्दं; मलहम; मरहम

**Linimentum.** See **Liniment.**

**Lining.** Covering. अस्तर; आवरण;

   **L. Membrane,** covering membrane. अस्तर कला; आवरक झिल्ली

**Linseed.** Flax seed; linum. अलसी; तीसी

**Lint.** Linen well scraped for dressing sores and wounds. लिंट; नरम रेशमी पट्टी, जो घावों की मरहम पट्टी करने के काम आती है

**Linum.** See **Linseed.**

**Lip.** One of the two borders of the mouth; labium oris. अधर; ओष्ठ; होंठ;

    **Cleft L.,** hare-lip. खण्डोष्ठ

**Lipaemia.** See **Lipemia.**

**Liparia.** Corpulency. स्थूलता; मोटापा

**Lipase.** A fat-splitting enzyme. लाइपेज; वसा बिखेरने वाला एक पाचक रस

**Lipectomy.** Surgical removal of fatty tissue. वसाऊतक-उच्छेदन; वसोतकोच्छेदन

**Lipemia.** Presence of fat in the blood; lipaemia. वसारक्तता; रक्त में चर्बी की बढ़ी हुई मात्रा;

    **Alimentary L.,** relatively transient lipemia occurring after the ingestion of foods with a large content of fat; post-prandial lipemia. भोजनोत्तर वसारक्तता;

    **Postprandial L.,** see **Alimentary Lipemia.**

**Lipid.** Fat-like; lipide. वसाभ; चर्बी जैसा; वसासम; चर्बी से मिलता-जुलता

**Lipide.** See **Lipid.**

**Lipocele.** Adipocele. मेदोमयबृद्धि

**Lipocere.** Adipocere. वसासिक्थ

**Lipocyte.** A fat-storing stellate cell (fat-cell) in the liver. वसाकोशिका

**Lipodystrophia.** See **Lipodystrophy.**

**Lipodystrophy.** Disturbed fat metabolism; lipodystrophia. वसादुष्पुष्टि; चर्बीपाचनदोष

**Lipogenesis.** Production of fat; adipogenesis. वसाजनन

**Lipogenic.** Relating to lipogenesis; adipogenic; adipogenous; lipogenous. वसाजनक

**Lipogenous.** See **Lipogenic.**

**Lipoid.** Resembling fat; fat-like; adipoid. वसाभ; वसासम; चर्बी जैसा या चर्बी से मिलता-जुलता

**Lipolysis.** The chemical breaking down of fat. वसापघटन; वसापजनन; वसालयन; चर्बी का रासायनिक विघटन

**Lipolytic.** Relating to, or causing lipolysis. वसापघटनी; वसालयी

**Lipoma.** A fatty tumour. वसार्बुद; चर्बी की रसौली

**Lipomatoid.** Resembling a lipoma. वसार्बुदाभ; चर्बी की रसौली जैसा

**Lipomatosis.** The production of a lipoma. वसार्बुदता

**Lipophilic.** Capable of being dissolved in lipids. वसारागी

**Liposis.** Adiposis. वसामयता; मेदुरता; fatty infiltration. वसीय अन्तःस्यन्दन

**Liposoluble.** Fat-soluble. वसाविलेय

**Liposphaxia.** Absence or cessation of the pulse. नाड़ीस्पन्दरोध; नाड़ीस्पन्द का अभाव

**Lipothymia.** Faintness. मूर्च्छावस्था; बेहोशी

**Lipotropic.** Having an affinity for lipids. वसाप्रेरक

**Lipotropy.** Affinity of basic dyes for fatty tissue. वसाप्रेरण

**Lippitude.** A puriform exudation from the margins of the eyelids; lippitudo. वर्त्मव्रणता; पलकों के किनारों पर घाव बन जाना

**Lippitudo.** See **Lippitude.**

**Lipuria.** The presence of fat in the urine. वसामेह; पेशाब में चर्बी जाना

**Lipuric.** Relating to lipuria. वसामेह सम्बन्धी

**Liquefacient.** An agent producing liquefaction. द्रावक; तरल करने वाला

**Liquefaction.** A conversion into liquid. द्रवण; द्रावण; द्रवीकरण; तरलीकरण

**Liquid.** A flowing substance. द्रव; द्रव्य; तरल (पदार्थ)

**Liquor.** Wine; a liquid solution. लिकर; मदिरा; उदक (द्रव्य); शराब;

   **L. Amnii,** fluid by which the foetus is surrounded before birth. गर्भोदक; उल्वोदक;

   **L. Sanguinis,** the fluid portion of the blood. रक्त-द्रव

**Lisping.** A defect of speech with imperfect pronunciation. अस्फुटवाक्; बोलने में अपूर्ण उच्चारण का दोष

**Lithaemia.** An excess of uric acid in the blood; lithemia. अतियूरिकाम्लरक्तता; अतिमिहयाम्लता; रक्त में यूरिक (मिहेय) अम्ल की अधिकता

**Lithagog.** See **Lithagogue.**

**Lithagogue.** An agent that expels calculi; lithagog. अश्मनिस्सारक; पथरी निकालने वाला

**Lithates.** A combination in lithic acid with a base. मूत्रक्षार

**Lithectomy.** See **Lithotomy.**

**Lithemia.** See **Lithaemia.**
**Lithiasis.** Formation of calculus. अश्मरीयता; अश्मरचना; पथरी बनना
**Lithic.** Pertaining to a stone. अश्मरीय; पथरी सम्बन्धी;
   L. Acid, a principle which is constantly present in the healthy urine; uric acid. लिथिक अम्ल; मूत्राम्ल:
   L. Diathesis, the tendency to gout. गठिया-प्रवणता
**Lithoclast.** See **Lithotrite.**
**Lithodialysis.** See **Litholysis.**
**Lithogenesis.** Formation of calculi. अश्मरीजनन
**Lithogenous.** Calculus forming. अश्मरीजनक
**Litholapaxy.** The removal of a crushed stone by irrigation. वस्तिअश्मरीभंजन; मूत्राशय की पथरी तोड़ कर निकालना.
**Lithology.** The science of the nature of calculi. अश्मविज्ञान
**Litholysis.** The dissolution of a stone in the bladder; lithodialysis. अश्मलयन; अश्मविघटन
**Lithonephrotomy.** Incision of the kidney for removal of the calculus. वृक्काश्मरीहरण
**Lithopaedion.** A calcified foetus in the uterus or abdominal cavity; lithopedion. अश्मगर्भ; गर्भाशय अथवा उदर गह्वर में कैल्सीभूत भ्रूण
**Lithopedion.** See **Lithopaedion.**
**Lithotomy.** The operation of opening the bladder to remove a stone; lithectomy. मूत्रााशय-अश्मरीहरण; वस्ति-अश्मरीहरण;
   **Suprapubic L.**, that in which the incision is made above the pubis. अधिजघनमूत्राशय-अश्मरीहरण
**Lithotripsy.** See **Lithotrity.**
**Lithotrite.** An instrument for performing lithotrity; lithoclast. वस्ति-अश्मरीभंजक; मूत्राशय-पथरी को तोड़ने के लिये प्रयुक्त किया जाने वाला यंत्र
**Lithotrity.** The crushing of a stone in the bladder; lithotripsy. वस्ति-अश्मरीभंजन; मूत्राशय-पथरी को तोड़ना अथवा चूर-चूर करना
**Lithous.** Stony; calculous. अश्मवत्; पथरी जैसा
**Lithuresis.** See **Lithuria.**
**Lithuria.** The lithic acid diathesis, in which the urine contains lithates or urates of soda; lithuresis. मूत्रक्षारमेह; पेशाब में मूत्रक्षार जाना
**Litmus.** A vegetable pigment used as an indicator of acidity or alkanity. लिटमस; शैवाल; नीलवर्ण काई; अम्लता या क्षारता का सूचक वनस्पति वर्णक;

**L. Paper,** bibulous paper impregnated with litmus. लिटमस पेपर; लिटमस पत्र; शैवाल पत्र

**Litter.** A stretcher for carrying the sick or wounded. स्ट्रेचर; लिट्टर; मरीजों अथवा घायलों को ले जाने के लिये प्रयुक्त की जाने वाली टिकटी

**Little's disease.** Congenital spastic paraplegia. सहजसंस्तम्भी अधरांगघात; पेशियों का आजन्म ऐंठनयुक्त अर्धांगघात

**Live.** Living; animate. सप्राण; जीवित

**Livedo.** The liver. यकृत्; जिगर; a small bluish spot in a tissue. नीललांछन, विशेष रूप से किसी ऊतक पर

**Liver.** The glandular viscus that secretes bile. यकृत्; जिगर;
  **Amyloid L.,** enlargement of the liver due to the deposition of an albuminous substance. श्वेतसारिक यकृत्; मण्डाभ यकृत्;
  **Fatty L.,** yellow discolouration of the liver due to fatty degeneration of the parenchymal cells. वसा-यकृत्;
  **Floating L.,** an easily displaced liver. चल यकृत्;
  **Hobnail L.,** one marked with nail-like projections from atrophic cirrhosis. कीलकी यकृत्;
  **Nutmeg L.,** one with a peculiar mottled appearance, occurring in heart disease, amyloid degeneration, etc. जायफली यकृत्;
  **L. Extract,** a solution of the anti-anaemic factors of fresh liver. यकृत् सार; ताजे जिगर से निर्मित एक रक्ताल्परोधक घोल;
  **L. Spots,** chloasma. विवर्णलांछन; चम्बल रोग

**Livid.** Black and blue; of a lead-colour. श्याव; नील; नीला; नीलाभ

**Lividity.** The state of being livid. श्यावता; नीलापन

**Lixiviation.** The washing of wood-ashes to extract salts. निक्षालन; लवण-सार प्राप्त करने के लिये काष्ठ-क्षार धोना

**Loa-loa.** See **Loiasis.**

**Loathing.** Indifference. विरक्ति; घृणा; नफरत

**Lobar.** Pertaining to a lobe. खण्डीय; खण्ड सम्बन्धी

**Lobate.** Having lobes. खण्डता; divided into lobes. खण्डित; lobe-shaped. खण्डाकार

**Lobe.** A rounded part of an organ or viscus demarked by fissures or divisions. खण्ड; पालि;
  **Caudate L.,** the tail-like process of the liver. पुच्छक-केन्द्रक खण्ड;
  **Frontal L.,** that part of the cerebral hemisphere in front of the

# Lobe

central and above the brain fissures called Sylvian fissures. ललाट खण्ड;

**Hapatic L.,** the lobe of the liver. यकृत् खण्ड;

**Occipital L.,** caudal region of either hemicerebrum. पश्चकपाल खण्ड;

**Olfactory L.,** the rhinencephalon. घ्राण-खण्ड;

**Optic L.,** the optic lobes of the brain. अक्षि-खण्ड;

**Orbital L.,** the convolutions above the orbit. नेत्रगुहा खण्ड;

**Parietal L.,** that part of the cerebral hemisphere back of the central and above the Sylvian fissures. पार्श्विका खण्ड;

**Pyramidal L.,** the prominence of the cerebellum. पिरामिदी खण्ड;

**Quadrate L.,** the anterior and posterior crescentic lobes of the cerebellum combined; an oblong lobe on the inferior surface of the liver. चतुरस्र खण्ड;

**Temporal L.,** the part of the cerebral hemisphere lying below the Sylvian fissures. शंख खण्ड

**Lobectomy.** Excision of a lobe, as of the lung, urterus, etc. खण्डोच्छेदन, जैसे फुप्फुस, जरायु, आदि के किसी खण्ड को काट कर हटा देना।

**Lobelia.** A genus of herbs; Indian tobacco, used in spasmodic asthma. लोबेलिया; तम्बाकू के पत्ते

**Lobi.** Plural of **Lobus.**

**Lobitis.** Inflammation of a lobe. खण्डशोथ

**Lobotomy.** See **Leukotomy.**

**Lobular.** Like, pertaining to, or composed of lobules. खण्डाकार; खण्डकाकार; खण्ड सम्बन्धी

**Lobulate.** Divided into lobules; lobulated. खण्डकित

**Lobulated.** See **Lobulate.**

**Lobule.** A little lobe; lobulus. खण्डक; खण्ड; दलिका

**Lobuli.** Plural of **Lobulus.**

**Lobulus.** See **Lobule.**

**Lobus.** A lobe. खण्ड; पालि; दल;

**L. Caudatus,** the caudate lobe. पुच्छक-केन्द्रक खण्ड;

**L. Medius,** the middle lobe. मध्य खण्ड

**Local.** Pertaining to one spot or part. स्थानिक; स्थानीय

**Localization.** The determination of the seat of disease. स्थाननिर्धारण;

स्थानसंश्रय; स्थापन; रोगस्थलनिर्धारण

**Location.** Place. स्थान; जगह

**Locator.** An instrument or apparatus for finding the position of a foreign object in tissue. निर्धारित्र; लोकेटर

**Lochia.** Vaginal discharge after labour. सूतिस्राव; प्रसवोत्तर स्राव; जेर;

   **L. Alba,** the whitish flow that takes place from about the seventh day. श्वेत सूतिस्राव;

   **L. Cruentia,** the sanguineous flow of the first few days; lochia rubra. लोहितसूतिस्राव;

   **L. Rubra,** see **Lochia Cruentia.**

   **L. Serosa,** the serous discharge occurring about the fifth day. सीरमी सूतिस्राव

**Lochial.** Pertaining to the discharges which follow childbirth. सूतिस्रावी; सूतिस्राव सम्बन्धी

**Lochiometra.** Retention of lochia in the womb. सूतिस्रावपूरितगर्भ; गर्भाशय के अन्दर सूतिस्राव रुक जाना

**Lochiometritis.** Puerperal metritis; lochometritis. सूतिस्रावी गर्भाशयशोथ

**Lochioperitonitis.** Puerperal peritonitis. सूतिस्रावीपर्युदर्याशोथ

**Lochiorrhagia.** Profuse flow of lochia; lochiorrhea; lochiorrhoea. अतिसूतिस्राव; विपुल सूतिस्राव; अत्यधिक जेर निकलना

**Lochirorhea.** See **Lochiorrhagia.**

**Lochiorrhoea.** See **Lochiorrhagia.**

**Lochometritis.** See **Lochiometritis.**

**Loci.** Plural of **Locus.**

**Lock-jaw.** Tetanus or trismus; a rigidity of the muscles of the jaws, with violent spasm. हनुस्तम्भ; धनुस्तम्भ; धनुर्वात

**Locomotion.** Animal movement. चलन; गमन; गति

**Locomotive.** See **Locomtor.**

**Locomotor.** Relating to locomotion; locomotive. गतिज; गति विषयक;

   **L. Ataxia,** acute ascending paralysis; locomotor ataxy. गतिभंग; चलन-अक्षमता; गतिहीनता; उग्र-आरोही पक्षाघात;

   **L. Ataxy,** see **Locomotor Ataxia.**

**Locular.** Relating to a loculus. क्षुद्रगह्वर सम्बन्धी

**Loculate.** Divided into small cavities; loculated. लघुगह्वरों में विभक्त; छोटे-छोटे विवरों में बांटा हुआ

**Loculated.** See **Loculate.**

**Loculi.** Plural of **Loculus.**

**Loculus.** A small cavity or chamber. क्षुद्रगह्वर

**Locus.** A place. स्थान; स्थल; लोकस

**Locust.** A winged insect. टिड्डी

**Logaditis.** Inflammation of the sclera. श्वेतपटलशोथ; श्वेतपटल का प्रदाह

**Logagnosia.** Aphasia; loss of speech; logamnesia; logasthenia. वाचाघात; स्वरभंग

**Logagraphia.** Agraphia; loss of sensibility to write or express thoughts in writing. लेखन-अक्षमता

**Logamnesia.** See **Logagnosia.**

**Logaphasia.** Aphasia of articulation. उच्चारण-अक्षमता

**Logasthenia.** See **Logagnosia.**

**Logoneurosis.** A neurotic disorder of speech. वागतंत्रिका-विक्षिप्ति; वाक्तंत्रिका-विक्षति; शब्दोच्चारदोष

**Logopathia.** See **Logopathy.**

**Logopathy.** Any disorder of speech; logopathia. वाग्-विकृति; वाक्-विकृति; उच्चारण-विकार

**Logoplegia.** Complete paralysis of speech. वाचाघात; वाक्शक्तिलोप; वाग्शक्तिलोप

**Loiasis.** A specific form of filariasis; loa-loa. लोआ-लोआ; फाइलेरिया का एक विशिष्ट रूप

**Loin.** The lower part of the back; lumbus. कटि; कमर; पीठ का निचला भाग या हिस्सा

**Longa.** Long. दीर्घ; लम्बा

**Longanon.** Rectum. मलांत्र; मलाशय

**Longevity.** The length of the life. दीर्घायु; आयुकाल; चिरायु; दीर्घजीवन

**Longing.** Irresistible desire. उत्कट अथवा अप्रतिहत इच्छा

**Long-sighted.** Hypermetropic. दूरदृष्टि

**Long-sightedness.** Hypermetropia. दूरदृष्टिता

**Longitudinal.** Running lengthwise, in the direction of long axis of the body or any of its parts. अनुदैर्घ्य

**Longus.** Long. दीर्घ; लम्बा

**Loop.** A ligature band in a cord or other cylindrical body. लूप; पाश; फन्दा; छल्ला

**Loquacious.** Excessive talkative. अतिवाचाल; अत्यधिक बातूनी; बहुत ज्यादा बोलने वाला

**Loquacity.** Excessive talkativeness. अतिवाचालता; अत्यधिक बातूनीपन

**Lordoma.** See **Lordosis.**

**Lordosis.** Anterior convex curvature of the spine; lordoma. अग्रकुब्जता; रीढ़ की हड्डी का आगे की ओर झुकना

**Lotio.** See **Lotion.**

**Lotion.** A liquid preparation used for washing; lotio. घोल; लोशन; घाव साफ करने की दवाई

**Lotium.** A discharge. स्राव

**Loupe.** A magnifying glass used in ophthalmology. लूप; आवर्धक लेंस

**Louse.** Pediculus; a genus of parasitic insects. यूका; जूं

**Lousicide.** An agent which destroys the louse. यूकानाशी; जूंनाशी; यूकानाशक; जूंनाशक

**Lower Dilution.** In Homoeopathy, from mother tincture to 6th potency. निम्न तनूकरण

**Lozenge.** A sweet medicated tablet. चूष; मीठी गोली

**L.P.O.** Left posterior oblique. वाम पृष्ठ तिर्यक

**Lubb-dupp.** Words descriptive of the heart sound as appreciated in auscultation. लब-डप, लब-डप ध्वनि; हृद्ध्वनि

**Lubrication.** Making smooth or slippery. स्नेहन; कोमल या चिकना करना

**Lubricity.** Lasciviousness; lewdness. कामुकता; कामासक्ति

**Lucid.** Clear. स्वच्छ; चेतन; स्वस्थ; निर्मल; साफ;

 **L. Interval,** a sane period. स्वच्छ समयान्तराल; चेतन समयान्तराल

**Lucidity.** Clearness. निर्मलता; स्वच्छता; healthy. स्वस्थ

**Lues.** Syphilis. उपदंश; फिरंगी रोग; आतशक

**Luetic.** Syphilitic. उपदंशग्रस्त; आतशकग्रस्त

**Lumbago.** Pain in the lumbar region; rheumatic stiffness affecting the muscle of the loins. कटिवेदना; कमरदर्द; कटिवात

**Lumbar.** Pertaining to the loins, i.e. the lower part of the back. कटिपरक; कमर सम्बन्धी;

 **L. Abscess,** psoas abscess which forms besides the psoas muscle at the bottom of the abdomen. कटि-विद्रधि; कमर का फोड़ा;

 **L. Puncture,** the tapping of the spinal subarachnoid space in the lumbar region to remove cerebrospinal fluid for examination

**Lumbar**

or for relieving abnormal tension. कटिवेध; कटिवेधन; कटिभेदन; कटिभेद;

**L. Region,** the loins. कटि-प्रदेश; कमर;

**L. Vertebra,** one of the five vertebras immediately cephalad to the sacrum. कटि-कशेरुका

**Lumbi.** Plural of **Lumbus.**

**Lumbocolostomy.** The formation of a permanent opening into the colon via an incision through the lumbar region. कटिबृहदांत्रसम्मिलन

**Lumbocostal.** Pertaining to the loins and the ribs. कटिपर्शुकी; कमर तथा पसलियों सम्बन्धी

**Lumbosacral.** Pertaining to the loins and the sacrum. कटित्रिकी; कटित्रिक सम्बन्धी

**Lumbricidal.** Destructive to intestinal worms. कृमिनाशक

**Lumbricide.** An agent that kills intestinal worms. कृमिमारक; कृमिघाती

**Lumbricoides.** Large round worms infesting the bowels. गोलकृमि

**Lumbricosis.** Infestation with intestinal worms. कृमिरुग्णता

**Lumbricus.** A genus of intestinal worms. आन्त्रकृमि; अन्तड़ियों के कीड़े

**Lumbus.** See **Loin.**

**Lumen.** The space inside a tubular structure. अवकाशिका; कुहर; कोटर

**Lump.** A tumour, especially of breast. अर्बुद; स्तनार्बुद; रसौली

**Lumpectomy.** Surgical removal of a tumour from the breast. स्तनार्बुद-उच्छेदन

**Lumina.** Plural of **Lumen.**

**Lunacy.** Insanity. विक्षिप्ति; उन्माद; उन्मत्तता; पागलपन

**Lunar.** See **Lunate.**

**Lunate.** Semilunar; resembling a half moon; lunar. अर्धचन्द्राकार; नवचन्द्राकार

**Lunatic.** Insane; one affected with insanity. विक्षिप्त; पागल; उन्मादी; उन्मत्त; pertaining to insanity. पागलपन सम्बन्धी

**Lung.** One of the two organs of respiration. फफ्फुस; फेफड़ा;

**L. Fever,** pneumonia. निमोनिया; फुप्फुसपाक

**Lunula.** The semi-circular white area at the root of the nails. चन्द्रक; नखगर्त; नखचन्द्रिका

**Lunulae.** Plural of **Lunula.**

**Lupiform.** See **Lupoid.**

**Lupoid.** Resembling lupus; lupiform. लूपसाभ; लूपसवत्; त्वग्यक्ष्माभ

**Lupous.** Relating to lupus. त्वग्यक्ष्मा सम्बन्धी

**Lupus.** Tuberculosis of the skin, occurring in the form of reddish brown tubercles. त्वग्यक्ष्मा; चर्मक्षय; लूपस; त्वचायक्ष्मा; त्वक्षय;

**Erythematous L.,** see **Lupus Erythematosus.**

**L. Erythematosus,** a form not due to tubercle bacillus; erythematous lupus. रक्तिम त्वग्यक्ष्मा; रक्तिम लूपस;

**L. Vulgaris,** typical lupus. चर्मक्षय; त्वग्यक्ष्मा

**Luteum.** Yellow; luteus. पीत; पीला;

**Corpus L.,** yellow cellular mass in the ovary that forms after the Graafian follicle has erupted. पीत-पिण्ड

**Luteus.** See **Luteum.**

**Luxatio-erecta.** A dislocation of the shoulder-joint in which the head of humerus is in the axilla and the shaft is directed upward against the head of the patient. उदग्र सन्धिभ्रंश

**Luxation.** A dislocation; out of joint. सन्धिच्युति; सन्धिभ्रंश; हड्डी का जोड़ से उखड़ना या अपनी जगह से हट जाना

**Luxus.** Excess of anything. अधिक; dilatation. विस्फार; फैलाव

**Lying-in.** Being in childbed; the puerperal state. प्रसूता; सूतिका

**Lymph.** A gland of the body, separated by the blood, and carried by the lymphatic vessels. लसीका;

**L. Cell,** see **Lymphocyte.**

**L. Glands,** see **Lymph Nodes.**

**L. Nodes,** small glandular organs inserted in the lymph vessels at stratagic point where they can filter infection and so protect the remainder of the body; lymph nodules. लसीकापर्व

**L. Nodules,** see **Lymph Nodes.**

**Lymphadenectasis.** Dilatation of the lymph-channels. लसीकापर्वविस्फार; लसीकापर्वस्फीति

**Lymphadenectomy.** Excision of one or more lymph nodes. लसीकापर्वोच्छेदन

**Lymphadenitis.** Inflammation of a lymph node. लसीकापर्वशोथ

**Lymphadenography.** Radiography after opaque oil is injected into the centre of an enlarged lymph node. लसीकापर्वचित्रण

**Lymphadenoid.** Resembling a lymph node. लसीकापर्वाभ

**Lymphadenoma.** Hodgkin's disease. लसीकापर्वार्बुद; scrofula. गण्डमाला;कण्ठमाला

**Lymphadenopathy.** Any disease of the lymph nodes. लसीकापर्वविकृति

**Lymphadenosis.** Overgrowth of lymphatic glands. लसीकाग्रन्थिलता

**Lymphagog.** See **Lymphagogue**.

**Lymphagogue.** Any substance capable of increasing the flow of lymph; lymphagog. लसीकावर्धक

**Lymphangial.** Relating to a lymphatic vessel. लसीकावाहिकीय; लसीकावाहिका सम्बन्धी

**Lymphangiectasia.** See **Lymphangiectasis**.

**Lymphangiectasis.** A dilatation of the lymph-vessels; lymph angiectasia; lymphectasia. लसीकावाहिकास्फीति

**Lymphangiectomy.** Excision of a lymphatic vessel. लसीकावाहिनी-उच्छेदन

**Lymphangiitis.** See **Lymphangitis**.

**Lymphangiography.** A description of the lymphatics. लसीकावाहिनीचित्रण

**Lymphangiology.** Study of the lymphatics; lymphology. लसीकावाहिकाविज्ञान

**Lymphangioma.** A tumour of the lymphatic vessels. लसीकावाहिकार्बुद

**Lymphangiophlebitis.** Inflammation of the lymphatic vessels and the veins. लसीकावाहिकाशिराशोथ

**Lymphangioplasty.** Replacement of lymphatics by artificial channels. लसीकावाहिनीसंधानकर्म

**Lymphangiotomy.** A dissection of lymphatics. लसीकावाहिका-उच्छेदन

**Lymphangitis.** Inflammation of the lymph vessels; lymphangiitis; lymphatitis. लसीकावाहिनीशोथ

**Lymphatic.** Pertaining to, conveying or containing lymph. लसीकापरक; लसीकावाहिका सम्बन्धी; sluggish, as of temperament. लसीकाप्रधान;

L. Glands, lymph nodes. लसीकापर्व;

L. Leukaemia, leukemia of lymphatic origin. लसीकाश्वेतरक्तता;

L. System, fine tubes pervading the body. temperament लसीकाजाल; लसीका-प्राणली;

L. Vessel, a circulatory network of vessels which drain and

distribute the lymphs (body glands). लसीकावाहिका; लसवाहिका

**Lymphatitis.** See **Lymphangitis.**

**Lymphectasia.** See **Lymphangiectasis.**

**Lymphoblast.** A young immature cell that matures into a lymphocyte; lymphocytoblast. लसीकाकोशिकाप्रसू

**Lymphoblastoma.** Malignant lymphoma in which single or multiple tumours arise from lymphoblast in lymph nodes. लसीकाकोशिकाप्रसू-अर्बुद

**Lymphocyte.** A white cell formed in the lymph nodes; a lymph cell. लसीकाकोशिका; लसकोशिका

**Lymphocythaemia.** An excess of lymphocytes in the blood; lymphocythemia; lymphocytosis. लसकोशिकाबहुलता; लसीकाकोशिकाबहुलता

**Lymphocythemia.** See **Lymphocythaemia.**

**Lymphocytic.** Pertaining to, or characterized by lymphocytes. लसीकाकोशिकीय

**Lymphocytoblast.** See **Lymphoblast.**

**Lymphocytoma.** A circumscribed nodule or mass of mature lymphocytes. लासीकाकोशिकार्बुद

**Lymphocytopenia.** See **Lymphopenia.**

**Lymphocytosis.** See **Lymphocythaemia.**

**Lymphodermia.** A disease of the cutaneous lymphatics. त्वग्वाहिकारोग

**Lymphoedema.** Excess of fluid in the tissues from obstruction of lymph vessels. लसीकाशोफ

**Lymphoepithelioma.** Rapidly growing malignant pharyngeal tumour. लसीकाउपकलार्बुद

**Lymphogenic.** See **Lymphogenous.**

**Lymphogenous.** Producing lymphs; lymphogenic. लसीकोत्पादक

**Lymphogranuloma Inguinale.** A tropical venereal disease caused by a virus; lymphogranuloma venereum. वंक्षणलसीकाकणिकागुल्म; रतिजलसीकाकणिकागुल्म

**Lymphogranulomatosis.** Hodgkin's disease. लसीकाकणिकागुल्मता

**Lymphogranuloma Venereum.** See **Lymphogranuloma Inguinale.**

**Lymphoid.** Resembling a lymph. लसीकाभ; लसीकावत्; लसीका-सदृश

**Lymphology.** See **Lymphangiology.**

**Lymphoma.** A tumour arising from the lymphoid tissue in the body. लसीकार्बुद

**Lymphopenia.** A reduction in the number of lymphocytes in the circulating blood; lymphocytopenia. लसीकाकोशिकाल्पता

**Lymphopoiesis.** Formation of lymphocytes. लसीकाकोशिकाजनन

**Lymphopoietic.** Pertaning to, or characterized by lymphopoiesis. लसीकाकोशिकाजनक; लसीकाकोशिकीय

**Lymphorrhagia.** A flow of lymph from a ruptured lymphatic; lymphorrhea; lymphorrhoea. लसीकास्राव

**Lymphorrhea.** See **Lymphorrhagia.**

**Lymphorrhoea.** See **Lymphorrhagia.**

**Lymphosarcoma.** A tumour made up of lymphatic and sarcomatous tissue. लसीकासार्कार्बुद

**Lymphotomy.** A dissection of the lymphatics. लसीका-उच्छेदन

**Lypothemia.** Severe mental prostration from grief; lypothymia. मनस्ताप; मानसिक सन्ताप

**Lypothymia.** See **Lypothemia.**

**Lysin.** A cell-dissolving substance in the blood. लाइसिन; रक्त के अन्दर एक कोशिका-विलेय पदार्थ

**Lysinogen.** An antigen that stimulates the formation of a specific lysin. लाइसिनजन

**Lysinogenic.** Having the property of lysinogen. लाइसिनजनक

**Lysis.** Gradual decline of a disease. अपघटन; संलयन; लयन; रोग का उत्तरोत्तर ह्रास

**Lysogen.** Something capable of inducing lysis. संलयनजन

**Lyssa.** Rabies; hydrophobia.; lyssa canina; lyssophobia. अलर्क; जलातंक

**Lyssin.** A specific virus of hydrophobia. एक विशिष्ट अलर्क विषाणु; लाइसिन

**Lyssophobia.** See **Lyssa.**

**Lyterian.** Termination of a disease. रोगोन्मूलन; रोगमुक्ति

**Lytic.** Relating to a lysis. अपघटनी; अपघटन अथवा लयन विषयक; संलायी; लायी; लयनी; relating to the lysin. लाइसिनी; लाइसिन सम्बन्धी

# M

**Macerate.** To soften by steeping or soaking. मसृण; द्रवनिवेशन करना

**Maceration.** Steeping in fluids. मसृणन; द्रवनिवेशन; द्रवसंमर्दन; तरल पदार्थों के अन्दर भिगाना या गलाना

**Macies.** Atrophy; leanness; wasting. अपक्षय; शोष

**Macrencephalia.** See **Macrocephaly**.

**Macrencephaly.** See **Macrocephaly**.

**Macro-.** Prefix meaning large. 'बृहत्', 'महा', 'अति' तथा 'स्थूल' के रूप में प्रयुक्त उपसर्ग

**Macrobiosis.** Long life; longevity. दीर्घायु

**Macroblast.** A large erythrocyte. बृहत्प्रसू; दीर्घप्रसू

**Macroblepharia.** The state of having abnormally large eyelids. बृहत्वर्त्मता; बड़ी-बड़ी पलकें

**Macrocephalia.** See **Macrocephaly**.

**Macrocephaly.** Overdevelopment of the head; macrencephalia; macrencephaly; macrocephalia; megacephaly; megalocephaly. बृहत्शीर्षता; महाशिरस्कता; दीर्घकपालीयता

**Macrocheilia.** Excessive development of the lips. बृहतोष्ठता; होंठों का अत्यधिक विकास होना

**Macrocheiria.** Large size of the hands; macrochiria; magalocheiria; megalochiria. बृहत्हस्तता; हाथों का बड़ा आकार होना

**Macrochiria.** See **Macrocheiria**.

**Macrocolon.** A sigmoid colon of unusual length. बृहदान्त्रता

**Macrocornea.** See **Megalocornea**.

**Macrocranium.** An enlarged skull. बृहत्करोटिता

**Macrocyte.** A giant blood-corpuscle in pernicious anaemia. बृहत्लोहितकोशिका; बृहत्पुटी

**Macrocythaemia.** The presence of macrocytes in the blood; macrocythemia; macrocytosis. बृहत्लोहितकोशिकारक्तता

**Macrocythemia.** See **Macrocythaemia**.

**Macrocytosis.** See **Macrocythaemia**.

**Macrodactylia.** See **Macrodactyly**.

**Macrodactyly.** Congenital overgrowth of fingers; macrodactylia; megadaclyly. बृहदांगुलिता; उँगलियों का जन्म से ही बड़ा रहना

**Macrodont.** Large-toothed; megadont. बृहद्दन्ती; बड़े दान्तों वाला

**Macrodontia.** The state of having abnormally large teeth; megadontia; megadontism; megalodontia; megalodontism. बृहद्दन्तता

**Macrogamete.** The mature female cell in propagative reproduction in sporozoa. बृहत्युग्मक; बृहत्जन्यु; नारीजन्यु; दो संयुग्मियों में से बड़ा संयुग्मी

**Macrogametocyte.** The enlarged merozoite before maturation into the female cell in propagative reproduction in sporozoa. बृहत्युग्मकजनक; बृहत्युग्मककोशिका; बृहत्जननकोशिका, बृहद्युग्मकता

**Macrogenitosomia.** Excessive development of genital body. बृहत्लिंगता

**Macroglossia.** Excessive development of the tongue; megaloglossia; pachyglossia. बृहत्जिह्वा; जीभ का अत्यधिक बढ़ना

**Macrognathia.** Enlargment or elongation of the jaw. बृहत्हनुता

**Macromastia.** Abnormally large breasts. बृहत्स्तनता; असाधारण रूप से बड़े हुये स्तन

**Macronucleus.** A large nucleus. बृहत्केन्द्रक; दीर्घकेन्द्रक

**Macronychia.** Excessive development of nails. दीर्घनखता

**Macropenis.** An abnormally large penis; megalopenis. बृहत्शिश्न; बृहत्लिंग

**Macrophage.** A large nucleated leukocyte; macrophagus. बृहत्भक्षककोशिका

**Macrophagus.** See **Macrophage.**

**Macrophthalmia.** Abnormally large eyes; magalophthalmus; megophthalmus. बृहद्नेत्रता; महानेत्रता

**Macropia.** See **Macropsia.**

**Macropodia.** Abnormal size of the feet; megalopodia. बृहत्पादता; पैरों का असाधारण रूप से बढ़ना

**Macroprosopia.** A large face out of proportion to the size of cranial vault. बृहदाननता; महाननता

**Macropsia.** Any disease of the eye in which objects appear enlarged; macropia; megalopsia. बृहत्दृष्टिता; आँखों का ऐसा रोग जिसमें प्रत्येक वस्तु बड़ी दिखाई देती है

**Macroscopic.** Relating to macroscopy; megascopic. महावीक्षणीय

**Macroscopy.** Examination of the objects with the naked eye. महावीक्षण

**Macrosomatia.** See **Macrosomia.**

**Macrosomia.** Oversize of the body; macrosomatia. बृहत्कायता; महाकायता; शरीर का अत्यधिक बढ़ा हुआ आकार

**Macrostoma.** Congenital fissure at the angle of the mouth, producing a large opening; macrostomia. बृहत्मुखद्वार

**Macrostomia.** See **Macrostoma.**

**Macrotia.** Abnormally large ears. बृहत्कर्णता; असाधारण रूप से बढ़े हुए कान

**Macula.** A spot; macule. बिन्दु; घनीफुल्ली; चकत्ता; चित्ती; दाग; धब्बा;

    **M. Corneae,** corneal opacity. स्वच्छमण्डल-अपारदर्शिता;

    **M. Cribrosa,** a name for the perforation of the fossa hemispherica for the passage of the filament of the auditory nerve. चालनीवत् बिन्दु;

    **M. Lutea,** the yellow spot of the retina. पीत बिन्दु

**Maculae.** Plural of **Macula.**

**Macular.** Pertaining to, or composed of a macula. बन्दव; चित्तीदार

**Maculate.** Spotted. बिन्दुकित; चित्तीदार; दाग वाला; धब्बेदार

**Maculated.** Spotted. चित्तीदार; दागवाला; बिन्दुकित; धब्बेदार

**Maculation.** A spotted condition. बिन्दुकन; चित्तीदार अवस्था

**Macule.** See **Macula.**

**Maculo-papular.** The presence of macules and raised palpable papules (spots) of the skin. चित्ती-पिटकीय; चित्तीदार तथा पिटकमय

**Maculopathy.** Any pathological condition of the macula lutea (yellow spot). पीतबिन्दुविकृति

**Mad.** Insane; rabid. विक्षिप्त; पागल

**Madarosis.** Loss of the eyelashes; milphosis. पक्ष्मशात; वर्त्माभाव; पलकों का अभाव

**Madefaction.** Making moist. आर्द्रीकरण

**Madescens.** Half wet or moist. अल्पार्द्र; dampness. सीलन

**Madness.** Insanity. विक्षिप्ति; पागलपन

**Madura-foot.** Pustules on the foot, endemic in India; mycetoma. मदुरापाद; कवकगुल्म

**Magenta.** A rich purplish-red coal-tar dye. मंजिष्ठा

**Maggot.** The larva-form of fly. मैगट; कीटार्भक; किसी मक्खी का लार्वा-रूप

**Maggot-pimples.** Acne. मुहासे; फुन्सियाँ

**Magnesia.** An oxide of magnesium; magnesium. मैग्नीशिया; मैग्नीशियम-ऑक्साइड; एक प्रकार का सफेद चूर्ण

**Magnesium.** See **Magnesia**.

**Magnet.** Load-stone. चुम्बक; लोहे को आकर्षित करने वाला पदार्थ-विशेष

**Magnetic.** Possessing the properties of magnetism. चुम्बकीय;

   **M. Field,** the space permeated by the magnetic lines of force surrounding a permanent magnet or coil of wire carrying electric current. चुम्बक-क्षेत्र

**Magnetism.** The power of magnet to attract or repel other masses. चुम्बकशक्ति; चुम्बकीय आकर्षण शक्ति; चुम्बकत्व

**Magnetotherapist.** One versed in magneto-therapy. चुम्बक-चिकित्सक

**Magnetotherapy.** The magnetic treatment of a disease. चुम्बक-चिकित्सा; चुम्बक द्वारा रोगोपचार करना

**Magnification.** The enlarging power of a microscope. आवर्धन; सूक्ष्मदर्शीयंत्र की आवर्धी शक्ति

**Magnum.** Large or great. महा; बड़ा

**Main en griffe.** Claw-hand. नखरहस्त;

   **M. Succulente,** oedema of the hands. हस्तशोफ; हाथों का शोफ

**Major.** Greater. बृहत्; बड़ा; बड़ी

**Mal-.** Prefix meaning ill or bad. 'रुग्णता' का अर्थ देने वाला उपसर्ग

**Mal.** Sickness; a disease. रोग; बीमारी; रुग्णता;

   **M.de mer,** sea-sickness. समुद्री रुग्णता; सामुद्रिक रुग्णता;

   **M.- praxis,** see **Malpractice.**

   **Grand M.,** major epilepsy. महापस्मार; महामिर्गी;

   **Petit-m.,** minor epilepsy. मृदु-अपस्मार; हल्की मिर्गी

**Mala.** The cheek. गाल; हनु; गण्ड; जबड़ा; the cheek-bone. गाल की हड्डी

**Malabsorption.** Poor or disordered absorption. अपावशोषण

**Malacia.** Softening of a part; malacosis. मृदुता; किसी भाग की कोमलता;

   **Spinal M.,** see **Myelitis.**

**Malacosis.** See **Malacia.**

**Maladjustment.** Bad or poor adaptation to any environment;

malalignment. कुसमंजन; कुसमायोजन

**Malady.** A disease, discomfort or disability. रोग; बीमारी; रुग्णता; रोगावस्था

**Malaise.** A feeling of uneasiness or discomfort. व्यग्रता; व्याकुलता; बेचैनी; घबराहट

**Malalignment.** See **Maladjustment**.

**Malar.** Pertaining to, or belonging to the cheeks. हनु अथवा गण्ड सम्बन्धी;
   **M. Bone,** the cheek-bone. हन्वस्थि; गण्डास्थि; जबड़े अथवा गाल की हड्डी;
   **M. Point,** the most prominent point in the outer surface of the malar bone. गण्ड-बिन्दु

**Malaria.** A febrile disease caused by a blood parasite. विषमज्वर; मलेरिया;
   **Quarten M.,** with a paroxysm on every fourth day. चतुर्थक मलेरिया; हर चौथे दिन आने वाला बुखार;
   **Quotidian M.,** occurring daily. दैनिक मलेरिया; रोज आने वाला (मलेरिया) ज्वर
   **Tertian M.,** with a paroxysm on every third day. तृतीयक मलेरिया; हर तीसरे दिन आने वाला बुखार

**Malarial.** Pertaining to malaria. विषमज्वरीय; मलेरिया सम्बन्धी;
   **M. Cachexia,** chronic malarial poisoning. विषमज्वरीय क्षीणता;
   **M. Fever,** the periodic fever of malaria; marsh fever. विषमज्वर; मलेरिया;

**Malariologist.** An expert in the study of malaria. मलेरियाविज्ञ; मलेरियाविज्ञानी

**Malassimilation.** Incomplete, faulty or imperfect assimilation. दु:सात्मीकरण; दु:स्वांगीकरण; अपूर्ण आत्मीकरण या स्वांगीकरण

**Maldevelopment.** Incomplete, faulty or imperfect development. कुविकास; अपूर्ण विकास; दुर्विकास

**Maldigestion.** Incomplete or impaired digestion. कुपाचन; पाचन की गड़बड़ी

**Male.** One of, or pertaining to, the impregnating sex. पुरुष; नर; नृ; पुरुष अथवा नर सम्बन्धी

**Malefern.** Filix Mas. मेलफर्न

**Malformation.** A wrong or improper formation, as of a part or organ of the body. कुरचना; रचनाविकार; विकृत-रचना

**Malfunction.** Disordered, inadequate or abnormal function. दुष्क्रिया;

अनुचित अथवा अस्वाभाविक क्रिया

**Malic Acid.** The acid of apples, pears, etc. मैलिक एसिड; सेबों, नासपातियों, आदि का अम्ल

**Malignancy.** The state of being bad to worse. दुर्दमता; संघातकता; सांघातिकता

**Malignant.** Virulent; dangerous; a term used to great severity of a disease. दुर्दम; घातक; संघातक; संघाती; सांघातिक

**Malingerer.** One feigning injury or illness. छलरोगी; कपटरोगी

**Malingering.** The intentional faking of disease. छलरुग्णता; बीमारी का बहाना बनाना; बीमारी या तकलीफ को बढ़ा-चढ़ा कर बताना

**Malis.** A parasitic cautaneous disease. चर्मरोग; मैलिस; एक परजीवी त्वक् रोग

**Malleable.** Capable of being shaped by being beaten or by pressure. आघातवर्ध्य; नम्य

**Malleation.** Chorea with hammering of the hands. लास्य; नर्तन रोग

**Mallei.** Plural of **Malleus.**

**Melleolar.** Pertaining to malleolus. गुल्फिक; गुल्फ सम्बन्धी

**Malleoli.** Plural of **Malleolus.**

**Malleolus.** A hammer head-shaped process of bones. गुल्फ; टखने का जोड़;

    **External M.,** see **Lateral Malleolus.**

    **Internal M.,** see **Medial Malleolus.**

    **Lateral M.,** external malleolus; the lower end of the fibula. बाह्य-गुल्फ; बहिर्गुल्फ

    **Medial M.,** internal malleolus; a process on the inner surface of the lower end of the tibia. अन्तर्गुल्फ; अन्त:गुल्फ

**Mallet.** Hammer. मुद्गर; हथौड़ी

**Malleus.** A small hammer-shaped bone of the internal ear. कर्णास्थि; हथौड़े के आकार जैसी कान की छोटी हड्डी

**Malnutrition.** The poor assimilation of nutrition. कुपोषण; पोषणतत्वाभाव

**Malocclusion.** Failure of the upper and lower teeth to meet properly when the jaws are closed; any diviation from a normal occlusion. कुधारणा

**Malpighian Bodies.** Small corpuscles found in the kidney;

Malpighi's bodies. वृक्क-कण; गुर्दे में पाये जाने वाले क्षुद्र कण

**Malpighi's Bodies.** See **Malpighian Bodies.**

**Malposition.** A wrong position. कुस्थिति; गलत स्थिति

**Malpractice.** Injurious and improper practice; malpraxis. दुश्चिकित्सा; दुष्टाचार; अनाचार; हानिप्रद एवं अनुचित चिकित्सा

**Malpresentation.** A faulty presentation. कुप्रस्तुति; कदुदय

**Malrotation.** Failure during embryonic development of normal rotation of all or any portion of the intestinal tract. कुघूर्णन

**Malt.** Partially fermented barley-seed, the starch being converted into grape-sugar. माल्ट; अनाज का सीरा

   **M. Sugar,** see **Maltose.**

**Maltose.** A sugar derived from the action of diastase on barley; malt sugar. माल्टोस; माल्ट शर्करा

**Malum.** A disease. रोग; बीमारी; रुग्णता

**Malunion.** Incomplete union, or union in a faulty position. कुसम्मिलन; पूरी तरह न मिलना या जुड़ना

**Mamelon.** A nipple. चूचुक

**Mamilla.** See **Mammilla.**

**Mamma.** The breast; the milk-secreting organ. स्तन; कुच

**Mammae.** Plural of **Mamma.**

**Mammal.** Animal that suckles its young. स्तनपायी

**Mammalgia.** Mastodynia; mastalgia; pain in the breast. स्तनार्ति; स्तनपीड़ा

**Mammalia.** The highest form of vertebrates. स्तनीवर्ग

**Mammaplasty.** Any plastic operation of the breast. स्तनसंघान

**Mammary.** Relating to the breast. स्तनविषयक; स्तन सम्बन्धी;

   **M. Abscess,** gathered breast; abscess of mammae. स्तन-विद्रधि;

   **M. Gland,** the milk-secreting gland. स्तन-ग्रन्थि

**Mammectomy.** Removal of the breast; mammotomy; mastectomy. स्तन-उच्छेदन

**Mammiform.** Of the form of the female breast; breast-shaped; mammose. स्तनाकार; स्तनरूप

**Mammilla.** A nipple; mamilla. चूचुक; कुचाग्र; स्तनवृन्त; a small papilla. क्षुद्र-अंकुरक

**Mammillae.** Plural of **Mammilla.**

**Mammillaplasty.** Any plastic operation on the nipples. चूचुकसंधान

**Mammillary.** Like a nipple. चूचुकाभ; चूचुक जैसा; स्तनाकार

**Mammilliform.** Of the form of a nipple. चूचुकरूप; चूचुकाकार

**Mammillitis.** Inflammation of the nipple. चूचुकशोथ

**Mammitis.** Inflammation of the breasts; mastitis. स्तनशोथ; स्तनों का प्रदाह; कुचशोथ

**Mammogram.** A radiograph of the breasts. स्तनचित्र

**Mammography.** X-ray examination of the breast after injection of an opaque agent; mastography. स्तनचित्रण

**Mammose.** See **Mammiform.**

**Mammotomy.** See **Mammectomy.**

**Mandible.** The lower jaw; mandibula. अधोहनु; निचला जबड़ा

**Mandibula.** See **Mandible.**

**Mandibular.** Pertaining to the lower jaw. अधोहनुज; निचले जबड़े सम्बन्धी

**Mane.** Morning. प्रातः; प्रातःकाल; सुबह

**Mange.** A skin disease of animals. खाज; पशुखाज; पशुओं को होने वाली चमड़ी की एक बीमारी

**Mania.** Raving or furious madness. उन्माद; व्यसन; उन्मत्तता; पागलपन; झक; सनक;

   **Alcoholic M.,** acute mania of alcoholic origin. मद्यज उन्माद;

   **Dancing M.,** an epidemic of choreic or convulsive movements. लास्योन्माद;

   **Epileptic M.,** a maniacal outburst in an epileptic. अपस्मारी उन्माद;

   **Puerperal M.,** a form sometimes following childbirth. प्रासूतिक उन्माद;

   **Transitory M.,** frenzied attacks of short duration. क्षणिक उन्माद;

   **M. a potu,** delirium tremens; trembling delirium. कम्पोन्माद; मदात्यय; मदिरोन्माद

**Maniac.** An insane person; manic. विक्षिप्त; उन्मत्त; उन्मादी; पागल; झक्की; सनकी

**Maniacal.** Having the nature of madness. उन्मत्त; उन्मादी

**Manic.** See **Maniac.**

**Manifest.** Clear or evident; obvious; plain. व्यक्त; अभिव्यक्त; स्पष्ट

**Manifestation.** Revelation; display or disclosure of characteristic signs or symptoms of an illness. अभिव्यक्ति

**Manipulation.** The mode of handling anything, or conducting an operation by hand. हस्तशल्य; हस्तोपचार; हाथों द्वारा किया जाने वाला उपचार

**Manometer.** An instrument for estimating the pressure exerted by the liquids and the gases. दाबमापी; दाबमापकयंत्र; तरल पदार्थों तथा गैसों के दबाव को मापने वाला यंत्र

**Mantoux Reaction.** See **Mantoux Test.**

**Mantoux Test.** A form of tuberculin test that injects the test material between the layers of the skin; Mantoux reaction. माण्टू परीक्षण; माण्टू जांच

**Manual.** Pertaining to, or performed by the hands. हस्त सम्बन्धी; हस्तकृत; हाथों का; हाथों से किया जाने वाला

**Manubria.** Plural of **Manubrium.**

**Manubrium.** The upper bone or portion of the sternum. उरोस्थि; वक्ष के ऊपर की हड्डी;

**M. Sterni,** the upper segment of the sternum. उरोस्थि-मुष्ठि

**Manufactory.** Factory. विनिर्माणशाला; निर्माणी

**Manufacture.** Preparation of things by hand or machinery on a large scale. विनिर्माण; निर्माण; उत्पादन

**Manus.** The hand. हस्त; हाथ; हस्तांग

**Manustupration.** See **Masturbation.**

**Maple Syrup Urine Disease.** A birth defect in body chemistry, involving defective amino–acid metabolism. सहज शरीर दोष; शरीर का कोई जन्मजात दोष

**Marantic.** See **Marasmic.**

**Marasmatic.** Affected with marasmus. सुखण्डीग्रस्त; शोषग्रस्त; सूखा रोग से पीड़ित

**Marasmic.** Pertaining to marasmus; marantic. सुखण्डी अथवा शोष सम्बन्धी

**Marasmus.** Atrophy; wasting away from various causes, especially in children. सुखण्डी; शोष; सूखा रोग

**Marc.** The refuge of fruit after extraction of juice. छूँछ

**Margin.** A border, or edge of any surface; margo. परिसीमा; सीमा; उपान्त; हाशिया

**Marginal.** Pertaining to, or at the border of. सीमा सम्बन्धी

**Margination.** Adhesion of leukocytes to the walls of the blood vessels in the first stage of inflammation. परिसराश्रयण

**Margines.** Plural of **Margo.**

**Margo.** See **Margin.**

**Margosa.** The Indian neem tree. नीम

**Marigold.** A plant of the genus **Calendula** bearing a yellow flower. गेंदा

**Mark.** A sign. चिन्ह;
 **Mother's M.,** naevus. मातृचिन्ह; मातृन्यच्छ; तिल

**Marrow.** A fatty substance in the cavities of long cylindrical bones; medulla osseum. मज्जा; अस्थिमज्जा; लम्बी हड्डियों की चर्बी;
 **Bone-m.,** that inside the bones. अस्थिमज्जा; हड्डियों के अन्दर विद्यमान चर्बी या गूदा;
 **Spinal M.,** the spinal cord. मेरुमज्जा; सुषुम्ना

**Marsh.** A tract of low land covered with water. दलदल;
 **M. Fever,** malarial fever. दलदल ज्वर; विषमज्वर; मलेरिया

**Martial.** Containing iron. लौहयोगिक; लौहमिश्रित

**Martin's Bandage.** An Indian rubber-bandage for varicose veins. मार्टिनी पट्टी; उभरी हुई शिराओं को बांधने के लिये प्रयुक्त की जाने वाली रबड़ की एक पट्टी

**Mascule.** Male or belonging to the male sex. पुरुष अथवा पौरुष सम्बन्धी; resembling a man. पुरुषाभ

**Masculine.** Relating to, or marked by the characteristics of male sex. पुरुष सम्बन्धी अथवा पुरुष जैसा

**Masculinity.** The characteristics of a male. पुंवत्ता; पुंस्त्व

**Masculinization.** Attainment of male characteristics. पुंस्त्वभवन

**Mask.** A bandage covering the face. मास्क; अवगुंठन; मुखावरण; नाक और मुँह ढकने का नकाब

**Masochism.** A form of sexual perversion which delights in cruel treatment, punishing the same. परपीड़ितकामुकता; परपीड्यकामुकता; परपीड़नकामुकता

**Masochist.** The passive party in the practice of masochism. परपीड़नकामुक

**Mass.** A collection of matter. समूह; पुंज; संहति; लुगदी; ढेर

**Massa.** The compound or lump from which the pills are formed. औषधिपिण्ड, जिससे गोलियाँ तैयार की जाती हैं

**Massage.** Stroking, kneading, for the relief of pain or muscular stiffness. मर्दन; मालिश;

**Cardiac M.,** manual rhythmic compression of the ventricles to maintain the circulation. हृत्मर्दन

**Massaging.** The performance of massage; massering. मालिश करना; मर्दन कार्य करना

**Massering.** See **Massaging.**

**Massive.** Heavy. भारी; पुंजल

**Massotherapy.** Treatment by, or therapeutic use of massage. मर्दनोपचार; मालिश द्वारा की जाने वाली चिकित्सा

**Mastadenitis.** Inflammation of the mammary glands. स्तनग्रन्थिशोथ; स्तनग्रन्थियों का प्रदाह

**Mastadenoma.** A benign tumour of the breast. स्तनार्बुद; स्तन की गांठ

**Mastalgia.** Pain in the breast. स्तनार्ति; स्तनवेदना; स्तन-पीड़ा

**Mastaluxe.** Swollen or enlarged female breasts. बृहदाकारस्तन; विवर्धित अथवा सूजे हुए स्तन

**Mastatrophy.** Atrophy of the breasts. स्तनशोष; स्तनों का सूखना

**Mastectomy.** Surgical removal of the breast; mammectomy; mammotomy; mastotomy. स्तन-उच्छेदन; स्तन को काट कर हटा देना

**Masticate.** To perform mastication; to chew. चर्वण करना; चबाना

**Mastication.** The act of chewing. चर्वण; चबाना

**Masticatory.** A remedy to be chewed. चर्वणीय (औषधि); चबाई जाने वाली (औषधि); relating to mastication. चर्वण सम्बन्धी

**Mastigophora.** One of the classes of protozoa. एककोशीय; एककोशिक; प्रारम्भिक जीव

**Mastitis.** Inflammation of the breasts; mammitis. स्तनशोथ; स्तनातिपूरण; स्तनों का प्रदाह

**Mastodynia.** Neuralgia and hyperaesthesia of the mammary glands; mammalgia. स्तनवेदना; स्तनपीड़ा

**Mastography.** See **Mammography.**

**Mastoid.** Shaped like a nipple. चूचुकाकार; the mastoid process of the temporal bone. कर्णमूल;

    **M. Abscess,** an abscess of the mastoid cells. कर्णमूल विद्रधि;

    **M. Bone,** see **Mastoid Process.**

    **M. Cells,** cells in the mastoid process; mastoid sinuses. कर्णमूल कोशिकाएं;

    **M. Gland,** the parotid gland. कर्णमूल ग्रन्थि;

**M. Process,** mastoid bone; the nipple-like projection of the petrous part of the temporal bone. कर्णमूलास्थि;

**M. Sinuses,** see **Mastoid Cells.**

**Mastoidectomy.** Drainage of the mastoid air-cells and excision of the diseased tissue. कर्णमूल-उच्छेदन

**Mastoiditis.** Inflammation of the mastoid cells. कर्णमूलशोथ; कर्णमूलकोशिकाशोथ; कर्णमूल-प्रदाह

**Mastoidotomy.** Incision into the mastoid process of the temporal bone. कर्णमूलछेदन

**Mastology.** A treatise on the breasts. स्तनप्रकरण; स्तनविज्ञान; दुग्ध-ग्रन्थियों का अध्ययन

**Mastoncus.** A tumour or swelling of the breasts. स्तनार्बुद

**Mastopathy.** Any disease of the breasts. स्तनरोग

**Mastopexy.** Plastic surgery to affix sagging breasts in a more elevated and normal position; mazopexy. स्तनस्थिरीकरण

**Mastoplasty.** Any plastic operation on the breasts. स्तनसंधान

**Mastoptosis.** Sagging of the breasts. स्तनपात; स्तनों का लटक जाना

**Mastosis.** A tumour of the breast. स्तनार्बुद; स्तन की रसौली

**Mastotomy.** See **Mastectomy.**

**Masturbation.** Production of venereal orgasm by friction with hand; onanism; manustupration. हस्तमैथुन; हथरस

**Materia Medica.** The science dealing with the origin, action and dosage of the drugs. मैटीरिया मेडिका; भेषज-निघंटु; औषध-निघंटु

**Maternal.** Pertaining to the mother. मातृ-आगत; माता से सम्बन्धित

**Maternity.** According to the rules of the motherhood. प्रसूति; मातृत्व

**Matrices.** Plural of **Matrix.**

**Matricide.** Killing of one's mother. मातृहत्या

**Matrix.** A mold; the cavity in which anything is formed. आधात्री; आधारक; the uterus. जरायु; गर्भाशय

**Matrixitis.** Onychia. नखशोथ; नाखुनों का प्रदाह

**Matron.** A midwife. मैट्रन; धात्री; धातृ

**Matter.** Pus collected in or emitted from an abscess, pustule, etc. स्राव; पीब; पूय; substance. पदार्थ; द्रव्य;

**Gray M.,** the regions of the brain and spinal cord made up of the cell bodies and dendrites of the nerve cells; gray substance;

substantia grisea. धूसर पदार्थ; धूसर द्रव्य;

**White M.,** the regions of the brain and spinal cord composed of nerve fibres; white substance; substantia alba. श्वेत पदार्थ; श्वेत द्रव्य

**Maturation.** Ripening. परिपक्वता; परिपाक; achievement of full development or growth. प्रौढ़ता

**Matured.** Fully developed. परिपक्व; पक्व; प्रौढ़

**Maw-worm.** The tape-worm. केंचुवा; स्फीत-कृमि; फीता-कृमि

**Maxilla.** One of the upper jaw-bones; upper jaw. ऊर्ध्वहनु; ऊपर वाला जबड़ा; ऊर्ध्वहन्वस्थि

**Maxillae.** Plural of **Maxilla.**

**Maxillary.** Referring or relating to one of the upper jaw-bones or the hollow or the sinus in that bone. ऊर्ध्वहनुज; ऊर्ध्वहन्वास्थिक; ऊपर वाले जबड़े से सम्बन्धित

**Maxillotomy.** Incision of the maxilla. ऊर्ध्वहनुच्छेदन

**Maximal.** Greatest. इष्टतम; अधिकतम

**Maximum.** The highest or the largest quantity. अधिकतम; अधिकाधिक; उच्चतम

**Mazoitis.** Mastitis; inflammation of the breast. स्तनशोथ; स्तनप्रदाह

**Mazopexy.** See **Mastopexy.**

**M.D.** Doctor of Medicine. एमo डीo

**Meal.** Food consumed at regular intervals or at a specific time. भोजन; आहार

**Mean.** The average or general tendency of a set of values. माध्य; माध्यम

**Measles.** Rubeola Morbilli; an eruptive disease of childhood. रोमान्तिका; खसरा

**Measly.** Resembling measles. रोमान्तिकाभ; रोमन्तिका-संक्रमित; खसरा जैसा

**Meat.** The flesh of animals, including poultery, that is used for food. मांस

**Meatal.** Pertaining to a meatus. कर्णकुहरीय; कर्णकुहर सम्बन्धी;

 **M.-plasty,** plastic operation on a meatus. कर्णकुहरसंधान

**Meatoplasty.** A plastic operation on a meatus. कर्णकुहरसंधान

**Meatorrhaphy.** Closing by suture of the wound made by performing a meatotomy. मूत्रमार्गमुखसीवन

**Meatoscope.** A speculum for examining a meatus. कुहरदर्शी

**Meatoscopy.** Instrumental examination of a meatus, especially the meatus of the urethra. कुहरदर्शन

**Meatotomy.** Cutting of the urinary meatus. मूत्रमार्गमुखछेदन

**Meatus.** A passage; an opening. कुहर; द्वार; छेद; मुख; नलिकापथ;
   **M. Acustis Externus,** see **Meatus Auditorius.**
   **M. Acustis Internus,** the internal canal leading through the petrous portion of the temporal bone and containing the facial and auditory nerves and vessels. अन्तःकर्णकुहर;
   **M. Auditorius.,** the external auditory canal; meatus acustis externus. बाह्य कर्णकुहर;
   **M. Urinarius,** external orifice of the urethra. मूत्रमार्ग-मुख

**Mechanical.** Pertaining to a machine; also acting by physical power. यान्त्रिक; भौतिक

**Mechanics.** The science of the action of the forces in promoting motion or equilibrium. यान्त्रिकी

**Mechanism.** The means by which an effect is obtained. क्रियाविधि; involuntary and constant response to a stimulus. प्रक्रिया

**Mechanotherapy.** The application of mechanical means to the treatment of injury or disease. यांत्रिक-चिकित्सा; यंत्रोपचार

**Meconin.** See **Meconine.**

**Meconine.** A neutral substance in opium; meconin. अफीम का सत; मेकोनिन

**Meconism.** Poisoning by opium. अफीम-विषाक्तता

**Meconium.** The first faeces of an infant voided shortly after birth. जातविष्ठा; नवजात शिशु का प्रथम मल; opium. अफीम

**Media.** The middle coat of an artery. (वाहिका)मध्यास्तर

**Medial.** Pertaining to, or near the middle. मध्यवर्ती; अभिमध्य

**Median.** The middle or mesial. मध्यम; माध्यिका; मध्यस्थ; समविभाजक;
   **M. Line,** an imaginary line from the crown of the head to the feet supposed to divide the body into two equal parts. मध्यस्थ रेखा; समविभाजक रेखा

**Mediastinal.** Pertaining to the mediastinum. मध्यस्थानिकीय; मध्यस्थानिका सम्बन्धी

**Mediastinitis.** Inflammation of the mediastinum. मध्यस्थानिकाशोथ; मध्यस्थानिका-प्रदाह

**Mediastinography.** Radiography of the mediastinum. मध्यस्थानिकाचित्रण

**Mediastinopericarditis.** Combined inflammation of the pericardium and mediastinum. मध्यस्थानिकापरिहृद्शोथ

**Mediastinoscope.** The endoscope for inspection of the mediastinum through a suprasternal incision. मध्यस्थानिकादर्शी

**Mediastinoscopy.** Exploration of the mediastinum through a suprasternal incision. मध्यस्थानिकादर्शन

**Mediastinotomy.** Incision into the mediastinum. मध्यस्थानिकाछेदन

**Mediastinum.** The space between the lungs. मध्यस्थानिका; मध्यावकाश

**Medical.** Pertaining to the medicine or treatment. आयुर्विज्ञानीय; भेषजीय; चिकित्सीय; वैद्यक; चिकित्सा सम्बन्धी;

> **M. Certificate,** a certificate given to a patient about his sickness. चिकित्सा प्रमाण-पत्र;
>
> **M. Ethics,** the rules govering the medical profession. चिकित्साचार; उपचार संहिता;
>
> **M. Jurisprudence,** forensic medicine or science; legal medicine. व्यवहार आयुर्विज्ञान; वैद्यक न्यायशास्त्र; न्यायवैद्यक;
>
> **M. Science,** the science that treats of medicine. आयुर्विज्ञान; चिकित्साविज्ञान

**Medicament.** A remedy or medicine. औषधि; औषधद्रव्य; a medicinal application. औषधीय विलेपन

**Medicamentosus.** Concerning drugs. औषधीय; औषध सम्बन्धी

**Medicate.** To permeate with medicinal substance. औषधयुक्त करना

**Medicated.** Permeated with a drug or medicine. औषधयुक्त

**Medication.** Drugs taken internally or applied externally. औषधप्रयोग; औषध-प्रदान; औषध

**Medicatrix.** Healing or curing. विरोहण; उपचार करना; इलाज करना;

> **M. Naturae,** the natural healing. स्वविरोहण

**Medicinal.** Having the qualities of, or pertaining to a medicine. रोगनिवारक; भेषजीय

**Medicine.** The science and art of healing, and preventing diseases. आयुर्विज्ञान; चिकित्सा-शास्त्र; a drug or remedy. औषध; औषधि; भेषज;

> **Clinical M.,** pertaining to the study of disease by the bedside of the patient. नैदानिक आयुर्विज्ञान;

**Forensic M.**, the relations of medicine to law; legal medicine; medical jurisprudence; state medicine. व्यवहार आयुर्विज्ञान; न्यायवैद्यक; वैद्यक न्यायशास्त्र;

**Legal M.**, see **Forensic Medicine.**

**Patent M.**, see **Proprietary Medicine.**

**Preventive M.**, that branch of medical science which aims at the prevention of disease. निरोधक आयुर्विज्ञान;

**Proprietary M.**, one the manufacture of which is limited or controlled by an owner, because of a patent, a copyright or secrecy as regards its constitution or method of manufacture; patent medicine. एकायत्त औषध;

**State M.**, see **Forensic Medicine.**

**Veterinary M.**, the field concered with the disease and health of animal species other than man. पशु आयुर्विज्ञान

**Medicolegal.** Pertaining to the forensic medicine. न्यायवैद्यकीय; न्यायवैद्यक; व्यवहार आयुर्विज्ञान सम्बन्धी

**Medicus.** A physician. चिकित्सक; वैद्य; हकीम

**Medium.** A substance used in bacteriology for the growth of organisms; a means. माध्यम;

**Contrast M.**, any material relatively opaque to x-rays, such as barium, used in rediography to visualize the stomach, intestine or other organ. विभेदक माध्यम;

**Culture M.**, a substance used for the cultivation, isolation, identification, or storage of micro-organism. सम्वर्ध माध्यम

**Medius.** The middle finger. माध्यमिका; बीच वाली उँगली

**Medulla.** The marrow in verious cavities. अन्तस्था; मज्जा; प्रान्तस्था; अस्थि-गह्वरों के अन्दर रहने वाला कोमल पदार्थ;

**M. Oblongata,** part of the brain within the cranium; nervous system of the senses. पश्चकपाल-अन्तस्था; मेरु-मज्जा;

**M. Ossium,** the bone-marrow; the tissue filling the cavities of the bones. अस्थि-मज्जा;

**M. Ossium Flava,** yellow bone-marrow. पीत अस्थि-मज्जा;

**M. Ossium Rubra,** red bone-marrow. लोहित अस्थि-मज्जा;

**M. Spinalis,** the spinal cord. मेरु-अन्तस्था; सुषुम्ना;

**M. Suprarenalis,** adrenal medulla; inner portion of the adrenal gland. अधिवृक्क प्रान्तस्था;

**Adrenal M.**, see **Medulla Suprarenalis.**

**Medullae.** Plural of **Medulla.**

**Medullar.** Pertaining to the medulla; medullary. अन्तस्था सम्बन्धी; मज्जा सम्बन्धी

**Medullary.** See **Medullar.**

  **M. Canal,** the hollow interior of long bones. अस्थि-नाल; तंत्रिका-नाल;

  **M. Ray,** the cortical bundle of uriniferous tubules. मज्जा-रश्मि

**Medullated.** Provided with, or having a medulla. मज्जावृत्त

**Medullectomy.** Excision of any medullary substance. मज्जा-उच्छेदन; अन्तस्था-उच्छेदन

**Medullitis.** Inflammation of marrow. मज्जाशोथ

**Megacephalic.** Large-headed; megalocephalic; megacephalous; megalencephalic. महाशिरस्क; दीर्घकपालिक; बहुत बड़े सिर वाला

**Megacephalous.** See **Megacephalic.**

**Megacephaly.** See **Macrocephaly.**

**Megacolon.** Condition of dilated and elongated colon. महाबृहदान्त्र; बड़ी आन्त की फैली हुई अवस्था

**Megadactyly.** See **Macrodactyly.**

**Megadont.** See **Macrodont.**

**Megadontia.** See **Macrodontia.**

**Megadontism.** See **Macrodontia.**

**Megakaryoblast.** Precursor of a megakaryocyte. महामूललोहितकोशिकाप्रसू

**Megakaryocyte.** A cell having a large nucleus; megalokaryocyte. महामूललोहितकोशिका

**Megalencephalic.** See **Megacephalic.**

**Megalgia.** Very severe pain. अत्युग्रवेदना

**Megaloblast.** A large-sized blood-corpuscle. महालोहितकोशिकाप्रसू

**Megalocephalic.** See **Megacephalic.**

**Megalocephaly.** See **Macrocephaly.**

**Megalocheiria.** See **Macrocheiria.**

**Megalochiria.** See **Macrocheiria.**

**Megalocornea.** Abnormal prominence of the cornea; macrocornea. महास्वच्छपटल; स्वच्छमण्डल का असाधारण उभार

**Megalocyte.** A large non-nucleated red blood cell. महालोहितकोशिका

**Megalodontia.** See **Macrodontia.**

**Megalodontism.** See **Macrodontia.**

**Megalogastria.** Abnormal size of stomach. उदरविस्फार; आमाशय का असाधारण आकार

**Megaloglossia.** See **Macroglossia.**

**Megalohepatia.** Enlargement of the liver; hapatomegaly. महायकृत्ता

**Megalokaryocyte.** See **Megakaryocyte.**

**Megalomania.** Insanity with delusional ideas of personal greatness or exaltation. महोन्माद; ऐसा पागलपन जिसमें रोगी स्वयं को एक महान व्यक्ति समझता है

**Megalopenis.** See **Macropenis.**

**Megalophthalmus.** See **Macrophthalmia.**

**Megalopodia.** See **Macropodia.**

**Megalopsia.** See **Macropsia.**

**Megaloureter.** Increase in the diameter of the ureter. महागवीनी

**Megarectum.** Extreme dilatation of the rectum. महामलांत्र

**Megascopic.** See **Macroscopic.**

**Megasema.** Abnormal enlargement of orbital index. दीर्घनेत्रकोटरता; नेत्रकोटर का अत्यधिक बढ़ जाना

**Megophthalmus.** See **Macrophthalmia.**

**Megrim.** Migraine; one-sided headache. अर्धकपाली; आधे सिर का दर्द; आधासीसी का दर्द

**Meibomian Glands.** Sebaceous glands lying in grooves on the inner surface of the eyelids, their ducts opening on the free margins of the lids. मीबोमी ग्रन्थियाँ; पलकों की वसा ग्रन्थियाँ

**Meibomianitis.** Inflammation of the Meibomian glands; meibomitis. मीबोमीग्रन्थिशोथ; पलकों की वसा-ग्रन्थियों का प्रदाह

**Meibomitis.** See **Meibomianitis.**

**Mel.** Honey; the substance deposited in the comb by honey-bee. मधु; शहद

**Mela.** A probe. सलाई; शलाका

**Melaena.** Black, tar-like stools. रुधिरकालामल; तारकोल जैसा काला पखाना

**Melancholia.** See **Melancholy.**

**Melancholic.** One affected with melancholia. विषादग्रस्त; खिन्न

**Melancholy.** A state of sadness; melancholia. विषाद; खिन्नता

**Melanic.** Relating to melanoma. मेलेनी; मेलेनिन-अर्बुद सम्बन्धी

**Melanin.** A dark pigment occurring naturally, though in varying amounts, in skin or in body parts, such as eyes, hair, etc. मेलेनिन; आँखों, बालों, आदि में प्रकट होने वाला एक काला वर्णक

**Melanism.** Unusually marked, diffused, melanin pigmentation of body hair. मेलेनिनता

**Melanocarcinoma.** See **Melanoma**.

**Melanocyte.** A dark-coloured wandering cell. मेलेनिनकोशिका; एक काले रंग की भ्रमण-कोशिका

**Melanoderma.** A black skin discolouration. कृष्णविसर्प; त्वक्मेलेनिनता; श्यामक्षत

**Melanodermic.** Relating to, or marked by melanoderma. कृष्णविसर्पीय

**Melanoglossia.** The presence of blackish patches on the tongue; black tongue. कृष्णजिह्वा

**Melanoma.** A malignant growth arising from pigmental tissue, usually a certain type of skin mole; melanocarcinoma. मेलेनोमा; मेलेनिन-अर्बुद

**Melanonychia.** Black pigmentation of the nails. श्यामनखता; नाखुनों का काला पड़ जाना

**Melanosarcoma.** A form of malignant melanoma. मेलेनिनसार्काबुद; दुर्दम मेलेनिन-अर्बुद

**Melanosis.** An abnormal deposit of black matter in the various parts of the body. मेलेनिनता; मेलेनिनमयता; श्यामक्षत; काले-काले घाव

**Melanuria.** Melanin in the urine. मेलेनिनमेह; पेशाब में मेलेनिन विद्यमान रहना

**Melia Azadirachta.** Azadirachta indica. नीम

**Melitis.** Inflammation of the cheeks. कपोलशोथ; गालों का प्रदाह

**Melituria.** Diabetes mellitus. मधुमेह; glycosuria. शर्करामेह

**Mellitus.** A derivative from Latin for honey; applied to sweet taste of urine in diabetes. मधु; शहद

**Diabetes M.,** see under **Diabetes**.

**Meloncus.** A tumour on the cheek. कपोलार्बुद; गाल पर उत्पन्न होने वाली कोई रसौली

**Member.** Limb. अंग; a functional part. कोई क्रियात्मक भाग या अंश

**Membra.** Plural of **Membrum**.

**Membrana**

**M. Basilaris,** see **Basilar Membrane.**

**Membrana.** A membrane. कला; झिल्ली;

**M. Flaccida,** the triangular portion of the tympanic membrane, called Shrapnell's membrane. श्लथ कला; श्रैपनेल कला; कान की झिल्ली का त्रिकोणक भाग;

**M. Granulosa,** the cellular layer lining a Graafian vesicle. कणिका कला;

**M. Sterni,** the membrane covering the sternum. उरोस्थि कला; छाती को ढक कर रखने वाली झिल्ली;

**M. Synovialis,** see **Synovial Membrane.**

**M. Tympani,** the thin semi-transparent membrane which covers the cavity of the drum of the ear; tympanic membrane. कर्णपटह; कर्णपट-गह्वर को ढक कर रखने वाली अर्ध-पारदर्शक झिल्ली

**Membrane.** A thin flexible substance investing many internal and some external parts of the body. कला; झिल्ली; पर्दा;

**Basement M.,** a thin layer that intervenes between epithelium and connective tissue. आधारक कला;

**Basilar M.,** the delicate membrane of the cochlea; membrana basilaris. आधार कला; आधारी कला;

**Cell M.,** the cell-wall. कोशिका-कला; कोशिका-प्राचीर;

**Cloacal M.,** the ventral wall of the cloaca of the embryo. अवस्कर कला;

**Drum M.,** see **Tympanic Membrane.**

**False M.,** diphtheritic membrane. अयथार्थ कला; रोहिणी-कला; कूट-कला;

**Mucous M.,** the lining or the cavities communicating with external air, as lining of the mouth, intestines, etc. श्लेष्म कला; श्लैष्मिक झिल्ली;

**Otolith M.,** membrane formed of otoliths and a mesh-work of fibrous tissue in the utricle and saccule. कर्णबालुका कला;

**Peridental M.,** see **Periodontal Membrane.**

**Periodontal M.,** a fibrous layer covering the cement of teeth; peridental membrane. परिदन्त कला; दन्त-मज्जा को ढक कर रखने वाला तन्तु-आवरण;

**Pupillar M.,** that which closes the foetal pupil. तारा कला; भ्रूण-पटल को बन्द रखने वाली झिल्ली;

**Serous M.**, a connective tissue-sheet lubricated with slippery serum. सीरमी कला;

**Shrapnell's M.**, see **Membrana Flaccida**.

**Synovial M.**, that lining articular ends of bones and inner surface of joint ligaments; membrana synovialis. श्लेषक कला;

**Thyrohyoid M.**, the membrane joining the thyroid cartilage and the hyoid bone. अवटुकण्ठिका कला; अवटु-उपास्थि एवं कण्ठास्थि को मिलाने वाली झिल्ली;

**Tympanic M.**, the membrane separating the external ear from the middle ear; drum membrane. कर्ण-कला; कर्णपटह; बाह्यकर्ण को मध्यकर्ण से अलग करने वाली झिल्ली;

**Virginal M.**, the hymen. योनिच्छद;

**Vitelline M.**, the true cell-membrane of the ovum. पीतक कला

**Membraniform.** Of the appearance of a membrane; membranoid. कलारूप; झिल्लीरूप

**Membranoid.** See **Membraniform**.

**Membranous.** Pertaining to, or consisting of membrane. कलामय; झिल्लीयुक्त; कला अथवा झिल्ली सम्बन्धी

**Membrum Muliebre.** The clitoris. भगशिश्निका

**Membrum Virile.** The penis. शिश्न; लिंग

**Menarche.** When the menstrual periods commence and other bodily changes occur. रजोदर्शन

**Menarcheal.** Relating to the menarche; menarchial. रजोदर्शन सम्बन्धी

**Menarchial.** See **Menarcheal**.

**Mendosus.** False. मिथ्या; अयथार्थ; कूट; incomplete. अपूर्ण

**Menidrosis.** Vicarious menstruation through sweet glands. स्वेदग्रन्थ्यार्तव; स्वेदग्रन्थियों से होने वाला ऋतुस्राव

**Menier's Disease.** Disturbed hearing and balance due to the disease of inner ear; hereditary vertigo; Meniere's syndrome. आनुवंशिक भ्रमि; मेनियर रोग

**Meniere's Syndrome.** See **Meniere's Disease**.

**Meningeal.** Pertaining to the meninges. तानिकीय; मस्तिष्कावरणीय; मस्तिष्कावरण सम्बन्धी

**Meninges.** The surrounding membranes of the brain and the spinal cord. तानिका; मस्तिष्कावरण; मस्तिष्कावरक झिल्लियां. Plural of **Meninx**.

**Meningioma.** A slowly growing fibrous tumour arising in the

## Meningiomata

meninges. तानिकार्बुद; मस्तिष्कावरणार्बुद; मस्तिष्कावरक झिल्ली की रसौली

**Meningiomata.** Plural of **Meningioma.**

**Meningis.** See **Meninx.**

**Meningism.** Hysteric pseudomeningitis; meningismus. वातोन्मादी कूटमस्तिष्कावरणशोथ

**Meningismus.** See **Meningism.**

**Meningitic.** Pertaining to the meningitis. तानिकाशोथज; मस्तिष्कावरणशोथज; मस्तिष्कावरणशोथ सम्बन्धी

**Meningitidis.** Plural of **Meningitis.**

**Meningitis.** Inflammation of the covering membrane of the brain and the spinal cord. मस्तिष्कावरणशोथ; तानिकाशोथ; मस्तिष्कावरक झिल्ली का प्रदाह;

**Basilar M.,** meningitis at the base of brain. आधारी तानिकाशोथ;

**Cerebral M.,** that affecting the membranes of the brain. प्रमस्तिष्क तानिकाशोथ; मस्तिष्ककलाशोथ; तानिकाकलाशोथ; मस्तिष्कावरक झिल्ली का प्रदाह;

**Cerebrospinal M.,** that affecting the membranes of the brain and cord; meningococcal meningitis. मस्तिष्कमेरुतानिकाशोथ;

**Meningococcal M.,** see **Cerebrospinal Meningitis.**

**Serous M.,** acute meningitis with secondary external hydrocephalus. सीरमी तानिकाशोथ;

**Spinal M.,** meningitis of the spinal cord. मेरुरज्जु तानिकाशोथ;

**Tubercular M.,** inflammation of the pia of the brain with effusion of lymph and pus; tuberculous meningitis. यक्ष्मज मस्तिष्कावरणशोथ;

**Tuberculous M.,** see **Tubercular Meningitis.**

**Meningocele.** A protrusion of meninges. मस्तिष्कावरण-हर्निया

**Meningocerebritis.** See **Meningoencephalitis.**

**Meningoencephalitis.** Inflammation of the brain and its membranes; meningocerebritis. तानिकामस्तिष्कशोथ; तानिकामस्तिष्क-प्रदाह; मस्तिष्क तथा उसकी झिल्लियों का प्रदाह

**Meningogastralgia.** Neuralgia of the stomach. उदरार्ति; उदरशूल; पेटदर्द

**Meningomyelitis.** Inflammation of the spinal cord and its membranes. तानिकामेरुरज्जुशोथ; मेरुरज्जु तथा उसकी झिल्लियों का प्रदाह

**Meningomyelocele.** See **Myelomeningocele.**

**Meninx.** Meningis; a membrane. कला; आवरण; झिल्ली; तानिका;

singular of **Meninges**.

**Meniscectomy.** The removal of a semilunar cartilage of the knee-joint, following injury and displacement. नवचन्द्रकोच्छेदन; जानु-सन्धि की अर्धचन्द्राकार उपास्थि को काट कर हटा देना

**Menisci.** Plural of **Meniscus**.

**Meniscus.** A semilunar cartilage, particularly in the knee-joint. नवचन्द्रक; जानु-सन्धि की अर्धचन्द्राकार उपास्थि

**Menopausal.** Associated with, or occasioned by menopause. रजोनिवृत्ति सम्बन्धी

**Menopause.** Cessation of the menstrual flow; change of life; climacterics; menopausia. रजोनिवृत्ति; वय:सन्धि

**Menopausia.** See **Menopause**.

**Menophania.** The very first menses. प्रथमार्तव; प्रथम रजोदर्शन

**Menorrhagia.** Excessive menstruation; excessive haemorrages; menostaxis. अत्यार्तव; अतिरज:; अतिरक्तस्राव; ऋतुस्राव के दौरान प्रचुर रक्तस्राव होना

**Menorrhalgia.** Dysmenorrhoea. कष्टार्तव; ऋतुस्राव के दौरान पेट में बहुत तेज दर्द होना

**Menorrhea.** The menstrual flow; menorrhoea. आर्तव; ऋतुस्राव; मासिक धर्म; रजोधर्म

**Menorrhoea.** See **Menorrhea**.

**Menostasis.** Suppression of menses; amenorrhoea. रजोरोध; ऋतुरोध

**Menostaxis.** See **Menorrhagia**.

**Menses.** The periodical or monthly flow of women; the courses; catamenia; menorrhea; menstruation. आर्तव; ऋतुस्राव; रजोधर्म; मासिक धर्म

**Menstrua.** Plural of **Menstruum**.

**Menstrual.** Pertaining to menses; menstruous. ऋतुस्रावी; आर्तव अथवा ऋतुस्राव सम्बन्धी;

    **M. Colic,** uterine colic due to menstruation. आर्तवशूल; ऋतुशूल;

    **M. Flux,** the menses. ऋतुस्राव; आर्तव

**Menstruation.** See **Menses**.

    **Vicarious M.,** bleeding from the nose, or other parts of the body when the menstruation is abnormally suppressed. उन्मार्गी ऋतुस्राव; अपथप्रवृत्तार्तव; अनुकल्प रज:; योनि के बदले किसी अन्य द्वार से ऋतुस्राव होना

**Menstruous.** See **Menstrual.**

**Menstruum.** A solvent. विलायक

**Mensuration.** The act of measuring. विस्तारकला; मापनकार्य; मापने की क्रिया

**Mentagra.** A herpetic eruption on the chin. चिबुक-विसर्प; ठोढ़ी का विसर्प (दाद)

**Mental.** Pertaining to the mind. मानसिक; relating to the chin; genial; genian. चिबुक अथवा ठोढ़ी सम्बन्धी;

**M. Deficiency,** lowered mental capacity. मानसिक दुर्बलता

**Mentalis.** The levator labii inferioris muscle. अधरउन्नमनिकापेशी

**Menti.** Plural of **Mentum.**

**Mephitic.** Poisonous; noxious. विषाक्त; विषैला; foul. दुर्गन्धित; बदबूदार

**Mentum.** The chin. अधोहनु; चिबुक; ठोढ़ी

**Meralgia.** Neuralgia of the thigh. ऊर्वार्ति; ऊरुपीड़ा; जांघ का दर्द

**Mercurial.** Pertaining to the mercury. पारदीय; पारे की; पारद सम्बन्धी

**Mercurialism.** Toxic effects of mercury on the body; hydrargyrum. पारदात्यय; पारदविषण्णता

**Mercury (Hg.).** A white, heavy liquid metal. पारद; पारा

**Meridrosis.** Local perspiration. स्थानिकस्वेदन; एकांगीस्वेदन; किसी स्थान-विशेष पर पसीना होना

**Merocele.** Femoral hernia. ऊरु-हर्निया; और्वी हर्निया; और्विक हर्निया

**Merozoite.** Any segment resulting from splitting up of the schizont in the asexual form of protozoa reproduction. खण्डजाणु; अंशाणु; मेरोजाइट

**Mesa.** The genitalia. जननेन्द्रियां; जननांग; प्रजननांग

**Mesaortitis.** Inflammation of the middle coat of the aorta. महाधमनीमध्यास्तरशोथ; महाधमनी के मध्य अस्तर का प्रदाह

**Mesarteritis.** Inflammation of the middle coat of an artery. धमनीमध्यास्तरशोथ; धमनी के मध्य अस्तर का प्रदाह

**Mesencephalic.** Pertaining to the mid-brain. मध्यमस्तिष्कीय; मध्यमस्तिष्क सम्बन्धी

**Mesencephalon.** The mid-brain. मध्य-मस्तिष्क

**Mesencephalotomy.** Surgical incision of the mid-brain. मध्यमस्तिष्कछेदन

**Mesenchyma.** The embryonic mesoderm; mesenchyme.

उपकलाहीनमध्यजनस्तर; भ्रूणमध्यजनस्तर

**Mesenchymal.** Relating to the mesenchyma. भ्रूणमध्यजनस्तर सम्बन्धी

**Mesenchyme.** See **Mesenchyma.**

**Mesenteric.** Pertaining to the mesentery or fibrous tissue supporting the bowels. आंत्रयोजनीय; मध्यांत्र सम्बन्धी;

   **M. Glands,** the lymphatic glands of the mesentery. आंत्रयोजनी ग्रन्थियाँ

**Mesenteritis.** Inflammation of mesentery. आंत्रयोजनीशोथ; मध्यांत्रशोथ; मध्यांत्र का प्रदाह

**Mesenterium.** See **Mesentery.**

**Mesentery.** A membrane in the cavity of the abdomen, which sustains and encompasses the intestines; mesenterium. आंत्रयोजनी; मध्यांत्र; आन्तों को बांधने वाली एक झिल्ली

**Mesh.** A net-work, e.g. of vessels or nerves. जालाक्षि

**Mesial.** Middle or median. अभिमध्य; मध्य; बीच में स्थित

**Mesion.** The conjugate median plane of the body; meson. मध्यतल; शरीर को बायें-दायें दो सममित भागों में बाँटने वाला अनुविक्षेप

**Mesmerism.** Animal magnetism. सम्मोहनविज्ञान; सम्मोहनविद्या

**Mesoblast.** The middle layer of the blastoderm; mesoderm. पूर्वमध्यजनस्तर; कोरक-चर्म का मध्य अस्तर; अन्तर्जन तथा बहिर्जन अस्तरों के बीच का भाग

**Mesocardia.** Plural of **Mesocardium.**

**Mesocardium.** The layers of splanchnic mesoderm which support the heart of the embryo. हृद्योजनी

**Mesocephal.** See **Mesocephalic.**

**Mesocephalic.** Mesocephal; partaining to mid-brain. मध्यमस्तिष्क सम्बन्धी; having a medium-sized head. मध्यम आकार के सिर वाला

**Mesocolic.** Pertaining to the mesocolon. बृहदांत्रयोजनी से सम्बन्धित

**Mesocolon.** The mesentery of the colon. बृहदांत्रयोजनी;

   **M. Sigmoideum,** pelvic mesocolon. श्रोणि-बृहदांत्रयोजनी

**Mesoderm.** See **Mesoblast.**

**Mesodont.** Having medium-sized teeth. मध्यदन्ती; मध्यम आकार के दान्तों वाला

**Mesoduodenum.** The mesentery of the primitive duodenum. आद्यग्रहणीयोजनी

# Mesogaster

**Mesogaster.** The same as **Mesogastrium**.

**Mesogastrium.** In embryo, the mesentery in relation to the dilated portion of the enteric canal, which is the future stomach. जठरयोजनी

**Mesometritis.** Inflammation of mesometrium. गर्भाशययोजनीशोथ; गर्भाशयपेशीअस्तरशोथ; गर्भाशयपेशीशोथ; पृथुस्नायुशोथ

**Mesometrium.** The broad ligament. गर्भाशयपेशीअस्तर; गर्भाशययोजनी; गर्भाशयपेशी; पृथुस्नायु

**Meson.** See **Mesion**

**Mesorchium.** The fold of peritoneum holding the foetal testes before their descent. वृषणयोजनी; भ्रूण के वृषणों को थाम कर रखने वाला उदरावरणीय अस्तर

**Mesorectum.** Peritoneal fold connecting rectum with sacrum. मलाशययोजनी; मलांत्र तथा त्रिकास्थि को जोड़ने वाला उदरावरणीय अस्तर

**Mesorrhine.** With a medium nasal index. मध्यनासा; मध्यम आकार के नाक वाला

**Mesosalpinx.** The upper part of the broad ligament. डिम्बवाहिनीयोजनी; पृथुस्नायु का ऊपरी भाग

**Mesosigmoid.** With a medium orbital index; the mesocolon of sigmoid colon. अवग्रहान्त्रयोजनी

**Mesosigmoiditis.** Inflammation of the sigmoid colon. अवग्रहान्त्रयोजनीशोथ

**Mesosigmoidopexy.** Surgical fixation of mesosigmoid. अवग्रहान्त्रयोजनीस्थिरीकरण

**Mesothelia.** Plural of **Mesothelium**.

**Mesothelial.** Relating to the mesothelium. मध्यकला सम्बन्धी

**Mesothelioma.** Any tumour developed from the mesothelium. मध्यकलार्बुद; मध्यकला से विकसित होने वाली कोई भी रसौली

**Mesothelium.** A special mesoderm lining the embryonic body cavity. मध्यकला; भ्रूणगह्वर को ढक कर रखने वाला एक विशेष प्रकार का मध्यजनस्तर

**Mesovaria.** Plural of **Mesovarium**.

**Mesovarium.** Paritoneal fold joining the ovary with the broad ligament. डिम्बग्रन्थियोजनी; डिम्बाशय को पृथुस्नायु के साथ जोड़ने वाला उदरावरणीय अस्तर

**Metabasis.** A change of any kind. परिवर्तन

**Metabolic.** Pertaining to metabolism. चयापचयी; चयापचय सम्बन्धी

**Metabolin.** Any substance produced during metabolism. चयापचयोत्पाद; मेटाबोलिन

**Metabolism.** The process of transferring food-stuff into tissue elements and energy for use in the body growth, repair and general function. चयापचय; उपापचय; शरीर की वह क्रिया जिससे भोजन ऊतक-तत्वों में परिणित होता है

**Metabolite.** A substance formed in metabolism. चयापचयज; चयापचयक

**Metacarpal.** Pertaining to metacarpus. करभिकास्थिक; करभिकास्थि सम्बन्धी

**Metacarpophalangeal.** Pertaining to the metacarpus and the phalanges. करभिका-अंगुल्यस्थिक; कलाई और उँगलियों की हड्डियों से सम्बधित

**Metacarpus.** The five bones which form the palm of hand between the wrist and fingers. करभ; करभिकायें; कलाई और उँगलियों के मध्य स्थित हड्डियाँ; करभिकास्थियां

**Metachromasia.** See **Metachromatism.**

**Metachromatic.** Relating to metachromatism. विविधरंजकता सम्बन्धी

**Metachromatism.** Any natural or artificial colour change; metachromasia. विविधरंजकता; रंगों में स्वाभाविक अथवा कृत्रिम परिवर्तन होना

**Metachysis.** The transfusion of blood. रक्ताधान; शरीर में रक्त डालना

**Metacyesis.** Extra-uterine gestation. परागर्भाशय-सगर्भता

**Metal.** A substance, as gold, silver, iron, etc. धातु, जैसे सोना, चांदी, लोहा, आदि

**Metallic.** Pertaining to a metal. धात्विक; धातव; धातु का

**Metalloid.** Resembling a metal. धात्वाभ; धातुवत्; उपधातु; धातु जैसा

**Metamere.** A primitive body-segment. विखण्ड; आदिकायांश; अनुखण्ड

**Metamorphism.** Transformation; structural change. कायान्तरण; रूपान्तरण

**Metamorphosia.** A visual defect with an apparent distortion of objects; metamorphosis. रूपान्तराभास; विरूपदृष्टिता; ऐसा दृष्टिदोष जिसमें प्रत्येक वस्तु टेढ़ी दिखाई देती है

**Metamorphosis.** See **Metamorphosia.**

**Metamyelocyte.** A myelocyte somewhat like a granular leukocyte in form. उत्तरकणिकाश्वेतकोशिका; मध्यमज्जाकोशिका

**Metanephroi.** Plural of **Metanephros.**

**Metanephron.** See **Metanephros.**

**Metanephros.** The posterior segment of the foetal renal organ; metanephron. पश्चवृक्कप्रसू; भ्रूण-वृक्कांग का पिछला खण्ड

**Metaphase.** That period in karyokinesis during which the chromatin loops split in two. मध्यावस्था; उत्तर-स्थिति; विभाजी-स्थिति

**Metaphyses.** Plural of **Metaphysis.**

**Metaphysis.** The growth zone between the metaphysis and diaphysis during development of a bone. अस्थिकाण्डकोटि

**Metaplasia.** Conversion of one tissue into another. इतरविकसन; इतरविकास; एक ऊतक का दूसरे ऊतक में बदलना

**Metaplastic.** Relating to metaplasia. इतरविकास सम्बन्धी

**Metastases.** Plural of **Metastasis.**

**Metastasis.** Removal or transfer of disease from one part of the body to another. स्थलान्तरण; स्थलान्तर; विक्षेप; विक्षेपण; रोग का किसी एक अंग से दूसरे अंग में स्थानान्तरण होना

**Metastatic.** Pertaining to metastasis. विक्षेपी; स्थलान्तरणीय

**Metasyphilis.** Congenital syphyilis, having no local signs or lesions. सहज उपदंश; जन्मजात उपदंश

**Metatarsal.** Relating to the metatarsus, or to one of the metatarsal bones. प्रपदिकीय

**Metatarsalgia.** Pain in the metatarsus. प्रपदिकार्ति; पैर के तलुवे की हड्डियों में दर्द

**Metatarsectomy.** Excision of the metatarsal. प्रपदिका-उच्छेदन

**Metatarsi.** Plural of **Metatarsus.**

**Metatarsophalangeal.** Pertaining both to the metatarsus and the phalanges. प्रपद-अंगुल्यस्थिक; पैर के तलुवे की हड्डियों तथा उँगली की हड्डियों से सम्बन्धित

**Metatarsus.** The distal portion of the foot between the ankle and the toes including five metatarsal bones. प्रपदिका; पैर की हड्डियां, जो उँगलियों और टखने के मध्य स्थित रहती हैं व जिसमें पैर के तलुवे की पांच हड्डियां भी सम्मिलित हैं

**Metathalamus.** The posterior part of the thalamus. पश्चचेतक

**Metathesis.** Transposition, especially of a disease process. व्यत्यास; a changing of places. स्थलान्तरण

**Metencephal.** See **Metencephalon.**

**Metencephalon.** The after-brain or the caudal portion of the brain; metencephal. अनुमध्यमस्तिष्क; मस्तिष्क का पुच्छल भाग

**Meteorism.** Gas in the abdominal cavity; meteorismus. आध्मान; अफारा

**Meteorismus.** See **Meteorism.**

**Meter(m).** A measure of length. मीटर

**Method.** The mode or manner, or orderly sequence of events of a process or procedure. पद्धति; रीति; तरीका

**Metopic.** Relating to the forehead or interior portion of the cranium. ललाटीय

**Metopion.** The midddle point of a line joining the frontal protuberances. ललाटबिन्दु

**Metra.** The uterus or womb. गर्भाशय; जरायु; बच्चेदानी

**Metralgia.** Pain in the womb; hysteralgia. गर्भाशयार्ति; जरायुशूल

**Metrectopia.** Displacement of the womb. जरायुभ्रंश; गर्भाशयच्युति

**Metritis.** Inflammation of the womb or uterus. गर्भाशयशोथ; जरायुशोथ; जरायु-प्रदाह

**Metrocarcinoma.** Cancer of the uterus. जरायुकैंसर; गर्भाशयकर्कटता

**Metrocele.** Henia of the uterus. जरायुस्त्रंस; गर्भाशय का हर्निया

**Metrocolpocele.** Protrusion of the womb into the vagina. अन्तर्योनिगर्भाशयस्त्रंस; गर्भाशय का योनि के अन्दर तक फैल जाना

**Metrocyte.** Mother cell. मातृकोशिका

**Metrodynia.** Pain in the uterus. जरायुशूल; जरायुपीड़ा; गर्भाशयवेदना

**Metrofibroma.** A uterine fibroma. जरायुतन्त्वर्बुद; गर्भाशयतन्त्वर्बुद

**Metromania.** Nymphomania. कामोन्माद (स्त्रियों में)

**Metropathia.** Any uterine disease; metropathy. जरायुविकृति; गर्भाशयविकृति; बच्चेदानी की कोई बीमारी;

  **M. Haemorrhagica,** with constant bleeding. रक्तस्रावी गर्भाशयविकृति

**Metropathy.** See **Metropathia.**

**Metroperitonitis.** Inflammation of the peritoneum of the womb. गर्भाशयावरणशोथ; जरायुकलाशोथ

**Metrophlebitis.** Inflammation of the uterine veins. गर्भाशयशिराशोथ; जरायुशिराशोथ

**Metroplasty.** Any plastic operation on the uterus; uteroplasty. गर्भाशयसंधान; जरायुसंधान

**Metroptosis.** Uterine displacement. जरायुभ्रंश; गर्भाशयच्युति

**Metrorrhagia.** Discharge of excessive black blood from the womb. रक्तप्रदर; अतिकालार्तव

**Metrorrhexis.** Rupture of the womb. गर्भाशयविदर

**Metrorrhea.** Any morbid uterine discharge; metrorrhoea. अत्यार्तव; अत्यधिक रज:स्राव होना

**Metrorrhoea.** See **Metrorrhea**.

**Metrosalpingitis.** Inflammation of the uterus and one or both Fallopian tubes. जरायुडिम्बवाहिनीशोथ; गर्भाशयडिम्बवाहिनीशोथ

**Metrosalpingography.** Radiography of the uterus and oviducts. जरायुडिम्बवाहिनीचित्रण; गर्भाशयडिम्बवाहिनीचित्रण

**Metroscope.** An instrument for examining the womb. जरायुजांचदर्शी; गर्भाशयजांचदर्शीयंत्र

**Metroscopy.** The examination of the womb with the metroscope. गर्भाशयजांच; जरायुजांच; जरायुदर्शन

**Metrostaxis.** A bloody oozing from the uterus. सततार्तव; अतिचक्रिकार्तव; जरायु से निरन्तर रक्तस्राव होते रहना

**Metrostenosis.** A narrowing of the uterine cavity. जरायुसंकीर्णन; गर्भाशयसंकीर्णन

**Metrotomia.** See **Metrotomy**.

**Metrotomy.** Hysterectomy; metrotomia; excision of the uterus. जरायु-उच्छेदन; गर्भाशय-उच्छेदन

**M.H.D.** Minimum haemolytic dose. न्यूनतम रक्तसंलायी मात्रा

**Miasm.** Sigular of **Miasms**.

**Miasma.** The miasm. विषदोष

**Miasmata.** See **Miasms**.

**Miasmatic.** Pertaining to miasms. विषदोषज; विषदोष सम्बन्धी

**Miasms.** Hahnemann's psora, sycosis, syphilis and poisonous influence from the atmosphere; miasmata. विषदोष, जिन्हें कच्छु, उपदंश एवं प्रमेह विषों के रूप में जाना जाता है

**Mica.** A mineral, called **Abhrak**. अभ्रक

**Micaceous.** Composed of crumbs, or mica. अभ्रकनिर्मित; अभ्रकमय; अभ्रकमिश्रित

**Micrencephaly.** See **Microcephaly**.

**Micro-.** Prefix meaning small. 'सूक्ष्म', 'अल्प' तथा 'लघु' के रूप में प्रयुक्त उपसर्ग

M.D.F.-21

**Microanatomy.** Microscopic anatomy. सूक्ष्मसंरचनाविज्ञान; histology. ऊतकविज्ञान

**Microangiopathy.** Thickening and reduplication of basement membrane in blood vessels. सूक्ष्मवाहिकाविकृति

**Microbe.** A micro-organism. सूक्ष्मजीव; जीवाणु

**Microbial.** Relating to a microbe or microbes; microbic. सूक्ष्मजीव अथवा सूक्ष्मजीवों सम्बन्धी

**Microbic.** See **Microbial**.

**Microbicidal.** Destructive of microbes; microbicide. सूक्ष्मजीवनाशी; जीवाणुनाशक

**Microbicide.** See **Microbicidal**.

**Microbiologic.** Relating to microbiology. सूक्ष्मजैविकी अथवा सूक्ष्मजीवविज्ञान सम्बन्धी

**Microbiologist.** One who specializes in microbiology. सूक्ष्मजीवविज्ञानी

**Microbiology.** The science of micro-organisms. सूक्ष्मजीवविज्ञान; सूक्ष्मजैविकी

**Microbiotic.** Having a short life. अल्पजीवी; अल्पायु

**Microblast.** A small red corpuscle. लघुलोहितकोशिकाप्रसू

**Microblepharia.** Condition of having abnormally small eyelids; microblepharism; microblepharon. लघुवर्त्मता; पलकें छोटी होना

**Microblepharism.** See **Microblepharia**.

**Microblepharon.** See **Microblepharia**.

**Microcephalic.** Having a small head. लघुशिरस्क; छोटे सिर वाला

**Microcephaly.** The state of having a small head; micrencephaly. लघुशिरस्कता

**Microcheilia.** Abnormal smallness of the lips; microchilia. लघुओष्ठता; होंठ छोटे रहना

**Microcheiria.** Abnormal smallness of the hands; microchiria. लघुहस्तता; हाथ छोटे रहना

**Microchilia.** See **Microcheilia**.

**Microchiria.** See **Microcheiria**.

**Micrococci.** Plural of **Micrococcus**.

**Micrococcus.** A genus of schizomycetes. सूक्ष्मगोलाणु

**Microcyte.** An undersized red blood cell found in the anemic blood. लोहितकोशिका

**Microcythaemia.** Abnormal smallness of the blood corpuscles; microcythemia. सूक्ष्मलोहितकोशिकारक्तता

**Microcythemia.** See **Microcythaemia.**

**Microcytic.** Pertaining to the microcytes. लघुलोहितकोशिकीय; लघुलोहितकोशिकाओं सम्बन्धी

**Microcytosis.** An increased number of microcytes in the circulating blood. लघुलोहितकोशिकाबहुलता

**Microdactyly.** Abnormal shortness of the fingers or toes. लघु-अंगुलिता; उँगलियां छोटी रहना

**Microdont.** Having small teeth. लघुदन्ती; सूक्ष्मदन्ती; छोटे दांतों वाला

**Microdontia.** Abnormal smallness of teeth. लघुदन्तता; दांत छोटे रहना

**Micrognathia.** Abnormal smallness of the jaw, especially of the lower one. लघु-अधोहनुता; निचले जबड़े की लघुता

**Microgonioscope.** An instrument for measuring minute angles. सूक्ष्मकोणदर्शी (यंत्र); छोटे-से-छोटे कोणों को मापने वाला यंत्र

**Micrography.** See **Microscopy.**

**Microgyria.** Smallness of the cerebral convolutions. लघुकर्णकता

**Microlith.** A minute calculus. सूक्ष्माश्मरी; छोटी-सी पथरी

**Microlithiasis.** Formation, presence, or discharge of minute concretions or gravels. सूक्ष्माश्मरीयता; छोटी-छोटी सी पथरियां बनना, विद्यमान रहना, अथवा उनका स्राव होना

**Micrology.** The science of microscopic objects. सूक्ष्मविज्ञान; अणुविज्ञान; सूक्ष्मविद्या; सूक्ष्मदर्शीविज्ञान

**Micromastia.** Abnormally small size of the breasts. लघुस्तनता; स्तन छोटे रहना

**Micrometer.** An instrument for microscopic measurement. सूक्ष्ममापी

**Micrometry.** The use of micrometer. सूक्ष्ममिति

**Micromyelia.** Abnormal smallness of the spinal cord. लघुमेरुरज्जुता; सुषुम्ना का असाधारण रूप से छोटा होना

**Micron.** A millionth part of a metre. माइक्रोन; एक मीटर का लाखवाँ भाग

**Micronychia.** Abnormal smallness of the nails. लघुनखता; नाखुन छोटे रहना

**Micro-organism.** A general term covering microscopic form, such as germs, viruses, etc. सूक्ष्माणु; सूक्ष्मजीव; सूक्ष्मांगी

**Micropenis.** An abnormally small penis; microphallus. लघुशिश्नता; शिश्न छोटा रहना

**Microphallus.** See **Micropenis.**

**Microphone.** An instrument for magnifying sounds. ध्वनिवर्धकयंत्र; माइक्रोफोन; ध्वनिविस्तारकयंत्र

**Microphotograph.** A microscopic photograph; a photomicrograph. सूक्ष्मदर्शीफोटोग्राफ; सूक्ष्मदर्शीचित्र

**Micropodia.** Abnormally small feet. लघुपादता; पैर छोटे रहना

**Micropsia.** A visual defect with apparent diminution of objects. लघुदृष्टिता; ह्स्वदृष्टिता; प्रत्येक वस्तु छोटी दिखाई देना

**Micropus.** Abnormal smallness of a leg. टांग का असाधारण रूप से छोटा रहना

**Micropyle.** An opening in the ovum for the entrance of the spermatozoon. वीजाण्डद्वार; अणुछिद्र; अणुद्वार; वह छिद्र जिसमें शुक्राणु प्रवेश करता है

**Microscope.** An instrument for examining small objects. सूक्ष्मदर्शीयंत्र; अणुवीक्षणयंत्र;

> **Binocular M.,** one with divergent oculars, one for each eye. द्विनेत्र-सूक्ष्मदर्शी (यंत्र)

**Microscopic.** Very small. अतिसूक्ष्म; minute. लघु; सूक्ष्म; pertaining to microscope. सूक्ष्मदर्शीयंत्र सम्बन्धी

**Microscopical.** The same as **Microscopic.**

**Microscopy.** The use of microscope; micrography. सूक्ष्मदर्शिकी; सूक्ष्मदर्शन

**Microsome.** With a small orbital index. लघुनेत्रगुहा

**Microsomia.** Dwarfishness; abnormal smallness of the body. वामनता; बौनापन

**Microstoma.** Abnormal smallness of mouth. लघुमुखद्वार; मुख का असाधारण रूप से छोटा होना

**Microsurgery.** Use of the binocular operating microscope during the performance of operations, usually oral. सूक्ष्मशल्यकर्म

**Microtia.** Abnormal smallness of the ears. लघुकर्णता; कानों का असाधारण रूप से छोटा होना

**Miction.** See **Micturition.**

**Microtome.** Instrument for making thin sections of tissues for microscopic examination. सूक्ष्मछिद्रक

**Micturition.** The act of voiding urine; miction; urination. मूत्रण; मूत्रोत्सर्जन

**Midbrain.** The mesencephalon. मध्यमस्तिष्क

**Midget.** Dwarf. वामन; बौना

**Midgut.** The embryonic bowel forming the jejunum and ileum. आद्यमध्यान्त्र

**Midriff.** The diaphragm; a muscular dome stretched across the body and separating the cavity of the abdomen from the cavity of the thorax or chest. व्यवधायकपेशी; मध्यच्छद

**Midwife.** A woman obstetrician. प्रसूति सहायिका; धातृ; धात्री; दाई; बच्चा जनाने वाली; सेविका

**Midwifery.** Obstetrics. प्रसूतिविज्ञान; प्रसूतिविद्या; प्रसूतितंत्र

**Migraine.** A severe type of headache, often one-sided and sometimes accompanied by visual disturbances. अर्धकपाली; आधासीसी का दर्द; आधे सिर का दर्द

**Migrating.** Everchanging; moving from place to place. परिभ्रमी; भ्रमणशील; स्थान बदलने वाला

**Mildew.** The common name for any one of a number of minute fungi destructive to living plants, food, etc. फफूंदी; कवक

**Miliaria.** A disorder of the sweat glands with obstruction of their ducts; miliary fever; sudamina. कंगुविस्फोट; धर्मरजिका; स्वेदराजिका;

   **M. Purpurea,** scarlet rash. आरक्त कंगुस्फोट

**Miliary.** Like millet-seeds, as a miliary eruption. कंगु; विकिरत;

   **M. Fever,** see **Miliaria.**

   **M. Gland,** the sebaceous gland of the skin. विकिरित ग्रन्थि;

   **M. Tuberculosis,** a form in which tuberculous nodules are widely dissiminated throughout the organs and tissues of the body. कंगु-यक्ष्मा

**Milieu.** Environment; surrounding. वातावरण

**Milk.** The secretion of the mammary glands. दुग्ध; दूध;

   **M. Abscess,** the abscess of the breast. स्तन-विद्रधि; स्तन का फोड़ा;

   **M. Crust,** the crusta lactea of children in one of the several varieties of eczema. दुग्ध निर्मोक;

   **M. Leg,** see **Phlegmasia Alba Dolens.**

   **M. Sugar,** lactose. दुग्ध-शर्करा

**Millar's Asthma.** A spasm of the glottis occurring in children during the first dentition. मिल्लर-दमा; बच्चों का श्वास रोग

**Mille.** One thousand. सहस्र; एक हजार

**Millepede.** An insect having many feet. बहुपादीकीट; असंख्य पैरों वाला कीड़ा

**Millesimal.** A thousandth part. सहस्रमलव; हजारवाँ भाग;
   **Fifty M.,** half of a thousandth part. शतार्धसहस्रमलव;

**Milligram (Mg).** One thousandth of a gram. मिलिग्राम

**Millimeter (Mm).** One thousandth of a meter. मिलिमीटर

**Milliliter (Ml).** One thousandth of a liter. मिलिलिटर

**Milphosis.** See **Madarosis.**

**Milt.** The spleen. प्लीहा; तिल्ली

**Mimetic.** Imitative; false. कूट; मिथ्या

**Mimic.** To imitate or simulate. नकल उतारना

**Mind.** The organ of consciousness. मन; चित्त

**Mineral.** A metallic substance found in nature. खनिज; खान से निकलने वाला पदार्थ

**Miner's Anaemia.** Cachexia. क्षीणता; दुर्बलता; कमजोरी; hookworm disease. स्फीतकृमि-रुग्णता

**Minim.** About a drop. लगभग एक बूंद; मिनिम; 1/60th part of a fluidram. एक ड्राम का साठवां भाग

**Minimal.** The least required. अल्पतम; न्यूनतम; अल्पिष्ठ

**Minimum.** The smallest amount. अल्पतम; न्यूनतम; अल्पिष्ठ;
   **M.Haemolytic Dose,** see **M.H.D.**

**Minor.** Small; lesser; minus. लघु; छोटा

**Minus.** See **Minor.**

**Miosis.** See **Myosis.**

**Miotic.** Pertaining to miosis; myotic. तारासंकोचक; तारासंकोची

**Misandria.** Fear of men. पुरुषभीति; नृभीति; मर्दों का डर

**Misanthropy.** Hatred of man and society. मनुष्य और समाज से घृणा

**Miscarriage.** Abortion; premature labour. गर्भपात; गर्भस्राव

**Misce.** Mix; a direction placed on prescriptions. मिश्रण करो; मिलाओ

**Miserable.** Worse. बदतर; बहुत खराब

**Misfit.** Unfit. अयुक्त; अयोग्य

**Misinterpretation.** Wrong interpretation. दुर्निरूपण

**Misogamy.** Aversion to marriage. विवाह से अरुचि

**Misogany.** Aversion to, or hatred of women. स्त्रियों से अरुचि या घृणा

**Misopedia.** Aversion to, or hatred of children; misopedy. बच्चों से अरुचि या घृणा

**Misopedy.** See **Misopedia.**

**Mist.** Filmy appearance before the eyes. धूमिका; धूमिलता; धुंध; mixture. मिश्रण

**Mistura.** A mixture; abbreviation : **Mist.** मिश्रण; मिक्सचर

**Mitchell's Disease.** Erythromelalgia; acromelalgia; red neuralgia. रक्तिमशःखार्ति

**Mite.** A minute parasitic insect. सूक्ष्मपरजीवी; सूक्ष्मकीट; किलनी; किल्ली; the louse. यूका; जूं

**Miticide.** An agent which destroys mites or lice. सूक्ष्मकीटनाशी; यूकानाशी; जूंमार

**Mitigate.** Palliate. शमन करना

**Mitoses.** Plural of **Mitosis.**

**Mitosis.** A complicated method of cell division occurring in specialized cells. सूत्रीविभाजन; विषमकोशिकाविभाजन

**Mitotic.** Relating to mitosis. सूत्रीविभाजक; सूत्रीविभाजन सम्बन्धी; marked by mitoses. सूत्रीविभाजनीय

**Mitral.** Denoting a structure resembling the shape of a headband. द्विकपर्दी;

   **M. Murmur,** murmur produced at the mitral valve. द्विकपर्दी मर्मर;

   **M. Orifice,** left atrioventricular aperture. द्विकपर्दी मुख;

   **M. Regurgitation,** backflow of blood from the left ventricle into the left atrium. द्विकपर्दी प्रत्यावहन;

   **M. Stenosis,** narrowing orifice of the mitral valve. द्विकपर्दी संकीर्णता;

   **M. Valves,** the two triangular valves of the systematic heart, situated between the left ventricle and auricle. द्विकपर्दी कपाट; बायें निलय और अलिन्द के मध्य स्थित दो त्रिकोणक कपाट

**Mixture.** A mutual corporation, preparation, or combination of several substances. मिश्रण; मिक्सचर

**M.L.D.** Minimum lethal dose. अल्पतम घातक मात्रा

**M.M.R.** Mass miniature radiography. सामूहिक लघु एक्स-रे चित्रण

**Mnemonics.** Memory-culture; the art of improving memory. स्मृति-सहायकविज्ञान

**M.O.** Medical Officer. चिकित्सा अधिकारी

**Moan.** To utter a sound expressive of suffering. कराहना

**Moaning.** Lamenting. कराह

**Mobile.** Movable. चल; गतिशील

**Mobility.** The quality of being easily moved. चलता; गतिशीलता

**Modality.** The condition of being better or worse, including various forms of sensations. रूपात्मकता; बहुलता; वृत्ति

**Mode.** Way; manner; custom; style. प्रणाली; तरीका; पद्धति

**Modification.** The act of modifying. रूपान्तरण; रूपान्तर

**Modioli.** Plural of **Modiolus**.

**Modiolus.** The axis of the cochlea of the ear. कर्णावर्तमध्याक्ष

**Modo-dicto.** As directed. निर्देशानुसार

**Modus.** A method or a mode. तरीका; पद्धति; प्रणाली;

    **M. Operandi,** the method of performing an act. कार्य-पद्धति; कार्य-प्रणाली; काम करने का तरीका

**Mogilalia.** Stammering speech. तुतलाना; हकलाना

**Moist.** Slightly wet; damp. आर्द्र; नम

**Moisture.** A moderate degree of wetness. आर्द्रता; नमी

**Mol.** See **Mole**.

**Molar.** A double tooth which bruises or grinds. चर्वणक; चबाने वाला;

    **M. Teeth.,** the six teeth in each jaw in permanent set which grind or bruise the solids put into the mouth. चर्वणक दन्त; चर्वण दन्त; ठोस पदार्थों को चबाने वाले दान्त

**Molasses.** The thick syrup drained from sugar in the process of refining. शीरा

**Mold.** Fungus which produces spores. कवकच्छद; फफूंदी; mould; a cast; shape. सांचा; ढांचा

**Mole.** A brownish spot on the skin; mol. तिल; न्यच्छ;

    **Carneous M.,** see **Fleshy Mole**.

    **Fleshy M.,** a blood-mole which has assumed a fleshy appearance; carneous mole. मांस-तिल

**Molecular.** Pertaining to molecules. आणविक; अणु सम्बन्धी;

    **M. Weight,** weight of a molecule attained by totalling the atomic weight of its contituent atoms. आणविक भार

**Molecule.** The smallest quantity of a substance. अणु; किसी पदार्थ की सूक्ष्मातिसूक्ष्म मात्रा

**Molimen.** An effort; the laborious performance of a normal function. प्रयत्न; प्रयास; कोशिश

**Molimina.** Plural of **Molimen.**

**Mollities.** A softening. मृदुता; कोमलता;

   **M. Medula Spinalis,** softening of the spinal marrow. मेरुमज्जा-मृदुता; मेरुमज्जा की कोमलता;

   **M. Ossium,** softening of the bones, originating in the cells of nutrition. अस्थि-मृदुता; हड्डी की कोमलता

**Molluscuous.** Relating to, or resembling molluscum. कोमलार्बुद सम्बन्धी अथवा कोमलार्बुदाभ

**Molluscum.** A chronic skin disease with pulpy tumours. कोमलार्बुद; कोमल अर्बुदों से युक्त चमड़ी का एक चिरकारी रोग;

   **M. Contagiosum,** a skin disease with hard, round nodules containing semi-liquid material; molluscum epitheliale. सांसर्गिक कोमलार्बुद;

   **M. Epitheliale,** see **Molluscum Contagiosum.**

   **M. Fibrosum,** a cutaneous disease with the development of fibro-cellular masses; molluscum simplex. तान्तव कोमलार्बुद; तन्तुमय कोमलार्बुद;

   **M. Simplex,** see **Molluscum Fibrosum.**

**Momentum.** The quantity of the motion of the body obtained by multiplying its mass by its velocity. संवेग; गति प्रदान करने वाली शक्ति; बल; जोर

**Monad.** A primary cell or germ. कोई प्राथमिक कोशिका या जीवाणु

**Monarthritis.** Arthritis of a single joint. एकलसंधिशोथ; किसी अकेले जोड़ का प्रदाह

**Mongolism.** A severe form of mental, bodily and other organic deficiencies. मंगोलता

**Monitor.** A device that provides a specific data for a given series of events, operations and circumstances. मॉनीटर

**Monitoring.** Sequential recording. मापक क्रिया; क्रमिक लेखन

**Monkshood.** Aconite. वत्सनाभ

**Monoblast.** An immature cell that develops into a monocyte. एककेन्द्रककोशिकाप्रसू

**Monocellular.** Having but one cell. एककोशिकीय

**Monochromatic.** Having but one colour. एकवर्णी

**Monochromatism.** The state of having or exhibiting only one colour. एकवर्णकता

**Monocular.** Having but one eye. एकाक्षिक; एकनेत्री

**Monoculus.** The name of a bandage adapted to cover only one of the eyes. नेत्रपट्टिका; मोनोकुलस; एक प्रकार की पट्टी जिससे एक आँख ही बन्द की जाती है

**Monocyte.** A mononuclear cell. एककेन्द्रकश्वेतकोशिका

**Monocytopenia.** Diminution in the number of monocytes in the circulating blood. एककेन्द्रकश्वेतकोशिकाल्पता

**Monocytosis.** Abnormal increase in the number of monocytes in the circulating blood. एककेन्द्रकश्वेतकोशिकाबहुलता

**Monogenesis.** Asexual reproduction. एकोद्भववाद; अलिंगीजनन; एकलिंगीजनन

**Monolocular.** Having one cell. एककोशिकीय

**Monomania.** Mental aberration on one point. एकोन्माद; एकलोन्माद

**Mononeuritis.** Inflammation of a side nerve. एकलतंत्रिकाशोथ; किसी अकेली नाड़ी का प्रदाह

**Mononuclear.** With a single nucleus. एककेन्द्रक; एककेन्द्री

**Mononucleosis.** An infectious disease of young adults and adolescents, sometimes called **kissing disease.** एककेन्द्रक-श्वेतकोशिकता; चुम्बनरुग्णता

**Monophobia.** A morbid fear of being left alone. एकान्तभीति; एकाकीपन का भय

**Monophyletic.** Originating from a single source. एकस्त्रोतोद्भव

**Monoplegia.** Paralysis of only one limb. एकांगघात; केवल एक अंग का पक्षाघात होना

**Monopodia.** The condition of having only one foot, usually due to the fusion of both feet. एकपादी

**Monopus.** Having only one foot by birth. सहजएकपादी; आजन्म एकपादी; जन्म से ही एक पैर वाला

**Monosaccharide.** A simple sugar that cannot be decomposed by hydrolysis. मोनोसैकेराइड; एक प्रकार की सामान्य चीनी

**Monovular.** Uniovular; the condition of having one ovum. एकडिम्बी

**Monoxide.** Any oxide having only one atom of oxygen. मोनॉक्साइड; ऑक्सीजन का मात्र एक अणुयुक्त ऑक्साइड

**Mons.** An anatomical eminence or single elevation above the level of the surface. जघन

**Mons Pubis.** See **Mons Veneris.**

**Mons Veneris.** The eminence formed by the pad of fat which lies over the pubic bone in the female; mons pubis. जघन-शैल

**Monster.** A teratism; a foetus being with abnormal development or superfluity or deficiency of parts or some vice of conformation. राक्षस; दैत्य; विरूप भ्रूण

**Monstrosity.** The condition of being a monster. राक्षसीवृत्ति; अतिविरूपता

**Montes.** Plural of **Mons.**

**Monthly Course.** Catamenia; menses. आर्तव; ऋतुस्राव; रज:; मासिकधर्म; रजोधर्म

**Monticuli.** Plural of **Monticulus.**

**Monticulus.** A protuberance; any slight rounded projection above a surface. प्रोद्वर्ध

**Mood.** The emotional state of an individnal. भावदशा; मूड

**Morbid.** Diseased; sickly; unsound; a term applied to unnatural conditions and appearances. विकृत; अस्वस्थ; रुग्ण; रोगी; बीमार;

   **M. Anatomy,** the anatomy of the diseased organs. विकृत अंगरचना; रुग्ण अंगों की रचना

**Morbidity.** A diseased state. विकृति; अस्वस्थता; रुग्णता

**Morbific.** Causing disease; pathogenic. विकृतिजन्य; रोगजनक

**Morbilli.** Measles; rubeola; rubella. रोमान्तिका; खसरा

**Morbilliform.** Resembling measles. रोमान्तिकाभ; खसरा जैसा

**Morbus.** A disease or illness. विकृति; विकार; बीमारी; रोग; रुग्णता;

   **M. Anglicus,** rickets. अस्थि-विकृति; अस्थि-विकार; रिक्केट;

   **M. Caducus,** epilepsy; morbus major; morbus sacer. अपस्मार; मिर्गी;

   **M. Coeruleus,** blue disease; cyanosis. श्यावता; नील रोग;

   **M. Coxarius,** hip-joint disease. नितम्बसन्धि रोग; कूल्हे के जोड़ों की बीमारी;

   **M. Cucullaris,** pertussis; whooping cough. कूकर कास; काली खाँसी;

   **M. Haemorrhagica Neonatorum,** a haemorrhagic affection of the newborn; morbus maculosus neonatorum. नवजात शिशु को होने वाला रक्तस्रावी रोग;

**M. Maculosus Hemorrhagicus,** purpura haemorrhagica. रक्तचित्तिता;

**M. Maculosus Neonatorum,** see **Morbus Haemorrhagica Neonatorum.**

**M. Major,** see **Morbus Caducus.**

**M. Sacer,** see **Morbus Caducus.**

**M. Virgineus,** chlorosis. हरित्पाण्डु रोग;

**M. Vulpis,** alopecia. खल्वाटता; गंजापन;

**M. Regius,** jaundice. कामला; पीलिया;

**M. Saltatorius,** chorea. लास्य; नर्तन रोग; नाचने की बीमारी;

**M. Tuberculosis Pedis,** madura foot. मदुरापाद; कवक-गुल्म

**Morcellation.** An act of dividing; the removal of a tumour or foetus by fragments; morcellement. खण्डांश; निष्कासन; विभाजन क्रिया

**Morcellement.** See **Morcellation.**

**Mordant.** A substance used to fix a stain. रंगबंधक; रंगस्थापक

**Morgue.** Mortuary; a dead-house; a place for holding dead bodies for identification and burial. शवकक्ष; शवगृह; मुरदाघर

**Moria.** Simple dementia. मनोभ्रंश; foolishness. मूर्खता; बेवकूफ़ी; dullness of comprehension. ज्ञानशून्यता; नासमझी

**Moribund.** Dying; at the point of death. मरणासन्न; मृयमाण; मृत्प्राय

**Morning Sickness.** Nausea and vomiting occurring every morning on rising and constituting one of the characteristic symptoms of pregnancy. प्रातःवमन; सगर्भोत्क्लेश; सगर्भकालीन मितली और वमन

**Moron.** A stupid person. जड़मति; क्षीणबुद्धि; बेवकूफ

**Moronity.** Stupidity; mental retardation. क्षीणबुद्धिता; जड़ता; बेवकूफ़ी

**Morphea.** A cutaneous lesion characterized by widespread sclerosis of the skin. त्वक्काठिन्य; चमड़ी की दूर-दूर तक होने वाली कठोरता

**Morphia.** A pain-dulling drug derived from opium; morphin; morphine. मॉर्फिया; अफीम का सत

**Morphin.** See **Morphia.**

**Morphine.** See **Morphia.**

**Morphinism.** Addiction to morphine. मॉर्फियात्यय; अत्यधिक मॉर्फिया लेने की आदत

# Morphogenesis

**Morphogenesis.** The genesis of form and the structure of various organs and parts of the body. अंगजनन; अंगोद्भव; संरचना विकास

**Morphologic (al).** Relating to morphology. आकृतिक; आकारिकी सम्बन्धी

**Morphology.** The science which deals with the form and structure of living things. आकारिकी; आकृतिविज्ञान; आकारविज्ञान; रूपविज्ञान

**Mors.** Death; mortis. मृत्यु; मौत

**Morsus.** A bite. दंश; डंक

**Mortal.** Liable to death. नश्वर; मृत्यु को प्राप्त होने वाला; नष्ट होने वाला

**Mortality.** Death. मृत्यु; मर्त्यता;

  **M. Rate,** the death-rate; proportion of deaths in a place. मृत्यु-दर

**Mortar.** A laboratory vessel used for pulverizing. खरल; ओखली; ऊखल

**Mortification.** Death of a part of the body; gangrene. कोथ; शरीर के मांस का सड़ना अथवा गलना

**Mortis.** See **Mors.**

**Mortuary.** A morgue; a dead-house. शवकक्ष; शवगृह; मुरदाघर; relating to death or burial. मृत्यु अथवा दाहकर्म सम्बन्धी

**Morula.** The mulberry mass of the ovum at a certain stage of cell-segmentation. कलल; कोशिकापुंज; वीर्याणुपुंज; डिम्बविभाजन में प्रथम ठोस गोलाकार आकृति

**Morulation.** Formation of the morula. कलल अथवा कोशिकापुंज बनने सम्बन्धी

**Morvan's chorea.** Fibrillary contractions of the muscles of the calves and the posterior portion of the thigh; Morvan's disease. मोर्वन लास्य; मोर्वन रोग

**Morvan's disease.** See **Morvan's chorea.**

**Moschus.** Musk. कस्तूरी

**Mosquito.** A blood-sucking insect, including **Anopheles,** responsible for transmitting many diseases including malaria, filariasis, yellow fever, dengue, etc. मच्छर; मशक

**Moth.** Chloasma; pigmentation of the skin. चर्मवर्णकता

**Mother.** The female parent. माँ; माता; मातृ; original. मूल;

  **M. Cell,** a multiplying cell. मातृ-कोशिका;

  **M. Tincture,** the first diluted solution of a medicinal substance. मूलार्क; अर्क

**Mother's Mark.** Naevus. न्यच्छ; तिल

**Motile.** Capable of spontaneous motion or movement. चर; स्वत:; गतिशील रहने की योग्यता रखने वाला

**Motility.** The moving power. चरता; स्वत:गतिशीलता

**Motion.** Evacuation of bowels. मलोत्सर्ग; मलोत्सर्जन; movement. गति; चाल;

   **M. Sickness,** an illness caused due to motion in trains, automobiles, ships, planes, buses, etc. गतिरुग्णता; वाहनरुग्णता

**Motor.** Causing motion; a part or centre that induces movements, as nerves or muscles. प्रेरक; गतिजनक;

   **M. Nerve,** the nerve concerned with, causing, or pertaining to motion. प्रेरक तंत्रिका

**Mottle.** The arrangment of coloured spots. कर्बुर; चितकबरा

**Mottled.** Marked with spots of different colours. कर्बुरित; चित्तीदार; चितकबरा; बदरंग; विभिन्न रंगों के धब्बों से युक्त

**Mould.** Multicellular fungus. फफूंदी; कवकच्छद; a cast; shape सांचा; ढांचा

**Moulding.** The compression of the foetal head during its passage through the genital tract in labour. शिरोघटन; घटन; ढालन

**Moult.** A crust. निर्मोक; पपड़ी

**Moulting.** Crusting. निर्मोकन; निमोचन; पपड़ियाना

**Mountain.** A very high hill. मेरु; पर्वत; पहाड़;

   **M. Fever,** see **Mountain Sickness.**

   **M. Sickness,** tachycardia and dyspnoea due to low oxygen content of rarefied air at the high altitudes; mountain fever. मेरु-ज्वर; पहाड़ी बुखार

**Mouth.** The cavity which contains tongue and teeth. मुख; मुँह;

   **M.- stick,** a device for use by persons who have no functioning hands. मुख-दण्ड;

   **M.-wash,** a pleasant preparation useful for rinsing mouth, but of no medicinal value. मुखधावन; मुखधावक

**Movement.** A motion; an action. गति; चाल; संचलन; क्रिया; stool; defecation. मल; पाखाना;

   **Amoeboid M.,** that produced by the protrusion of processes of protoplasm. अमीबाभ गति;

   **Circus M.,** rapid circular movement. चक्रिल गति; तेज वृत्ताकार गति;

   **Foetal M.,** that of the foetus in utero. भ्रूण गति; गर्भाशय के अन्दर बच्चे की हरकत

**Muciferous.** Producing mucus; muciparous. श्लेष्मोत्पादक; आँव पैदा करने वाला

**Muciform.** Resembling mucus; mucoid. श्लेष्माभ

**Mucilage.** The solution of a gum in water. श्लेषक; चेप; लेस; गोंद

**Mucilaginous.** Like mucilage; ropy. लेसदार; चेपदार; चिपचिपा

**Mucin.** An albuminoid constituent of mucus. श्लेष्मरस; श्लेष्मा का अन्नसार जैसा घटक या उपादान

**Muciparous.** See **Muciferous**.

**Mucitis.** Inflammation of the mucous membrane. श्लेष्मकलाशोथ; श्लैष्मिक झिल्ली का प्रदाह

**Mucocele.** Mucous tumour or polypus. श्लेष्मार्बुद; enlarged lacrimal sac. श्लेष्मपुटिका; श्लेष्मपुटी; विवर्धित अश्रुनली

**Mucoenteritis.** Inflammation of the mucous coat of the intestines. श्लेष्मान्त्रशोथ; आन्तों की श्लैष्मिक झिल्ली का प्रदाह

**Mucoid.** Resembling mucus or mucous tissue. श्लेष्माभ; श्लेष्मऊतकाभ; श्लेष्मा या श्लैष्मिक ऊतक से मिलता-जुलता

**Mucolytics.** Drugs which soften mucus and so reduce viscosity of secretion from the respiratory tract. श्लेष्मसंलायी औषधियाँ; श्लेष्मा को नरम करने वाली दवाइयाँ

**Mucomembranous.** Relating to a mucous membrane. श्लैष्मिक झिल्ली सम्बन्धी

**Mucopurulent.** Of the nature of the mingled mucus and pus. श्लेष्मपूयाभ; कफ और पीब जैसा

**Mucopus.** Mucus with pus. श्लेष्मपूय; पीब के साथ श्लेष्मा

**Mucosa.** A mucous membrane. श्लेष्मकला; श्लैष्मिक झिल्ली

**Mucose.** See **Mucous**.

**Mucous.** Pertaining to, or resembling mucus; mucose. श्लैष्मिक; श्लेष्माभ;

   **M. Cyst,** cyst that secretes mucus. श्लेष्म-पुटी; श्लेष्मा छोड़ने वाली पुटी;

   **M. Membrane,** the lining or the cavities communicating with the external air, as lining of mouth, intestines, etc. श्लेष्मकला; श्लैष्मिक झिल्ली;

   **M. Tumour,** a myxoma. श्लेष्मार्बुद; श्लैष्मिक रसौली

**Mucoviscidosis.** A congenital hereditary disease with failure of development of normal mucous-secreting glands, sweat glands and pancreas. श्लेष्मश्यानरुग्णता; ग्रन्थियों के सामान्य बहाव को रोकने वाला एक जन्मजात तथा वंशगत रोग

**Mucus.** The viscid fluid secreted by mucous glands. श्लेष्मा; आँव

**Muliebria.** The female genital organs. स्त्रीजननांग

**Multi-.** Prefix signifying many. 'बहु' के रूप में प्रयुक्त उपसर्ग

**Multicapsular.** Having many capsules. बहुसम्पुटीय; अनेक सम्पुटों वाला

**Multicellular.** Composed of many cells. बहुकोशिकीय; अनेक कोशिकाओं से बना हुआ

**Multifetation.** A pregnancy with more than two foetus; multifoetation. बहुभ्रूणगर्भता; दो से अधिक भ्रूण वाला गर्भ

**Multifid.** Divided into many parts; multifide. बहुशाखी; अनेक भागों में विभक्त

**Multifide.** See **Multifid.**

**Multifoetation.** See **Multifetation.**

**Multiform.** Having many forms or shapes; polymorphic. बहुरूपी

**Multigravida.** A woman who has borne many children; multipara. बहुप्रजाता; बहुप्रसूता; बहुप्रसवा; कई बच्चों को जन्म देने वाली माता

**Multilobar.** Having several lobes; multilobate; multilobed. बहुखण्डीय; अनेक खण्डों वाला

**Multilobate.** See **Multilobar.**

**Multilobed.** See **Multilobar.**

**Multilobular.** Having many lobules. बहुखण्डकीय; अनेक खण्डकों वाला

**Multilocular.** Having many cells or compartments. बहुकोष्ठकी; बहुकोशिकी; अनेक कोशिकाओं अथवा खण्डों वाला

**Multinuclear.** Having many nuclei. बहुकेन्द्रकी; असंख्य केन्द्रों वाला

**Multipara.** See **Multigravida.**

**Multiparity.** Production of several children at a birth. बहुप्रसविता; एक बार में ही असंख्य बच्चों को जन्म देने की अवस्था

**Multiple.** Having many parts or relations. बहु; बहुत से; असंख्य;

**M. Sclerosis,** a nervous system disease of many symptoms, due to deterioration and hardening of brain and nerve tissues. बहुकाठिन्य; स्नायुप्रणाली का एक रोग, जिसमें मस्तिष्क तथा तंत्रिकाओं के ऊतक कठोर हो जाते हैं

**Mummification.** The dessication of a tissue so that it resembles a mummy in colour and texture. ममीकरण; ममीभवन; dry gangrene. शुष्क कोथ

**Mumps.** A virus infection of the parotid or salivary glands, sometimes affecting the sex glands, the female breasts and the pancreas; parotitis. कर्णपूर्वग्रन्थिशोथ; कर्णमूलग्रन्थिशोथ; कनफेड़; गलसुआ

**Mural.** Pertaining to the wall of a cavity, organ or vessel. भित्तिक; किसी गुहा, अंग या वाहिका-प्राचीर सम्बन्धी

**Murmur.** A gentle blowing auscultatory sound. मर्मर; सरसराहट; श्वास के साथ निकलने वाली एक ध्वनि;

    **Aortic M.,** a murmur produced at the aortic orifice. महाधमनी-मर्मर

    **Arterial M.,** the sound made by the arterial current. धमनी-मर्मर;

    **Cardiac M.,** any adventitious sound heard over the heart; heart murmur. हृद्-मर्मर

    **Continuous M.,** a murmur heard without interruption throughout systole and into diastole. सतत मर्मर;

    **Diastolic M.,** a cardiac murmur occurring during the diástole. अनुशिथिलन मर्मर;

    **Endocardial M.,** one produced within the heart-cavities. हृदयान्त मर्मर;

    **Exocardial M.,** one produced outside of the heart-cavities. हृद्-बाह्य मर्मर;

    **Friction M.,** a sound due to the rubbing of two inflamed surfaces upon each other. घर्षण मर्मर;

    **Functional M.,** one due to excited action of the heart or resulting from anaemia; innocent murmur; inorganic murmur. क्रियात्मक मर्मर;

    **Haemic M.,** a sound due to changes in the amount or quality of the blood and not to organic lesions. अरक्तक मर्मर; रक्ताल्प मर्मर;

    **Heart M.,** see **Cardiac Murmur.**

    **Indirect M.,** a sound due to blood flowing in a direction contrary to normal. अप्रत्यक्ष मर्मर;

    **Innocent M.,** see **Functional Murmur.**

    **Inorganic M.,** see **Functional Murmur.**

    **Mitral M.,** the sound produced at the mitral valve. द्विकपर्दी मर्मर;

    **Musical M.,** one with a musical quality. संगीत मर्मर;

    **Obstructive M.,** a murmur caused by narrowing of one of the valvular orifices. रोधज मर्मर;

**Presystolic M.**, a cardiac murmur occurring just before systole. प्रकुंचनपूर्व मर्मर;

**Pulmonary M.**, a murmur produced at the pulmonary orifice of the heart. फुप्फुस-मर्मर;

**Regurgitant M.**, one due to the blood flowing backward into the ventricle. प्रत्यावहन मर्मर;

**Systolic M.**, that occurring during the systole. प्रकुंचन मर्मर;

**Vesicular M.**, a fine, normal, inspiratory, auscultatory sound heard over the chest. कोष्ठकी मर्मर

**Musca Domestica.** The common house-fly. घरेलू मक्खी; गृहमक्षिका

**Muscae Volitantes.** Spots before eyes. दृष्टिचित्तिता; आँखों के आगे चित्तियाँ दिखाई देना

**Muscle.** Flesh; musculus; the fleshy part of the body which causes motion, or by which movements are accomplished. पेशी; मांस-पेशी; गतिप्रदायक शरीर का मांसल भाग;

**Abductor M.**, muscle that draws away from the midline; musculus abductor. अपावर्तक पेशी;

**Adductor M.**, muscle that draws toward the midline; musclus adductor. अपवर्तनी पेशी;

**Antagonistic M.**, one having an opposite function. विरोधी पेशी;

**Arytenoid M.**, one originating from the muscular process of the arytenoid cartilage of the larynx and narrows the vocal cord; musculus arytenoideus. अनुप्रस्थ पेशी;

**Biceps M.'s**, the muscles of the arms and the thigh. प्रगण्ड पेशियां;

**Brachial M.**, one originating from lower two-thirds of the anterior surface of the humerus and flexes forearms; musculus brachialis. प्रगण्डिका पेशी;

**Cardiac M.**, the muscle of the heart; myocardium muscle. हृत्पेशी; हृद्पेशी·

**Ciliary M.**, smooth muscle of the ciliary body, consisting of circular and radiating fibres, and changes shape of lens in process of accommodation; musculus ciliaris. रोमक पेशी; रोमिका पेशी;

**Coracobrachial M.**, that originating from coracoid process of the scapula and adducts and flexes the arms; musculus coracobrachialis. तुण्डप्रगण्डिका पेशी;

# Muscle

**Cremaster M.,** one that raises testicle. वृषण-उत्कर्षिका पेशी;

**Cruciate M.,** the muscle in which the bundles of muscle fibres cross in an x-shaped configuration. स्वस्तिक पेशी;

**Digastric M.,** muscle that lowers th jaw; musculus digastricus. द्विपिण्डिका पेशी;

**Extensor M.,** muscle that extends a part. प्रसारिणी पेशी;

**Flexor M.,** muscle that bends a part. आकुंचनी पेशी;

**Intrinsic M.,** a muscle that has both its origin and insertion within a structure. अन्तस्थ पेशी;

**Involuntary M.,** muscle not under conscious control. अनैच्छिक पेशी;

**Myocardiac M.,** see **Cardiac Muscle.**

**Striated M.,** muscle fibres that possess alternate light and dark bands or striation; striped muscle. रेखित पेशी;

**Striped M.,** see **Striated Muscle.**

**Unstriated M.,** muscle without markings; unstriped muscle. अरेखित पेशी;

**Unstriped M.,** see **Unstriated Muscle.**

**Voluntary M.,** muscle whose action is controlled by wish. ऐच्छिक पेशी

**Muscular.** Pertaining to the muscles. मांसल; पेशी सम्बन्धी;

**M. Asthenopia,** weak or painful vision due to strain of ocular muscles. पेशी अवसाद;

**M. Dystrophy,** a disease in which the muscle tissue gradually wastes away; myodystrophy. पेशी-अपविकास;

**M. Fibre,** the fleshy fibre that forms the body of the muscles. पेशी-तन्तु;

**M. Reflex,** a deep or tendon reflex. पेशी-प्रतिवर्त;

**M. System,** the muscles of the body taken together. पेशी-जाल; पेशी-तंत्र;

**M. Tumour,** a myoma. पेशी-अर्बुद; पेश्यर्बुद

**Muscularis.** The muscular coat of an organ. पेशिका; पेशीकला; पेशी-अस्तर;

**M. Mucosae,** the layer of non-striated muscular tissue in mucous membranes. श्लेष्मल पेशिका; श्लेष्मल पेशीकला

**Musculature.** A set of muscles. पेशीसमूह; पेशीविन्यास; पेशीसंस्थान

**Musculi.** Plural of **Musculus.**

**Musculi Pectinati.** Small muscular columns on the inner surface of the auricular appendix of the heart. कंकतिका पेशिकायें

**Musculocutaneous.** Pertaining to the muscle and the skin. पेशीत्वचीय; पेशीत्वग्परक; पेशी एवं त्वचा सम्बन्धी

**Musculomembranous.** Composed of muscle and membrane. पेशीकलामय; पेशी एवं कला द्वारा संरचित

**Musculoskeletal.** Referring the framework of the body including muscles and skeleton. पेशीकंकालीय

**Musculus.** A muscle. पेशी; मांस-पेशी;

   **M. Abductor,** see **Abductor Muscle.**

   **M. Adductor,** see **Adductor Muscle.**

   **M. Arytenoideus,** see **Arytenoid Muscle.**

   **M. Brachialis,** see **Brachial Muscle.**

   **M. Ciliaris,** see **Ciliary Muscle.**

   **M. Coracobrachialis,** see **Coracobrachial Muscle.**

   **M. Digastricus,** see **Digastric Muscle.**

**Mushroom.** The edible members of the fungus tribe are so called. छत्रक; खुम्भी

**Musiotherapy.** Treatment of mental diseases by means of music. संगीतोपचार

**Musk.** Moschus. कस्तूरी

**Mustard.** Crushed seeds of the mustard plant which can be used orally as an emetic, externally as a counterirritant. सर्षप; सरसों

**Mutable.** Subject to change; fickle. उत्परिवर्ती; अस्थिर; चंचल

**Mutagen.** Any agent that causes production of a mutation. उत्परिवर्तजन

**Mutagenesis.** Production of mutation. उत्परिवर्तजनन

**Mutagenic.** Having the power to cause mutations. उत्परिवर्तजनक

**Mutant.** A cell which is the result of a genetic change. उत्परिवर्ती; पैत्रिक लक्षणों से भिन्न

**Mutation.** A change in presentation of a foetus. उत्परिवर्तन; भ्रूणपरिवर्तन

**Mute.** Dumb; a person who has no faculty of speech. मूक; गूंगा;

   **Deaf-m.,** unable to hear and speak. मूक-बधिर; गूंगा-बहरा

**Mutilation.** The loss of a member or portion of the body. छिन्नभिन्नता; व्यंगीकरण

**Mutism.** Dumbness. मूकता; गूंगापन

**Muttering.** Uttering with imperfect articulation. बड़बड़ाना; बड़बड़ाहट

**Myalgia.** Pain in the muscles; cramp; myodynia. पेश्यार्ति; पेशीशूल; पेशी का दर्द

**Myasthenia.** Muscular debility. पेशीदौर्बल्य; पेशीदुर्बलता;

   **M. Congenita,** muscular weakness by birth. सहज पेशीदुर्बलता; पेशियों की जन्मजात कमजोरी;

   **M. Gravis,** severe muscular weakness of a specific type. गभीर पेशीदुर्बलता

**Myatonia.** Absence of a muscular tone; myatony. पेशी-अतानता; पेशियों में तानता का अभाव;

   **M. Congenita,** that of infant. सहज पेशी-अतानता; पेशियों की आजन्म अतानिक अवस्था

**Myatony.** See **Myatonia.**

**Myatrophy.** See **Myoatrophy.**

**Mycete.** A fungus. कवक

**Mycetism.** See **Mycetismus.**

**Mycetismus.** Mushroom-poisoning; mycetism. छत्रकविषण्णता; छत्रकविषाक्तता

**Mycetoma.** See **Madura-foot.**

**Mycobacterium.** Small slender rod bacteria containing gram-positive rods. यक्ष्माणु; छोटे-छोटे लम्बे गोल दण्डाणु;

   **M. Leprae,** the causative agent of leprosy or leprous lesions; Hansen's bacillus. कुष्ठाणु;

   **M. Tuberculosis,** a species that causes tuberculosis; Koch's bacillus. यक्ष्माणु

**Mycocyte.** A mucous cell. कवकश्वेतकोशिका; श्लेष्मकोशिका

**Mycologist.** One versed in mycology. कवकविज्ञानी

**Mycology.** The science of fungi. कवकविज्ञान; कवक और उनसे उत्पन्न रोगों सम्बन्धी विज्ञान

**Mycosis.** The presence of parasitic fungi in the body, as well as the disease caused by them. कवकता; कवक द्वारा उत्पन्न रुग्णता

**Mydriasis.** Dilatation of the pupils. ताराविस्फार; आँखों की पुतलियाँ फैल जाना

**Mydriatic.** An agent causing mydriasis. ताराविस्फार; आँखों की पुतलियां फैलाने वाला कारक

**Myectomy.** Excision of a muscle. पेशी-उच्छेदन; पेशीकर्तन

**Myelalgia.** Pain in the spinal cord. मेरुमज्जाशूल; मेरुमज्जार्ति; सुषुम्ना का दर्द

**Myelencephalitis.** Inflammation of the medulla oblongata. मेरुरज्जुमस्तिष्कशोथ; मेरुरज्जुमस्तिष्क-प्रदाह

**Myelencephalon.** The medulla oblongata. पश्चकपाल-अन्तस्था; the cerebrospinal axis. मस्तिष्कमेरु-अक्ष; पुरोरज्जुमस्तिष्क

**Myelin.** The white fatty substance constituting the medullary sheath of a nerve. माइलिन; वह श्वेत पदार्थ जो स्नायु-मज्जा के आवरण का घटक होता है

**Myelinic.** Pertaining to myelin. माइलिनी; माइलिन सम्बन्धी

**Myelitis.** An acute inflammation of the whole or of any part of the substance of the spinal cord; spinal malacia. मेरुरज्जुशोथ; मज्जाशोथ; मेरुरज्जुमृदुता;

 **Ascending M.,** that in which the inflammation travels up the cord. आरोही मेरुरज्जुशोथ;

 **Descending M.,** that in which the inflammation travels downward. अवरोही मेरुरज्जुशोथ;

 **Disseminated M.,** one in which there are several foci. विकीर्ण मेरुरज्जुशोथ;

 **Transverse M.,** that extending across the cord. अनुप्रस्थ मेरुरज्जुशोथ

**Myeloblast.** Immature bone-marrow cell that develops into a myelocyte. मेरुरज्जुप्रसू

**Myeloblastoma.** Tumour containing myeloblasts. मेरुरज्जुप्रसू-अर्बुद

**Myeloblastosis.** Presence of many myeloblasts in the blood tissue, or both. मेरुरज्जुप्रसूरक्तता अथवा मेरुरज्जुप्रसू-ऊतिता, या दोनों अवस्थायें

**Myelocele.** A form of spina bifida with spinal cord protrusion. सुषुम्नाविस्फार; मेरुरज्जुतानिका-हर्निया

**Myelocyte.** The nucleus of a cell of gray matter. प्राक्कणिकाश्वेतकोशिका

**Myelofibrosis.** Formation of fibrous tissue within the bone-marrow and cavity; myeloid metaplasia. मज्जातन्तुमयता; अस्थिमज्जा एवं अस्थि-गह्वर के अन्दर तन्तु-ऊतक का निर्माण होना

**Myelogenesis.** Development of bone-marrow. अस्थिमज्जाजनन; मज्जाजनन

**Myelogenic.** Produced in or by bone-marrow; myelogenous. मज्जाजनक; अस्थिमज्जाजनक

**Myelogenous.** See **Myelogenic.**

**Myelography.** Skiagraphy of the spinal cord for diagnostic purposes. मेरुरज्जुचित्रण

**Myeloid.** Resembling marrow; medullary. मज्जाभ; मज्जावत्;

  **M. Metaplasia,** see **Myelofibrosis.**

**Myeloma.** A tumour of medullary substance. मज्जाबुर्द

**Myelomalacia.** A primary non-inflammatory and apparently idiopathic softening of the spinal cord. मेरुरज्जुमृदुता; सुषुम्ना की कोमलता

**Myelomatosis.** Plasma cells neoplasia which can manifest as myeloma, tumours in bones, a diffuse change throughout the marrow or as extramedullary lesion. मज्जाबुर्दता; दुर्दम मज्जाबुर्दता

**Myelomeningocele.** Spina bifida with portion of cord and membranes protruding; meningomyelocele. मेरुरज्जुतानिका-हर्निया; सुषुम्नापुटी

**Myelon.** The spinal cord. मेरुरज्जु; सुषुम्ना

**Myeloparalysis.** Paralysis of the spinal cord. मेरुरज्जुघात; सुषुम्नाघात

**Myelopathic.** Relating to myelopathy. सुषुम्नाविकृति अथवा मेरुरज्जु विकृति सम्बन्धी

**Myelopathy.** Any disease of the spinal cord. मेरुरज्जुविकृति; सुषुम्नाविकृति

**Myelophthisis.** Wasting or atrophy of the spinal cord. मज्जाक्षीणता; सुषुम्नाक्षीणता

**Myelosclerosis.** Sclerosis of the spinal cord. सुषुम्नाकाठिन्य; मज्जाकाठिन्य

**Myelosis.** The formation of a medullary tumour. मज्जामयता; मज्जाबुर्दता

**Myelotomy.** Incision of the spinal cord. मेरुमज्जाछेदन

**Myenteric.** Relating to the myenteron. आंत्रपेशी-अस्तर सम्बन्धी

**Myenteron.** The muscular coat of the intestine. आंत्रपेशीअस्तर; आंत्रपेश्यावरण

**Myitis.** Inflammation of a muscle. पेशीशोथ; पेशी-प्रदाह

**Myoatrophy.** Muscular atrophy; myatrophy. पेशीशोष

**Myocardia.** See **Myocardium.**

**Myocardiac.** See **Myocardial.**

**Myocardial.** Pertaining to muscular tissues of the heart;

**myocardiac.** हृद्पेशिज; हृद्पेशीय; हृदय के पेशी-ऊतकों से सम्बन्धित

**Myocarditis.** Inflammation of the muscular substance of the heart. हृद्पेशीशोथ; हृत्पेशीशोथ; हृद्पेशी का प्रदाह

**Myocardium.** The muscular mass of the heart; myocardia. हृद्पेशी; हृत्पेशी; हृदय का पेशीपिण्ड

**Myoclonus.** Clonic contractions of individual or goups of muscles. पेशी-अवमोटन

**Myocolpitis.** Inflammation of the uterine muscle. जरायुपेशीशोथ; गर्भाशयपेशीशोथ

**Myocyte.** A muscle cell. पेशीकोशिका

**Myodemia.** Fatty degeneration of muscle-tissue. वसीय पेशी व्यपजनन; वसापेशी-अपजनन; पेशी-ऊतक का वसापजनन

**Myodynia.** Pain in the muscle; myalgia. पेशीशूल; पेश्यार्ति; पेशीवेदना

**Myodystrophy.** Muscular dystrophy. पेशी-अपविकास; पेशीशोष

**Myofibroma.** A combined myoma and fibroma. पेशीतन्तुअर्बुद; पेशीतन्त्वर्बुद; एक मिश्र पेशी-अर्बुद एवं तन्तु-अर्बुद

**Myofibrosis.** Excessive connective tissue in a muscle. पेशीतन्तुमयता; किसी पेशी में संयोजी-ऊतक की अधिकता

**Myogenesis.** Formation of a muscle. पेशीजनन

**Myogenic.** Originating in muscle. पेशीजनक; पेशीजनित; relating to the origin of muscle cells or fibres. पेशी-कोशिकाओं अथवा पेशी-तन्तुओं सम्बन्धी

**Myogenous.** The same as **Myogenic.**

**Myogram.** A tracing of a muscle contraction on the myograph. पेशीलेख

**Myograph.** An instrument for taking tracings of muscular contractions. पेशीलेखी(यंत्र)

**Myographic.** Relating to a myogram, or the record of a myograph. पेशीलेख अथवा पेशीलेखन सम्बन्धी

**Myography.** A description of the muscles. पेशीलेखन

**Myoid.** Resembling muscle. पेशीवत्; पेशी जैसा

**Myokymia.** Continuous fibrillary contractions of the muscles of the extremities. पेशीतन्तुस्फुरण; हाथ-पांव की पेशियों की स्फुरणशील सिकुड़न

**Myolipoma.** A combined muscular and fatty tumour. पेशीवसार्बुद; मिश्र पेशी-अर्बुद तथा वसार्बुद

**Myology.** The science of the nature, function, structure, and diseases

**Myolysis**          **696**

of the muscles. पेशीप्रकरण; पेशीविज्ञान; पेशियों की प्रकृति, क्रिया, बनावट तथा रोगों का वैज्ञानिक अध्ययन

**Myolysis.** The disintegration of muscle-tissue. पेशीलयन; पेशी-अपघटन

**Myoma.** A tumour made up of the muscular element. पेश्यर्बुद; पेशी-तत्व से निर्मित कोई रसौली

**Myomalacia.** Morbid softening of a muscle. पेशीमृदुता; पेशी-विशेष की कोमलता

**Myomatous.** Of the nature of, or pertaining to a myoma. पेश्यर्बुदीय; पेशी-अर्बुदीय

**Myomectomy.** Removal of uterine myoma by abdominal section. पेश्यर्बुदोच्छेदन; गर्भाशयपेश्यर्बुदोच्छेदन; जरायुपेश्यर्बुदोच्छेदन

**Myometritis.** Inflammation of the uterine muscle. गर्भाशयपेशीशोथ; जरायुपेशीशोथ; जरायुपेशी का प्रदाह; गर्भाशयपेशी का प्रदाह

**Myometrium.** Muscular wall of the womb. गर्भाशयपेशीअस्तर; गर्भाशयपेशीप्राचीर; जरायुपेशीप्राचीर; जरायुपेशीअस्तर

**Myon.** A muscle; a muscular unit. पेशी

**Myonecrosis.** Necrosis of muscle. पेशीगलन

**Myoneural.** Pertaining to muscle and nerve. पेशी एवं स्नायु सम्बन्धी; पेशीतंत्रिकापरक

**Myoneuralgia.** Neuralgic pain in a muscle. पेशीतंत्रिकार्ति

**Myonosus.** Any disease of the muscles. पेशीविकृति; पेशियों का कोई रोग

**Myopalmus.** Muscular twitching. पेशीस्फुरण

**Myoparalysis.** Muscular paralysis. पेशीघात; पेशियों का पक्षाघात

**Myoparesis.** Slight paralysis of a muscle. आंशिकपेशीघात

**Myopathic.** Pertaining to myopathy. पेशीवैकृत; पेशीविकृतिक

**Myopathy.** Any disease of the muscles. पेशीविकृति; पेशियों का कोई रोग

**Myope.** A short-sighted person. निकटदृष्टि

**Myopia.** Near-sightedness. निकटदृष्टिता; दूर की चीज न दिखाई देने का रोग

**Myopic.** Affected with, or pertaining to myopia. निकटदृष्टिक; निकटदृष्टि सम्बन्धी

**Myoplastic.** Ralating to the plastic surgery of a muscle. पेशीसंधानकर्म सम्बन्धी

**Myoplasty.** Plastic operation on muscle. पेशीसंधानकर्म

**Myorrhexis.** The rupture of a muscle. पेशीविदर; किसी पेशी में फट कर दरार पड़ जाना

**Myosarcoma.** A malignant tumour derived from muscle. पेशीसार्कार्बुद; पेशीसार्कोमा; किसी पेशी की सांघातिक रसौली

**Myosclerosis.** Hardening of muscles. पेशीकाठिन्य

**Myosis.** A permanent contraction of the eye; miosis. तारासंकोच; अक्षिपेशीसंकोच; आँखों की स्थाई सिकुड़न

**Myositis.** Inflammation of the muscular tissues. पेशीशोथ; पेशी के ऊतकों का प्रदाह; पेशीविकृति;

   **M. Fibrosa,** a form accompanied by infiltration of fibrous tissue. तन्तुकर पेशीविकृति;

   **M. Ossificans,** a form associated with ossification of the connective tissue. अस्थिकर पेशीविकृति

**Myospasm.** Spasmodic muscular contraction. पेशी-उद्वेष्ट

**Myotalgia.** A painful cramp. पेश्यार्ति; पेशीशूल

**Myotic.** See **Miotic.**

**Myotome.** An instrument for cutting a muscle. पेशीछिद्रक; पेशीकर्तक

**Myotomy.** The dissection of muscles. पेशी-उच्छेदन; पेशीकर्तन

**Myotonia.** Tonic muscular spasm. पेशीतानता; पेशी की तानिक उद्वेष्टता;

   **M. Congenita,** a disease characterized by tonic spasms of voluntary muscles. सहज पेशीतानता; ऐच्छिक पेशियों की तानिक उद्वेष्टता के साथ होने वाला रोग

**Myringa.** The ear-drum or tympanic membrane; myrinx. कर्णपटह; कर्णकला; कर्णपटल; कान का पर्दा

**Myringectomy.** See **Myringodectomy.**

**Myringitis.** Inflammation of the membrana tympani. कर्णपटहशोथ; कर्णकलाशोथ; कान के पर्दे का प्रदाह

**Myringodectomy.** Excision of part or all of the membrana tympani; myringectomy. कर्णपटह-उच्छेदन; कान का पर्दा काट कर हटा देना

**Myringoplasty.** Plastic operation on the tympanic membrane. कर्णपटहसंधानकर्म

**Myringotome.** A delicate instrument for incising the tympanic membrane. कर्णपटहछिद्रक; कर्णपटहछेदक

**Myringotomy.** Incision of the tympanic membrane. कर्णपटहछेदन

**Myrinx.** See **Myringa.**

**Myristica.** A genus of trees; also the seeds of the nutmeg. जायफल

**Myrobalans.** The fruit of **Terminalia Bellerica,** used in diarrhoea. हरीतकी; हर

**Myxadenitis.** Inflammation of the mucous glands. श्लेष्मग्रन्थिशोथ; श्लैष्मिक ग्रन्थियों का प्रदाह

**Myxedema.** Clinical syndrome of hypothyroidism; myxoedema. श्लेष्मशोफ; अवटु-अल्पक्रियता का नैदानिक संलक्षण या चिन्ह; मिक्सिडीमा

**Myxoedema.** See **Myxedema.**

**Myxoid.** Like mucus. श्लेष्माभ; श्लेष्मवत्; श्लेष्मा जैसा

**Myxoma.** A connective tissue tumour composed largely of mucoid material. श्लेष्मार्बुद

**Myxopoiesis.** Mucus production. श्लेष्मोत्पादन

**Myxoviruses.** Name for the influenza group of viruses. श्लेष्मविषाणु

**Myster.** The nose. नासिका; नाक

# N

**Nacreous.** Lustrous, like mother of pearls. मुक्तास्फोटी; शुक्तिपुट; मोती जैसा चमकीला

**NAD.** No abnormality detected. निर्विकार; नीरोग

**Naevo-lipomata.** Naevus. न्यच्छ; तिल; fatty tumour. वसार्बुद

**Naevus.** A mole; nevus. न्यच्छ; तिल;

    **N. Meterni,** spots or marks of various kinds on children at birth; mother's mark; naevus maternus. मातृ-न्यच्छ; आजन्म न्यच्छ; जन्मजात तिल;

    **N. Maternus,** see **Naevus Meterni.**

    **N. Unius Lateralis,** a congenital naevus that occurs in streaks or linear bands on one side of the body. एकपार्श्वी न्यच्छ;

    **N. Venosus,** one chiefly of veins. शिरामय न्यच्छ; शिरा-न्यच्छ;

    **Capillary N.,** one involving the capillaries of the skin. केशिका-न्यच्छ;

    **Cutaneous N.,** a naevus of the skin. त्वक्-न्यच्छ; चर्म-न्यच्छ;

**Facial N.**, a naevus of the face. आनन-न्यच्छ; चेहरे का तिल

**Nail.** The horny lamina covering the back of the terminal phalanx of each finger or toe; unguis. नख; नाखुन; कील; नखर;

    **N.-bed**, the cavity for the lodgment of the nail. नख-शय्या;

    **N.-fold**, the redundant tissue around the base and edge of a nail. नख-वलि;

    **Ingrowing N.**, overlapping of the nail by the flesh, with ulceration. अन्तर्वर्धी नख;

**Naja.** A genus of venomous serpents, which includes cobras. नागविष; फणिधर सर्प; फनदार सांप

**Naked.** Unclothed. नग्न; नंगा;

    **N. Eye**, the eye unaided by a microscope. प्रत्यक्ष; बिना किसी सूक्ष्मदर्शीयंत्र की सहायता के

**Nanism.** Dwarfishness. वामनता; बौनापन

**Nano.** Dwarf. वामन; बौना

**Nanoid.** Dwarflike. वामनवत्; बौने जैसा

**Nanous.** Dwarfish; nanus. वामन; बौना

**Nanus.** See **Nanous**.

**Nape.** See **Nape of neck.**

**Nape of neck.** The back part of the neck. ग्रीवापृष्ठ; गुद्दी; मन्या; गर्दन का पिछला भाग

**Narcissism.** Self-love. स्वरूपकामुकता; आत्ममोह; आत्मरति; आत्मासक्ति; स्वयं में ही अधिक रुचि लेना

**Narcoanalysis.** Analysis of mental content under light anaesthesia, usually an intravenous barbiturate. तन्द्राविश्लेषण

**Narcolepsy.** An irresistible tendency to go to sleep; hypnolepsy. तन्द्रालुता; आवेशिक निद्रा; औंघाई

**Narcose.** In a condition of stupor. मूर्च्छित; बेहोश; गहरी नींद में सोया हुआ

**Narcosis.** Sleep or general anaesthesia produced by some narcotic drugs; narcotism. सुषुप्ति; स्वापकता; मादकता; मद; नशा; निद्रावहन; स्वापक-व्यसन

**Narcosynthesis.** The building up of a clearer mental picture of an incident involving the patient by reviving memories of it under light anaesthesia. तन्द्रा-मनःसंश्लेषण

**Narcotherapy.** Psychotherapy conducted with the patient under the influence of a sedative or narcotic. निद्रोपचार

**Narcotic.** An opiate; anything inducing sleep. स्वापक; मादक अथवा नशीला पदार्थ या नशीली औषधि

**Narcotin.** An active principle of opium; narcotine. अफीम का एक सक्रिय सारघटक; नारकोटिन

**Narcotine.** See **Narcotin.**

**Narcotism.** See **Narcosis.**

**Nares.** Plural of **Naris.**

**Naris.** The nostril; an aperture of the nose. नासापक्षक; नासारन्ध्र; नासागह्वर; नथुना

**Naristillae.** Nasal drop. नासाबिन्दु

**Nasal.** Pertaining to the nose. नासापरक; नाक सम्बन्धी;

   **N. Bones,** two small bones forming the arch of the nose. नासिकास्थियां; नासास्थियां; नाक की दो चापाकार हड्डियां;

   **N. Cartilage,** the cartilage of the nose. नासिका-उपास्थि; नासा-उपास्थि;

   **N. Cavity,** cavity between floor of the cranium and roof of mouth. नासा-गह्वर; नथुना;

   **N. Fossa,** the nasal passage. नासा-खात; नासिका-खात;

   **N. Septum,** the wall between the two nasal cavities. नासा-पट

**Nascent.** The newborn. नवजात; नवप्रसूत

**Nasi.** The nose. नासिका; नाक;

   **N. Ossa,** the two nasal bones. नासिकास्थियां; नासास्थियां; नाक की दो हड्डियां;

   **Alae N.,** the wings of the nose. नासा-पक्षक

**Nasiform.** Of the form of nose. नासिकाकार; नाक के आकार जैसा

**Nasion.** The point on the skull at which the nasofrontal suture is cut across by the median anteroposterior plane. नासामूलबिन्दु

**Nasitis.** Inflammation of the nose. नासाशोथ; नासिकाशोथ; नाक का प्रदाह

**Nasoantritis.** Inflammation of the nose and of the antrum of Highmore. नासाकोटरशोथ; नासिकाविवरों का प्रदाह; नासाविवरशोथ

**Nasology.** The science or study of the nose. नासिकाविज्ञान; नाक का वैज्ञानिक अध्ययन

**Nasopalatine.** Pertaining to the nose and the palate. नाक तथा तालु सम्बन्धी

**Nasopharyngeal.** Pertaining to the nose and the pharynx. नाक तथा ग्रसनी सम्बन्धी

**Nasopharyngitis.** Inflammation of the nose and the pharynx. नासाग्रसनीशोथ; नाक और ग्रसनी का प्रदाह

**Nasopharyngolaryngoscope.** A fiberoptic endoscope used to visualize the upper airways and the pharynx. नासाग्रसनीस्वरयंत्रदर्शी; नाक, ग्रसनी एवं स्वरयंत्र की जांच में प्रयुक्त होने वाला यंत्र

**Nasopharyngoscope.** An electrically lighted instrument for examining the throat, behind the nose. नासाग्रसनीदर्शी; नासाग्रसनीजांचयंत्र; नाक एवं ग्रसनी की जांच में प्रयुक्त होने वाला यंत्र

**Nasopharynx.** The portion of the pharynx above the soft palate. नासाग्रसनी; कोमल तालु के ऊपर स्थित ग्रसनी भाग

**Nasoscope.** Instrument for examination of the nasal cavity; rhinoscope. नासादर्शी (यंत्र)

**Nasoseptitis.** Inflammation of the nasal septum. नासापटशोथ; नासापट-प्रदाह

**Nasosinusitis.** Inflammation of the nasal accessory sinuses. नासाविवरशोथ; नासा-गह्वरों का प्रदाह

**Nasus.** The nose. नासिका; नाक

**Natal.** Relating to the nates. नितम्बों अथवा कूल्हों सम्बन्धी; pertaining to parturition. प्रसव सम्बन्धी; a native. अधिवासी; मूल-निवासी

**Natality.** The birth-rate. जन्मदर; जन्म-संख्या

**Natant.** Swimming; floating. तैरना

**Nates.** Buttocks; two projections of the body on which we sit. नितम्ब; चूतड़; कूल्हे

**Nature.** The essential or original character of a thing. स्वभाव; प्रकृति

**Naturopath.** A practitioner of healing cult which relies on so-called natural methods, i.e. diet, air, sun, water, etc. प्राकृतिक चिकित्सक

**Naturopathy.** Treatment by natural means, like heat, light, water, diet, etc. प्राकृतिक चिकित्सा; भौतिक उपायों द्वारा रोगोपचार करना

**Naupathia.** Sea-sickness. समुद्री रुग्णता; सामुद्रिक रुग्णता; नौवहन-रुग्णता

**Nausea.** A desire to vomit; sickness of stomach. मितली; मिचली; मतली; मचली; उत्क्लेश;

**N. Gravidarum,** morning sickness. सगर्भोत्क्लेश; सगर्भकालीन मिचली

**N. Navalis,** sea-sickness. समुद्री रुग्णता; सामुद्रिक रुग्णता; नौकायन रुग्णता; नौवहन-रुग्णता

**Nauseant.** A substance that produces nausea. उत्क्लेशक; मितली पैदा करने वाला

**Nauseated.** Affected with nausea. मितलीग्रस्त; मिचलीग्रस्त

**Nauseous.** Producing nausea; disgusting. उत्क्लेशी; वमनकारी

**Navel.** Umbilicus. नाभि; सुण्डी;

   **N.- string,** the umbilical cord. नाभिबन्ध; नाभिरज्जु; नाल; आवलनाल

**Navicular.** Boat-shaped. नौकाभ; नौकाकार; नाव जैसे आकार का;

   **N. Fossa,** the name of a small cavity within the fourchette. नौकाभ खात; नौकाकार गुहा; नौगह्वर

**Nearsight.** Myopic. निकटदृष्टि

**Nearsightedness.** Myopia. निकटदृष्टिता; दूर की चीजें न दिखाई देने का रोग

**Nearthrosis.** A false joint; neoarthrosis. अयथार्थ सन्धि; कूटसन्धि; कृत्रिम सन्धि; नकली जोड़; abnormal articulation. विषम सन्धि

**Nebula.** Slight haziness on the cornea. हल्की फुल्ली; अर्धस्वच्छता; नीहारिका; बदली; धुँधलापन; a cloudy suspension in the urine. धूमिल मूत्रता

**Nebulae.** Plural of **Nebula.**

**Nebuliser.** An atomiser; an apparatus for converting a liquid into a fine spray; nebulizer. कणित्र; तरल पदार्थ को सूक्ष्म कणों में बदलने वाला यंत्र

**Nebulizer.** See **Nebuliser.**

**Necator.** Ankylostoma, a genus of nematode hookworms. अंकुशमुखीकृमि; केंचुवा

**Neck.** The part of the body between the head and the trunk. ग्रीवा; गर्दन, सिर और धड़ को मिलाने वाला भाग;

   **Stiff-n.,** wry-neck; torticollis. मन्यास्तम्भ;

   **Wry-n.,** see **Stiff-neck.**

**Necrobiosis.** Molecular death of a part. जीवोतिगलन; किसी अंग की आणविक मृत्यु

**Necrobiotic.** Pertaining to, or characterized by necrobiosis. जीवोतिगलन सम्बन्धी; जीवोतिगलनीय

**Necrocytosis.** Death of the cells. कोशिकाक्षय; कोषाणुओं का क्षय; कोषों या कोशिकाओं की मृत्यु

**Necrogenic.** Relating to, living in, or having origin in dead matter; necrogenous. मृत्युजनक

**Necrogenous.** See **Necrogenic.**

**Necrology.** A treatise on death. मृत्युविज्ञान; मृत्युप्रकरण; मृत्यु सम्बन्धी अध्ययन

**Necrolysis.** Necrosis and dissolution of tissue. ऊतिलयन

**Necromania.** A morbid tendency to take interest in dead bodies or in death. मृत्योन्माद; शवोन्माद

**Necrophagous.** Living on dead bodies. मृतभक्षी; शवभक्षी; मरे हुए जीवों को खा कर जीवित रहने वाला

**Necrophilia.** Sexual intercourse with a dead body. शवमैथुन; मृतक के साथ सम्भोग करना

**Necrophobia.** Morbid fear of a dead body. शवभीति; शवातंक; शव या मृतक देखकर भयभीत होना

**Necropneumonia.** Gangrene of the lung. फुफ्फुसकोथ; फुफ्फुस-परिगलन

**Necropsy.** The examination of dead-body; necroscopy. शव-परीक्षा; मृत-शरीर की जांच करना; मरणोत्तर जांच

**Necroscopy.** See **Necropsy.**

**Necrosis.** Mortification of the body parts. परिगलन; अस्थिगलन; अस्थिक्षय; ऊतकक्षय;

   **Coagulative N.,** a form marked by formation of fibrin; fibrinous necrosis. आतंची परिगलन; फाइब्रिन-रचना के साथ होने वाला परिगलन;

   **Colliquative N.,** necrosis marked by the formation of a liquid; liquefactive necrosis. द्रवणशील परिगलन; द्रव्य रचना के साथ होने वाला परिगलन;

   **Fat N.,** necrosis of fatty tissue occurring in small white areas. वसा-परिगलन; लघु श्वेत क्षेत्रों में प्रकट होने वाला वसा-ऊतक का परिगलन;

   **Fibrinous N.,** see **Coagulative Necrosis.**

   **Liquefactive N.,** see **Colliquative Necrosis.**

   **Mercurial N.,** that due to chronic mercurial poisoning. पारदी परिगलन; पारद के अपव्यवहार के कारण होने वाला परिगलन;

   **Moist N.,** that in which the dead tissue is moist and soft. आर्द्र परिगलन, जिसमें मृत-ऊतक नम और कोमल होता है;

   **Superficial N.,** necrosis affecting the portion of bone just beneath the periosteum. उपरिस्थ परिगलन; अस्थ्यावरण के ठीक नीचे जब हड्डी प्रभावित हो कर गलने लगती है

**Necrospermia.** The discharge of semen containing non-motile spermatozoa. मृतशुक्राणुता; अचल शुक्राणुओं से युक्त वीर्यपात होना

**Necrotic.** Pertaining to necrosis. परिगलन अथवा अस्थिगलन सम्बन्धी

**Necrotomy.** The dissection of dead body or excision of dead bones or tissues. गलितास्थिछेदन; शव-व्यच्छेदन; विविक्तांशनिष्कासन

**Need.** Something required or wanted; a requisite. आवश्यकता; जरूरत

**Needle.** A slender, sharp-pointed instrument for stitching, ligaturing, suturing, puncturing or passing a ligature around an artery, or for injection or aspiration. सूची; सुई

**Needle-holder.** An instrument for grasping needle in suturing; needle-carrier; needle-driver; needle-forceps. सूचीघर

**Needling.** Puncturing with a needle. सूचीकरण; विपाटन

**Nagative.** The opposite of positive; not affirmative. ऋण; ऋणात्मक; अग्राही

**Negativism.** An active refusal to cooperate. नकारात्मकता; ऋणात्मकता; अग्राहिता

**Nemanthelminthes.** A species of worms including the round and the thread worms. गोल एवं सूत्र कृमि; चनूने

**Nematoblast.** A spermatoblast. वीर्याणुकोशिकाप्रसू; दंशककोशिकाप्रसू

**Nematocidal.** See **Nematocide**.

**Nematocide.** An agent that destroys nematodes. सूत्रकृमिनाशक; सूत्रकृमियों को नष्ट करने वाला पदार्थ

**Nematoda.** See **Nematodes**.

**Nematodes.** Thread-like creatures or worms that have two sexes and an intestinal canal; nematodas. सूत्रकृमि; धागे जैसे जीव अथवा कृमि, जिनके दो लिंग तथा एक आंत होती है

**Nematodiasis.** Infection with nematodes. सूत्रकृमिसंक्रमण

**Nematoid.** Resembling a thread. सूत्राभ; सूत्रवत्; धागे जैसा; a threadworm. सूत्रकृमि; धागे जैसा कृमि

**Neo-.** Prefix meaning new. 'नव' के रूप में प्रयुक्त उपसर्ग

**Neoarthrosis.** See **Nearthrosis**.

**Neocerebellum.** The large lateral portion of the cerebellar hemisphere. नवानुमस्तिष्क

**Neocortex.** See **Neopallium**.

**Neodiathermy.** A short-wave diathermy. लघुतरंगऊष्मापार्य;

लघु-विद्युत्धाराओं द्वारा शरीर की सिकाई करना

**Neologism.** A specially coined word, often Meaningless. नवशब्द; अनर्थक शब्द; व्यर्थशब्दरचना

**Neomembrane.** A false membrane. कूटकला; अयथार्थ झिल्ली

**Neonatal.** Pertaining to the newborn. नवजात (शिशु) सम्बन्धी

**Neonate.** A newborn baby upto one month old. नवजात (शिशु)

**Neonatology.** The scientific study of the newborn. नवजात (शिशु) विज्ञान; नवजात (शिशु) का वैज्ञानिक अध्ययन

**Neonatorum.** Pertaining to the newborn. नवजात (शिशु) सम्बन्धी

**Neopallium.** The cerebral hemisphere with the exception of the rhinencephalon; neocortex. नवप्रावारक

**Neoplasia.** The process of the formation of neoplasms. अर्बुद-रचना; नवगुल्म; नवार्बुद

**Neoplasm.** A new growth or tumour. नवोत्पत्ति; गुल्म; अर्बुद; रसौली

**Neoplastic.** Newly formed, as the matter which fills up a wound. नवोत्पादित

**Neostriatum.** The caudate nucleus and putamen considered together. नवरेखीपिण्ड

**Neothalamus.** The lateral and dorsomedial nuclei of the thalamus. नवचेतक

**Nephralgia.** Pain in the kidney. वृक्कार्ति; वृक्कशूल; गुर्दे का दर्द

**Nephric.** Renal; relating to kidney. वृक्कपरक; वृक्क सम्बन्धी

**Nephritic.** Pertaining to nephritis. वृक्कशोथज; वृक्कशोथ समबन्धी

**Nephritides.** Plural of **Nephritis.**

**Nephritis.** Inflammation of the kidney; Bright's disease. वृक्कशोथ; गुर्दे का प्रदाह;

> **Interstitial N.,** nephritis in which interstitial connective tissue is chiefly affected. अन्तरालीय वृक्कशोथ;
>
> **Suppurative N.,** one in which an abscess is formed in the kidney. पूतिज वृक्कशोथ; सपूय वृक्कशोथ

**Nephritogenetic.** Producing nephritis. वृक्कशोथजनक; गुर्दे का प्रदाह पैदा करने वाला

**Nephrocalcinosis.** Multiple areas of calcification within the kidney substances. वृक्ककैल्सीमयता

**Nephrocapsectomy.** Excision of the capsule of the kidney; nephrocapsulectomy. वृक्कसम्पुटोच्छेदन

**Nephrocapsulectomy.** See **Nephrocapsectomy.**

**Nephrocele.** Hernia of the kidney. वृक्कहर्निया; गुर्दे का हर्निया

**Nephrocoloptosis.** Prolapse of the kidney and the colon. वृक्क-बृहदांत्रच्युति; गुर्दे तथा बड़ी आन्त का अपने स्थान से हट जाना

**Nephrogenetic.** See **Nephrogenic.**

**Nephrogenic.** Arising in the kidney or giving rise to kidney tissue; nephrogenetic; nephrogenous. वृक्कजनक; वृक्कजन्य

**Nephrogenous.** See **Nephrogenic.**

**Nephrography.** A description of the kidney. वृक्कचित्रण

**Nephroid.** Resembling a kidney; reniform; kidney-shaped. वृक्काभ; गुर्दे जैसा

**Nephrolith.** A stone in the kidney. वृक्काश्मरी; गुर्दे की पथरी; मूत्रपथरी

**Nephrolithiasis.** Formation of renal stone. वृक्काश्मरता; गुर्दे की पथरी बनना

**Nephrolithotomy.** Incision of the kidney for calculus. वृक्काश्मरीहरण; वृक्काश्मरीछेदन

**Nephrology.** The science of the kidneys. वृक्कविज्ञान; वृक्कों अर्थात् गुर्दों का वैज्ञानिक अध्ययन

**Nephrolysis.** Surgical detachment of an inflamed kidney or destruction of renal cells. वृक्कलयन

**Nephrolytic.** Pertaining to nephrolysis. वृक्कलयन सम्बन्धी; causing nephrolysis. वृक्कलयनकारी

**Nephroma.** A tumour arising from kidney tissue. वृक्कार्बुद

**Nephromalacia.** A morbid softening of the kidneys. वृक्कमृदुता; गुर्दों की कोमलता

**Nephromegaly.** Abnormal enlargement of one or both kidneys. अतिवृक्कता

**Nephrons.** Those physiological units of the kidney which are active in producing the urine. वृक्काणु; वृक्क; गुर्दे; वृक्कांग; वृक्काणुप्रसू

**Nephropathy.** Kidney disease; renopathy; nephrosis. वृक्कविकृति; गुर्दे का रोग; अपवृक्कता

**Nephropexy.** The fixation of a floating kidney. वृक्कस्थिरीकरण

**Nephroptosis.** Downward displacement of the kidney. वृक्कभ्रंश;

वृक्कच्युति; परिभ्रमीवृक्क; गुर्दे की निम्नाभिमुखी स्थानच्युति

**Nephropyelitis.** Nephritis and pyelitis both. वृक्कगोणिकाशोथ; वृक्क तथा गोणिका का प्रदाह

**Nephropyeloplasty.** A plastic operation on the pelvis of kidney. वृक्कगोणिकासंधान (कर्म)

**Nephropyosis.** Suppuration of the kidney. वृक्कपूयता; वृक्कपूतिता

**Nephros.** Nephron. वृक्काणुप्रसू; वृक्क; गुर्दा; वृक्काणु; वृक्कांग

**Nephrosclerosis.** Renal insufficiency from hypertensive vascular disease. वृक्ककाठिन्य; गुर्दों की कठोरता

**Nephrosclerotic.** Pertaining to, or causing nephrosclerosis. वृक्ककाठिन्य सम्बन्धी या वृक्ककाठिन्यकारी

**Nephrosis.** See **Nephropathy.**

**Nephrotic.** Pertaining to nephrosis. अपवृक्कीय; वृक्कविकृति सम्बन्धी

**Nephrostomy.** Incision of the kidney. वृक्कछेदन; वृक्कछिद्रीकरण

**Nephrotoxic.** Any substance which inhibits or prevents the functions of kidney cells or causes their destruction. वृक्कविषकर; वृक्कविषण्णता पैदा करने वाला पदार्थ; nephrolytic. वृक्कलयनकारी

**Nephroureterectomy.** Excision of the kidney and ureter. वृक्कगवीनी-उच्छेदन; गुर्दे और मूत्रनली को काट कर हटा देना

**Nephroureterocystectomy.** Surgical removal of kidney, ureter and bladder. वृक्कगवीनीमूत्राशय-उच्छेदन; गुर्दे, मूत्रनली तथा मूत्राशय को काट कर निकाल देना

**Nerve.** A bundle of fibres, conveying the impulses of movement and sensation to and from the organs. स्नायु; तंत्रिका; नाड़ी;

   **Afferent N.,** one transmitting impulses from periphery to the centre; centripetal nerve. अभिवाही तंत्रिका;

   **Articular N.,** a branch of a nerve supplying a joint. संधि-तंत्रिका; संधि-स्नायु;

   **Calorific N.,** a nerve, the stimulation of which increases the heat of the parts to which it is distributed; thermic nerve. ऊष्माजनक तंत्रिका;

   **Centripetal N.,** see **Afferent Nerve.**

   **Centrifugal N.,** see **Efferent Nerve.**

   **Cranial N.,** a nerve arising directly from the brain, making its exit through a foramen of the skull. कपाल तंत्रिका;

   **Depressor N.,** any afferent nerve, the stimulation of which

**Nerve**

depresses the vasomotor centre. रक्तदाबह्रासी तंत्रिका;

**Efferent N.,** one carrying impulses from the centre to the periphery; centrifugal nerve. अपवाही तंत्रिका;

**Motor N.,** one containing only or chiefly motor fibres. प्रेरक तंत्रिका;

**Parasympathetic N.,** one of the nerves of the parasympathetic nervous system. परानुकम्पी तंत्रिका;

**Peripheral N.,** any nerve that connects the brain or spinal cord with peripheral receptors or effectors. परिसरीय तंत्रिका;

**Pressor N.,** an efferent nerve, the irritation of which stimulates the vasomotor centre. रक्तदाबवर्धक तंत्रिका;

**Secretory N.,** an efferent nerve, the accumulation of which causes glandular activity. स्रावी तंत्रिका;

**Sensory N.,** an afferent nerve conveying impulses that are processed by the central nervous system. संवेदी तंत्रिका;

**Spinal N.,** one making its exit through an intervertebral foramen. मेरुतंत्रिका;

**Sympathetic N.,** one of a system distributed to the blood vessels and viscera. अनुकम्पी तंत्रिका;

**Thermic N.,** see **Calorific Nerve.**

**Trophic N.,** one that presides over nutrition. पोषी तंत्रिका;

**Vasoconstrictor N.,** one effecting the contraction of the blood vessels and viscera. वाहिका-संकीर्णक तंत्रिका;

**Vasodilator N.,** one the stimulation of which causes dilation of vessels. वाहिकाविस्फारक तंत्रिका;

**N. Grafting,** the insertion of a piece of nerve-tissue into another nerve. तंत्रिका निरोपण

**Nervi.** Plural of **Nervus.**

**N. Nervorum,** small nerves supplying the nerve sheaths. तंत्रि-तंत्रिकायें; सूक्ष्म-स्नायु; लघु-तंत्रिकायें

**Nervimotor.** Relating to a motor nerve; neurimotor. प्रेरक-स्नायु सम्बन्धी

**Nervine.** A medicine which acts on the nerve. स्नायु-औषधि; स्नायुजाल को प्रभावित करने वाली औषधि

**Nervous.** Relating to a nerve. स्नायविक; स्नायुमूलक; तंत्रिका संबंधी; abnormally excitable. अति-उत्तेजनाशील; अत्यन्त अधीर;

**N. Centre,** the brain, spinal marrow and ganglion. स्नायु-केन्द्र;

**N. Debility,** neurasthenia. स्नायुदौर्बल्य; तंत्रिकावसाद;

**N. System,** the nerves of the body taken together. स्नायु-प्रणाली; स्नायुजाल; नाड़ी मण्डल

**Nervousness.** An acute term covering almost anything for which no other cause can be found. स्नायविकता; अधीरता; hypochondriasis. रोगभ्रम

**Nervus.** A nerve. स्नायु; तंत्रिका; नाड़ी

**Nettle-rash.** A popular term to describe urticaria. शीतपित्त; पित्ती; जुलपित्ती; छपाकी

**Network.** A structure bearing a resemblance to a woven fabric or net. जाली

**Neural.** Relating to nerves. स्नायविक; नाड़ीपरक; स्नायु सम्बन्धी

**Neuralgia.** Pain in the neve; neurodynia. तंत्रिकार्ति; तंत्रिकाशूल; स्नायुशूल; नाड़ीशूल

**Neuralgic.** Pertaining to neuralgia. स्नायुशूलपरक; स्नायुशूल, नाड़ीशूल अर्थात् तंत्रिकाशूल सम्बन्धी

**Neurapraxia.** Temporary loss of function in peripheral nerve fibres. तंत्रिका-अल्पक्रियता; परिसरीय स्नायु-तन्तुओं की क्रिया की अस्थायी हानि

**Neurasthenia.** An outmonded term for chronic fatigue and weakness. तंत्रिकावसाद; स्नायुदौर्बल्य; तंत्रिकादौर्बल्य

**Neurasthenic.** Relating to neurasthenia. तंत्रिकावसादी; तंत्रिकावसाद सम्बन्धी; one affected with neurasthenia. तंत्रिकावसादग्रस्त

**Neurataxia.** Ataxia of cerebrospinal origin. तंत्रिकावसाद; प्रमस्तिष्कमेरुमूलक गतिभंग

**Neuraxon.** An axis-cylinder process. अक्षतंतु

**Neure.** See **Neurocyte.**

**Neurectasia.** See **Neurectasis.**

**Neurectasis.** Surgical stretching of a nerve; neurectasia. तंत्रिकाविस्फार; स्नायुविस्फार

**Neurectomy.** Excision of whole or part of a nerve. तंत्रिकोच्छेदन; किसी स्नायु या उसके किसी अंश को काट कर हटा देना

**Neurectopia.** Displacement of a nerve from its normal position. तांत्रिका-अस्थानता; स्नायुच्युति

**Neurenteric.** Pertaining to the embyonic neural canal and intestinal tube. तंत्रिकांत्रज; तंत्रिका एवं आंत्र सम्बन्धी

**Neurilemma.** The sheath incasing a nerve; neurolemma. तंत्रिकाच्छद; तंत्रिकावरण

**Neurilemmitis.** Inflammation of neurilemma. तंत्रिकाच्छदशोथ; तंत्रिकावरणशोथ

**Neurilemmoma.** A tumour of neurilemma; neurinoma. तंत्रिकाच्छदार्बुद

**Neurimotor.** See **Nervimotor.**

**Neurin.** The matter of which the nervous system is composed; neurine. न्यूरिन; स्नायुजाल-निर्माणक पदार्थ

**Neurine.** See **Neurin.**

**Neurinoma.** See **Neurilemmoma.**

**Neuritic.** Pertaining to neuritis. तंत्रिकाशोथज; स्नायु-प्रदाह सम्बन्धी

**Neuritis.** Inflammation of nerve. तंत्रिकाशोथ; स्नायु-प्रदाह;

   **Alcoholic N.,** that due to alcoholism. मद्यज तंत्रिकाशोथ;

   **Ascending N.,** that which travels from the periphery centrad. आरोही तंत्रिकाशोथ;

   **Descending N.,** that advancing from the brain or spinal cord forward the periphery. अवरोही तंत्रिकाशोथ;

   **Diabetic N.,** a polyneuritis seen in diabetes. मधुमेहज तंत्रिकाशोथ;

   **Endemic N.,** beriberi. स्थानपदिक तंत्रिकाशोथ; बेरी-बेरी;

   **Facial N.,** peripheral paralysis of the facial nerve. आनन तंत्रिकाशोथ;

   **Interstitial N.,** that affecting the connective tissue of a nerve trunk. अन्तरालीय तंत्रिकाशोथ;

   **Leprotic N.,** that due to the bacillus of leprosy; leprous neuritis. कुष्ठज तंत्रिकाशोथ;

   **Leprous N.,** see **Leprotic Neuritis.**

   **Optic N.,** that affecting the optic nerve. दृष्टि-तंत्रिकाशोथ;

   **Pressure N.,** that due to compression. दाब-तंत्रिकाशोथ;

   **Retrobulbar N.,** that of the optic nerve posterior to the eyeball. गोलकपश्च-तंत्रिकाशोथ;

   **Sciatic N.,** sciatica. आसन-तंत्रिकाशोथ; गृध्रसी; सायटिका;

   **Toxic N.,** one due to alcoholism, lead-poisoning, arsenic poisoning or some other poisons. विषण्ण तंत्रिकाशोथ

**Neuro-.** Prefix meaning nerve. 'तंत्रिका' के रूप में प्रयुक्त उपसर्ग

**Neuroanatomy.** The anatomy of the nervous system. तंत्रिकाशारीर; स्नायुजाल-रचना

**Neuroarthropathy.** Any disease of the nerve-joints. तंत्रिकासन्धिविकृति; स्नायु-जोड़ों का कोई रोग

**Neuroblast.** A primitive nerve cell. तंत्रिकाकोशिकाप्रसू; कोई प्रारम्भिक स्नायुकोशिका

**Neuroblastoma.** Malignant tumour arising in adrenal medulla from tissue of sympathetic origin. तंत्रिकाकोशिकाप्रसूअर्बुद

**Neurochorioretinitis.** Combined inflammation of the optic nerve, choroid and retina. तंत्रिकारंजितपटलदृष्टिपटलशोथ; दृष्टितंत्रिका, रंजितपटल तथा दृष्टिपटल का मिश्र प्रदाह

**Neurochoroiditis.** Combined inflammation of the choroid coat and optic nerve. तंत्रिकारंजितपटलशोथ; रंजितपटल तथा दृष्टितंत्रिका का मिश्र प्रदाह

**Neurocyte.** A nerve-cell including all its processes; neure; neuron. तंत्रिकाकोशिका; स्नायुकोशिका

**Neurocytolysis.** Destruction of neurons. तंत्रिकालयन

**Neurocytoma.** A tumour of the nerve cell, usually ganglionic. तंत्रिकाकोशिकार्बुद; स्नायुकोशार्बुद; स्नायु-कोशिका की रसौली

**Neurodendrite.** Dendrite; neurodendron. पार्श्वतन्तु

**Neurodendron.** See **Neurodendrite.**

**Neurodermatitis.** A neurotic dermatitis with itching; neurodermatosis. तंत्रिकात्वक्शोथ; स्नायुचर्म के प्रदाह के साथ खुजली होना; स्नायुत्वक्शोथ

**Neurodermatosis.** See **Neurodermatitis.**

**Neurodocitis.** Inflammation of nerve roots from pressure of the bony canal through which they pass. सम्पीडनतंत्रिकाशोथ; सम्पीडनस्नायुशोथ

**Neurodynamic.** Pertaining to nervous energy. तंत्रिका-ऊर्जा सम्बन्धी

**Neurodynia.** Neuralgia. तंत्रिकाशूल; स्नायुशूल; स्नायुवेदना; स्नायुपीड़ा

**Neuroectoderm.** The embryonic tissue that gives rise to nerve tissue. तंत्रिकाबहिर्जनस्तर

**Neuroectodermal.** Relating to the neuroectoderm. तंत्रिकाबहिर्जनस्तरीय; तंत्रिकाबहिर्जनस्तर सम्बन्धी

**Neuroepithelioma.** A relatively rare tumour of neuroepithelium in a nerve of special sense. तंत्रिका-उपकलार्बुद

**Neuroepithelium.** Specialized nerve epithelium constituting end-organs of nerves of special sense, as the rods and cones of the retina. तंत्रिका-उपकला; स्नायु-उपकला

**Neurofibroma.** A combined neuroma and fibroma. तंत्रिकातन्तु-अर्बुद; स्नायुतन्तु-अर्बुद; मिश्र स्नायु-अर्बुद एवं तन्तु-अर्बुद

**Neurofibromas.** Plural of **Neurofibroma.**

**Neurofibromata.** Plural of **Neurofibroma.**

**Neurofibromatosis.** Multiple neurofibromas; neuromatosis. तंत्रिकातंतु-अर्बुदता

**Neurogenesis.** The formation of nerve tissue. तंत्रिकाजनन; स्नायु-ऊतक की रचना

**Neurogenetic.** See **Neurogenic.**

**Neurogenic.** Neurogenetic; neurogenous; originating within or forming nervous tissue. तंत्रिकाजन्य; तंत्रिकाजनक; relating to neurogenesis. तंत्रिकाजनन सम्बन्धी

**Neurogenous.** See **Neurogenic.**

**Neuroglia.** The reticulated framework of the substance of the brain and the spinal cord. तंत्रिकाबन्ध

**Neuroglial.** Relating to neuroglia; neurogliar. तंत्रिकाबन्धीय; तंत्रिकाबन्ध सम्बन्धी

**Neurogliar.** See **Neuroglial.**

**Neuroglioma.** A glioma having nerve-cells. तंत्रिकाबन्धार्बुद; स्नायुबन्धार्बुद

**Neurohypophysis.** The posterior portion of the pituitary gland. तंत्रिकापीयूषिका

**Neuroid.** Resembling a nerve or nerve substance. स्नायुवत्; तंत्रिकाभ; किसी स्नायु अथवा स्नायु-पदार्थ से मिलता-जुलता

**Neurolemma.** See **Neurilemma.**

**Neuroleptanalgesia.** Anaesthetic technique in which major agents are a neuroleptic and an analgesic drug, allowing patient to retain ability to cooperate. मनोवियोजी-असंवेदनता

**Neuroleptics.** Drugs acting on the nervous system. मनोवियोजी-औषिधिवर्ग; स्नायु-प्रणाली को प्रभावित करने वाली औषधियां

**Neurologist.** One versed in neurology. तंत्रिकाविज्ञानी; स्नायुविज्ञानी

**Neurology.** The medical specialty concerned with the physical diseases of the brain and nerves. तंत्रिकाविज्ञान; स्नायुविज्ञान

**Neurolysin.** An antibody causing destruction of ganglion and cortical cells; neurotoxin. तंत्रिकालयनक; तंत्रिकाविषज

**Neurolysis.** The exhaustion of the nerve. तंत्रिकालयन; तंत्रिका-अपघटन; स्नायु-अपघटन

**Neurolytic.** Relating to neurolysis. तंत्रिकालयन सम्बन्धी

**Neuroma.** A tumour found on a nerve trunk or mass. तंत्रिकार्बुद;

**Acoustic N.**, a tumour of eighth cranial nerve. श्रवण तंत्रिकार्बुद;

**Amputation N.**, one of the stumps at the end of a divided nerve; false neuroma; traumatic neuroma. अंगोच्छेदनतंत्रिकार्बुद;

**Cystic N.**, a false neuroma with the formation of cysts. पुटीय तंत्रिकार्बुद;

**False N.**, see **Amputation Neuroma.**

**Plexiform N.**, the development of multiple fibromatous tumours along the course of one or more nerves, attended with hyperplasia of the nerve-fibres. जालरूप तंत्रिकार्बुद;

**Traumatic N.**, see **Amputation Neuroma.**

**Neuromalacia.** A softening of nerve tissue. तंत्रिकामृदुता; स्नायु-ऊतक की कोमलता

**Neuromatosis.** See **Neurofibromatosis.**

**Neuromatous.** Affected with neuroma. तंत्रिकार्बुदग्रस्त

**Neuromere.** A segment or division of the neuron. मेरुरज्जुखण्ड; तंत्रिकाकोशिका का विखण्डन अथवा विभाजन

**Neuromeric.** Pertaining to a neuromere. मेरुरज्जुखण्डीय; मेरुरज्जुखण्ड सम्बन्धी

**Neuromuscular.** Pertaining to both nerves and the muscles. तंत्रिकापेशी सम्बन्धी

**Neuromyelitis.** Neuritis combined with spinal cord inflammation; myeloneuritis. तंत्रिकासुषुम्नाशोथ

**Neuromyopathy.** Any disease of the nerves and muscles. तंत्रिकापेशी-विकृति; तंत्रिकाओं एवं पेशियों का कोई रोग

**Neuromyositis.** A combined neuritis and myositis. तंत्रिकापेशीशोथ; तंत्रिकाओं तथा पेशियों का मिश्र प्रदाह

**Neuron.** A nerve cell; neurocyte; neurone. तंत्रिकाकोशिका

**Neuronal.** Pertaining to a neuron. तंत्रिकाकोशिकीय अथवा तंत्रिकाकोशिका सम्बन्धी

**Neurone.** See **Neuron.**

**Neuronophagia.** The destruction of neurones by phagocytes; neuronophagy. तंत्रिकाकोशिकाभक्षण

**Neuronophagy.** See **Neuronophagia.**

**Neuroparalysis.** Paralysis resulting from disease of nerve supplying the affected part. तंत्रिकाघात; स्नायुघात

**Neuropathic.** Relating to the diseases of the nervous system. स्नायुरोग अथवा तंत्रिकाविकृति सम्बन्धी

**Neuropathogenesis.** The origin or causation of a disease of the nervous system. तंत्रिकाविकृतिजनन

**Neuropathology.** Treatise on nerve disease. तंत्रिकाविकृतिविज्ञान; स्नायुरोगप्रकरण

**Neuropathy.** Any disease of the nervous system. तंत्रिकाविकृति; स्नायुरोग; स्नायु-प्रणाली का कोई रोग

**Neuropharmacology.** The branch of pharmacology dealing with drugs that affect the nervous system. तंत्रिकाभेषजगुणविज्ञान; भेषजविज्ञान की वह शाखा जो उन औषधियों के व्यवहार का वर्णन करती है जो स्नायु-प्रणाली को प्रभावित करती हैं

**Neurophysiology.** Physiology of the nervous system. तंत्रिकाभौतिकी; तंत्रिकाभौतिकविज्ञान

**Neuroplasm.** The granular interstitial substance cementing the fibrillas of an axis-cylinder. तंत्रिकाद्रव्य

**Neuroplasty.** Surgical repair of a nerve. तंत्रिकासंधान

**Neuroplegia.** Peralysis of a nerve. तंत्रिकाघात; स्नायुघात; किसी नाड़ी का पक्षाघात

**Neuroplegic.** Relating to neuroplegia. तंत्रिकाघाती; तंत्रिकाघात सम्बन्धी

**Neuropore.** A small opening at the anterior extremity of the primary telencephalon. तंत्रिकारन्ध्र; तंत्रिकाछिद्र

**Neuropraxia.** A state of nerve in which, due to trauma, the conduction is blocked across a point, but the continuity of the nerve is not interrupted. तंत्रिकाक्षति

**Neuroretinitis.** Inflammation of the optic nerve and retina. तंत्रिका-दृष्टिपटलशोथ; दृष्टितंत्रिका एवं नेत्रपटल का प्रदाह

**Neurosarcoma.** A malignant tumour of the nervous system. तंत्रिकासार्कार्बुद

**Neurosis.** An abnormal way of meeting a situation; an emotional disorder; mania. विक्षिप्ति; पागलपन;

   **Axiety N.,** chronic abnormal distress and worry to the point of panic; anxiety state. चिन्ता विक्षिप्ति;

   **Cardiac N.,** anxiety concerning the state of the heart. हृत्विक्षिप्ति;

**Occupation N.**, one of a class of spasmodic and coordinative disturbances, mainly of functional origin, affecting groups of muscles used in special work or movements; occupational neurosis; professional neurosis. व्यवसायज विक्षिप्ति; व्यावसायिक विक्षिप्ति;

**Occupational N.**, see **Occupation Neurosis.**

**Professional N.**, see **Occupation Neurosis.**

**Traumatic N.**, any functional nervous disorder following an accident or traumatic injury. अभिघातज विक्षिप्ति

**Neurosthenia.** Excessive nervous power. प्रबृद्ध स्नायुशक्ति; बढ़ी हुई स्नायुशक्ति

**Neurosurgeon.** A surgeon specializing in neurosurgery. तंत्रिकाशल्यचिकित्सक

**Neurosurgery.** Surgery of the nervous system. तंत्रिकाशल्यविज्ञान; तंत्रिकाशस्त्रकर्म; स्नायु-जाल की शल्यचिकित्सा

**Neurosyphilis.** Syphilitic infection of brain or spinal cord or both. तंत्रिकातंत्र-उपदंश; स्नायुतंत्र-उपदंश

**Neurotic.** Affected with neurosis. विक्षिप्त; स्नायविक; पागल; relating to neurosis. विक्षिप्ति सम्बन्धी

**Neurotomy.** Dissection of the nerves, or division of a nerve. तंत्रिकोच्छेदन; तंत्रिकाविच्छेदन; तंत्रिका-कर्तन

**Neurotoxin.** See **Neurolysin.**

**Neurotripsy.** The crushing of a nerve. तंत्रिकासंदलन; किसी स्नायु का कुचलना

**Neurotrophic.** Pertaining to the nutritive influence of nerves. तंत्रिकापोषित; तंत्रिकाबृद्धि अथवा स्नायुपोषण सम्बन्धी

**Neurotrophy.** The nutritive influence of nerves. तंत्रिकापोषण; स्नायुपोषण

**Neurotropic.** Having an affinity for the nervous system. तंत्रिकाप्रेरित

**Neurotropism.** The attraction or repulsion exercised upon regenerating nerve-fibres; neurotropy. तंत्रिकारोग

**Neurotropy.** See **Neurotropism.**

**Neutral.** Possessing neither acid nor basic properties. उदासीन; क्रियाशून्य; impotent. नपुंसक

**Neutralization.** Rendering ineffective of any action, process or potential. उदासीनीकरण; निराकरण

**Neutralize.** To render inactive or negative. निष्क्रिय करना; उदासीनीकरण करना

**Neutropenia.** Subnormal number of neutrophiles in the peripheral blood. उदासीनरागीकोशिकाल्पता; परिसरीय रक्त में उदासीनरागी-कोशिकाओं की कमी;

    **Malignant N.,** an aplastic anaemia with an acute febrile course and high mortality. दुर्दम उदासीनरागीकोशिकाल्पता

**Neutrophil.** See **Neutrophile.**

**Neutrophile.** A cell or histological element that is readily stained by neutral anilin dyes; neutrophil. उदासीनरागी; उदासीनरागीकोशिका

**Nevi.** Plural of **Nevus.**

**Nevoid.** Like a nevus; nevous. न्यच्छाभ; न्यच्छवत्; तिल जैसा

**Nevous.** See **Nevoid.**

**Nevus.** See **Naevus.**

**Newborn.** See **Neonate.**

**N.F.** National Formulary. राष्ट्रीय सूत्रसंहिता

**Niacin.** Nicotinic acid. निकोटिन अम्ल; नियासीन

**Nicotin.** A poisonous alkaloid of tobacco; nicotine. निकोटिन; तम्बाकू से प्राप्त एक विषैला क्षार

**Nicotine.** See **Nicotin.**

**Nicotinic.** Pertaining to nicotin. निकोटिनी; निकोटिन सम्बन्धी;

    **N.Acid,** one of the essential food factors of Vitamin 'B' Complex. निकोटिन अम्ल

**Nicotinism.** Morbid effects from the excessive use of tobacco. निकोटिनविषण्णता; तम्बाकू के अपव्यवहार से होने वाली रुग्णता

**Nictation.** See **Nictitation.**

**Nictitation.** Winking ; a nictation. नेत्रोन्मीलन; पलकें झपकना

**Nidal.** Relating to a nidus or nest. उद्गम केन्द्र अथवा नीड़ सम्बन्धी

**Nidation.** Implantation of the early embryo in the uterine mucosa. डिम्बारोपण; जरायुकला के अन्दर भ्रूण का स्थान ग्रहण करना

**Nidi.** Plural of **Nidus.**

**Nidus.** A focus of infection. उद्गमकेन्द्र; a cluster or nestlike structure. नीड़; घोंसला

**Night-blindness.** Sightlessness during night. नक्तान्धता; रतौंधी; निशान्धता; रात को न दिखाई देने का रोग

**Nightmares.** Terrifying dreams of being unable to cry or escape from a seemingly impending evil. दु:स्वप्न

**Nightshade.** Belladonna. बेलाडौना; अंगूरशेफा

**Night-sweat.** Excessive sweating during night. रात्रिस्वेद; नक्तस्वेद; रात में पसीना होना

**Night-terror.** A disorder allied to nightmares in which a child awakes screaming in fright. निशाभीति; निशातंक; रात को डर लगना

**Night-walking.** Somnambulism; walking in sleep; noctambulation. निद्राभ्रमण; निद्राचलन; सोते-सोते उठकर चल देना

**Nigricans.** Blackish. श्यामल; श्याम; काला-काला

**Nigrites.** Blackness. श्यामलता; कालापन

**Nipple.** Papilla mammae; the conical eminence in centre of each breast, containing the outlets of the milk ducts. चूचुक; स्तन का अगला भाग, जिससे दूध बाहर निकलता है

**Nisus.** The contraction of the diaphragm and abdominal muscles for the expulsion of faeces. मध्यच्छदोदरपेशीसंकोच; मध्यच्छद एवं उदरपेशियों की सिकुड़न; the monthly course of a woman. ऋतुस्राव; आर्तव

**Nit.** The egg of the head-louse, attached to the human hair or clothing. लिक्षा; लीख

**Nitrate.** The salt of nitric acid; nitrite. जवाखार या शोराम्ल का लवण;
 Silver N., lunar caustic; nitrate of silver. सिल्वर नाइट्रेट;
 N. of silver, see Silver Nitrate.

**Nitric Acid.** Dangerous caustic, occasionally used in testing urine for certain bacteria. शोरा अम्ल; जवाखार; नाइट्रिक एसिड

**Nitrification.** The formation of nitrates, especially that due to the action of certain bacteria. नाइट्रीकरण; नाइट्रीभवन

**Nitrite.** See **Nitrate.**

**Nitrogen.** A colourless element. नाइट्रोजन; नेत्रजन

**Nitrogenisation.** A conversion into nitrogen. नाइट्रोजनीकरण; नाइट्रोजनीभवन; नाइट्रोजन-प्रवेशन

**Nitrogenised.** Combined with nitrogen; nitrogenous. नाइट्रोजनीभूत; नाइट्रोजनीकृत; नाइट्रोजनयुक्त

**Nitrogenous.** Relating to nitrogen or containing nitrogen. नाइट्रोजन सम्बन्धी या नाइट्रोजनयुक्त

**Nitrometer.** An apparatus for gas analysis. नाइट्रोजनमापी

**Noct.** In the night; nocte. रात को

**Noctalbuminuria.** Presence of albumin in urine during night. नक्तान्नसारमेह; रात को पेशाब में अन्नसार जाना

**Noctambulation.** See **Night-walking.**

**Nocte.** See **Noct.**

**Nocte maneque.** Night and morning. रात्रि एवं प्रातः; रात को और सुबह

**Noctiphobia.** A morbid dread of night. निशाभीति; नक्तभीति; रात में डर लगना

**Nocturia.** Excessive urine at night. निशामेह; रात को बहुत पेशाब होना

**Nocturnal.** Occurring at night. निशाकालीन; रात्रिकालीन; रात को प्रकट होने वाला;

**N. Blindness,** night blindness. निशान्धता; नक्तान्धता; रतौंधी; रात को न दिखाई देने का रोग;

**N. Emission,** an involuntary discharge of semen during sleep; nocturnal pollution; spermatorrhoea. शुक्रमेह; रात्रिस्खलनता;

**N. Pollution**, see **Nocturnal Emission.**

**Nodal.** Relating to any node. पर्विका अथवा पर्व (गांठ) सम्बन्धी

**Node.** A swelling or protuberance; nodosa; nodus. पर्विका; पर्व; गांठ; गूमड़; गूमड़ी;

**Lymph N.,** round or oval reddish bodies, from a pin-head to small bean in size on the lymph vessels in certain regions. लसीका-पर्व

**Nodi.** Plural of **Nodus.**

**Nodosa.** See **Node.**

**Nodose.** See **Nodular.**

**Nodosities.** Plural form of **Nodosity.**

**Nodosity.** A concretion, especially calcareous, as in gout. पर्विलता; पर्विकता

**Nodular.** Like a node; nodose. पर्विल; पर्ववत्; पर्व जैसा

**Nodule.** A small node or excrescence; nodulus. पर्विका; लघुपर्व; छोटी सी गांठ

**Nodulus.** See **Nodule.**

**Nodus.** See **Node.**

**Noma.** A synonym for ulcerative or gangrenous stomatitis. मुखकोथ; कोथजमुखपाक;

**N. Pundendi,** see **Noma Vulvae.**

**N. Vulvae,** ulceration of vulva; noma pudendi. भगकोथज व्रण

**Nomenclature.** A system of technical names. नामकरण; नामपद्धति

**Nomogram.** The representing of correlations by graphs. सामान्य मानकलेख

**Nonabsorbable.** That which is not capable of being absorbed. अनवशोषणीय; शोषण के अयोग्य

**Nonadherent.** Not connected to adjacent organs. अचिप्य; न चिपकने वाला

**Non Compos Mentis.** Of unsound mind. असमाहित-चित्त; मन्दबुद्धि; जड़बुद्धि

**Nonigravida.** Pregnant for the ninth time. नवमगर्भा; नवीं बार गर्भवती होने वाली स्त्री

**Nonimmunity.** Lack of protection against disease; aphylaxia. अरोगक्षमता

**Nonipara.** A women, who has born nine children. नवमप्रसूता; नौ बच्चों को जन्म देने वाली स्त्री

**Nonviable.** Incapable of life. जीवन-अक्षम; जीने के अयोग्य; मृत; of independent existence. स्वतंत्र अस्तित्व वाला

**Norm.** See **Norma**.

**Norma.** Norm; Model. प्रतिरूप; नमूना; normal. सामान्य; rule. नियम; a standard or ideal for a specific group. किसी विशिष्ट वर्ग के लिये एक मानक या आदर्श

**Normae.** Plural of **Norma**.

**Normal.** As it ought to be; according to rule or type. सामान्य; स्वाभाविक; स्वस्थ

**Normoblast.** A blood-corpuscle of normal size. लोहितकोशिकाप्रसू; सामान्य आकार की रक्तकणिका; सामान्यलोहितकोशिका

**Normochromia.** Normal colour. सामान्य रंग; एक स्वाभाविक रंग

**Normocyte.** A normoblast. सामान्यलोहितकोशिका; लोहितकोशिकाप्रसू

**Normocytosis.** A normal state of the corpuscular elements of the blood. सामान्यलोहितकोशिकता

**Normothermia.** Normal body temperature. शरीर का सामान्य तापमान रहना

**Nose.** Nosus; the organ of smell. नासिका; नासा; नाक; घ्राणेन्द्रिय;
   **N.-bleed,** expistaxis. नासारक्तस्रवण; नकसीर फूटना;
   **Saddle N.,** a nose with markedly depressed bridge. पर्याण नासा

**Nosocomium.** A hospital. अस्पताल; चिकित्सालय

**Nosode.** Any disease product. रोगविषनिर्मित औषधि; नसोड

**Nosogenesis.** The development and progress of a disease; nosogeny; nosopoietic; pathogenesis. रोगजनन; रोग का विकास होना या रोग बढ़ना

**Nosogenic.** Relating to nosogenesis or nosogeny; pathogenic. रोगजनक

**Nosogeny.** See **Nosogenesis**.

**Nosography.** A description of the disease. रोगवर्णन

**Nosologic.** Relating to nosology. रोगों के वैज्ञानिक वर्गीकरण से सम्बन्धित

**Nosology.** The scientific classification of diseases; nosonomy; nosotaxy. रोगवर्गीकरणविज्ञान; रोगों का वैज्ञानिक वर्गीकरण

**Nosonomy.** See **Nosology**.

**Nosophobia.** An abnormal dread of disease. रोगभीति; रोगातंक

**Nosopoietic.** See **Nosogenesis**.

**Nosotaxy.** See **Nosology**.

**Nostalgia.** Home-sickness. गृहातुरता; घर लौटने की अधीरता

**Nostril.** The aperture of the nose. नासारन्ध्र; नासापक्षक; नासाद्वार; नथुना

**Nostrum.** A quack or secret medicine. गुप्तौषध; पेटेण्ट दवा

**Nosus.** The nose. नासिका; नासा; नाक

**Notal.** Dorsal; pertaining to the back. पीठ सम्बन्धी; पृष्ठीय; पृष्ठज

**Notalgia.** Pain in the back. पृष्ठवेदना; पृष्ठशूल; कमरदर्द

**Notch.** A depression or indentation on the margin of a bone. भंगिका; खांच; दनदाना; कटाव; दर्रि;

> **Cardiac N.,** a deep notch between the oesophagus and fundus of the stomach. अभिहृद्फुप्फुसभंगिका;

> **Dicrotic N.,** the notch in the pulse tracing which precedes the second or dicrotic wave. द्विस्पन्दी भंगिका;

> **Jugular N.,** one forming the posterior boundary of the jugular foramen. जुगुलर भंगिका;

> **Nasal N.,** an uneven interval between the internal angular processes of the frontal bone. नासा भंगिका

**Notifiable.** Worthy of notice. सूच्य; सूचित करने योग्य

**Notochord.** The primitive back-bone. पृष्ठदण्ड; आद्यपृष्ठवंश; मेरुदण्ड

**Notochordal.** Relating to notochord. पृष्ठदण्ड अथवा मेरुदण्ड सम्बन्धी

**Notomyelitis.** Inflammation of the spinal cord. सुषुम्नाशोथ; मेरुरज्जुशोथ; मेरुरज्जु-प्रदाह; मेरुदण्ड का प्रदाह

**Nourishment.** Nutrition. पोषण

**Noxious.** Poisonous; injurious; harmful. विषाक्त; हानिकारक

**Nubile.** Sexually mature; fit for marriage. विवाह-योग्य

**Nucha.** The nape of neck. पश्चग्रीवा; गर्दन का पिछला भाग

**Nuchal.** Relating to the nape of neck. पश्चग्रीवा अथवा गर्दन के पिछले भाग सम्बन्धी

**Nuclear.** Pertaining to the nucleus. केन्द्रकी; केन्द्रक सम्बन्धी

**Nuclei.** Plural of **Nucleus.**

**Nuclein.** A nitrogenous constituent of cell nuclei. न्यूक्लीन; कोशिका-केन्द्रकों में पाया जाने वाला एक नेत्रजन घटक

**Nucleoiod.** See **Nucleoliform.**

**Neucleolar.** Relating to nucleolus. उपकेन्द्रक सम्बन्धी

**Nucleoli.** Plural of **Nucleolus.**

**Nucleoliform.** Resembling a nucleolus; nucleoiod; nucleoloid. उपकेन्द्रकाभ

**Nucleoloid.** See **Nucleoliform.**

**Nucleolus.** A small granule in the interior of the nucleus. उपकेन्द्रक; केन्द्रक के अन्दर पाई जाने वाली एक छोटी कणिका

**Nucleoplasm.** The ground-substance of the nucleus of a cell. कोषरस; केन्द्रकद्रव्य

**Nucleus.** A mass of protoplasm; the executive centre of a muscle or organ; the germ of a new cell. केन्द्रक;

   **Arcuate N.**, the nucleus located on the ventral and medial aspects of the pyramid in the medulla oblongata. चापाकार केन्द्रक;

   **Cuneate N.**, an elongated mass of gray matter in the external posterior column of postoblongata. कीलक केन्द्रक;

   **Hypothalamic N.**, see **Nucleus Hypothalamicus.**

   **Olivary N.**, the nucleus of the olivary body. वर्तुलिका केन्द्रक;

   **Pontine N.**, the gray matter of the pons; nucleus pontis. पोंस केन्द्रक;

   **N. Hypothalamicus**, the hypothalamic nucleus; one of the nuclei occuring in four groups found in hypothalamus. अधःश्चेतक केन्द्रक;

   **N. Pontis**, see **Pontine Nucleus.**

**Nude.** Naked. नग्न; नंगा

**Nulligravida.** See **Nullipara.**

**Nullipara.** A woman who has not born any child; nulligravida. बंध्या; बांझ; अप्रसवा

**Nulliparity.** The condition of being nulliparous. बंध्यता; बांझपन; अप्रसविता

**Nulliparous.** Never having given birth to a child. बंध्या; बांझ; अप्रसवा

**Numbness.** Anaesthesia; a lack of sensation. सुन्नपन; स्पर्शज्ञानहीनता

**Nummular.** Coin-shaped; nummularis. सिक्काभ; नाणकाभ; सिक्के के आकार का

**Nummularis.** See **Nummular.**

**Nun's murmur.** A humming sound heard over the large veins at the root of the neck in healthy persons. भिनभिनाहट

**Nurse.** One who is professionally trained and takes care of the sick. परिचारिका; धाय; नर्स; to suckle; to give suck to an infant. स्तनपान कराना;

N. Midwife, one licenced with both for midwifery and nursing. धाय-परिचारिका

**Nursery.** Department of a hospital where the newborns are cared for. शिशुपालनगृह; शिशुसदन; नर्सरी

**Nursing.** Feeding an infant at the breast. स्तनपान कराना; to take care of the sick. परिचर्या (करना); रोगी की देख-भाल करना

**Nutgall.** An excrescence on the leaves of **Quercus Lusitanica,** caused by the deposited ova of an insect. माजूफल

**Nutmeg.** See **Myristica.**

N. Liver, one with a peculiar mottled appearance. जायफली यकृत्

**Nutrient.** A nutritious substance. पोषक; पौष्टिक पदार्थ

**Nutriment.** Nourishing foods which repair the waste of the system. पोषणाहार; पौष्टिकाहार; पौष्टिक पदार्थ; पोषाहार

**Nutriology.** The scienfitic study of the nutritious substances. पोषणिकी; पोषणप्रकरण; पोषणविज्ञान

**Nutrition.** The process of promoting growth, or repairing the losses of the system. पोषण

**Nutritious.** Nourishing; capable of sustaining life; affording nutrition; nutritive. पौष्टिक; पुष्टिकर; पोषक

**Nutritive.** See **Nutritious.**

**Nux Vomica.** The nuts of **Strychnos nux vomica** from which strychnine is obtained. नक्स वोमिका; कुचला

**Nyctalgia.** Pain occurring during the night. रात्रिशूल; रात्रिकालीन पीड़ा; निशार्ति

**Nyctalope.** Affected with night blindness. नक्तान्ध; निशान्ध; ऐसा रोगी जिसे रात में दिखाई नहीं देता

**Nyctalopia.** Night blindness. नक्तान्धता; निशान्धता; रतौंधी; रात को दिखाई न देने का रोग

**Nyctophobia.** A morbid fear of darkness. निशाभीति; अंधकारभीति

**Nycturia.** Nocturnal urinary incontinence. निशामेह; निशामूत्रण; नक्तमेह; रात्रिमूत्रण

**Nympha.** One of the labia minora. लघुभगोष्ठ; क्षुद्रभगोष्ठ

**Nymphae.** Plural of **Nympha**.

**Nymphas.** Plural of **Nympha**.

**Nymphectomy.** Surgical removal of hypertrophied nymphae. लघुभगोष्ठ-उच्छेदन; क्षुद्रभगोष्ठ-उच्छेदन

**Nymphitis.** Inflammation of labia minora. क्षुद्रभगोष्ठशोथ; लघुभगोष्ठशोथ; लघुभगोष्ठ का प्रदाह

**Nymphomania.** Excessive sexual desire in woman. स्त्रीकामोन्माद; स्त्रियों में पाया जाने वाला कामोन्माद

**Nymphomaniac.** A victim of nymphomania; nymphomaniacal. कामोन्मादग्रस्त (स्त्री)

**Nymphomaniacal.** Nymphomaniac. कामोन्मादग्रस्त (स्त्री); relating to nymphomania. स्त्री-कामोन्माद सम्बन्धी

**Nystagmus.** Oscillatory movement of the eyeball. अक्षिदोलन; नेत्रकम्प; Rotatory N., partial rolling of the eyeball around the visual axis. घूर्णी अक्षिदोलन

**Nyxis.** Pricking. चुभन; piercing. चुभनशील; puncture. छिद्र; paracentesis. परावेधन

# O

**Oak.** A tree of genus **Quercus**. शाहबलूत; बाँज; बलूत; ओक

**Oakum.** A surgical dressing of shredded rope. सन्न-पट्टिका

**Oat.** Grain or seed of a cereal grass used as a food. सामान्य यव अथवा जई

**Oat-meal.** A meal prepared by grinding the grains of the **Avena Sativa** or common oat. यविकाचूर्ण; जई का दलिया

**Oath.** A solemn attestation or affirmation. शपथ; कसम

**Obdormition.** Numbness of an extremity due to pressure on sensory nerve. बाह्यांगी सुन्नपन

**Obeliac.** Relating to the obelion. शिखाबिन्दु सम्बन्धी;
   Morbid O., the condition of weighing atleast twice the ideal weight. द्विगुण स्थूलता

**Obelion.** The sagittal suture between the parietal foramen. शिखाबिन्दु

**Obese.** Extremely fat or corpulent. स्थूल; स्थूलकाय

**Obesity.** Overweight, mainly due to fat rather than the bone and muscle; corpulency. स्थूलता; मेदुरता; पीनता; मोटापा

**Obituary.** Pertaining to death or death-news; death-notice. निधन-समाचार; निधन-सूचना; मृत्यु-समाचार; मृत्यु सम्बन्धी समाचार

**Object Blindness.** An inability to comprehend objects seen. बिम्बान्धता

**Objective.** Belonging to the object. वस्तुपरक; अभिदृश्यक; belonging what is external to man. परानुभूत;
   **O. Symptoms,** symptoms apparent to physical means of diagnosis. परानुभूत लक्षण

**Obligate.** Compelled to act in a given manner. अधिबद्ध; आग्रही; अविकल्प; अपरिहार्य

**Oblique.** Slanting; deviating from the perpendicular. बक्र; तिर्यक; तिरछा; टेढ़ा

**Obliquity.** The condition of being slanting, or inclined. बक्रता; तिर्यकता; तिरछापन; टेढ़ापन

**Obliteration.** Extinction, or complete occlusion of a part by degeneration. अभिलोपन; उच्छेद; व्यामर्श; विरूपण

**Oblivion.** Forgetfulness; failure of memory. विस्मृति; विस्मरण; स्मृतिलोप; याद न रहना

**Oblongata.** Medulla oblongata; part of the brain within the cranium; nervous system of the senses. पश्चकपाल-अन्तस्था; मेरुमज्जा; ज्ञानेन्द्रियां

**Obscure.** Hidden or indistinct. अदृश; अस्पष्ट; to make less distinct or to hide. दृष्टिगोचर होने में रुकावट डालना

**Observation.** The examination of a thing. पर्यवलोकन; पर्यविक्षण; प्रेक्षण; जांच-कार्य

**Obsession.** The neurotic mental state of having an uncontrollable desire to dwell on an idea or an emotion. मनोग्रस्ति; मनोद्वेग; possesion by a demon. प्रेतबाधा

**Obstetric.** Relating to midwifery; obstetrical. प्रसूति सम्बन्धी; प्रासूतिक

**Obstetrical.** See **Obstetric.**

**Obstetrician.** A qualified doctor who practises the science and art of obstetrics. प्रसूतिविज्ञानी; धातृविज्ञानी; धातृविद्याविशारद

**Obstetrics.** Medical speciality concerned with the care of a pregnant woman and her delivery; midwifery. प्रसूतिविज्ञान; धातृविज्ञान; धातृविद्या

**Obstinate.** Intractable; not yielding to arguments. दुराग्रही; ढीठ; refractory. अननुसारी; दुश्चिकित्स्य

**Obstipation.** Constipation; costiveness; obstructio alvi. मलबद्धता; कोष्ठबद्धता; कब्ज

**Obstructed.** Stopped up or closed, as a way or passage. रुद्ध; अवरुद्ध; बाधित

**Obstructio Alvi.** See **Obstipation.**

**Obstruction.** The blocking of canal of an opening. अवरोध; व्यारोध; अवरुद्धता; बाधा; रुकावट

**Obstruent.** That which obstructs or prevents a normal discharge from the bowels. मलरोधक; मलावरोधक; obstructing; blocking; clogging; any agent causing obstruction. अवरोधक; रोधक

**Obtund.** To dull or blunt. कुन्द कर देना

**Obturation.** Obstruction or occlusion. अवरोध; अन्तर्रोध; बाधा; रुकावट

**Obturator.** That which obstructs a cavity or opening. गवाक्ष; किसी गह्वर में रुकावट डालने वाला

**Obtuse.** Blunt; dull; not sharpened. कुन्द; धारहीन; खुंडा; dull, especially in intellect. मंद (बुद्धि)

**Obtusion.** Dullness of sensibility; a blunting. मंदसंवेद्यता; संवेदनामंदता; अतीक्ष्णता; सुन्नता

**Occipital.** Concerned with the back of the head, called occiput. पश्चकपालिक; पश्चकपालीय; सिर के पिछले भाग से सम्बन्धित;

   **O. Bone,** characterized by large hole through which spinal cord passes. पश्चकपालास्थि; सिर के पीछे वाली हड्डी;

   **O. Lobe,** the posterior portion of the cerebral hemisphere. पश्चकपालखण्ड; मस्तिष्क का पिछला खण्ड

**Occipitis.** Plural of **Occiput.**

**Occipitofacial.** Relating to the occiput and the face. सिर के पिछले भाग तथा चेहरे से सम्बन्धित; पश्चकपालाननीय

**Occipitofrontal.** Relating to the occiput and the forehead or the frontal lobe of the cerebral cortex. पश्चकपाल एवं ललाट अथवा प्रमस्तिष्क प्रांतस्था के अगले खण्ड सम्बन्धी

**Occipitomental.** Relating to occiput and chin. पश्चकपाल एवं हनु (ठोढ़ी) सम्बन्धी

**Occiput.** The back part of the head. पश्चकपाल; गुद्दी; सिर का पिछला भाग

**Occlude.** To close or bring together. अधिधारित करना; भींचना

**Occlusal.** Pertaining to occlusion or closure of an opening. किसी द्वार को रुद्ध या बंद कर देने सम्बन्धी

**Occlusion.** The closure of the opening of a tube or duct. अधिधारण; अन्तर्रोध; संरोध; रोध; नाड़ीरोध

**Occlusive.** Serving to close. पूर्णावरोधक; पूर्णतया बंद कर देने वाला; concerning occlusion. अन्तर्रोध सम्बन्धी

**Occulomotor.** The third nerve which moves the eyes. नेत्रप्रेरक (तंत्रिका); आँखों को चलायमान रखने वाली खोपड़ी की तीसरी तंत्रिका (नाड़ी)

**Occult.** Hidden; secret. गुप्त; अदृश; अप्रत्यक्ष; अदृश्य;

   **O. Blood,** blood in such minute quantity that it can be recognized only by microscopic examination or by chemical means. अदृश्य रक्त

**Occupation.** A holding, tenure, possession, an employment, business, vocation, pursuit, etc. व्यवसाय; व्यावृत्ति;

   **O. Disease,** see **Occupational Disease.**

**Occupational.** Belonging to an occupation. व्यावसायिक; व्यावृत्तिक;

   **O. Disease,** one of the consequences of the occupation of a patient; occupation disease. व्यावसायिक रोग;

   **O. Therapy,** the use of occupation, usually manual, for therapeutic or remedial purpose in mental and physical disorders. व्यावसायिक रोगोपचार; व्यावसायिक चिकित्सा

**Octan.** Recurring every eighth day. अठवारा (ज्वर); आठवें रोज आने वाला (बुखार)

**Ocular.** Relating to the eyes. चाक्षुष; नेत्रों सम्बन्धी;

**O. Spectres,** imaginary objects floating before the eyes. नेत्रचित्तिता; आँखों के आगे तैरती काल्पनिक वस्तुएं

**Ocularist.** One skilled in correcting the general derangement of the eyes, including its design, fabrication, fitting of artificial eyes, and making of prostheses associated with the appearance or functions of the eyes. नेत्रविज्ञानी; नेत्रविज्ञानवेत्ता

**Oculi.** Plural of **Oculus.**

**Oculist.** An eye physician; an ophthalmologist. नेत्ररोगविशेषज्ञ; नेत्रविज्ञानी; नेत्ररोगचिकित्सक

**Oculography.** A method of recording eye-position and eye-movements. नेत्रगतिलेखन

**Oculogyria.** The limits of rotation of the eyeballs. नेत्रपरिभ्रमण

**Oculogyric.** Referring to movements of the eyeballs. नेत्रपरिभ्रमी

**Oculomotor.** Relating to the movements of the eyeballs. नेत्रप्रेरक; नेत्रगोलकों की गतियों से सम्बन्धित;

   **O. Nerve,** the third cranial nerve which moves the eye and supplies the upper eyelid. नेत्रप्रेरक तंत्रिका

**Oculus.** The eye; the organ of vision, consisting of the eyeball and the optic nerve. नेत्र; चक्षु; अक्षि; आँख;

   **O. Dexter,** the right eye. दक्षिणाक्षि; दायां नेत्र; दाईं आँख;

   **O. Sinister,** the left eye. बामाक्षि; बायां नेत्र; बाईं आँख

**Odontagra.** Toothache; pain in the teeth; odontalgia. दंतार्ति; दंतशूल; दांत का दर्द

**Odontalgia.** See **Odontagra.**

**Odontalgic.** Allaying toothache. दंतवेदनाहर; दांत का दर्द कम करने वाली (औषधि); relating to, or marked by odontalgia. दंतशूल सम्बन्धी अथवा दंतशूलपरक

**Odontectomy.** Surgical removal of a tooth. दंतनिष्कर्षण; दंत-उच्छेदन; शल्यकर्म द्वारा दांत निकाल देना

**Odontiasis.** The cutting of the teeth. दंतोच्छेदन

**Odontic.** Pertaining to the teeth. दांतों सम्बन्धी; दंतपरक

**Odontitis.** Inflammation of the teeth-pulp. दंतशोथ; दंतमज्जाशोथ; दांतों का प्रदाह

**Odontoblast.** A columnar cell forming dentin. दंतकोशिकाप्रसू; दंतोत्पादककोशिका

**Odontoblastoma.** A tumour composed principally of odontoblast. दंतकोशिकाप्रसू-अर्बुद

**Odontocele.** An alveodental cyst. दंतउलूखल-पुटक

**Odontoclast.** A cell absorbing the root of the tooth. दंतमूलशोषक; दंतनाशक

**Odontogenesis.** The process of development of teeth; odontogeny; odontosis. दंतजनन; दांत विकसित होने की प्रक्रिया

**Odontogeny.** See **Odontogenesis.**

**Odontoid.** Resembling a tooth. दंताभ; दंतवत्; दांत जैसा; दंतोपम

**Odontolith.** The concretion which is deposited around the teeth. दंताश्मरी; दंतपथरी

**Odontologist.** A dentist or dental surgeon. दंतचिकित्सक; दंतविज्ञानी; दंतशल्यकर्मी

**Odontology.** Dentistry. दंतविज्ञान

**Odontolysis.** Loss or erosion of calcium from tooth. दंतापघटन

**Odontoma.** A tumour of the dental tissue. दंतार्बुद; दंत-ऊतकार्बुद; दंत-ऊतक की रसौली;

**Ameloblastic O.,** a neoplasm that contains enamel, dentin and odontogenic tissue that does not develop to form enamel. दंतवल्कप्रसू-अर्बुद;

**Complex O.,** an odontoma in which the epithelial and mesenchymal cells are completely differentiated. संकर दंतार्बुद; सम्मिश्र दंतार्बुद;

**Compound O.,** a developmental odontogenic anomaly comprising of two or more anomalous or miniature teeth. विवृत दंतार्बुद; संयुक्त दंतार्बुद; यौगिक दंतार्बुद;

**Coronary O.,** bony tumour at the crown of a tooth. शिखर दंतार्बुद; शीर्ष दंतार्बुद;

**Follicular O.,** bony shell in gums below the tooth margin, usually after the second dentition. कूपिक दंतार्बुद;

**Radicular O.,** an odontoma close to, or on the root of a tooth. दंतमूलार्बुद

**Odontoneuralgia.** Facial neuralgia caused by a carious tooth. दंततंत्रिकार्ति

**Odontonomy.** Dental nomenclature. दंतसज्ञा; दांतों की सजावट

**Odontopathy.** Any disease of the teeth. दंतविकृति; दांतों की कोई बीमारी

**Odontosis.** See **Odontogenesis.**

**Odontotherapy.** The treatment given for disease of the teeth. दंतोपचार; दंतचिकित्सा; दांतों का इलाज

**Odontotomy.** Cutting into the crown of a tooth. दंतोच्छेदन

**Odor.** See **Odour.**

**Odorant.** Something that stimulates the sense of smell. घ्राणशक्तिवर्धक; सूंघने की शक्ति बढ़ाने वाला (तत्व)

**Odoriferous.** Yielding an odour; odorous. गन्धमय; गन्धयुक्त; सगन्ध; खुशबूदार

**Odorous.** See **Odoriferous.**

**Odour.** Scent; smell; odor. गन्ध; सुगन्ध

**Odourless.** Without any smell. गन्धहीन

**Odynophagia.** Pain upon swallowing; dysphagia. कृच्छ्रनिगरण; निगरणकष्ट

**Oedema.** Accumulation of serum in cellular tissue; serous swelling; edema. शोफ; जलशोष; शोथ;

  **Cardiac O.,** a dependent oedema of the subcutaneous tissues in cardiac failure. हृदशोफ;

  **Hepatic O.,** is caused by osmotic pressure changes in the blood. यकृत्शोफ;

  **Pulmonary O.,** is a form of waterlogging of the lungs because of ventricular failure or mitral stenosis. फुप्फुसशोफ;

  **Renal O.,** results from disturbed kidney filtration in nephritis. वृक्कशोफ;

  **Subcutaneous O.,** is demonstrable by the 'pitting' produced by pressure of the finger. अधस्त्वक्-शोफ

**Oedematous.** Pertaining to oedema; edematous. शोफज; जलशोथज; जलशोथ अथवा शोफ सम्बन्धी

**Oesophageal.** Pertaining to the oesophagus; esophageal. ग्रासनली सम्बन्धी

**Oesophagectasia.** A dilated gullet (oesophagus); oesophagectasis; esophagectasia. ग्रासनलीविस्फार; ग्रासनली का फैल जाना

**Oesophagectasis.** See **Oesophagectasia.**

**Oesophagectomy.** Excision of part or the whole of the oesophagus; esophagectomy. ग्रासनली-उच्छेदन; ग्रासनली या उसके किसी भाग को काट कर हटा देना

**Oesophagitis**

**Oesophagitis.** Inflammation of oesophagus; esophagitis. ग्रासनलीशोथ; ग्रासनली का प्रदाह

**Oesophagoplasty.** A plastic operation on the oesophagus; esophagoplasty. ग्रासनलीसंधान

**Oesophagoscope.** An instrument for visualization of body cavities or organs; esophagoscope. ग्रासनलीदर्शी; ग्रासनलीगुहादर्शी

**Oesophagoscopy.** Examination of oesophagus with the help of an oesophagoscope; esophagoscopy. ग्रासनलीदर्शन; ग्रासनलीगुहादर्शी

**Oesophagotomy.** An incision into the oesophagus; esophagotomy. ग्रासनलीछेदन

**Oesophagus.** The gullet; passage from pharynx to stomach; esophagus. ग्रासनली; ग्रसनी से लेकर आमाशय तक का भाग

**Official.** Authorized by the pharmacopoea. अधिकृत (औषध); प्राधिकृत (औषध); शास्त्रोक्त (औषध); authoritative. शासकीय

**Officinale.** A chemical or pharmaceutical preparation regularly kept in a druggist's stock. आफीसिनेल; अपरिहार्य (औषध)

**O.H.** Abbreviation for **Omni Hora,** which means every hour. प्रति घण्टा; हर घण्टे में

**Oil.** A greasy liquid, not miscible with water. तेल; तैल; ऐसा तरल पदार्थ जो पानी के साथ नहीं घुलता;

    **Almond O.,** extracted from the seeds of almonds. बादाम तेल;

    **Castor O.,** a fixed oil from seeds of **Ricinus Communis,** used as a cathartic. कैस्टर आयल;

    **Coconut O.,** a semi-solid fat from the fruit of the palm. नारियल तेल;

    **Cod-liver O.,** fixed oil from the livers of the cod-fish. कॉडलिवर तेल; कॉडयकृत् तेल;

    **Croton O.,** fixed oil from the seeds of **Croton Tiglium;** oleum tigli. जमालगोटा तेल;

    **Essential O.,** see **Volatile Oil.**

    **Ethereal O.,** see **Volatile Oil.**

    **Gingeli O.,** sesame oil; til oil. तिल का तेल;

    **Nut O.,** derived from the ground-nuts. मूंगफली का तेल;

    **Olive O.,** a fixed oil from ripe olives; sweet oil. जैतून तेल; ऑलिव आयल;

    **Pea-nut O.,** fixed oil from pea-nuts. मूंगफली का तेल

Sweet O., see **Olive Oil.**

Til O., see **Gingeli Oil.**

**Volatile O.**, a substance of oily consistence, derived from a plant and characterized by aromatic odour and leaving no permanent stain on paper; essential oil; ethereal oil. वाष्पशील तेल

**Ointment.** Unguentum; a soft, fatty, medicated mixture. मरहम; मलहम; विलेपन; लेप

**Oleaginous.** Having the nature of oil. तेलीय; तैलीय; तैलाभ; तेल जैसा

**Olecranon.** The head of extremity of the elbow-joint. कूर्पर

**Oleic.** Relating to oil. तैलीय; तेल सम्बन्धी

**Oleum.** Oil. तेल; तैल;

    **O. Anisa,** an essential oil from anise. सौंफ तेल;

    **O. Olivae,** olive oil. जैतून तेल; ऑलिव आयल;

    **O. Ricini,** castor oil. कैस्टर आयल;

    **O. Sesami,** the til-oil; gingeli oil; sesame oil. तिल का तेल;

    **O. Tigli,** the croton oil. जमालगोटा तेल

**Olfaction.** The act of smelling or the sense of smell; osphresis. सूंघना; घ्राण-संवेदना; गंधज्ञान

**Olfactometer.** See **Osmometer.**

**Olfactory.** Pertaining to smelling; osphretic. घ्राण अथवा गन्ध सम्बन्धी;

    **O. Bulb,** the bulbous end of the olfactory nerve. घ्राण बल्ब; घ्राण कन्द;

    **O. Organ,** the nose. नाक; नासिका; नासा

**Oligaemia.** Diminished quantity of blood; oligemia. अल्परक्तता; रक्ताल्पता

**Oligaemic.** Affected with oligaemia; oligemic. अल्परक्ती; अल्परक्तक; रक्ताल्प

**Oligemia.** See **Oligaemia.**

**Oligemic.** See **Oligaemic.**

**Oligo-.** Prefix meaning deficiency or diminution. 'अल्प' के रूप में प्रयुक्त उपसर्ग

**Oligoamnios.** Deficiency in the amount of the amniotic fluid; oligohydramnion. उल्वतरलाल्पता

**Oligocardia.** Bradycardia. हृद्मंदता

**Oligocythaemia.** A deficiency of red corpuscles in the blood. रुधिर-कणिकाल्पता; रक्त में लाल कणों की कमी

**Oligocystic.** Consisting of only a few cysts. अल्पपुटीय

**Oligodactylia.** See **Oligodactyly.**

**Oligodactyly.** Congenital thinness or deficiency in number of digits; oligodactylia. अल्पांगुलिता

**Oligodipsia.** Abnormal absence of thirst. तृष्णालोप; तृष्णाभाव; प्यास का अभाव; प्यास न लगना

**Oligodontia.** Abnormal smallness of teeth. तघुदंतता;

**Oligogalactia.** Slight or scanty secretion of milk. अल्पदुग्धस्राव

**Oligohydramnion.** See **Oligoamnios.**

**Oligomenorrhea.** See **Oligomenorrhoea.**

**Oligomenorrhoea.** Scanty menstruation; oligomenorrhea. अल्पार्तव; ऋतुस्राव की अत्यल्प मात्रा

**Oligophrenia.** Mental deficiency. मन्दबुद्धिता; अल्पबुद्धिता; जड़बुद्धिता

**Oligopnea.** See **Oligopnoea.**

**Oligopnoea.** Deficient respiration; oligopnea. अल्पश्वसन

**Oligoptyalism.** Scanty salivation. अल्पलारता; लाराल्पता

**Oligoria.** An abnormal disliking of a person or thing. अरुचि

**Oligospermia.** Deficiency of spermatozoa in the semen; oligozoospermia. अल्पशुक्राणुता; वीर्य में शुक्राणुओं की कमी होना

**Oligotrophia.** See **Oligotrophy.**

**Oligotrophy.** Deficient nutrition; oligotrophia. अल्पपोषण

**Oligozoospermia.** See **Oligospermia.**

**Oliguria.** Scantiness of urine. अल्पमूत्रता; मूत्राल्पता; पेशाब की कमी

**Oliva.** An olive-shaped grey body behind the anterior pyramid of the medulla oblongata. वर्तुलिका

**Olivae.** Plural of **Oliva.**

**Olivary.** Relating to an olive, or shaped like an olive. जैतूनाकार; वर्तुलिका अथवा जैतून सम्बन्धी

**Olive.** The olive tree or its fruits. जैतून;

    **O. Oil,** see **Oleum Olivae.**

**Omagra.** Gout of the shoulders. स्कन्धवात; कंधों का गठिया

**Omalgia.** Neuralgia of the shoulders. स्कन्धार्ति; स्कन्धशूल; कन्धों का दर्द

**Omarthritis.** Inflammation of the shoulder-joints. स्कन्धसन्धिशोथ; कन्धों के जोड़ों का प्रदाह

**Omenta.** Plural of **Omentum.**

**Omental.** Relating to omentum; epiploic. वपा सम्बन्धी

**Omentectomy.** Excision of the omentum. वपा-उच्छेदन

**Omentitis.** Inflammation of the omentum. वपाशोथ; वपाजाल-प्रदाह

**Omentofixation.** See **Omentopexy.**

**Omentopexy.** Fixation of the omentum to the abdominal wall or an adjacent organ; omentofixation; epiplopexy. वपास्थिरीकरण

**Omentotomy.** Incision of the omentum. वपाछेदन

**Omentum.** A fold of peritoneum or serous covering of the bowels. वपा; वपाजाल; पेट का पर्दा जो उदरस्थ आशयों को जठर के साथ जोड़ता है

**Omitis.** Inflammation in, or on the shoulders. स्कन्धशोथ; कंधे का प्रदाह

**Omni Bihora.** After every two hours. प्रति दो घण्टे बाद; हर दो घण्टे बाद; दो-दो घण्टे में

**Omni Hora.** Every hour. प्रति घण्टा; एक-एक घण्टे में

**Omni Mane.** Every morning. नित्य प्रात:; रोज सुबह

**Omni Nocte.** Every night. नित्य रात्रि; रोज रात को

**Omnivorous.** Living on food of all kinds. सर्वहारा; हर प्रकार के भोजन पर जीवनयापन करने वाला

**Omohyoid.** Pertaining to the scapula and the hyoid. अंसकण्ठिकी; स्कन्धफलक एवं कण्ठिका सम्बन्धी

**Omphalectomy.** Excision of the umbilicus. नाभि-उच्छेदन

**Omphalelcosis.** Ulceration at the umbilicus. नाभिव्रण

**Omphalic.** Pertaining to the umbilicus. नाभिपरक; नाभि सम्बन्धी

**Omphalitis.** Inflammation of the umbilicus. नाभिशोथ; नाभि का प्रदाह

**Omphalocele.** Umbilical hernia. नाभिवर्ध्म; नाभितुण्ड; नाभिस्फोट; नाभि-हर्निया

**Omphaloenteric.** Relating to the umbilicus and the intestine. नाभि एवं आंत्र सम्बन्धी

**Omphalomesenteric.** Pertaining to the umbilicus and mesentery. नाभिआंत्रयोजनिक; नाभि एवं आंत्रयोजनी सम्बन्धी

**Omphalophlebitis.** Inflammation of the umbilical veins. नाभिशिराशोथ

**Omphalorrhagia.** Bleeding from the umbilicus. नाभिरक्तस्त्रवण; नाभि से खून बहना

**Omphalorrhexis.** Rupture of the umbilical cord during childbirth. नाभिरज्जुविदर

**Omphalos.** The umbilicus. नाभि

**Omphalotomy.** Cutting of the umbilical cord at birth. नाभिरज्जु-उच्छेदन

**Onanism.** Masturbation; incomplete coition. हस्तमैथुन; अपूर्णमैथुन; आत्मव्यभिचार

**Onanist.** One who is addicted to onanism. आत्मव्यभिचारी

**Oncogenesis.** Origin and growth of a neoplasm. अर्बुदजनन; रसौली बनना

**Oncogenic.** Causing, inducing or being suitable for the formation and development of a neoplasm; oncogenous. अर्बुदजनक

**Oncogenous.** See **Oncogenic.**

**Oncologist.** A specialist in oncology. अर्बुदविज्ञानी

**Oncology.** The science of tumours. अर्बुदविद्या; अर्बुदविज्ञान; अर्बुदप्रकरण

**Oncolysis.** Destruction of a neoplasm. अर्बुदलयन; अर्बुदापघटन

**Oncolytic.** Pertaining to, characterized by, or causing oncolysis. अर्बुदलयनिक; अर्बुदापघटनीय

**Oncoma.** A tumour. अर्बुद; रसौली

**Oncometer.** An instrument for measuring the size of a tumour. अर्बुदमापी

**Oncosis.** Formation of tumour. अर्बुदोत्पत्ति; अर्बुदरचना

**Oncotic.** Relating to, or caused by oncosis. अर्बुदोत्पत्ति सम्बन्धी

**Oncotomy.** Incision of a boil, abscess or tumour. अर्बुदछेदन

**Oneirodynia.** Nightmare. दु:स्वप्न; restlessness in sleep. अशान्त निद्रा; बेचैन नींद

**Oniomania.** A morbid desire to buy everything. क्रयोन्माद; खरीदारी करने का पागलपन

**Ontogeny.** The history of individual development. व्यक्तिवृत्त; जीवविकास का इतिहास

**Onychalgia.** Pain in the nails. नखार्ति; नखशूल

**Onychatrophia.** Atrophy of nails; onychatrophy. नखशोष

**Onychatrophy.** See **Onychatrophia.**

**Onychectomy.** Surgical removal of nails. नख-उच्छेदन

**Onychia.** Chronic inflammation of matrix of a nail; whitlow. नखशोथ; अंगुलबेढ़ा; अंगुल्याग्रप्रदाह; चिप्य

**Onychitis.** Inflammation of the soft parts about nails; onyxitis. नखमांसशोथ; नखशोथ; नाखून के चारों ओर के नरम भागों का प्रदाह

**Onychocryptosis.** Ingrowing of the nail. नखान्त:बृद्धि; नाखुन के नीचे किसी प्रकार की नवोत्पत्ति होना; अन्त:नखोत्पत्ति

**Onychogryposis.** Thickening and curvature of the nails. नखबक्रता; नखशृंगता; नाखुनों का मोटा और टेढ़ा-मेढ़ा होना

**Onychoid.** Resembling a nail. नखाभ; नखवत्; नाखून से मिलता-जुलता

**Onycholysis.** Loosening of the nails. नखलयन; नखापघटन

**Onychoma.** A tumour arising from the nail or nail-bed. नखार्बुद

**Onychomycosis.** A parasitic disease of the nails. नखकवकता; नखदद्रु; नाखुनों का एक परजीवी रोग

**Onychopathy.** Any disease of the nails; onychosis. नखविकृति

**Onychophagia.** See **Onychophagy.**

**Onychophagy.** Biting of the nails; onychophagia. नखचर्वणता; दान्तों से नाखुन कुतरना

**Onychoplasty.** A corrective or plastic operation of the matrix of the nail. नखसंधान

**Onychosis.** See **Onychopathy.**

**Onychotomy.** Incision into a nail. नखछेदन

**Onyx.** A nail; unguis. नख; नाखुन

**Onyxis.** A sinking or ingrowing of the nail into the flesh. अन्त:नखोत्पत्ति; सहजअन्तवर्धीनख; नाखुन के अन्दर मांस बढ़ना

**Onyxitis.** See **Onychitis.**

**Oocyst.** The envelope which surrounds the cell. युग्मकपुटी; सम्पुटित युग्मक; कोशिका को घेर कर रखने वाला आवरण

**Oocyte.** An ovum before it has left a Graafian follicle. डिम्बाणुजनकोशिका; पूर्वडिम्बकोशिका;

    **Primary O.,** an oocyte during its growth phage and prior to completion of the first maturation division. प्राथमिक डिम्बाणुजनकोशिका;

    **Secondary O.,** an oocyte resulting from first maturation division. द्वित्तीयक डिम्बाणुजनकोशिका

**Oogamous.** Generated by means of an ovum. डिम्बजनक; डिम्बाणुजनक

**Oogenesis.** The production and formation of ova in ovary; ovigenesis. डिम्बजनता; डिम्बपरिपक्वता; डिम्बोत्पति एवं रचना

**Oogenetic.** Producing ova; ovigenetic. डिम्बजनक

**Oogonia.** Plural of **Oogonium.**

**Oogonium.** The primitive egg mother cell, from which the oocytes are developed. डिम्बाणुप्रसूजन

**Ookinete.** The actively motile fertilized cell. चलयुग्मक; सक्रिय चलनिषिक्त-कोशिका

**Oophoralgia.** Pain in the ovaries. डिम्बाशयशूल; डिम्बाशयार्ति; डिम्बाशयपीड़ा

**Oophorectomy.** Excision of an ovary; ovariectomy; ovariotomy. डिम्बाशयोच्छेदन; डिम्बग्रन्थि-उच्छेदन; डिम्बाशय-उच्छेदन; डिम्बाशय को काट कर निकाल देना

**Oophoritis.** Inflammation of an ovary; ovaritis. डिम्बाशयशोथ; डिम्बाशय-प्रदाह

**Oophorocystectomy.** Excision of an ovarian cyst. डिम्बाणुपुटी-उच्छेदन

**Oophoroma.** A tumour of the ovary. डिम्बाशयार्बुद; डिम्बग्रन्थि की कोई रसौली

**Oophoromania.** Insanity from ovarian disease. डिम्बाशयविकृतिजविक्षिप्ति; डिम्बाशय के किसी रोग के कारण होने वाला पागलपन

**Oophoron.** Ovary. डिम्बाशय; डिम्बग्रन्थि

**Oophoropexy.** Surgical fixation of an ovary. डिम्बाशय-सम्मिलन; डिम्बग्रन्थि-सम्मिलन

**Oophoroplasty.** Plastic operation upon an ovary. डिम्बाशयसंधान; डिम्बग्रन्थिसंधान

**Ooplasm.** The protoplasmic portion of the ovum; ovoplasm. डिम्बद्रव्य

**Oosperm.** A fertilized ovum. जननाणु; निषिक्त-डिम्ब

**Ootid.** A ripe ovum after first maturation has been completed and the second has begun. डिम्बाणुप्रसू

**Opacity.** Imperviousness to light. अपार्यता; अपारदर्शिता; अपारभासिता; पारान्धता; धुँधलापन; फुल्ली

**Opaque.** Non-transparent; impervious to light. अपारदर्शी; अपारभासी; पारान्ध; धुँधला

**O.P.D.** Out-patient Department. बहिरंग रोगी विभाग

M.D.F.-23

**Opening.** An orifice. मुख; द्वार; छिद्र; छेद; विवर

**Operation.** Any act performed with instrument by the hands of a surgeon; any surgical procedure, or operative technique. शल्यकर्म; शस्त्रकर्म; शल्यक्रिया; शल्योपचार; चीर-फाड़; ऑपरेशन

**Operative.** Pertaining to an operation. शल्यक्रियात्मक; शल्योपचारक; शल्यचिकित्सा सम्बन्धी; active. सक्रिय; effective. प्रभावी

**Operator.** One who performs surgical operations. शल्यकर्मी

**Opercula.** Plural of **Operculum.**

**Opercular.** Relating to an operculum. प्रच्छद सम्बन्धी

**Operculum.** A lid or cover. प्रच्छद; आच्छद; छद; पलक; आवरण; ढक्कन

**Ophthalmalgia.** Pain in the eye. नेत्रशूल; चक्षुशूल; नेत्रार्ति; आँख में दर्द होना

**Ophthalmia.** Inflammation of the eye; ophthalmitis. नेत्राभिष्यन्द; नेत्रप्रदाह; आँख आना; आँख दुखना; नेत्रशोथ;

    **Phlyctenular O.,** conjunctivitis marked by the formation of vesicles in the epithelial layer of the cornea or conjunctiva. अलजीय नेत्राभिष्यन्द;

    **O. Neonatorum,** opthalmia of the newborn. नवजात नेत्राभिष्यन्द

**Ophthalmic.** Pertaining to the eye. नेत्र सम्बन्धी; नेत्रीय; one affected with ophthalmia. नेत्राभिष्यन्दग्रस्त

**Ophthalmist.** See **Ophthalmologist.**

**Ophthalmitis.** Inflammation of the eye; ophthalmia. नेत्रशोथ; नेत्र-प्रदाह; नेत्राभिष्यन्द; आँख आना; आँख दुखना

**Ophthalmo-.** Prefix signifying the eye. 'नेत्र', 'चक्षु' अथवा 'अक्षि' के रूप में प्रयुक्त उपसर्ग

**Ophthalmocele.** Protrusion of the eyeball. नेत्रगोलकविस्फार; अक्षिगोलकविस्फार; नेत्रगोलक का बाहर की ओर फैल जाना

**Ophthalmocopia.** Eye-fatigue; eye-strain; asthenopia. नेत्रावसाद; आँखों का थक जाना

**Ophthalmodiaphnoscope.** Instrument for examining the interior of the eye. नेत्रपार्श्वप्रदीपक

**Ophthalmodynamometer.** Instrument for determining pressure in ophthalmic arteries. नेत्ररक्तदाबमापी

**Ophthalmodynamometry.** Use of an ophthalmodynamometer. नेत्ररक्तदाबमिति

**Ophthalmodynia.** Violent inflammatory pain in the eye. नेत्रवेदना; नेत्रपीड़ा; आँख में प्रचण्ड प्रदाहक पीड़ा होना

**Ophthalmograph.** An instrument for recording the movement of the eyes during reading. नेत्रगतिलेखी

**Ophthalmography.** A description of the eye. नेत्रगतिलेखन; आँख की गतियों का वर्णन

**Ophthalmolith.** A calculus of the lacrimal duct; dacryolith. नेत्राश्मरी; नेत्रपथरी

**Opthalmologist.** One who studies ophthalmology; ophthalmist. नेत्रविज्ञानी; नेत्ररोगविशेषज्ञ

**Ophthalmology.** The medical specialty concerned with the diseases of the eyes and conversation of the vision. नेत्रविज्ञान; नेत्ररोगविज्ञान; चक्षुरोगविज्ञान

**Ophthalmomalacia.** An abnormal softness of the eye. नेत्रमृदुता; आँख की अस्वाभाविक कोमलता

**Ophthalmometer.** An instrument for measuring the eye, especially the amount of corneal curvature. नेत्रस्वच्छवैषम्यमापी; नेत्र की किरण-बक्रता या अपवर्तक शक्ति को मापने का यंत्र

**Ophthalmometry.** The use of ophthalmometer. नेत्रस्वच्छवैषम्यमिति; नेत्र की किरण-बक्रता या अपवर्तक शक्ति को मापना

**Ophthalmomyitis.** See **Ophthalmomyositis.**

**Ophthalmomyositis.** Inflammation of the extrinsic muscle of the eye; ophthalmomyitis. नेत्रपेशीशोथ; आँख की बाहरी पेशी का प्रदाह

**Ophthalmomyotomy.** Surgical section of one or more extrinsic muscles of the eye. नेत्रपेशीछेदन

**Ophthalmopathy.** Any disease of the eye. नेत्ररोग; चक्षुरोग; नेत्रविकृति; आँख का कोई रोग

**Ophthalmophacometer.** An instrument to ascertain how far the lens lies behind the cornea and to measure the two surfaces of the lens during rest, or during accommodation; ophthalmophakometer. नेत्रलेन्समापी; नेत्रलेन्समापकयंत्र

**Ophthalmophakometer.** See **Ophthalmophacometer.**

**Ophthalmoplasty.** Any plastic operation upon the eye. नेत्रसंधान

**Ophthalmoplegia.** Paralysis of ocular muscles. नेत्रपेशीघात; अक्षिपेशीघात; नेत्रघात; चक्षुस्तम्भ; आँख का लकवा;

 **Exophthalmic O.,** ophthalmoplegia of the eyeballs. बहिर्गताक्षि नेत्रपेशीघात;

**External O.**, see **Ophthalmoplegia Externa.**

**Internal O.**, see **Ophthalmoplegia Interna.**

**Partial O.**, ophthalmoplegia involving only one or two of the extrinsic or intrinsic ocular muscles. आंशिक नेत्रपेशीघात;

**Progressive O.**, gradual paralysis of all the muscles of both eyes. प्रगामी नेत्रपेशीघात; नेत्रों का मन्दगतिक पक्षाघात होना;

**Total O.**, see **Ophthalmoplegia Totalis.**

**O. Externa**, paralysis of the external muscles; external ophthalmoplegia. बाह्यनेत्रपेशीघात; बाहरी नेत्रपेशियों का पक्षाघात होना;

**O. Interna**, paralysis of the internal muscles; internal ophthalmoplegia. आन्तरिक नेत्रपेशीघात; अन्दरूनी नेत्रपेशियों का पक्षाघात होना;

**O. Totalis**, that involving the iris and ciliary body, as well as the external muscles; total ophthalmoplegia. सर्वनेत्रपेशीघात; नेत्रों के समस्त अवयवों का पक्षाघात होना

**Ophthalmoptosis.** Exophthalmos. नेत्रोत्सेध; बहिर्गताक्षि; आँखों का बाहर की ओर फैलना

**Ophthalmorrhagia.** Haemorrhage of the eyes. नेत्ररक्तस्राव; आँखों से रक्तस्राव होना

**Ophthalmorrhexis.** Rupture of an eyeball. नेत्रविदरण; नेत्रगोलक फट जाना

**Ophthalmos.** The eye. नेत्र; चक्षु; अक्षि; आँख

**Ophthalmoscope.** An arrangement of mirrors for illumination of the interior of the eye, as to judge of its condition, especially the retina. नेत्रदर्शी; नेत्रान्तदर्शी; नेत्रान्तवीक्षकयन्त्र; दृष्टिपटलदर्शी

**Ophthalmoscopy.** Examination of the interior of the eye with the help of opthalmoscope. नेत्रदर्शन; नेत्रान्तदर्शन; दृष्टिपटलदर्शन; चक्षुजांच; आँख के भीतरी भाग का निरीक्षण करना;

**Direct O.**, the method of the erect or upright image, the observer's eye and the ophthalmoscope being brought close to the eye of the patient. प्रत्यक्ष दृष्टिपटलदर्शन;

**Indirect O.**, the method of the inverted image, in which the observer's eye is placed about sixteen inches far from that of the patient, and a twenty diopter biconcave lens is held at a distance about two inches of the fundus. अप्रत्यक्ष दृष्टिपटलदर्शन

**Opiate.** A preparation of opium for producing sleep; it is commonly applied to any medicine capable of procuring sleep. निद्रावह; निद्राकारी; पीड़ाहर; वेदनाहर; अफीममिश्रित औषधि

**Opiomania.** A morbid desire for opium. अहिफेनोन्माद; अफीमोन्माद; अफीम खाने की अप्रतिहत इच्छा होना

**Opisthion.** The middle point of the posterior edge of the foramen magnum opening at the occipital bone. पश्चमध्यबिन्दु

**Opisthotic.** Relating to posterior parts of the ear apparatus. कर्णपश्चक; कर्णतंत्र के पिछले भागों से सम्बन्धित

**Opisthotonos.** Spasmodic bending backward of the body. बाह्यापतानक; बाह्यायाम; धनुर्वात; शरीर का पीछे की ओर झुक कर अकड़ जाना

**Opium.** The concrete juice of poppy. अहिफेन; अफीम

**Opiumism.** An opium-taking habit. अफीमात्यय; अहिफेनात्यय; अहिफेनिलता; अफीम के अपव्यवहार का कुफल

**Opobalsam.** Balsam of Mecca. गुग्गुल

**Opodeldoc.** Soap liniment. एक स्वफेनलेप; एक कर्पूरयुक्त साबुनी लिनिमेण्ट

**Opotherapy.** The treatment of diseases by the administration of animal organs or extract from them. रस-चिकित्सा; अंगरस-चिकित्सा

**Ophthalmolith.** A calculus of the eye. नेत्रपथरी; नेत्राश्मरी; आँख की पथरी

**Oppilition.** Obstruction. अवरोध; रुकावट; constipation. मलावरोध; कोष्ठबद्धता; मलबद्धता; कब्ज

**Oppression.** A sense of weight, especially about chest, impeding respiration. श्वासावरोध; श्वासरोध; छाती में भारीपन की अनुभूति

**Opsialgia.** Facial neuralgia. आननार्ति; आननशूल; चेहरे का दर्द

**Optesthesia.** Visual sensibility to light stimuli. दृष्टि-संवेदना

**Optic.** Pertaining to the sight or eye; optical. दृष्टिपरक; दृष्टिगत; चाक्षुष; अक्षिक; नैत्रिक; दृष्टि अथवा नेत्र सम्बन्धी;

  **O. Nerve,** the nerve of the second pair giving sensibility to the eye. नेत्र-तंत्रिका; चक्षु-तंत्रिका; अक्षि-तंत्रिका;

  **O. Thalamus,** the great posterior ganglion of the brain. अक्षि-चेतक; मस्तिष्क का पिछला तंत्रिका-उपकेन्द्र

**Optical.** See **Optic.**

**Optician.** A maker of lenses and optical instruments. काशित्रिक; नेत्रोपकरण-निर्माता

**Optics.** The science of light and vision. दृग्विद्या; प्रकाशिकी; प्रकाशविज्ञान; प्रकाश एवं दृष्टि सम्बन्धी विज्ञान

**Optimism.** A hopeful view of things. आशावाद; आशावादिता; आशावृत्ति

**Optimum.** The most desirable state of affairs. इष्टतम; श्रेष्ठ; सर्वोत्तम; अनुकूलतम;

   **O. Temperature,** the temperature that is suitable for a procedure or operation. इष्टतम तापमान; अनुकूलतम तापमान

**Optist.** One who refracts without drugs; optometerist; refractionist. दृष्टिमितिज्ञ; नेत्रापवर्तनमितिज्ञ; नेत्रापर्वतनविशेषज्ञ

**Optometer.** Instrument for measuring refractive power of eye. दृष्टिमापी; नेत्रापवर्तनमापी; नेत्रापवर्तनमापकयंत्र

**Optometerist.** See **Optist.**

**Optometry.** Use of an optometer; measurement of the visual refractive power. दृष्टिमिति; नेत्रापवर्तनमिति

**Optomyometer.** An instrument for determining the relative power of the extrinsic muscles of the eye. नेत्रपेशीमापी

**Ora.** Plural of **Os,** in case of mouth. मुख

**Oral.** Relating to the mouth. मुखी; मौखिक; मुख सम्बन्धी;

   **O. Surgery,** surgery in and about the mouth. मुखी शल्योपचार

**Orbicular.** Circular; spheric. वृत्ताकार; वर्तुलाकार; मण्डलाकार; गोल; गोलाकार

**Orbicularis.** A name given to muscles whose fibres encircle an orifice. वर्तुलपेशियाँ

**Orbit.** One of the two bony cavities in which the eyes are placed; orbita. नेत्रगुहा; नेत्रगह्वर; नेत्रकोटर; अक्षिकूप; कपाल का वह अस्थिकुहर जिसमें आँख स्थिर रहती है

**Orbita.** See **Orbit.**

**Orbitae.** Plural of **Orbit.**

**Orbital.** Relating to the orbit. नेत्रगह्वरीय; नेत्रकोटरीय; नेत्रगह्वर अथवा नेत्रकोटर सम्बन्धी

**Orbitalis.** The superior palpebral muscle. अक्षिका (पेशी)

**Orbitonometer.** An instrument for measuring the resistance of the eyeball on being pushed back into the orbit. नेत्रपश्चदाबमापी

**Orbitonometry.** Determining the displacement of the eyeball into the orbit by using the orbitonometer. नेत्रपश्चदाबमिति

**Orbitotomy.** Surgical incision into the eye. नेत्रगुहाछेदन

**Orchialgia.** Pain in the testicles. वृषणशूल; वृषण-पीड़ा

**Orchidectomy.** Castration of the male; orchiectomy. वृषणोच्छेदन; वृषण-उच्छेदन

# Orchidopexia 742

**Orchidopexia.** See **Orchidopexy.**

**Orchidopexy.** The suturing up of a testicle; orchidopexia. वृषणस्थिरीकरण

**Orchiectomy.** See **Orchidectomy.**

**Orchidotomy.** See **Orchotomy.**

**Orchiocele.** A tumour of the testicle. वृषणार्बुद; वृषणकोष की रसौली; scrotal hernia. वृषण-हर्निया; अण्डकोष का हर्निया

**Orchiopathy.** Any disease of the testicle. वृषणविकृति; अण्डकोष का कोई रोग

**Orchioplasty.** Plastic surgery of the testis. वृषणसंधान

**Orchiotomy.** Incision into a testis. वृषणछेदन

**Orchis.** The testicle. वृषणग्रन्थि; वृषण; अण्डकोष

**Orchises.** Plural of **Orchis.**

**Orchitis.** Inflammation of the testicle. वृषणशोथ; वृषणग्रन्थिशोथ; वृषण-प्रदाह; अण्डशोथ; अण्डग्रन्थिशोथ; अण्डकोष का प्रदाह

**Orchotomy.** Excision of a testicle; castration; orchidotomy. वृषणग्रन्थि-उच्छेदन; अण्डग्रन्थि-उच्छेदन; अण्डकोष-उच्छेदन

**Order.** An arrangement or sequence of events. क्रम; rule. नियम; procedure. तरीका

**Orderly.** A male attendant. अर्दली

**Organ.** Such structure to an organ as is essential to the carrying of some process. अंग; इन्द्रिय; शरीर की कोई क्रियाशील रचना

**Organic.** Relating to an organ. आंगिक; कायिक; denoting chemical substances containing the compounds of carbons. कार्बनिक; relating to an animal or vegetable organism. जैवी; जैव;

O. Disease, a disease accompanied by demonstrable changes in the body. आंगिक रोग

**Organa.** Plural of **Organum.**

**Organism.** Any living individual, whether plant or animal, considered as a whole. जीव

**Organization.** Orderly structure of parts. रचना; बनावट

**Organogenesis.** Formation of organs during development; organogeny. अंगजनन

**Organogenetic.** See **Organogenic.**

**Organogenic.** Relating to organogenesis; organogenetic. अंगजनन सम्बन्धी

**Organogeny.** See **Organogenesis.**

**Organology.** The science of the organs. अंगविज्ञान; अंगशास्त्र; अवयवविज्ञान

**Organon.** A system. प्रणाली; सिद्धान्त; तर्कशास्त्र; an organ; organum. अंग

**Organopathy.** The disease in an organ. अंगरोग; अंगविकृति; अंगविकार; the living economy. अवयवरुजा; the local application of drug. औषध-लेपन; औषधियों का स्थानिक प्रयोग

**Organotherapy.** The treatment of diseases by the administration of animal organs, or extracts from them. अंगरस-चिकित्सा

**Organotrope.** See **Organotropic.**

**Organotrophic.** Concerning the nutrition of the organ. अंगपोषी

**Organotropic.** Having affinity for certain organs; organotrope. अंगरागी; अंगप्रेरक

**Organum.** An organ. अंग

**Orgasm.** Highest point of excitement in sexual intercourse. कामोत्तेजना; कामोन्माद; रतिक्षण

**Orientation.** The location of one's position in a given environment. दिग्विन्यास; अभिविन्यास

**Orifice.** An opening or entrance; orificium; oris. द्वार; मुख; रन्ध्र; प्रवेशपथ;

   **Anal O.,** the anus. गुद; मलद्वार;

   **Cardiac O.,** opening of oesophagus into the stomach. हृद्द्वार; हृद्-रन्ध्र;

   **Mitral O.,** opening between the atrium and ventricle. द्विकपर्दी मुख; द्विकपर्दी रन्ध्र;

   **Pyloric O.,** opening from the stomach into the duodenum; pylorus. जठरनिर्गम

**Orificia.** Plural of **Orificium.**

**Orificial.** Pertaining to an orifice. मुखी; द्वार या मुख सम्बन्धी

**Orificium.** See **Orifice.**

**Origin.** The commencement, source or beginning. प्रारम्भ; उदय; उद्भव; उद्गम; मूलस्रोत

**Oris.** See **Orifice.**

**Ornithosis.** Disease acquired through birds. पक्षीजन्यरोग; पक्षियों द्वारा उत्पन्न होने वाला; रोग; parrot fever. शुक-ज्वर

**Orogenital.** Pertaining to the mouth and the external genital area. मुख एवं बाह्य-जननांगी क्षेत्र सम्बन्धी

**Orotherapy.** Whey-cure. तक्रचिकित्सा; तक्रोपचार; छाछ द्वारा की जाने वाली चिकित्सा

**Orthetics.** See **Orthotics**.

**Orthodontia.** The correction of irregularities of the teeth. दन्तवैषम्यसुधार; दन्ताजंव; दान्तों की सिधाई

**Orthodontics.** A branch of dentistry dealing with prevention and correction of irregularities of teeth. विषमदन्तविज्ञान; दान्तों के दोष को सुधारने सम्बन्धी विज्ञान

**Orthodontist.** A dentist who corrects irregularities of teeth. दन्तवैषम्यवेत्ता; दन्तवैषम्यविज्ञानी

**Orthopaedic.** Concerning orthopaedics or the correction of deformities; orthopedic. विकलांग; विकृतांग

**Orthopaedics.** The medical specialty concerned with the bones, joints and other supporting tissues; orthopedics. विकलांगविज्ञान; विकृतांगोपचार; अस्थियों, सन्धियों तथा अन्य पोषक ऊतकों से सम्बन्धित विशेष चिकित्सा पद्धति

**Orthopaedist.** One practising orthopaedic surgery; orthopedist. विकलांगविज्ञानी; विकृतांगचिकित्सक

**Orthopaedy.** The science that treats of deformities of bones, joints, and other supporting tissues; orthopedy. विकलांगचिकित्सा; विकृतांगोपचार; अस्थियों, सन्धियों तथा अन्य पोषक ऊतकों के दोषों से सम्बन्धित विज्ञान

**Orthopedic.** See **Orthopaedic**.

**Orthopedics.** See **Orthopaedics**.

**Orthopedist.** See **Orthopaedist**.

**Orthopedy.** See **Orthopaedy**.

**Orthophoria.** A tending of the visual lines in parallelism. नेत्रअविचलनप्रवृत्ति

**Orthophoric.** Relating to orthophoria. नेत्रअविचलनप्रवृत्ति सम्बन्धी

**Orthopnea.** Difficult respiration relieved only in an upright position; orthopnoea. ऊर्ध्वस्थश्वसन; ऋजुश्वासता; लेट कर सांस लेने की अशक्तता

**Orthopnoea.** See **Orthopnea**.

**Orthostatic.** Caused by the upright position. ऊर्ध्वस्थस्थितिज

**Orthotics.** The science concerned with the making and fitting of orthopaedic appliances; orthetics. कृत्रिमअंगविज्ञान

**Orthotist.** One skilled in orthotics. कृत्रिमअंगविज्ञानी; कृत्रिमअंगवेत्ता

**Orthotonos.** A tetanic cramp in which the body is held straight. समतान; एक धनुष्टम्भी ऐंठन जिसमें शरीर सीधा तन जाता है

**O.S.** Oculus sinister; left eye. बामाक्षि; बायां नेत्र; बाईं आँख

**Os.** The mouth. मुख, मुँह; bone; ossis. अस्थि; हड्डी; an opening into a hollow organ or canal. द्वार; छिद्र;

**O. Calcis,** the bone of the tarsus which forms the heel. गुल्फास्थि; गुल्फिकास्थि; एड़ी की हड्डी;

**O. Coccygeus,** the small bone at the end of the vertebral column; coccyx. पुच्छास्थि; गुदास्थि; अनुत्रिक;

**O. Coxae,** the innominate bone. श्रोणि;

**O. Femoris,** the thigh bone; femur. ऊर्विका; ऊरु-अस्थि; ऊर्वस्थि; जांघ की हड्डी;

**O. Frontale,** the large single bone forming the forehead and the upper margin and roof of the orbit on either side; frontal bone. ललाटास्थि; माथे की हड्डी;

**O. Humeri,** the humerus. प्रगण्डिका;

**O. Hyodeum,** U-shaped bone at the base of the tongue; hyoid bone. कण्ठिकास्थि;

**O. Innominatum,** the innominate or hip-bone. श्रोणि; नितम्बास्थि;

**O. Ischii,** the ischium. आसनास्थि; नितम्बास्थि; कूल्हे की हड्डी;

**O. Pubis,** the pubic bone. जघनास्थि; जांघ की हड्डी;

**O. Temporale,** the temporal bone. कर्णपटास्थि; कनपट्टी की हड्डी;

**O. Unguis,** the lacrimal bone. अश्रु-अस्थि; अश्रुग्रन्थि की हड्डी;

**O. Uteri,** the entrance of the womb. जरायुमुख

**Oscedo.** Yawning. जम्भाई; जम्हाई

**Oscheal.** Relating to scrotum; scrotal. वृषणकोषीय; वृषणकोष सम्बन्धी

**Oscheitis.** Inflammation of scrotum; oschitis. वृषणकोषप्रदाह; वृषणकोषशोथ; अण्डकोषशोथ; अण्डकोषप्रदाह; अण्डकोष का प्रदाह

**Oscheocele.** Scrotal hernia. वृषणकोष-हर्निया; अण्डकोष-विस्फार

**Oscheoplasty.** Plastic repair of the scrotum; scrotoplasty. वृषणसंधान

**Oscheoma.** A tumour of the testicle; oscheoncus. वृषणार्बुद; अण्डकोष की रसौली

**Oscheoncus.** See **Oscheoma.**

**Oschitis.** See **Oscheitis.**

**Oscillation.** A swimming or vibration. दोलन; प्रदोलन; थिरकन; कम्पन

**Oscillometer.** An apparatus for measuring oscillation of any kind. दोलनमापी

**Oscillometry.** Use of an oscillometer. दोलनमिति

**Oscitation.** The act of yawning or gaping. तन्द्रा; सुस्ती; जम्भाई; जम्हाई

**Oscula.** Plural of **Osculum.**

**Osculation.** The act of kissing. चुम्बन; अधिस्पर्श

**Osculum.** A small aperture. लघुछिद्र; छोटा-सा छेद; निर्गमद्वार

**Osmics.** The science of olfaction. घ्राणविज्ञान

**Osmium.** A rare metal associated with platinum and iridum. गुर्धातु; गुरुधातु; एक भूरे रंग की धातु

**Osmolar.** See **Osmotic.**

**Osmolarity.** The osmotic pressure exerted by a substance in aqueous solution. परासारिता; परासरणीप्रभाव

**Osmometer.** Instrument for testing the sense of smell; olfactometer. घ्राणसंवेदनामापी; घ्राणसंवेदनामापकयंत्र; one for velocity of osmotic force. रसाकर्षमापी; परिसरणमापी; परासरणमापी

**Osmosis.** The passage of substance in solution through animal membranes. रसाकर्षण; परासरण; अभिसरण; प्रसरण

**Osmotic.** Pertaining to osmosis; osmolar. रसाकर्षी; परासरणी; परासरणीय

**Osphresis.** See **Olfaction.**

**Osphresiology.** The science of odours, or sense of smell. घ्राणविज्ञान

**Osphretic.** See **Olfactory.**

**Ossa.** Plural of **Os** in case of bone.

**Osseous.** Bony; osteal. अस्थिमय; अस्थिवत्; अस्थ्याभ; हड्डी जैसा

**Ossicle.** Any small bone; bonelet; ossiculum. अस्थिका; लघ्वास्थि; छोटी हड्डी

**Ossiculum.** See **Ossicle.**

**Ossiferous.** Bearing or producing bone-tissue; ossific. अस्थितन्तुजनक; अस्थिजन; अस्थिमय; अस्थिज

**Ossific.** See **Ossiferous.**

**Ossification.** The formation of bony matter; ostosis. अस्थीभवन; अस्थीकरण; अस्थिविकास; हड्डी बनना

**Ossifluent.** Breaking down and softening of the bony tissues. अस्थिदौर्बल्य; अस्थिमृदुता; हड्डियों की कमजोरी और कोमलता

**Ossify.** To change into bone. अस्थीकरण करना या होना; अस्थीभवन होना या करना

**Ossis.** Bone. अस्थि; हड्डी

**Ostalgia.** Pain in bone; ostealgia; osteodynia. अस्थ्यार्ति; अस्थिशूल; अस्थिपीड़ा; अस्थिवेदना; हड्डी में दर्द

**Osteal.** See **Osseous.**

**Ostealgia.** See **Ostalgia.**

**Ostectomy.** Excision of a bone. अस्थि-उच्छेदन; अस्थ्युच्छेदन; हड्डी को काट कर निकाल देना

**Osteitis.** Inflammation of the bone; ostitis. अस्थिशोथ; अस्थिप्रदाह; हड्डी का प्रदाह;

**Caseous O.,** tuberculous caries of bone. यक्ष्मज अस्थिक्षय;

**Condensing O.,** see **Osteosclerosis.**

**Sclerosing O.,** see **Osteosclerosis.**

**O. Deformans,** a rarefying osteitis in which the bones become deformed from pressure. विरूपक अस्थिविकृति

**Ostempyesis.** Suppuration in bone. अस्थिपूतिता

**Osteo-.** Prefix denoting reference to the bone. 'अस्थि' के रूप में प्रयुक्त उपसर्ग

**Osteoarthritis.** The common, usually non-crippling form of arthritis due to aging; osteoarthrosis. अस्थिसन्धिशोथ; जोड़ों के आस-पास की प्रदाहयुक्त सूजन

**Osteoarthropathy.** Any disease of the bony articulations. अस्थिसन्धिविकृति; हड्डी के जोड़ों का कोई रोग

**Osteoarthrosis.** See **Osteoarthritis.**

**Osteoarthrotomy.** Excision of a bone-joint. अस्थिसन्धि-उच्छेदन; हड्डी का जोड़ काटना

**Osteoblast.** Cell concerned with forming new bone material and repairing the old. अस्थिकोशिकाप्रसू; अस्थिप्रसू; हड्डी बनाने वाला तत्व

**Osteoblastic.** Relating to the osteoblast. अस्थिकोशिकाप्रसू सम्बन्धी

**Osteoblastoma.** A benign tumour of osteoblasts. अस्थिकोशिकाप्रसू-अर्बुद

**Osteocampsia.** Abnormal curvature of bone. अतिअस्थिबक्रता; हड्डी का अस्वाभविक टेढ़ापन होना

**Osteochondritis.** Combined inflammation of bone and cartilage. अस्थ्युपास्थिशोथ; अस्थि एवं उपास्थि दोनों का मिश्र प्रदाह;

**O. Deformans Juvenilis,** false pain in the hip; pseudocoxalgia. कूटनितम्बार्ति; कूल्हे की अयथार्थ पीड़ा

**Osteochondroma.** A bony and cartilaginous tumour. अस्थ्युपास्थि-अर्बुद

**Osteochondromata.** Plural of **Osteochondroma.**

**Osteoclasia.** The therapeutic fracture of bones; osteoclasis; osteoclasty. अस्थिभंजन; अस्थि-उच्छेदन

**Osteoclasis.** See **Osteoclasia.**

**Osteoclast.** Cell which eliminates bone tissue not needed for skeletal strength and efficiency. अस्थि-अवशोषीकोशिका; वह कोशिका जो अस्थि-ऊतक का शोषण कर उसे छिन्न-भिन्न कर देती है; an instrument used to break a deformed bone to correct the deformity. अस्थिभंजक

**Osteoclastoma.** A tumour of the osteoclasts; giant cell tumour. अस्थि-अवशोषीकोशिकार्बुद; अस्थिअवशोषीकोशिका की रसौली

**Osteoclasty.** See **Osteoclasia.**

**Osteocope.** Pain in the bones; boneache. अस्थिपीड़ा; अस्थिवेदना; हड्डियों में दर्द

**Osteocyte.** A bone-cell carrying on continuous maintenance activity within the bone. अस्थिकोशिका

**Osteodynia.** Pain in the bone; ostealgia. अस्थिवेदना; अस्थिपीड़ा; हड्डी में दर्द होना

**Osteodystrophia.** Faulty growth of bone; osteodystrophy. अस्थिदुष्पोषण; हड्डी का दोषपूर्ण विकास

**Osteodystrophy.** See **Osteodystrophia.**

**Osteofibroma.** A benign tumour of bony and fibrous tissues. अस्थितंतु-अर्बुद; अस्थितंत्वर्बुद

**Osteofibrosis.** Fibrosis of bone. अस्थितंतुता

**Osteogen.** A soft substance from which bone is developed. अस्थिजन; कोई कोमल पदार्थ जिससे हड्डी का विकास होता है

**Osteogenetic.** See **Osteogenic.**

**Osteogenic.** Bone-producing; osteogenetic; osteogenous. अस्थिजनक

**Osteogenesis.** The development and formation of bone; osteogeny; osteosis. अस्थिजनन; हड्डी बनना और उसका विकास होना

**Osteogenous.** See **Osteogenic.**

**Osteogeny.** See **Osteogenesis.**

**Osteography.** The descriptive anatomy of bones. अस्थिवर्णन

**Osteoid.** Having the nature of bone. अस्थ्याभ; अस्थिरूप; अस्थिवत्; अस्थ्याकार; osseous tissue prior to calcification. अस्थिकल्प

**Osteology.** Science of the anatomy, structure and function of bones. अस्थिप्रकरण; अस्थिविज्ञान

**Osteolysis.** The absorption of bone. अस्थिलयन; अस्थ्यपघटन

**Osteolytic.** Destructive of bone. अस्थिलायी; अस्थिनाशक; हड्डी नष्ट करने वाला

**Osteoma.** Any bone-tumour. अस्थ्यर्बुद; हड्डी की रसौली

**Osteomalacia.** A morbid softening of bones. अस्थिमृदुता; हड्डियों का नरम पड़ जाना

**Osteomyelitis.** Inflammation commencing in the marrow of bone. अस्थिमज्जाशोथ; अस्थिमज्जा का प्रदाह

**Osteonecrosis.** Necrosis of bones. अस्थिगलन; हड्डियों का गलना

**Osteoneuralgia.** Neuralgia of bones. अस्थ्यार्ति; अस्थिशूल; हड्डियों में दर्द होना

**Osteopath.** A practitioner of osteopathy; osteopathist. अस्थिरोगविज्ञानी; अस्थिरोगचिकित्सक; अस्थिरोगों की चिकित्सा करने वाला

**Osteopathia.** See **Osteopathy.**

**Osteopathic.** Pertaining to osteopathy. अस्थिरोगचिकित्सा सम्बन्धी

**Osteopathist.** See **Osteopath.**

**Osteopathy.** Any disease of bone; osteopathia. अस्थिरोग; अस्थिविकार; हड्डी का कोई रोग

**Osteopenia.** See **Osteoporosis.**

**Osteoperiostitis.** Inflammation of both bone and periosteum. अस्थि-पर्यस्थिशोथ; हड्डी और उसकी झिल्ली का प्रदाह

**Osteopetrosis.** A spotty calcification of the bones which fracture spontaneously; marble bone. अस्थि-अश्मरता; अस्थ्यश्मरता; हड्डियों का चित्तीदार कैल्सीभवन होना, जिसके कारण वे स्वयमेव टूटती रहती हैं

**Osteophyte.** A bony outgrowth or nodosity. अस्थि-उद्वर्ध

**Osteoplastic.** Relating to osteoplasty or bony formation. अस्थिसंधानक; अस्थिसंधान सम्बन्धी

**Osteoplasty.** Any plastic operation of bone. अस्थिसंधान

**Osteopoikilosis.** Mottled or spotted bones. घनबिन्दुकित-अस्थिता

**Osteoporosis.** Change of compact into cancellous bone-tissue; osteopenia. अस्थि-सुषिरता

**Osteopsathyrosis.** Unusual bone fragility. अपूर्ण-अस्थिजनन

**Osteorrhaphy.** A bone-suture; osteosuture. अस्थिसीवन

**Osteosarcoma.** A sarcomatous tumour growing from bone. अस्थिसार्कार्बुद; हड्डी की कैंसराभ रसौली

**Osteosclerosis.** Induration of bone; condensing osteitis; sclerosing osteitis. अस्थिकाठिन्य; हड्डियों की कठोरता

**Osteosis.** See **Osteogenesis.**

**Osteosuture.** See **Osteorrhaphy.**

**Osteotome.** A bone-saw. अस्थिविच्छेदक; हड्डी काटने वाली आरी

**Osteotomy.** Division or cutting of a bone. अस्थिविच्छेदन; हड्डी काटना;

    **Cuneiform O.,** removal of wedge of bone. कीलाकार अस्थिविच्छेदन;

    **Linear O.,** simple division of a bone. रेखी अस्थिविच्छेदन

**Osteum.** A bone. अस्थि; हड्डी

**Ostia.** Plural of **Ostium.**

**Ostincae.** Orifice of the womb; os uteri. जरायुमुख; गर्भाशयमुख

**Ostitis.** See **Osteitis.**

**Ostium.** The mouth of a tubular passage. मुख; मुखिका; अपवाहीरन्ध्र; आयस्क; छिद्र; द्वार;

    **Abdominal O.,** see **Ostium Abdominale.**

    **O. Abdominale,** the abdominal or distal orifice of the Fallopian tube; abdominal ostium. उदरमुख; डिम्बवाहिनी उदरमुख;

    **O. Frontale,** ostium of frontal sinus. ललाट-विवर छिद्र;

    **O. Primum,** the passage-way beneath the septum of the atria of the embryonic heart. प्राथमिक रन्ध्र;

    **O. Secundum,** the opening near the dorsal attachment of the septum of the atria of the embryonic heart. द्वितीयक रन्ध्र;

    **O. Vaginae,** the external orifice of the vagina. योनिद्वार; योनिमुख

**Ostoid.** Osseous; bony. अस्थ्याभ; अस्थिवत्; हड्डी जैसा

**Ostosis.** See **Ossification.**

**Os uteri.** The entrance of the womb. जरायुमुख; गर्भाशय-मुख

**O.T.** Occupational therapy. व्यावसायिक चिकित्सा; Operation Theatre. आपरेशन थियेटर; शल्यकर्मशाला

**Otalgia.** Pain in the ear. कर्णशूल; कर्णार्ति; कर्णपीड़ा; कान में दर्द

**Othelcosis.** Ulceration of the ear. कर्णव्रणता; कान के अन्दर घाव बनना

**Otic.** Pertaining to the ear; oticus. कर्णपरक; कान सम्बन्धी

**Oticus.** See **Otic**.

**Otitic.** Pertaining to otitis. कर्णशोथज; कर्णशोथ सम्बन्धी

**Otitis.** Inflammation of the ear. कर्णशोथ; कान का प्रदाह

   **Furuncular O.**, the formation of furuncles in the external meatus. पनसिका-कर्णशोथ;

   **O. Externa**, inflammation of the skin of the external auditory canal. बाह्यकर्णशोथ; कान के बाहरी भाग का प्रदाह;

   **O. Interna**, labyrinthitis. आन्तरकर्णशोथ; आभ्यन्तरकर्णशोथ;

   **O. Media**, inflammation of the middle ear cavity. मध्यकर्णशोथ; कान के मध्य भाग का प्रदाह

**Otoconia.** See **Otolith**.

**Otoconium.** See **Otolith**.

**Otocyst.** The embryonic auditory vesicle. श्रवणपुटी

**Otodynia.** Pain in the ear. कर्णार्ति; कर्णशूल; कान का दर्द; कर्णवेदना; कर्णपीड़ा

**Otogenic.** Having its origin in the ear; otogenous. कर्णजनक

**Otogenous.** See **Otogenic**.

**Otography.** A description of the ear. कर्णरचनालेख; कर्णवृतान्त

**Otolith.** A granule of calcium carbonate in the labyrinth of ear; otoconia; otoconium. कर्णबालुका; कर्णकण; कर्णपथरी

**Otologic.** Referring to the diseases of the ear or the ears. कर्णविकृतिक; कर्णरोग सम्बन्धी

**Otologist.** One specializing in the functions and diseases of the ear. कर्णरोगविज्ञानी; कर्णरोगचिकित्सक; कर्णविशेषज्ञ

**Otology.** The science which deals with the structure, function and diseases of the ear. कर्णरोगविज्ञान; कर्णविज्ञान; कानों की बनावट, क्रिया तथा बीमारियों सम्बन्धी विज्ञान की शाखा

**Otomycosis.** The presence of, or the condition caused by fungus in the external ear. कर्णकवकता; कवक द्वारा उत्पादित बाह्य-कर्ण की अवस्था

**Otoncus.** An aural tumour. कर्णार्बुद; कान की रसौली

**Otopathy.** Any disease of the ear. कर्णरोग; कर्णविकृति; कान का रोग

**Otoplasty.** Reparative or plastic surgery of the ears to correct their defects and deformities. कर्णसंधान

**Otopolypus.** A polyp occurring in the ear. कर्णपुर्वंगक; कर्णपालिप

**Otorrhagia.** Haemorrhage from the ear. कर्णरक्तस्राव; कान से खून बहना

**Otorrhea.** A discharge of serous mucus or purulent fluid from the ear; otorrhoea. कर्णस्राव; कान बहना

**Otorrhoea.** See **Otorrhea**.

**Otosclerosis.** Sclerosis of the tissues of the labyrinth and middle ear. कर्णगहनसम्पुटकाठिन्य

**Otoscope.** An instrument for examining ear. कर्णदर्शी; कर्णवीक्षकयंत्र; कान की जांच के लिये प्रयुक्त किया जाने वाला यंत्र

**Otoscopy.** Examination of the ear with otoscope. कर्णदर्शन; कर्णवीक्षण; कान की जांच करना

**Ototomy.** The dissection of the ear. कर्णोच्छेदन; कर्ण-उच्छेदन; कर्णविच्छेदन

**Oturia.** A urinary discharge from the ear. कर्णमूत्रस्राव; कर्णमेह; कान से मूत्रस्राव होना

**Ounce.** Eight drachms; two table spoonful. औंस; आठ ड्राम; दो चाय के चम्मचों की मात्रा के बराबर

**Outer.** External. बाह्य; बहि:; बाहरी

**Outlet.** The place or means by which anything is let out; a passage outwards. बहिर्गम; निकास; निर्गम मार्ग; मुख; द्वार

**Outpatient.** One who is treated at, but not detained in a hospital. बहिरंगरोगी; अस्पताल में बाहर से आने वाला रोगी

**Outpatient Department.** See **O.P.D.**

**Outpatient Service.** Care of patients in hospital clinics without admitting to a hospital bed. बहिरंगरोगी सेवा

**Output.** That which is produced, ejected or excreted in a specified period of time. निष्याद; निकास; निर्गम

**Ova.** Plural of **Ovum**.

**Oval.** Egg-shaped. डिम्बाकार; अण्डाकार;

    **O. Foramen,** aperture between the auricles of the foetal heart. अण्डाकार छिद्र; डिम्बाकार छिद्र

**Ovalis.** Ovular. अण्डाकार; डिम्बाकार

**Ovaltine.** A proprietary food beverage. ओवल्टिन; एक पौष्टिक आहार

**Ovaralgia.** Ovarian neuralgia; ovarialgia. डिम्बाशयशूल; डिम्बग्रन्थिशूल; डिम्बार्ति

**Ovaria.** The ovaries, whence the ova passes through the Fallopian tubes into the womb. डिम्बग्रन्थियाँ; डिम्बवाहीनलियाँ; अण्डद्रव्य

**Ovarial.** See **Ovarian.**

**Ovarialgia.** See **Ovaralgia.**

**Ovarian.** Pertaining to the ovaries; ovarial; ovaricus. डिम्बाशयी; अण्डाशयी; डिम्बग्रन्थियों सम्बन्धी

**Ovaricus.** See **Ovarian.**

**Ovariectomy.** Excision of an ovary; ovariotomy; oophorectomy. डिम्बग्रन्थि-उच्छेदन; डिम्बग्रन्थि को काट कर हटा देना

**Ovariocentesis.** Puncture of an ovary or an ovarian cyst. डिम्बछेदन; डिम्बपुटीछेदन

**Ovariocyesis.** Ovarian pregnancy. डिम्बगर्भ

**Ovariosalpingitis.** Inflammation of the ovary and the oviduct. डिम्बग्रंथिडिम्बवाहिनीशोथ; डिम्बाशय एवं डिम्बवाहीनली का प्रदाह

**Ovariotomy.** See **Ovariectomy.**

**Ovarious.** Ovular. डिम्बाकार; अण्डाकार

**Ovaritis.** Inflammation of an ovary. डिम्बग्रन्थिशोथ; डिम्बाशयशोथ; अण्डाशयशोथ; डिम्बाशय अथवा अण्डाशय का प्रदाह

**Ovarium.** See **Ovary.**

**Ovary.** One of the two generative glands in female containing the ova or the germ-cell; ovarium. डिम्बग्रन्थि; डिम्बाशय; अण्डाशय; मादाजननग्रन्थि

**Overdose.** Too great a dose. अतिमात्रा; बृहद्मात्रा; बढ़ी हुई मात्रा

**Overextension.** Excessive extension. अतिप्रसार; अत्यधिक फैलाव

**Overflow.** The continuous escape of liquids. अतिस्राव; अत्यधिक बहाव

**Ovicidal.** Causing death of an ovum. डिम्बमारक

**Ovicide.** Destructive of ova. डिम्बनाशक; अण्डाणुनाशक

**Oviduct.** The Fallopian tube; ductus ovaricus. डिम्बाहिनी; डिम्बवाहीनली

**Ovification.** The production of ova. डिम्बजनन; अण्डोत्पादन

**Oviform.** Oval; egg-shaped; ovoid. डिम्बाकार; अण्डाकार; डिम्बाभ; अण्डाभ

**Ovigenesis.** See **Oogenesis.**

**Ovigerous.** Bearing eggs; oviparous. डिम्बजनक; अण्डज; अण्डे देने वाला

**Oviparous.** See **Ovigerous.**

**Ovoid.** See **Oviform.**

**Ovoplasm.** See **Ooplasm.**

# Ovular

**Ovular.** Like an ovum. डिम्बाकार; अण्डाकार; pertaining to an ovum. डिम्बाशय अथवा अण्डाशय सम्बन्धी

**Ovulation.** The maturation and escape of ova. डिम्बक्षरण; डिम्बोत्सर्जन

**Ovulatory.** Relating to ovulation. डिम्बक्षरण सम्बन्धी

**Ovum.** The female reproductive cell; an egg. डिम्ब; अण्डाणु; स्त्री-बीजकोशिका; मादाजननकोशिका

    **Blighted O.**, an impregnated ovum arrested in its development; pathologic ovum. लीन डिम्ब; विकृतिक डिम्ब;

    **Holoblastic O.**, the ova in which the entire yolk undergoes segmentation. विदलित डिम्ब;

    **Pathologic O.**, see **Blighted Ovum.**

**Oxalate.** A salt of oxalic acid. ऑक्सैलेट; पिष्ट; एक तिग्मीय पदार्थ

**Oxaluria.** The presence of calcium oxalate in the urine. पिष्टमेह; मूत्र में कैल्शियम ऑक्सैलेट विद्यमान रहना

**Oxidation.** The chemical process of uniting with oxygen, or burning; oxidization. उपचयन; जारण

**Oxide.** A compound of oxygen with another element or a radical; oxyde. जारेय; जारक एवं अन्य तत्वों अथवा प्रांगारिक मूल का मिश्रण; ओषजन का सम्मिश्रण

**Oxidization.** See **Oxidation.**

**Oxyde.** See **Oxide.**

**Oxyesthesia.** Hyperesthesia; abnormal acuteness of sensation. अतिसम्वेदिता; बढ़ी हुई सम्वेदनशीलता

**Oxygen.** One of the gaseous elements which acts as a supporter of life and combustion. ऑक्सीजन; प्राणवायु

**Oxygenation.** Addition of oxygen to any chemical or physical system. ऑक्सीकरण

**Oxygenator.** Artificial 'lung', as used in heart surgery. ऑक्सीजनित्र

**Oxylalia.** Abnormally rapid speech. तीव्रवाक्; द्रुतवाक्

**Oxyntic.** Rendering acid. अम्लस्रावी; अम्लजनक

**Oxyopia.** Excessive acuteness of vision. तीक्ष्णदृष्टि; दृष्टि की अत्यधिक तीक्ष्णता

**Oxyphile.** See **Oxyphilic.**

**Oxyphilic.** Readily stained with acid dyes; oxyphile; oxyphilous. अम्लवर्णरागी

**Oxyphilous.** See **Oxyphilic.**

**Oxysalt.** A salt of an oxyacid (oxygenated acid). जारलवण

**Oxytocic.** An agent promoting uterine contraction. गर्भाशयसंकोचक; जरायुसंकोचक; जरायु की सिकुड़न बढ़ाने वाला पदार्थ; hastening parturition. प्रसवकारक; an abortive. गर्भपातक; गर्भस्त्रावक

**Oxyuriasis.** Disease manifestation from infection with oxyuris (pinworm). सूत्रकृमिरोग

**Oxyuricide.** A drug fatal to oxyuris. सूत्रकृमिनाशक; सूत्रकृमियों को नष्ट करने वाली औषधि

**Oxyuris.** A genus of nematode worms. कृमि;
   **O. Vermicularis,** the ascaris or thread worm. सूत्रकृमि

**Oz.** Ounce. औंस; आठ ड्राम

**Ozaena.** A foetid nasal ulceration and discharge; ozena. पीनस; पूतिनासा; व्रणग्रस्त नाक से दुर्गन्धित स्राव होना

**Oze.** Stench. दुर्गन्ध; बदबू

**Ozena.** See **Ozaena.**

**Ozone.** A peculiar modification of oxygen which exists in very poor atmospheres. प्रजारक; रोगाणुओं एवं संक्रमण को नष्ट करने वाला द्रव्य

**Ozostomia.** A foul odour from the mouth. दुर्गन्धित श्वास; मुख से बदबूदार श्वास निकलना

# P

**Pabular.** Pertaining to diet. आहार्य; आहारविषयक; भोजन सम्बन्धी

**Pabulous.** Nutritious. आहारसम्पन्न; पौष्टिक

**Pabulum.** Food; anything nutritive. खाद्य; आहार; भोजन; पौष्टिक पदार्थ

**Pacemaker.** Any rhythmic centre that establishes a pace of activity. गतिचालक; गतिप्रेरक

**Pachaemia.** Thickening of the blood; pachemia. रक्तघनता; खून गाढ़ा होना

**Pachemia.** See **Pachaemia.**

**Pachyacria.** Acromegaly. अतिकायता

**Pachyblepharon.** Thick eyelids. स्थूलवर्त्म; मोटी पलकें

# Pachycephalia

**Pachycephalia.** A thick skull; pachycephaly. स्थूलशीर्ष; स्थूलकपाल; स्थूलकरोटि; मोटी खोपड़ी

**Pachycephalic.** Relating to, or marked by pachycephalia. स्थूलशीर्ष सम्बन्धी अथवा स्थूलशीर्षी

**Pachycephalous.** Having a thick skull; pachycephalus. स्थूलशीर्षी; बृहन्मुण्डी; स्थूलकपाली; जिसकी खोपड़ी की हड्डियाँ मोटी हों

**Pachycephalus.** See **Pachycephalous.**

**Pachycephaly.** See **Pachycephalia.**

**Pachydactylia.** Thickening of the fingers or toes; pachydactyly. स्थूलांगुलिता; उँगलियां मोटी होना अथवा नाखुन मोटे होना

**Pachyderma.** Thickening of the skin; elephantiasis; pachydermia; pachydermatosis. गजचर्मता; दृढ़चर्मता; स्थूलचर्मता; त्वक्स्थूलता; चमड़ा मोटा होने का रोग

**Pachydermatosis.** See **Pachyderma.**

**Pachydermatous.** Thick-skinned. स्थूलचर्मधारी; स्थूलचर्म; गजचर्म; घनत्वक्; मोटी खाल का

**Pachydermia.** See **Pachyderma.**

**Pachyemia.** See **Pachyhemia.**

**Pachyemic.** Having thick blood; pachyemous. स्थूलरक्तक; स्थूलरक्तधारी

**Pachyemous.** See **Pachyemic.**

**Pachygastrous.** Having a large abdomen. स्थूलउदर

**Pachyglossia.** An unusual thickening of the tongue. स्थूलजिह्वा; जिह्वास्थूलता; जीभ का मोटा होना

**Pachyhemia.** Thickening of the blood; pachyemia. स्थूलरक्तता; रक्तस्थूलता; खून का गाढ़ा होना

**Pachymeningitis.** Inflammation of the dura mater. दृढ़तानिकाशोथ; दृढ़तानिका-प्रदाह;

P. Externa, that affecting the external layer of the dura. बाह्य-दृढ़तानिकाशोथ;

P. Interna, that involving the internal layer of the dura. आभ्यन्तर दृढ़तानिकाशोथ

**Pachymeningopathy.** Any disease of the dura mater. दृढ़तानिकारोग

**Pachymeninx.** The dura. दृढ़तानिका

**Pachymeter.** An instrument for measuring the thickness of the body. स्थूलित्र; स्थूलतामापी; स्थूलतामापीयंत्र; मोटाईमापकयंत्र

**Pachyonychia.** Abnormal thickness of the fingernails or toenails. स्थूलनखता; उँगलियों के नाखुनों का असाधारण रूप से मोटा होना;

**P. Congenita,** the congenital thickening of the nails. सहजस्थूलनखता; नाखुनों का जन्मजात मोटा होना

**Pachypodous.** Having thick feet. स्थूलपाद

**Pachytic.** Fat. स्थूल; मोटा

**Pachyotous.** Having thick ears. स्थूलकर्ण; मोटे कानों वाला

**Pack.** A moist blanket placed around the patient; wet-pack. आर्द्रवस्त्रावेष्टन; आर्द्रवस्त्रावेष्टनोपचार; पैक;

**Wet-p.,** see **Pack.**

**Pad.** A small, flat cushion to apply or relieve pressure on a part or fill a depression. उपधान; कवलिका; गद्दी; तह

**Paederasty.** Sexual intercourse with boys per anus; pederasty; sodomy. गुदमैथुन; गुदामैथुन; लौंडेबाजी

**Paediatrician.** A specialist in children's disease; pediatrician. बालचिकित्साविज्ञानी; बालरोगविज्ञानी; शिशुस्वास्थ्यविज्ञानी; बच्चों की बीमारियों की चिकित्सा करने वाला

**Paediatrics.** The branch of science dealing with the children; pediatrics; paediatry. बालचिकित्साविज्ञान; बालरोग-विज्ञान; कौमार-भृत्य; शिशुस्वास्थ्यविज्ञान

**Paediatry.** See **Paediatrics.**

**Paedology.** The science of childhood; pedology. बालविज्ञान; शिशुचिकित्साशास्त्र

**Pain.** The sensation of discomfort, arising from injury or disease of any of the nerves of the body; algia. वेदना; पीड़ा; दर्द; आर्ति; शूल; कष्ट; संताप;

**Aching P.,** deep-rooted pain. गभीर वेदना;

**Acute P.,** a short, sharp, cutting pain. तीव्र वेदना; तीव्र पीड़ा; उग्र पीड़ा;

**After-p.,** pain following labour from contraction of uterus. प्रसवोत्तर वेदना;

**Bearing-down P.,** labour-like pain. प्रवहण वेदना; प्रसव जैसी पीड़ा;

**False P.,** a pain in the later stage of pregnancy, like labour pain. मिथ्याप्रसव वेदना; कूटप्रसव वेदना;

**Girdle P.,** painful sensation resembling the tightening of a cord around the waist. मेखलावेदना; कटिवेदना; कमरदर्द;

# Pain

**Labour P.,** rhythmical uterine contraction at child-birth. प्रसव वेदना;

**Menstrual P.,** dysmenorrhoea. कष्टार्तव; ऋतुशूल; दर्दनाक ऋतुस्राव होना;

**P. Receptor,** bare nerve endings in the tissue cells of the skin and other organs, though not present everywhere in the body. वेदनाग्राही; वेदनाग्राहक; पीड़ाग्राही; पीड़ाग्राहक

**Painless.** Without pain. वेदनारहित; दर्दहीन; पीड़ाहीन; कष्टहीन

**Painter's Colic.** Lead poisoning. आंत्रशूल; सीसा-विषण्णता; रंगसाजों को होने वाला उदरशूल

**Paired Organs.** Organs of which the body has a pair, such as eyes, kidneys, sex glands, lungs, ears, etc. युग्मांग; युगलांग; जोड़ों वाले अंग, जैसे नेत्र, वृक्क, जनन-ग्रन्थियाँ, फुफ्फुस, कर्ण, आदि

**Palatable.** Tasty. स्वादिष्ट; रसीला

**Palatal.** See **Palatine.**

**Palate.** The partition separating the cavity of the mouth from that of nose; palatum. तालु; काकुद;

**P.-bone,** that helping to form the outer wall of the nose. तालवस्थि; तालु की हड्डी;

**Artificial P.,** a plate used to close a fissure in the palate. कृत्रिम तालु;

**Bony P.,** see **Hard Palate.**

**Cleft P.,** a congenital cleft between the palatal bones, which leaves a gap in the root of the opening directly into the nose; palatoschisis. खण्ड-तालु;

**Hard P.,** the front part of the roof of the mouth formed by the two palatal bones; bony palate. कठोर तालु;

**Soft P.,** the velum palati, situated at the posterior end of the palate and consisting of muscle covered by mucous membrane. मृदु तालु; कोमल तालु

**Palati.** Plural of **Palatum.**

**Palatiform.** Shaped like the palate. तालुरूप; ताल्वाकार; तालुवत्; ताल्वाभ; तालु जैसा

**Palatine.** Belonging to the palate; palatal. तालव; तालु सम्बन्धी;

**P. Arches,** the bilateral double pillars of arch-like folds formed by the descent of the soft palate as it meets the pharynx. तालु-चाप;

**P. Bone,** the palate bone. ताल्वस्थि; तालु की हड्डी;

**P. Membrane,** the membrane of the roof of the mouth. तालु-कला; तालु को ढक कर रखने वाली झिल्ली

**Palatitis.** Inflammation of the palate. तालुशोथ; तालु का प्रदाह

**Palatoglossal.** Pertaining to the palate and the tongue. तालु तथा जीभ सम्बन्धी

**Palatognathus.** Cleft or fissured palate. खण्ड-तालु

**Palatograph.** An instrument for recording the movement of the palate. तालुगतिलेखी (यंत्र)

**Palatopharyngeal.** Pertaining to both the palate and pharynx. तालु तथा ग्रसनी सम्बन्धी

**Palatoplasty.** Plastic surgery of the palate. तालुसंधान

**Palatoplegia.** Paralysis of the palate. तालुघात; तालु का पक्षाघात; तालु का लकवा

**Palatoplegic.** Belonging to palatoplegia. तालुघात सम्बन्धी

**Palatorrhaphy.** Suture of a cleft-palate. तालुसीवन

**Palatoschisis.** Cleft-palate. खण्ड-तालु

**Palatum.** See **Palate.**

**Pale.** Deficient in intensity of colour. पीला; निष्प्रभ; निस्तेज; धुँधला

**Palilalia.** Constant repetition of a sentence; paliphrasia. निरर्थकपुनरुक्ति; किसी वाक्य को निरर्थक दोहराते जाना

**Palindromia.** The recurrence of a disease. रोग की पुनरावृत्ति

**Palindromic.** Recurring. पुनरावर्ती; बार-बार प्रकट होने वाला

**Palingenesis.** Rebirth; regeneration. पुनर्जनन; फिर से जन्म लेना या होना

**Paliphrasia.** See **Palilalia.**

**Palliate.** To sooth or mitigate a disease. रोगोपशमन करना; रोगदमन करना

**Palliation.** The treatment which improves the patient's feelings without curing disease. रोगोपशमन; रोगदमन

**Palliative.** A medicine which mitigates or lessens the severity of a disease or of suffering without being curative. प्रशामक; रोगोपशामक; रोगदमनकारी

**Pallid.** Pale. पीला; पाण्डु; पाण्डुर

**Pallidectomy.** Destruction of a predetermined section of globus pallidus. पाण्डुगोलकोच्छेदन

# Pallidity

**Pallidity.** See **Pallidness**.

**Pallidness.** Paleness; pallidity. पीलापन; पाण्डुरता; पाण्डुता

**Pallidum.** See **Pallidus**.

**Pallidus.** Pale; pallid; pallidum. पीला; पाण्डुर; पाण्डु; मुरझाया हुआ; Globus P., pale section within the lenticular nucleus of the brain. पाण्डुरगोलक

**Pallium.** The fissured portion of each cerebral hemisphere. प्रावार

**Pallor.** Unusual paleness; deathlike paleness. पीलिमा; पाण्डुता; अस्वाभाविक पीलापन;

P. Luteus, see **Pallor Virginum**.

P. Virginum, chlorosis; unusual paleness in girls at puberty; pallor luteus. अरक्तता; रक्ताल्पता; अल्परक्तता; हरितपाण्डुता

**Palm.** The anterior or flexor surface of the hand. करतल; हथेली

**Palma Christi.** The castor-oil plant. एरण्ड; कैस्टर आयल का पौधा

**Palmar.** Belonging to the palm of the hand. करतल अथवा हथेली सम्बन्धी; करतलगत

**Palmaris.** Muscles of the palms of the hand. करतलपेशियाँ; हथेली की पेशियाँ

**Palmate.** Shaped like palms. करतलाकार; हथेलियों जैसा

**Palmature.** A union of fingers. जालीयत उँगलियां; झिल्लीदार उँगलियां

**Palmistry.** The art of foretelling events by the marks of the palms of the hands. हस्तरेखाविज्ञान

**Palmus.** Palpitation. हृदय की क्षेपक गति; twitching; throbbing; स्पन्दन; the palm. हथेली

**Palpable.** Capable of being palpated. परिस्पृश्य; संस्पृश्य; परिस्पर्शन योग्य

**Palpate.** To explore with the hand. परिस्पर्शन करना; संस्पर्शन करना

**Palpation.** The method of examining disease by pressing upon or touching the diseased part. परिस्पर्शन; संस्पर्शन

**Palpebra.** The eyelid; palpebrum. नेत्रच्छद; वर्त्म; पक्ष्म; पलक

**Palpebrae.** Plural of **Palpebra**.

**Palpebral.** Belonging to the eyelids. नेत्रच्छदीय; वर्त्मीय; पक्ष्मीय; पलकों सम्बन्धी

**Palpebration.** The act of winking. अक्षिनिमेष

**Palpebrum.** See **Palpebra**.

**Palpitant.** Pulsating; beating. स्पन्दनशील; धड़कने वाला

**Palpitation.** Quickened action of the heart, in which it beats too rapidly and too strongly. स्पन्दन; धड़कन;

**P. Cordis,** palpitation of the heart. हृत्स्पन्द; हृदय की धड़कन; दिल की धड़कन

**Palsy.** The popular term for paralysis, especially if there is shaking and trembling associated with it. घात; अंगघात; पक्षाघात; फालिज;

**Bell's P.,** see **Facial Palsy.**

**Facial P.,** facial hemiparesis from oedema of the seventh (facial) cranial nerve; Bell's palsy. आननघात; चेहरे का फालिज;

**Lead P.,** paralysis of the muscles of the arm due to lead-poisoning. सीसक अंगघात; बाहों की पेशियों का सीसाविषजनित पक्षाघात;

**Shaking P.,** paralysis agitans. सकम्प अंगघात

**Pampiniform.** Having the form of a tendril. प्रतानाकार

**Pan-.** Prefix signifying all or everything. 'सर्व', 'सब', 'प्रत्येक' 'पूर्ण' के रूप में प्रयुक्त उपसर्ग

**Panacea.** A remedy claimed to be curative in all diseases; a quack remedy. सर्वौषधि; रामबाण; सर्वव्याधिहर; सारे रोगों की अचूक दवा

**Panangiitis.** Inflammation involving all the coats of a blood vessel. वाहिकास्तरशोथ

**Panaria.** See **Panaritium.**

**Panaris.** See **Panaritium.**

**Panaritium.** Whitlow; paronychia; panaria; panaris; phlegmonous inflammation of a finger or toe. चिप्प; परिनखशोथ; अंगुलबेढ़ा; हाथ या पैर की उँगली का सपूय प्रदाह

**Panarteritis.** Inflammation of all the structures of an artery. पूर्णधमनीशोथ; धमनी की सम्पूर्ण संरचनाओं का प्रदाह

**Panarthritis.** Inflammation of all the structures of a joint. पूर्णसन्धिशोथ; जोड़ की सम्पूर्ण संरचनाओं का प्रदाह

**Pancarditis.** Inflammation of all the structures of the heart. पूर्णहृद्शोथ; हृदय की सम्पूर्ण संरचनाओं का प्रदाह

**Pancolectomy.** Excision of the entire colon. पूर्णबृहदांत्रोच्छेदन; बड़ी आंत को पूरी तरह निकाल देना

**Pancreas.** The principal digestive gland situated below and behind the stomach. अग्न्याशय; क्लोमग्रन्थि; पाचकग्रन्थि

**Pancreata.** Plural of **Pancreas.**

**Pancreatalgia.** Pain in the pancreas. अग्न्याशयशूल; क्लोमग्रंथिशूल

**Pancreatectomy.** Excision of a part or the whole of the pancreas. अग्न्याशयोच्छेदन; क्लोमग्रन्थि-उच्छेदन

**Pancreatic.** Pertaining to the pancreas. अग्न्याशयिक; क्लोमग्रन्थि अथवा अग्न्याशय सम्बन्धी;

    **P. Fluid,** the fluid secreted by the pancreas; pancreatic juice. अग्न्याशय रस;

    **P. Juice,** see **Pancreatic Fluid.**

**Pancreaticoduodenal.** Relating to the pancreas and the duodenum. अग्न्याशय तथा ग्रहणी सम्बन्धी

**Pancreaticosplenic.** Relating to the pancreas and the spleen. अग्न्याशय तथा प्लीहा सम्बन्धी

**Pancreatin.** A mixture of enzymes obtained from the pancreas. अग्न्याशयजन्यकिण्व; अग्न्याशयरसनिर्मित एक खमीर

**Pancreatitis.** Inflammation of the pancreas. अग्न्याशयशोथ; क्लोमग्रन्थिशोथ; पाचक-ग्रन्थि का प्रदाह

**Pancreatogenic.** See **Pancreatogenous.**

**Pancreatogenous.** Of pancreatic origin; formed in the pancreas; pancreatogenic. अग्न्याशयजनक; अग्न्याशयजनित

**Pancreatography.** A radiological visualization of pancreas. अग्न्याशयचित्रण

**Pancreopathy.** Diseases of the pancreas. अग्न्याशयविकार

**Pancytopenia.** Describes peripheral blood picture, when red cells, granular white cells and platelets are reduced, as occurs in suppression of bone-marrow function. पूर्णरक्तकोशिकाहीनता

**Pandemic.** A wide spread epidemic. विश्वमारी; महामारी; सार्वलौकिक; देशान्तरगामी

**Pandiculation.** Yawning; the act of stretching the limbs. अंगड़ाई; जम्हाई; कसमसाहट

**Panencephalitis.** A diffuse inflammation of the brain. विसरितमस्तिष्कशोथ

**Pang.** Suffocative of the breast; a sharp momentary pain. यंत्रणा; यातना; तीव्र क्षणिक पीड़ा;

    **Breast P.,** angina pectoris. हृद्शूल; हृच्छूल; हृदयार्ति

**Panhysterectomy.** An old term for removal of the uterus and adnexa, more accurately described as a total hysterectomy. पूर्णगर्भाशयोच्छेदन

**Panic.** A violent and unreasoning anxiety and fear. आतंक; संत्रास; भय; भीति; डर

**Panicula.** A swelling or tumour. सूजन या अर्बुद

**Panis.** Bread. रोटी

**Panivorous.** Living on bread. रोटीभोजी; रोटी पर पलने वाला

**Panni.** Plural of **Pannus.**

**Panniculi.** Plural of **Panniculus.**

**Panniculitis.** Inflammation of the panniculus adiposus of the abdominal wall. अधस्त्वकस्तरशोथ; अधस्त्वक्वसास्तरशोथ

**Panniculus.** A membrane or layer. अधस्त्वकस्तर; कला; झिल्ली; आवरण;

  **P. Adiposus,** the layer of subcutaneous fat. अधस्त्वक्वसास्तर;

  **P. Carnosus,** the layer of muscular fibres by means of which the skin is moved. अधस्त्वक्पेशी-अस्तर;

  **P. Hymeneus,** the hymen. योनिच्छद; सतीच्छद;

  **P. Subtilis,** the pia mater. मृदु-तानिका;

  **P. Transversus,** the diaphragm. मध्यच्छद

**Pannosity.** Softness of the skin. त्वग्मृदुता; चमड़ी की कोमलता

**Pannus.** A membrane of granular tissue covering an articular cartilage in rheumatoid arthritis and the cornea in trachoma. पैनस; नाखूना

**Panochia.** Bubo. क्षत; गांठ; गिल्टी

**Panophthalmia.** See **Panophthalmitis.**

**Panophthalmitis.** Inflammation of all the tissues; panophthalmia. सर्वनेत्रशोथ; समस्त ऊतकों का प्रदाह

**Panosteitis.** Inflammation of all the constituents of a bone. पूर्णअस्थिशोथ; हड्डी के सारे घटकों का प्रदाह

**Panotitis.** Inflammation of the entire ear. पूर्णकर्णशोथ

**Panphobia.** Groundless fear of everything. सर्वभीति; प्रत्येक वस्तु के प्रति निरर्थक भय

**Pansinusitis.** Inflammation of all paranasal sinuses on one or both sides. पूर्णवायुविवरशोथ; पूर्णनासाविवरशोथ; सम्पूर्ण परानासावायुविवरों का प्रदाह

**Panting.** Difficulty of breathing; dyspnoea. श्वासकष्ट; श्वास फूलना; हाँफना

**Papilla.** A minute nipple-shaped eminence. अंकुरक; फुन्सी; गूमड़ी; optic disc. अक्षिबिम्ब;

## Papilla

**Anal P.'s,** epithelial projections on the edges of the anal valves. गुदांकुरक;

**Dermal P.'s,** those on the skin. त्वक्-अंकुरक;

**Filiform P.,** any one of the very slender papillae at the tip of the tongue. सूची-अंकुरक;

**P. Duodeni,** the duodenal papilla. ग्रहणी-अंकुरक;

**P. Lacrimalis,** the papilla of the lacrimal duct at the inner canthus of the eye. अश्रु-अंकुरक;

**Papillae, Papillas.** Plurals of **Papilla.**

**P. Conicae,** the cone-shaped papillae. शंक्वाकार अंकुरक;

**P. Filiformes,** numerous elongated conical projections on the dorsum of the tongue; filiform papillae. सूत्री अंकुरक

**Papillary.** Like a papilla. अंकुरकवत्; अंकुराभ; belonging to the papilla. अंकुरक सम्बन्धी

**Papilledema.** See **Papilloedema.**

**Papilliform.** Shaped like a papilla. अंकुराकार; अंकुरकरूप; अंकुरक; अक्षिबिम्बाभ अथवा अक्षिबिम्ब के आकार का

**Papillitis.** Most usually inflammation of optic disc, otherwise inflammation of a papilla. अक्षिबिम्बशोथ अथवा अंकुरकशोथ

**Papilloedema.** Oedema of the optic disc, indicative of increased intracranial pressure; papilledema. अक्षिबिम्बशोफ

**Papilloma.** A simple tumour arising from a non-glandular epithelial surface. अंकुरकार्बुद

**Papillomatosis.** The formation of papillomas. अंकुरकार्बुदता

**Papillomatous.** Belonging to papilloma. अंकुरकार्बुदीय

**Papillotomy.** Incision into a papilla. अंकुरकछेदन

**Pappus.** The first downy beard on the cheeks and chin. रोमगुच्छ; लोमगुच्छ

**Paprika.** The pepper. मिर्च; काली मिर्च

**Pap-test.** Short form for **Papniculao,** named after the discoverer. It consists of the smear specimen of the body secretion for the early detection of cancer. पैप-जांच; कैंसर के निदानार्थ की जाने वाली एक जांच विधि

**Papular.** Abounding in pimples; consisting of papules. पिटिकीय; फुंसियों से युक्त; फुंसीदार; relating to papules. पिटिकाओं सम्बन्धी

**Papulation.** The formation of papules. पिटिकाभवन; फुंसियां बनना

**Papule.** A small swelling on the skin; a pimple. पिटिका; फुन्सी

**Papulopustular.** Pertaining to both papules and pustules. पिटकों तथा फुन्सियों सम्बन्धी

**Papulosis.** The occurrence of numerous widespread papules. पिटिकमयता; असंख्य फुंसियां प्रकट हो जाना

**Papyraceous.** Resembling paper. कागज जैसा

**Par-.** Prefix signifying similarity. 'समता' तथा 'साम्य' के रूप में प्रयुक्त उपसर्ग

**Par.** A pair, especially a pair of cranial nerves. युगल; जोड़ा (खास तौर से कपालतंत्रिकाओं का जोड़ा)

**Para-.** Prefix signifying beyond, beside, near, etc. 'परा' तथा 'अप' के रूप में प्रयुक्त उपसर्ग

**Parablepsia.** Perverted vision. विपर्यस्त दृष्टि

**Parabulia.** Perversion of will. विपर्यस्त इच्छा

**Paracentesis.** The withdrawal of fluid from its closed cavity by insertion of a hollow needle or canula. परावेधन

**Paracentetic.** Relating to paracentesis. परावेधनीय; परावेधन सम्बन्धी

**Paracentral.** Near a centre. पराकेन्द्रिक; पराकेन्द्रीय; किसी केन्द्र के पास

**Paracolitis.** Inflammation of the peritoneal coat of the colon. पराबृहदांत्रशोथ

**Paracusia.** See **Paracusis.**

**Paracusis.** Disordered hearing; paracusia. अपश्रवण; श्रवणदोष

**Paracystitis.** Inflammation of the connective tissue and other structures about the urinary bladder. परामूत्राशयशोथ

**Paradidymis.** A body on the spermatic cord above the epididymis. परावृषण

**Paradoxia.** A contradictory statement. असंगत कथन; विरोधी वक्तव्य

**Paradoxic.** Contradictory; paradoxical. विरोधाभासी

**Paradoxical.** See **Paradoxic.**

**Paraesthesia.** Any abnormality of a sensation; paresthesia; dysesthesia. अपसंवेदन; संवेदना में किसी प्रकार की अस्वाभाविकता

**Paraffin.** A white, waxy, crystalline hydrocarbon from coal-tar, wood, petroleum, etc. पैराफिन; मृदुवसा; एक प्रकार का हल्का विरेचक

**Paraganglia.** Plural of **Paraganglion.**

**Paraganglioma.** A condition in which there is a tumour of the adrenal medulla, or of the structurally similar tissues associated with the sympathetic chain. परागण्डिकार्बुद

**Paraganglion.** A small roundish body containing chromaffin cells. परागण्डिका

**Paraglossa.** Swelling or hypertrophy of the tongue. जिह्वापांग; बहिर्जिह्वा; जीभ की सूजन या बृद्धि

**Paragrammatism.** See **Paraphasia.**

**Paralalia.** A disorder of articulation. उच्चारणदोष; अपउच्चारण

**Paralexia.** Aphasic inability to read. उच्चारण-अक्षमता; पढ़ कर बोलने की असमर्थता

**Parallax.** The apparent displacement of an object due to a change in the observer's position. लम्बन

**Paralysed.** Affected with palsy. पक्षाघातग्रस्त; लकवाग्रस्त; फालिजग्रस्त

**Paralysis.** Palsy; a loss of sensations, motion, function and sometimes intellect, affecting one or more parts of the body. पक्षाघात; अंगघात; घात; लकवा; फालिज;

**Ascending P.,** a form of paralysis marked by loss of motor power in the legs, gradually extending upwards. आरोही अंगघात; नीचे से ऊपर की ओर बढ़ता हुआ पक्षाघात;

**Bulbar P.,** a form due to the degeneration of the nuclei of origin of the nerves arising in the oblongata. मेरुशीर्षघात; मेरुशीर्ष का पक्षाघात;

**Cerebral P.,** that due to brain-lesion. प्रमस्तिष्क अंगघात;

**Compression P.,** paralysis due to compression of a nerve. सम्पीडन अंगघात;

**Conjugate P.,** paralysis of one or more of the external muscles of the eye. संयुग्म नेत्रघात;

**Crossed P.,** paralysis of an arm on one side and of a leg on the other. व्यत्यस्त अंगघात; एक ओर की भुजा तथा दूसरी ओर की टांग का पक्षाघात;

**Facial P.,** a paralysis of the muscles or the face. आननपेशीघात; चेहरे की पेशियों का पक्षाघात;

**General P.,** an organic disease of the brain, marked by progressive loss of power and deterioration of the mind, ending in dementia and death. व्यापक अंगघात; सार्वदैहिक पक्षाघात;

**Infantile P.,** poliomyelitis; obstetric paralysis. शिशु-अंगघात; पोलियो; बच्चों को होने वाला पक्षाघात;

**Mixed P.**, combined motor and sensory paralysis. मिश्र-अंगघात;

**Motor P.**, loss of power of muscular contraction. प्रेरक अंगघात;

**Obstetric P.**, see **Infantile Paralysis**.

**Pseudobulbar P.**, a symmetric lesion of the halves of the cerebrum, producing paralysis of the lips, tongue, larynx, or pharynx. कूटमेरु-शीर्षघात;

**Reflex P.**, that sometimes following the wound of a nerve. प्रतिवर्त अंगघात;

**Sensory P.**, loss of sensation. सम्वेदी अंगघात;

**Spastic P.**, that associated with rigidity of the muscles and heightened tendon-reflexes. संस्तम्भी अंगघात;

**P. Agitans**, shaking palsy; Parkinson's disease; Parkinsonism. सकम्प अंगघात; कम्पायन पक्षाघात;

**P. Illeus**, paralysis of the intestinal muscles so that the bowel contents cannot pass onwards even though there is no mechanical obstruction. आंत्रपेशीघात; आंत्रपेशियों का पक्षाघात

**Paralytic.** Pertaining to paralysis. घातज; पक्षाघाती; पक्षाघात सम्बन्धी

**Paramastitis.** Inflammation of the tissues lying deep to the mammary glands. परास्तनशोथ

**Paramedical.** Service related to medicine and performed by technically trained persons. पराचिकित्सीय; पराचिकित्सकीय;

**P. Personnel**, technically trained persons performing medical services. पराचिकित्सा-कर्मचारी; पराचिकित्साकर्मी

**Paramenia.** Disordered menstruation. आर्तव-विकार; विकृतार्तव; सदोष ऋतुस्राव; मासिकधर्म की गड़बड़ी

**Parametria.** Plural of **Parametrium**.

**Parametritis.** Inflammation of the pelvic connective tissue. परागर्भाशयसंयोजीऊतकशोथ; श्रोणिसंयोजक ऊतकों का प्रदाह

**Parametrium.** The connective tissue immediately surrounding the uterus. परागर्भाशयसंयोजीऊतक

**Paramnesia.** The common illusion of feeling as if one had already undergone the experience that may be passing. अपस्मृति

**Paramyoconus-multiplex.** A nervous disease with clonic spasms of the voluntary muscles. बहुपरापेश्यवमोटन

**Paramyotonia.** Defective muscular tonicity. परापेशीतानता; पेशियों की दोषपूर्ण तानता;

**Paramyotonia**

**Congenital P.,** see **Paramyotonia Congenita.**

**P. Congenita,** a family disease characterized by tonic spasm; congenital paramyotonia. सहज परापेशीतानता; पेशियों का आजन्म तानिक उद्वेष्ट

**Paranasal.** Near the nasal cavities, as the various sinuses. परानासीय; परानासिक; नथुनों अथवा नासा-गह्वरों के पास

**Paranoia.** A chronic form of insanity with delusions. पौरानोइया; मिथ्याभ्रम के साथ होने वाली विक्षिप्ति का जीर्ण रूप

**Paranoid.** Pertaining to the type of mental illness in which suspicion plays an important role. संविभ्रमी; चित्तविक्षेपी

**Paraoesophageal.** Near the oesophagus. पराग्रासनलीय; ग्रासनली के पास

**Paraparesis.** Partial paralysis of the lower extremities. आंशिक निम्नांगघात; निम्नांगों का आंशिक पक्षाघात

**Paraparetic.** Relating to paraparesis. आंशिक निम्नांगघात सम्बन्धी

**Paraphasia.** Aphasic confusion of words; paragrammatism; paraphrasia. वाग्विकार; वाग्वैकल्य; अपवाक्; स्खलितवाक्

**Paraphimosis.** Retraction of the prepuce behind the glans penis so that the tight ring of the skin interferes with the blood flow in the glans. शिश्नमुण्डच्छदसंकीर्णन; लिंगमुण्डच्छदसंकीर्णन

**Paraphonia.** Change of voice; abnormal condition of the voice. स्वरविकार; स्वरपरिवर्तन; ध्वनि की अस्वाभाविक अवस्था

**Paraphrasia.** See **Paraphasia.**

**Paraplegia.** Paralysis of both sides of the body. अधरांगघात; पादसंस्तम्भन; शरीर के दोनों पार्श्वों का पक्षाघात;

**Spastic P.,** lateral sclerosis. संस्तम्भी अधरांगघात

**Paraplexia.** A mild form of apoplexy. मृदुअपसन्न्यास; रक्ताघात की हल्की अवस्था

**Parapraxia.** Defective performance of purposive acts. चेष्टाविपर्यय

**Pararectal.** Near the rectum. परामलाशयी; मलांत्र के पास

**Pararenal.** Near the kidney. परावृक्कीय; गुर्दे के पास

**Parasitaemia.** Parasites in the blood; parasitemia. परजीवीरक्तता; रक्त में परजीवी विद्यमान रहना

**Parasitemia.** See **Parasitaemia.**

**Parasites.** Animals which live in or on the bodies of other animals, such as intestinal worms. परजीवी; अन्य जीवों के अन्दर पलने वाले जीव

**Parasitic.** Relating to the parasites; parasitical. पारजैविक; परजीवीय; परजीवियों सम्बन्धी;

**P. Growths,** excrescenses like cancerous tumours, tubercles, etc. परजीवी गुल्म; कर्कटाबुर्द; गुलिकाबुर्द जैसा उभार

**Parasitical.** See **Parasitic.**

**Parasiticidal.** See **Parasiticide.**

**Parasiticide.** An agent which destroys parasites; parasiticidal. परजीवीनाशक; परजीवियों को नष्ट करने वाला

**Parasitism.** The state of being infested with parasites. परजीविता

**Parasitologist.** A specialist in parasitology. परजीवीविज्ञानवेत्ता

**Parasitology.** The science of parasites. परजीवीविज्ञान

**Parasitosis.** Infestation with parasites. परजीवीरुग्णता

**Parasternal.** Near the sternum. परा-उरोस्थिक; उरोस्थि के पास

**Parasympathetic.** Those nerves which reverse the action of the sympathetic nerves; also a part of the autonomic nervous system. परानुकम्पी; स्वैच्छिक स्नायु-जाल का एक भाग

**Parasympathomimetic.** Relating to an agent having an action resembling that caused by stimulation of parasympathetic nervous system. परानुकम्पी-अनुकारी

**Parathyroid.** Four small endocrine glands lying close to, or embedded in the posterior surface of the thyroid gland. परावटु; अवटुग्रन्थि के पिछले भाग में स्थित चार छोटी-छोटी ग्रन्थियां

**Parathyroidectomy.** Excision of one or more parathyroid glands. परावटु-उच्छेदन

**Paratonsillar.** Near the tonsils. परागलतुण्डिकीय; गलतुण्डिकाओं के पास

**Paratracheal.** Near the trachea. पराश्वासनलीय; श्वासनली के पास

**Paratyphoid Fever.** A variety of enteric fever, but less severe and prolonged than typhoid. परांत्रिक ज्वर; आंत्रिक ज्वर का एक मृदु रूप

**Paraumbilical.** Near the umbilicus. परानाभिक; परानाभीय; नाभि के पास

**Paraurethral.** Near the urethra. परामूत्रपथीय; परामूत्रमार्गी; मूत्रमार्ग के पास

**Paravaginitis.** Inflammation of the connective tissue alongside the vagina. परायोनिशोथ

**Paravertebral.** Near the spinal column. पराकशेरुकीय; मेरुदण्ड के पास

**Paraxial.** An organism parasitic upon animal. उपाक्षीय; पराक्षीय

**Parenchyma.** The distinguishing tissue of the gland contained and supported by the connective tissue from work or strain. सार—ऊतक; सारूतक; मृदु—ऊतक; मृदूतक

**Parenchymal.** Relating to parenchyma. मृदूतकीय; सारऊतकीय

**Parenchymatitis.** Inflammation of the parenchyma. सारूतकशोथ; मृदूतकशोथ

**Parenteral.** Not via the alimentary tract. आन्त्रेतर

**Paresis.** Partial or slight paralysis. आंशिकघात; हल्का-सा पक्षाघात

**Paretic.** Pertaining to paresis. आंशिकघात सम्बन्धी; affected with paresis. आंशिकघातग्रस्त; आंशिक पक्षाघात से पीड़ित

**Paresthesia.** See **Paraesthesia.**

**Pareunia.** Coitus; sexual intercouse. मैथुन; रति; सम्भोग

**Paries.** Parts forming the walls or units of cavities. प्राचीर; भित्ति; दीवार

**Parietal.** Relating to a wall. पार्श्विक; भित्तिक; भित्तीय; किसी प्राचीर सम्बन्धी; **P. Bone,** the bone forming the cranial sides and roof. पार्श्विकास्थि; कपालपार्श्व एवं कपालभित्ति की रचना करने वाली हड्डी;
**P. Lobe,** the cerebral lobe. पार्श्विक खण्ड; प्रमस्तिष्क खण्ड; सिर का अगला खण्ड

**Parietes.** Plural of **Paries.**

**Parity.** Condition of a woman with regard to the number of children she has borne. प्रसविता

**Parkinsonism.** A brain disease affecting the nerves and through them the muscles, with stiffness and trembling; paralysis agitans; Parkinson's disease. पार्किन्सनता; सकम्प अंगघात; कम्पनयुक्त अंगघात; तंत्रिकाओं तथा पेशियों का एक रोग

**Parkinson's Disease.** See **Parkinsonism.**

**Parodinia.** See **Parodynia.**

**Parodynia.** Morbid or painful labour; parodinia. कष्टप्रसव; दर्दनाक प्रसव

**Paronychia.** A whitlow; panaritium. परिनखशोथ; चिप्य; अंगुलबेढ़ा; उपनखपाक; नाखुन की सूजन

**Paronychial.** Relating to the paronychia or the nail-fold; panaritium. परिनखशोथ; चिप्य अथवा उपनख सम्बन्धी

**Paroophoron.** See **Parovarium.**

**Parorexia.** Perverted sense of taste. अपरुचि; विरसता; बदला हुआ स्वाद

**Parosmia.** Perverted sense of smell. घ्राणविकृति; विपर्यस्तघ्राणता; परिवर्तित घ्राणसम्वेदना

**Parosteitis.** Inflammation of the outer surface of the periosteum; parostitis. पर्यस्थिशोथ; पर्यस्थिकलाशोथ; अस्थ्यावरण के बाहरी तल का प्रदाह

**Parostitis.** See **Parosteitis.**

**Parotic.** Near or beside the ear. पराकर्ण; कान के पास

**Parotid.** Near the ear. कर्णमूलीय; कान के पास; कर्णमूल; कर्णपूर्व;

    **P. Gland,** the salivary gland situated in front of and below the ear. कर्णमूलग्रन्थि; कर्णपूर्वग्रन्थि

**Parotidectomy.** Excision of the parotid gland. कर्णमूलग्रन्थि-उच्छेदन; कर्णमूलग्रन्थि को काट कर हटा देना

**Parotiditis.** Inflammation of the parotid glands; mumps; parotitis. कर्णमूलग्रन्थिशोथ; कर्णपूर्वग्रन्थिशोथ; कनफेड़; कनपेड़

**Parotitis.** See **Parotiditis.**

**Parous.** Having born a child or many children. प्रजाता; एक बच्चे या कई बच्चों को जन्म देने वाली स्त्री

**Parovarian.** Near the ovary. पराडिम्बग्रन्थिक; डिम्बग्रन्थि के पास; pertaining to the parovarium. पराडिम्बग्रन्थि सम्बन्धी

**Parovarium.** A few scattered rudimentary tubules in the broad ligament between the epoophoron and the uterus; paroophoron. पराडिम्बग्रन्थि

**Paroxysm.** Intermittent attack, as of a disease. प्रवेग; दौरा; आक्रमण; रोगावेग; a sharp spasm or convulsion. उग्राक्षेप; उग्र-उद्वेष्ट

**Paroxysmal.** Coming on in attacks or paroxysms. प्रवेगी; दौरे के रूप में प्रकट होने वाला

**Parrot Disease.** See **Parrot Fever.**

**Parrot Fever.** A virus infection transmitted by birds, especially the parrots and related species; parrot disease; ornithosis. शुक-ज्वर; पक्षियों, विशेष रूप से तोतों द्वारा फैलने वाला एक विषाणु रोग

**Pars.** A part, or portion of a structure. भाग; अंश;

    **P. Laryngea Pharyngis,** the laryngeal part of the pharynx. ग्रसनी का स्वरयंत्रज भाग

**Part.** See **Pars.**

**Partes.** Plural of **Pars.**

**Partes Aequales.** Equal parts. समभाग

**Parthenogenesis.** A form of asexual reproduction in which female reproduces its kid without fecundation by male. अनिषेकजनन

**Partial.** Relating to a part only. आंशिक; मात्र एक भाग सम्बन्धी

**Particle.** A very small piece or portion of anything. कण

**Parturient.** A woman who has recently given birth to a child. प्रसूता; प्रसवमाना

**Parturifacient.** Medicines inducing or promoting labour. प्रसूतिकर; प्रसवकारी

**Parturition.** Labour; childbirth; the act of giving birth to a child; partus. प्रसव; प्रसूति; बच्चे को जन्म देने की क्रिया

**Partus.** See **Parturition.**

**Parulis.** Gumboil; inflammation, swelling or abscess in the gum. मसूढ़ा फूलना; मसूढ़े के अन्दर प्रदाह, सूजन या फोड़ा होना

**Parvule.** A granule or pellet. गुलिका; कण; गोली

**Passa.** A whitlow. चिप्प; अंगुलबेढ़ा

**Passage.** A duct, channel, pore or opening. पथ; द्वार; नली; a secretion. निस्सरण; उत्सर्जन

**Passion.** Intense emotion. अतिभावुकता; उग्र मनोद्वेग

**Passive.** Inactive. निष्क्रिय; शैरिक; submissive. समर्पणशील

**Paste.** Any sort of sticky substance. गोंद; लेप; लेई; a soft compound of medicine. पेस्ट

**Pasteurisation.** See **Pasteurization.**

**Pasteurism.** Vaccination. टीका; टीकाकरण

**Pasteurization.** The heating of milk to destroy disease-causing germs, named after Louis Pasteur, its originator; pasteurisation. पैस्चुरीकरण; निर्जीवाणुकरण; रोगोत्पादक जीवाणुओं को ताप द्वारा नष्ट करने की प्रक्रिया

**Pasteurized.** Heated according to the method of Louis Pasteur. पैस्चुरीकृत; निर्जीवाणुकृत

**Pastpointing.** A diagnostic point for brain disease. अपनिर्देशन

**Patch.** An irregular spot or area. चित्ती; धब्बा; पैच; क्षेत्र;

**Mucous P.**, a lesion of syphilis observed on mucous membranes. श्लेष्मल धब्बा; श्लेष्मकलाओं पर उपदंश का एक घाव

**Patch-test.** A means of determining skin sensitivity or general allergy, used in diagnosis and as a test for safety of hair dyes. पैच-टेस्ट; पैच-जांच

**Patella.** A round sesamoid bone in front of knee; the knee-cap जानुका; जान्वस्थि; जानुफलक; घुटने की चौड़ी हड्डी

**Patellae.** Plural of **Patella.**

**Patellar.** Pertaining to a patella. जानुफलक अथवा जान्वस्थि सम्बन्धी

**Patellectomy.** Excision of the patella. जानुका-उच्छेदन

**Patelliform.** Of the form of patella. जानुकारूप; जानुकाकार; घुटने की चौड़ी हड्डी जैसा

**Patency.** The condition of being open. एकस्वत्व

**Patent.** Open; not closed or occluded. व्यक्त; एकस्व; विवृत; सच्छिद्र

**Pathema.** A morbid condition. रोगावस्था; विकृतावस्था; पीड़ितावस्था

**Pathematology.** See **Pathology.**

**Pathetic.** Causing an emotion, especially of sorrow or pity. मार्मिक; मर्मस्पर्शी; हृदयग्राही

**Pathic.** Diseased. रुग्ण; रोगग्रस्त; relating to a disease. रोग सम्बन्धी

**Pathogen.** Any disease-producing agent. विकृतिजन; रोगजन; कोई रोगोत्पादक पदार्थ

**Pathogenesis.** The origin and development of a disease; pathogeny. विकृतिजनन; रोगजनन; किसी रोग का जन्म और विकास

**Pathogenetic.** Causing disease; pathogenic. रोगजनक; रोगजन्य; विकृतिजनक; विकारी; रोगमूलक; बीमारी पैदा करने वाला

**Pathogenic.** See **Pathogenetic.**

**Pathogenicity.** The condition of being pathogenic or of causing disease. विकृतिजनकता; रोगजनकता

**Pathogeny.** See **Pathogenesis.**

**Pathognomonic.** Distinctive of a special disease. विकृति-व्याधिज्ञापक; रोगनिदानात्मक; विशिष्ट व्याधिज्ञापक

**Pathognomy.** The science of the signs by which a disease is recognised. रोगचिन्हविज्ञान

**Pathography.** Description of a disease. रोगवर्णन

**Pathologic.** Pathological; resulting from disease. विकृतिजन्य; वैकृत; relating to pathology. विकृतिविज्ञान सम्बन्धी; morbid; diseased. रुग्ण; बीमार

**Pathological.** See **Pathologic.**

**Pathologist.** A specialist in pathology. विकृतिविज्ञानी; रोगविज्ञानी; रोगों का ज्ञाता; विकृतिविज्ञान का विशेषज्ञ

**Pathology.** That part of medicine which treats of the cause, nature, etc. of a disease; pathematology. विकृतिविज्ञान; रोगविज्ञान; विकृति; रोग के कारण, स्वभाव आदि से सम्बन्धित विज्ञान;

   **Cellular P.,** that which makes the cells the basis of all vital phenomena. कोशिकाविकृति; कोशिकारोगविज्ञान;

# Pathology

**Experimental P.**, the study of morbid processes artificially induced in animals. प्रायोगिक विकृतिविज्ञान

**Pathophobia.** A morbid fear of disease. रोगभीति; रोगातंक; बीमारी का डर

**Pathophysiology.** Derangement or alteration of function seen in disease. विकारी-शरीरक्रिया

**Patient.** One who is suffering from or under treatment of any disease. रोगी; बीमार; मरीज; रुग्ण

**Pator Narium.** The cavities of the nose. नासाछिद्र; नासा-गह्वर; नथुने

**Patulous.** Expanded; open. विवृत; खुला हुआ या फैला हुआ

**Paunch.** The abdominal cavity and its contents. उदरगह्वर और उसके पदार्थ

**Pause.** Temporary stop. विराम

**Pavor.** Fright. भय; भीति; डर; आतंक;

   **P. Nocturnus,** nightmare. निशाभीति; निशातंक

**P.C.** Abbreviation for **Post-cebum.**

**Peanut.** The fruit of **Arachis Hypogoea.** मूंगफली; मटर

**Pearl.** A small hollow sphere of thin glass containing a medicinal fluid for inhalation. मुक्ता; मोती; cataract. मोतियाबिन्द

**Peccant.** Morbid; unhealthy. रुग्ण; अस्वस्थ; producing disease. रोगजनक

**Pectinate.** Resembling a comb. कंकतदन्त; कंकताकार; कंघे जैसे दान्त

**Pectiniform.** Comb-shaped. कंकताकार; कंकतरूप; कंघे जैसा

**Pectora.** Plural of **Pectus.**

**Pectoral.** Pertaining to the breast. वक्षीय; उरस्त्राणीय; वक्ष सम्बन्धी

**Pectoralis.** The muscle of the breast. वक्षपेशी; छाती की पेशी

**Pectori.** In the chest. वक्ष में; छाती में

**Pectoriloquy.** The distinct transmission of articulate speech to the ear on auscultation. वक्षध्वनि; परिश्रवणध्वनि

**Pectus.** The chest. वक्ष; छाती;

   **P. Carinatum,** pigeon-chest; chicken-breast. कपोतवक्ष; उन्नतोरोस्थिक वक्ष;

   **P. Excavatum,** funnel chest; pectus recurvatum. कीपवक्ष;

   **P. Recurvatum,** see **Pectus Excavatum.**

**Pedal.** Relating to the foot. पदिक; पादक; पैर सम्बन्धी

**Pederast.** One who practises pederasty. गुदमैथुनकारी; लौंडेबाज

**Pederasty.** See **Paederasty.**

**Pedes.** Plural of **Pes.**

**Pedialgia.** Pain in the foot. पादशूल; पादार्ति; पैर का दर्द

**Pediatric.** Relating to pediatrics. बालरोगविज्ञान सम्बन्धी

**Pediatrician.** A children disease specialist; paediatrician. बालरोगविशेषज्ञ; बालरोगविज्ञानी; बालरोगचिकित्सक

**Pediatrics.** The medical speciality concerned with the diseases of the children, upto the age of 18 years; paediatrics; paediatry; pediatry. बालरोगविज्ञान; बालरोगचिकित्सा; कौभारभृत्य

**Pediatry.** See **Pediatrics.**

**Pedicle.** The stalk of attachment of a tumour. वृन्त; डण्ठल जैसी बनावट

**Pedicterus.** Jaundice of the newborn. शिशुकामला; नवजात शिशु को होने वाला पीलिया

**Pedicular.** Relating to lice. यूका अथवा जूं सम्बन्धी

**Pediculi.** Plural of **Pediculus.**

**Pediculicide.** An agent which destroys the lice. यूकानाशी; जूंनाशक; जूंमार (औषधि)

**Pediculosis.** The symptoms produced by lice. यूकोपसर्ग; यूकारोग; जूं से होने वाली बीमारी;

   **P. Pubis,** the pubic louse. जघन यूका

**Pediculus.** A genus of lice; the louse. यूका; जूं;

   **P. Capitis,** the head louse. शिरोयूका; शिरोयूकोपसर्ग;

   **P. Corporis,** the body louse. वस्त्रयूका; देहयूका; काययूकोपसर्ग;

   **P. Humanus Corporis,** the same as **Pediculus Corporis.**

   **P. Pubis,** the pubic louse. जघन यूका

**Pediform.** Shaped like a foot. पादवत्; पैर जैसा

**Pedodontics.** Treating the teeth of the children. शिशुदन्तचिकित्सा

**Pedodontist.** A dentist who practices pedodontics. शिशुदन्तचिकित्सक

**Pedology.** See **Paedology.**

**Peduncle.** A stalk-like structure, often acting as a support. वृन्त; वृंतक; बन्धन; रज्जु;

   **Cerebellar P.,** the white cord of the cerebrum. अनुमस्तिष्क वृंतक; अनुमस्तिष्क रज्जु;

**Cerebral P.'s,** three pairs of stout bundles of nerve-fibres connecting the cerebellum with the other chief parts of the brain. प्रमस्तिष्क वृन्तक

**Peduncular.** Pertaining to peduncle. वृन्तीय; वृन्त सम्बन्धी

**Pedunculated.** Having a peduncle. वृन्तमय; वृन्तीय

**Peeling.** Desquamation. विशल्कन; शल्कन; छिल्का उतरना

**Peer.** An associate of about equal age. समवय युगल; contemporary. समकालीन; समकालिक

**Pelage.** The hairy system of the body. लोम-प्रणाली; शरीर का केश-जाल

**Pelioma.** A livid spot in typhoid fever. नीलचित्तिता; आंत्रिक ज्वर में प्रकट होने वाले नीले धब्बे

**Peliosis.** Purpura. चित्तिता;

 **P. Haemorrhagica,** see **Purpura Haemorrhagica.**

**Pellagra.** A cutaneous disease almost confined to the northern parts of Italy. वल्कचर्म; त्वक्-परूषता; रौद्रा; पेलाग्रा

**Pellagragenic.** Producing pellagra. वल्कचर्मजनक; पेलाग्राजनक

**Pellagrous.** Relating to pellagra. वल्कचर्म सम्बन्धी

**Pellet.** A little pill. गुटिका; वटी; टिक्की

**Pellicle.** A thin film or membrane. सूक्ष्मावरण; पटल; सूक्ष्मकला; झिल्ली

**Pelma.** See **Planta.**

**Pelopathy.** Mud treatment. कीचोपचार; गारे-कीचड़ द्वारा की जाने वाली चिकित्सा

**Pelves.** Plural of **Pelvis.**

**Pelvic.** Relating to the pelvis. श्रोणि सम्बन्धी; गोणिकीय; पेडू का;

 **P. Girdle,** the ring of bones which forms the hips and lower abdominal area. श्रोणि-बन्ध; गोणिका-बन्ध

**Pelvimeter.** An instrument, especially devised to measure the pelvic diameter. श्रोणिमापी; गोणिकामापी

**Pelvimetry.** The measurement of the dimensions of the pelvis. श्रोणिमिति; गोणिकामिति

**Pelviotomy.** See **Pubiotomy.**

**Pelvis.** A basin-shaped bony cavity forming the lower portion of the abdomen. श्रोणि; गोणिका; वस्तिप्रदेश; पेडू;

 **Android P.,** a masculine or funnel-shaped pelvis; male type pelvis. पुंवत् श्रोणि;

**Beaked P.**, pelvis with the pelvis bones laterally compressed and pushed forward so that the outlet is narrow and long. चंचुवत् श्रोणि;

**Contracted P.**, a pelvis with less than normal measurements in any diameter. संकुचित श्रोणि;

**False P.**, large pelvis; pelvis major. कूट श्रोणि; मिथ्या श्रोणि;

**Large P.**, see **False Pelvis**.

**Male Type P.**, see **Android Pelvis**.

**Obstetrical P.**, see **True Pelvis**.

**Osteomalacic P.**, one marked by lessening of the transverse and oblique diameters and by great increase of the antero-posterior diameters. अस्थिमृदुतायुक्त श्रोणि;

**Rachitic P.**, one with sinking in and forward of the sacrovertebral angle and flaring outward of the iliac crests. रिक्केटी श्रोणि;

**Small P.**, see **True Pelvis**.

**Split P.**, one with congenital separation of the symphysis pubis. विपाटित श्रोणि;

**True P.**, the part below the iliopectineal line; obstetric pelvis; small pelvis; pelvis minor. यथार्थ श्रोणि; वास्तविक श्रोणि;

**P. Major**, see **False Pelvis**.

**P. Minor**, see **True Pelvis**.

**Pemphigus.** A disease of the skin with an eruption of bullas. पेम्फीगस नामक चर्म रोग; बिम्बिका; फफोला; छाला

**Pendulous.** Hanging down. दोलायमान; लम्बित; नीचे की ओर लटका हुआ

**Penetrating.** Entering beyond surface. वेधी; अन्तर्वेधी; अन्तर्विष्ट

**Penile.** Pertaining to the penis. शिश्न सम्बन्धी

**Penis.** The male organ of copulation. शिश्न; लिंग

**Penitis.** Inflammation of the penis. शिश्नशोथ; लिंग-प्रदाह

**Penology.** The science of crime, its punishment and prevention. दण्डशास्त्र; दण्डविज्ञान; अपराधविज्ञान

**Pentadactyl.** See **Pentadactyly**.

**Pentadactyly.** Having five fingers; pentadactyl. पंचांगुलिक

**Pentavalent.** Having a valence of five. पंचसंयोजी

**Pepsin.** A peculiar digestive principle which, with the gastric juice, forms the digestive solvent of the stomach; pepsine. पेप्सिन; पाचकरस; जठर-रस का पाचक किण्व; पित्त का एक प्रमुख अंश

**Pepsine**

**Pepsine.** See **Pepsin**.
**Peptic.** Adding digestion. पाचक; अग्निवर्धक;
   **P. Ulcer,** ulcer in the stomach or duodenum. उदरव्रण; ग्रहणीव्रण; आंत या पेट का फोड़ा अथवा घाव
**Per-abdomen.** Through the abdomen. उदर द्वारा; उदर-प्रवेशी
**Per-anum.** See **Per-anus**.
**Per-anus.** Through the anus; per-anum. गुदा-प्रवेशी; मलद्वार से
**Percept.** The mental product of a sensation. सम्वेदना; सम्बोध; अनुभूति; प्रतिबोध
**Perception.** Receiving of an impression through the senses. प्रत्यक्ष ज्ञान; अवगम; बोध; अनुभूति
**Perceptivity.** Ability to receive impressions. बोधगम्यता; अनुभूतिक्षमता
**Percolate.** To subject to percolation. परिस्राव; रिसना
**Percolation.** The process by which the fluid slowly passes through a hard but porous substance. परिस्रवण; रिसाव
**Percolator.** A long conic vessel used in percolation. परिस्रावित्र; पर्कोलेटर; परिस्रवण प्रक्रिया में प्रयुक्त एक लम्बा शंक्वाकार पात्र
**Percuss.** To perform percussion on. परिताड़न करना; समाहत करना
**Percussion.** The mode of examining diseases by striking upon or even diseased parts and judging by the sounds made thereby. परिताड़न; समाहनन;
   **Auscultatory P.,** auscultation of the chest or other parts at the same time when the percussion in made. परिश्रवणीय; परिताड़न;
   **Palpatory P.,** finger percussion concerned with the resistance of the tissues under the finger as well as upon the sound elicited. परिस्पर्शनीय परिताड़न
**Percussor.** An instrument for performing percussion. परिताड़नयंत्र
**Percutaneous.** Through unbroken skin. त्वचाप्रवेशी; चमड़ी से
**Perforans.** Penetrating; perforating. छिद्रिल; सछिद्र; छिद्रित
**Perforate.** To pierce with holes. छिद्र करना; वेधना; छेद करना
**Perforated.** Pierced with holes. विद्ध; छिद्रित; सछिद्र
**Perforation.** An opening or a penetrating wound. वेधन; छिद्रण; वेध; छिद्र
**Perforator.** An instrument to open the skull. पर्फोरेटर; वेधक; छिद्रक
**Perfusion.** Isolating the circulation in a limited portion of the body

for the purpose of treating cancer in that area with highly potent drugs. निवेशन; द्रवनिवेशन; रक्तनिवेशन

**Peri-.** Prefix signifying around or about. 'परि' के रूप में प्रयुक्त उपसर्ग

**Periadenitis.** Inflammation of soft tissues surrounding the glands. परिलसीकापर्वशोथ; ग्रन्थि-ऊतकों का प्रदाह

**Perianal.** Surrounding the anus. परिगुदीय; गुदा के आस-पास का

**Periaortitis.** Inflammation of the tissues around aorta. परिमहाधमनीशोथ; महाधमनी को घेर कर रखने वाले ऊतकों का प्रदाह

**Periappendicitis.** Inflammation of peritoneum around the appendix. परिउपांत्रशोथ; उपांत्र के इर्द-गिर्द उदरावरण का प्रदाह

**Periarterial.** Surrounding an artery. परिधमनिक; किसी धमनी के आस-पास का

**Periarteritis.** Inflammation of the outer convering of the arteries. परिधमनीशोथ; धमनियों के बाहरी आवरण का प्रदाह

**Periarthritis.** Inflammation of the structures surrounding a joint. परिसन्धिशोथ; सन्धि-आवरण का प्रदाह

**Periarticular.** Surrounding a joint. परिसन्धिक; किसी सन्धि के आस-पास का

**Periaxial.** See **Periaxonic.**

**Periaxonic.** Around an axis; periaxial. पर्यक्षतन्तुक; किसी अक्ष के चारों ओर का

**Peribronchitis.** Inflammation of the tissues surrounding the bronchi or bronchial tubes. परिश्वसनिकाशोथ

**Pericardectomy.** Surgical removal of pericardium; pericardiectomy. परिहृदुच्छेदन; हृदयावरण-उच्छेदन; हृदयावरण को काट कर हटा देना

**Pericardia.** Plural of **Pericardium.**

**Pericardiac.** Pertaining to the pericardium; pericardial. हृदयावरक; हृदयावरण सम्बन्धी

**Pericardial.** See **Pericardiac.**

**Pericardiectomy.** See **Pericardectomy.**

**Pericardiocentesis.** The withdrawal of fluid from the pericardial sac by insertion of a hollow needle or cannula. परिहृद्वेधन

**Pericardiotomy.** An incision of the pericardium. हृदयावरणछेदन; परिहृद्छेदन

**Pericarditic.** Relating to pericarditis. परिहृद्शोथ सम्बन्धी

**Pericarditis.** Inflammation of the pericardium. परिहृद्शोथ; हृदयावरणशोथ; हृदय की झिल्ली का प्रदाह;
**Adhesive P.**, that in which the two layers of pericardium tend to adhere. आसंजी हृदयावरणशोथ;
**Dry P.**, a form without effusion. शुष्क हृदयावरणशोथ;
**Fibrinous P.**, a form in which the membrane is covered with fibrinous exudate. फाइब्रिनी हृदयावरणशोथ;
**Purulent P.**, that in which the fluid becomes purulent. सपूय हृदयावरणशोथ;
**Visceral P.**, the epicardium; the layer attached to the heart. आशयिक हृदयावरणशोथ
**Pericardium.** The fibroserous membrane covering the heart. परिहृद्; हृदयावरण
**Pericellullar.** Around a cell. परिकोशीय; परिकोशिकीय; कोशिका के चारों ओर
**Perichondral.** Relating to perichondrium. उपास्थ्यावरण सम्बन्धी
**Perichondritis.** Inflammation of the perichondrium. पर्युपास्थिशोथ; उपास्थि-आवरण का प्रदाह
**Perichondrium.** A membrane around a cartilage. पर्युपास्थि; उपास्थि-आवरण; उपास्थ्यावरण
**Pericolic.** Around the colon. परिबृहदान्त्रिक; बृहदान्त्र के चारों ओर का
**Pericolitis.** Inflammation of the tissues around the colon; pericolonitis. परिबृहदान्त्रशोथ; बृहदान्त्रावरण का प्रदाह
**Pericolonitis.** See **Pericolitis.**
**Pericolpitis.** Inflammation around the vagina; perivaginitis. परियोनिशोथ
**Pericorneal.** Surrounding the cornea. परिकनीनिकी; कनीनिका के आस-पास का
**Pericranitis.** Inflammation of the pericranium. परिकपालशोथ
**Pericranium.** The periosteum of the cranium. परिकपाल; कपालावरण
**Pericystic.** Surrounding the urinary bladder, the gall-bladder or a cyst; perivesical. परिआशयिक; परिपुटीय
**Pericystitis.** Inflammation of the tissues around the bladder. परिपुटीशोथ; मूत्राशय-ऊतकों का प्रदाह
**Pericyte.** One of the slender, relatively undifferentiated, connective

tissue cells in close relationship to the outside of the capillary walls. परिकोशिका

**Peridental.** Around a tooth. परिदन्तीय; दान्त के चारों ओर

**Periderm.** Around the skin; periderma. परित्वक्; त्वचा के चारों ओर का

**Periderma.** See **Periderm.**

**Perididymis.** The serous coat investing the testes. परिवृषणकोशकला; वृषणों को ढक कर रखने वाली सीरमी कला

**Perididysmitis.** Inflammation of the perididymis. परिवृषणकोशकलाशोथ

**Peridiverticulitis.** Inflammation of tissues around an intestinal diverticulum. परिविपुटीशोथ

**Perifollicular.** Around the follicele. परिपुटकीय; पुटक के चारों ओर का

**Perifolliculitis.** Inflammation of the area surrounding the hair follicles. परिपुटकशोथ; परिलोमपुटकशोथ

**Perigastric.** Surrounding the stomach. परिजठरीय; आमाशय के चारों ओर का

**Perigastritis.** Inflammation of the peritoneal coat of the stomach. परिजठरशोथ; जठरावरणशोथ; पर्यामाशयशोथ; आमाशयावरक झिल्ली का प्रदाह

**Periglottis.** The mucous membrane of the tongue. परिजिह्वा; जिह्वावरण; जीभ की श्लेष्मकला

**Perihepatitis.** Inflammation of the serous covering of the liver. परियकृत्शोथ; यकृतावरणशोथ; यकृत् की सीरमी कला का प्रदाह

**Perijejunitis.** Inflammation around the jejunum. परिमध्यांत्रशोथ

**Perikarya.** Plural of **Perikaryon.**

**Perikaryon.** The cytoplasm of a neuron. परिकेन्द्रकद्रव्य

**Perilaryngitis.** Inflammation of the tissues around the larynx. परिस्वरयंत्रशोथ

**Perilymph.** The fluid contained in the internal ear, between the bony and membranous labyrinth; perilympha. परिलसीका; परिलसीकावाहिनी

**Perilympha.** See **Perilymph.**

**Perimetria.** Plural of **Perimetrium.**

**Perimetritis.** Inflammation of the peritoneal covering of the uterus. परिगर्भाशयऊतिशोथ; जरायु-आवरक झिल्ली का प्रदाह

**Perimetrium.** Peritoneal covering of the uterus. परिगर्भाशय; गर्भाशयपर्यस्तर; जरायु-आवरक झिल्ली

# Perinatal

**Perinatal.** Occurring at, or pertaining to the time of birth. प्रसवकालीन; प्रसव के दौरान प्रकट होने वाला या उससे सम्बन्धित

**Perinea.** Plural of **Perineum.**

**Perineal.** Relating to the perineum. मूलाधारीय; उत्सर्गांतरालीय; मूलाधार से सम्बन्धित

**Perineoplasty.** Plastic surgery of the perineum. मूलाधारसंधान

**Perineorrhaphy.** The operation for the repair of a torn perineum. मूलाधारसीवन

**Perineotomy.** A perineal incision made during the birth of a child when the vaginal orifice does not stretch sufficiently; episiotomy. मूलाधारछेदन

**Perinephric.** Surrounding the kidney. परिवृक्कीय; वृक्क के पास का

**Perinephritis.** Inflammation of the tissue around the kidney. परिवृक्कशोथ; गुर्दे के आस-पास वाले ऊतक का प्रदाह

**Perineum.** The external surface of the perineal body, lying between vulva and anus in females and scrotum and anus in males. मूलाधार; उत्सर्गांतराल; मलद्वार और अण्डकोष का निचला भाग

**Perineuritis.** Inflammation of a perineurium. परितंत्रिकाशोथ; तंत्रिकावरण का प्रदाह

**Perineurium.** A sheath investing a funiculus of a nerve fibre. परितंत्रिका; तंत्रिकावरण

**Period.** An interval of time; one of the stages of a disease. काल; युग; अवधि; प्रक्रम;

**Incubation P.,** the period between implantation of a contagium and the appearance of a disease; latent period. उद्भवन काल;

**Latent P.,** see **Incubation Period.**

**Menstrual P.,** the menses; monthly period. आर्तवकाल; ऋतुकाल;

**Monthly P.,** see **Menstrual Period.**

**Periodic.** Recurring after definite intervals. कालिक; नियतकालिक; आवर्ती

**Periodicity.** Recurring at regular intervals. आवर्तिता; आवर्तता; कालक्रम

**Periodontal.** Around a teeth. परिदन्तीय; दान्तों के चारों ओर का

**Periodontia.** Plural of **Periodontium.**

**Periodontics.** Treatment of the diseases of the tissues around the teeth. दन्तूतकोपचार; दन्त-ऊतकचिकित्सा; परिदन्तोपचार; दान्तों के समीपवर्ती ऊतकों के रोगों की चिकित्सा

**Periodontist.** A dentist who specializes in periodontics. दन्तोतक-चिकित्सक; दन्तोतकोपचारक

**Periodontitis.** Inflammation of the membrane of a tooth-socket; Rigg's disease. परिदन्तशोथ; दन्तावरणशोथ; दन्तकोटर-कला का प्रदाह; रिग्ग रोग

**Periodontium.** A fibrous envelope of the cementum. परिदन्त; दन्तावरण

**Periodontosis.** Wasting away of the bone surrounding the teeth, resulting in consequent looseness of teeth. दन्तक्षय; दान्तों की समीपवर्ती हड्डी का क्षय

**Periorbit.** The periosteum of the orbit. परिनेत्रगुहा

**Periossium.** See **Periosteum**.

**Periostea.** Plural of **Periosteum**.

**Periosteal.** Pertaining to periosteum. पर्यस्थिक; अस्थ्यावरणीय; पर्यस्थिकला सम्बन्धी

**Periosteitis.** Inflammation of the periosteum; periostitis. पर्यस्थिकलाशोथ; अस्थ्यावरणशोथ; अस्थि-आवरक झिल्ली का प्रदाह

**Periosteoma.** A hard growth near the bone. पर्यस्थिकलार्बुद; हड्डी के पास उत्पन्न होने वाला कोई कठोर गुल्म

**Periosteum.** A fibrous membrane investing bones; periossium. अस्थ्यावरण; पर्यस्थिकला; हड्डियों को ढक कर रखने वाली तन्तु-कला

**Periostitis.** See **Periosteitis**.

**Peripancreatitis.** Inflammation of the peritoneal coat of the pancreas. पर्यग्न्याशयशोथ

**Peripheral.** Away from the centre, as the nerves and blood vessels in the arms and legs. परिसरीय; प्रान्तस्थ; केन्द्र से दूर

**Periphery.** The bounding line. परिसर; उपान्त

**Periphlebitis.** Inflammation of the outer coat of a vein. परिशिराशोथ; शिरावरणशोथ; शिरा की बाहरी झिल्ली का प्रदाह

**Peripleuritis.** Inflammation around the pleura. परिफुफ्फुसावरणशोथ; फुफ्फुसावरण के आस-पास का प्रदाह

**Peripneumonia.** Inflammation of the substance of the lungs. परिफुफ्फुसपाक; फुफ्फुस-पदार्थ का प्रदाह

**Periproctitis.** Inflammation around the rectum and anus; perirectitis. परिमलांत्रशोथ; मलाशय एवं गुदा के चारों ओर का प्रदाह

**Periprostatitis.** Inflammation of the tissues surrounding the prostate. परिपुरःस्थग्रन्थिशोथ

**Perirectitis.** See **Periproctitis.**

**Perirenal.** Around the kidney. परिवृक्कीय; गुर्दे के चारों ओर का

**Perisalpingitis.** Inflammation around the the oviduct. परिडिम्बवाहिनीशोथ; डिम्बवाहिनी के चारों ओर का प्रदाह

**Perisalpinx.** The peritoneal covering of the uterine tube. परिडिम्बवाहिनी

**Perisplenitis.** Inflammation of the peritoneal coat of the spleen and of the adjacent structures. परिप्लीहाशोथ; प्लीहा तथा उसके निकटवर्ती भागों की आवरक झिल्ली का प्रदाह

**Peristalsis.** Wave-like motion, as of oesophagus, stomach and intestines, which keeps the food material moving; peristole. पुरःसरण; क्रमाकुंचन; लहर जैसी गति

**Peristaltic.** Pertaining to peristalsis. पुरःसरणीय; क्रमाकुंचक;
  **P. Action,** the undulation or vermicular movement of the intestines in their convolutions. पुरःसरणीय क्रिया; क्रमाकुंचक क्रिया

**Peristole.** See **Peristalsis.**

**Perisystole.** An interval between the dilatation and contraction of the heart. परिप्रकुंचन; हृदय के फैलने और सिकुड़ने के बीच की अवधि

**Peritectomy.** See **Peritomy.**

**Peritomy.** Excision of a portion of conjunctiva at the edge of the cornea to prevent vascularization of a corneal ulcer; peritectomy. परिच्छेदन

**Peritonea.** Plural of **Peritoneum.**

**Peritoneal.** Relating to the peritoneum. उदरावरणीय; उदरावरण सम्बन्धी

**Peritoneopathy.** Any disease of the peritoneum. पर्युदर्यरोग; उदरावरणरोग

**Peritoneoplasty.** Loosening adhesions and covering the raw surfaces with peritoneum to prevent reformation. पर्युदर्यासंधान; उदरावरणसंधान

**Peritoneoscope.** An instrument for performing laparoscopy. पर्युदर्यादर्शी; उदरावरणदर्शीयंत्र

**Peritoneoscopy.** Laparoscopy. पर्युदर्यादर्शन; उदरावरणदर्शन

**Peritoneotomy.** Incision of the peritoneum. पर्युदर्याच्छेदन; उदरावरणछेदन

**Peritoneum.** A thin, smooth membrane that invests the whole internal surface of the abdomen and the organs contained in that cavity. पर्युदर्या; उदरावरण

**Peritonitis.** Inflammation of the peritoneum. पर्युदर्याशोथ; उदरावरणशोथ; उदरावरण का प्रदाह;

**Adhesive P.**, that with adhesion between the parietal and visceral layers; plastic peritonitis. आसंजी पर्युदर्याशोथ;

**Plastic P.**, see **Adhesive Peritonitis.**

**Tuberculous P.**, that due to the deposit of miliary tubercles upon the peritoneum. यक्ष्मज पर्युदर्याशोथ

**Peritonsillar.** Around the tonsil. गलतुण्डिका के चारों ओर का;

**P. Abscess**, quinsy. परिगलतुण्डिका-विद्रधि

**Peritonsillitis.** Inflammation of the connective tissue above and behind the tonsil. परिगलतुण्डिकाशोथ

**Perityphlitis.** Inflammation around the caecum. पर्यन्धान्त्रशोथ; परिअन्धान्त्रशोथ; अन्धान्त्र के चारों ओर का प्रदाह

**Periumbilical.** Surrounding the umbilicus. परिनाभिक; नाभि के आस-पास का

**Periureteral.** Around the ureters; periureteric. परिमूत्रनलीय; परिगवीनीय; मूत्रनलियों के चारों ओर का

**Periureteric.** See **Periureteral.**

**Periureteritis.** Inflammation of the tissues about a ureter. परिमूत्रनलीशोथ

**Periurethral.** Around the urethra. परिमूत्रपथीय; मूत्रमार्ग के चारों ओर का

**Periurethritis.** Inflammationof the tissues about the urethra. परिमूत्रपथशोथ

**Perivaginal.** Around the vagina. परियोनिक; योनि के चारों ओर का

**Perivaginitis.** See **Pericolpitis.**

**Perivascular.** Around a blood vessel. परिवाहिकीय; किसी रक्त-वाहिका के चारों ओर का

**Perivesical.** See **Pericystic.**

**Perivisceritis.** Inflammation surrounding any viscus or viscera. पर्यंतरांगशोथ; अंतरांगों को प्रभावित करने वाला प्रदाह

**Perleche.** An intertrigo at the angle of the mouth with maceration, fissuring or crust formation. परलेश

**Permeability**

**Permeability.** In physiology, the ability of the cell membranes to allow salts, glucose, urea and other soluble substances to pass into and out of the cells from the body fluids. अन्तर्गम्यता; पारगम्यता

**Pernasal.** Performed through the nose. नासाप्रवेशी; नाक द्वारा दिया जाने वाला

**Pernicious.** Fatal; highly destructive. प्रणाशी; घातक; मारक;

**P. Anaemia,** results from the inability of the bone-marrow to produce normal red cells because of the deprivation of a protein released by gastric glands. प्रणाशी अरक्तता; घातक अरक्तता; सांघातिक अरक्तता

**Pernio.** A chilblain. शीतदंश; तुषारदंश; बिवाई फटना

**Perniosis.** Chronic chilblains. जीर्ण शीतदंश; बिवाइयाँ फटने की पुरानी बीमारी

**Perodactyly.** A congenital condition charaterized by deformed fingers or toes. विरूपांगुलिता; उँगलियों का आजन्म टेढ़ा-मेढ़ा होना

**Peroneal.** Pertaining to the fibula. बहिर्जंघिकीय; बहिर्जंघिका सम्बन्धी

**Per-oral.** Through the mouth. मुखी; मुखप्रवेशी; मुख द्वारा दिया जाने वाला

**Per-os.** By the mouth. मुखप्रवेशी; मुखी; मुख द्वारा

**Perosis.** Defective formation. सदोषरचना; अपसामान्य रचना; दोषपूर्ण रचना

**Peroxide.** An oxide with the highest amount of oxygen. अतिजारेय; पैरोक्साइड

**Per-rectum.** By the rectum. मलान्त्रप्रवेशी; मलांत्र द्वारा

**Perseveration.** A mental symptom consisting of an apparent inability of the patient's mind to detach itself from one idea to another with normal speed. सतत-प्रसक्ति; अकारण प्रसक्ति

**Personal.** Individual. व्यक्तिगत; वैयक्तिक; निजी

**Personality.** The various mental attitude-characteristics which distinguish a person. व्यक्तित्व

**Perspiration.** Sweating. स्वेदन; स्वेद; पसीना

**Per-tubam.** Through a tube. नलिकाप्रवेशी; नली द्वारा

**Pertussis.** Whooping cough; tussis convulsiva. कूकरकास; काली-खाँसी

**Per-urethram.** Through the urethra. मूत्रपथप्रवेशी; मूत्रमार्ग द्वारा

**Peruvian Bark.** Cinchona. कुनीन-वृक्ष की छाल

**Perversion.** The state of being turned away from the normal course. विपर्यास; वामता; उलट-फेर;

**Sexual P.**, unnatural sexual intercourse. लैंगिक विपर्यास; अस्वाभाविक सम्भोग

**Pervert.** One who has turned from the right way. विपर्यस्त; पथभ्रष्ट

**Pervious.** Permitting penetration. प्रवेश्य; पारगम्य

**Pes.** A foot or foot-like structure. पद; पाद; पैर या पैर जैसा;

   **P. Anserina**, see **Pes Anserinus**.

   **P. Anserinus**, a plexus of facial nerves; pes anserina. आननस्नायुजाल; स्नायु-पेशियों का तंत्रिका-जाल;

   **P. Calcaneous**, club-foot, the heel alone touching the ground. अवनत-पार्ष्णिपाद;

   **P. Cavus**, the hollow foot when the longitudinal arch of the foot is accentuated; claw-foot. नखरपाद; उन्नतचापपाद;

   **P. Equinus**, club-foot, the patient walking on his toes. उन्नत-पार्ष्णिपाद;

   **P. Planus**, valgus foot; flat foot. सपाटपाद; चपटापाद;

   **P. Valgus**, club-foot with eversion of the foot. बहिर्नतपाद;

   **P. Varus**, club-foot with inversion of the foot. अन्तर्नतपाद

**Pessary.** An instrument placed in the vagina to support the uterus; a vaginal suppository; pessum. पिधा; योनिवर्ति; गर्भाशयधारकवलय; पेस्सरी

**Pessum.** See **Pessary**.

**Pest.** The plague; pestilence. प्लेग; महामारी; विनाशकारी; जनपदमारी

**Pesticides.** Substances which kill pests. विनाशक; जीवनाशी

**Pestiferous.** Destructive. घातक; विनाशक; सांघातिक

**Pestilence.** Any deadly epidemic disease. विनाशकारी; जनपदमारी; महामारी

**Pestle.** An instrument for pounding, used in a mortar. मुद्गर; मूसली; मूसल

**Petechia.** Singular of **Petechiae**.

**Petechiae.** Small subcutaneous haemorrhages; purple spots on the skin. रुधिरांक; रुधिरचिन्ह

**Petechial.** Pertaining to petechia. रुधिरांकी; रुधिरांक सम्बन्धी

**Petiolate.** Stalked or pedunculate; petiolated; petioled. सवृन्त

**Petiolated.** See **Petiolate**.

**Petioled.** See **Petiolate**.

# Petitmal

**Petitmal.** Minor epilepsy, in which the momentary loss of consciousness is characteristic. पेटीमाल; मृदु-अपस्मार; मिर्गी का हल्का दौरा

**Petrified.** Deprived of vitality. अश्मीभूत; प्राणहीन; निष्प्राण

**Petroleum.** Rock-oil, called **Petrol.** पेट्रौल

**Petromastoid.** The petrous and mastoid portions of the temporal bone. अश्मकर्णमूल

**Petrosa.** The petrous portion of the temporal bone. अश्मास्थि

**Petrosae.** Plural of **Petrosa.**

**Petrosal.** Pertaining to the petrous bone; petrous. अश्मास्थिक; अश्मास्थि सम्बन्धी

**Petrositis.** Inflammation of the petrous portion of the temporal bone. अश्मास्थिशोथ

**Petrous.** Resembling a stone. अश्माभ; अश्मवत्; पत्थर जैसा; petrosal. अश्मास्थिक

**P. Bone,** the lower pyramidal portion of the temporal bone; petrous portion. अश्मास्थि;

**P. Portion,** see **Petrous Bone.**

**Peyer's glands.** The clustered glands of intestines. आंत्रजाल; पीयर ग्रंथियाँ; आन्तों की घुंघराली ग्रन्थियाँ

**Peyer's patches.** Flat patches of lymphatic tissues situated in the small intestine but mainly in the ileum. पीयर चित्तियाँ

**Phacoanaphylaxis.** Hypersensitiveness to protein of the crystalline lens. लेंस-तीव्रग्राहिता

**Phacocele.** Hernia of the lens. लेंस-हर्निया

**Phacomalacia.** Softening of the lens. लेंसमृदुता

**Phacoscope.** An instrument for observing the changes in the crystalline lens during accommodation. लेंसदर्शी

**Phagedaena.** Gangrenous ulceration; corroding ragged sores; phagedena. विनाशीव्रण; आशुप्रसारीव्रण; भक्षीव्रण; कोथमयव्रण; शीघ्र सड़ने वाला घाव

**Phagedena.** See **Phagedaena.**

**Phagedenic.** Belonging to the corroding ragged sores. विनाशीव्रण सम्बन्धी

**Phagedenoma.** A phagedenic ulcerous tumour. विनाशीव्रणार्बुद

**Phagocyte.** A white blood cell which destroys bacteria and tissue debris. भक्षककोशिका; भक्षकाणु; जीवाणुभक्षी; जीवाणुनाशक

**Phagocytic.** Pertaining to phagocytes. भक्षककोशिकीय; भक्षककोशिकाओं सम्बन्धी

**Phagocytosis.** The engulfment by phagocytes of foreign or other particles or cells harmful to the body. भक्षककोशिकाक्रिया

**Phalangeal.** Pertaining to phalanges. अंगुलास्थिक; उँगलियों की हड्डियों से सम्बन्धित

**Phalanges.** The small bones of the fingers and toes. अंगुलिपर्व; अंगुल्यस्थियाँ; उँगलियों की छोटी हड्डियाँ

**Phalanx.** Singular of **Phalanges.**

**Phallalgia.** Pain in the penis; phallodynia. लिंगवेदना; शिश्नपीड़ा; शिश्नार्ति; लिंगशूल

**Phallectomy.** Surgical removal of the penis. शिश्नोच्छेदन; शिश्न को काट कर हटा देना

**Phalli.** Plural of **Phallus.**

**Phallic.** Relating to, or resembling penis. शिश्न सम्बन्धी अथवा शिश्नवत्

**Phallitis.** Inflammation of the penis. शिश्नशोथ

**Phallodynia.** See **Phallalgia.**

**Phalloplasty.** Reparative or plastic surgery of the penis. शिश्नसंधान

**Phallotomy.** Surgical incision into the penis. शिश्नछेदन

**Phallus.** An artificial penis. कृत्रिमशिश्न; नकली लिंग

**Phantasm.** An optic illusion. दृष्टिभ्रम; मृगमरीचिका

**Phantasia.** See **Phantasy.**

**Phantasy.** Imagination where images or chains of images are directed by the desire or pleasure of the thinkers, normally accompanied by feeling of unreality; phantasia. स्वैरकल्पना

**Phantom.** An apparition; a phantasm. आभासी; छाया;

 **P. Tumour,** a distension from wind. आभासी अर्बुद; छायार्बुद

**Pharbitis Seeds.** Ipomea Hederacea. कालादाना

**Pharmaceutical.** Pertaining to drugs and pharmacy. भेषजिक; औषधीय; औषध-निर्माण सम्बन्धी

**Pharmaceutics.** Pertaining to the art of preparing or compounding medicines. भेषजिकी; औषधनिर्माणविज्ञान

**Pharmaceutist.** See **Pharmacist.**

**Pharmacist.** A person trained in handling of drugs and compounding of prescription as licensed by the state; pharmaceutist. भेषजज्ञ; औषध-विक्रेता

**Pharmacodynamics.** The science that relates to the action of the drugs. भेषजक्रियाविज्ञान

**Pharmacogenetic.** Produced by drugs. औषधिजनित

**Pharmacogenetics.** The study of genetically determined variations in responses to drugs. भेषजप्रकरण

**Pharmacognosis.** See **Pharmacognosy.**

**Pharmacognosy.** Deals with the source, preparation, dosages, etc. of drugs; pharmacognosis. औषध-प्रकृतिविज्ञान

**Pharmacologist.** One versed in the study of pharmacology. भेषजगुणविज्ञानी; भेषजगुणविज्ञानवेत्ता; औषधप्रभावविद्

**Pharmacology.** The science of drugs in all their relations. भेषजगुणविज्ञान; औषधियों का वैज्ञानिक अध्ययन

**Pharmacopoea.** The work containing a test of accepted drugs and establishing standards for their strength, purity, together with directions for making preparations from them; pharmacopoeia. भेषजकोश; भेषजसंहिता

**Pharmacopoeal.** Relating to pharmacopoea; pharmacopoeial. भेषजकोश सम्बन्धी

**Pharmacopoeia.** See **Pharmacopoea.**

**Pharmacopoeial.** See **Pharmacopoeal.**

**Pharmacy.** The act of preparation and dispensing drug. भेषजी; फार्मेसी

**Pharyngalgia.** Pain in the pharynx; pharyngodynia. ग्रसनीशूल; ग्रसनीपीड़ा

**Pharyngeal.** Pertaining to the pharynx. ग्रसनी सम्बन्धी

**Pharyngectomy.** Removal of a part of pharynx. ग्रसनी-उच्छेदन; ग्रसनी के किसी भाग को काट कर हटा देना

**Pharyngemphraxis.** A pharyngeal obstruction. ग्रसनीरोध

**Pharynges.** Plural of **Pharynx.**

**Pharyngismus.** See **Pharyngospasm.**

**Pharyngitis.** Inflammation of the pharynx. ग्रसनीशोथ; गलकोषप्रदाह;
   **Atrophic P.**, a form attended with atrophy of the mucous membrane; pharyngitis sicca. शोषी ग्रसनीशोथ; शुष्क ग्रसनीशोथ; ग्रसनी का शुष्क प्रदाह;

Catarrhal P., that attended by copious secretion. अभिष्यन्दी ग्रसनीशोथ; प्रतिश्यायी ग्रसनीशोथ;
Granular P., the chronic form with granular bodies on the mucous membrane. कणिकामय ग्रसनीशोथ;
P. Sicca, see Atrophic Pharyngitis.
**Pharyngodynia.** Pain in the pharynx; pharyngalgia. ग्रसनीशूल; ग्रसनीपीड़ा
**Pharyngoepiglottic.** Pertaining to the pharynx and epiglottis; pharyngoepiglottidean. ग्रसनी एवं कण्ठच्छद सम्बन्धी
**Pharyngoepiglottidean.** See Pharyngoepiglottic.
**Pharyngoepiglottis.** The pharynx and epiglottis. ग्रसनीकण्ठच्छद; ग्रसनी तथा कण्ठच्छद
**Pharyngoglossal.** Relating to the pharynx and the tongue. ग्रसनी एवं जिह्वा सम्बन्धी
**Pharyngolaryngeal.** Pertaining to the pharynx and the larynx. ग्रसनीस्वरयंत्रज; ग्रसनी तथा स्वरयंत्र सम्बन्धी
**Pharyngolaryngectomy.** Surgical removal of the pharynx and the larynx. ग्रसनीस्वरयंत्र-उच्छेदन; ग्रसनी तथा स्वरयंत्र को काट कर हटा देना
**Pharyngolaryngitis.** Inflammation of the pharynx and larynx. ग्रसनीस्वरयंत्रशोथ; ग्रसनी तथा स्वरयंत्र का प्रदाह
**Pharyngology.** The science of the pharyngeal mechanism, functions and diseases. ग्रसनीविज्ञान; ग्रसनी की बनावट, क्रिया तथा रोगावस्थाओं सम्बन्धी विज्ञान
**Pharyngomycosis.** Fungal invasion of the mucous membrane of the pharynx. ग्रसनीकवकता
**Pharyngopathy.** Any disease of the pharynx. ग्रसनीरोग
**Pharyngoplasty.** Any plastic operation of the pharynx. ग्रसनीसंधान
**Pharyngoplegia.** Paralysis of the pharynx. ग्रसनीघात; गलकोष का पक्षाघात
**Pharyngorhinitis.** Inflammation of the mucous membrane of the pharynx and the nasal mucosae. ग्रसनीनासाशोथ
**Pharyngoscope.** An instrument for examining the pharynx. ग्रसनीदर्शकयंत्र; ग्रसनीदर्शी
**Pharyngoscopy.** Examination of the pharynx. ग्रसनीदर्शन
**Pharyngospasm.** Spasm of the pharynx; pharyngismus. ग्रसनी-उद्वेष्ट; ग्रसनीआकर्ष; गलकोष की ऐंठन
**Pharyngostenosis.** Stricture of the pharynx. ग्रसनीसंकीर्णता

**Pharyngotomy.** The operation of opening into the pharynx. ग्रसनीछेदन

**Pharyngotonsillitis.** Inflammation of the pharynx and tonsils. ग्रसनी-गलतुण्डिकाशोथ; ग्रसनी तथा गलतुण्डिकाओं का प्रदाह

**Pharyngotympanic.** Relating to the pharynx and the middle ear. ग्रसनी तथा मध्यकर्ण सम्बन्धी

**Pharynx.** The space at the back of the mouth generally called the "throat" which extends upward to meet the nasal cavities and is continuous with the larynx going downward. ग्रसनी; गलकोष

**Phase.** One of the stages in which a thing appears during its course of change or development. प्रावस्था

**Phenic.** Obtained from coal-tar. कोलतार से प्राप्त प्रांगविक पदार्थ;

**P. Acid,** see **Phenol.**

**Phenol.** Carbolic acid; a powerful antiseptic widely used as a 1 in 20 solution; phenic acid. फ़ीनौल; दर्शव; प्रांगविक अम्ल; कार्बोलिक एसिड; फेनिक एसिड

**Phenomena.** Plural of **Phenomenon.**

**Phenomenon.** A symptom; an occurrence of any sort in relation to a disease. लक्षण; घटनाक्रम; घटनाचक्र

**Phenotype.** Persons of like characteristics though of different heredity. समलक्षणी; ऐसे व्यक्ति जिनमें भिन्न पैत्रिकता होते हुए भी समान लक्षण मिलते हैं

**Phenyl.** An organic radical found in carbolic acid. फेनिल; फिनाइल; प्रांगविक अम्ल में पाया जाने वाला एक जैवी तत्त्व

**Phial.** A small glass-bottle; a vial. काचकूपिका; लघुकूपी; छोटी शीशी

**Phiala.** A phial. शीशी; काचकूपिका; लघुकूपी

**Philtra.** Plural of **Philtrum.**

**Philtrum.** The vertical groove in the middle of the upper lip. ओष्ठखात

**Phimoses.** Plural of **Phimosis.**

**Phimosis.** Narrowness of the opening of the prepuce, preventing it from being drawn over the glans; phymosis; capistration. निरुद्धप्रकाश; निरुद्धमणि; शिश्नमुख की अतिसूक्ष्मता

**Phimotic.** Relating to phimosis. निरुद्धप्रकाश अर्थात् शिश्नमुख की अतिसूक्ष्मता सम्बन्धी

**Phisiotherapy.** See **Physiotherapy.**

**Phlebectasia.** The dilatation of a vein; phlebectasis. शिराविस्फार; किसी शिरा का फूलना

**Phlebectasis.** See **Phlebectasia.**

**Phlebectomy.** Excision of a segment of a vein; venectomy. शिरा-उच्छेदन; किसी शिरा को काट कर हटा देना

**Phlebemphraxis.** Venous thrombosis. शिराघनास्त्रता

**Phlebitis.** Inflammation of a vein. शिराशोथ; शिराप्रदाह

**Phlebogram.** A radiograph of venous system. शिरालेख; शिराचित्र

**Phlebograph.** A venous sphygmograph; an instrument for making a tracing of the venous pulse. शिरालेखी

**Phlebography.** X-ray examination of the venous system; venography. शिराचित्रण

**Phlebolite.** See **Phlebolith.**

**Phlebolith.** A vein-stone; calcareous concretion in a vein; phlebolite. शिराश्मरी; शिरा में किसी प्रकार की पथरी बनना

**Phlebolithiasis.** The formation of venous phleboliths. शिराश्मरीयता; शिराओं में पथरी बनना

**Phlebology.** The science of veins. शिराविज्ञान; नाड़ीविज्ञान

**Phlebosclerosis.** Abnormal hardening of a vein. शिराकाठिन्य; नाड़ी की कठोरता

**Phlebostasis.** Venostasis. शिरास्थैर्य

**Phlebostenosis.** Narrowing of the lumen of a vein. शिरासंकीर्णता

**Phlebothrombosis.** Thrombosis in a vein. शिराघनास्त्रता; शिरा के अन्दर थक्का बन जाना

**Phlebotome.** A lancet for bleeding. शिराच्छेदक; शिराच्छिद्रक; रक्तस्राव के निमित्त प्रयुक्त किसी शिरा में छेद करने वाली सुई

**Phlebotomy.** Venesection; incision of a vein. शिराच्छेदन; शिरावेध; शिराशल्यता; किसी शिरा में छेद करना

**Phlegm.** Mucus matter ejected from the fauces and secreted on the lungs. श्लेष्मा; बलगम; कफ

**Phlegmasia.** Acute and severe inflammation. शोथ; प्रदाह;

**P. Alba Dolens,** milk-leg; an acute oedema, especially of leg from venous obstruction; milk-leg. श्वेतपादशोथ; शिरारोध के कारण टांग में तीव्र शोफ प्रकट हो जाना;

**P. Cerulea Dolens,** cyanosis of the foot caused by thrombosis of the veins of a limb. नीलपादशोथ; घनास्त्रता के कारण पैर नीला पड़ जाना

**Phlegmatic.** Cold, heavy, dull, as a phlegmatic temperament or constitution. श्लेष्मज; श्लेष्मल; कफोत्पादक

**Phlegmon.** A boil; suppurative inflammation of areolar tissue. शोथव्रण; अर्बुद; फोड़ा; अवकाशी ऊतक का सपूयशोथ

**Phlegmonic.** Pertaining to inflammation in the cellular tissue, with swelling; phlegmonous. श्लेष्मोत्पन्न; अर्बुदी; दाहक; सूजन के साथ प्रदाह

**Phlegmonous.** See **Phlegmonic.**

**Phleps.** A vein. शिरा; नाड़ी

**Phlogistic.** Inflammatory. शोथकर; शोथकारी; प्रदाहक

**Phlogosis.** Inflammation. शोथ; प्रदाह; दर्द के साथ सूजन

**Phlyctena.** A vesicle with serous contents; a blister. फफोला; सद्रव क्षुद्रकोष; छाला

**Phlyctenula.** A minute vesicle or phlyctenule. सूक्ष्मक्षुद्रकोष; छोटा-सा फफोला या छाला

**Phlyctenulae.** Plural of **Phlyctenula.**

**Phlyctenular.** Having the nature of phlyctenula. अलजीय; स्फोटक

**Phlyctenule.** A minute blister or vesicle, unusually occurring on the conjunctiva or the cornea; phlysis. सूक्ष्मक्षुद्रकोष; छोटा-सा फफोला

**Phlysis.** See **Phlyctenule.**

**Phobia.** A morbid fear, with or without foundation in relation to disease, as cancer-phobia, hydrophobia, photophobia, etc. भीति; आतंक; संत्रास; भय; डर

**Phobiac.** Relating to phobia. आतंक, भय अथवा डर सम्बन्धी

**Phonal.** Relating to sound or to the voice. ध्वनि अथवा आवाज सम्बन्धी

**Phonation.** The emission of vocal sounds. ध्वनन; ध्वनि-निस्सारण; ध्वनि-उच्चार; शब्दोच्चार

**Phonatory.** Concerning utterance of vocal sounds. ध्वनिका; ध्वनि-निस्सारक; relating to phonation. ध्वनि-निस्सारण अथवा शब्दोच्चार सम्बन्धी

**Phonetic.** Relating to speech or to the voice. वक्तव्य अथवा आवाज सम्बन्धी

**Phonetics.** The study of vocal sounds. ध्वनिविज्ञान

**Phonic.** Pertaining to the voice. ध्वनिपरक; ध्वनिक; ध्वनि सम्बन्धी

**Phonocardiogram.** A graphic record of heart sounds. हृद्ध्वनिलेख

**Phonocardiograph.** An instrument for graphically recording the heart sounds. हृद्ध्वनिलेखयंत्र

**Phonocardiography.** The graphic record of heart sounds and murmurs by electric reproduction. हृद्ध्वनिलेखन

**Phonoreceptor.** A receptor for sound stimuli. ध्वनिग्राही

**Phoria.** The relative direction assumed by the eyes by binovular fixation of a given object. विचलनप्रवृत्ति

**Phorology.** Science dealing with the disease agents or carriers. रोगवाहकविज्ञान

**Phosphate.** Any salt of phosphatic acid. स्फुर-अम्ल; फास्फेट; भास्वरी लवण अथवा क्षार

**Phosphatic.** Consisting of, or containing phosphates. भास्वरी; स्फुर-अम्लीय; फास्फेटी

**Phosphaturia.** An excess of phosphates in the urine. स्फुर-अम्लमेह; फास्फेटमेह

**Phosphenes.** Subjective light-sensations from pressure on the eyeballs. प्रकाशवलय

**Phosphorescence.** The property of shining in the dark without the evolution of heat. स्फुरदीप्ति

**Phosphorus.** A non-metallic, poisonous and highly inflammable element. भास्वर; फास्फोरस

**Photalgia.** Pain in the eyes from exposure to intense light; photodynia. दीप्तिनेत्रशूल; प्रकाशाक्षिशूल

**Photic.** Relating to light. प्रकाश सम्बन्धी

**Photobiotic.** Living in the light exclusively. प्रकाशजीवी; मात्र रोशनी के सहारे जीवित रहने वाला प्राणी

**Photochemical.** Chemical changes brought about by light. प्रकाश-रासायनिक; रोशनी द्वारा लाया गया रासायनिक परिवर्तन

**Photochemistry.** The science of the chemistry of light. प्रकाशरसायन (शास्त्र)

**Photodynia.** See **Photalgia.**

**Photogenic.** Light producing. प्रकाशजनक

**Photolysis.** Decomposition of a chemical compound by the action of light. प्रकाशलयन

**Photomania.** Delirium produced by the action of intense light. प्रकाशोन्माद; अतिप्रकाशजनित प्रलाप

**Photometer**

**Photometer.** An instrument for measuring the intensity of light. प्रकाशमापी; प्रकाश की तीव्रता को मापने का यंत्र

**Photometry.** The measurement of the intensity of light. प्रकाशमिति; प्रकाश की तीव्रता मापना

**Photomicrograph.** The photograph of an enlarged microscopic object. सूक्ष्मदर्शी-फोटोग्राफ

**Photophobia.** Dread of light, owing to extreme sensibility of retina. प्रकाशभीति; प्रकाशसंत्रास; प्रकाश-असह्यता; रोशनी से आतंकित रहना

**Photophobic.** Relating to photophobia. प्रकाशभीति सम्बन्धी

**Photopsia.** Subjective sensations of light; photoptosia; photopsy. प्रकाशाभास; प्रकाशानुभूति

**Photopsy.** See **Photopsia**.

**Photoptosia.** See **Photopsia**.

**Photosensitive.** Sensitive to light, as pigments in the eye. प्रकाशसुग्राही; रोशनी के प्रति सम्वेदनशील

**Phototherapy.** Treatment of diseases by means of light rays; light treatment. प्रकाशचिकित्सा; प्रकाशोपचार

**Phren.** The diaphragm. मध्यच्छद; the mind. मन; चित्त

**Phrenalgia.** Pain in the diaphragm. मध्यच्छदार्ति

**Phrenasthenia.** Paraparesis of diaphragm. आंशिकमध्यच्छदपात; मध्यच्छद का आंशिक पक्षाघात; weakness of mind. मनोदौर्बल्य; मानसिक दुर्बलता

**Phrenemphraxis.** Crushing of a section of phrenic nerve; phreniclasia. मध्यच्छदतंत्रिकासंदलन

**Phrenesis.** Delirium; frenzy. प्रलाप; उन्मत्तता

**Phrenetic.** Maniacal; delirious. विक्षिप्त; उन्मत्त; मतान्ध; सनकी

**Phrenic.** Relating to the diaphragm, or mind. मध्यच्छद अथवा मन सम्बन्धी

**Phreniclasia.** See **Phrenemphraxis**.

**Phrenicocolic.** Pertaining to the diaphragm and colon. मध्यच्छद एवं बृहदान्त्र सम्बन्धी

**Phrenitis.** Inflammation of the diaphragm or the brain. मध्यच्छद अथवा मस्तिष्क का प्रदाह

**Phrenoplegia.** Paralysis of the diaphragm. मध्यच्छदाघात; मध्यच्छद का पक्षाघात

**Phrenospasm.** Spasm of the diaphragm. मध्यच्छदाकर्ष; मध्यच्छद की ऐंठन

**Phrynoderma.** Dryness of the skin. त्वक्रूक्षता; मेकत्वचा; त्वचा की रूक्षता

**Phthiriasis.** Condition of being infested with lice. चीलरप्रवणता

**Phthisic.** Consumptive. यक्ष्माग्रस्त; क्षयग्रस्त; तपेदिक से पीड़ित

**Phthisical.** Relating to phthisis. यक्ष्मा अर्थात् क्षय सम्बन्धी

**Phthisis.** A wasting away of the body or any part of the body; pthisis. यक्ष्मा; क्षय; तपेदिक; टी० बी०;

   **P. Acutus,** acute or galloping consumption. उग्रक्षय; यक्ष्मा की तीव्र अवस्था;

   **P. Bulbi,** progressive atrophy of the eyeball. नेत्रक्षय;

   **P. Laryngea,** laryngeal tuberculosis. स्वरयंत्रक्षय; स्वरयंत्र की टी० बी०;

   **P. Mesenterica,** consumption of the bowels. आंत्रक्षय; आंतों की टी० बी०;

   **P. Nodosa,** miliary tuberculosis of the lungs. कर्बुरित फुप्फुसक्षय;

   **P. Pulmonalis,** pulmonary tuberculosis. फुप्फुसक्षय; फेफड़े की टी० बी०;

**Phylogenesis.** The evolutionary development of any plant or animal species; phylogeny. जातिवृत्त

**Phylogenetic.** Relating to phylogenesis; phylogenic. जातिवृत्त सम्बन्धी

**Phylogenic.** See **Phylogenetic.**

**Phylogeny.** See **Phylogenesis.**

**Phymosis.** See **Phimosis.**

**Physaliform.** Like a bubble or small bleb. बुद्बुदाकार; बुलबुले जैसा

**Physic.** The science of medicine. औषधविज्ञान; उपचारविज्ञान; चिकित्साविज्ञान; body. शरीर

**Physical.** Relating to the physic or the body. भौतिक; शारीरिक;

   **P. Medicine,** the use of physical agents in treating diseases, such as light, heat, water, massage, exercise, etc. भौतिक चिकित्सा;

   **P. Trait,** morphological trait. शारीरिक लक्षण

**Physician.** One who treats diseases or patients. चिकित्सक; कायचिकित्सक; वैद्य

**Physicist.** One skilled in physics. भौतिकविज्ञानी; a physician. चिकित्सक; वैद्य

**Physicochemical.** Pertaining to the physics and chemistry. भौतिकी तथा रसायनविज्ञान सम्बन्धी

**Physics.** The science of inorganic matters and its forces. भौतिकविज्ञान; भौतिकी; अजैवी पदार्थों तथा उनकी शक्तियों से सम्बन्धित विज्ञान

**Physiochemical.** Pertaining to physiology and chemicals. शरीरवृत्ति तथा रसायनविज्ञान सम्बन्धी

**Physiologic.** See **Physiological**.

**Physiological.** In accordance with natural process of the body; physiologic. शरीरक्रियात्मक; शरीरवृत्तिक

**Physiologist.** A specialist in physiology. शरीरक्रियाविज्ञानी

**Physiology.** The science of the functions of the body. शरीरक्रियाविज्ञान; शरीरवृत्ति

**Physiotherapeutic.** Pertaining to physiotheraphy. भौतिकचिकित्सा सम्बन्धी

**Physiotherapist.** A physician who specializes in physical medicine. भौतिकचिकित्सक; भौतिकचिकित्साशास्त्री

**Physiotherapy.** Treatment based on physical agents: light, heat, electricity, massage, vibration, water, exercise, etc.; phisiotherapy. भौतिकचिकित्सा; प्राकृतिकचिकित्सा

**Physique.** The physical make up of a living being. शारीरिकगठन; देहविन्यास

**Physometra.** A gaseous uterine enlargement. वायुगर्भाशयता; जरायुविस्फार

**Physon.** Flatulence. आध्मान; अफारा; पेट फूलना

**Phytoid.** Resembling a plant. पौधे जैसा

**Phytology.** The science which treats of the vegetable kingdom. वनस्पतिविज्ञान; वनस्पति जगत से सम्बन्धित विज्ञान

**Phytosis.** A parasitic disease. उद्भिद्-व्याधि; परजीवीजन्यरोग; परजीवियों द्वारा होने वाली रुग्णता

**Pia.** See **Piamater**.

**Pial.** Pertaining to the piamater. मृदुतानिका सम्बन्धी

**Piamater.** The innermost layer of the meninges; pia. मृदुतानिका; मृदुकला; मस्तिष्कावरण का सबसे अन्दर वाला अस्तर

**Piar.** Fat; corpulent. स्थूलकाय; मोटा

**Pica.** Desire for extraordinary articles of food. दोहद; किसी विशेष प्रकार के भोजन की इच्छा

**Piedra.** A disease of the hair due to micrococci. केशकवकोपसर्ग; सूक्ष्मगोलाणुओं द्वारा उत्पन्न होने वाली बालों की बीमारी

**Pigeon-chest.** A narrow chest; bulging anteriorly in the breast in one region. कपोतवक्ष; कबूतर जैसी छाती वाला

**Pigment.** Colouring matter in the skin, hair and eyes, as bile pigment. वर्णक; रंजक;

**Bile P.**, colouring matter in the bile. पित्तवर्णक

**Pigmentary.** Pertaining to pigment. वर्णक अथवा रंजक सम्बन्धी

**Pigmentation.** Colouration of the skin or tissues by a deposit of pigment. वर्णकता; वर्णकयुक्तता; रंजकता; रंज्यता

**Pigmented.** Coloured, as the result of a deposit of pigment. रंजकित

**Pilar.** See **Pileous.**

**Pileous.** Hairy; pilar. सशिरोरुह; केशयुक्त; रोमिल

**Piles.** Haemorrhoids; painful tumours around or within the anus. अर्श; बवासीर;

**Blind P.**, haemorrhoids which do not bleed. शुष्कार्श; वातार्श; सूखी बवासीर

**Pili.** Plural of **Pilus.**

**Pill.** A small sugar-coated pellet or pilule; pilula. गोली; वटी; गुटिका

**Pillar.** A supporting part or process. स्तम्भ

**Pilomotor Nerve.** One of the tiny nerves attached to the hair follicles. रोमहर्षणी तंत्रिका; रोमहर्षक तंत्रिका

**Pilonidal.** Containing hair. रोमयुक्त; लोमयुक्त

**Pilorum.** The hair; pilus. रोम; लोम; केश; बाल

**Pilosebaceous.** Pertaining to the hair follicle and the sebaceous gland opening into it. केशत्वग्वसीय; केशपुटकों तथा उनके अन्दर खुलने वाली वसा-ग्रन्थि सम्बन्धी

**Pilula.** A small, spheric, medicinal mass; a pill. गोली; वटी; गुटिका

**Pilule.** See **Pill.**

**Pilus.** Hair. केश; बाल; लोम; रोम

**Pimelitis.** Inflammation of the adipose tissue. वसा-ऊतकशोथ; वसोतकशोथ

**Pimelosis.** Adiposis वसामयता; fatty degeneration. वसापजनन

**Pimple.** A small pustule, boil or papule. फुन्सी; पुटिका; मुहासा

**Pinched.** Like a pea in shape and size. चणकाकार; चने या मटर के दाने के आकार का

**Pink Disease.** Acrodynia; a disease of the infants thought to be the result of mercury poisoning. शिशुशाखावेदना; पारदविषण्णता के कारण होने वाला एक शिशु रोग

**Pink-eye.** A popular name for contagious conjunctivitis. संक्रमीनेत्रश्लेष्मलाशोथ

**Pinna.** The part of the ear which is external to the head; the auricle. कर्णपाली; अलिन्द

**Pinnae.** Plural of **Pinna.**

**Pinocytosis.** The imbibition of liquids by cells. अवशोषीकोशिकता

**Pint.** The eighth part of a gallon. पिंट; ग्यारह छटांक के लगभग

**Pinworm.** Seatworm; a member of the genus of **Enterobius** or related genera nematodes in the unit of oxyuridae. सूचीकृमि

**Pipe.** A tube or tube-like structure. नली; नलिका; प्रणाल

**Pipet.** A small graduated tube for taking up liquid; pipette. सूक्ष्मनली

**Pipette.** See **Pipet.**

**Piriform.** Pear-shaped. नाशपातीरूप; नाशपाती के आकर का

**Pisciform.** Of the form of a fish. मत्स्यरूप; मीनरूप; मछली जैसा

**Pisiform.** Pea-shaped. चणकाकार; चने या मटर के दाने जैसा

**Pit.** A hollow fovea. गर्त; गर्तक; विवर;

   **P. of stomach,** epigastrium. उदरगर्त; अधिजठर

**Pitch.** A black solid substance formed by boiling tar. तारकोल

**Pitchman.** A promoter, usually posing as a health lecturer, for food fads or other forms of quackery. कुवैद्य; नीमहकीम

**Pith.** The marrow of bones. मज्जा; अस्थिमज्जा; the centre of a hair. लोमकेन्द्र

**Pithing.** The destroying of the central nervous system by piercing the brain and cord; decerebration. मस्तिष्कसुषुम्नावेधन

**Pitting.** Making an identation in dropsical tissues. दाबगर्तक; दाबनिम्नता

**Pituitary Body.** See **Pituitary Gland.**

**Pituitary Extract.** Vasopressin, formed in the hypothalamus and passes down the nerves in the pituitary stalk to be stored in the posterior lobe of the pituitary gland. पीयूषिका-रस

**Pituitary Gland.** The principal gland of internal secretion located under the middle of lower surface of the brain; pituitary body. पीयूषिका-ग्रन्थि

**Pituitrin.** A brand of pituitary. पिटुइट्रिन

**Pityriasis.** A scaly eruption of the skin. तुषाभशल्कन; अपशल्कितत्वग्शोथ; सिध्म; मरा-मांस; एक चर्मरोग; चमड़ी का एक पपड़ीदार उद्भेद;

**P. Alba,** seborrhoeic dermatitis. श्वेततुषाभशल्कन;

**P. Capitis,** dendruff. रूसी; फास;

**P. Circinata,** see **Pityriasis Rosea.**

**P. Rosea,** a form with scaly red patches; pityriasis circinata. गुलाबी तुषाभशल्कन;

**P. Rubra,** a form with general scaliness and redness. रक्तिम तुषाभशल्कन

**Placebo.** An inert drug given to satisfy the patient. कूटभेषज; रोगी की संतुष्टि के लिये दी जाने वाली निष्क्रिय औषधि

**Placenta.** The special organ which nourishes the unborn. अपरा; गर्भनाल; जरायुनाल; बीजांडासन;

**Adherent P.,** an abnormal adherence of placenta to the uterine wall after child-birth. अभिलग्न अपरा;

**Annular P.,** see **Placenta Annularis.**

**Battledore P.,** the insertion of the cord in the margin of the placenta. परिसरनाल अपरा;

**Duplex P.,** one divided into two parts. द्विगुणित अपरा; द्विगुण अपरा;

**Incarcerated. P.,** one retained by irregular contraction of the uterus. बद्ध अपरा;

**Retained P.,** one not expelled by the uterus after labour. अनिर्गत अपरा;

**P. Annularis,** one extending around the interior of the uterus in the form of a belt; annular placenta. वलयाकार अपरा;

**P. Membranacea,** one abnormally thin. कलामय अपरा;

**P. Praevia,** presentation of the placenta before the foetus. सम्मुखी अपरा;

**P. Succenturiata,** an accessory growth in the placenta. सहखंडी अपरा

**Placental.** Pertaining to placenta. गर्भनालीय; जरायुवी; अपरा सम्बन्धी;

**P. Insufficiency,** inefficiency of the placenta. अल्पनाभिरज्जुता; अपरा की मन्द क्रिया

**Placentation.** The form and mode of attachment of the placenta. अपराविकास; बीजांडन्यास

**Placentitis.** Inflammation of the placenta. अपराशोथ; गर्भनालशोथ; जरायुनालशोथ; जरायुनाल-प्रदाह

**Placentography**

**Placentography.** X-ray examination of the placenta by injection of opaque substance. अपराचित्रण

**Placodes.** Cellular thickening of the ectoderm which contributes to the development of certain nerve structures. स्थाली

**Plagiocephaly.** An asymmetrical craniostenosis due to premature closure of the lamboid and coronal sutures on one side, characterized by an oblique deformity of the skull. असममितशीर्षता

**Plague.** A severe epidemic caused due to rat-infection. प्लेग; ताऊन;

**Bubonic P.**, the usual form of plague marked by inflammatory enlargement of the lymphatic glands in the groin, axillae or other parts. ग्रन्थिल प्लेग;

**Haemorrhagic P.**, the haemorrhagic form of bubonic plague. रक्तस्रावी प्लेग;

**Pneumonic P.**, a frequently fatal form in which there are areas of pulmonary consolidation, with chill, pain in side, bloody expectoration and high fever. फुप्फुसी प्लेग

**Plane.** A smooth surface. तल; कोमल तल

**Planimeter.** A kind of perimeter. क्षेत्रफलमापी; परिमितिक

**Planoconcave.** Flat on one side and concave on the other. समतलावतल

**Planoconvex.** Flat on one side and convex on the other. समतलोत्तल

**Planta.** The sole of the foot; pelma. पादतल; पदतल; पैर का तलुवा

**Plantae.** Plural of **Planta.**

**Plantar.** Pertaining to the sole of the foot. पदतलीय; पदतल सम्बन्धी

**Plantaris.** An extensor muscle of the foot. पादतल; पदतल; जंघा-उपपिण्डिका; पैर की प्रसारक पेशी

**Plaque.** A flat plate or area. चकत्ता

**Plasm.** See **Plasma.**

**Plasma.** The serum or liquid portion of the blood; plasm. प्लाविका; रक्तरस; रक्त का सीरम या द्रव-अंश

**Plasmablast.** Precursor of the plasma cell. प्लाविकाप्रसू

**Plasmacyte.** Plasma cell; plasmocyte. प्लाविकाकोशिका

**Plasmalemma.** Cell membrane. कोशिकाकला

**Plasmapheresis.** Taking blood from a donor, separating the cellular elements from the plasma, then returning the red cells and repeating the whole process. प्लाविकाहरण

**Plasmatic.** Relating to plasma or protoplasm; plasmic. प्लाविकीय; रक्तरसीय; प्लाविका अथवा रक्तरस सम्बन्धी

**Plasmic.** See **Plasmatic.**

**Plasmocyte.** See **Plasmacyte.**

**Plasmodia.** Plural of **Plasmodium.**

**Plasmodium.** A large jelly-like mass formed by an aggregation of amoebas; a genus of protozoa. विषमज्वराणु; अमीबाभचय

**Plasmogene.** Bioplasm; living substance. कोशिकाद्रवजीव

**Plasmolysis.** Dessolution of cellular components. प्लाविकालयन

**Plaster.** A substance used in medical practice being made to adhere to the surface of the body. पट्टी; पलस्तर; प्लास्टर;

**Adhesive. P.,** resin plaster. आसंजी पलस्तर; चिपक पट्टी;

**Bandage P.,** a bandage stiffened with the plaster of Paris. पलस्तरयुक्त पट्टी;

**P. of Paris,** a mold cast upon the body to keep it rigid. पैरिस पलस्तर; प्लास्टर ऑफ पैरिस

**Plastic.** Easily moulded. सुघट्य; सुनम्य; प्लास्टिक;

**P. Operation,** see **Plastic Surgery.**

**P. Surgery,** surgery aimed at restoring the lost function, and in some instances improving personal appearance; plastic operation. सुघट्य शल्यचिकित्सा; प्लास्टिक सर्जरी

**Plasticity.** The state of being plastic. सुघट्यता; सुनम्यता; कायान्तरण-क्षमता

**Plasty.** Plastic operation. संधान; संधानकर्म

**Plate.** A flat metal bar for protecting fractured bones. प्लेट; पट्ट; पट्टिका;

**Auditory P.,** the bone plate forming the roof of the auditory meatus. श्रवण पट्टिका;

**End P.,** the terminal of a motor nerve in a muscular fibre. अन्त्य प्लेट; अन्त्य पट्टिका;

**Tympanic P.,** the bony sides and floor of the auditory meatus. मध्यकर्ण पट्टिका

**Platelet.** Thrombocyte. बिम्बाणु

**Platycephalus.** Having a broad, flat skull. चिपिटकपाल; चौड़ी, चपटी खोपड़ी वाला

**Platyelminthes.** See **Platyhelminthes.**

**Platyhelminthes.** Broad worms; flat worms; flukes; platyelminthes. चिपिटकृमि; पृथुकृमि; चौड़े कृमि

**Platypellic.** Having a broad pelvis; platypelvic. चिपिटश्रोणि; चपटी गोणिका वाली

**Platypelvic.** See **Platypellic.**

**Platyrrhine.** Having a broad and flat nose. चिपिटनासा; चौड़ी तथा चपटी नाक वाला

**Pledget.** A small flat compress of lint. फाहा; पतले वस्त्र का छोटा-सा चपटा सम्पीड

**Pleocytosis.** Increase of lymphocytes in the cerebrospinal fluid. मेरुद्रवकोशिकाबहुलता; अनुमस्तिष्कमेरु-द्रव्य में लस-कोशिकाओं की बृद्धि होना

**Pleomorphic.** Having several distinct forms; polymorphous. बहुरूपी; अनेक रूपों वाला

**Pleomorphism.** Denotes a wide range in shape and size of individuals in a bacterial population. बहुरूपता; विविधरूपता

**Pleomorphous.** See **Polymorphous.**

**Plethora.** Repletion; too great fullness of the blood vessels of the body, hence a plethoric habit of the body. अतिरक्तप्रवाह; रक्तबहुलता; अतिरक्तता

**Plethoric.** Oversupplied with blood; sanguine. रक्तबहुल, रक्तप्रधान

**Plethysmograph.** An instrument for measuring accurately the blood flow in the limbs. रक्तसंचारमापी

**Plethysmography.** Use of plethysmograph. रक्तसंचारमापन

**Plethysmometry.** Measuring the fullness of a hollow organ or vessel, as of the pulse. रक्तसंचारमिति

**Pleura.** Lining membrane of the thorax, covering also the lungs. परिफुफ्फुस; फुफ्फुसावरण; फेफड़े की झिल्ली

**Pleurae.** Plural of **Pleura.**

**Pleural.** Relating to the pleura. परिफुफ्फुसीय; फुफ्फुसावरणीय; पार्श्वक; फेफड़े की झिल्ली से सम्बन्धित;

P. Calculus, see **Pleurolith.**

**Pleuralgia.** Pain in the intercostal muscles. परिफुफ्फुसशूल; फुफ्फुसावरणशूल; फेफड़े की झिल्ली का दर्द

**Pleurectomy.** Excision of a part of the pleura. परिफुफ्फुस-उच्छेदन; फुफ्फुसावरण के किसी भाग को काट कर हटाना

**Pleurisy.** A disease marked by the inflammation of the pleura, with exudation into its cavity and upon its surface; pleuritis. फुफ्फुसावरणशोथ; परिफुफ्फुसशोथ; फेफड़े की झिल्ली का प्रदाह; प्लूरिसी;

**Adhesive P.,** see **Dry Pleurisy.**

**Diaphragmatic P.,** that restricted to the pleural surface of the diaphragm. मध्यच्छद-फुप्फुसावरणशोथ;

**Dry P.,** that attended with little or no effusion of the fluid; fibrinous pleurisy; pleurisy sicca. शुष्क फुप्फुसावरणशोथ;

**Fibrinous P.,** see **Dry Pleurisy.**

**Haemorrhagic P.,** that attended with bloody exudate. रक्तस्रावी फुप्फुसावरणशोथ;

**Interlobar P.,** that affecting the pleural layers between the lobes. अन्तराखण्डी फुप्फुसावरणशोथ;

**Wet P.,** pleurisy with effusion. आर्द्र फुप्फुसावरणशोथ; सद्रव-फुप्फुसावरणशोथ;

**P. Sicca,** see **Dry Pleurisy.**

**Pleuritic.** Affected with or pertaining to pleurisy. फुप्फुसावरणशोथग्रस्त; फुप्फुसावरणशोथ सम्बन्धी

**Pleuritis.** See **Pleurisy.**

**Pleurocele.** See **Pneumatocele.**

**Pleurodynia.** Pain in the intercostal muscles; pleuralgia. पार्श्ववेदना कूटफुप्फुसावरणशोथ; फुप्फुसावरणशूल

**Pleurogenic.** Of pleural origin or beginning in the pleura; pleurogenous. परिफुप्फुसजनक

**Pleurogenous.** See **Pleurogenic.**

**Pleurography.** Radiography of the pleural cavity. परिफुप्फुसचित्रण

**Pleurohepatitis.** Hepatitis with extension of the inflammation at the neighbouring portion of the pleura. परिफुप्फुसयकृत्शोथ; फुप्फुसावरण तथा यकृत् का प्रदाह

**Pleurolith.** A concretion in the pleural cavity; pleural calculus. परिफुप्फुसाश्मरी

**Pleuropericarditis.** Inflammation of the pericardium of the pleura. परिफुप्फुसपरिहृदशोथ

**Pleuropneumonia.** Inflammation of the pleura and the lungs; pleuropneumonitis. फुप्फुसावरण-फुप्फुसप्रदाह; फुप्फुसावरणफुप्फुसशोथ

**Pleuropneumonitis.** see **Pleuropneumonia.**

**Pleuropulmonary.** Relating to the pleura and lung. फुप्फुसावरण तथा फुप्फुस सम्बन्धी

**Pleurothotonous.** A tetanic lateral bending of the body. पार्श्वायाम; शरीर का धनुष जैसा आड़ा-तिरछा मुड़ना

**Pleurotomy**

**Pleurotomy.** Incision of the pleura; thoracotomy. वक्षछेदन; परिफुफ्फुसछेदन

**Plexectomy.** Surgical incision of a plexus. जालिकाछेदन

**Plexiform.** Resembling a plexus. जालरूप; जालकरूप; जालिकारूप

**Plexitis.** Inflammation or irritation of plexus. जालिकाशोथ

**Plexus.** A network of the nerves or vessels. जाल; जालिका; जालक; स्नायुजाल; नाड़ीजाल; तन्तुजाल;

**Aortic P.**, a nerve plexus on each side and in front of the abdominal aorta; one surrounding the thoracic aorta. महाधमनी-जालिका; महाधमनी-जाल;

**Brachial P.**, one in the lower part of the neck, reaching to the axilla. प्रगण्ड-जालिका; प्रगण्ड-जाल;

**Celiac P.**, formed of numerous nervous filaments, and situated in the abdomen. कुक्षि-जालिका; कुक्षि-जाल;

**Cervical P.**, one opposite the four upper vertebras. ग्रैव-जालिका; गर्दन का नाड़ीजाल; ग्रीवा-जाल;

**Coccygeal P.**, one on the dorsal surface of the coccyx and caudal end of the sacrum. अनुत्रिक-जालिका; अनुत्रिक-जाल;

**Gastric P.**, a branch of the celiac plexus accompanying the gastric artery. जठर-जालिका; जठर-जाल;

**Hepatic P.**, a branch of the celiac plexus attending the hepatic artery to the liver. यकृत्-जालिका; यकृत्-जाल;

**Hypogastric P.**, one before the promontory of the sacrum. अधोजठर-जालिका;

**Lumbar P.**, one formed by the anterior divisions of the lumbar spinal nerves in the psoas muscle. कटि-जालिका; कटि-जाल;

**Lymphatic P.**, a network of lymphatic capillaries, usually without valves, that open into one or more larger lymphatic vessels; plexus lymphaticus. लसीका जाल;

**Ovarian P.**, a venous plexus in the broad ligament; a nerve plexus distributed to the ovaries. डिम्बग्रन्थि-जालिका;

**Parotid P.**, the pes anserinus. कर्णपूर्व-जालिका; कर्णमूल-जालिका;

**Patellar P.**, one in front of the patella. जानुका-जालिका;

**Pelvic P.**, one at the side of the rectum and bladder, distributed to the viscera of the pelvis and plexuses of the pelvis. श्रोणि-जालिका; श्रोणि-जाल;

**Pharyngeal P.**, nerve plexuses supplying in pharynx. ग्रसनी-जालिका; ग्रसनी-जाल;

**Phrenic P.**, one accompanying the phrenic arteries. मध्यच्छद-जालिका;

**Prostatic P.**, one occupying the sides of the prostate. पुरःस्थग्रन्थि-जालिका;

**Pterygoid P.**, a plexus of veins which accompanies the internal maxillary artery between the pterygoid muscles. पक्षाभ जालिका;

**Pulmonary P.**, one of two autonomic plexuses, anterior and posterior, at the hilus of each lung; plexus pulmonalis. फुप्फुस-जाल;

**Renal P.**, one near the renal artery. वृक्क-जालिका; वृक्क-जाल;

**Sacral P.**, one ventrad of the sacrum. त्रिक-जालिका; त्रिक-जाल;

**Solar P.**, network of the nerves lying upon the vertebral column, the aorta and the pillars of the diaphragm. सौर-जालिका; सौर-जाल;

**Splenic P.**, one around the splenic artery. प्लीहा-जालिका; प्लीहा-जाल;

**Tympanic P.**, one in the tympanum. मध्यकर्ण-जालिका;

**Uterine P.**, a venous plexus on the walls of the uterus. गर्भाशय-जालिका; जरायु-जाल;

**Vaginal P.**, a nerve plexus supplying the walls of the vagina. योनि-जालिका; योनि-जाल;

**Vesical P.**, one surrounding the vesical arteries. मूत्राशय-जालिका;

**P. Lymphaticus**, see **Lymphatic Plexus**.

**P. Pulmonalis**, see **Pulmonary Plexus**.

**Plexuses.** Plural of **Plexus**.

**Plica.** A fold. वली; पुटक; झुर्री; तह;

**P. Fimbriata**, a fold of mucous membrane having a fringed free edge on either side of the frenum linguae. झल्लरी-पुटक;

**P. Lacrimalis**, a fold of mucous membrane guarding the lower opening of the nasolacrimal duct; lacrimal fold. अश्रु-पुटक;

**P. Palmatae**, radiating folds in the mucous membrane of the cervix. करतलाकार पुटक;

**P. Polonica**, a matting of the hair with swelling and bleeding. लोमपुटक; रोमगुच्छ;

**P. Seminularis**, a mucous fold at the inner canthus of the eye. अर्धचन्द्रकपुटक;

**P. Spiralis,** the spiral valve of the gall-bladder. सर्पिल पुटक;

**P. Triangularis,** a fold of mucous membrane covering the supratonsillar fossa. त्रिकोण पुटक

**Plicae.** Plural of **Plica.**

**Plication.** An operation for reducing the size of a hollow viscus by taking folds or tucks in walls. वलीकरण

**Plombage.** Extrapleural compression of the tuberculous lung cavity. रिक्तीभरण

**Plumbago.** Graphites. ग्रैफाइटिस; सीसा

**Plumbism.** Lead-poisoning. सीसात्यय; सीसाविषण्णता

**Plumbum.** Lead; a soft, bluish white metal. सीसा; एक कोमल, नीली-श्वेत धातु

**Pluriglandular.** Pertaining to several glands; multiglandular; polyglandular. बहुग्रन्थिक; अनेक ग्रन्थियों सम्बन्धी

**Pluripara.** A woman who has given birth to several children. बहुप्रसवा; बहुत से बच्चों को जन्म देने वाली स्त्री

**Pluripotent.** Having the capacity to affect more than one organ or tissue; pluripotential. बहुशक्तिक

**Plurisegmental.** Having several segments. बहुखंडांशी; अनेक खण्डों वाला

**Pneograph.** See **Pneumograph.**

**Pneumarthrosis.** A collection of air or gas in a joint. संधिवातसंचय; किसी जोड़ पर हवा या गैस का जमाव होना

**Pneumatic.** Pertaining to gases or to respiration. वायवी; वायुमय; वायुरूप; गैसों अथवा श्वास सम्बन्धी

**Pneumatocele.** Gaseous hernia of the lung or other parts; pneumocele; pleurocele. वायुपुटी; फेफड़े या अन्य भागों का हर्निया

**Pneumatogram.** See **Pneumogram.**

**Pneumatograph.** See **Pneumograph.**

**Pneumatography.** See **Pneumography.**

**Pneumatology.** The science of respiration. श्वासविज्ञान

**Pneumatosis.** Morbid accumulation of gas in any part of the body. वायुपुटिता; शरीर के किसी भाग में गैस का अधिक जमाव होना

**Pneumaturia.** The passage of flatus with urine, usually as a result of bladder-bowel fistula. वायुमेह; पेशाब के साथ हवा निकलना

**Pneumectomy.** See **Pneumonectomy.**

**Pneumo.** The lung. फुप्फुस; फेफड़ा

**Pneumocele.** See **Pneumatocele.**

**Pneumococcal.** Relating to the pneumococcus. क्लोमगोलाणुक; क्लोमगोलाणु सम्बन्धी

**Pneumococcemia.** The presence of pneumococci in the blood. क्लोमगोलाणुरक्तता; रक्त में क्लोमगोलाणु होना

**Pneumococci.** Plural of **Pneumococcus.**

**Pneumococcosis.** Infection with pneumococci. क्लोमगोलाणुरुग्णता

**Pneumococcosuria.** Presence of pneumococci or their specific capsular substance in the urine. क्लोमगोलाणुमेह

**Pneumococcus.** A coccal bacterium arranged characteristically in pairs. क्लोमगोलाणु;

**Rheumatoid P.**, fibrosing alveolitis occurring in patients suffering from rheumatoid arthritis. आमवातज क्लोमगोलाणु; आमवाती क्लोमगोलाणु

**Pneumoconioses.** Plural of **Pneumoconiosis.**

**Pneumoconiosis.** Dust disease; fibrosis of the lungs caused by long continued inhalation of dust in industrial occupations; calcicosis; pneumokoniosis. फुप्फुसधूलिमयता; फेफड़ों की तन्तुमयता

**Pneumodilation.** Dilation or dilatation of the lungs. फुप्फुसविस्फार; फेफड़ों का फैलाव

**Pneumoencephalogram.** X-ray picture of the cerebral ventricles after injection of air. मस्तिष्कवायुवीचित्र; वायुमस्तिष्कचित्र

**Pneumoencephalography.** Radiographic examination of cerebral ventricles after injection of air by means of a lumbar cisternal puncture. मस्तिष्कवायुवीचित्रण; वायुमस्तिष्कचित्रण

**Pneumogastric.** Belonging to the lungs and the stomach. फुप्फुसजठरीय; फुप्फुस एवं आमाशय सम्बन्धी

**Pneumogram.** The tracing or graphic record obtained with the pneumograph; pneumatogram. श्वसनलेख; फुप्फुसगतिलेख

**Pneumograph.** An instrument for recording chest movement; pneumatograph; pneograph. श्वसनीलेखी; फुप्फुसगतिलेखी

**Pneumography.** Description of the lungs; pneography; pneumatography. फुप्फुसचित्रण

**Pneumokoniosis.** See **Pneumoconiosis.**

**Pneumolith.** A calculus in the lungs. फुप्फुसाश्मरी; फेफड़े की पथरी

**Pneumolithiasis.** Formation of calculi in the lungs. फुप्फुसाश्मरीयता; फेफड़ों में पथरियां बनना

**Pneumolysis.** Separation of the two pleural layers or the outer pleural layer from the chest wall to collapse the lung. फुप्फुसलयन; फुप्फुस-अपघटन; फुप्फुसापघटन

**Pneumomediastinum.** Escape of air into the mediastinal tissues. वातमध्यस्थानिका

**Pneumomycosis.** A fungus infection of the lung; pneumonomycosis. फुप्फुसकवकता; फेफड़े का कवक-रोग

**Pneumon.** The lung. फुप्फुस; फेफड़ा

**Pneumonectomy.** Excision of a lung; pneumectomy. फुप्फुसोच्छेदन; फेफड़ा काट कर हटाना

**Pneumonia.** Inflammation of the lungs; pneumonitis. फुप्फुसपाक; फुप्फुसशोथ; फेफड़ों का प्रदाह; निमोनिया;

Acute. P., see **Lobar Pneumonia.**

Aspiration P., the due to the inspiration of irritant substance into the lung. चूषण फुप्फुसपाक;

Bronchial P., bronchopneumonia. श्वसनीफुप्फुसपाक;

Central P., acute pneumonia beginning in the interior of a lobe of the lung. मध्यवर्ती फुप्फुसपाक;

Chronic P., see **Interstitial Pneumonia.**

Double P., lobar pneumonia involving both lungs. द्विगुण फुप्फुसपाक; डबल निमोनिया;

Fibroid P., see **Interstitial Pneumonia.**

Hypostatic P., a kind occurring in the weak or aged, affecting the lower posterior portions of the lung. अधःस्थितिक फुप्फुसपाक;

Interstitial P., that marked by the increase of interstitial connective tissue; chronic pneumonia; fibroid pneumonia. अन्तरालीय फुप्फुसपाक;

Lobar P., acute pneumonia, most often due to a specific microorganism; acute pneumonia. खण्डीय फुप्फुसपाक; खण्ड-फुप्फुसपाक;

Lobular P., bronchopneumonia. खण्डकीय फुप्फुसपाक; श्वसनी-फुप्फुसपाक;

Massive P., Lobar pneumonia with the filling of air-cells, bronchi, or even the entire lung with fibrinous exudation. सामूहिक फुप्फुसपाक;

**Migratory P.**, a form involving one lobe after another; wandering pneumonia; pneumonia migrans. भ्रमणशील फुप्फुसपाक;
**Rheumatic P.**, pneumonia occurring in severe rheumatic fever. आमवातज फुप्फुसपाक; आमवाती फुप्फुसपाक;
**Wandering P.**, see **Migratory Pneumonia**.
**P. Migrans**, see **Migratory Pneumonia**.
**Pneumonic.** See **Pulmonary**.
**Pneumonitis.** Inflammation of the lung tissues; pneumonia. फुप्फुसपाक; फुप्फुसशोथ; फुप्फुसीय ऊतकों का प्रदाह
**Pneumonomycosis.** A fungus-infection of the lungs. फुप्फुसकवकता; फेफड़ों का कवक-रोग
**Pneumonopathy.** Any morbid condition of the lungs. फुप्फुसविकृति; फेफड़ों की रुग्ण अवस्था
**Pneumopericardium.** Presence of gas in the pericardial sac. वायुहृदयावरण
**Pneumoperitoneum.** Air or gas in the peritoneal cavity. वायुपर्युदर्या; उदरावरण में वायु अथवा गैस विद्यमान रहना
**Pneumopleuritis.** Inflammation of the lungs and pleura. फुप्फुसपरिफुप्फुसशोथ; फेफड़ों तथा उनकी झिल्ली का प्रदाह
**Pneumopyothorax.** See **Pneumothorax**.
**Pneumoradiography.** Radiographic examination of the lungs after injection of air. फुप्फुसवायुचित्रण
**Pneumothorax.** Gas or air in the pleural cavity; pneumopyothorax; aerothorax. वातिलवक्ष; वातवक्ष
**Pneumoventriculography.** Examination of the cerebral ventricles by x-ray after injection of air directly. निलयवायुचित्रण
**Pock.** A pustule of small-pox. स्फोट; पिटक; चेचक का दाना;
   **P.-mark.** the mark of pit left from small-pox. पिटक-चिन्ह; चेचक का दाग
**Podagra.** Gout of the foot. पादवात; पैर का गठिया
**Podalgia.** Pain in the feet; pododynia. पादार्ति; पादशूल; पैरों में दर्द
**Podalic.** Relating to the feet. पैरों सम्बन्धी
**Podiatry.** Treatment of the foot. पादचिकित्सा; पैर का इलाज
**Podocyte.** An epithelial cell of the renal glomerulus attached to the outer surface of the glomerular basement membrane of the cytoplasmic foot process; foot cell. पादकोशिका

**Pododynia.** See **Podalgia.**

**Podogram.** An imprint of the sole of the foot. पदतलचित्र; पादतलचित्र

**Pogonion.** The anterior middle point of the chin. चिबुकाग्रबिन्दु; ठोढ़ी का अगला बीच वाला बिन्दु

**Poikiloblast.** See **Poikilocyte.**

**Poikilocyte.** Abnormally shaped erythrocyte; poikiloblast. विषमलोहितकोशिका; अस्वाभाविक आकार की लोहितकोशिका

**Poikilocythemia.** See **Poikilocytosis.**

**Poikilocytosis.** Presence of poikilocytes in the peripheral blood; poikilocythemia. असमकोशिकता

**Poikilothermal.** See **Poikilothermic.**

**Poikilothermic.** Adapting body temperature to environment; poikilothermic. असमतापी; विषमतापी

**Point.** A sharp end of any object. नोक; चोंच; a small area or spot. बि-दु; चिन्ह; a stage or condition reached. अंक;

**Dew P.,** the temperature at which dew forms. ओसांक;

**Freezing P.,** the degree of cold at which a liquid becomes solid. हिमांक;

**McBurney's P.,** a point above the anterior superior spine of the ilium and the umbilicus where the pressure of fingers cause pain in case of acute appendicitis. मैकबर्नी बिन्दु;

**Melting P.,** the degree of temperature at which fusible solids begin to melt. गलनांक;

**Nodal P.,** the centre of curvature of a spheric lens or refracting surface, through which rays of light pass, joining conjugate points. निर्नति बिन्दु

**Poison.** A toxic agent. विष; गरल; कालकूट; हलाहल; जहर;

**P. Ivy,** skin irritation due to toxic oils in this wild plant. सिरपेंची विषण्णता; सिरपेंची विष;

**P. Nut,** the **Strychnos nux vomica,** that affords Strychnine. कुचला; कुचला विष;

**P. Oak,** skin irritation due to toxic oils in this common wild plant. बलूत विषण्णता; बलूत विष

**Poisoning.** The administration of poison. विष देना; the state of being poisoned. विषण्णता; विषाक्तता;

**Blood P.**, septicemia; pyemia. पूतिजीवरक्तता; रक्तविषण्णता; रक्तविषाक्तता;

**Food P.**, poisoning in which the active agent is contained in the ingested food. खाद्यविषण्णता; खाद्यविषाक्तता; आहारविषाक्तता

**Poisonous.** Toxic; toxicant; pertaining to, or caused by a poison. विषाक्त; जहरीला; विषैला

**Polar.** Pertaining to a pole. ध्रुवीय; ध्रुव सम्बन्धी; having poles. ध्रुवों वाला

**Polarisation.** Referring to light, a condition in which the vibrations take place in one plane; it reduces glare in glasses and mirrors; polarization. ध्रुवीकरण; विद्युदग्राच्छादन

**Polarity.** The state of having poles. ध्रुवता

**Polarization.** See **Polarisation.**

**Pole.** One of the two points in a magnet, called South Pole and North Pole, or at the extremities of the axis of an organ or body, or on a sphere at the greatest distance from its equator; polus. ध्रुव; छोर; कोटि

**Poli.** Plural of **Polus.**

**Policlinic.** See **Polyclinic.**

**Poliencephalitis.** See **Polioencephalitis.**

**Polio.** Abbreviated term for **Poliomyelitis.**

**Polioencephalitis.** Inflammation of the cerebral gray matter; poliencephalitis. पोलियोमस्तिष्कशोथ; मस्तिष्क के भूरे पदार्थ का प्रदाह

**Poliomyelitis.** Infantile paralysis; implantation of the gray matter of the cord. पोलियो; पोलियोमेरुरज्जुशोथ; धूसरमज्जाशोथ; शिशुअंगघात

**Poliosis.** Grayness of the hair. पालित्य; बालों का भूरापन

**Poliovirus Hominis.** The virus responsible for causing poliomyelitis. पोलियोविषाणु

**Pollen.** The male cells of certain plant, distributed by the wind. पराग; पुष्परज; रेणु

**Pollenosis.** Allergic condition arising from sensitization to pollen. परागरुग्णता

**Pollex.** The thumb or great toe. हस्तांगुष्ठ अथवा पादांगुष्ठ; हाथ या पैर का अंगूठा;

**P. Pedis,** the great toe. पादांगुष्ठ; पैर का अंगूठा

**Pollices.** Plural of **Pollex.**

**Pollution.** The spoiling of a natural resource, such as air or water by noxious or dangerous contaminants. प्रदूषण; दूषण

**Polus.** A pole. ध्रुव

**Poly-.** Prefix signifying many. 'बहु' तथा 'अति' के रूप में प्रयुक्त उपसर्ग

**Polyadenitis.** Inflammation of many lymph nodes. बहुग्रन्थिशोथ; अनेक लसीका पर्वों का प्रदाह

**Polyarteritis.** Inflammation of many arteries. बहुधमनीशोथ; बहुत-सी धमनियों का प्रदाह;
 **P. Nodosa,** aneurysmal swelling and thrombosis occurring in the affected vessels. पर्विल बहुधमनीशोथ

**Polyarthralgia.** Pain in several joints. बहुसन्धिशूल; अनेक जोड़ों में दर्द

**Polyarthric.** Having many joints; polyarticular; multiarticular. बहुसन्धिक; अनेक जोड़ों वाला

**Polyarthritis.** Inflammation of several joints at the same time. बहुसन्धिशोथ; अनेक सन्धियों का प्रदाह

**Polyarticular.** See **Polyarthric.**

**Polyblast.** A general term designating the various cells seen in newly developing connective tissue. बहुकेन्द्रकप्रसू

**Polycholia.** Excessive secretion of bile. अतिपित्तनिस्सरण; पित्त का अधिक मात्रा में रिसना

**Polychrest.** Having many virtues; medicine useful for many diseases. बहुप्रयुक्त; अनेक रोगों में प्रयुक्त की जानी वाली औषधि

**Polychromasia.** Quality of having many colours. बहुवर्णकता

**Polychromatic.** Many coloured; multicoloured. बहुवर्णकी; बहुरंगी; अनेक रंगों वाला

**Polychromatophilia.** A tendency of certain cells to stain with basic and acid dyes, or a condition characterized by the presence of many red blood cells that have an affinity for acid, basic or neutral stains. बहुवर्णरागिता

**Polyclinic.** A large general hospital; policlinic. सर्वोपचारगृह; चिकित्सालय

**Polycoria.** An eye with more than one pupil. बहुतारा

**Polycyesis.** Multiple pregnancies. बहुगर्भता

**Polycystic.** Composed of many cysts. बहुपुटीय; असंख्य पुटियों से निर्मित

**Polycythaemia.** See **Polycythemia.**

**Polycythemia.** Increase in the number of circulating red blood corpuscles; polycythaemia. बहुलोहितकोशिकारक्तता; लोहितकोशिकाबहुलता; प्राथमिक अतिलोहितकोशिकारक्तता

**Polydactyl.** Having many fingers or toes; polydactylism; polydactyly. बहुअंगुलिता

**Polydactylism.** See **Polydactyl.**

**Polydactyly.** See **Polydactyl.**

**Polydipsia.** Constant and excessive thirst with dryness of mouth. बहुतृषा; अतिपिपासा; अत्यधिक प्यास लगना

**Polyemia.** Abundance of blood; polyhemia. बहुरक्तता; रक्त की अत्यधिक बढ़ी हुई मात्रा

**Polyeuria.** Excessive secretion of urine; polyuria. बहुमूत्रता; अत्यधिक मूत्रस्राव होना

**Polygalactia.** Excessive secretion of milk, especially at the weaning period. अतिस्तन्यता; बहुस्तन्यता

**Polygenesis.** Producing many offsprings. बहुजननता; बहुद्भववाद

**Polyglandular.** See **Pluriglandular.**

**Polygraph.** An instrument which records pulses simultaneously. बहुस्पन्दलेखी; बहुलेखी

**Polyhedral.** Having many surfaces or blades. बहुफलकीय

**Polyhemia.** See **Polyemia.**

**Polyhydramnios.** An excessive amount of polyamniotic fluid. अत्युल्वोदकता

**Polyhidrosis.** See **Polyidrosis.**

**Polyidrosis.** Excessive sweating; polyhidrosis. अतिस्वेदन; अत्यधिक पसीना

**Polymasia.** See **Polymastia.**

**Polymastia.** Condition of having more than two breasts; polymasia. बहुस्तनता

**Polymenorrhea.** Excessive menstrual flow; polymenorrhoea. बहुआर्तव; लघुचक्री आर्तव; ऋतुस्राव की अधिकता

**Polymenorrhoea.** See **Polymenorrhea.**

**Polymer.** A substance of high molecular weight. पॉलीमर; बहुलक

**Polymerism.** Having many parts. बहुलकता; अनेक अंश अथवा भाग होने की अवस्था

**Polymerization.** A reaction in which a molecular weight product is produced by successive additions. बहुलकीकरण

**Polymorphic.** See **Polymorphous.**

**Polymorphism.** The condition of being polymorphous. बहुरूपता

**Polymorphonuclear.** Having a many-shaped or lobulated nucleus. बहुरूपीकेन्द्रक

**Polymorphous.** Having many forms; polymorphic; pleomorphic; pleomorphous. बहुरूपी; अनेक रूपों वाला

**Polymyalgia.** Pain in several muscle groups. बहुपेश्यार्ति; असंख्य पेशी-समूहों में दर्द;

**P. Rheumatica,** a syndrome occurring in elderly people comprising of a crippling ache in the shoulders, pelvic girdle muscles and spine, with pronounced morning stiffness and a raised E.S.R. आमवातज बहुपेश्यार्ति; आमवाती बहुपेश्यार्ति

**Polymyositis.** Inflammation of many muscles at a time. बहुपेशीशोथ; अनेक पेशियों का प्रदाह

**Polyneuralgia.** Neuralgia of several nerves simultaneously. बहुतंत्रिकार्ति; बहुतंत्रिकाशूल

**Polyneuritis.** Multiple neuritis. बहुतंत्रिकाशोथ; अनेक नाड़ियों का प्रदाह

**Polyneuropathy.** A disease process involving a number of peripheral nerves. बहुतंत्रिकाविकृति

**Polyoncosis.** Formation of multiple tumours. बहुअर्बुदता

**Polyonychia.** Presence of supernumerary nails on fingers and toes. बहुनखता

**Polyopia.** Multiple vision. बहुदृष्टिता; बहुदृष्टि

**Polyorrhymenitis.** See **Polyserositis.**

**Polyp.** An abnormal growth of soft tumour, commonly found in the nose, uterus, rectum, etc.; polypus. पुर्वंगक; पालिप

**Polypectomy.** Surgical removal of a polyp. पुर्वंगक-उच्छेदन; पुर्वंगक को काट कर हटाना

**Polyphagia.** Excessive eating; bulimia. अतिक्षुधा; अत्यधिक भोजन करना; अतिभक्षण

**Polypharmacy.** A prescription indicating the use of many drugs at the same time. बहुभेषजी

**Polyphonic.** Having many voices. बहुध्वनिक; असंख्य ध्वनियों वाला

**Polyphyletic.** Derived from more than one source. बहूद्भवी

**Polyplegia.** Paralysis of several muscles. बहुपेशीघात; असंख्य पेशियों का पक्षाघात

**Polypi.** Plural form of **Polyp.**

**Polypoid.** Resembling a polyp. पुर्वंगकाभ; पुर्वंगक जैसा

**Polyposis.** A condition in which there are numerous polypi in an organ. बहुपुर्वंगकता; किसी अंग में असंख्य पुर्वंगक होना

**Polypus.** See **Polyp.**

**Polysarca.** Overfatness; obesity; corpulency. बहुस्थूलता; अत्यधिक मोटापा

**Polyserositis.** Inflammation of several serous membranes; polyorrhymenitis. बहुसीरमीकलाशोथ; असंख्य सीरमी कलाओं का प्रदाह

**Polysinusitis.** Simultaneous inflammation of two or more sinuses. बहुविवरशोथ

**Polytendinitis.** Inflammation of several tendons. बहुकण्डराशोथ

**Polythelia.** Having more than one nipple. बहुचूचुकता; एक से अधिक चूचूक होना

**Polyuresis.** See **Polyuria.**

**Polyuria.** Excessive secretion of urine; polyeuria; polyuresis. बहुमूत्रता; अत्यधिक पेशाब होना

**Polyvalent.** Having a combining value greater than two atoms of a univalent element. बहुसंयोजक

**Pompholyx.** Vesicular skin eruptions on the feet or hands. पादचर्मस्फोट; हस्तचर्मस्फोट

**Pons.** A process or bridge of tissue connecting two parts. संयोजक अंश अथवा अंग

**Pontes.** Plural of **Pons.**

**Ponticulosis.** See **Ponticulus.**

**Ponticulus.** A small pons; ponticulosis. कर्णकण्टक; सूक्ष्मांग

**Pool.** A collection of blood in any region of the body. संचय; रक्तसंचय

**Popliteal.** Pertaining to the ham of knee. जानुपृष्ठीय; जानुपृष्ठ सम्बन्धी

**Popliteus.** The popliteal muscle. जानुपृष्ठपेशी; घुटने के पीछे की पेशी

**Pore.** The orifice of the absorbing and exhaling vessels. छिद्र; रोमकूप; रोमछिद्र; लोमरन्ध्र

**Porencephalia.** A condition marked by the presence of depressions on the surface of the brain; porencephaly. सुषिरमस्तिष्कता; सरन्ध्रमस्तिष्कता

**Porencephaly.** See **Porencephalia.**

**Pori**. Plural of **Porus**.

**Poriform**. Resembling a pore. रोमकूपाभ; लोमरन्ध्राभ; रोमछिद्रवत्

**Poroses**. Plural of **Porosis**.

**Porosis**. The formation of callus. घट्टा; किण

**Porosity**. The condition of a body containing pore, as a sponge. सरन्ध्रता; रन्ध्रमयता; छिद्रिलता

**Porous**. Having pores. रन्ध्रिल; छिद्रिल

**Porrigo**. Favus of the scalp; scald-head; ringworm. दद्रु; दाद; मण्डलकुष्ठ; खोपड़ी की चमड़ी का एक रोग;

**P. Capitis**, scald-head. करोटि-प्रदाह; करोटिशोथ; मण्डलकुष्ठ; दद्रु; दाद;

**P. Favosa**, a large, soft, flat and straw-coloured pustule. दीर्घाकार, कोमल, चपटी और तिनके के रंग की फुंसी

**Porta**. The depression of an organ at which the vessels enter and leave. प्रतिहार; द्वार;

**P. Hepatis**, the transverse fissure through which the portal vein, hepatic artery and bile ducts pass on the undersurface of the liver. यकृत् प्रतिहार

**Portae**. Plural of **Porta**.

**Portal**. Relating to the porta. प्रतिहारी; प्रतिहार सम्बन्धी;

**P. System**, four large veins two mesenteric, one splenic and one gastric. प्रतिहार-प्रणाली; प्रतिहार-जाल;

**P. Vein**, one conveying blood into the liver. प्रतिहारी शिरा

**Portio**. A portion; a part. भाग; अंश;

**P. Cervicis**, see **Portio Vaginalis**.

**P. Dura**, the facial nerve. ललाट-तंत्रिका; चेहरे की स्नायु;

**P. Vaginalis**, the portion of the cervix projecting into the vagina; portio cervicis. योनिगतगर्भाशयग्रीवा भाग

**Portion**. A part or section; portio. भाग; अंश

**Portiones**. Plural of **Portio**.

**Portogram**. X-ray of portal vein after splenic puncture and injection of radio-opaque liquid, or after injection of radio-opaque liquid into the portal vein at operation. प्रतिहारीचित्र

**Portography**. Radiographic delineation of the portal material introduced into the spleen or into the portal vein. प्रतिहारीचित्रण

**Porus**. A pore. छिद्र; लोमकूप; a callosity. घट्टा; किण; त्वचा की कठोरता

**Position.** Posture. स्थिति; आसन; दशा; attitude. प्रवृत्ति; झुकाव;
   **Dorsal P.**, that in which the patient lies on the back. अधिपृष्ठ-स्थिति;
   **Genu-cubital P.**, see **Knee-elbow Position.**
   **Genupectoral P.**, see **Knee-chest Position.**
   **Knee-chest P.**, a prone position resting on the knees and upper part of the chest; genupectoral position. जानुवक्षासन;
   **Knee-elbow P.**, one in which the patient rests upon the knees and elbows with the head upon the hand; genu-cubital position. जानुकूर्परासन;
   **Obstetric P.**, see **Recumbent Position.**
   **Recumbent P.**, that in which the patient lies on the left side with the right thigh and knee drawn up; obstetric position. श्यान-स्थिति
**Posititio.** The same as **Position.**
**Positive (+).** Affirmative; definite; opposed to negative. ग्राही; धन; धनात्मक
**Posological.** Relating to posology. औषधिमात्राविज्ञान सम्बन्धी
**Posology.** The science of medicinal doses. औषधिमात्राविज्ञान; औषधिमात्रिकी
**Post-.** Latin preposition meaning after, behind, or posterior. 'उत्तर' एवं 'पश्च' के रूप में प्रयुक्त प्रत्यय;
   **P.-abortal,** after abortion. गर्भपातोत्तर; गर्भस्रावोत्तर;
   **P.-anaesthetic,** after anaesthesia. निश्चेतनोत्तर;
   **P.-anal,** behind the anus. गुदपश्च; मलद्वार के पिछले भाग से सम्बन्धित;
   **P.-axial,** behind the axis. अक्षपश्च;
   **P.-cebum,** after a meal; post-cibal; post-cibus. भोजनोत्तर; भोजनोपरान्त; भोजन के बाद;
   **P.-central,** behind the central fissure. मध्यपश्च;
   **P.-cibal,** see **Post-cebum.**
   **P.-cibus,** see **Post-cebum.**
   **P.-coital,** after coitus. संगमोत्तर; सम्भोगोत्तर
   **P.-convulsive,** occurring after a convulsion. आक्षेपोत्तर;
   **P.-diphtheritic,** following an attack of diphtheria. रोहिणीरोगोत्तर;
   **P.-encephalitic,** following an attack of encephalitis. मस्तिष्कशोथोत्तर;
   **P.-epileptic,** following an epileptic seizure. अपस्मारोत्तर; मिर्गी के दौरे के बाद;

**P.-febrile,** occurring after a fever. ज्वरोत्तर; ज्वर के बाद प्रकट होने वाला;

**P.-ganglionic,** situated after a collection of nerve cells (ganglion) as a post-ganglionic nerve fibre. गण्डिकापश्च;

**P.-menopausal,** occurring after the menopause has been established. रजोनिवृत्त्योत्तर; रजोनिवृत्ति काल के बाद;

**P.-mortem,** after death, usually inferring dissection of the body. मरणोत्तर; मृत्यु के बाद;

**P.-mortem Examination,** autopsy. मरणोत्तर जांच; शव परीक्षा;

**P.-nasal,** situated behind the nose and in the nasopharynx. नासापश्च; नाक के पीछे;

**P.-natal,** after delivery. प्रसवोत्तर;

**P.-operative,** after operation. शल्यकर्मोत्तर;

**P.-partum,** after a birth or parturition. प्रसवोत्तर; जन्मोत्तर;

**P.-prandial,** following a meal. भोजनोत्तर; भोजन के बाद;

**P.-vaccinal,** after vaccination. टीकोत्तर; टीका लगने के बाद

**Posterior.** Behind in position; the back part of anything. पृष्ठ; पश्च; पिछली ओर का;

**P. Chamber,** the space between the iris and the lens. पश्च-कक्ष; पश्च-प्रकोष्ठ;

**P. Nares,** the opening of the nostrils into the gullet. पश्च-नासा; नथुनों का पिछला भाग

**Posterolateral.** Behind and to one side. पश्चपार्श्व; पश्चपार्श्विक

**Posthioplasty.** Reparative or plastic surgery of the prepuce. शिश्नमुण्डच्छदसंधान

**Posthitis.** Inflammation of the prepuce. शिश्नमुण्डच्छदशोथ; लिंगमुण्डचर्म का प्रदाह

**Posthumous.** Occurring after death; applied to a child born after the death of his father. पितृमरणोत्तर; पिता की मृत्यु के बाद

**Postomania.** Delirium tremens. कम्पोन्माद

**Postponing.** When the paroxysms recur after the regular time. अनियतकालिक

**Postulate.** A well-known law. अभ्युपगम; अभ्युधारण; सुपरिचित विधान

**Postural.** Pertaining to the posture. स्थितिज; स्थिति सम्बन्धी

**Posture.** Position. संस्थिति; स्थिति; आसन; attitude. प्रवृत्ति; झुकाव

**Potable.** Suitable for drink. पेय; पीने योग्य

**Potash.** An alkaline substance obtained from wood-ashes. पोटाश; लकड़ी की राख से प्राप्त एक क्षार पदार्थ

**Potassium.** The basic element of potash. पोटैशियम; पोटाशियम; पोटाश का मूल सार;

  **P. Bromide,** bromide of potash, widely used as a mild sedative. पोटैशियम ब्रोमाइड;

  **P. Chloride,** chloride of potash; a mild antiseptic used in mouth washes and gargles. पोटैशियम क्लोराइड;

  **P. Citrate,** an alkaline diuretic, widely used in cystitis. पोटैशियम साइट्रेट;

  **P. Hydroxide,** caustic potash. पोटैशियम हाइड्रॉक्साइड;

  **P. Iodide,** used as an expectorant in bronchitis and asthma. पोटैशियम आयोडाइड;

  **P. Permangnate,** purple crystals with powerful disinfectant and deodorizing properties. पोटैशियम परमैंगनेट

**Potency.** Power; efficacy; the strength to which a medicine is diluted. शक्ति; पोटेंसी; क्षमता

**Potent.** Denoting potency; powerful. शक्तिशाली

**Potentiation.** In chemotherapy, a degree of synergism that is greater than additive. प्रवलीकरण

**Potion.** A draft; potus. घूंट

**Pott's disease.** Spinal caries; spinal tuberculosis. मेरुक्षय; spondylitis. कशेरुकासन्धिशोथ

**Potus.** See Potion.

**Pouch.** Pocket; a pocket-shaped cavity. कोष्ठ; धानी; बीजकोष; जेब;

  **P. of Douglas,** recto-uterine pouch. मलाशययोनिकोष्ठ

**Poultice.** Cataplasm. उपनाह; प्रलेप; लेई; पुल्टिस

**Powder.** A dry mass of minute separate particles of any substance. चूर्ण; विचूर्ण; पावडर;

  **Aromatic P.,** a mixture of nutmeg, ginger, cinnamon and cardamom. सुवासित चूर्ण

**Power.** Capacity. क्षमता; potency. शक्ति

**Pox.** Any eruptive disease, like small-pox, great-pox (syphilis) and chicken-pox. स्फोट; फुन्सी;

**Chicken-p.,** varicella. लघु मसूरिका; छोटी माता;
**Great-p.,** syphilis. उपदंश;
**Small-p.,** variola. मसूरिका; चेचक
**P.P.B.** Positive pressure breathing. धन दाब श्वसन
**Practice.** The exercise of any professional practice. वृत्ति; व्यवसाय;
**Medical P.,** practice of medicine. चिकित्सा व्यवसाय
**Practitioner.** A medical practitioner; a physician. चिकित्सक; चिकित्सा व्यवसायी; वैद्य; हकीम
**Praecordial.** See **Precordial.**
**Pre-.** Prefix signifying before. 'पुरः', 'पुरा', 'प्राक्' तथा 'पूर्व' के रूप में प्रयुक्त उपसर्ग
**Preanaesthesia.** Before anaesthesia; preanesthesia. प्राक्निश्चेतना; निश्चेतनापूर्व; संज्ञाहरणपूर्व; सम्वेदनाहरणपूर्व
**Preanaesthetic.** Preliminary drug given to facilitate induction of general anaesthesia; preanesthetic. प्राक्संज्ञाहारी (औषधि)
**Preanesthesia.** See **Preanaesthesia.**
**Preanesthetic.** See **Preanaesthetic.**
**Preaxial.** Anterior to the transverse body-axis. पुरोक्ष
**Precancerous.** Referring to body condition which might favour the development of cancers, such as chronic sores, irritations and exposure to substances known to cause cancer. प्राक्कैंसर; कैंसरपूर्व; कैंसर प्रकट होने से पहले
**Precarious.** Irrational. तर्कहीन; निराधार; कल्पित; पराश्रित; असंगत
**Precentral.** In front of the central fissure. पुरःकेन्द्रक
**Precipitate.** A substance separated by precipitation. अवक्षेप; प्रक्षेप; निस्साद; तलछट
**Precipitation.** The process of throwing down solids from the liquids that hold them in solution; sediment-like substance. अवक्षेपण; प्रक्षेपण; निस्सादन; अवपतन
**Precocious.** Before the usual time. कालपूर्व; नियत समय से पहले
**Precocity.** Rapid development before the usual time. कालपूर्वप्रौढ़ता; कालपूर्वपक्वता; नियत समय से पूर्व होने वाला द्रुत विकास
**Precordia.** The area of chest overlying the heart; precordium. पुरोहृद्; हृदय के ऊपर स्थित वक्ष-प्रदेश
**Precordial.** Pertaining to the area of the chest immediately over

the heart; praecordial. पुरोहृदीय; पुरोहृद् सम्बन्धी

**Precordis.** The forepart of the chest overlying the heart. पुरोहृद्; हृदय के ऊपर स्थित वक्ष का अगला भाग

**Precordium.** See **Precordia**.

**Precuneus.** The anterior horn of the lateral ventricle. पुरःकीलक

**Precursory.** Preceding and indicative of something to follow as precursory symptoms; forerunner. पुरःसर; पूर्वगामी; पुरोवर्ती; अग्रणी; अग्रदूत

**Prediabetes.** Potential disposition to diabetes mellitus. मधुमेहपूर्व; मधुमेह प्रकट होने से पहले

**Prediastole.** The interval in the cardiac rhythm immediately preceding the diastole. अनुशिथिलनपूर्व

**Predigestion.** Artificial digestion of protein or amylolysis before digestion takes place in the body. पाचनपूर्व; पाचन से पहले

**Predisposing.** Conferring a tendency to disease. प्रवर्तनपूर्व; स्ववृत्तिक; रोगप्रवण

**Predisposition.** A condition of special susceptibility to a disease. पूर्वप्रवृत्ति; रोगप्रवणता; रोग के प्रति विशेष सुग्राह्यता

**Pre-eclampsia.** A condition characterized by albuminuria, hypertension and oedema, arising usually during the later part of pregnancy. प्राक्गर्भक्षेपक; सगर्भता के अन्तिम दिनों में अन्नसारमेह, उच्चरक्तदाब तथा शोफ की अवस्था

**Prefrontal.** Situated in the anterior portion of the frontal lobe of the cerebrum. मस्तिष्काग्र; मस्तिष्क के अगले खण्ड में स्थित

**Preganglionic.** Preceding or in front of a collection of the nerve-cells (ganglion). गण्डिकापूर्व; पाक्गण्डिकीय

**Pregnancy.** Gestation; being with a child right from conception to parturition, normally 40 weeks or 280 days. सगर्भता; सगर्भावस्था; गर्भधारण; गर्भावस्था; गर्भ;

**Abdominal P.,** see **Extra Uterine Pregnancy**.

**Ampullary P.,** tubal pregnancy situated near the mid-portion of the oviduct. कलशिका सगर्भता,

**Cornual P.,** that occurring in one of the horns of a two-horned uterus. शृंगी सगर्भता;

**Ectopic P.,** see **Extra Uterine Pregnancy**.

**Extra Uterine P.,** the development of the ovum outside of the cavity of the uterus; abdominal pregnancy; ectopic pregnancy. अस्थानिक सगर्भता;

**False P.,** see **Pseudocyesis.**

**Interstitial P.,** the development of the ovum in the part of the oviduct that passes through the wall of the uterus; intramular pregnancy. अन्तरालीय सगर्भता;

**Intramular P.,** see **Interstitial Pregnancy.**

**Multiple P.,** more than one foetus in the uterus. बहुसगर्भता;

**Ovarian P.,** development of an impregnated ovum in an ovarian follicle; ovariocyesis. डिम्बग्रंथीय सगर्भता;

**Phantom P.,** see **Pseudocyesis.**

**Tubal P.,** that within an oviduct. डिम्बवाहिनी सगर्भता

**Pregnant.** A female bearing within her the product of conception; gravid. सगर्भा; गर्भवती; गर्भिणी

**Premature.** Occurring before the proper time. कालपूर्व; अपक्व; अपरिपक्व; अकालपरिणत; असमय;

**P. Baby,** where the birth-weight is less than 2.5 kg. (5-1/2 lbs.) and, therefore, special treatment is needed. अकाल शिशु;

**P. Beat,** extra-systole. द्रुत-स्पन्द; कालपूर्व प्रकुंचन;

**P. Labour,** expulsion of the foetus before 280 days of gestation. कालपूर्व प्रसव; अकाल प्रसव; अपरिपक्व प्रसव

**Prematurity.** The state of being premature. कालपूर्वता

**Premaxillary.** In front of the maxilla. ऊर्ध्वहनुज

**Premedication.** Drugs given before the administration of another drug, e.g. those given before an anaesthetic. पूर्वऔषध-प्रयोग

**Premenstrual.** Preceding menstruation. प्रागार्तव; ऋतुस्राव से पहले

**Premolars.** The eight bicuspid teeth, two on each side of each jaw lying between the molars. अग्रचर्वणक दन्त

**Premonitory.** Giving previous warning or notice, as the premonitory symptoms of a disease; prodromal. पूर्वसूचक; पूर्वबोधी

**Premorbid.** Preceding the occurrence of a disease. रोगपूर्व

**Premunition.** Infection immunity. ससंक्रमणप्रतिरक्षा; ससंक्रमणरोगक्षमता

**Prenatal.** Occurring before child-birth. प्रसवपूर्व; जन्मपूर्व; प्रसव से पहले

**Preoperative.** Before an operation. शस्त्रकर्मपूर्व; शल्यक्रिया अथवा शल्यकर्म से पहले

**Preparalysis.** Before the onset of an attack of paralysis. पक्षाघातपूर्व; पक्षाघात से पहले

**Preparation.** To make a thing ready for use as a medicine. योग; योगनिर्माण; उपक्रम; विरचना; तैयारी

**Prepatellar.** In front of the knee-cap. पुरोजानुक

**Prepuberal.** See **Prepubertal.**

**Prepubertal.** Before puberty; prepuberal. यौवनपूर्व

**Prepuce.** The foreskin of the penis; preputium. शिश्नमुण्डच्छद; लिंगमुण्डच्छद

**Preputia.** Plural of **Preputium.**

**Preputial.** Pertaining to the prepuce. शिश्नमुण्डच्छदीय

**Preputium.** See **Prepuce.**

  **P. Clitoridis,** the external fold of the labia minora forming a cap over the clitoris. भगशिश्निकामुण्डच्छद

**Prerenal.** Before or in front of the kidney. वृक्काग्र; गुर्दे के अगले भाग में

**Presbyacousia.** See **Presbyacusis.**

**Presbyacusia.** See **Presbyacusis.**

**Presbyacusis.** Senile deafness; presbyacousia; presbyacusia; presbykousis. जरा-वधिरता

**Presbykousis.** See **Presbyacusis.**

**Presbyopia.** Farsightedness; long-sightedness due to old age. जरादूरदृष्टि

**Presbyopic.** Suffering from presbyopia. जरादूरदृष्टिक

**Prescribe.** Making of a prescription. औषध-निर्देशन

**Prescriber.** A physician who prescribes medicines. औषधनिर्देशक

**Prescription.** The formula written by a physician for his patient. औषधपत्र; नुस्खा

**Presenile.** See **Presenility.**

**Presenility.** A condition occurring before the senility is established; presenile. जरापूर्व; बुढ़ापे से पहले प्रकट होने वाली अवस्था

**Presentation.** The part of the body of the foetus which is in advance during birth. प्रस्तुति; उदय;

  **P. of foetus,** the part that presents itself at birth. भ्रूण-प्रस्तुति; भ्रूणोदय;

**Breech p. of foetus,** that of the buttocks. नितम्ब-प्रस्तुति; स्फिक्-प्रस्तुति; नितम्बोदय;

**Vertex p. of foetus,** that of the head. शीर्ष-प्रस्तुति; शीर्षोदय

**Preservative.** Tending to keep from decay. परिरक्षक; परिरक्षी

**Presphygmic.** Preceding the occurrence of the arterial pulse. स्पन्दपूर्व

**Pressor.** A substance which raises the blood pressure; hypertensor. रक्तदाबवर्धक; रक्तदाब बढ़ाने वाला पदार्थ

**Pressoreceptor.** Baroreceptor. दाबग्राही

**Pressure.** A stress or force acting in any direction against resistance. दबाव; दाब; weight. भार; tension. तनाव;

**P. Area,** the bony prominence of the body over which the flesh of bedridden patients is nuded of its blood supply. दाब क्षेत्र;

**P. Point,** a place at which an artery passes over a bone, against which it can be compressed to stop bleeding. दाब बिन्दु;

**P. Sore,** a decubitus ulcer, arising from continual compression of the flesh over a bony prominence. दाब क्षत.

**Abdominal P.,** pressure surrounding the bladder. उदर दाब;

**Blood P.,** the pressure or the tension of the blood within the arteries, maintained by the contraction of left ventricle. रक्त दाब;

**Diastolic P.,** the lowest blood pressure reached during any given ventricular cycle. अनुशिथिलन दाब;

**Osmotic P.,** pressure that is applied to a solution to prevent the passage into it of solvent when solution and pure solvent are separated by a perfectly semipermeable membrane. परासरण दाब;

**Pulse P.,** the variation in blood pressure occurring during the cardiac cycle. नाड़ी दाब;

**Systolic P.,** the highest blood pressure reached during any given ventricular cycle. प्रकुंचन दाब

**Presystole.** The period preceding the systole or contraction of the heart-muscle. पूर्वप्रकुंचन; हृद्य की पेशी सिकुड़ने से पहले का समय

**Presystolic.** Pertaining to presystole. पुरःप्रकुंचनीय; पूर्वप्रकुंचन सम्बन्धी

**Preterm Delivery.** Premature labour. अकालप्रसव; नियत समय से पहले होने वाला प्रसव

**Preventive.** Prophylactic; warding off. निरोधक; निवारक

**Prevertebral.** In front of the vertebra. पूर्वकशेरुकीय; पूर्वकशेरुक; कशेरुका के सामने

**Prevesical.** Anterior to the bladder. अग्रगवीनी

**Priapism.** Involuntary erection of penis. अविरत शिश्नोत्थान; अविरत लिंगोद्रेक

**Pricking.** A pain compared to the sensation of being pricked. चुभन; वेदना

**Prickle.** A hard, hair-like, epidermal outgrowth. शूक; तीक्ष्णवर्ध;
   **P. Cell,** an epidermal cell furnished with radiating processes which connect with similar cell. शूक कोशिका

**Prickly Heat.** Summer rash; miliaria. घमौरी; अम्हौरी; अंघौरी; धर्मराजिका; कंगुविस्फोट

**Primae Viae.** The stomach and the bowel. आमाशय तथा आंतें

**Primal.** First or primary. प्रथम अथवा प्राथमिक; primordial. आद्य

**Primary.** First; initial. प्राथमिक; प्रारम्भिक; आद्य; पूर्ववर्ती; main; principal. मुख्य;
   **P. Complex,** the initial tuberculous infection in a person, usually in lungs. प्रारम्भिक फुप्फुसक्षय; फुप्फुसीय यक्ष्मा की प्रारम्भिक अवस्था

**Primigravida.** A woman who is pregnant for the first time. प्रथमगर्भी; प्रथम बार गर्भ धारण करने वाली स्त्री

**Primipara.** A woman giving birth to her first child. प्रथमप्रसवा; प्रथम बार प्रसव होने वाली स्त्री

**Primiparity.** The condition of being a primipara. एकप्रसविता; प्रथमप्रसविता

**Primitive.** First in point of time; original. आद्य; पूर्वग; प्रारम्भिक; मूल

**Primordial.** Primitive; original; primordius. आद्य; पूर्वग; प्रारम्भिक; मूल

**Primordium.** An organ or structure in its earliest state. आद्यांग; किसी अंग या बनावट की मूल अवस्था

**Primordius.** See **Primordial.**

**Primum.** Primary; primus. प्राथमिक; मुख्य

**Primus.** See **Primum.**

**Princeps.** A chief or main artery. प्रधान अथवा प्रमुख धमनी

**Principal.** Cardinal; chief; main. प्रमुख; प्रधान; मुख्य

**Principes.** Plural of **Princeps.**

**Principle.** A chemic compound. रासायनिकमिश्रण; a theory. तत्त्व; सिद्धान्त; नियम; a constituent. घटक;

**Principle**

**P. of Medicine,** a basis for a system of medicine. वैद्यक-सिद्धान्त; उपचार-नियम; चिकित्सा के सिद्धान्त

**Privates.** The external genitals; private parts. बाह्य-जननांग

**P.R.N.** Abbreviation for **Pro-re-nata.**

**Probe.** A small instrument for examining wounds. प्रोब; एषणी; घावों की जांच में काम आने वाला एक छोटा-सा यंत्र

**Procedure.** Method; technique. पद्धति; रीति; नियम; तरीका; तकनीक

**Process.** A method; phenomena, प्रक्रम; प्रक्रिया; a prolongation or prominence of a part. प्रवर्ध;

**Acromial P.,** see **Acromion Process.**

**Acromion P.,** the process at the summit of the scapula; acromial process. अंसकूट प्रवर्ध;

**Ciliary P.,** circularly arranged choroidal foldings continuous with the iris in front; processus ciliaris. रोमक प्रवर्ध;

**Infundibular P.,** see **Infundibuliform Process.**

**Infundibuliform P.,** the cremasteric process of the transversalis fascia; infundibular process. कीपाकार प्रवर्ध;

**Jugular P.,** a process of the occiput behind the jugular foramen. ग्रीवा प्रवर्ध;

**Lacrimal P.,** one of the inferior turbinated bones articulating with the lacrimal bone. अश्रु प्रवर्ध;

**Mammilary P.,** the tubercle on each superior articular process of a lumbar vertebra. चूचुक प्रवर्ध;

**Mastoid P.,** a conic projection at the base of the mastoid portion of the temporal bone. कर्णमूल प्रवर्ध;

**Maxillary P.,** a thin plate of bone descending from the ethmoid process; processus maxillaris. ऊर्ध्वहनु प्रवर्ध;

**Nasal P.,** a thick, triangular process forming part of the lateral wall of the nose; processus nasalis. नासा प्रवर्ध;

**Odontoid P.,** that of the axis which articulates with the atlas. दन्ताभ प्रवर्ध;

**Olecranon P.,** the olecranon. कूर्पर प्रवर्ध;

**Pterygoid P.,** one from the palate bone and one from the sphenoid bone; processus pterygoideus. पक्षाभ प्रवर्ध;

**Sphenoidal P.,** a thin plate, directed upward and inward from the vertical plate of the palate bone. जतूक प्रवर्ध;

**Spinous P.**, the backward projection from the middle of the posterior part of the arch of a vertebra; processus spinosus. कशेरुकाकण्टक प्रवर्ध;

**Transverse P.**, a process projecting outward from each side of a vertebra; processus transversalis. अनुप्रस्थ प्रवर्ध;

**Vocal P.**, the anterior angle of the arytenoid cartilage. स्वर प्रवर्ध;

**Xiphoid P.**, the ensiform cartilage; processus xiphoideus. उरोस्थि प्रवर्ध

**Processus.** Process. प्रवर्ध; प्रक्रिया; प्रक्रम;

**P. Ciliaris**, see **Ciliary Process.**

**P. Cochleariformis**, a bony plate separating the canal for the Eustachian tube from the tensor tympani muscle. कर्णावर्तरूपी प्रवर्ध;

**P. Maxillaris**, see **Maxillary Process.**

**P. Nasalis**, see **Nasal Process.**

**P. Pterygoideus**, see **Pterygoid Process.**

**P. Spinosus**, see **Spinous Process.**

**P. Transversalis**, see **Transverse Process.**

**P. Xiphoideus**, see **Xiphoid Process.**

**Procidentia.** Complete prolapsus of the uterus; bearing down of the womb or the lower bowels. पूर्णजरायुभ्रंश; गर्भाशयपूर्णभ्रंश; जरायुभ्रंश; गर्भाशयच्युति; गर्भाशय अथवा निचली आंतों का अपने स्थान से हट जाना

**Procreate.** To beget; to produce by the sexual act. जन्मदेना; जनना; पैदा करना

**Procreation.** Reproduction. प्रजनन; जनन

**Procreative.** Having the power to procreate or beget. जननक्षम; प्रजननक्षम

**Proctagra.** Pain in the anus or rectum. मलद्वार अथवा मलाशय का दर्द

**Proctalgia.** The presence of pain in the anal or the rectal region. गुदार्ति; मलांत्रशूल

**Proctectasia.** Dilatation of anus or rectum. गुदाविस्फार या मलांत्रविस्फार

**Proctectomy.** Excision of the rectum. मलांत्र-उच्छेदन; मलांत्र को काट कर हटा देना

**Proctitis.** A catarrhal inflammation of the rectum; rectitis. मलाशयशोथ; मलांत्र-प्रदाह; मलांत्रशोथ;

**Granular P.**, acute inflammation of the rectum. कणिका मलांत्रशोथ; मलांत्र का उग्र प्रदाह

**Proctocolectomy.** Surgical excision of the rectum and the colon. मलांत्रबृहदांत्र-उच्छेदन; मलांत्र एवं बृहदांत्र को काट कर हटा देना

**Proctocolitis.** Inflammation of the rectum and the colon. मलांत्रबृहदांत्रशोथ; मलांत्र एवं बृहदांत्र का प्रदाह

**Proctodaeum.** See **Proctodeum**.

**Proctodea.** Plural of **Proctodeum**.

**Proctodeum.** The primitive anus; proctodaeum. आद्यगुद; आद्यगुहा; पश्चांत्र

**Proctodynia.** Pain in the anus or rectum; proctalgia. मलद्वार अथवा मलांत्र का दर्द

**Proctologic.** Relating to proctology. गुदारोगविज्ञान सम्बन्धी

**Proctology.** The medical specialty concerned with the anus and rectum and their diseases. गुदारोगविज्ञान

**Proctoparalysis.** Paralysis of the anus. गुदाघात; मलद्वार का पक्षाघात

**Proctopexy.** Surgical fixation of a prolapsing rectum; rectopexy. गुदास्थिरीकरण; मलाशयस्थिरीकरण

**Proctoplasty.** Reparative or plastic surgery of the anus, or of the rectum; rectoplasty. गुदासंधान; मलांत्रसंधान

**Proctoptosia.** Prolapse of the rectum and anus; proctoptosis. मलांत्रगुदाभ्रंश; मलाशय तथा मलद्वार की स्थानच्युति

**Proctoptosis.** See **Proctoptosia**.

**Proctoscope.** An instrument for examining the rectum. मलाशयदर्शी; मलाशय की जांच करने के लिये प्रयुक्त किया जाने वाला उपकरण

**Proctoscopy.** Ocular inspection of the rectum. मलाशयदर्शन; मलांत्र की प्रत्यक्ष जांच करना

**Proctosigmoiditis.** Inflammation of the rectum and the sigmoid colon. मलांत्र-अवग्रहांत्रशोथ; मलाशय-अवग्रहांत्रशोथ

**Proctosigmoidoscope.** An instrument for examining the rectum and sigmoid colon. मलाशय-अवग्रहांत्रदर्शी; मलांत्र एवं अवग्रहांत्र की जांच के लिये प्रयुक्त किया जाने वाला यंत्र

**Proctosigmoidoscopy.** Direct inspection through a sigmoidoscope of the rectum and sigmoid colon. मलाशय-अवग्रहांत्रदर्शन

**Proctotomy.** Incision of the rectum. मलांत्रछेदन

**Prodromal.** Premonitory; indicating the approach of a disease;

prodromic. प्रारम्भिक; प्राथमिक; पूर्ववर्ती; पूर्वरूप; पूर्वरूपी; प्राक्रूपी

**Prodrome.** A forerunner or sign of disease. प्राथमिक अथवा प्रारम्भिक लक्षण

**Prodromic.** See **Prodromal.**

**Product.** Something produced. उत्पाद; उपज; पदार्थ; गुणनफल

**Productive.** Generating. उत्पादक; उत्पादनकारी; उर्वर

**Proerythroblast.** Pronormoblast; the earliest cells that show differentiation in the direction of erythrocyte formation. प्राक्लाहितकोशिकाप्रसू

**Profunda.** Deep-seated; profundus. गभीर; गहन; गहरा

**Profundus.** See **Profunda.**

**Profuse.** Excessive. विपुल; प्रचुर; अत्यधिक

**Progeny.** Offspring; descendents. संतति; संतान; फल; परिणाम

**Progeria.** A combining infantilism and senility. कालपूर्वजरा; शिशुता एवं बृद्धावस्था का मिश्रित रूप; समय से पहले ही बुढ़ापा आ जाना

**Progestational.** Before or favouring pregnancy. गर्भपूर्व

**Proglossis.** Tip of the tongue. जिह्वानोक; जीभ की चोंच

**Prognathic.** See **Prognathus.**

**Prognathism.** The state of being prognathus. उद्गतहनुता; उद्गति

**Prognathous.** See **Prognathus.**

**Prognathus.** Having projecting jaws; prognathic; prognathous. उद्गतहनु

**Prognosis.** A forecast as to the probable result of an attack of a disease. पूर्वानुमान; प्राग्ज्ञान; फलानुमान; भावीफल

**Prognostic.** Relating to, or concerning with prognosis. अग्रसूचक; पूर्वचिन्हात्मक

**Progressive.** Going forward. प्रगामी; वर्धमान;

   **P. Locomotor Ataxia,** inability to walk steadily. प्रगामीचलन-अक्षमता; सीधे चलने की अयोग्यता

**Projection.** A pushing out बहिर्वेशन; a prominence. उत्सेध; the act of throwing forward. प्रक्षेपण; प्रक्षेप

**Prolactin.** Hormone secreted in the anterior pituitary gland. It acts only on the pregnant woman's breasts preparing them for milk production. स्तनप्रेरक; स्तनजनक; प्रोलैक्टिन

**Prolapse.** To fall or sink down. भ्रंश; स्थानच्युति; च्युति;

**Prolapse**

**Anal P.**, falling down of the anus; prolapsus ani. गुदाभ्रंश; मलद्वार की स्थानच्युति;

**Rectal P.**, falling down of the rectum; prolapsus recti. मलाशयभ्रंश; मलांत्र की स्थानच्युति;

**Uterine P.**, displacement or falling down of the uterus; prolapsus uteri. जरायुभ्रंश; गर्भाशय की स्थानच्युति;

**Vaginal P.**, protrusion of the upper part of the vagina into the lower; prolapsus vaginae. योनिभ्रंश; योनि की स्थानच्युति

**Prolapsus.** Falling down, as of a womb, anus or rectum; prolapse. भ्रंश; स्थानच्युति;

**P. Ani**, see **Anal Prolapse**.

**P. Recti**, see **Rectal Prolapse**.

**P. Uteri**, see **Uterine Prolapse**.

**P. Vaginae**, see **Vaginal Prolapse**.

**Proliferate.** Increase by cell division. प्रफलन करना; आत्मपुनर्जनन करना

**Proliferation.** The production of similar form, especially of cells and morbid cysts. प्रफलन; प्रोद्भवन; प्रचुरोद्भवन

**Proliferative.** See **Proliferous**.

**Proliferous.** Bearing many youngs; proliferative. प्रफली; प्रफलनशील; बहुजनक; अबन्ध्य

**Prolific.** Fruitful; productive; multiplying abundantly. बहुप्रज; अबन्ध्य; प्रजननशील

**Prominence.** An elevation. उत्सेध

**Promontory.** A projection, prominence or elevation. प्रोतुंग; उत्सेध

**Pronation.** Turning the ventral surface downward. अवतानन; अलिन्दतल का नीचे को मुड़ना

**Pronator.** That which pronates. अवताननक

**Prone.** Face downwards. अधोमुखस्थिति; नीचे की ओर झुका हुआ मुख; inclined to. प्रवण; प्रवृत्त

**Pronephron.** See **Pronephros**.

**Pronephros.** The premordial kidney; pronephron. आद्यपूर्ववृक्क

**Pronormoblast.** See **Proerythroblast**.

**Prootic.** In front of the ear. पुरःकर्ण

**Prophase.** Anaphase. पूर्वावस्था

**Prophylactics.** Agents designed to ward off a possible invasion of disease. रोगनिरोधी; प्रतिषेधक; रोगहारी; रोगनिरोधक; रोग के सम्भावित आक्रमण को रोकने वाले पदार्थ

**Prophylaxes.** Plural of **Prophylaxis.**

**Prophylaxis.** The preventive treatment or medicine. रोगनिरोध; रोगरोधन; अनागत व्याधि चिकित्सा; रोगरोधक चिकित्सा

**Proprietary Name.** The patented brand name or trade mark. एकायत्त नाम अथवा ट्रेड मार्क (व्यापार चिन्ह)

**Proprioceptive.** Capable of receiving stimuli originating in muscles, tendons and other internal tissues. प्रग्राही; ऊतकसम्वेदी

**Proprioceptor.** One of the varieties of sensory end organs in muscles, tendons and joint capsules. प्रग्राहक

**Proptosis.** Forward protrusion, especially of an eyeball. नेत्रोत्सेध; नेत्रगोलक का आगे की ओर फैलना

**Proptotic.** Referring to proptosis. नेत्रोत्सेधी

**Propulsion.** The leaning forward of the body, as if pushed. प्रणोदन; नोदन

**Pro-re-nata.** According to circumstances. Abbreviation: **P.R.N.** आवश्यकतानुसार; समयानुसार; परिस्थितियों के अनुसार

**Prosencephalon.** The forebrain; the fore-part of the anterior primary vesicle. अग्रमस्तिष्क; मस्तिष्क का अगला भाग

**Prosopalgia.** Neuralgia of the face; prosoponeuralgia. आननशूल; ललाटशूल; चेहरे की तंत्रिकाओं का दर्द

**Prosopalgic.** Relating to prosopalgia. आननशूल सम्बन्धी

**Prosopectasia.** Enlargement of the face. आननबृद्धि

**Prosoponeuralgia.** See **Prosopalgia.**

**Prosopoplegia.** Facial paralysis. आननघात; चेहरे का पक्षाघात

**Prosopoplegic.** Relating to facial paralysis. आननघात सम्बन्धी

**Prosospasm.** Involuntary twitching of the facial muscles; facial tic. आननपेशी-उद्वेष्ट

**Prostata.** See **Prostate Gland.**

**Prostatalgia.** Pain in the prostate gland; prostatodynia. पुरःस्थग्रन्थिशूल; पुरःस्थग्रन्थि की पीड़ा

**Prostate.** See **Prostate Gland.**

**P. Gland,** the gland which surrounds the bladder opening in the male; prostata; prostate. पुरःस्थग्रन्थि; पौरुष-ग्रन्थि

**Prostatectomy**

**Prostatectomy.** Surgical removal of the prostate gland. पुर:स्थग्रन्थिउच्छेदन; पुर:स्यग्रंथ्युच्छेदन; पुर:स्योच्छेदन; पुर:स्थग्रन्थि को काट कर हटाना

**Prostatic.** Relating to the prostate gland. पुर:स्थग्रन्थिक; पुर:स्थग्रन्थि सम्बन्धी;

**P. Fluid,** the fluid secreted by the prostate gland. पुर:स्थद्रव; पुर:स्थग्रन्थि द्वारा नि:स्रावित द्रव्य

**Prostatitis.** Inflammation of the prostate gland. पुर:स्थशोथ; पुर:स्थग्रन्थिशोथ; शिश्नग्रन्थिशोथ; पुर:स्थग्रन्थि का प्रदाह

**Prostatocystitis.** Inflammation of the prostate and the bladder. पुर:स्थग्रंथिमूत्राशयशोथ

**Prostatodynia.** See **Prostatalgia.**

**Prostatolith.** A prostatic calculus; a concretion formed in the prostate gland. पुर:स्थग्रन्थि-अश्मरी

**Prostatolithotomy.** Incision of the prostate for removal of a calculus. पुर:स्थग्रन्थि-अश्मरी-उच्छेदन

**Prostatomegaly.** Enlargement of the prostate gland. पुर:स्थग्रन्थिबृद्धि

**Prostatorrhea.** See **Prostatorrhoea.**

**Prostatorrhoea.** A thin, gleety urethral discharge from the prostate gland; prostatorrhea. पुर:स्यातिस्राव; पुर:स्थग्रन्थि से पतला प्रमेहज स्राव होना

**Prostheses.** Plural of **Prosthesis.**

**Prosthesis.** An artificial substitute for a missing part. कृत्रिम-अंग; नकली अंग

**Prosthetic.** Relating to a prosthesis or an artificial part. कृत्रिम-अंग सम्बन्धी

**Prosthetics.** The branch of surgery which deals with prostheses. कृत्रिम-अंगविज्ञान; शल्यविज्ञान की कृत्रिम-अंगों सम्बन्धी शाखा

**Prothetist.** One skilled in constructing and fitting prostheses. कृत्रिमांगविज्ञानी

**Prostitution.** Indiscriminate sexual intercourse. वेश्यावृत्ति; गणिकावृत्ति; लैंगिक व्यभिचार; अवैध संगम करना

**Prostration.** Extreme nervous exhaustion. अवसाद; अवसन्नता

**Protanomalopia.** See **Protanopia.**

**Protanomalopsia.** See **Protanopia.**

**Protanopia.** A defect in a first constituent, essential for colour vision, as in red blindness; protanomalopia; protanomalopsia. लालवर्णान्धता; लाल रंग पहचानने की अयोग्यता

**Protective.** An antiseptic dressing. संरक्षी; रक्षात्मक; कोई पूतिरोधक पट्टी

**Protein.** A food substance based on compounds of nitrogen essential for body growth and maintenance, found mainly in the meats, fish, eggs, poultry, cheese and the leguminous vegetables. प्रोटीन; मांसजातीय खाद्य पदार्थ

**Proteinuria.** Protein in the urine. प्रोटीनमेह; पेशाब में प्रोटीन जाना; albuminuria. अन्नसारमेह

**Proteolysis.** The breaking down of proteins into simpler substances. प्रोटीनलयन; प्रोटीन-अपघटन

**Proteometabolism.** Protein metabolism. प्रोटीन-चयापचय

**Protodiastolic.** Early diastolic; relating to the beginning of cardiac diastole. आद्यानुशिथिलन

**Protopathic.** The term applied to a less sensibility, as opposed to epicritic. स्थूलस्पर्शसंवेदी; अल्पसंवेदी; स्थूलस्पर्शी

**Protoplasm.** The living matter of cells and tissues. जीवद्रव्य; कोशिकाओं तथा ऊतकों का सजीव पदार्थ

**Protoplasmic.** Relating to the protoplasm. जीवद्रव्यीय; जीवद्रव्य सम्बन्धी

**Prototype.** An original type or model. प्राग्रूप; आदिरूप; मूलरूप

**Protozoa.** A class of unicellular animal organism. प्रजीवाणु; शुक्राणु; बीजाणु

**Protozoal.** Relating to protozoa. प्रजीवाणुक; जीवाणुओं अथवा शुक्राणुओं सम्बन्धी

**Protozoon.** Singular of **Protozoa.**

**Protractor.** A surgical instrument. प्रसारक; प्रोट्रैक्टर; एक शल्योपकरण; **P. Muscle,** a muscle drawing forward. प्रसारक पेशी

**Protrude.** Thrust forward; to cause to project. फैलना; फैलाना; उभरना; उभारना; बहि:सरण होना; उद्वर्तन होना

**Protrusion.** Thrust or projecting forward or outward. उद्वर्तन; बहि:सरण; उत्क्रमण; फैलाव

**Protuberance.** A swelling, projection or tumour of the body; protuberantia. प्रोद्वर्ध; शोथ; स्फीति; गिल्टी; उभार; फुलाव; सूजन

**Protuberantia.** See **Protuberance.**

**Proud Flesh.** Excessive granulation. अतिकणांकुरण

**Proving.** A homoeopathic test for the effect of a drug. प्रमाणीकरण; सिद्धीकरण

**Provocative.** An agent which excites appetite or passion. प्रोत्तेजक; उत्तेजक; प्रेरक

**Proximal.** See **Proximate.**

**Proximate.** Nearest; next in order; proximal. सन्निकट; निकटस्थ; समीपस्थ

**Prurigo.** A chronic papular skin disease with intense itching. कण्डूपिटिक; त्वचा पर तेज खाज मारते छोटे-छोटे दाने

**Pruritic.** Pertaining to the pruritus. प्रखर खाज अथवा प्रचण्ड खुजली सम्बन्धी

**Pruritus.** Intense itching. कण्डू; प्रखर खाज; प्रचण्ड खुजली;

   **Senile P.,** see **Pruritus Senilis.**

   **P. Ani,** itching of the anus. गुदकण्डू; मलद्वार की खुजली;

   **P. Senilis,** itching associated with degenerative changes in the skin of the aged; senile pruritus. जरा कण्डू; बुढ़ापे में होने वाली प्रचण्ड खुजली;

   **P. Vulvae,** itching of the vulva. भगकण्डू; योनिद्वार की खुजली

**Pseud-.** See **Pseudo-.**

**Pseudarthrosis.** See **Pseudoarthrosis.**

**Pseudo-, Pseud-.** Prefixes meaning false. 'कूट' अथवा 'मिथ्या' के रूप में प्रयुक्त उपसर्ग

**Pseudoamenorrhoea.** False amenorrhoea. कूट-अनार्तव; प्रच्छन्नार्तव; प्रच्छन्न ऋतुस्राव

**Pseudoanaemia.** False anaemia. कूट-अरक्तता

**Pseudoankylosis.** False ankylosis. कूटसन्धिग्रह

**Pseudoangina.** False angina. कूटहृद्शूल

**Pseudoarthrosis.** A false joint, due to an ununited fracture; pseudarthrosis. कूटसन्धि; आभासी सन्धि

**Pseudocartilage.** False cartilage. कूट-उपास्थि

**Pseudocast.** False cast. कूटनिर्मोक

**Pseudochorea.** A spasmodic affection resembling chorea. कूटलास्य

**Pseudocoxalgia.** False pain in the hip. कूटनितम्बार्ति; कूल्हे में क्षणिक पीड़ा

**Pseudocrisis.** A rapid reduction of body temperature resembling a crisis, followed by fever. कूट-संकट

**Pseudocyesis.** The existence of the signs and symptoms of pregnancy in a woman who believes that she is pregnant, when, in fact, this is not so; phantom pregnancy; false pregnancy. कूट-सगर्भता; गर्भाभास; मिथ्यागर्भ

**Pseudocyst.** False or adventitious cyst. कूटपुटी; कूटकोशिका

**Pseudodiphtheria.** False diphtheria. कूट-रोहिणी; कूट-डिप्थेरिया

**Pseudodiphtheritic.** Pertaining to false diphtheria. कूट-रोहिणिक; कूट-रोहिणी सम्बन्धी

**Pseudofracture.** A condition in which an x-ray shows formation of new bone with thickening of periosteum at the site of injury to bone. कूट-अस्थिभंग

**Pseudohematuria.** False hematuria. कूट-रक्तमेह

**Pseudohermophrodite.** A person in whom the gonads of one sex are present, while the external genitalia comprise those of the opposite sex. कूट-उभयलिंगी

**Pseudohermaphroditism.** Spurious hermaphroditism. कूट-उभयलिंगिता

**Pseudohypertrophic.** Giving a false appearance of enlargement. कूट-अतिबृद्धिक

**Pseudohypertrophy.** Increase in size of a part due to overgrowth of an unimportant tissue. कूट-अतिबृद्धि

**Pseudoicterus.** Discolouration of the skin not due to bile pigment; pseudojaundice. कूटकामला

**Pseudojaundice.** See **Pseudoicterus.**

**Pseudoleukemia.** Hodgkin's disease; a disease resulting in chronic anaemia or more properly anaemic cachexia, associated with the blood changes, symptoms of the spleen and other glandular tissues and organs, especially the lymphatic glands. कूटश्वेतरक्तता; कूटअतिश्वेतकोशिकारक्तता

**Pseudologia.** False speech. कूटभाषण; मिथ्याभाषण;
  P. Phantastica, a constitutional tendency to tell and defend fantastic lies plausibly. विकारी मिथ्याभाषण

**Pseudomania.** Feigned insanity. कूट-उन्माद; कूट-विक्षिप्ति

**Pseudomembrane.** A false membrane. कूटकला; अयथार्थ झिल्ली

**Pseudomucin.** A gelatinous substance (not mucin) found in some ovarian cysts. कूटश्लेष्मरस; डिम्ब-पुटियों में पाया जाने वाला एक चिपचिपा पदार्थ

**Pseudoparalysis.** False paralysis. कूट-अंगघात

**Pseudoparesis.** A condition marked by the papillary changes, tremors and speech disturbances. कूट-आंशिकघात

**Pseudoparkinsonism.** The signs and symptoms of paralysis agitans when they are not postencephalitic. कूटसकम्प-अंगघात

**Pseudoparturition.** False labour. कूटप्रसव; मिथ्याप्रसव

**Pseudoplegia.** False paralysis. कूट-अंगघात

**Pseudopodia.** False legs. कूटपाद

**Pseudopsora.** False psora. कूटकच्छु

**Pseudosycosis.** False sycosis. कूटप्रमेह

**Pseudosyphilis.** False syphilis. कूट-उपदंश

**Pseudotuberculosis.** A condition simulating tuberculosis. कूटयक्ष्मा

**Psilosis.** Depilation. केशोन्मूलन; thrush. मुखव्रण

**Psittacosis.** Parrot fever. शुकरोग; शुकज्वर; an infectious disease of birds. पक्षियों को होने वाला एक संक्रामक रोग

**Psoas.** One of the two muscles of the loins. कटि; नितम्ब; कूल्हा; कमर;
   P. Abscess, lumbar abscess. कटि-विद्रधि; कमर का फोड़ा
   P. Muscle, the muscle of the loin. कटिलम्बिनी; नितम्ब-पेशी

**Psoasitis.** Inflammation of the muscles of the back or lumbar region. नितम्बपेशीशोथ; नितम्बपेशी का प्रदाह

**Psora.** Itch; scabies; one of the three Hahnemann's chronic miasms called psora, syphilis and sycosis. कच्छु; कच्छुविष; खाजरोग; खुजली

**Psoriasis.** A chronic disfiguring disease of the skin in which erythromatous areas are covered with adherent scales. विचर्चिका; अपरस

**Psoric.** Affected with psora. कच्छुविषग्रस्त; खाजरोग से पीड़ित; relating to psora. कच्छुविषज; कच्छुविष सम्बन्धी

**Psoritic.** Pertaining to psoriasis. विचर्चिका अथवा अपरस सम्बन्धी

**Psychasthenia.** Mental fatigue. मनोवसाद; मनोदौर्बल्य; मानसिक थकान

**Psychiatrics.** See **Psychiatry.**

**Psychiatrist.** A doctor of medicine with advance training and experience in the diseases of mind and disturbances in the emotions. मनोरोगचिकित्सक; मनोरोगविज्ञानी

**Psychiatry.** The medical specialty concerned with the diseases of mind and problems of emotional character; psychiatrics. मनोरोगविज्ञान; मनोविकारविज्ञान; मनोविकारिकी

**Psychic.** Of the mind. मानसिक; दिमागी; any sensitive person. संवेदनशील व्यक्ति

**Psychical.** Concerned with soul or mind. मानसिक; मनोविषयक; मनोपरक

**Psychoanalysis.** A division of psychiatry that involves prolonged exploration of the patient's personality. मनोविश्लेषण; मनोगहन

**Psychoanalyst.** A psychotherapist or psychiatrist, trained in psychoanalysis and applying its methods in the treatment of emotional disorders; psychotherapist. मनोविश्लेषक

**Psychoanalytic.** Pertaining to psychoanalysis. मनोविश्लेषण सम्बन्धी

**Psychodynamics.** The science of the mental processes, especially of the causative factors in mental activity. मनोविज्ञान

**Psychogenesis.** The development of the mind. मनोविकास

**Psychogenic.** Arising from the mind. मनोजात; मानसिक; आधिज

**Psychologic.** See **Psychological.**

**Psychological.** Pertaining to psychology; psychologic. मनोवैज्ञानिक; मनोविज्ञान सम्बन्धी

**Psychologist.** A person, not a physician, who has been trained in the study of human behaviour and psychology. मनोविज्ञानी; मनोमितिज्ञ

**Psychology.** The study of the behaviour of an organism in its environment. मनोविज्ञान; मानसिकी

**Psychometrics.** See **Psychometry.**

**Psychometric.** Measurement of the duration and force of mental processes. मनोमितिक

**Psychometry.** The measurement of the time required for cerebration; psychometrics. मनोमिति

**Psychomotor.** Causing movement by the will; motor effect of psychic or cerebral activity. मन:प्रेरक; मनोप्रेरक; मन को प्रेरित करने वाला

**Psychoneurosis.** Mental neurosis. मनस्तंत्रिकाविक्षिप्ति; मनोविक्षिप्ति

**Psychoneurotic.** Insane; of unsound mind. विक्षिप्त; पागल; relating to psychoneurosis. मनोविक्षिप्ति सम्बन्धी

**Psychopath.** One who is morally irresponsible. मनोविकृत; विकृतमनस्क

**Psychopathia.** See **Psychopathy.**

**Psychopathology.** The pathology of abnormal mental processes. मनोविकृति; अस्वाभाविक मानसिक क्रियाओं सम्बन्धी विज्ञान

**Psychopathy** 840

मनोविकृति; अस्वाभाविक मानसिक क्रियाओं सम्बन्धी विज्ञान
**Psychopathy.** Any disease of the mind; psychopathia. मनोविकार; मनोरोग; पागलपन; कोई मानसिक रोग

**Psychophysics.** A branch of experimental psychology dealing with the study of stimuli and sensation. मनोभौतिकी

**Psychoses.** Plural of **Psychosis.**

**Psychosis.** A specific mental illness arising in the mind itself, as opposed to neurosis. मनोविक्षिप्ति; पागलपन

**Psychosomatic.** A term describing a disease in which the mental or emotional influences produce or aggravate physical changes. मन:कायिक; मन:शारीरिक

**Psychosurgery.** The treatment of mental disorders by operation upon the brain, e.g. lobotomy. मन:शल्यचिकित्सा

**Psychotherapist.** See **Psychoanalyst.**

**Psychotherapy.** Treatment aimed at helping the patient solve his psychic and emotional problems. मनोरोगचिकित्सा; मनोरोगोपचार

**Psychotic.** Affected with, or relating to mental disorder. मनोविक्षिप्त; मनोविकारी अथवा मनोविकार सम्बन्धी

**Pterion.** The point of junction of sphenoid, frontal, temporal and parietal bones. पक्षकबिन्दु

**Pterygium.** A triangular thickening of bulbar conjunctiva extending from inner canthus toward the cornea. प्रस्तारी-अर्म; कन्दी नेत्रश्लेष्मला की त्रिकोणक स्थूलता

**Pterygoid.** Resembling a wing; wing-shaped. पक्षाभ; पंख जैसा

**Pterygomaxillary.** Pertaining to the maxilla and pterygoid process. पक्षाभऊर्ध्वहनुज

**Pterygopalatine.** Pertaining to the pterygoid process and the palate bone. पक्षाभतालुज

**Pthisis.** See **Phthisis.**

**Ptilosis.** Falling off of the eyelashes. वर्त्मरोमपात; पलकों के केश गिरना

**Ptomaine.** The food. खाद्य; भोजन; आहार;
  **P. Poisoning,** food poisoning. खाद्य-विषण्णता; खाद्य-विषाक्तता

**Ptoses.** Plural of **Ptosis.**

**Ptosis.** A drooping of the upper eyelids from paralysis; blepharoplegia; blepharoptosis. वर्त्मपात; पलकों का पक्षाघात; ऊपर की पलकों का गिरना

**Ptotic.** Pertaining to ptosis. वर्त्मपाती; पलकें गिरने सम्बन्धी

**Ptyalagogue.** Sialagogue. लालावर्धक; लारवर्धक

**Ptyalectasis.** Sialectasis. लालावाहिकास्फीति

**Ptyalin.** An amylolytic ferment of saliva. लाला; लार

**Ptyalism.** Excessive secretion of saliva. अतिलालास्रा<sub>i</sub>ग्ता; अतिलारमयता

**Ptyalolith.** Salivary calculus. लालाश्मरी; लारपथरी

**Puberal.** Pertaining to puberty. यौवनपरक; तारुणीय; यौवनावस्था सम्बन्धी

**Pubertas Praecox.** Sexual precocity; premature sexual development. कालपूर्वयौन

**Puberty.** The period of life in which young people of both sexes are fit to marry and to procreate; pubescence. यौवनारम्भ; तारुण्यगमन; वयस्कता

**Pubes.** Plural of **Pubis.**

**Pubescence.** See **Puberty.**

**Pubescent.** Concerning pubescence. रोमिल

**Pubic.** Relating to the pubes. पुरोनितम्बीय; जघन अथवा शिश्नरोम सम्बन्धी; **P. Bone,** os pubis. जघनास्थि; जांघ की हड्डी

**Pubiotomy.** Cutting the pubic bone to facilitate delivery of live child; pelviotomy. जघनछेदन; गोणिकोच्छेदन

**Pubis.** The mons veneris; the hairy region covering the pubic bone. जघनरोम; जांघ के बाल; शिश्नरोम

**Pubofemoral.** Pertaining to the os pubis and femur. जघन एवं ऊरु सम्बन्धी

**Puboprostatic.** Pertaining to the pubis and prostate. जघन एवं पुर:स्थ सम्बन्धी

**Pubovesical.** Pertaining to the pubis and bladder. जघन एवं वस्ति सम्बन्धी

**Pudenda.** Plural of **Pudendum.**

**Pudendal.** Relating to the pudendum; pudic. बाह्यजननांग सम्बन्धी; बाह्यजननांगी

**Pudendum.** The femal external genital. गुह्य; बाह्यजननांग

**Pudic.** See **Pudendal.**

**Puerile.** Pertaining to the childhood. बालपन; बाल्यावस्था; बाल्यकालीन; बचपन सम्बन्धी

**Puerpera.** A parturient woman, who is giving or has recently given birth to a child. सूतिका; प्रसूता

**Puerperal.** Belonging to, or following childbirth. प्रसूतिक; प्रसवोत्तर; प्रसूति सम्बन्धी

**Puerperia.** Plural of **Puerperium.**

**Puerperium.** The puerperal state. प्रसूतिकाल; सूतिकावस्था; प्रसवोत्तरकाल

**Pulex.** A genus of fleas that infests man and many animals. पिस्सू

**Pulicide.** A chemical agent destructive to fleas. पिस्सूनाशी

**Pulmo.** The lung; pulmon; pulmonis. फुप्फुस; फेफड़ा

**Pulmoflator.** Apparatus for inflation of lungs. फुप्फुसविस्फारक; फेफड़े फैलाने वाला उपकरण

**Pulmon.** See **Pulmo.**

**Pulmonary.** Pertaining to the lungs; pulmonic; pneumonic. फुप्फुसीय; फुप्फुसी; फेफड़ों सम्बन्धी

**Pulmonic.** See **Pulmonary.**

**Pulmonis.** See **Pulmo.**

**Pulmonitis.** Inflammation of the lung. फुप्फुसशोथ; फेफड़े का प्रदाह

**Pulp.** The soft matter of certain organs. मज्जा; दन्तमज्जा; the soft part of a fruit. गूदा;

  **Dental P.**, found in the cavity of the teeth. दन्तमज्जा; दन्तगह्वरों में पाया जाने वाला गूदा;

  **Digital P.**, elastic, soft prominence on the palmar or plantar surface of the last phalanx of a finger or toe. अंगुलिमज्जा

**Pulpa.** Pulp. मज्जा; गूदा;

  **P. Dentalis**, the dental pulp; pulpa dentis. दन्तमज्जा; दन्तगह्वरों में पाया जाने वाला गूदा;

  **P. Dentis**, see **Pulpa Dentalis.**

**Pulpal.** Relating to the pulp. मज्जा अथवा गूदा सम्बन्धी

**Pulpectomy.** Removal of the entire pulp structure of a tooth. दन्तमज्जा-उच्छेदन

**Pulpitis.** Inflammation of the dental pulp. दन्तमज्जाशोथ; दन्तमज्जा का प्रदाह

**Pulpotomy.** Pulp amputation. मज्जा-उच्छेदन

**Pulpy.** Resembling a pulp; pultaceous. मज्जावत्; मज्जाभ; गूदा जैसा

**Pulsatile.** Beating; throbbing; pulsating. स्पन्दनशील; स्पन्दनमान; स्पन्दी

**Pulsating.** See **Pulsatile.**

**Pulsation.** Throbbing or beating, as of the pulse or heart. स्पन्दन; धड़कन

**Pulse.** The beat or throbbing of the heart and arteries, usually felt at the wrist above the ball of the thumb; pulsus. नाड़ी; नब्ज; नाड़ीस्पन्द;

**Anacrotic P.,** one of the sygmographic tracing which is marked by notches in the ascending limb; anadicrotic pulse. उत्स्पन्दी नाड़ी;

**Anadicrotic P.,** see **Anacrotic Pulse.**

**Bounding P.,** one of the large volume and force. उत्प्लावी नाड़ी;

**Capillary P.,** an intermittent filling and emptying of the skin-capillaries. केशिकास्पन्द;

**Catacrotic P.,** a pulse that is repeated in the line of descent once or thrice. विषमावरोही नाड़ी;

**Collapsing P.,** pulse feebly striking the finger, then subsiding abruptly and completely. अवसादी नाड़ी; निपाती नाड़ी;

**Dicrotic P.,** one with excessive recoil wave. द्विस्पन्दी नाड़ी;

**Intermittent P.,** one in which one or more beats are dropped. सविरामी नाड़ी;

**Irregular P.,** one in which the beats occur at irregular intervals. अनियमित नाड़ी;

**Thready P.,** a weak, usually rapid and scarcely perceptible pulse. क्षीण नाड़ी;

**Venous P.,** one that occurs in vein. शिरास्पन्द; शिरानाड़ी;

**P. Rate,** the number of pulsations in an artery in a minute. नाड़ी दर

**Pulsus.** A pulse. नाड़ी; नब्ज

**Pultaceous.** See **Pulpy.**

**Pulver.** A powder; pulveratum. चूर्ण; विचूर्ण

**Pulveratum.** See **Pulver.**

**Pulverisable.** Capable of being converted into powder. चूर्णनीय; विचूर्णनीय; चूर्ण में बदलने योग्य

**Pulverisation.** The act of reducing to a powder; pulverization. चूर्णन; विचूर्णन; संपेषण; पीसना; भुरभुरा करना

**Pulverization.** See **Pulverisation.**

**Pulvinar.** Posterior eminence of the optic thalamus. चेतकपश्चान्त

**Pulvis.** A powder. चूर्ण; विचूर्ण

**Pump.** An apparatus for drawing liquids from a reservoir. पम्प; उदंचिका; पिचकारी;

# Pump

**Breast P.,** a suction instrument for withdrawing milk from the breast. स्तन-उदंचिका; ब्रेस्ट-पम्प; स्तन-पम्प;

**Stomach P.,** an apparatus for removing the contents of the stomach by suction. आमाशय-उदंचिका; स्टोमक-पम्प; आमाशय-पम्प

**Puncta.** Plural of **Punctum.**

**Punctata.** Dotted or spotted; punctate. बिन्दुकित; कर्बुरित;

**P. Lachrymalis,** the orifice or the lachrymal canals of the eye. अश्रुद्वार; अश्रुनलीमुख

**Punctate.** See **Punctata.**

**Punctum.** A point; a minute spot. बिन्दु; रन्ध्रक; धब्बा;

**P. Lacrimale,** minute orifices of the lacrimal canals upon the eyelids near the inner canthus. अश्रुरन्ध्रक;

**P. Proximum,** the point nearest the eye at which an object can be seen distinctly. निकट बिन्दु;

**P. Remotum,** the farthest point at which an object can be distinctly seen with the eye in repose. दूर-बिन्दु

**Puncture.** A perforated wound made with a sharp, fine instrument. वेध; वेधन; छिद्र; छिद्रण; भेदन; to make a whole with a small, sharp pointed object. बारीक छेद कर देना;

**Lumbar P.,** the tapping of the spinal subarachnoid space in the lumbar region to remove cerebrospinal fluid for examination or for the relief of abnormal tension; spinal puncture. कटिवेध; कटिवेधन;

**Spinal P.,** see **Lumbar Puncture.**

**Pungent.** Powerful; pricking; biting; acrid. तीक्ष्ण; तीखा; तिक्त; कटु

**Pupa.** The stage of insect metamorphosis following the larva and preceding the image (an image or shadow). प्यूपा

**Pupae.** Plural of **Pupa.**

**Pupil.** The aperture of the eye through which light passes; pupilla. तारा; पटल; पुतली;

**Argyll Robertson's P.,** a form of iridoplegia, characterized by loss of reflexes to light with normal pupillary contraction on accommodation and convergence. आर्गाइल राबर्टसन तारा

**Pupilla.** See **Pupil.**

**Pupillae.** Plural of **Pupilla.**

**Pupillary.** Pertaining to the pupil. पटल, तारा अथवा पुतली सम्बन्धी

**Pupillometer.** An instrument for measuring the diameter of the pupil. तारामापी

**Pupillometry.** Measurement of the pupil. तारामिति

**Pupilloplegia.** A condition in which the pupil reacts slowly to light stimuli. आंशिकताराघात

**Pupilloscopy.** Retinoscopy. तारादर्शन

**Pure.** Unstained; unalloyed. शुद्ध; विशुद्ध; असली; ख़ालिस

**Purgation.** Evacuation of the bowels. विरेचन; रेचन

**Purgative.** A drug causing evacuation of fluid faeces. विरेचक; रेचक; दस्तावर दवाई

**Puriform.** Having the form and appearance of pus or matter. पूयाभ; पूयवत्; पीब जैसा; मवाद जैसा

**Purify.** To cleanse. शोधन करना; परिशोधन करना; शुद्ध करना

**Purin Bodies.** Constituents of proteins, most common in red meats and internal glandular organs. प्यूरिन-पिण्ड; प्रोटीन पदार्थों के घटक

**Purpura.** A blood condition which causes bleeding under the skin and into other tissues, such as joints; land scurvy; peliosis. चित्तिता;

  P. Haemorrhagica, a grave form with mucous haemorrhages; peliosis haemorrhagica. रक्तचित्तिता; नीलारुणरुजा

**Purpuric.** Pertaining to purpura. रक्तचित्तिता अथवा नीलारुणरुजा सम्बन्धी

**Purulent.** Consisting of pus-like matter. सपूय; पीबयुक्त; मवादयुक्त

**Puruloid.** Resembling pus. पूयाभ; पीब जैसा

**Pus.** A yellowish, white liquid matter found in abscesses, wounds, etc. पूय; पीब; मवाद

**Pusher.** A seller of illegal narcotic drugs. कुवैद्य; स्वापक विक्रेता

**Pustula.** Pustule. पूयस्फोट; पकी हुई फुंसी

**Pustula Maligna.** A gangrenous focus due to bacillus anthrax. दुर्दम पूयस्फोट

**Pustulant.** An agent causing pustulation. सपूय; पूतिजन्य; पूतिजनक; पीब अथवा मवाद पैदा करने वाला

**Pustular.** Consisting of, or appearing as pustules, as in small-pox. पूयस्फोटिकाभ; फुन्सी जैसा दिखाई देने वाला

**Pustule.** An elevation of the skin, having an inflamed base, and containing pus; a pimple. पूयस्फोटिका; फुंसी;

**Malignant P.,** anthrax. आंगारव्रण; नासूर

**Putamen.** The external layer of the lenticular nucleus. कवच

**Putrefaction.** Decay and destruction of the organised matter of decomposition. पूतीभवन; पूयन; पीब पड़ना; मवाद बनना

**Putrefactive.** Causing or pertaining to putrefaction. पूतिजन्य; पूयोत्पादक; पूतिगन्धी

**Putrescence.** Rottenness; decay. पूतिरक्तता; पूतीभवन; क्षय; दुर्गन्ध; सड़ान्ध

**Putrescent.** Becoming putrid or pertaining to the putrefaction process. पूतिमान; विगलित; गला-सड़ा

**Putrid.** Decomposed; offensively rotten. विघटित; दुर्गन्धित; गला-सड़ा

**Putrillage.** Rotten material. पूतिद्रव्य; मवाद; पूय; पीब

**Pyaemia.** A grave form of septicaemia in which pyogenic bacteria lodge and grow in distant organs; pyemia. पूयरक्तता; पूतिरक्तता; खून में पीब विद्यमान रहना

**Pyarthrosis.** Pus in a joint cavity. पूयसन्धि; पूतिसन्धि; सन्धिपूतिता

**Pyelectasia.** See **Pyelectasis.**

**Pyelectasis.** Dilatation of the renal pelvis; pyelectasia. वृक्कगोणिकाविस्फार; वृक्कगोणिका का फैलना

**Pyelitis.** Inflammation of the pelvis of the kidney (renal pelvis). वृक्कगोणिकाशोथ; वृक्कपूयार्ति; वृक्कवस्ति का प्रदाह

**Pyelocystitis.** Pyelitis with cystitis. वृक्कगोणिकामूत्राशयशोथ; वृक्कगोणिकाशोथ के साथ मूत्राशयशोथ होना

**Pyelogram.** A radiograph of the renal pelvis and ureter; pyelograph. गोणिकाचित्र

**Pyelograph.** See **Pyelogram.**

**Pyelography.** Radiographic visualization of the renal pelvis and the ureter. वृक्कगोणिकामूत्रनलीचित्रण

**Pyelolithotomy.** The operation for removal of a stone from the renal pelvis. वृक्कगोणिकाश्मरीहरण; वृक्कगोणिका से पथरी निकालने के लिये किया जाने वाला ऑपरेशन

**Pyelonephritis.** Inflammation of the pelvis of the kidney. वृक्कगोणिकाशोथ; वृक्कगोणिका का प्रदाह

**Pyelonephrosis.** Any disease of the renal pelvis. गोणिकापवृक्कता

**Pyeloplasty.** A plastic operation of the pelvis of the kidney. वृक्कगोणिकासंधान

**Pyeloscopy.** Fluoroscopic observation of the pelvis and calices of the kidney. वृक्कगोणिकादर्शन

**Pyemesis.** Vomiting of pus. पूतिवमन; पीब की कै होना

**Pyemia.** See **Pyaemia.**

**Pyesis.** The formation of pus; suppuration. पूतिरचना; पूतित्ता

**Pygmy.** A physiologic dwarf. बौना; पिग्मी

**Pyknosis.** A condensation and reduction in size of the cell or its nucleus. केन्द्रकसंघनन; श्यानकेन्द्रता; संहतीकरण

**Pylephlebitis.** See **Pylophlebitis.**

**Pylophlebitis.** Acute inflammation of the portal vein; pylephlebitis. उग्रप्रतिहारीशिराशोथ; प्रतिहारी शिरा का उग्र प्रदाह

**Pyloralgia.** Painful spasm of the pylorus. जठरनिर्गमशूल; जठरनिर्गम की दर्दनाक ऐंठन

**Pylori.** Plural of **Pylorus.**

**Pyloric.** Pertaining to the pylorus. जठरनिर्गमीय; जठरनिर्गम सम्बन्धी;

   **P. Sphincter,** muscles surrounding the opening at the lower end of the stomach. जठरनिर्गमसंकोची;

   **P. Stenosis,** narrowing of the pylorus due to scar tissue formed during the healing of a duodenal ulcer. जठरनिर्गमसंकीर्णता; जठरनिर्गम की सिकुड़न

**Pyloristenosis.** Stricture or narrowing of the orifice of the pylorus; pylorostenosis. जठरनिर्गमसंकीर्णता

**Pyloritis.** Inflammation of the pylorus. जठरनिर्गमशोथ; जठरनिर्गम का प्रदाह

**Pyloromyotomy.** Incision of the pyloric sphincter muscle. जठरनिर्गमसंकोचीछेदन

**Pylorospasm.** Spasm of the pyloric muscle. जठरनिर्गमाकर्ष; जठरनिर्गमपेशी की ऐंठन

**Pylorostenosis.** See **Pyloristenosis.**

**Pylorotomy.** Incision of the pylorus. जठरनिर्गमछेदन

**Pylorus.** Lower orifice of the stomach. जठरनिर्गम; आमाशय का निचला द्वार

**Pyocolpos.** Pus in the vagina. योनिपूतिता; योनि के अन्दर पीब पड़ना

**Pyoderma.** Chronic cellulitis of the skin, manifesting itself in granulation tissue, ulceration, colliquative necrosis or vegetative lesion; pyodermia. त्वक्पूतिता; त्वक्पूयता; पूयत्वग्रोग; त्वचा में पीब पड़ना

**Pyodermia.** See **Pyoderma.**

**Pyogenesis.** Formation of pus. पूतिजनन; पीब अथवा मवाद बनना

**Pyogenic.** Pus-forming. पूतिजनक; पूतिजन्य; pertaining to the formation of-pus. पूतिजनन सम्बन्धी

**Pyoid.** Resembling pus. पूयाभ; पीब अथवा मवाद जैसा

**Pyometra.** A collection of pus in the womb. पूयगर्भाशयता; गर्भाशयपूतिता; जरायु के अन्दर पीब पड़ना

**Pyon.** Pus. पूय; पूति; पीब; मवाद

**Pyonephritis.** Suppurative inflammation of the kidney. वृक्कपूतिशोथ

**Pyonephrosis.** Suppuration within the kidney. वृक्कपूतिता; पूयवृक्कता; गुर्दे में पीब पड़ना

**Pyopericarditis.** Pericarditis with purulent effusion. सपूयहृद्यावरणशोथ; पीब बनने के साथ हृदयावरण का प्रदाह होना

**Pyoperitonitis.** Suppurative inflammation of the peritoneum. सपूयउदरावरणशोथ

**Pyophthalmia.** Purulent ophthalmia; pyophthalmitis. सपूयनेत्रश्लेष्मलाशोथ; सपूयनेत्राभिष्यन्द

**Pyophthalmitis.** See **Pyophthalmia.**

**Pyorrhea.** See **Pyorrhoea.**

**Pyorrhoea.** A discharge of pus, usually from the teeth sockets; pyorrhea. पूयस्राव; पूतिस्राव; पायरिया; दन्तपूतिता

**Pyosalpingitis.** Suppurative inflammationof the Fallopian tube. सपूयडिम्बवाहिनीशोथ

**Pyosalpinx.** A Fallopian tube containing pus. पूयडिम्बवाहिनी; डिम्बावाही नली में पीब भरना

**Pyosis.** The formation of pus; suppuration. पूयरचना; पूतिरचना; पूयनिर्माण; पीब अथवा मवाद बनना

**Pyramid.** Any conic eminence of an organ. शंकु; सूचीस्तम्भ; पिरामिद

**Pyramidal.** Applied to some conical shaped eminences in the body. शंक्वाकार; शुण्डाकार; सूचीस्तम्भीय; पिरामिदी

**Pyretic.** Causing or pertaining to fever. ज्वरकारी अथवा ज्वर सम्बन्धी

**Pyretogenetic.** See **Pyrogenic.**

**Pyretogenic.** See **Pyrogenic.**

**Pyretogenous.** See **Pyrogenic.**

**Pyrexia.** An elevation of temperature; fever. ज्वर; बुखार

**Pyrogen.** A substance capable of producing a pyrexia. ज्वरकारी; ज्वरोत्पादक; बुखार पैदा करने वाला पदार्थ

**Pyrogenic.** Causing fever; pyretogenetic; pyretogenic; pyretogenous. ज्वरजन्य; ज्वरजनक

**Pyrolysis.** Decomposition of a substance by heat. तापलयन

**Pyromania.** Fire mania; mania for setting fires. अग्न्योन्माद; दहनोन्माद; आग लगाने का पागलपन

**Pyrophobia.** Morbid dread of fire. अग्निभीति; आग का डर

**Pyrosis.** Water-brash; heart-burn; pain in the region of the stomach and vomiting of watery fluid. अम्लिकोद्गार; हृद्दाह; आमाशय में पीड़ा होने के साथ पनीला वमन होना

**Pyrotic.** Burning; caustic. दाहक; ज्वलनकारी; acidic. अम्लज; अम्लकर; relating to pyrosis. हृद्दाह सम्बन्धी

**Pyuria.** Presence of pus in the urine. पूतिमेह; पेशाब में मवाद जाना

# Q

**Q-angle.** Obtuse angle, formed by patellar tendon and patellar ligament. Q- ऐंगल; Q-कोण

**Q.D.** Quaque die; every day. प्रतिदिन; हर रोज

**Q-fever.** See **Quartan Fever.**

**Q.H.** See **Quaque Hora.**

**Q.D.S.** Quarter in die sumendum; take four times a day. दिन में चार बार लें

**Q.D. or Q.I.D.** See **Quarter in die.**

**Q.L.** See **Quantum Libet.**

**Q.M.** See **Quaque Matin.**

**Q.P.** See **Quantum Placent.**

**Q.Q.H.** See **Quaque Quarta Hora.**

**Q.S.** See **Quantum Sufficiat.**

**Quack.** A person, usually not a physician, who pretends to have the medical knowledge and experience which he does not possess, for the purpose of defrauding patients for his own profit. कुवैद्य; नीमहकीम

**Quackery.** Treating the sick without the knowledge of medicine. कुवैद्यकी; नीमहकीमी

**Quacksalver.** One who 'quaks' (sells) his salves; a medical huckster. कुवैद्य; नीमहकीम

**Quad.** Abbreviated form of **Quadriceps, Quadrilateral, Quadrant, Quadriplegia.**

**Quadrangular.** Having four angles. चतुष्कोणीय; चतुष्कोणक;

Q. Lobe, a region forming the superior portion of each cerebellar hemisphere. चतुष्कोणीय खण्ड;

Q. Membrane, the upper portion of the elastic membrane of the larynx. चतुष्कोणीय कला

**Quadrans.** A quarter; quadrant. चौथाई

**Quadrant.** See **Quadrans.**

**Quadrate.** Square. चतुरस्र; वर्गाकार;

Q. Lobe, a small lobe of the liver. चतुरस्र खण्ड; यकृत् का एक छोटा सा खण्ड

**Quadriceps.** The 'Q' extensor femoris muscle of the thigh which possesses four heads. चतुःशिरस्क; चार सिरों वाली (पेशी)

**Quadrigemina.** The superior portion of midbrain. चतुष्टय

**Quadrigeminal.** Fourfold. चतुष्टय; चार भागों वाला;

Q. Bodies, the four rounded eminences situated under the callosum. चतुष्टयपिण्ड

**Quadrilateral.** Having four sides. चतुर्भुज; चार भुजाओं वाला

**Quadrilocular.** Having four chambers, cavities or spaces. चतुष्कोटरीय

**Quadripara.** See **Quartipara.**

**Quadriplegia.** Paralysis of all the four limbs. चतुरंगघात; चारों अंगों का पक्षाघात

**Quadriplegic.** Pertaining to, or affected with quadriplegia. चतुरांगघात सम्बन्धी या चतुरांगघातग्रस्त

**Quadruped.** A four-footed animal. चतुष्पादी; चौपाया; चार पैरों वाला

**Quadruplet.** One of four children born at one birth. चतुर्ज

**Qualitative.** Pertaining to the quality; qualitive. गुणात्मक; गुण सम्बन्धी

**Qualitive.** See **Qualitative.**

**Quality.** That which constitutes or characterizes a thing. गुण; धर्म; स्वभाव

**Qualmish.** Sick at the stomach; affected with nausea and languor. वमनेच्छु; उद्विग्न; मिचली तथा आलस से पीड़ित

**Qualmishness.** Nausea and languor. मतली; मितली; मिचली; उद्विग्नता

**Quanta.** Plural of **Quantum.**

**Quantitative.** Pertaining to the quantity; quantitive. मात्रात्मक; मात्रामूलक; मात्रा सम्बन्धी

**Quantitive.** See **Quantitative.**

**Quantity.** Any amount. मात्रा; प्रमात्रा; परिमाण

**Quantum.** A certain definite amount; the supposed atom of light. मात्रा; प्रमात्रा; परिमाण;

  **Q. Libet,** see **Quantum Vis.**

  **Q. Placent,** as may be thought desirable. इच्छानुसार;

  **Q. Sufficiat,** sufficient quantity. पर्याप्त मात्रा;

  **Q. Vis,** as much as you like; quantum libet. जितना चाहो

**Quaque Hora.** After every hour. हर घण्टे बाद

**Quaque Matin.** Every morning. नित्य प्रात:; रोज सुबह

**Quaque Quarta Hora.** After every four hour. हर चार घण्टे बाद

**Quarantine.** The period of isolation for preventing the spread of communicable disease. संगरोध; संगरोधन; अन्य लोगों से दूर रखना

**Quart.** The fourth part of a gallon. क्वार्ट; चौथाई गैलन; एक गैलन का चौथाई भाग

**Quartan.** Having a paroxysm every 72 hours or every fourth day. चतुर्थक; हर ७२ घण्टे में या चौथे दिन प्रकट होने वाला;

  **Q- Fever,** an infectious fever transmitted from cattle, sheep and goats, or by ticks and carried by air and breathed in. चतुर्थक ज्वर; हर चौथे दिन प्रकट होने वाला बुखार

**Quarter in die.** Four times a day. Q.D.; Q.I.D. दिन में चार बार

**Quarternary.** Denoting a chemical compound containing four

**Quartipara**

elements. चार तत्त्वों या मूलकों द्वारा निर्मित; fourth in order. क्रम में चौथा

**Quartipara.** A woman pregnant for the fourth time; quadripara. चतुर्गर्भा; चतुष्गर्भा; चौथी बार गर्भ धारण करने वाली स्त्री

**Quercus Infectoria.** A genus of trees, the oak. माजूफल वृक्ष

**Quickening.** First perceptible movement of a foetus in the uterus. प्रथम गर्भस्पन्दन, जिसमें मां को गर्भाशय के अन्दर भ्रूण की गति पहली बार महसूस होती है

**Quicklime.** Calcium Oxide. कलीचूना; अनबुझा चूना

**Quicksilver.** Mercury. पारद; पारा

**Quiescent.** Becoming quiet. शान्त; निश्चल; निष्क्रिय; क्रियाशून्य

**Quinic.** Antipyretic. विज्वरिक; विज्वरीय; pertaining to quinine. कुनीन सम्बन्धी;

   **Q. Fever,** a fever with cutaneous eruptions, occurring among workmen making quinine. कुनीन-ज्वर

**Quinine.** A medicine prepared from cinchona. कुनीन; सिनकोना से तैयार की जाने वाली औषधि

**Quininism.** Bad effects of abusing quinine, e.g. headache, noises in the ears and partial deafness, disturbed vision, nausea, etc. कुनीनात्यय; कुनीन-विषण्णता; कुनीन का सेवन करने के फलस्वरूप उत्पन्न होने वाली बीमारियाँ

**Quinsy.** An acute severe inflammation of the tonsils with fever. परिगलतुण्डिका-विद्रधि; कण्ठपाक; गलप्रदाह; सपूयगलतुण्डिकाशोथ

**Quintipara.** A woman who has born five children. पंचजाता; पांच बच्चों को जन्म देने वाली स्त्री

**Quintan.** An intermittent fever returning every fifth day. पंचक; हर पांचवें रोज़ प्रकट होने वाला सविराम ज्वर

**Quiver.** Shiver. कांपना

**Quiz.** An informal examination in a medical subject. क्विज; चिकित्सा-विज्ञान सम्बन्धी अनौपचारिक परीक्षा

**Quode vide.** In order of alphabetical arrangements. वर्णक्रमानुसार

**Quotid.** Daily. नित्य; हर रोज़

**Quotidian.** Daily, as a quotidian ague, having a paroxysm every day. दैनिक; हर रोज़ प्रकट होने वाला

**Quotient.** The number of times one amount contained in another. भागफल; भजनफल

**Q. V.** Abbreviation for **Quantum vis and Quode vide.**

# R

**R̸.** Symbol of **Recipe.**

**Rabic.** Concerning rabies. अलर्क अथवा जलातंक सम्बन्धी

**Rabid.** Suffering from or infected with. अलर्कग्रस्त; जलातंकग्रस्त; पागल

**Rabies.** A serious virus infection transmitted from many wild and domesticated animals to man; hydrophobia; madness arising from the bite of a rabid dog. अलर्क; जलातंक

**Race.** A class of animals or individuals having common somatic inherited characteristics. जाति

**Racemose.** Resembling a bunch of grapes. गुच्छित; गुच्छेदार; गुच्छाकृतिक; अंगूर के गुच्छे से मिलता-जुलता

**Raches.** Vertebral column. कशेरुकादण्ड; कशेरुकाखण्ड; मेरुदण्ड; सुषुम्ना

**Rachial.** Spinal; relating to spine; rachidial; rachidian. मेरुदण्ड सम्बन्धी

**Rachialgia.** Pain in the spine. मेरुदण्डार्ति; मेरुशूल; सुषुम्नार्ति; रीढ़ की हड्डी का दर्द

**Rachicentesis.** Lumbar puncture; rachiocentesis. कटि-छिद्रण; मेरु-छिद्रण

**Rachides.** Plural of **Rachis.**

**Rachidial.** See **Rachial.**

**Rachidian.** See **Rachial.**

**Rachigraph.** A graph for recording the curves of the vertebrae. कशेरुकालेख

**Rachiocentesis.** See **Rachicentesis.**

**Rachiocysis.** Effusion of water in the spinal cord. मेरुदण्डद्रवता; मेरुदण्डजलता; रीढ़ की हड्डी में पानी भर जाना

**Rachiodynia.** Pain in the spinal cord. मेरुमज्जार्ति; मेरुशूल; सुषुम्नार्ति; मेरुमज्जा का दर्द

**Rachioscoliosis.** Lateral curvature of spine. पार्श्वकुब्जता; मेरुदण्ड की एकपार्श्वी बक्रता

**Rachiotomy.** Excision of a vertebral lamina. कशेरुकाफलक-उच्छेदन

**Rachises.** Plural of **Rachis**.

**Rachis.** The spinal column. कशेरुकादण्ड; मेरुदण्ड; सुषुम्ना; रीढ़ की हड्डी

**Rachischisis.** A cleft in the vetebral column. मेरुनलिकाविदर

**Rachitic.** Pertaining to rachitis or affected with rickets; rickety. बालास्थिविकारी; रिक्केटी; रिक्केटरोगग्रस्त;

**Rachitis.** Ricket; inflammatory disease of the vertebral column. कशेरुकादण्डशोथ; मेरुशोथ; रिक्केट; अस्थिबक्रता

**Rackitogenic.** Producing or causing rickets. रिक्केटजनक

**Rachotomy.** Excision of the vertebral column. कशेरुका-उच्छेदन; कशेरुकोच्छेदन; कशेरुका-खण्ड को काट कर हटाना

**Radectomy.** See **Radiectomy**.

**Radial.** Pertaining to the radius. बहिप्रकोष्ठीय; बहिप्रकोष्ठ सम्बन्धी; radiating. विकिरणकारी; बिखराने वाला

**Radiant.** Diverging from a centre, as rays. विकीर्ण; विकिरणी; उज्ज्वल; चमकदार

**Radiate.** To spread out in all directions from a centre. विकीर्ण होना या करना; बिखराना

**Radiating.** Diverging from a common centre. विकिरणकारी; बिखराने या बिखरने वाला

**Radiatio.** Radiation. विकिरण; बिखराव;

   R. Acustica, see **Acoustic Radiation**.

   R. Optica, see **Optic Radiation**.

   R. Pyramidalis, see **Pyramidal Radiation**.

**Radiation.** The invisible energy rays given off by x-ray, radium and other chemicals when exposed to radioactivity. विकिरण; बिखराव;

   **Acoustic R.**, a tract of fibres extending from the medial geniculate body to the superior and transvers temporal gyri; radiatio acustica; auditory radiation. श्रवणतन्तु-विकिरण;

   **Auditory R.**, see **Acoustic Radiation**.

   **Optic R.**, a strand of fibres continuous with those of the corona radiata, derived mainly from the pulvinar, the geniculate bodies and the optic tract, and radiating into occipital lobes; radiatio optica. दृष्टितन्तु-विकिरण;

**Pyramidal R.**, white fibres passing from the cortex to the pyramidal tract; radiatio pyramidalis. पिरामिदी विकिरण;

**Thalamic R.**, tracts of fibres from the optic thalami that radiate into the hemispheres. चेतकतन्तु-विकिरण

**Radectomy.** See **Radiectomy.**

**Radiationes.** Plural of **Radiatio.**

**Radical.** Pertaining to the root or origin. मूलक; जड़ अथवा मूल सम्बन्धी

**Radices.** Plural of **Radix.**

**Radicle.** Any one of the smallest branches of a vessel or nerve. मूलांकुर; तंत्रिकामूल; शिरामूल; शाखिका

**Radicotomy.** See **Rhizotomy.**

**Radicula.** A spinal nerve root. मेरुस्नायुमूल

**Radicular.** Pertaining to a radicle. मूलोद्भवी; मूलक

**Radiculectomy.** See **Rhizotomy.**

**Radiculitis.** Inflammation of the nerve root. तंत्रिकामूलशोथ; शिरामूलशोथ; स्नायुमूल का प्रदाह

**Radiculoganglionitis.** Inflammation of the nerve root and the ganglion. तंत्रिकामूलगण्डिकाशोथ; तंत्रिकामूल एवं गण्डिका का प्रदाह

**Radiculotomy.** See **Rhizotomy.**

**Radiectomy.** Surgical removal of one or more roots of a multirooted tooth; root amputation; radectomy; radisectomy. दंतमूलोच्छेदन; दंतमूल-उच्छेदन

**Radii.** Plural of **Radius.**

**Radioactive.** Giving off penetrating rays due to spontaneous breaking up of atoms. विघटनाभिक; रेडियोधर्मी; विकिरणशील; रेडियोएक्टिव

**Radioactivity.** The power of spontaneous emission of rays having chemic and electric properties. विघटनशीलता; रेडियोधर्मिता; विकिरणशीलता

**Radiocarpal.** Relating to the radius and the carpus. बहि:प्रकोष्ठिका एवं मणिबन्ध सम्बन्धी

**Radiodermatitis.** Dermatitis due exposure to radiation. विकिरणत्वक्शोथ

**Radiogram.** See **Radiograph.**

**Radiograph.** The finished printed x-ray picture; radiogram; skiagram; skiagraph. विकिरणचित्र; क्ष-रश्मिचित्र

**Radiographer.** X-ray technician. विकिरणचित्रकार; क्ष-रश्मिचित्रकार; एक्स-रेचित्रकार; रेडियोग्राफर

**Radiography.** The art of making radiographs; skiagraphy. विकिरणचित्रण; रक्स-रेचित्रण; क्ष-रश्मिचित्रण

**Radioisotope.** An unstable isotope that decays to a stable state by emitting radiation. विकिरण-समस्थानिक

**Radioimmunity.** Lessened sensitivity to radiation. विकिरणक्षमता

**Radiolesion.** A lesion caused by radiation. विकिरणविक्षति

**Radiologic.** Pertaining to radiology; radiological. विकिरणविज्ञान सम्बन्धी

**Radiological.** See **Radiologic.**

**Radiologist.** A specialist in x-ray diagnosis. विकिरणविज्ञानी; एक्स-रेविद्; क्ष-रश्मिविज्ञानी

**Radiology.** The branch of medicine concerned with radioactive substances; roentgenology. विकिरणविज्ञान

**Radioluscent.** Partially penetrable by x-rays or other forms of radiation. विकिरणपारभासी

**Radiomimetic.** Produces effects similar to those of radiotherapy. विकिरण-अनुकारी; रेडियो-अनुकारी

**Radisectomy.** See **Radiectomy.**

**Radiosensitive.** Affected by x-rays. विकिरणसुग्राही

**Radiotherapist.** A specialist in the treatment of diseases by x-rays. विकिरण-चिकित्सक; विकिरणवेत्ता; विकिरण-चिकित्साविज्ञानी

**Radiotherapy.** Treatment by means of x-rays, radium and other radioactive substances. विकिरणचिकित्सा; रेडियोचिकित्सा

**Radioulnar.** Pertaining to the radius and ulna. बहिरन्त:प्रकोष्ठकी; bones of forearm. बाजुओं की हड्डियाँ

**Radium.** A source of radiation useful in treating diseases. रेडियम

**Radius.** The bone on the outer side of the forearm. बहि:प्रकोष्ठिका; त्रिज्या; रेडियस

**Radix.** A root; the primary or beginning portion of a part or organ buried in tissue or by which it arises from another structure. मूल; जड़; उद्गम

**Raisins.** Dried grapes. शुष्कद्राक्षा; दाख; मुनक्का; सूखे अंगूर

**Rale.** Rattle or rhoncus; a bubbling sound heard in the bronchi in diseases; wheezing. आगन्तुक ध्वनि; फेफड़े की बुद्बुद् करती हुई आवाज; राल;

**Gurgling R.,** coarse sound heard over trachea nearly filled with secretion. घर्घर राल;

**Sonorous R.,** a snoring sound produced by a projecting mass of viscid secretion in a large bronchus. सुस्वनिक राल

**Rami.** Plural of **Ramus.**

**Ramification.** Extension in a branch-like form, as of an artery. प्रशाखन; बहुशाखन

**Ramitis.** Inflammation of a ramus. प्रशाखाशोथ

**Ramollissement.** Softening of an organ or part. अंगमृदुता; शरीर के किसी अंग या भाग की कोमलता

**Ramus.** A branch of an artery, vein or nerve. प्रशाखा, जैसे धमनी, शिरा या नाड़ी की शाखा;

**R. Anastomoticus,** a blood vessel that interconnects the neighbouring vessels; anastomotic branch. सम्मिलनी प्रशाखा;

**R. Communicans,** a branch from the anterior root of the spinal nerve to the sympathetic chain of the ganglia. संगमी प्रशाखा

**Rancescent.** Becoming sour or rancid. खट्टा होना; विरस होना

**Rancid.** Foetid or musty smell. विरस; कटु; पूतिगन्धी; दुर्गन्धित

**Randomisation.** Random sampling. यादृच्छिक प्रतिचयन

**Ranine.** Pertaining to the undersurface of the tongue जिह्वाधस्तलीय; जीभ के निचले तल सम्बन्धी; relating to frog. मेंढक अथवा दादुर सम्बन्धी

**Ranula.** A tumour under the tongue. अधःजिह्वापुटी; जीभ के नीचे उत्पन्न रसौली या गिल्टी

**Ranular.** Pertaining to a ranula. अधःजिह्वापुटीय; जीभ के नीचे उत्पन्न रसौली या गिल्टी से सम्बन्धित

**Rape.** Act of sexual intercourse with a women by force and against her will. बलात्संग; बलात्कार; किसी स्त्री से जबरदस्ती सम्भोग करना

**Raphe.** A seam, suture, ridge or crease; rhaphe. सन्धिरेखा; सीवनी; तुन्नसेवनी

**Raptus.** Any sudden attack of a disease. आकस्मिकरोगावेग; अचानक ही किसी रोग का आक्रमण होना

**Rarefaction.** An act or process of making a substance less dense. विरलीकरण; विरलीभवन; विरलन

**Rash.** An eruption on the skin. विस्फोट; पित्तिका; दाना;

**Nettle R.,** urticaria. शीतपित्त; छपाकी; जुलपित्ती; पित्ती;

**R. Fever,** scarlet fever; scarletina. रक्तज्वर; आरक्तज्वर

**Raspatory.** An instrument used for scraping a bone. रैस्पेटरी; हड्डी खुरचने के लिये प्रयुक्त किया जाने वाला यंत्र

**Rate.** A record of the measurement of an event or process in terms of its relation to some fixed standard. दर;

**Basal Metabolic R. (BMR),** heat production at the lowest level of cell chemistry in the waking state; basal metabolism. आधारी चयापचय दर;

**Birth R.,** the precise number of births for a year related to an exact population and place. जन्म-दर;

**Death R.,** see **Mortality Rate.**

**Erythrocytes Sedimentation R.,** see **E.S.R.**

**Fatality R.,** see **Mortality Rate.**

**Mortality R.,** the ratio of the total number of deaths to the total population of a given community; death rate; fatality rate. मृत्यु-दर;

**Pulse R.,** rate of the pulse recorded as beats per minute. नाड़ी-दर;

**Respiratory R.,** frequency of breathing, recorded as the number of breaths per minute. श्वास-दर;

**Sedimentation R.,** the sinking velocity of blood cells. अवसादन दर

**Ratio.** An expression of the relationship of one quantity to another. अनुपात

**Rational.** Reasonable; opposed to empiric. युक्तिसंगत; तर्कसंगत

**Rauwolfia.** The root of an Indian plant, called **Sarpagandha.** सर्पगंधा

**Ray.** A line of light or heat proceeding from a luminous point. किरण; रश्मि; प्रकाशरेखा; अर्;

**Alpha R.'s,** rays composed of positively charged particles of helium derived from atomic disintegration of radioactive elements. अल्फा किरणें;

**Beta R.'s,** negatively charged electrons expelled from atoms of disintegrating radioactive elements. बीटा किरणें;

**Gamma R.'s,** heterogenous vibrations caused by electronic disturbance in atoms of radioactive elements during their disintegration. गामा किरणें;

**Roentgen R.'s,** x-rays discovered by Wilhem Konrad Roentgen, which have a penetrative power through opaque substance; x-rays. रायंटजन किरणें; क्ष-किरणें;

**X-r.'s,** see **Roentgen Rays.**

**Raynaud's Disease.** Paroxysmal spasm of the digital arteries, producing pallor, or cyanosis of fingers or toes, and occasionally resulting in gangrene. रेनाड रोग; उँगली की धमनियों की दौरे के रूप में प्रकट होने वाली ऐंठन

**Ray's Mania.** Moral insanity. नैतिक विक्षिप्ति; रे-उन्माद

**R.B.C.** Red blood cell or count. लोहित रुधिर कोशिका अथवा लोहित रुधिर गणन; लाल रक्त कोशिका अथवा लाल रक्त गणन

**Reaction.** Responsive action; effect. प्रतिक्रिया; अभिक्रिया; प्रभाव

**Reactionary.** Anything producing reaction. प्रतिक्रियात्मक; अभिक्रियात्मक

**Reactivate.** To render active again. प्रतिक्रियाशील करना; अभिक्रियाशील करना; पुन: क्रियाशील या सक्रिय करना

**Reactivation.** Making something or some process active again. पुनर्क्रियाशीलता; अभिक्रियाशीलता

**Reactivative.** Capable of being reactivated; to reactivate. प्रतिक्रियाशील; अभिक्रियाशील; पुन:क्रियाशील

**Reactive.** To make active again. पुन: सक्रिय करना

**Reactivity.** The process of reacting. पुनर्संक्रियता

**Reagent.** An agent capable of producing a chemical reaction. अभिकर्म; अभिकर्मक; प्रतिक्रियाशील द्रव्य अथवा शक्ति

**Rebreathing.** Inhalation of part or all of gases previously exhaled. पुनश्वर्सन

**Recalcification.** The restoration to the tissues of lost calcium salts. पुनर्कैल्सीकरण; पुनर्कैल्सीभवन

**Recanalisation.** Spontaneous restoration of the continuity of the lumen of any occluded duct or tube. पुनर्नलीकरण

**Receiver.** A vessel for receiving distillation products. आदायक; ग्राही; संग्राही

**Receptacle.** See **Receptaculum.**

**Receptacula.** Plural of **Receptaculum.**

**Receptaculum.** Reservoir; a receptacle. आधान; पात्र

**Receptor.** Sensory afferent nerve-endings capable of receiving and transmitting stimuli. ग्राहक; ग्राही;

   **R. Cells,** specialized cells that collect information for the organism. ग्राही कोशिकायें; शरीर से आदेश संग्रह करने वाली विशिष्ट कोशिकायें

**Recess.** See **Recessus.**

**Cochlear R.**, see **Recessus Cochlearis**.

**Elliptical R.**, see **Recessus Ellipticus**.

**Recession.** A withdrawal or retreating of tissue. प्रतिसार; प्रतिगमन

**Recessive.** Lacking control; not dominant. अप्रभावी; प्रभावहीन

**Recessiveness.** The quality of being recessive. अप्रभाविता; प्रभावहीनता

**Recessus.** A recess; a small hollow or indentation. दरी;

**R. Cochlearis**, a small depression in the vestibule of the internal ear; the cochlear recess. कर्णावर्त दरी;

**R. Ellipticus**, the fossa hemielliptica; the elliptical recess. दीर्घवृत्त दरी

**Recipe.** The caption of a prescription, which means take. Symbol: ℞. नुस्ख़ालेखन में 'लीजिये' के निर्देशार्थ प्रयुक्त संकेत चिन्ह

**Reclination.** The act of lying down. अधोविलम्बन; लेटने की क्रिया

**Reclining.** Lying down; recumbent. अध:शायी; लेटी हुई

**Recovery Room.** Area provided with equipment and nursing needed to care for patients immediately after surgical operation. उपलब्धि कक्ष; रिकवरी रूम

**Recta.** Plural of **Rectum**.

**Rectal.** Pertaining to rectum. मलाशयी; मलांत्रीय; मलाशय सम्बन्धी

**Rectalgia.** Pain in the rectum. मलाशयार्ति; मलांत्रशूल; मलांत्र की पीड़ा

**Rectectomy.** Rectotomy; incision for stricture of the rectum. मलांत्र छेदन

**Rectification.** Purification of a substance. शोधन; परिशोधन; किसी पदार्थ को शुद्ध करना

**Rectified.** Made more pure, or stronger. शोधित; परिशोधित; शुद्ध किया गया

**Rectify.** To correct. सुधार करना; ठीक या सही करना; to purify or refine by distillation. शोधन करना; परिशोधन करना

**Recti-minores.** Two muscles of the head. सिर की दो पेशियाँ

**Rectitis.** Inflammation of the rectum. मलाशयशोथ; मलांत्रशोथ; मलाशय का प्रदाह

**Rectocele.** Prolapse of the rectum. मलाशयभ्रंस; मलाशयभ्रंश; मलांत्र की स्थानच्युति

**Rectopexia.** See **Rectopexy**.

**Rectopexy.** Fixation of the rectum; rectopexia. मलाशयस्थिरण

**Rectoplasty.** Proctoplasty; plastic surgery on the anus and the rectum. गुद-मलाशयसंधान

**Rectoscope.** An instrument for examining the rectum. मलाशयदर्शी; मलांत्र की जांच के लिये प्रयुक्त किया जाने वाला यंत्र

**Rectoscopy.** Examination of the rectum. मलाशयदर्शन; मलांत्र की जांच करना

**Rectosigmoid.** Pertaining to the rectum and sigmoid portion of the colon. मलाशयअवग्रहांत्रज; मलांत्र एवं अवग्रहांत्र सम्बन्धी

**Rectosigmoidectomy.** Surgical removal of the rectum and sigmoid colon. मलांत्र-अवग्रहांत्रोच्छेदन; मलाशय तथा अवग्रहांत्र को काट कर हटा देना

**Rectostenosis.** Stricture of the rectum; proctostenosis. मलाशयसंकीर्णता

**Rectotomy.** See **Rectectomy.**

**Rectouterine.** Pertaining to the rectum and uterus. मलाशय एवं गर्भाशय सम्बन्धी

**Rectovaginal.** Pertaining to the rectum and vagina. मलाशय एवं योनि सम्बन्धी

**Rectovesical.** Pertaining to the rectum and bladder. मलाशय एवं मूत्राशय सम्बन्धी

**Rectum.** The termination of the intestines at the fundament so called, the outlet being termed as anus; the lower part of the large intestine. मलाशय; मलांत्र

**Rectus.** Straight; name of certain muscles. सीधी; सरल; कुछ पेशियों के नाम, जिन्हें सरल पेशियाँ कहा जाता है

**Recumbent.** In a lying down posture; leaning against another part. अधःशायी; अर्धशायित; परिवलित; किसी दूसरे अंग का सहारा लेकर लेटी हुई स्थिति

**Recuperate.** To recover health and strength; to recover. पुनर्स्वास्थ्यलाभ होना या करना

**Recuperation.** Convalescence; return to health. पुनर्स्वास्थ्यलाभ; उल्लाघ; आरोग्यलाभ

**Recurrence.** A return; relapse. पुनरावृत्ति; पुनरावर्तन; पुनरुक्ति; आवर्तन

**Recurrent.** Constantly returning; relapsing. पुनरावर्ती; प्रत्यावर्ती; आवर्ती; आवर्तक;

   **R. Fever,** relapsing fever. आवर्ती ज्वर

**Recurvation.** A backward bending or flexure. प्रतिवर्तन

**Recurved.** Bent backward. प्रतिवर्तित; पीछे की ओर मुड़ी हुई

**Red.** A colour resembling blood. लाल; लोहित; रक्तिम; खून से मिलता-जुलता रंग;

**R. Blood Cells,** minute, circular discs floating in the blood which carry oxygen to the tissues and carbondioxide away from them. लाल रक्त कोशिकायें; लोहित रक्त कोशिकायें;

**R. Corpuscles,** the same as **Red Blood Cells.**

**R. Gown,** small red spots like flea-bites, which cover the infant all over like a gown, otherwise term "red-gum". रक्तचित्तिता;

**R. Gum,** a red papular eruption of infants. शिशुरक्तचित्तिता;

**R. Marrow,** found in the intestines of cancellous bones. लोहितमज्जा; रक्तमज्जा

**Redressement.** Correction of deformity. क्षतिपूर्ति करना; निवारण करना

**Reduce.** To weaken. घटाना; कम करना; to decompose. अपचयन करना

**Reducible.** Capable of being decomposed or reduced. अपचेय; घटाया या कम किया जाने वाला

**Reduction.** The bringing or putting back into its place; restoration to a normal situation; repositioning. पुनःस्थापन; पुनर्स्थापन

**Reduplicated.** Doubled. द्विरावृत्त; पुनरावृत्त; दोहराया गया

**Reduplication.** The doubling of the paroxyms in certain forms of intermittent fever. द्विरावृत्ति; पुनरावृत्ति

**Refine.** To purify; to free from impurities. शुद्ध करना; परिष्कार करना; परिमार्जित करना

**Reflection.** A bending back; throwing back a ray of light or radiant energy from surface; reflexion. पश्चनति; परावर्तन; पीछे की ओर मुड़ना

**Reflector.** A mirror for reflecting light. परावर्तक

**Reflex.** An involuntary response in which a stimulus is received by a nerve transmitted and finally translated into muscular activity - all in a fraction of seconds, reflected or thrown back. प्रतिवर्त; परावर्तित क्रिया;

**Abdominal R.,** contraction of muscles about the umbilicus on the downward stroking of the side of the abdomen. औदरिक प्रतिवर्त; उदर-प्रतिवर्त

**Anal R.,** a contraction of the sphincter ani on anal irritation. गुद-प्रतिवर्त;

**Auditory R.**, any reflection occurring in response to sound. श्रवण-प्रतिवर्त;

**Ciliospinal R.**, pupillary dilatation from rubbing the skin of the neck. रोमकमेरु-प्रतिवर्त;

**Corneal R.**, closure of the eyelid from irritation of the conjunctiva. स्वच्छपटल-प्रतिवर्त;

**Cranial R.**, any brain reflex. मस्तिष्क-प्रतिवर्त;

**Cremasteric R.**, contraction of the cremaster muscle from the stimulation of the skin of the thigh. वृषण-उत्कर्षिका प्रतिवर्त;

**Crossed R.**, movement of parts opposite to parts excited. विपक्ष प्रतिवर्त;

**Deep R.**, one developed by the percussion of a tendon of bone. गभीर प्रतिवर्त;

**Knee-r.**, a sudden contraction of the anterior muscles of the thigh; knee-jerk; patellar reflex; quadriceps reflex. जानु-प्रतिवर्त;

**Laryngeal R.**, on coughing an irritation of the fauces and larynx. स्वरयंत्र-प्रतिवर्त;

**Paradoxic R.**, dilatation of pupil on stimulation of retina by light. विरोधाभासी प्रतिवर्त;

**Patellar R.**, see **Knee-reflex**.

**Pharyngeal R.**, irritation of pharynx on swallowing. ग्रसनी-प्रतिवर्त;

**Plantar R.**, contraction of toes on striking the sole of the foot. पादतल-प्रतिवर्त;

**Pupillary R.**, contraction of the iris on exposure of the retina to light. तारा-प्रतिवर्त;

**Quadriceps R.**, see **Knee-reflex**.

**Spinal R.**, any reflex emanating from a centre in the spinal cord. मेरु-प्रतिवर्त;

**Superficial R.**, one that is developed by irritation of the skin. उपरिस्थ प्रतिवर्त;

**Tendon R.**, muscle reflex action. कण्डरा-प्रतिवर्त;

**R. Arc**, the mechanism necessary for a reflex action. प्रतिवर्त-चाप

**Reflexion.** See **Reflection.**

**Reflexogenic.** Causing a reflex; reflexogenous. प्रतिवर्तजनक

**Reflexogenous.** See **Reflexogenic.**

**Reflexograph.** An instrument for graphically recroding a reflex. प्रतिवर्तलेखी

**Reflexometer.** An instrument for measuring the force necessary to excite a reflex. प्रतिवर्तमापी

**Reflux.** A backward flow. प्रतिवाह; पश्चवाह; उद्गीरण

**Refract.** To bend back. परावर्तन करना; पीछे की ओर मोड़ना

**Refractile.** Capable of being bent back. परावर्तक; पीछे की ओर मोड़ देने योग्य

**Refraction.** The behaviour of light-rays passing from mediums of different densities. अपवर्तन; परावर्तन; वक्रीकरण;

Double R., the power possessed by certain substances of dividing a ray of light, and thus producing a double image of an object. द्विगुण अपवर्तन;

Dynamic R., the static refraction of the eye, plus that secured by the action of the accommodative apparatus. गतिक अपवर्तन;

Error of r., any refractive disturbance. अपवर्तन दोष;

Index of r., the refractive capacity of any medium as compared with that of the air. अपवर्तन सूचकांक;

Static R., that of the eye when accommodation is at rest. स्थैतिक अपवर्तन

**Refractionist.** One who corrects ametropia. दृष्टिमितिज्ञ; नेत्रापवर्तनमितिज्ञ

**Refractive.** Pertaining to refraction; refrigent. परावर्ती; अपवर्तन सम्बन्धी

**Refractometer.** An instrument for measuring refraction of the eye. अपवर्तनांकमापी; नेत्रापवर्तन मापने का यंत्र

**Refractometry.** Measurement of the refractive index or using the refractometer for determining the refractive error of the eye. अपवर्तनांकमिति

**Refractory.** Resistant to treatment; obstinate; intractable. दुश्चिकित्स्य; दु:साध्य

**Refrigent.** The same as **Refraction.**

**Refrigerant.** Cooling; an agent having cooling properties. प्रशीतक; शैत्यकारी; तापहर

**Refrigeration.** The act of cooling, or reducing fever. प्रशीतन; तापहरण; ठण्डा करने की क्रिया

**Refrigerator.** An ice-chest. प्रशीतित्र; रेफ्रिजरेटर

**Regenerate.** To produce. पुनर्जनन करना; to renew. पुनर्नवीकरण करना

**Regeneration.** A new growth or repair of lost tissues. पुनर्जनन; पुनरुद्भवन

**Regimen.** The methodic use of food; also called diet regimen. आहारविधान; पथ्यापथ्यनियम

**Regio.** See **Region.**

**Region.** A part or division of the body; regio. प्रदेश; क्षेत्र; कोई सीमाबद्ध अंश;

    **Abdominal R.,** the topographical subdivision of the abdomen. उदर प्रदेश;

    **Ciliary R.,** the part of the eye occupied by the ciliary body. रोमक प्रदेश;

    **Epigastric R.,** median region of the abdomen above the umbilical and between hypochondriac regions. अधिजठर प्रदेश;

    **Hypochondriac R.,** lateral region of the abdomen above a line passing through the tips of the tenth rib. अध:पर्शुक प्रदेश;

    **Hypogastric R.,** a median abdominal region below the umbilical and between the inguinal regions. अधोजठर प्रदेश;

    **Iliac R.'s,** see **Inguinal Regions.**

    **Inguinal R.'s,** the lowest lateral abdominal regions below a line passing through the highest point of iliac crest; iliac regions. वंक्षण प्रदेश;

    **Lumbar R.,** abdominal region on each side of the umbilical region. कटि-प्रदेश;

    **Perineal R.,** that of the perineum. मूलाधार प्रदेश;

    **Precordial R.,** the surface of the chest covering the heart. पुरोहृद्-क्षेत्र;

    **Umbilical R.,** the median abdominal region. नाभि-प्रदेश

**Regional.** Pertaining to a region. प्रादेशिक; क्षेत्रीय

**Regiones.** Plural of **Ragio.**

**Regression.** Return of the symptoms or relapse of a disease. प्रतिक्रमण; परावर्तन; प्रत्यागमन; लक्षणों की पुनरावृत्ति होना

**Regressive.** Retreating. प्रतिक्रमी; प्रतिगामी; प्रत्यागमनशील

**Regular.** Normal, or conforming to the rule. नियमित; विधिवत्; सुव्यवस्थित; स्वाभाविक

**Regurgitant.** Flowing backward; regurgitating. प्रत्यावह; प्रत्यावाही; ऊर्ध्वनिक्षेपी

**Regurgitate.** To be pushed back; to rise from the stomach back into the mouth, as food or drink. ऊर्ध्वनिक्षेप होना या करना; उगलना

**Regurgitating.** See **Regurgitant.**

**Regurgitation.** Return of food or drink from the stomach. ऊर्ध्वनिक्षेप; प्रत्यावहन; खाद्य अथवा पेय पदार्थों का आमाशय से मुँह के रास्ते वापस आना; backward flow. प्रतिवाह

**Rehabilitation.** Restoration to the best possible functioning state after serious illness or injury. पुनरुत्थान; पुनर्वास

**Reimplantation.** Replacement of a part that has been removed from the body. पुनर्स्थापन; निष्कासित अंग को पुन: जोड़ना

**Reinfection.** Infection a second time. पुनर्संक्रमण

**Reinoculation.** Inoculation a second time. पुनर्टीकाकरण

**Rejuvenation.** A return of the youthful condition or to the normal. पुनर्यौवन; कायाकल्प

**Relapse.** The return of a disease soon after convalescence. पुनरावृत्ति; आवृत्ति

**Relapsing.** Recurring. पुनरावर्ती; आवर्ती; पुन: प्रकट होने वाला;
    **R. Fever,** epidemic remittent, bilious remittent, mild yellow fever, etc. पुनरावर्ती ज्वर; आवर्ती ज्वर

**Relationship.** The state of being related, associated or connected. सम्बन्ध

**Relaxant.** That which reduces tension. शिथिलकर; श्लथक; तनाव कम करने वाला

**Relaxation.** Loosening, as relaxation of the bowels. शिथिलन; शिथिलता; श्रान्ति; ढीलापन

**Relief.** Deliverance from sickness; amelioration. आराम; उपशम; ह्रास

**Relieve.** To free wholly or partly. मुक्त करना; छुटकारा दिलाना

**Remanence.** Retentivity; the quality of being retentive. धारणशीलता

**Remedial.** Affording a remedy or cure; having the nature of a remedy. प्रतिकारक; उपचारक; आरोग्यकारक; आरोग्यकारी

**Remedy.** A medicine which restores health or lessens disease. उपचार; औषध

**Remission.** A lessening in severity; the period of abatement in fever. विसर्ग; विच्छेद; ज्वरविरामकाल; तीव्रता का ह्रास

**Remittent.** A disease which presents remissions, but does not entirely cease as distinguished from intermittent, in which there are periods of complete cessation of symptoms. अल्पविरामी; अर्धविसर्गी; स्वल्पविरामी; थोड़ा-सा अन्तर देकर प्रकट होने वाला

**Remote.** The more distant. दूरवर्ती; दूरस्थ; सुदूर

**Ren.** Kidney. वृक्क; गुर्दा;

   **R. Mobilis,** movable or floating kidney. चल वृक्क

**Renal.** Belonging to the kidneys. वृक्कों अर्थात् गुर्दों सम्बन्धी;

   **R. Calculus,** stone in the kidney; renal stone. वृक्काश्मरी; गुर्दे की पथरी;

   **R. Stone,** see **Renal Calculus.**

**Renes.** Plural of **Ren.**

**Renicapsule.** A suprarenal body. अधिवृक्क-पिण्ड

**Reniform.** Having the form or shape of kidney. वृक्काकार; वृक्काभ; गुर्दे जैसा

**Renin.** An enzyme, found only in the kidney cortex. रेनिन; मूत्रपिण्ड में पाया जाने वाला एक पदार्थ

**Renipuncture.** Puncture of the renal capsule. वृक्कसम्पुट-छिद्रण

**Renitis.** Inflammation of the kidneys. वृक्कशोथ; वृक्कप्रदाह; गुर्दों का प्रदाह

**Rennet.** A gastric ferment curdling milk. वसातंच; जमा हुआ दूध

**Rennin.** Milk curdling enzyme of gastric juice. रेन्निन; दूध को दही में बदलने वाला पदार्थ

**Renogenic.** Originating in or from the kidney. वृक्कजनित

**Renogram.** X-ray of renal shadow following injection of opaque medium, demonstrated in aortograph series. वृक्कलेख; गुर्दे की छाया का एक्स-रे

**Renography.** Radiography of the kidney. वृक्कविकिरणलेख

**Renomegaly.** Enlargement of the kidney. अतिवृक्कता; गुर्दे का आकार बढ़ जाना

**Renopathy.** Any disease of the kidney. वृक्करोग; गुर्दे की बीमारी

**Repair.** Restoring sound health, or healing processes. विरोहण; आरोग्यलाभ

**Repellent.** Capable of driving off or repelling; repulsive. विकर्षक; दूर हटा देने वाला अथवा अलग कर देने वाला

**Repercolation.** A repeated percolation. पुनःस्रवण; पुनःपरिस्रवण

**Repercussion.** Drawing back; repelling. प्रतिप्रभाव; प्रतिघात; प्रतिकार

**Repertory.** An index to the symptoms of diseases and their remedies, in which they are arranged in an orderly manner so

**Repetatur**

that they may be found without trouble. रिपर्टरी; चयनिका; भैषज्यचयनिका

**Repetatur.** Repeat. दुहराइये; दोहराइये

**Replantation.** Replacement of an organ or part back in its original site and re-establishing its circulation; re-implantation. पुन:रोपण; पुनर्रोपण

**Repletion.** The condition of being full. परिपूर्णावस्था; परिपूर्णता; प्रतिपूर्ति

**Replication.** Refolding or duplication of a part. प्रतिकृत्ति

**Reposition.** Replacement of a part. पुनर्स्थापन; नियोजन; निक्षेप; प्रत्यंगरोपण

**Repositioning.** See **Reduction**.

**Repositor.** An instrument for replacing a part. पुनर्स्थापित्र; पुन:स्थापी; पुनर्स्थापी

**Repression.** Suppression. दमन; उपशमन

**Reproduce.** To bring-forth an offspring. जनन करना; सन्तान पैदा करना

**Reproduction.** Regeneration. जनन; सन्तानोत्पत्ति

**Reproductive.** Pertaining to reproduction. जननीय; जनन सम्बन्धी

**Repulsive.** See **Repellent**.

**Resect.** To cut off; to excise a segment of a part. काट देना

**Resection.** Surgical excision. उच्छेदन; काटकर निकाल फेंकना

**Reservoir.** See **Receptaculum**.

**Resident.** A house officer, generally a doctor, attached to a hospital for clinical training after the internship. निवासी चिकित्सक

**Residua.** Plural of **Residuum**.

**Residual.** Remaining after a disease or any injury, as 'residual debility'. अवशिष्ट; अवशेषांगी

**Residue.** Remainder; rest; that which remains; residuum. अवशिष्ट; अवशेष; शेष; बाकी

**Residuum.** See **Residue**.

**Resin.** A mixture of complex organic substances which can occur naturally or be manufactured synthetically. रेजिन; राल; सर्जास; यक्षधूप

**Resinous.** Having the nature of a resin. रेजिनी; रालवत्

**Resistance.** Power of resisting; a passive force exerted in opposition to another and active force. प्रतिरोध

**Resolution.** Disappearance of a tumour or inflammation by a gradual process, without suppuration. शमन; विभेदन; शोथोपशमन; decomposition. विघटन; absorption. अवशोषण

**Resolvent.** That which causes solution of tissues. विलायक; शोथ अथवा प्रदाहनाशक औषधि या विलेपन

**Resonance.** A sound heard on percussing the chest or on ausculting chest during speech. अनुनाद; अनुकम्पन; सन्दोलन; प्रतिनाद;

**Tympanitic R.,** that heard on percussion over intestines and large lung cavities within walls. आध्मानी अनुनाद;

**Vesicular R.,** the normal pulmonary note. कोष्ठकी अनुनाद;

**Vocal R.,** the sound heard on auscultation of the chest during ordinary speech. श्रव्यवाक् अनुनाद

**Resonant.** Giving a vibrant sound on percussion. अनुनादी; प्रतिनादी; प्रतिनादित

**Resorption.** To absorb again. पुनःशोषण; पुनर्शोषण; पुनश्चूषण; पुनर्ग्रहण

**Respirable.** Suitable for respiration. श्वसनयोग्य; श्वासयोग्य; श्वास-प्रश्वास लेने योग्य

**Respiration.** The act of breathing; inhaling and exhaling air by the lungs. श्वसन; श्वास-प्रश्वास; श्वास; सांस;

**Abdominal R.,** respiration carried on by the diaphragm and abdominal muscles. उदरीय श्वसन; औदरिक श्वसन;

**Artificial R.,** artificial production of normal respiratory movements. कृत्रिम श्वसन; कृत्रिम रूप से श्वास पैदा करना;

**Bronchial R.,** a blowing respiration of the high pitch. श्वसनिका-श्वसन;

**Cutaneous R.,** the giving off of carbondioxide and taking up of oxygen through the skin. त्वक्श्वसन;

**Laboured R.,** difficult respiration. कष्टश्वसन; कष्टश्वास

**Respirator.** A device using alternate pressure and vacuum to help the patient's breath when they have had a paralysis due to illness or injury. श्वासित्र; श्वासयंत्र; श्वसनित्र

**Respiratory.** Pertaining to respiration; referring to the breathing organs. श्वास सम्बन्धी;

**R. Tract,** the part of the spinal cord whence the nerves of respiration take their rise. श्वासनली

**Response.** An action or movement due to the application of a stimulus. अनुक्रिया; प्रतिवेदन

**Rest.** Remainder. अवशिष्ट; शेष; repose after exertion. विश्राम

**Restitution.** A return to the normal condition. प्रत्यावर्तन; प्रत्यानयन; पुनर्स्थापन

**Restless.** Agitated mentally. व्यग्र; व्याकुल; बेचैन

**Restlessness.** Agitation due to mental or arterial disturbances. व्यग्रता; व्याकुलता; बेचैनी

**Restoration.** Recovery or renewal of health. समुत्थान; प्रत्यावर्तन; आरोग्यलाभ

**Restorative.** An agent restoring health and strength. शक्तिदाता; रोगनाशक; स्वास्थ्य एवं शक्ति प्रदान करने वाला

**Restraint.** Intervention, such as to prevent a maniacal patient from doing harm to himself or others. निग्रह

**Resuscitate.** To revive; to restore to life after apparent death. पुनर्जीवन देना; पुनर्जीवित करना

**Resuscitation.** Reviving from apparent death, as from drowning; revivification. पुनरुज्जीवन; पुनर्जीवन; पुनरुत्थान; होश में लाना या आना

**Retained.** Kept from departure or escape. प्रतिधृत; रुद्ध

**Retardation.** Delay; hinderance. विलम्बन; मन्दन; मन्दता; अवरुद्धता; अवरोध;

   **Mental R.,** subaverage intellectual functioning; amentia. बुद्धि-मन्दता

**Retarded.** Not developed in a normal way; dwarf; subnormal growth. विलम्बित; अल्पविकसित; अपूरित

**Retching.** An unsuccessful attempt at vomiting. वमनोद्रेक; उबकाई

**Rete.** A network of nerve fibres. जाल; जाली; पेशीजाल;

   **R. Mucosum,** the innermost layer of the epidermis. श्लेष्म जाल;

   **R. Testis,** one formed in the mediastinum testis. वृषण जाल

**Retention.** Stopping of natural discharges, as of urine, etc. रोध; रोधन; अवरोधन; अवधारण; धारण; रुकावट

**Retentive.** Having the power to retain. रोधी; धारक; प्रतिधारी; अवरोधक

**Retentivity.** See **Remanence.**

**Retia.** Plural of **Rete.**

**Retial.** Of the nature of a rete. जालीय; जालप्रकृति का

**Reticula.** Plural of **Reticulum.**

**Reticular.** Resembling a net; net-like; reticulated. जालीय; जालवत्; जालाकार; जालीदार; जाल जैसा; जालीरूप

**Reticulated.** See **Reticular.**

**Reticulation.** The presence or formation of a reticulum or network. जालिकाभवन

**Reticulocyte.** A net-like or meshed erythrocyte. जाललोहितकोशिका

**Reticulocytosis.** Excess of reticulocytes in the blood; reticulosis. जाललोहितकोशिकाबहुलता

**Reticuloendothelial System.** A widely scattered system of cells, of common ancestry and fulfilling many vital function, e.g. defence against infection, antibody, blood cells and bile pigment formation, etc. जालीयअन्तःकला प्रणाली; कोशिकाओं का एक विस्तारपूर्वक बिखरा हुआ जाल

**Reticuloendotheliosis.** Proliferation of the reticuloendothelium in any of the organs or tissues. जालीयअन्तःकलाकोशिकता

**Reticuloendothelium.** The cells making up the reticuloendothelial system. जालीयअन्तःकलाकोशिका

**Reticulosis.** See **Reticulocytosis.**

**Reticulum.** A fine network, formed by cells or formed of certain structures within cells or of connective tissue fibres between cells. जाल; जालिका; जाली

**Retifera.** A roundworm. गोलकृमि

**Retiform.** Net-shaped. जालवत्; जालाकार; जालरूप

**Retina.** The layer of light-sensitive nervous cells at the back of the inner surface of the eyeball which makes vision possible. दृष्टिपटल; नेत्रपटल; चक्षुपटल; अक्षिपट; अक्षिपटल

**Retinacula.** Plural of **Retinaculum.**

**Retinaculum.** A band holding back a part. उपबन्धनी

**Retinal.** Pertaining to the retina. अक्षिपटीय; चक्षुपटलीय; नेत्रपटलीय; नेत्रपटल सम्बन्धी

**Retinitis.** Inflammation of the retina. दृष्टिपटलशोथ; नेत्रपटलशोथ; दृष्टिपटल-व्यपजनन; नेत्रपटल-प्रदाह;
R. Pigmentosa, retinal sclerosis with atrophy and pigmentation. वर्णंकित दृष्टि-पटलव्यपजनन

**Retinoblastoma.** A malignant tumour of the neuroglial element of the retina, occurring exclusively in children. दृष्टिपटलप्रसूअर्बुद; कनीनिका की एक सांघातिक रसौली

**Retinochoroiditis.** Inflammation of both retina and choroid. दृष्टिरंजितपटलशोथ; कनीनिका एवं रंजितपटल का प्रदाह

**Retinopathy.** Any non-inflammatory disease of the retina. दृष्टिपटलविकृत्ति; कनीनिका का कोई प्रदाहरहित रोग

**Retinopexy.** Formation of chorioretinal adhesions surrounding a retinal tear for correction of retinal detachment. नेत्रपटलस्थिरण; दृष्टिपटलस्थिरण

**Retinoscope.** An instrument for the detection of refractive errors by illumination of retina using a mirror. दृष्टिपटलदर्शी; नेत्रापवर्तनमापी

**Retinoscopy.** The objective method of determining eye refraction by the character of reflected images. दृष्टिपटलदर्शन; नेत्रापवर्तनमापन

**Retort.** A vessel with a long neck in distillation. कांचपत्र; बकयंत्र; करमडेग; आसवन क्रिया के लिये प्रयुक्त किया जाने वाला शीशे का बर्तन

**Retractable.** See **Retractile.**

**Retractile.** Capable of being drawn back; retractable. आकुंचनशील; संकोचनीय; पीछे की ओर खिंच जाने योग्य

**Retraction.** The act of drawing back. प्रत्याकुंचन; आकुंचन; प्रतिगमन; संकोचन; निवर्तन; पीछे की ओर खींचने की क्रिया

**Retractor.** An instrument for drawing back the lip of the wound. प्रतिकर्षक; निवर्तित्र; घाव की चमड़ी पीछे खींचने वाली एक चिमटी; muscle that draws a part backward. आकुंचक (पेशी)

**Retreatment.** Treatment for the second time. पुनर्चिकित्सा; पुनर्संसाधन; दूसरी बार इलाज करना

**Retro-.** Prefix meaning backward or behind. 'प्रत्यक्', 'प्रत्यग्', 'पश्च' अथवा 'प्रति' के रूप में प्रयुक्त उपसर्ग

**Retrobulbar.** Of the back of the eyeball. पश्चनेत्रगोलकीय; प्रत्यगक्षिगोलकी; आँख की पुतली के पीछे वाला

**Retrocaecal.** Pertaining to the back of the cecum; retrocecal. प्रत्यक्-उण्डुकीय; अंधान्त्र के पिछले भाग सम्बन्धी

**Retrocecal.** See **Retrocaecal.**

**Retrocedent.** Disappearing from the surface; going back. प्रतिवर्ती; स्थानान्तरगामी; स्थान बदलने वाला

**Retrocession.** A retrograde movement; a going back; a relapse. प्रत्यावर्तन; प्रत्यागमन; पीछे को मुड़ना

**Retroflexed.** Bent backward. पश्चनत; पीछे की ओर झुका हुआ

**Retroflexion.** A bending or flexing backward. पश्चकुंचन; प्रत्यग्बक्रण; पीछे की ओर मुड़ना या मोड़ना

**Retrograde.** Receding or going backward. पश्चगतिक; पश्चगामी; प्रतिगामी

**Retrography.** A reversal of the order of writing. प्रतिलेख

**Retrogression.** A retrograde movement. प्रतिगमन; विपरीत गति

**Retroperitoneal.** Behind the peritoneum. प्रत्यक्-पर्युदर्यिक; उदरावरण के पीछे

**Retropharyngeal.** Behind the pharynx. प्रत्यक्-ग्रसनिक; ग्रसनी के पीछे

**Retropulsion.** Driving or turning back. पश्चसरण; पीछे की ओर चलना या मुड़ना

**Retroscope.** A speculum for rectal examination. प्रतिदर्शी; पश्चदर्शी; मलांत्रदर्शी; मलांत्रवीक्षकयंत्र

**Retrospection.** Morbid dwelling on the past. पश्चावलोकन; बीते हुए दिनों की याद में ही डूबा रहना

**Retroversion.** A turning back. पश्चनति; प्रत्यइ्नति; पीछे की ओर मुड़ना

**Reunion.** Joining again. पुन:संयोग; प्रतिसंयोग; पुनरेकन; दुबारा जुड़ना

**Revaccination.** Second or repeated vaccination. पुनर्टीकाकरण; दुबारा या बार-बार टीका लगाना

**Revellent.** Derivative; causing revulsion; revulsive. प्रत्युत्तेजक; प्रत्युत्तेजनकारी

**Reversal.** A turning in the opposite direction. उत्क्रमण; परिवर्तन

**Reversion.** A return to the original type. उत्क्रमण; प्रत्यावर्तन; परावर्तन; परिवर्तन; मूल रूप में वापस जाना

**Revivification.** See **Resuscitation.**

**Revulsion.** Diverting a disease from one part of the body to another. प्रत्युत्तेजन; रोग को शरीर के किसी एक भाग से दूसरे में स्थानान्तरित करना

**Revulsive.** See **Revellent.**

**Rhabdomyolysis.** An acute, fulminating, potentially fatal disease of skeletal muscle. रेखीपेशीलयन

**Rhabdomyoma.** A rare form of myoma containing striated muscular fibre. रेखीपेश्यर्बुद

**Rhabdomyosarcoma.** A malignant neoplasm derived from skeletal muscle; rhabdosarcoma. रेखीपेशीसार्कोमा; रेखी-सार्कोमा

**Rhabdosarcoma.** See **Rhabdomyosarcoma.**

**Rhachialgia.** Pain in the spine of the neck. ग्रीवामेरुशूल; backache. पृष्ठवेदना

**Rhachitis.** A constitutional disease of childhood marked by the increased cell growth of the bones, deficiency of earthy matter, deformities and changes in the liver and the spleen; rickets; rachitis. बालास्थिविकार; अस्थिविकार; हड्डी का दोष; रिक्केट

**Rhacoma.** Excoriating; chapping, निस्त्वचनीय; विदरण; pendulous scrotum. लम्बित अण्डकोष; लम्बित वृषणकोष

**Rhagade.** A fissure or chap in the skin or mucous membranes. परिद्वारक्षतचिन्ह; विदर; चमड़ी या श्लैष्मिक झिल्लियों की फटन

**Rhagades.** Plural of **Rhagade.**

**Rhagadia.** Plural of **Rhagade.**

**Rhaphe.** See **Raphe.**

**Rhegma.** A laceration or fracture. विदारण; अस्थिभंग; a rent or fissure. विदर

**Rheocord.** See **Rheostat.**

**Rheology.** The study of the deformation and flow of material. स्रावविज्ञान; स्रवणविज्ञान; धाराविज्ञान

**Rheometer.** A galvamometer. विद्युत्धारामापी

**Rheometry.** The measurement of the electric current or blood flow. विद्युत्धारामिति; रक्तस्रावमिति

**Rheostat.** An instrument for measuring the resistance of an electric current, or for adding any known resistance to an electric circuit; rheocard. धारानियंत्रक

**Rheum.** Catarrhal discharge. प्रतिश्यायी स्राव; a genus of plant. रियूम

**Rheumarthrosis.** Rheumatism of the joints. संधिवात

**Rheumatalgia.** Rheumatic pain. वातवेदना; आमवातार्ति; आमवाती दर्द

**Rheumatic.** Pertaining to the rheumatism. आमवाती; आमवात सम्बन्धी;

    **R. Diathesis,** a constitutional tendency to rheumatism. आमवाती प्रवणता;

    **R. Fever,** an acute, severe illness, usually the same as rheumatism. आमवात-ज्वर

**Rheumatism.** An acute disease with painful inflammation and swelling of one or more joints and often with endocarditis. आमवात; जोड़ों का दर्दनाक प्रदाह तथा सूजन;

    **Articular R.,** involves the soft tissues and includes fibrositis, lumbago, etc. सन्धि-आमवात; सन्धिवात;

    **Gonorrhoeal A.,** arthritis associated with urethritis. प्रमेहज आमवात;

**Inflammatory R.**, acute rheumatism with a tendency to valvular heart-disease. प्रदाहक आमवात;

**Lumbar R.**, lumbago. कटिवेदना;

**Muscular R.**, muscular pain with or without fever and other rheumatic symptoms. पेशी-आमवात; पेशीवात;

**Palindromic R.**, that of the recurring nature. पुनरावर्ती आमवात

**Rheumatoid.** Resembling rheumatism. आमवाताभ; आमवात सदृश; आमवात जैसा; गठियारूप;

**R. Arthritis,** a disease of unknown etiology, characterized by a chronic polyarthritis, mainly affecting the smaller peripheral joints. गठियारूप सन्धिशोथ; जोड़ों का गठियारूप प्रदाह

**Rheumatologist.** A specialist in the diagnosis and treatment of rheumatic condition. आमवातरोगविज्ञानी

**Rheumatology.** The science or the study of rheumatic disease. आमवातविज्ञान; आमवात रोग का वैज्ञानिक अध्ययन

**Rh-Factor.** A characteristic of blood which is of importance in pregnancy. र-फैक्टर; रक्त की विशेष अवस्था जिसकी महत्ता का अंकन सगर्भता के दौरान किया जाता है

**Rhin.** The nose. नासा; नाक; नासिका

**Rhinal.** Pertaining to, or belonging to the nose. नाक सम्बन्धी

**Rhinalgia.** Pain in the nose; rhinodynia. नासार्ति; नासिकार्ति; नाक का दर्द

**Rhinarium.** The nasal region. नासाप्रदेश; नासिकाप्रदेश

**Rhinencephalic.** Relating to the rhinencephalon. घ्राणमस्तिष्कीय; घ्राणमस्तिष्क सम्बन्धी

**Rhinencephalon.** The olfactory lobe of the brain. घ्राणमस्तिष्क; मस्तिष्क का घ्राणी खण्ड

**Rhinial.** Relating to olfaction. घ्राणी; घ्राणीय; घ्राण सम्बन्धी

**Rhinion.** The point at the lower end of the suture between the nasal bones. नासामूलबिन्दु; नासास्थिबिन्दु

**Rhinitis.** Inflammation of the mucous membrane of the nose. नासाशोथ; नासिका-प्रदाह;

**Acute R.,** coryza; cold in the head. प्रतिश्याय; सर्दी-जुकाम;

**Allergic R.,** rhinitis associated with hay fever. प्रत्यूर्जित नासाशोथ;

**Atrophic R.,** that followed by atrophy of the mucous membrane. शोषी नासाशोथ; नाक की झिल्ली का सूखा प्रदाह;

**Hypertrophic R.,** that marked by the hypertrophy of the nasal mucous membrane. अधिबृद्ध नासाशोथ; नाक की श्लेष्म कला की अतिबृद्धि के साथ प्रदाहक अवस्था;

**Purulent R.,** chronic rhinitis in which pus formation is excessive. सपूय नासाशोथ; पूतित नासाशोथ

**Rhinobyon.** A nasal plug or tampon. नासा पिचु; नाक बंद करने के लिये प्रयुक्त किया जाने वाला डाट

**Rhinocleisis.** See **Rhinostenosis.**

**Rhinodynia.** See **Rhinalgia.**

**Rhinogenous.** Originating in the nose. नासामूलक; नासाजनित

**Rhinolalia.** A nasal tone of the voice, due to nasal defect. अनुनासिकतादोष; अनुनासिकवाक्;

**R. Aperta,** that due to undue pustulousness of the posterior nares. असंवृत्तीय अनुनासिकतादोष;

**R. Clausa,** that due to undue closure of the posterior nares. रोधज अनुनासिकतादोष

**Rhinolite.** See **Rhinolith.**

**Rhinolith.** A nasal calculus; a stone in the nose; rhinolite. नासाश्मरी; नाक की पथरी

**Rhinolithiasis.** The formation of nasal calculus. नासाश्मरीयता

**Rhinologist.** A specialist in the diseases of the nose. नासिकारोगविज्ञानी; नासारोगविज्ञानी; नासारोगविशेषज्ञ

**Rhinology.** The science of the nose and its diseases. नासिकारोगविज्ञान; नासारोगविज्ञान; नासाज्ञान

**Rhinometer.** An instrument for measuring the nose. नासामापी

**Rhinonecrosis.** Necrosis of the nasal bone. नासास्थिगलन

**Rhinopathy.** Disease of the nose. नासाविकृति; नाक का रोग

**Rhinopharyngitis.** Inflammation of both nose and pharynx. नासाग्रसनीशोथ; नाक और ग्रसनी का प्रदाह

**Rhinophonia.** A nasal tone in speaking. अनुनासिकवाक्

**Rhinophyma.** Nodular enlargement of the skin of the nose. नासाबृद्धि; नाक की चमड़ी बढ़ कर कठोर हो जाना

**Rhinoplasty.** Any plastic operation on the nose. नासासंधान; नासिकासंधान

**Rhinopolypus.** Nasal polyp; a polypus of the nose. नासापुर्वंगक; नाक का पॉलिप

**Rhinorrhagia.** The same as **Epistaxis.**

**Rhinorrhea.** A mucous discharge from the nose; rhinorrhoea. नासास्राव; नाक से श्लैष्मिक स्राव होना

**Rhinorrhoea.** See **Rhinorrhea.**

**Rhinoscleroma.** A stony hardness of the skin and mucous membrane of the nose. नासाकठिनार्बुद; नाक की चमड़ी तथा श्लेष्म-कला की पत्थर जैसी कठोरता

**Rhinoscope.** An instrument for examining the nose. नासिकादर्शी; नासिकाजांचयंत्र

**Rhinoscopy.** The examination of the nasal fossas. नासिकादर्शन

**Rhinostenosis.** Nasal obstruction; rhinocleisis. नासारोध

**Rhinotomy.** Any cutting operation of the nose. नासा-उच्छेदन; नासाकर्तन

**Rhizome.** A subterranean stem. प्रकन्द

**Rhizotomy.** Surgical division of a root, usually the posterior root of a spinal nerve; radicotomy; radiculectomy; radiculotomy. मेरुतंत्रिकामूलछेदन; मेरुतंत्रिकामूलनिष्क्रियण

**Rhombencephalon.** The hind-brain. पश्चमस्तिष्क; मस्तिष्क का पिछला भाग

**Rhomboid.** Diamond-shaped. हीरकाकार; हीरकरूप; हीरे के आकार जैसा

**Rhonchal.** See **Rhonchial.**

**Rhonchi.** Plural of **Rhonchus.**

**Rhonchial.** Relating to the rhoncus; rhonchal. कण्ठ की खड़खड़ाहट अथवा घरघराहट सम्बन्धी

**Rhonchus.** See **Rhoncus.**

**Rhoncus.** A rattling in the throat; rhonchus. कण्ठ की खड़खड़ाहट अथवा घरघराहट

**Rhubarb.** The direct root of Chinese **Rheum Officinale.** रेवन्दचीनी

**Rhus.** A genus of shrubs. पौधों की एक जाति;

   R. **Toxicodendron,** poison oak or ivy, a powerful local irritant. बलूत-विष; सिरोंचा-विष;

   R. **Venenata,** poison ash. क्षार-विष

**Rhythm.** A measured periodic movement. ताल; एक नपी-तुली नियतकालिक गति; अनुक्रम;

   **Gallop R.,** a form of heart's action in which the cardiac sounds

# Rhythmic

occur in groups of three. बल्गित ताल; हृदय की क्रिया का एक रूप जिसमें हृद्ध्वनि तीन समूहों में प्रकट होती है

**Rhythmic.** Pertaining to the rhythm; rhythmical. तालबद्ध; क्रमबद्ध; ताल सम्बन्धी;

**R. Chorea**, a form of chorea in which the movements occur at regular intervals. तालबद्ध लास्य

**Rhythmical.** See **Rhythmic**.

**Rib.** Costa; one of the bones inclosing the chest; one of a series of 12 pairs of narrow, curved bones extending laterally and anteriorily from sides of thoracic vertebrae and foming a part of the skeletal thorax. पर्शुका; पसली;

**False R.**, one of the five lower ribs not attached directly to the sternum. कूट-पर्शुका;

**Floating R.**, one of the two lower ribs on either side that are not attached anteriorly. चल-पर्शुका;

**True R.**, one of the seven upper ribs attached to the sternum. यथार्थ पर्शुका

**Riboflavine.** A constituent of Vitamin 'B' Complex, found generally in green vegetables, liver, kidneys, wheat germ, milk, eggs and cheese. रिबोफ्लैविन; विटामिन 'बी' कॉम्प्लेक्स का एक घटक

**Rice-water Stool.** The stool of Asiatic cholera. माण्डाभ मल; हैजाजनित दस्त

**Ricin.** A toxic albuminoid from castor-oil bean. रिसिन; एरण्ड की फलियों से प्राप्त होने वाला अन्नसार

**Ricinin.** A crystalline alkaloid from castor-oil. रिसिनिन; एरण्ड की फलियों से प्राप्त होने वाला एक मणिभ रवेदार पदार्थ

**Ricinus.** A genus of plants furnishing castor-oil. एरण्ड का पौधा

**Rickets.** Rachitis; a constitutional disease of childhood, marked by the increased cell-growth of the bones, deficiency of earthy matter, deformities and changes in the liver and the spleen. रिक्केट; बालास्थिविकार; अस्थिवक्रता; हड्डियों का टेढ़ापन

**Rickettsia.** Unknown organism found in typhus. रिक्केट्टसिया; मोहज्वर में पाया जाने वाला एक जीवाणु

**Rickettsiae.** Plural of **Rickettsia**.

**Rickety.** Affected with rickets. रिक्केट्ग्रस्त; रिक्केट रोग से पीड़ित; बालास्थिविकारग्रस्त

**Ricord's chancre.** The parchment-like initial lesion of syphilis. उपदंश का चर्मपटतुल्य प्रारम्भिक घाव

**Rider's bone.** A bony formation in the leg-muscles from riding. घुड़सवारों की टांगों की पेशियों में होने वाली अस्थिरचना

**Ridge.** A linear elevation (usually rough). कटक

**Riggs' disease.** See **Periodontitis.**

**Right.** Opposite to left; dextral. दक्षिण; दायाँ; दाईं;

**Rigid.** Stiff. कठोर; दृढ़; अकड़ी हुई

**Rigidity.** Stiffness; immobility or inflexibility. कठोरता; दृढ़ता; अकड़न; ऐंठन

**Rigor.** Stiffness; rigidity. काठिन्य; अकड़न; कठोरता; sudden sense of chilliness. शीतकम्प; कम्पकम्पी; कम्पन;

   **R. Mortis,** the rigidity of the body after death. मृत्युज काठिन्य; मृत्यु के बाद होने वाली कठोरता;

   **Postmortem R.,** the same as **Rigor Mortis.**

**Rima.** A fissure or furrow; rime. रेखाछिद्र; विदर;

   **R. Glottidis,** the opening between the vocal bands; rima vocalis. कण्ठ-रेखाछिद्र;

   **R. Vestibuli,** the interval between the false vocal folds. प्रघाण रेखाछिद्र;

   **R. Vocalis,** see **Rima Glottidis.**

**Rime.** See **Rima.**

**Rimose.** Fissured; marked by cracks. विदरित; फटा हुआ

**Rimula.** A small fissure. क्षुद्र-विदर

**Ring.** A circular opening. वलय; छल्ला; अंगूठी; वृत्ताकार मुख

**Ring-knife.** A circular or oval ring with internal cutting edge for shaving off tumours in the nasal and other cavities. गुहार्बुदछुरिका; रिंग-नाइफ

**Ringworm.** A fungus infection of the skin, hair and nails; herpes circinatus. दद्रु; दाद; मण्डलकुष्ठ; चमड़ी का एक कवक रोग

**Risus.** Laughter-like. हास्यानुकारी;

   **R. Sardonicus,** the spastic grin of tetanus. हास्यानुकारी मुखभंग

**R.M.P.** Registered Medical Practitioner. पंजीकृत चिकित्सक

**Robertson's Bullock-heart Media.** Cooked meat media; administering medicine through cooked meat. पक्वमांस माध्यम

**Robertson's pupil.** The same as **Argyll Robertson's pupil.**

**Roborant.** Tonic; strengthening. बलवर्धक; शक्तिदायक

**Rock-fever.** Malta fever. चट्टान-ज्वर; माल्टा-ज्वर; माल्टा-द्वीप में होने वाला ज्वर

**Rock-salt.** Common salt found in masses or beds. खनिजलवण; सेंधा नमक

**Rod.** A straight cylindrical formation. शलाका; छड़

**Roentgen Rays.** Invisible light rays which penetrate the most solids. रौंटजन किरणें; रायंटजन किरणें

**Roentgenism.** Disease from misuse of x-ray or roentgen rays. रौंटजनता; रायंटजनता; एक्स-रेरुग्णता

**Roentgenogram.** Skiagraphic radiograph. रौंटजनचित्रण; विकिरणचित्रण

**Roentgenography.** Skiagraphy; radiography. रौंटजनलेख; विकिरणलेख

**Roengenology.** See **Radiology.**

**Roger's disease.** The presence of a congenital abnormal communication between the two ventricles of the heart; ventricular septal defect. रॉगर रोग

**Rollet's Chancre.** Mixed chancre. रौल्लेट शैंकर; मिश्र कठिनार्बुद

**Roominess.** Specific volume. विशिष्ट-आयतन

**Root.** The base or place of origin; radix. मूल; जड़; आधार; आधारिक; मूलस्थानिक;

   **R. Amputation,** see **Radiectomy.**

**Rosacea.** A skin disease which shows on flush areas of the face, especially in women at menopause; acne rosacea. गुलाबचर्मता; गुलाबी मुहासे

**Rosae.** A genus of the plants of the order of rosacea. गुलाब

**Rose.** The same as **Rosae;** a term applied to erysipelas from its colour. गुलाबी विसर्प;

   **R. Catarrh,** see **Rose Cold.**

   **R. Cold,** hay-fever; rose-catarrh. तृणपुष्प ज्वर; परागज ज्वर;

   **R. Hips,** the fruit or seed of a rose, used in pharmacy and promoted by food faddists. गुलाब का बीज;

   **R. Rash,** scarlet-rash; roseola. गुलाबी दाना; लाल खसरा

**Roseola.** Rose-rash; scarlet-rash. लाल खसरा; गुलाबी दाना; muscular erythemia. पेशी-त्वग्रक्तिमा

**R. Infantum,** a non-contagious roseola in infants. असंक्रामी स्फोटक

**Rostellum.** A small beak. शीर्षांग; तुण्डक; छोटी चोंच; क्षुद्रचंचु

**Rostra.** Plural of **Rostrum.**

**Rostral.** Relating to a rostrum. चंचु सम्बन्धी

**Rostrate.** Beaked; having a beak or hook. चंचुक

**Rostrum.** A projection or ridge; a beak. चंचु; तुण्ड

**Rot.** Decay; decomposition. विगलन; क्षय

**Rotation.** Turning on the axis. घूर्णन; परिभ्रण; परिक्रमण

**Rotator.** A muscle having the action of turning a part. आवर्तनी पेशी; किसी भाग को मोड़ने वाली पेशी

**Rotula.** The knee-pan or patella. जान्वस्थि; घुटने की चौड़ी हड्डी

**Rotular.** Pertaining to the patella. जान्वस्थिक; जान्वस्थि सम्बन्धी

**Roughage.** Coarse food containing much indigestible vegetable fibre composed of cellulose. रूक्षांश; रेशा; अनाज का चोकर आदि

**Rouleaux.** A row of red blood cells, resembling a roll of coins. गुल्ली; लाल रक्त कोशिकाओं की पंक्ति

**Round Ligament.** Ligamentus teres hepatis, i.e. the round ligament of the liver, the remains of umbilical vein. गोलबन्धन

**Roundworm.** An intestinal worm, called ascaride, which infects children, usually through contact with infected pets, especially dogs and cats. गोलकृमि; केंचुवा

**Rub.** Friction encountered in moving one body over another. घर्षण; घीसना; रब; घर्षध्वनि

**Rubefacient.** An agent that reddens the skin. रक्तिमकारी

**Rubefaction.** Erythema of the skin. रक्तचर्मता; त्वग्रक्तिमा

**Rubella.** Infectious fever of childhood, resembling mild measles; German measles, lasting for one day. रूबेला; जर्मन रोमान्तिका अथवा खसरा

**Rubeola.** Red measles lasting for five days; an exanthematous contagious disease of children; also called **Rubeola Vulgaris.** रोमान्तिका; खसरा;

**R. Vulgaris,** see **Rubeola.**

**Rubia Cordifolia.** A genus of plants. मंजीठ

**Rubigo.** Rust. जंग

**Rubor.** Erythema. रक्तिमा; redness. लाली

**Ructus.** The belching of wind from the stomach. उबकाई; डकार

**Rudiment.** An organ or structure that is incompletely developed; the first indication of a structure in the course of ontogeny; rudimentum. मूलांग; आद्यावशेष

**Rudimenta.** Plural of **Rudiment.**

**Rudimentary.** Undeveloped; not formed. मूलांगी; आद्यांगिक; अल्पवर्धित; अविकसित

**Rudimentum.** See **Rudiment.**

**Ruga.** A wrinkle. झुर्री; वलय

**Rugae.** Plural of **Ruga.**

**Rugose.** Wrinkled; rugous; marked by rugae. झुर्रीदार; वलयी

**Rugosity.** The condition of being in wrinkles. झुर्रियां पड़ना; वलयन

**Rugous.** See **Rugose.**

**Rule.** Criterion. नियम; standard. मानक; guide. मार्गदर्शक

**Rumbling.** A low gurgling in the stomach. गुड़गुड़ाहट; गड़गड़ाहट

**Ruminant.** An animal that chews the cud (sheep, cow, deer, etc.). चतुष्पदी पशु, जैसे भेड़, गाय, हिरन, आदि जो खाने या चरने के बाद जुगाली करते हैं; रोमन्थक (पशु)

**Rumination.** Remastication of swallowed food. रोमन्थन; निगले हुए भोजन का पुनर्चर्वण

**Rump.** The end of the back-bone. पुट्ठा; the buttocks. कूल्हे; नितम्ब

**Rundown.** Weak; debilitated. क्षीण; दुर्बल; कमजोर

**Rupia.** A syphilitic eruption with incrusted foul ulcers. रूपिया; उपदंश; उपदंश का एक पपड़ीदार विस्फोट; yaws. फफोले; याज

**Rupture.** A break of any organ or soft part. विदर; छिद्र; फटन; हर्निया

# S

**Sac.** Bag; a cyst; a pouch. कोश; नली; थैली;

**Lacrimal S.,** the dilated upper portion of the lacrimal duct; lachrymal sac. अश्रुनली;

**S. Lac,** abbreviated form of **Saccharum Lactis.**

**Lachrymal S.,** see **Lacrimal Sac.**

**S.-shaped,** see **Sacciform.**

**Saccadic.** Jerky. क्षेपक; क्षेपीय; झटकेदार

**Saccate.** Relating to a sac. कोशीय; कोश सम्बन्धी

**Saccharated.** Containing sugar. शर्करित; शर्करायुक्त; शर्करालिप्त; शर्करीय

**Saccharephidrosis.** Sweet perspiration. मधुस्वेद; मीठा पसीना

**Sacchariferous.** Containing sugar. शर्करित; शर्करायुक्त; शर्करालिप्त; शर्करीय

**Saccharification.** Conversion into sugar. शर्करीकरण; शर्करीभवन

**Saccharimeter.** See **Saccharometer.**

**Saccharin.** A well known sugar substitute, containing sugar. सैक्रीन; सैकेरिन; कोलतार शक्कर

**Saccharine.** Relating to sugar. शर्करा सम्बन्धी; sweet. मीठा; मीठी

**Saccharolytic.** Capable of breaking down a sugar molecule. शर्करालायी

**Saccharometer.** An instrument for estimating the amount of sugar in a solution; saccharimeter. शर्करामापी; किसी घोल में शर्करा को मापने का यंत्र

**Saccharose.** Cane-sugar; sucrose. शर्करा; इक्षुशर्करा; ईख से निर्मित शर्करा (चीनी)

**Saccharum.** Sugar; sucrose. शर्करा; चीनी;

   **S. Album,** white sugar. श्वेत-शर्करा;

   **S. Lactis,** sugar of milk, or milk-sugar; lactose. दुग्ध-शर्करा; लैक्टोस

**Sacci.** Plural of **Saccus.**

**Sacciform.** Of the form of a sac; saccular; sacculated; sac-shaped; pouched. कोशाकार; कोशरूप

**Saccular.** Like a sac. लघुकोशाभ; लघुकोशाकार; pertaining to a sac. लघुकोशीय; लघुकोश सम्बन्धी; sacciform; sacculated; sac-shaped. कोशाकार; कोशरूप

**Sacculated.** See **Sacciform.**

**Saccule.** A small sac; sacculus. लघुकोश; क्षुद्रनली

**Sacculus.** See **Saccule.**

**Saccus.** A sac. कोश; नली; थैली;

   **S. Endolymphaticus,** a sac of the duramater in the aqueduct of the vestibule. अन्तरुदक कोश;

**Saccus**

S. **Lachrymalis,** see **Saccus Lacrimalis.**

S. **Lacrimalis,** the lacrimal sac; saccus lachrymalis. अश्रुकोश; अश्रुनली

**Sachral.** Situated in, or related to sacrum; sacral. त्रिकास्थिज; त्रिकज; त्रिकास्थि सम्बन्धी

**Sachralgia.** Pain in the sacrum; sacralgia; sacrodynia. त्रिकार्ति; त्रिकशूल; त्रिकास्थिशूल

**Sacral.** See **Sachral.**

**Sacralgia.** See **Sachralgia.**

**Sacrectomy.** Resection of a portion of the sacrum to facilitate an operation. त्रिक-उच्छेदन

**Sacro-.** A term applied to parts connected with the sacrum. 'त्रिक' शब्द के रूप में प्रयुक्त उपसर्ग

**Sacrococcygeal.** Pertaining to the sacrum and the coccyx. त्रिकानुत्रिकीय; त्रिक एवं अनुत्रिक सम्बन्धी

**Sacrocoxalgia.** Pain in the sacrum and the coccyx. त्रिकानुत्रिकार्ति; त्रिक एवं अनुत्रिक का दर्द

**Sacrocoxitis.** Inflammation of the sacroiliac joint; sacroiliac disease. त्रिकानुत्रिकसन्धिशोथ; त्रिक एवं अनुत्रिक के जोड़ का प्रदाह

**Sacrodynia.** See **Sacralgia.**

**Sacroiliac.** Pertaining to the sacrum and the ileum. त्रिकश्रोणिफलकीय; त्रिक एवं श्रोणिफलक सम्बन्धी;

S. **Disease,** see **Sacrocoxitis.**

**Sacrolumbar.** Pertaining to the sacrum and the loins. त्रिककटीय; त्रिककटिज; त्रिककटि सम्बन्धी अथवा त्रिकास्थि तथा कमर सम्बन्धी

**Sacrum.** The triangular bone above the coccyx. त्रिक; त्रिकास्थि; पुच्छास्थि के ऊपर एक त्रिकोणक हड्डी

**Saddle.** Anything shaped like a seat, as of a rider's seat to be placed on the horse's back, a seat of bicycle, etc. पर्याण; काठी;

S.**-back,** anterior curvature of the spine. अग्रकुब्जता;

S.**-joint,** a concavo-convex articulation. अवतलोत्तल सन्धि;

S.**-nose,** one with flattened bridge of nose, often a sign of congenital syphilis. पर्याणनासा; काठीरूप नासिका; काठी जैसी नाक

**Sadism.** The obtaining of pleasure from inflicting pain, violence or degradation on another person, or the sexual partner. परपीडनकामुकता; दूसरे साथी को कष्ट देकर उसके साथ लैंगिक सम्भोग करना

**Sadist.** One who takes pleasure in sadism. परपीडनकामुक; दूसरे साथी को पीड़ा देकर लैंगिक सम्भोग करने वाला

**Sadistic.** Pertaining to, or characterized by sadism. परपीडनकामुकता सम्बन्धी; sadist. परपीडनकामुक

**Sadness.** An emotional feeling of dejection and melancholy. उदासी

**Safflower.** A genus of plants. कुसुम्भ; करड़ी

**Saffron.** Crocus sativus; the stigmas of flowers are emmenagogue. केसर; केसरी

**Sage.** A starchy fecula from certain plants. साबूदाना; सागू

**Sage-femme.** A midwife. धातृ; दाई

**Sagittal.** Resembling an arrow. शराभ; बाण जैसा; antero-posterior. अग्र-पश्च; सममितार्धी; मध्यतल; आगे-पीछे

**Sal.** A salt. लवण; नमक;

**S. Ammonia,** aromatic solution of ammonia. नौसादर

**Salaceous.** Lustful, or inciting to lust. कामुक; व्यभिचारी

**Salacity.** Strong venereal desire. अतिकामोद्रेक; सम्भोग की प्रबल इच्छा

**Saliferous.** Containing saline; salty. लवणमय; लवणयुक्त; नमकीन

**Saline.** Containing or pertaining to salt; salty. लवणयुक्त; लवण सम्बन्धी; सैलाइन

**Salinometer.** An instrument for measuring the quantity of salt in a solution. लवणमापी; किसी घोल में नमक की मात्रा मापने का यंत्र

**Saliva.** The spittle; the secretion of the salivary glands of the mouth which aids mastication, swallowing, etc. लाला; लार; थूक

**Salivant.** Stimulating the flow of saliva; salivatory. लालाकारी; लालास्रावक; लारोत्पादक; लारजन्य; लार के बहाव को उद्दीप्त करने वाला

**Salivary.** Pertaining to the saliva. लारमय; लार वाला; लार सम्बन्धी;

**S. Calculus,** a stone formed in the salivary ducts. लालाश्मरी; लारपथरी;

**S. Glands,** six in number and located three on each side of the mouth; they secrete the saliva which moistens the food during chewing and begins the digestive process. लाला-ग्रन्थियाँ; लार-ग्रन्थियाँ

**Salivation.** Production of an excessive flow of saliva, as by mercury. लालास्रवण; लालास्राव; लारस्राव; लारमयता

**Salivator.** An agent causing salivation. लालानिस्सारक; लारनिस्सारक; लार पैदा करने वाला पदार्थ

**Salivaroty.** See **Salivant.**

**Salk Vaccine.** A preparation of killed poliomyelitis virus and as an antigen to produce active artificial immunity to poliomyelitis. साक वैक्सीन; पोलियोरोधी टीका

**Sallow.** Pallid. पाण्डुरवर्ण; पाण्डुवर्ण; पीतवर्ण; पीला

**Salmonella.** A genus of bacteria belonging to the family of **Enterobacteriaceae,** causing gastroenteritis and enteric fever. साल्मोनेला; एण्टीरोवैक्टीरियाई परिवार का एक जीवाणु जो जठरांत्रशोथ एवं आंत्रिक ज्वर का कारण होता है

**Salpingectomy.** Excision of a Fallopian tube. डिम्बवाहिनी-उच्छेदन; अण्डाणुनाल-उच्छेदन; डिम्बवाही नली को काट कर हटा देना

**Salpinges.** Plural of **Salpix.**

**Salpingitic.** Relating to salpingitis. डिम्बवाहिनीशोथ सम्बन्धी

**Salpingitis.** Inflammation of the Fallopian tube. डिम्बवाहिनीशोथ; अण्डाणुनालशोथ; डिम्बवाही नली का प्रदाह;

**Interstitial S.,** that with excessive formation of connective tissue. अन्तरालीय डिम्बवाहिनीशोथ;

**Purulent S.,** salpingitis with secretion of pus instead of mucus or serum; suppurative salpingitis. पूयस्रावी डिम्बवाहिनीशोथ;

**Suppurative S.,** see **Purulent Salpingitis.**

**Salpingogram.** Radiological examination of tubal patency by injecting an opaque substance into the uterus and along the tubes. डिम्बवाहिनीचित्र

**Salpingography.** Radiographic imaging of the uterine tubes after injection of a radio-opaque substance. डिम्बवाहिनीचित्रण

**Salpingolithiasis.** The formation of a calculus in the Fallopian tube. डिम्बवाहिनी-अश्मरीयता; डिम्बवाही नली के अन्दर पथरी बनना

**Salpingolysis.** Surgical disruption of adhesions in the Fallopian tube. डिम्बवाहिनीलयन

**Salpingo-oophorectomy.** Excision of an ovary and the oviduct. डिम्बवाहिनीग्रन्थि-उच्छेदन

**Salpingo-oophoritis.** Inflammation of an ovary and tube; salpingo-ovaritis. डिम्बवाहिनीग्रन्थिशोथ

**Salpingo-ovaritis.** See **Salpingo-oophoritis.**

**Salpingoperitonitis.** Inflammation of both ovary and peritoneum. डिम्बवाहिनीपर्युदर्याशोथ; डिम्बवाहिनी एवं उदरावरण का प्रदाह

**Salpingopexy.** Surgical fixation of an oviduct. डिम्बवाहीनलीस्थिरीकरण

**Salpingoplasty.** Surgical repair of the Fallopian tube. डिम्बवाहीनलीसंधान

**Salpinx.** Fallopian tube; they are two in number; salpynx. डिम्बवाहिनी; अण्डाणुनाल; डिम्बवाही नली

**Salpynx.** See **Salpinx**.

**Salt.** Any union of a base with an acid; chloride of soda; sodium chloride. लवण; नमक

**Salting-in.** A conversion into salt. लवणन; नमक में बदलना

**Salting-out.** Making free from salt. लवणक्षेपण; नमकविहीन करना

**Salty.** See **Saliferous**.

**Salubrious.** Pertaining to health. स्वास्थ्य सम्बन्धी; healthful. स्वास्थ्यप्रद; आरोग्यकारी

**Salubrity.** The same as **Salubrious**.

**Salus.** Health. स्वास्थ्य

**Salutary.** Healthful; promoting health; wholesome. स्वास्थ्यप्रद; आरोग्यवर्धक; आरोग्यकारी

**Salve.** An ointment; an unguentum. मलहम; मरहम; अनुलेप

**Sample.** A specimen. प्रतिदर्श; नमूना

**Sanation.** The act of healing. विरोहण; विरोहण क्रिया

**Sanatoria.** Plural of **Sanatorium**.

**Sanatorium.** A special hospital for the treatment of tubercular patients. क्षयरोगचिकित्सालय; सैनेटोरियम

**Sanatory.** Health-giving; curative. स्वास्थ्यदायी; रोगमुक्तिकारी

**Sand.** Minute fragments of stone. बालुका; बालु; बालू; रेत; सिकता;
  **S.-bath,** hot sand for the immersion of a vessel. बालुका-ऊष्मक; बालु-ऊष्मक; सिकता-स्नान;
  **S.-fly,** responsible for short, sharp, pyrexial fever, called "sand-fly fever" of the tropics. बालु-मक्षिका;
  **S.-fly Fever,** fever caused due to sand-fly. बालु-मक्षिका ज्वर

**Sane.** Of sound mind. स्वस्थचित्त; संयत; प्रकृतिस्थ

**Sanguifacient.** Making blood; hemopoietic. रक्तनिर्माणक

**Sanguiferous.** Conveying blood. रक्तवाही; circulatory. रक्तसंचारी

**Sanguification.** Conversion of the chyle into the blood; hemopoiesis. रक्तनिर्माण; रक्तीकरण; रक्तीभवन; अन्नरस से बनने वाला रक्त

**Sanguifluxus.** Haemorrhage; abnormal bleeding. रक्तस्राव; खून बहना

**Sanguine.** Abounding with blood; of the nature of blood; bloody. रक्तवर्ण; आरक्त; रक्तपूर्ण; hopeful. आशावादी; cheerful; full of vitality. उल्लासमय; आह्लादित

**Sanguineous.** Plethoric; full of blood. रक्तप्रधान; रक्तबहुल; bloody. रक्तिम; रक्तमिश्रित; relating to blood. रक्त सम्बन्धी

**Sanguinolent.** Tinged with blood; bloody. रक्तरंजित; रक्तमिश्रित; सरक्त; रक्ताभ

**Sanguinopurulent.** Containing blood and pus. रक्तपूतियुक्त; रक्तपूतिमिश्रित

**Sanguis.** Blood. रक्त; खून

**Sanguivorus.** Blood-sucking. रक्तजीवी; रक्तचूषक; खून चूसने वाला

**Sanies.** A thin, often blood-stained purulent discharge from wounds on sores, hence sanious. पतला रक्तपूतिस्राव; पतली रक्तमिश्रित पीब बहना

**Sanious.** Ichorus and blood-stained. पूयरक्तक; तीखा एवं रक्तरंजित

**Sanitarium.** An older name for a mental disease hospital. मनोरोगचिकित्सालय; मानसिक रोगों के चिकित्सालय का पुराना नाम

**Sanitary.** Promoting or pertaining to health. आरोग्यवर्धक; स्वास्थ्यवर्धक; relating to cleanliness and health. स्वच्छता अथवा स्वास्थ्य सम्बन्धी; healthful. स्वस्थ

**Sanitation.** The proper disposal of all wastes and various matters and proper cleanliness in regard to foodstuff, environment, etc. स्वच्छता; समार्जन; सफाई

**Sanitization.** The sanitary arrangements; the process of making something sanitary. स्वच्छता-प्रबन्ध; सफाई का इन्तजाम

**Sanity.** The condition of soundness of mind, emotion and behaviour. स्वस्थचित्तता; विवेकशीलता

**Santalam Album.** White sandal wood. श्वेत चन्दनवृक्ष

**Santonica.** The flower heads of **Artemesia pauciflora;** levant wormseed; it is anthelmintic. किरमानी पुष्प

**Sap.** The vital juice circulating in plants. रस; पौधों में संचरणशील जैवी तत्व

**Saphena.** A name given to two large veins of the leg. जघनशिरा; टांग की दो बड़ी शिराओं के लिये प्रयुक्त नाम

**Sapientiaedentes.** Wisdom teeth; posterior molars. पृष्ठचर्वणक; अक्ल

दाढ़

**Sapo.** Soap; compound of a fatty acid with alkaline base. साबुन

**Saponaceous.** Containing or having the properties of soap. मेदुर; साबुनी; साबुन जैसा; साबुन वाला

**Saponification.** A conversion into soap. साबुनीकरण; साबुनीभवन; साबुन में बदलना

**Sapor.** Taste; relish. स्वाद; जायका

**Saporific.** Producing taste or flavour. सुस्वादु; जायकेदार; मजेदार

**Sapphism.** Unnatural sexual intercourse between women. स्त्रीसमलिंगकामुकता; स्त्रियों में समलिंगी कामुकता

**Sapraemia.** See **Sapremia**.

**Sapremia.** Blood poisoning; sapraemia. रक्तविषण्णता; पूतिरक्तता

**Saprodontia.** Caries of the teeth. कृमिदन्त; दन्तक्षरण; दन्तक्षय

**Saprogen.** Any micro-organism living on dead organic matter and causing putrefaction. पूतिजन

**Saprogenic.** Arising in decaying matter; saprogenous; saprozoic. पूतिजनक; पूतिकारक

**Saprogenous.** See **Saprogenic**.

**Saprophyte.** A plant deriving its substance from dead organic matter. मृतोपजीवी; मृतजीवी; मृतभक्षी

**Saprophytic.** Pertaining to saprophytes. मृतोपजीवीपरक; मृतजीवीपरक; मृतजीवियों सम्बन्धी

**Saprostomous.** Having a foul breath. दुर्गन्धित श्वास

**Saprozoic.** See **Saprogenic**.

**Sarchinae.** Small micro-organisms found in the stomach sometimes. सूक्ष्मातिसूक्ष्मजीवाणु

**Sarcina.** A genus of bacteria. घनगोलाणु

**Sarcitis.** Inflammation of the muscle tissues. पेशीऊतकशोथ; पेशीऊतकों का प्रदाह

**Sarco-.** Prefix meaning flesh. 'मांस' के रूप में प्रयुक्त उपसर्ग

**Sarcoblast.** Myoblast; embryonic cell that develops into a muscle cell. पेशीमांसप्रसू

**Sarcocele.** A fleshy tumour of the testicles. वृषणमांसार्बुद; वृषणार्बुद; वृषणों की एक मांसल रसौली

**Sarcode.** A name for animal protoplasm. सारकोड; जीवद्रव्य का एक नाम

**Sarcoid.** Resembling flesh; tumour. मांसार्बुदाभ; मांसल अर्बुद अथवा मांस की रसौली जैसा

**Sarcology.** The science of the soft tissue of the body. मृदूतिविज्ञान; शरीर के कोमल ऊतकों से सम्बद्ध विज्ञान

**Sarcoma.** A malignant cancerous tumour arising from a bone, muscle or other framework or the tissue in the body. भ्रूणार्बुद; ऊतकार्बुद; सार्कार्बुद; सार्कोमा

**Sarcomata.** Plural of **Sarcoma.**

**Sarcomatoid.** Resembling a sarcoma. सार्कोमाभ; सार्कार्बुदाभ; ऊतकार्बुदाभ

**Sarcomatosis.** A condition in which sarcomata are widely spread throughout the body. बहुऊतकार्बुद; वह अवस्था जिसमें सारे शरीर में दूर-दूर तक सार्कार्बुद फैले रहते हैं

**Sarcomatous.** Having the nature of sarcoma. सार्कार्बुदाभ; सार्कोमाभ; भ्रूणार्बुदाभ; ऊतकार्बुदाभ; मध्यजनस्तराभ

**Sarcopoietic.** Forming muscle. मांसनिर्माणक; पेशीनिर्माणक

**Sarcosis.** Abnormal growth of flesh. अतिमांसबृद्धि; अस्वाभाविक मांसबृद्धि; अत्यधिक मांस बढ़ना

**Sarcotic.** Producing flesh. मांसोत्पादक; मांस बढ़ाने वाला; relating to flesh. मांस सम्बन्धी

**Sarcous.** Fleshy. मांसल; मांसाभ; मांस जैसा; relating to muscular tissue. मांसोतक सम्बन्धी

**Sardonic.** A convulsive affection of the muscles of the face accompanying some spasmodic diseases. अनैच्छिक; निरंकुश; असंयत; चेहरे की मांस-पेशियों का एक आक्षेपी रोग

**Sardonicus.** Demoniac laughter; the spastic grin of tetanus; risus sardonicus. हास्यानुकारी मुखभंग

**Sarsaparilla.** The rhizome of **Smilax Officinalis** and other species of smilax. चोबचीनी

**Satellite.** A vein accompanying an artery. धमनीसहचराशिरा; अनुषंगीशिरा; धमनी के साथ-साथ चलती हुई शिरा

**Satellitism.** Mutualism; symbiosis. आनुषंगिकता; साहचर्य

**Satiety.** Fullness beyond desire, especially with food. तृप्ति; संतृप्ति

**Saturate.** To fill to excess. संतृप्त होना; संतृप्त करना

**Saturated.** Having all the chemic affinities satisfied. संतृप्त;

   **S. Solution,** solution containing as much of the solid drug material as can be dissolved. संतृप्त घोल

**Saturation.** The condition of holding in solution all of a solid, capable of being contained. संतृप्ति; संतृप्तीकरण

**Saturnine.** Pertaining to lead. सीसज; सीसा सम्बन्धी

**Saturnism.** See Saturnismus.

**Saturnismus.** Lead-poisoning; plumbism; saturnism. सीसाविष; सीसाजनित विषण्णता; सीसात्यय

**Satyriasis.** Excessive venereal desire in males. कामार्ति; अतिकामोद्रेक; पुरुषों में अतिकामुकता

**Savill's Disease.** Epidemic eczema. व्यापक छाजन; महामारीरूप छाजन; सैविल रोग

**Saw.** A surgical instrument for the excision of a bone. क्रकच; आरी

**Scab.** A crust formed over a wound or ulcer. शल्क; पर्पटी; खुरण्ड; पपड़ी; पामा; कण्डू

**Scabicidal.** Destructive to itch-mites. कण्डूपरजीवीनाशक; खाजपरजीवीनाशक

**Scabicide.** Lethal to itch-mites. कण्डूपरजीवीमारक; खाजपरजीवीमारक

**Scabies.** The itch, a contagious parasitic skin disease. कण्डू; खाज; खुजली; पामा;

S. **Vesicula Humida,** watery itch. सजल खुजली; सजल कण्डू

**Scabrities.** Abnormal thickening of the finger nails. नखस्थूलता; नाखुनों का अस्वाभाविक मोटापन

**Scala.** A bladder-like organ; the cochlear canal. अध:कुल्या; कोई आशयनुमा अंग

**Scald.** An injury caused by moist heat. तप्तद्रवदाहक्षत; तप्तद्रवदाह; भाप या गर्म पानी से जल कर बनने वाला घाव;

S.-**head,** inflammation of the scalp. शिरोवल्कशोथ; करोटिशोथ; खोपड़ी का प्रदाह

**Scale.** A thin crust covering the skin. पर्पटी; शल्क; पपड़ी; खुरण्ड; measurement. माप; to desquamate. पपड़ी उतरना या उतारना

**Scaled.** Crusted. पर्पटित; शल्कित; पपड़ीदार

**Scaling.** The formation of crusts. पर्पटीकरण; पर्पटीभवन; शल्कन; पपड़ियां बनना

**Scall.** A division of skin diseases, comprising of impetigo, eczema, psoriasis. पपड़ी; शल्क; पर्पटी; खुरण्ड; inflammation or irritation,

**Scalp**

followed by scab. प्रदाह; शोथ; खुजली; scald. तप्तद्रवदाहक्षत

**Scalp.** The integument covering the cranium. शिरोवल्क; शिरोस्थिचर्म; कपालावरण; करोटिच्छद

**Scalpel.** A small, straight knife of surgeon, which may or may not have detachable blades. छुरिका; छुरी

**Scalphocephalia.** See **Scalphocephaly.**

**Scalphocephalus.** See **Scalphocephaly.**

**Scalphocephaly.** A boat-shaped cranium; scalphocephalia; scalphocephalus; scaphocephalus; scaphocephaly. नौकाकार-करोटि; नौकाभकरोटि; नौकाभशिर; नाव जैसी खोपड़ी

**Scaly.** Covered with scales; squamous. शल्कमय; वल्काकृत; पर्पटित; पपड़ीदार

**Scanning.** Recording on a photographic plate, the emission of radioactive waves from a specific substance injected into the body. क्रमवीक्षण

**Scanty.** Deficient. अल्पमात्रिक; अल्प मात्रा में; बहुत कम मात्रा में

**Scaphocephalus.** See **Scalphocephaly.**

**Scaphocephaly.** See **Scalphocephaly.**

**Scaphoid.** Keel-shaped; shaped like a boat. नौकाभ; नौकाकार; नाव जैसे आकार का;

  **S. Abdomen,** the sunken appearance of the belly. नौकाभ उदर; पेट की नाव जैसी आकृति;

  **S. Bone,** the boat-shaped bone of the tarsus and carpus. नौकाभ-अस्थि; नाव जैसी हड्डी

**Scapi.** Plural of **Scapus.**

**Scapula.** A large, flat, triangular bone of the shoulder; the shoulder-blade. अंसफलक; स्कन्धफलक

**Scapulae.** Plural of **Scapula.**

**Scapulalgia.** Pain in the shoulder-blade. अंसफलकार्ति; स्कन्धफलकार्ति; स्कन्धफलक में दर्द होना

**Scapular.** Pertaining to the shoulder-blade. अंसफलकीय; स्कन्धफलकीय; स्कन्धफलक सम्बन्धी

**Scapulary.** A shoulder-bandage. स्कन्धबन्धनपट्ट; स्कन्धपट्टिका; कंधे पर बांधी जाने वाली पट्टी

**Scapulectomy.** Excision of the scapula. स्कन्धफलक-उच्छेदन;

अंसफलक-उच्छेदन

**Scapulopexy.** Operative fixation of the scapula to the chest-wall or to the spinous process of the vertebrae. अंसफलकस्थिरीकरण; स्कन्धफलकस्थिरीकरण

**Scapus.** A shaft or stem. स्तम्भ; तना

**Scar.** Cicatrix. क्षतचिन्ह; व्रणचिन्ह; घाव का निशान

**Scarf-skin.** The epidermis or outer layer of the skin; the cuticle. बाह्य-त्वचा; चर्म-झिल्ली

**Scarification.** The making of a series of small, superficial incisions or punctures in the skin. प्रच्छान; उत्पाटन; छिद्रण; छेदन

**Scarificator.** An instrument used in scarification. प्रच्छानक; छिद्रक; उत्पाटक

**Scarlatina.** An acute infectious and eruptive fever, called scarlet fever. रक्तज्वर; आरक्तज्वर; लोहितज्वर;

   **S. Anginosa,** a form with marked throat symptoms. गलार्ति-आरक्तज्वर;

   **S. Haemorrhagica,** a form accompanied by haemorrhage. रक्तस्रावी आरक्तज्वर;

   **S. Maligna,** a malignant form of scarlatina. दुर्दम आरक्तज्वर; सांघातिक रक्तज्वर;

   **S. Simplex,** the benign type of scarlatina. सरल आरक्तज्वर; सुदम आरक्तज्वर

**Scarlatinal.** Pertaining to scarlatina. आरक्तज्वरीय; आरक्तज्वर सम्बन्धी

**Scarlatiniform.** Resembling scarlatina; scarlatinoid. आरक्तज्वराभ; आरक्तज्वररूप; आरक्तज्वर जैसा

**Scarlatinoid.** See **Scarlatiniform.**

**Scarlatinous.** Having the nature of scarlatina. आरक्तज्वराभ; आरक्तज्वर जैसा

**Scarlet Fever.** See **Scarlatina.**

**Scatology.** The scientific study and analysis of the faeces. मलविज्ञान; मलप्रकरण

**Scatophagy.** Eating of excrements; coprophagy. मलभक्षण

**Scatoscopy.** Examination of the faeces. मलदर्शन

**Scent.** An emanation from living or dead tissues or materials that stimulates the olfactory sense. गंध; महक

**Schema.** A diagram or chart. डायाग्राम; चार्ट; a plan or scheme. योजना; परिकल्पना

**Schemata.** Plural of **Schema**.

**Schematic.** According to plan. योजनाबद्ध; कार्यप्रदर्शी

**Scheme.** A plan. योजना; व्यवस्था

**Schistocyte.** A segmentary blood corpuscle. विखण्डितलोहितकोशिका

**Schistosoma.** Bilharzia; a genus of blood flukes. शिस्टोसोमा; बिलहार्जिया

**Schizogony.** Reproduction by endogenous spore-formation. विखण्डीजनन

**Schizoid.** Pertaining to dementia praecox. विखण्डित मनस्कता सम्बन्धी; अन्तराबन्धी; resembling schizophrenia. विखण्डितमनस्कताभ

**Schizomycetes.** The fission fungi, bacteria. विखण्डी-कवक

**Schizont.** Any adult sporozoon which is multiplied by schizogony. खण्डप्रसू; विखण्डीजनन द्वारा बढ़ता हुआ कोई बीजाणु

**Schizonychia.** Splitting of the nails. विखंण्डितनखता

**Schizophasia.** Muttering and incomprehensible speech of schizophrenic persons; word salad. निरर्थक-शब्दोच्चारण

**Schizophrenia.** A mental disease characterized by disorganization of the patient's personality, often resulting in chronic life long ill-health and hospitalization. विखण्डित मनस्कता; विदलित चित्तवृत्ति

**Schizophrenic.** Pertaining to schizophrenia. विखण्डित मनस्कता सम्बन्धी; affected with schizophrenia. विखण्डितमनस्कताग्रस्त

**Schneiderian Membrane.** The lining membrane of the nose; nasal mucosa. नासा-कला; नाक की श्लैष्मिक झिल्ली

**Sciatic.** Pertaining to the large nerve running down the back of the thigh; sciatical. पृथुस्नायु सम्बन्धी; कटिस्नायु सम्बन्धी;

**S. Nerve,** the termination of the sacral or sciatic plexus. पृथुस्नायु; कटिस्नायु

**Sciatica.** Neuralgia of the parts supplied by the great sciatic nerve and its posterior cutaneous branches. गृध्रसी; पृथुस्नायुशूल; कटिस्नायुशूल; सायटिका

**Sciatical.** See **Sciatic**.

**Science.** Systematic knowledge. विज्ञान; शास्त्र;

**Medical S.,** science relating to the causes, diagnosis and treatment of diseases. आयुर्विज्ञान; चिकित्साविज्ञान; चिकित्साशास्त्र; उपचारविज्ञान

**Scientist.** One who is versed in science. वैज्ञानिक; विज्ञानी; वेत्ता

**Scirrhoid.** Resembling scirrhus. ग्रन्थ्यर्बुदाभ; ग्रन्थि-अर्बुद जैसा; सिर्संभ

**Scirrhoma.** See **Scirrhus**.

**Scirrhous.** Pertaining to scirrhus. ग्रन्थ्यर्बुद अथवा सिर्स सम्बन्धी

**Scirrhus.** Indolent, hard tumour; a form of cancer, principally affecting the breast; scirrhoma; scirrus. ग्रन्थ्यर्बुद; कठोर कैंसर; सिर्स

**Scirrus.** See **Scirrhus**.

**Scission.** A splitting, separation or division. विखण्डन; विलगन; विभाजन

**Sclera.** The white, tough membrane of the eyeball; sclerotica. श्वेतपटल; नेत्रगोलक की सफेद व ठोस कला (झिल्ली)

**Sclerae.** Plural of **Sclera**.

**Scleral.** Pertaining to the sclera. श्वेतपटलीय; श्वेतपटल सम्बन्धी

**Sclerectasis.** Protrusion of the sclera. श्वेतपटलविस्फार

**Sclerectoiridectomy.** Combined sclerectomy and iridectomy. श्वेतपटलपरितारिका-उच्छेदन

**Sclerectomy.** Excision of a portion of the sclera. श्वेतपटल-उच्छेदन

**Sclerema.** See **Scleroderma**.

**Sclerencephalia.** Hardening of the brain. मस्तिष्ककाठिन्य; मस्तिष्क की कठोरता

**Scleriasis.** Abnormal hardness of a part. कठोरता; कड़ापन

**Scleriritomy.** Incision of the sclera and iris. श्वेतपटलपरितारिकाछेदन; श्वेतपटल एवं परितारिका को छेदना

**Scleritis.** Inflammation of the sclera. श्वेतपटलशोथ; श्वेतपटल का प्रदाह

**Sclerodactylia.** See **Sclerodactyly**.

**Sclerodactyly.** Digital scleroderma; sclerodactylia. अंगुलि-त्वक्काठिन्य; उँगली की चमड़ी की कठोरता

**Scleroderma.** A chronic indurated skin; sclerema; scleroedema. त्वक्काठिन्य; त्वक्कठोरता

**Scleroedema.** See **Scleroderma**.

**Sclerogenous.** Producing hard or indurated tissue; causing sclerosis. काठिन्यजनक

**Scleroiritis.** Inflammation of the sclera and iris. श्वेतपटलपरितारिकशोथ; श्वेतपटल एवं परितारिका का प्रदाह

**Sclerokeratitis.** Cellular infiltration and inflammation of the sclera and the cornea. श्वेतपटलकनीनिकाशोथ

**Sclerokeratoiritis.** Inflammation of sclera, cornea and iris. श्वेतपटलकनीनिकापरितारिकाशोथ

**Scleromalacia.** A softening of the sclera. श्वेतपटलमृदुता; श्वेतपटल की कोमलता

**Sclerosing.** Undergoing sclerosis. काठिन्यकर

**Sclerosis.** A hardening of a tissue, as in a scar. काठिन्य; कठोरता; कड़ापन;

**Amyotrophic Lateral S.,** chronic anterior poliomyelitis combined with lateral sclerosis. पेशीशोषी पार्श्वपथ-काठिन्य;

**Disseminated S.,** arthropathy of tabes dorsalis. प्रसृत काठिन्य;

**Multiple S.,** multiple cerebrospinal sclerosis. बहुसृत काठिन्य;

**Vascular S.,** sclerosis of the walls of the blood vessels; arteriosclerosis. धमनी-काठिन्य; वाहिकाप्राचीर की कठोरता

**Sclerotic.** Pertaining to sclera; scleral. श्वेतपटल सम्बन्धी; hard; indurated. कठोर

**Sclerotica.** See **Sclera.**

**Sclerotitis.** Inflammation of the sclera; scleritis. श्वेतपटलशोथ; श्वेतपटल का प्रदाह

**Sclerotome.** A knife used in sclerotomy. श्वेतपटलछेदक

**Sclerotomy.** Incision of the sclera for relief of acute glaucoma prior to doing a decompression operation. श्वेतपटलछेदन

**Sclerous.** Hard; indurated. कठोर

**Scolex.** The head of a tapeworm by which it attaches itself to the intestinal wall. स्कोलेक्स

**Scolioma.** Curvature of the spine. मेरुवक्रता; कुब्जता; कूबड़पन

**Scoliosis.** Lateral curvature of the spine. पार्श्वकुब्जता; रीढ़ का एक ओर का टेढ़ापन

**Scoliotic.** Relating to scoliosis. पार्श्वकुब्जता सम्बन्धी

**Scoop.** Spoon-shaped surgical instrument. स्कूप

**Scorbiculus Cordis.** The pit of the stomach. उदरगर्त

**Scorbutic.** Pertaining to scurvy. शीताद सम्बन्धी; affected with scurvy. शीतादग्रस्त; producing scurvy; scorbutigenic. शीतादजनक

**Scorbutigenic.** See **Scorbutic.**

**Scorbutus.** Scurvy. शीताद; स्कर्वी

**Scotoma.** A dark spot in the visual field; blind spot. अन्धक्षेत्र; दृष्टि-क्षेत्र में एक काला धब्बा;

**Absolute S.,** scotoma with perception of light entirely absent. पूर्ण अन्धक्षेत्र;

**Annular S.,** a zone of scotoma surrounding the centre of the visual field. वृत्ताकार अन्धक्षेत्र;

**Negative S.,** a scotoma due to destruction of the retinal centre and not perceptible to the patient. अज्ञात अन्धक्षेत्र;

**Positive S.,** a scotoma perceptible to the patient as a dark spot. ज्ञात अन्धक्षेत्र;

**Relative S.,** a scotoma with only partial impairment of light perception. सापेक्ष अन्धक्षेत्र

**Scotomata.** Plural of **Scotoma.**

**Scotomatous.** Relating to scotoma. अन्धक्षेत्र सम्बन्धी

**Scotometer.** An instrument used in scotometry. अन्धक्षेत्रमापी

**Scotometry.** The locating and measurement of scotomata. अन्धक्षेत्रमापन; अन्धक्षेत्रमिति

**Scotopia.** See **Scotopic Vision.**

**Scotopic.** Poor light. मन्द-द्युति; तिमिर; धुँधला प्रकाश; धुँधली रोशनी;

**S. Vision,** the ability to see well in poor light; scotopia. मन्दद्युति-दृष्टि; धुँधले प्रकाश में भली-भांति दिखाई देना

**Scourge.** Any severe epidemic disease. उग्रमहामारी

**Scouring.** Purging; diarrhoea. रेचन; अतिसार; प्रवाहिका; पेचिश

**Scraping.** An abrading. आखुरण; खुरचन; खरोंच

**Scratch.** An abrasion. खरोंच; खुरचन

**Scratching.** Abrading. खरोंच; खरोंचना

**Screening.** Rapid superficial examination of groups of persons to identify those most in need of medical care. परेक्षण; अनुवीक्षण

**Scrobiculum.** See **Scrobiculus Cordis.**

**Scrobiculus Cordis.** The pit of the stomach; scrobiculum. उदरगर्त

**Scrofula.** A morbid constitutional state of the system characterized by indolent, glandular tumours that suppurate slowly, heal with difficulty and leave scars, etc. कण्ठमाला; गण्डमाला

**Scrofuloderma.** Cutaneous scrofula; scrofulodermia. यक्ष्मज त्वगलन; त्वगण्डमाला

**Scrofulodermia.** See **Scrofuloderma.**

**Scrofulosis.** A scrofulous condition, disease or diathesis; scrophulosis. कण्ठमाला रोग; गण्डमाला रोग की प्रवृत्ति

**Scrofulous.** Affected with scrofula. कण्ठमालाग्रस्त; गण्डमालाग्रस्त; pertaining to scrofula. कण्ठमाला अथवा गण्डमाला सम्बन्धी

**Scrophulosis.** See **Scrofulosis.**

**Scrota.** Plural of **Scrotum.**

**Scrotal.** Pertaining to the scrotum. अण्डकोशीय; अण्डकोश सम्बन्धी;

   **S. Hernia,** a protrusion of any of the contents of the abdomen into the scrotum; scrotocele. वृषणस्त्रंस; अण्डकोश का हर्निया;

   **S. Sac,** the scrotum. वृषणकोश; अण्डकोश

**Scrotectomy.** Excision of a part of scrotum. वृषणकोश-उच्छेदन; अण्डकोश-उच्छेदन

**Scrotitis.** Inflammation of the scrotum. वृषणकोशशोथ; अण्डकोशशोथ; वृषणकोश अथवा अण्डकोश का प्रदाह

**Scrotocele.** See **Scrotal Hernia.**

**Scrotum.** Bag holding the testes. वृषणकोश; अण्डकोश

**Scruple.** Twenty grains or one-third of a drachm. स्क्रुपल; बीस ग्रेन अथवा ड्राम का तीसरा भाग

**Scuba.** A self-contained underwater breathing apparatus; also used to refer to the sport of underwater diving and swimming. अधिजलश्वासयंत्र

**Scum.** An insolube layer which rises to the surface of a liquid. फेन; फफूंद; सेवाल; एक अविलेय परत जो किसी द्रव्य-तल के ऊपर जमता है

**Scurf.** Dandruff; the exfoliated epidermis of the scalp. रूसी; पपड़ी; शुष्क चर्म; wrinkle. झुर्री; वलय; कुंचन

**Scurfy.** Dry or wrinkled skin. शुष्कचर्म; झुर्रीदार चमड़ी; कुंचितचर्म

**Scurvy.** A nutritional disease, caused by dietetic errors and marked by weakness, anaemia, spongy gums, sometimes with ulceration of gums and haemorrhages into the skin and from mucous membrane. शीताद; स्कर्वी; पोषण-दोष के कारण होने वाला एक रोग

**Scuta.** Plural of **Scutum.**

**Scute.** A crescentic plate forming the outer wall of the portion of the tympanum above the antrum. प्रशल्कढाल; scutum. अवटूपास्थि

**Scutulum.** A favus-crust. चषकीपीतपर्पटी

**Scutum.** The thyroid cartilage. अवटूपास्थि; अवटु-उपास्थि

**Scybala.** Plural of **Scybalum**.

**Scybalous.** Consisting of scybala. बिष्ठाग्रन्थियुक्त; मलगांठयुक्त

**Scybalum.** Hard faeces in lumps. बिष्ठाग्रन्थि; मलगांठ; मल की कठोर गांठ; सुद्दा

**Scyphoid.** Cup-shaped. चषकाकार; प्याले के आकार जैसा

**Scythian Disease.** Atrophy of the male genitalia. लिंगशोष; शिश्नशोष; लिंग सूखना

**Scytitis.** Dermatitis. त्वक्शोथ; त्वचा का प्रदाह

**Seal.** To close firmly with an adhesive or waxy material. बन्द करना; सील लगाना

**Sea-sickness.** Nausea or vomiting caused by the motion of the vessel. नौकायन-रुग्णता; समुद्री-रुग्णता

**Seatworm.** Pinworm; oxyuris. सूत्रकृमि

**Sebaceous.** Oily; fatty; relating to fat. वसामय; चर्बीयुक्त; वसा सम्बन्धी

**Sebiferous.** See **Sebiparous**.

**Sebiparous.** Producing sebaceous matter; sebiferous. वसोत्पादक; वसा पैदा करने वाला पदार्थ

**Sebolith.** A concretion in sebaceous gland. वसाग्रन्थ्यश्मरी; वसाश्मरी; वसाग्रंथि की पथरी

**Seborrhagia.** See **Seborrhoea**.

**Seborrhea.** See **Seborrhoea**.

**Seborrheal.** See **Seborrhoeic**.

**Seborrhoea.** A disturbance of the oil glands in the skin; seborrhagia; seborrhea. त्वग्वसास्राव; त्वचा की वसा ग्रन्थियों का कोई दोष;

   **S. Capillitii,** that of the scalp; seborrhoea capitis. करोटिज त्वग्वसास्राव;

   **S. Capitis,** see **Seborrhea Capillitii**.

   **S. Corporis,** that of the trunk. कायिक त्वग्वसास्राव; दैहिक त्वग्वसास्राव; देहत्वग्वसास्राव;

   **S. Faciei,** that of the face. आनन त्वग्वसास्राव;

   **S. Oleosa,** that with oily contents. तैलत्वग्वसास्राव;

   **S. Sicca,** dry form with branny scales. शुष्क त्वग्वसास्राव

**Seborrhoeal.** See **Seborrhoeic**.

# Seborrhoeic

**Seborrhoeic.** Affected with seborrhoea; seborrhoic; seborrheal; seborrhoeal. त्वग्वसास्त्रावग्रस्त

**Seborrhoic.** See **Seborrhoeic.**

**Sebum.** The oily secretion from sebaceous glands in the skin. त्वग्वसा

**Secondary.** Second or inferior in order or time. द्वित्तीयक; गौण; अनुषंगी

**Secreta.** Substance discharged by a gland. उदासर्ग; ग्रन्थिस्राव; उत्सृष्ट अथवा निःसृत पदार्थ

**Secretagog.** See **Secretogogue.**

**Secrete.** To separate especially from the blood. निःसृत करना या होना

**Secretion.** The product of various organs of the body, as bile is the secretion of the liver. स्राव;

    **External S.**, that thrown out to the surface of an organ. बहिःस्राव;

    **Internal S.**, that not thrown out but absorbed by the blood. अन्तःस्राव

**Secretogog.** See **Secretogogue.**

**Secretogogue.** A substance having the property of stimulating a gland to increased activity; secretagog; secretogog. स्राववर्धक; स्राव बढ़ाने वाला

**Secretoinhibitory.** Restraining or curving secretion. स्रावरोधक; स्रावरोधी

**Secretomotor.** Stimulating secretion; secretomotory. स्रावप्रेरक

**Secretomotory.** See **Secretomotor.**

**Secretor.** That which performs secretion. स्रावक; स्रावी

**Secretory.** Relating to secretion or secretions. स्राव अथवा स्रावों सम्बन्धी

**Sectia.** See **Section.**

**Section.** A cut or division; dissection; sectio. छेदन; उच्छेदन; काटना

**Sectiones.** Plural of **Sectio.**

**Secundigravida.** A woman pregnant for the second time. द्विगर्भा; दूसरी बार गर्भवती होने वाली स्त्री

**Secundine.** After-birth; lochia. खेड़ी; जेरी; सूतिस्राव

**Secundipara.** A woman who has produced two infants at two separate times. द्विप्रसवा; दो बच्चों को अलग-अलग समय पर जन्म देने वाली स्त्री

**Secundiparity.** The state of being secundipara. द्विप्रसविता; दूसरी बार गर्भवती होने की अवस्था

**Secundis Horis.** Every two hours. हर दो घण्टे में

**Secundum Artem.** According to rule. नियमानुसार

**Sedation.** The producing of a sedative effect. शमन; प्रशमन; उपशमन; शीतलन

**Sedative.** Soothing; calming; an agent allaying irritability. शामक; उपशमनकारी; शान्तिदायक; प्रशामक

**Sedentary.** Accustomed to sit much; occupied in sitting. उपवेशनशील; निष्क्रिय; शारीरिक श्रम न करने सम्बन्धी

**Sediment.** The deposit from any liquid substance which sinks to the vessel when the same is allowed to stand. तलछट; तलौंछ

**Sedimentation.** A conversion into sediment. अवसादन; तलछटीकरण; तलछटीभवन;

**S. Rate,** laboratory test of speed at which erythrocytes settle. अवसादन दर

**Sedimentator.** A centrifuge. अपकेन्द्र

**Sedimentometer.** A photographic apparatus for the automatic recording of blood sedimentation rate. रक्त-अवसादनदरमापी; अवसादनदरमापी

**Seed.** See **Semen.**

**Segment.** A part of an organ or any other; a small piece; section; segmentum; lobe. खण्ड; खण्डांश

**Segmenta.** Plural of **Segment.**

**Segmental.** Pertaining to a segment or segmentation. खण्डांशीय; खण्डीय; खण्ड या खण्डांशीभवन सम्बन्धी

**Segmentation.** The process of forming segments. खण्डांशीभवन; खण्डीभवन; विदलन

**Segmentum.** See **Segment.**

**Segregation.** Removal of certain parts from a mass; separation. पृथक्करण; किसी पिण्ड से कुछ अंशों को अलग कर देना

**Segregator.** Separator; any instrument or device used for bringing about a separation of two substances, such as cream from milk. पृथक्कारी

**Seismocardiogram.** Cardiograph. हृत्स्पन्दलेख

**Seismocardiography.** Cardiography. हृत्स्पन्दलेखन

**Seizure.** A sudden attack of a disease, pain, or of symptoms, such as convulsions. ग्रह; आक्रमण

**Selection.** Choice. वरण; चयन; चुनाव
**Selene.** White spots on the nails. श्वेतनखता; नाखुनों पर सफेद धब्बे पड़ना
**Self.** Same; identical; own; personal. स्वत:; वैयक्तिक; निजी; स्व-;
  **S.-abuse,** masturbation; self-pollution. हस्तमैथुन; स्वमैथुन;
  **S.-fertilization,** self-impregnation. स्वसंसेचन; स्वनिषेचन
  **S.-impregnation,** see **Self-fertilization.**
  **S.-murder,** see **Suicide.**
  **S.-pollution,** see **Self-abuse.**
**Sella Turcica.** Pituitary fossa of sphenoid bone. पर्याणिका; जतूकास्थि का पीयूषिका खात
**Sellar.** Relating to the sella turcica. पर्याणिका सम्बन्धी
**Semeilogy.** Symptomatology. लाक्षणिकी; लाक्षणिकता
**Semen.** The fecundation fluid of the male containing spermatozoa. वीर्य; शुक्र; a seed. बीज
**Semens.** Plural of **Semen.**
**Semenuria.** Presence of semen in the urine; spermaturia. शुक्रमेह; पेशाब में वीर्य जाना
**Semicoma.** Condition bordering on the unconsciousness. अर्धसन्न्यास; अर्धमूर्च्छित अवस्था
**Semicomatose.** In a condition of impaired consciousness. अर्धसन्न्यासग्रस्त; अर्धमूर्च्छित
**Semiconscious.** Partly conscious. अर्धमूर्च्छित; अर्धचेतन
**Semilunar.** Shaped like a crescent or half moon. अर्धचन्द्राकार; नवचन्द्राकार
**Semina.** Plural of **Semen.**
**Seminal.** Pertaining to semen. शुक्र अथवा वीर्य सम्बन्धी
**Semination.** Introduction of semen into uterus. वीर्यरोपण; शुक्रसेचन
**Seminiferous.** Carrying or producing semen. शुक्रजनक; वीर्योत्पादक; वीर्यधारी
**Seminoma.** A malignant tumour of the testis. दुर्दम वृषणार्बुद; वृषणकोष का एक सांघातिक अर्बुद
**Semipermeable.** Used to describe a membrane which is permeable to some substance in solution, but not in others. अर्धपारगम्य
**Semis.** Half. अर्ध; आधा

**Senecio.** A genus of composite plants, several species of which are employed in medicine. पालितचूड़ा (पौधा)

**Senescence.** Chronicity. जीर्णता; चिरता; the state or process of growing old. जरा; बुढ़ापा

**Senescent.** Growing old. वृद्ध; बूढ़ा

**Senile.** Relating to senility; of old age; senilis. जराजन्य; जराकालीन; बृद्धावस्था का; बुढ़ापे का;

    **S. Deafness,** deafness due to old age. जराबधिरता; बुढ़ापे का बहरापन

**Senilis.** See **Senile.**

**Senilism.** Premature old age. कालपूर्व-जरा; अकाल-जरा

**Senility.** Old age. बृद्धावस्था; बुढ़ापा; the weakness of old age. जरा-दौर्बल्य; बुढ़ापे की कमजोरी

**Senna.** Leaves and pods of a purgative plant from Egypt and India. मार्कण्डी; स्वर्णपत्री; सनाय; एक रेचक पौधे की पत्तियां और फलियां; sennapod. सनायफली

**Sensation.** An impression conveyed by an afferent nerve to the sensorium; a feeling. सम्वेदन; सम्वेदना; संवेदना; अनुभूति

**Sense.** One of the perceptive faculties; feeling; sensation. ज्ञान; बोध; सम्वेद; संवेद;

    **Colour S.,** perception of various colours. वर्ण-बोध;

    **Light S.,** perception of degree of light. प्रकाश-बोध;

    **Muscular S.,** consciousness of muscular movements. पेशी-बोध;

    **Special S.,** one of the five senses related to the organs of sight, smell, hearing, taste and touch. विशेष ज्ञान

**Senses.** The perceptive faculties. ज्ञान; बोध; सम्वेद; संवेद

**Sensibility.** Faculty of receiving impressions. सम्वेदनशीलता; सम्वेद्यता; बोधगम्यता; प्रभावग्रहण की योग्यता

**Sensible.** Endowed with the sense of feeling; having reason. सम्वेदनशील; बोधगम्य; संज्ञावान

**Sensitive.** Capable of being sensitive, or susceptible. सम्वेदनशील; सुग्राही; सूक्ष्मग्राही; सुग्राही बनने योग्य

**Sensitivity.** The state of being sensitive. सम्वेदनशीलता; सुग्राहिता; सूक्ष्मग्राहिता

**Sensitization.** Rendering sensitive. सुग्राहीकरण; सुग्राहीभवन; सूक्ष्मग्राहीभवन; सूक्ष्मग्राहीकरण; सम्वेदनशील करना; immunization. प्रतिरक्षीकरण; रोगक्षमीकरण

**Sensitized.** Made sensitive. सुग्राहीकृत

**Sensoria.** Plural of **Sensorium.**

**Sensorial.** Pertaining to the sensorium. संवेदी; संवेदनाक्षेत्र सम्बन्धी

**Sensorimotor.** Pertaining to both sensation and motion. संवेदीप्रेरक; सम्वेदनाप्रेरक; संवेदना एवं गति सम्बन्धी

**Sensorium.** The common centre of sensation. संवेदनाक्षेत्र; संवेदना का प्रमुख केन्द्र

**Sensory.** Relating to sensation. संवेदी; सम्वेदी; अनुभूति सम्बन्धी

**Sentient.** Having sensation. संवेदनसमर्थ; संवेदनासमर्थ

**Sentiment.** Feeling in relation to one idea. मनोभाव; मनोवृत्ति

**Separation.** Disconnection; disunion. पृथक्करण; पृथक्भवन

**Separator.** An instrument for separating pericranium from the skull; separatory. पृथक्कारी; करोटि से करोटि-आवरण को अलग करने का यंत्र

**Separatory.** See **Separator.**

**Sepses.** Plural of **Sepsis.**

**Sepsis.** Putrefaction; septicemia; blood poisoning. पूतिता; रक्तपूतिता; रक्तविषण्णता; पूतिजीवरक्तता

**Septa.** Plural of **Septum.**

**Septal.** Pertaining to a septum. पटलीय; पटीय; पटल सम्बन्धी

**Septemia.** See **Septicaemia.**

**Septic.** Relating to sepsis. पूतिज; विषाक्त; विषण्ण; विषण्णता या विषाक्तता सम्बन्धी; capable of producing putrefaction. पूतिजन्य; caused by sepsis. पूति-उत्पादित

**Septicaemia.** An unhealthy condition of the blood; blood poisoning; septemia; septicemia. पूतिजीवरक्तता; रक्तपूतिता; रक्तविषण्णता; रक्त की दूषित अवस्था

**Septicemia.** See **Septicaemia.**

**Septicemic.** Pertaining to, or affected with septicemia. पूतिजीवरक्तक; रक्तपूतिता सम्बन्धी

**Septipara.** A woman pregnant for the seventh time. सप्तगर्भा; सातवीं बार गर्भवती होने वाली स्त्री

**Septomarginal.** Relating to the margin of a septum. पटपरिसरीय; पटपरिसर सम्बन्धी

**Septonasal.** Concerning the nasal septum. नासापट सम्बन्धी

**Septoplasty.** Plastic surgery of the nasal septum. नासापटसंधान

**Septostomy.** Surgical formation of an opening in a septum. नासापटछिद्रीकरण

**Septotomy.** Incision of a septum, especially of the nasal septum. नासापटछेदन

**Septula.** Plural of **Septulum**.

**Septulum.** A minute septum or partition. पटिका; क्षुद्रपट

**Septum.** A partition; a dividing membrane or wall. पट; पटल;

   **S. Lucidum,** the wall between the lateral ventricles of the brain; septum pellucidum. स्वच्छ-पट; मस्तिष्कपार्श्व-निलय का मध्यपट;

   **S. Nasi,** the nasal septum; the partition between the nostrils. नासा-पट; नाक के बीच का पर्दा;

   **S. Pectiniforme,** the imperfect septum between the erectile bodies of the penis and clitoris. कंकत-पट; शिश्न एवं भगशिश्निका के उत्तान-पिण्डों के बीच वाला अपूर्ण पट;

   **S. Pellucidum,** see **Septum Lucidum**.

   **S. Rectovaginale,** partition between the rectum and vagina; rectovaginal sptum. मलांत्रयोनि-पट;

   **S. Scroti,** that dividing the scrotum into two cavities; scrotal septum. वृषण-पट; वृषण को दो भागों में बांटने वाला पर्दा;

   **Nasal S.,** see **Septum Nasi**.

   **Rectovaginal S.,** see **Septum Rectovaginale**.

   **Scrotal S.,** see **Septum Scroti**.

**Sequel.** See **Sequela**.

**Sequela.** A morbid condition following as a consequence of another disease; sequel. अनुगम; परिणाम; फल; अनुप्रभाव; रोगोत्तर विकार

**Sequelae.** Plural of **Sequela**.

**Sequele.** The same as **Sequelae**.

**Sequester.** See **Sequestrum**.

**Sequestra.** Plural of **Sequestrum**.

**Sequestral.** Relating to sequestrum. विविक्त अथवा विविक्तांश सम्बन्धी

**Sequestration.** The formation of a sequestrum. विविक्तीभवन; the isolation of a patient. पृथक्भवन; पृथक्करण; रोगी को अलग रखना या करना

**Sequestrectomy.** Excision of a sequestrum. विविक्तोच्छेदन; विविक्तांश-उच्छेदन

**Sequestrum.** A fragment of a necrosed bone; sequester. विविक्त; विविक्तांश

**Sera.** Plural of **Serum.**

**Seralbumin.** The albumin of the blood. रसान्नसार; सीरमान्नसार; रक्तान्नसार

**Serial.** Following a regular order; arranged in rows. क्रम; पंक्तिबद्ध

**Series.** A line or row of things. अनुक्रम; श्रेणी; माला

**Seriflux.** A serous or watery discharge. सीरमीस्राव अथवा जलस्राव; रिसाव

**Serious.** Alarming. गम्भीर; अरिष्ट

**Serocolitis.** Inflammation of the serous coat of the colon. परिबृहदांत्रशोथ; बृहदांत्रावरणशोथ

**Seroenteritis.** Inflammation of the serous covering of the intestine; perienteritis. आंत्रावरणशोथ

**Serohepatitis.** Inflammation of the hepatic peritoneum. यकृतावरणशोथ; यकृतावरण का प्रदाह

**Serological.** Pertaining to serology. सीरमी; सीरमविज्ञान सम्बन्धी

**Serologist.** One who is versed in serology. सीरमविज्ञानी; सीरमविज्ञानविशेषज्ञ; सीरमविज्ञानवेत्ता; रक्तोदकविज्ञानी

**Serology.** The branch of science dealing with the study of sera. सीरमविज्ञान; रक्तोदकविज्ञान

**Seromembranous.** Relating to a serous membrane. सीरमीकला सम्बन्धी

**Seromucoid.** Resembling the serum and the mucus. सीरमश्लेष्माभ; सीरम तथा श्लेष्मा जैसा

**Seromucous.** Pertaining to both serum or mucus. सीरमश्लैष्मिक; सीरम तथा श्लेष्मा सम्बन्धी; composed of both serum and mucus. सीरमश्लेष्मनिर्मित

**Seropurulent.** Containing serum and pus. सीरमपूयमय; लसीपूयमय; रक्तमत्सुपूययुक्त

**Seropus.** Combined serum and pus; purulent serum. सीरमपूतिमय; सपूय सीरम

**Serosa.** A serous membrane. सीरमीकला

**Serosae.** Plural of **Serosa.**

**Serositis.** Inflammation of a serous membrane. सीरमीकलाशोथ; सीरमीकला का प्रदाह

**Serosity.** Having the quality of a serous fluid. मेदुरता; मेदस्विता; पतलापन

**Serosynovitis.** Synovitis with serous effusion. सीरमीश्लेषककलाशोथ; सीरमीस्राव के साथ श्लेषक कला का प्रदाह

**Serotherapy.** Treatment of diseases by the use of blood serum; serum therapy. सीरमचिकित्सा; रक्तोद-प्रयोग द्वारा की जाने वाली रोगों की चिकित्सा

**Serous.** Having the nature of serum, i.e. clear fluid without pus or matter. सीरमी; रक्तमत्सुवत्; रक्तोदकीय; relating to serum. सीरम सम्बन्धी;
  **S. Membrane,** one lining a cavity which has no communication with air. सीरमी कला

**Serpiginous.** Creeping or spread from part to part, as ringworm. सर्पिल; दद्रुसम; दाद जैसा रेंगने वाला

**Serpigo.** Ringworm; tinea. कक्ष्या; दद्रु; दाद; मण्डलकुष्ठ; herpes. हर्पीज; दाद

**Serrate.** Notched like a saw; dentate; serrated. दन्तुर; दान्तेदार; दन्तुरित

**Serrated.** See **Serrate.**

**Serration.** An identation, as in saw. दन्तुरण; क्रकचन; दान्तेदार किनारे की रचना

**Serrulate.** Marked with small serrations. सूक्ष्मक्रकचित; सूक्ष्मदन्तुरित

**Serum.** The liquid portion of the blood that separates from the red blood. सीरम; लस; रस; रक्तोद; रक्तमत्सु;
  **S. Therapy,** see **Serotherapy.**
  **Antitetanic S.** (ATS), serum given to counteract tetanus toxin. हनुस्तम्भरोधी सीरम; धनुर्वातरोधी सीरम;
  **Blood S.,** the clear liquid portion of serum without its fibrin and corpuscle; plasma. रक्तरस; प्लाविका

**Sesamoid.** Resembling a seed or grain. वर्तुलिकाभ; तिलाकार; कण्डराभ;
  **S. Bone,** a small bone developed in a tendon. कण्डरास्थि;
  **S. Cartilages,** the small cartilages in the nasal wings. वर्तुलिकास्थियाँ

**Sesamoiditis.** Inflammation of the sesamoid bones. कण्डरास्थिशोथ; कण्डरास्थि का प्रदाह

**Sessile.** Having no peduncle, but attached directly by a broad base. अवृन्त; निर्वृन्त

**Seventh pair of nerves.** The facial nerves; the cranial nerves; nervus facialis. आननतंत्रिकायें; चेहरे की नाड़ियाँ

**Severe**

**Severe.** Acute. प्रचण्ड; उग्र; तीव्र

**Sex-.** Prefix meaning six. 'षट्' के रूप में प्रयुक्त उपसर्ग

**Sex.** The quality which distinguishes between male and female. लिंग

**Sexdigital.** With six fingers or toes. षटंगुलिक; छ: उँगलियों वाला

**Sexing.** See Sexuality.

**Sexology.** The study of all aspects of sex and sexual behaviour. रतिविज्ञान; कामसूत्र

**Sextan.** Recurring every sixth day. षट्दिवसीय; हर छठवें दिन प्रकट होने वाला

**Sextaparte Horae.** Post cibus; ten minutes after meals. भोजन के दस मिनट बाद

**Sextis Horis.** Every six hours. हर छ: घण्टे में

**Sextuplets.** Six children born at one birth. षटक; एक साथ छ: बच्चे पैदा होना

**Sexual.** Relating to the sex. लैंगिक; यौन सम्बन्धी;

   **S. Intercourse,** coition. लैंगिक सम्भोग; रतिक्रिया; संगम;

   **S. Organs,** the organs of generation. जननांग; जननेन्द्रियां; गुप्तांग

**Sexuality.** The collective differences in which individuals make one male and another female; sexing. लिंग-निर्धारण

**Shaking.** Shivering. हल्लन; कम्पन; कम्प; संक्षोभ

**Shank.** A popular name for tibia or shin. जंघा

**Sheath.** A covering; an investing substance. आवरण; आच्छद; पिधान; vagina. योनि;

   **Arachnoid S.,** a delicate partition lying between the pial sheath and the dural sheath of the optic nerve. जालतानिका-आवरण; जालतानिकावरण;

   **Capillary S.,** lymph channel surrounding certain capillaries. केशिका-आवरण; केशिकावरण;

   **Dentinal S.,** the structure lining the dental canal. दन्त-आवरण; दन्तावरण;

   **Femoral S.,** the fascia covering the femoral vessel. औरवी आवरण; और्व्यावरण

   **Synovial S.,** the synovial membrane lining a passage through which tendon glides. श्लेषक आवरण; श्लेषकावरण

**Shelf Operation.** An open reduction of a congenital dislocation of hip-joint involving the use of a bone-graft. नितम्बसन्धिसंधान; शेल्फ ऑपरेशन

**Shield.** Any protecting device or screen, as a lead shield for protecting the operator from x-rays or a watchglass to protect the eye in case of gonorrhoeal ophthalmia. वर्म; शील्ड

**Shift.** Transfer. स्थानान्तरण; a change in position or direction. विस्थापन

**Shiga's bacillus.** One of the bacteria producing dysentery in the Middle and Far East. अमीबाणु; पेचिश पैदा करने वाला जीवाणु; शिगा बेसिलस

**Shin.** The anterior part of the leg. प्रजंघिका; शिखा; टांग का अगला भाग;

   **S. Bone,** the tibia; the medial bone of the foreleg. प्रजंघिकास्थि; पिण्डली की हड्डी

**Shingles.** Herpes zoster. विसर्पी छाजन; भैंसिया दाद; हर्पीज

**Ship-fever.** Typhus fever. मोह-ज्वर; तंत्रिका-ज्वर; नौवहन-ज्वर

**Shirodkar's operation.** Placing of a purse-string suture around an incompetent cervix during pregnancy and removed when labour starts. जरायुसंधान; गर्भाशयसंधान; शिरोदकर ऑपरेशन

**Shiver.** A slight chill or tremor. काम्पना; थरथराना

**Shivering.** Shaking with cold or fear. कम्पन; थरथराहट

**Shock.** Sudden or instantaneous depression of the vital power. आघात; प्रघात; स्तब्धता; क्षोभ;

   **S. Treatment,** electric current passed through the brain; also induced by injections. क्षोभ-चिकित्सा; आघातोपचार

**Shooting.** Like a quick, glancing sensation. तेज; गोली लगने जैसा

**Short-sight.** Myopic. निकटदृष्टि

**Shortsightedness.** Myopia; a condition of not being able to see very far; nearsightedness. निकटदृष्टिता

**Short-winded.** Difficult or oppressed breathing after or during exercise, often arising simply from fatness. श्वासकष्ट

**Shot.** A vernacular term for an injection; used also to denote a dose of narcotic. इंजेक्शन; अन्त:क्षेपण; स्वापक

**Shoulder.** The scapuloclavicular articulation and the adjacent parts. स्कन्ध; कन्धा; अंस;

   **S.-blade,** the scapula. स्कन्धफलक; अंसफलक;

   **S.-girdle,** formed by the clavicle and scapula on either side. स्कन्ध-पट्टी

**Show.** A popular term for the blood-stained vaginal discharge at the commencement of the labour. प्रसवसूचकस्राव; दर्श; the menses. आर्तव; ऋतुस्राव

**Shrapnell's membrane.** Membrana flaccida; the triangular portion of the tympanic membrane. श्लय-कला; कर्णपट का त्रिकोणक अंश; श्रैपनेल कला

**Shrill.** Acuteness of sound. कर्णवेधी; मर्मस्पर्शी; मर्मभेदी; तीव्र

**Shrub.** A low bushy tree. क्षुप; गुल्म; झाड़ी

**Shunt.** A term applied to the passage of blood through other than the usual channel. पार्श्वपथ

**Sialaden.** The salivary gland. लालाग्रन्थि; लारग्रन्थि

**Sialadenitis.** Inflammation of the salivary glands; sialoadenitis. लालाग्रन्थिशोथ; लारग्रन्थिशोथ; लारग्रन्थियों का प्रदाह

**Sialadenoncus.** A tumour of the salivary glands. लालाग्रन्थ्यर्बुद; लारग्रन्थियों की गिल्टी

**Sialagog.** See **Sialagogue.**

**Sialagogic.** Increasing the flow of saliva. लालावर्धक; लारवर्धक

**Sialagogue.** An agent increasing the flow of saliva; sialagog; sialogog; sialogogue; ptyalagogue. लालावर्धक; लारवर्धक

**Sialectasis.** Protrusion of the salivary ducts; ptyalectasis. लालावाहिकास्फीति

**Sialemesia.** Vomiting of saliva; sialemesis. लालावमन; लारवमन

**Sialemesis.** See **Sialemesia.**

**Sialic.** Salivary; relating to, or resembling saliva. लार सम्बन्धी अथवा लार जैसी

**Sialine.** Having the nature of the saliva. लाराभ; लार जैसा; concerning the saliva; salivary. लाला अथवा लार सम्बन्धी

**Sialisus.** Salivation; ptyalism. लालास्राव; लारस्राव

**Sialitis.** Inflammation of the salivary ducts. लालावाहिकाशोथ; लारनलियों का प्रदाह

**Sialoadenectomy.** Excision of the salivary gland. लालाग्रंथि-उच्छेदन; लारग्रंथि-उच्छेदन

**Sialoadenitis.** See **Sialadenitis.**

**Sialoadenotomy.** Incision of a salivary gland. लालाग्रंथिछेदन; लारग्रंथिछेदन

**Sialoangiectasis.** Dilatation of salivary ducts. लारनलिकाविस्फार; लालावाहिकाविस्फार

**Sialoangiitis.** Inflammation of a salivary duct; sialodochitis. लारनलिकाशोथ; लालावाहिकाशोथ

**Sialocele.** Ranula; cyst or tumour of a salivary gland. लालाग्रन्थ्यर्बुद; लालाग्रन्थिपुटी

**Sialodochitis.** See **Sialoangiitis.**

**Sialodochoplasty.** Reparative surgery of a salivary gland. लालाग्रन्थिसंधान

**Sialogenous.** Producing saliva. लालाजनक; लारजनक; लारोत्पादक

**Sialogog.** See **Sialagogue.**

**Sialogogue.** See **Sialagogue.**

**Sialogram.** Radiographic picture of the salivary glands and ducts. लालावाहिकाचित्र; लारवाहिकाचित्र

**Sialography.** Radiographic examination of the salivary glands and ducts after introducing radio-opaque material into the duct. लालावाहिकाचित्रण

**Sialoid.** Pertaining to, or resembling saliva. लार सम्बन्धी; लारवत्

**Sialolith.** A salivary calculus. लालावाहिकाश्मरी; लाराश्मरी

**Sialolithiasis.** The forming of salivary calculi. लालावाहिकाश्मरता; लाराश्मरता; लारपथरी

**Sialolithotomy.** Incision of a salivary gland or duct to remove a calculus. लालाग्रन्थिछेदन; लालावाहिकाछेदन

**Sialon.** The saliva. लाला; लार

**Sialorrhea.** Salivation; ptyalism; sialorrhoea. लालास्राव; लारस्राव

**Sialorrhoea.** See **Sialorrhea.**

**Sialostenosis.** Stricture of a salivary duct. लालावाहिकासंकीर्णन

**Sib.** Abbreviation for **Sibling.**

**Sibilant.** Making hissing sound; wheezing, as a rale. सीत्कारी; हिस्-हिस् की ध्वनि करती हुई; सुसकारने वाली

**Sibling.** One of a family by the same parents; abbreviated form : **Sib.** सहोदर

**Sicca.** Dry; siccum. शुष्क; सूखा हुआ

**Siccant.** Siccative; drying or that which dries. शुष्ककारी

**Siccative.** See **Siccant.**

**Siccum.** See **Sicca.**

**Sick.** The patient; ill; unwell; suffering from a disease. रोगी; बीमार; मरीज; nauseated. मितलीग्रस्त; मिचलीग्रस्त

**Sickly.** Diseased. अस्वस्थ; रुग्ण

**Sickness.** Disease. अस्वस्थता; रुग्णता; व्याधि;
  **Air-s.,** one caused due to an air journey; aviation sickness. उड्डयन अस्वस्थता;
  **Altitude S.,** a syndrome caused by low inspired oxygen pressure and characterized by nausea, headache, dyspnoea, malaise and sleeplessness. तुंगता अस्वस्थता;
  **Aviation S.,** see **Air-sickness.**
  **Car-s.,** one on account of journey by motor car, bus or any other road transport. वाहन-रुग्णता;
  **Falling S.,** epilepsy. अपस्मार; मिरगी; मिर्गी;
  **Green S.,** anaemia. रक्ताल्पता;
  **Morning S.,** nausea gravidarum; the nausea and vomiting of early pregnancy. प्रातःवमन; प्रातःअस्वस्थता;
  **Mountain S.,** see **Soroche.**
  **Sea-s.,** nausea or vomiting caused by the motion of a vessel. नौकायन-रुग्णता; समुद्री रुग्णता;
  **Sleeping S.,** a peculiar epidemic disease characterized by increasing somnolence. निद्रा-रोग; अत्यधिक नींद आने की बीमारी;
  **Train S.,** ailments caused by travelling in a rail. गति-अस्वस्थता; रेल-रुग्णता

**Side-chain.** Freedom from risk or infection; immunity. रोगक्षमता; प्रतिरक्षा

**Side-effect.** Any physiological change other than the desired one. अनुषंगी-प्रभाव

**Siderofibrosis.** Fibrosis associated with small foci in which iron is deposited. अयस्कतंतुता

**Siderosis.** Iron-colouring of the tissues. अयस्कता; अयसमयता; लोहमयता; लौहरंजनता; ऊतकों का लोहे जैसा रंग होना

**Siderotic.** Containing iron. अयस्कमय; अयसमय; लोहमय; लोहयुक्त

**Sig.** Abbreviation for **Signetur** or **Signa.**

**Sigh.** A prolonged deep inspiration. सिसकी; लम्बी सांस खींचना

**Sight.** Vision; the ability or faculty of seeing. दृष्टि; नजर;

**Far-s.**, rays of light focusing behind the retina; hypermetropia; hyperopia. दूरदृष्टि;

**Near-s.**, rays of light focusing before the retina; myopia. निकटदृष्टि

**Sigmoid.** Shaped like the letter 'S'. अवग्रहान्त्र; अवग्रह; अवग्रह रूपी; अवग्रहाकार; बक्र; अवग्राही;

**S. Cavities**, the two depressions on the head of the ulna for articulation with the radius and humerus. अवग्रह-गह्वर;

**S. Flexure**, the S-shaped portion of the colon above the rectum. अवग्रहांत्र-आनमन;

**S. Notch**, a deep depression between the coronoid and condyloid processes. अवग्राही खांच

**Sigmoidectomy.** Excision of the sigmoid colon. अवग्रहांत्र-उच्छेदन

**Sigmoiditis.** Inflammation of the colon. अवग्रहान्त्रशोथ; बृहदांत्रशोथ; बृहदांत्र का प्रदाह

**Sigmoidopexy.** Fixation of the sigmoid colon to a firm structure to correct the prolapse of the rectum. अवग्रहांत्र-स्थिरीकरण

**Sigmoidoproctostomy.** Establishment of an artificial anus by anastomosis of the sigmoid flexure with the rectum; sigmoidorectostomy. अवग्रहांत्रमलांत्रसम्मिलन

**Sigmoidorectostomy.** See **Sigmoidoproctostomy.**

**Sigmoidoscope.** Instrument for examining the sigmoid flexure. अवग्रहान्त्रदर्शी; अवग्रहान्त्र की जांच के लिये प्रयुक्त किया जाने वाला यन्त्र

**Sigmoidoscopy.** Visual inspection of the sigmoid flexure. अवग्रहान्त्रदर्शन; अवग्रहान्त्र की प्रत्यक्ष जांच करना

**Sigmoidostomy.** Establishment of an artificial anus by opening into the sigmoid colon. अवग्रहांत्रसम्मिलन

**Sign.** An evidence of disease or an abnormality. चिन्ह; निशान

**Signa.** See **Signetur.**

**Signal.** Direction sent from the brain. संकेत; इशारा

**Signetur.** The directions on a prescription; signa. सेवनविधि; औषधनिर्देश

**Silicate.** A salt of salicylic acid. सैकतीय

**Silicatosis.** See **Silicosis.**

**Silicosis.** A pathological condition of the lungs due to the inhalation of stone-dust; silicatosis; Maision's disease. सिकतामयता; पत्थरों की धूल को श्वास के साथ खींचने के कारण होने वाली फेफड़ों की विकृत अवस्था

**Silver.** Argentum; a metal of white lusturous colour. रजत; चांदी;

Sterling S., the pure silver. शुद्ध रजत; शुद्ध चांदी;

S. Nitrate, in the form of small sticks, used as a caustic for warts. सिल्वर नाइट्रेट

**Similia Similibus Curantur.** The homoeopathic "Law of Similars" or the doctorine expressing the cardinal principles of homoeopathy-"Let likes be cured by likes." सदृश विधान

**Similimum.** The remedy that corresponds most nearly to the existing symptoms of the patient. सदृशतम औषधि; रोगी के लक्षणों से समानता रखने वाली औषधि

**Simple.** Plain; not complicated; simplex. सरल; सादा

**Simples.** An old term for medicinal herbs. वनस्पतियाँ

**Simplex.** Simple. सरल; सादा

**Sinapis.** Mustard. सर्षप; सरसों;

S. Alba, white mustard. श्वेत सर्षप; सफेद सरसों;

S. Nigra, black mustard. श्याम सर्षप; काली सरसों

**Sinapism.** A mustard poultice or plaster. सर्षपोपनाह; सरसों का लेप

**Sinapized.** Mixed with mustard. सर्षपमय; सरसों के साथ मिला हुआ

**Sincipita.** Plural of **Sinciput.**

**Sincipital.** Relating to the sinciput. अग्रोपरिशीर्षी

**Sinciput.** The fore- and upper part of the head. अग्रोपरिशीर्ष; सिर का अगला और ऊपर वाला भाग

**Sinciputs.** Plural of **Sinciput.**

**Sinew.** A tendon or ligament. अस्थिमांसपेशी; कण्डरा; स्नायु

**Singer's node.** A small ovoid nodule on the edge of the vocal cord in singers. कण्ठ-पर्व; गले की गिल्टी

**Single.** See **Singular.**

**Singular.** Single. एकल

**Singulis Horis.** Every hour. प्रति घण्टा; हर घण्टे में

**Singultus.** Hiccough. हिक्का; हिचकी

**Sinistrad.** Towards the left side. बायीं ओर; वामस्थ; वामावर्त

**Sinistral.** Pertaining to the left side. वामस्थ; वामावर्त; वामपार्श्ववर्ती; बायाँ; बायीं ओर का

**Sinistrality.** Left-handedness, or left-sided. वामहस्तता अथवा वामपार्श्वता

**Sinistrocular.** Left-eyed; habitual use of left eye. वामनेत्री; बायीं ओर से देखने का आदी

**Sinistromanual.** Left-handed. वामहस्त

**Sinistropedal.** Left-footed. वामपाद

**Sinistrous.** Awkward; clumsy; unskilled. फूहड़; भोंडा; अनाड़ी; अदक्ष

**Sinogram.** Radiographic picture of a sinus. नाड़ीव्रणचित्र

**Sinum.** See **Sinus.**

**Sinuous.** Wavy; winding. सर्पिल; बक्र; पेंचदार; टेढ़ा-मेढ़ा

**Sinus.** A space or cavity, such as hollow in the bones of head and especially the nasal sinuses; sinum. विवर; खातिका; नाड़ीव्रण; शिरानाल; साइनस;

    **Aortic S.,** the space between each semilunar valve and the wall of the aorta. महाधमनी शिरानाल;

    **Cavernous S.,** a large sinus extending from the sphenoid fissure to the apex of the petrous bone. गह्वर शिरानाल;

    **Circular S.,** a venous sinus surrounding the pituitary body and communicating on each side with cavernous sinus. वर्तुल शिरानाल;

    **Coccygeal S.,** a fistula opening in the region of the coccyx. अनुत्रिक शिरानाल;

    **Coronary S.,** a large sinus in the transverse groove between the left auricle and the left ventricle of the heart. हृद्-शिरानाल;

    **Inferior Petrosal S.,** a large sinus arising from the cavernous sinus, running along the lower margin of the petrous bone, and joining the lateral sinus to form the internal jugular vein. निम्न-अश्म शिरानाल; निम्नाश्म-शिरानाल;

    **Laryngeal S.,** the ventricle of the larynx. स्वरयंत्र खातिका;

    **Lymph S.,** spaces in the parenchyma of a lymphatic gland between the pulp of the gland and the dilatations of the lymphatic vessels; lymphatic sinus. लसीका शिरानाल;

**Lymphatic S.,** see **Lymph Sinus.**

    **Maxillary S.,** antrum of Highmore; maxillary antrum; an air cavity in the body of maxilla, communicating with the middle meatus of the nose. ऊर्ध्वहनु-विवर;

    **Precervical S.,** a recess between the lowermost branchial arch and the trunk of the embryo. पश्चकपाल शिरानाल;

    **Renal S.,** the prolongation inward the hilum of the kidney. वृक्क खातिका;

    **Sphenoid S.,** the air-space in the body of the sphenoid bone communicating with the nasal cavity. जतूक विवर;

**Transverse S.,** one uniting the inferior petrosal sinus. अनुप्रस्थ शिरानाल;

**Uterine S.,** a small irregular vascular channel in the endometrium. जरायु शिरानाल; गर्भाशय शिरानाल

**Sinusitis.** Inflammation of a sinus. शिरानालशोथ; वायुविवरशोथ; गर्तदाह

**Sinusoid.** A dilated channel into which arterioles open in some organs and which take the place of the usual capillaries. शिरानालाभ; शिरानाल जैसा; resembling a sinus. शिरानाल से मिलता-जुलता

**Sinusotomy.** Incision into a sinus. शिरानालछेदन

**Si Opus Sit (SOS).** As may be needed; per requirement. आवश्यकतानुसार; यथावश्यक; आवश्यकता के अनुसार

**Sister.** Any registered nurse in a public or private hospital. परिचारिका; नर्स; सिस्टर

**Sitch-bath.** Hip-bath; sitz-bath. कटि-स्नान; नितम्ब-स्नान

**Site.** Location; place; position. स्थल; स्थान; स्थिति

**Sitiology.** See **Sitology.**

**Sitology.** A treatise on dietetics; sitiology. आहारविज्ञान; पथ्यविज्ञान; पथ्यशास्त्र

**Sitophobia.** Insanity with abhorrence of food. आहारभीति; आहारातंक; भोजनातंक; भोजनसंत्रास; आहारसंत्रास

**Situs.** See **Site.**

**S. Inversus,** visceral inversion; abnormal displacement of viscera to opposite side of the body, the liver being on the left side and the heart on the right. विपरीत स्थान

**Sitz-bath.** See **Sitch-bath.**

**Skeletal.** Relating to the skeleton. कंकालीय; अस्थिपंजरीय; अस्थिपंजर सम्बन्धी;

**S. Muscle,** one attached to the skeleton. कंकाल-पेशी;

**S. Tissue,** the tissue of the framework of the body. अस्थि-ऊतक

**Skeleton.** The bony framework of the body. पंजर; अस्थिपंजर; कंकाल; हड्डियों का ढांचा

**Skene's glands.** Two small glands at the entrance of the female urethra. स्कीन ग्रन्थियाँ; स्त्रीमूत्रपथ के प्रवेश-द्वार पर दो छोटी-छोटी ग्रन्थियाँ

**Skenitis.** Inflammation of the Skene's glands. स्कीनग्रन्थिशोथ; स्कीनग्रन्थियों का प्रदाह

**Skiagram.** The finished printed x-ray picture; skiagraph; actinogram; actinograph. एक्स-रेचित्र; क्ष-किरणचित्र; छायाचित्र
**Skiagraph.** See **Skiagram.**
**Skiascopy.** Retinoscopy. दृष्टिपटलदर्शन; fluoroscopy. प्रतिदीप्तिदर्शन
**Skin.** The external covering of the body; cutis. चर्म; त्वक्; त्वचा; चमड़ी; खाल
**Skull.** The bony framework of the head; calvaria. करोटि; खोपड़ी; S.-cap, the cranium. कपाल
**Sleep.** Period of rest where physiological activities and consciousness are diminished and voluntary muscles become inactive. सुप्ति; निद्रा; नींद;
  **S. Disease,** sleeping sickness. निद्रारोग;
  **S. Walking,** somnambulism. निद्राभ्रमण; सुप्तिभ्रमण; नींद में चलना
**Sleeping Sickness.** See **Sleep Disease.**
**Sleeplessness.** Insomnia; loss of sleep. अनिद्रा; निद्राभाव; नींद का अभाव
**Slide.** A glass slip for microscopic specimen. पट्टिका; काच-पट्टिका; स्लाइड
**Slimy.** Glutinous; gelatinous; tenacious. श्लैष्मिक; पंकिल; चिपचिपा
**Sling.** A suspending bandage for a limb. गोफन; लटकन
**Slit.** A narrow opening. विवर; छिद्र
**Slit-lamp.** In ophthalmology, an instrument consisting of a microscope combined with a rectangular light source. स्लिट-लैम्प
**Slough.** The separated dead matter in an ulceration. मृत्तोतक; निर्मोक; खुरण्ड; पपड़ी
**Sloughing.** The formation of sloughs. निर्मोकन; निर्मोक बनना; खुरण्ड बनना
**Sluggish.** Of slow movement. धीमा; मन्दगतिक
**Slumber.** Light sleep; cat-nap. ऊँघ; हल्की नींद; to butcher. वध करना; काटना
**Small Intestines.** The intestines that include duodenum, jejunum and ileum. लघ्वान्त्र; छोटी आन्तें; छोटी अन्तड़ियाँ
**Small-pox.** A serious and highly contagious virus disease; variola. मसूरिका; शीतला; चेचक; बड़ी माता
**Smear.** A film of material spread out on a glass slide for microscopic examination. लेपन; आलेप; लेप

**Smegma.** Sebaceous secretion about the penis or labia. शिश्नमल; भगोष्ठमल

**Smell.** The perception of odour. गन्ध; to scent, सूंघना; olfaction. घ्राण-संवेदना; गंधज्ञान

**Smelling Salt.** A mixture of compounds usually containing some form of ammonia; acts as a stimulant, when inhaled. सुगन्धित लवण

**Smooth.** Evenly spread; glossy. कोमल; मृदु

**Snap.** A short sharp sound; a click, said especially of heart sounds. स्फुटन

**Snare.** A surgical instrument with a wire loop at the end, used for removal of polypi. पाश; नाक के पॉलिप (पुर्वगकों) को हटाने के लिये प्रयुक्त किया जाने वाला एक शल्य-यंत्र

**Sneezing.** An explosive expulsion of air through the nasal passages and mouth. छींक

**Snore.** A noisy breathing in sleep or coma; snoring. निद्राघूर्णन; खर्राटे लेना; खर्राटे भरना

**Snoring.** See **Snore.**

**Snow-blindness.** Partial blindness from reflection of snow. हिमान्धता; बर्फीली चमचमाहट में ठीक न दिखाई देने का रोग

**Snuffles.** A catarrhal discharge from the nasal mucous membrane in infants. नासाश्लेष्मस्राव; शिशुओं की नाक की झिल्ली से निरन्तर पानी बहते रहना

**Soap.** See **Sapo.**

**Sob.** To weep with convulsive movements of the chest. सिसकियां भरना; सुबक-सुबक कर रोना

**Socia-parodites.** An occasional small separate lobe of the parotid gland. कर्णपूर्वग्रन्थि-विमुक्तांश

**Sociology.** The scientific study of interpersonal and intergroup social relationship. सामाजिकज्ञान; समाजविज्ञान

**Socket.** The hollow part of a joint. गर्त; गर्तिका; the proximal portion of a prosthesis into which the stump of an amputed extremity is fitted. सॉक्केट;

**S. of tooth,** the hollow place which receives and holds the tooth. दन्त-गर्त

**Soda.** The common sodium bicarbonate; soda-ash. साधारण सोडा; सामान्य सोडियम बाइकार्बोनेट या खाने का सोडा

**Sodae Biboras.** Borax; sodium borate. सुहागा; सोडियम बोरेट; सोडे बाइबोरस

**Sodium Bicarbonate.** Baking soda. बेकिंग सोडा; खाने का सोडा

**Sodium Borate.** Borax. सुहागा

**Sodium Chloride.** The common salt; chloride of soda. साधारण नमक; लवण

**Sodium Citrate.** An alkaline diuretic very similar to potassium citrate. सोडियम साइट्रेट

**Sodium Sulphate.** A poplur domestic purgative. सोडियम सल्फेट

**Sodomist.** One who practices sodomy; sodomite. लौंडेबाज

**Sodomite.** See **Sodomist.**

**Sodomy.** Sexual connection by the anus. गुदमैथुन; गुदामैथुन; लौंडेबाजी

**Soft.** Not bony or cartilaginous; gentle in action or motion. कोमल; मृदु;

   **S. Palate,** the rear portion of the roof of the mouth. मृदु तालु; कोमल तालु;

   **S. Sore,** the primary ulcer of genitalia, occurring in the venereal disease; chancroid. मृदुव्रण; मृदुक्षत; कोमल घाव

**Softening.** Malacia; a diminution of the natural and healthy consistence of organs. मृदुता; कोमलता;

   **S. of brain,** progressive dementia. मस्तिष्क-मृदुता; मनोभ्रंश

**Sol.** Abbreviation for **Solution.** घोल, विलेय, आदि के लिये प्रयुक्त होने वाला अंग्रेजी शब्द का संक्षिप्त रूप

**Solanum Tuberosum.** Potato. आलू

**Solar.** Relating to the sun or sun-light. सौर; सूर्य अथवा धूप या सूर्य की रोशनी सम्बन्धी;

   **S. Energy,** the light of heat from the sun which is capable of doing work, when properly harnessed. सौर ऊर्जा; सूर्य की गर्मी;

   **S. Plexus,** a large network of sympathetic nerve ganglia and fibres in the upper region of the abdomen extending from one adrenal gland to the other. सूर्य प्रतान; स्नायु गुच्छ; आमाशय के पीछे का तंत्रिकाजाल

**Solarium.** A sun-bath sanatorium. सूर्यरश्मिचिकित्सागृह; सूर्यस्नानगृह

**Sole.** The under-part or the plantar surface of the foot. पदतल; पैर का तलवा; main. मुख्य; प्रमुख

**Soleus.** A fish-shaped muscle of the calf of leg. पिण्डिका; पिण्डली की एक मछली के आकार जैसी पेशी

**Solid.** Hard; compact; firm; not fluid or gaseous. ठोस; दृढ़; कठोर

**Solidification.** A disorder of the lungs causing them to solidify. दृढ़ीभवन; फुप्फुसकाठिन्य; hepatization. यकृतीभवन

**Solitary.** Alone; single. एकाकी; एकल;

   **S. Glands,** small, flattened granular bodies found in the stomach and the intestines. एकल ग्रन्थियाँ

**Solitude.** Devoid of any other being. एकान्त

**Solium.** A variety of tapeworm. स्फीतकृमि; फीताकृमि; सोलियम

**Solubility.** The condition of being soluble. विलेयता; घुलनशीलता

**Solubilization.** Converting into solution. विलेयीकरण; घोल बनाना

**Soluble.** That which is dissolved in a fluid. विलेय; विलयशील; घुलनशील

**Solution.** A compound liquid. घोल; the diffusion of a solid substance in a liquid. विलयन;

   **Saline S.,** a solution of any salt; salt-solution. लवण घोल;

   **Salt-s.,** see **Saline Solution.**

   **Saturated S.,** one in which as much of the solid is dissolved as will be held in solution without depositing or floating. संतृप्त घोल

**Solvent.** That which dissolves a substance. विलायक; घोलने वाला पदार्थ

**Soma.** The body, including the head and neck, but without limbs. काय; देह; शरीर

**Somasthenia.** Weakness of the body; somatasthenia. कायदुर्बलता; देहदौर्बल्य; शारीरिक कमजोरी

**Somatagnosia.** Inability to identify the parts of the body. अंगज्ञानाभाव; अंगबोधहीनता

**Somatalgia.** Pain in the body; somatodynia. कायार्ति; देहशूल

**Somatasthenia.** See **Somasthenia.**

**Somatasthesia.** See **Somesthesia.**

**Somatic.** Pertaining to the body. कायिक; दैहिक

**Somatodynia.** See **Somatalgia.**

**Somatology.** Study of anatomy and physiology. देहविज्ञान; शरीर-रचना एवं क्रियाविज्ञान

**Somatopathy.** Disease of the body. शारीरिकरोग

**Somatoplasm.** The protoplasm of the body-cells. कायद्रव्य; शरीर की कोशिकाओं का द्रव्य

**Somatopleural.** Relating to the somatopleure. आद्यकायास्तरीय; आद्यकायास्तर सम्बन्धी

**Somatopleure.** The upper layer of the mesoblast. आद्यकायास्तर

**Somatopsychic.** Relating to both body and mind. कायमानसिक; मनोकायिक; देह एवं मन सम्बन्धी

**Somatotomy.** The anatomy of the human body. मानवशरीर-रचना

**Somatotherapy.** Therapy directed at bodily or physical disorders. कायचिकित्सा; भौतिक चिकित्सा

**Somatotrophic.** See **Somatotropic.**

**Somatotropic.** Having a stimulating effect on body growth; somatotrophic. कायपोषी

**Somesthesia.** Bodily sensation; somatesthesia. कायसंवेदना; कायिकसंवेदता; देहसंवेदना

**Somesthetic.** Pertaining to the body sensation. कायसंवेदी; देहसंवेदना सम्बन्धी

**Somite.** A mesoblastic segment. भ्रूणकायखण्ड; भ्रूणकाय; भ्रूणदेह

**Somnambulance.** See **Somnambulism.**

**Somnambulism.** Habitual walking in sleep; somnambulance. निद्राभ्रमण; निद्राचलन; नींद में चलना

**Somnambulist.** A person who walks in sleep. निद्राचर; स्वापचारी; नींद में चलने वाला

**Somnifacient.** A medicine for producing sleep. निद्रापक; निद्राजनक; स्वापक; नींद लाने वाली; निद्राकारी

**Somniferous.** Causing sleep; soporific. निद्राकर; सुप्तिकारक; नींद लाने वाली

**Somniloquence.** Talking in sleep; somniloquism. निद्रालाप; नींद में बोलना

**Somniloquism.** See **Somniloquence.**

**Somnipathy.** Any disorder of sleep. निद्रापकरोग

**Somnolence.** The condition of drowsiness. तन्द्रा; निद्रा; सुप्ति; ऊँघ; semiconscious. अर्धचेतन

**Somnolency.** Sleeping heaviness; a sort of coma. तन्द्रालुता; उनींदापन

**Somnolent.** Inclined to sleep. तन्द्रालु; निद्रालु; उनींदा

**Somnolentia.** A condition of incomplete sleep in which some faculties are excited and others are in repose. तन्द्रा; ऊँघ

**Somnolescent.** Inclined to sleep; drowsy. तन्द्रालु

**Sonorous.** Resonant; ringing. ध्वनिक; सुस्वनिक; प्रतिध्वनिपूर्ण

**Sopor.** Profound sleep. जड़िमा; गहन तन्द्रा

**Soporiferous.** Producing profound sleep. जड़िमाकारी; निद्राकारी; निद्रापक; निद्राजनक; स्वापक; नींद लाने वाला

**Soporific.** An agent which induces profound sleep. निद्रावह; तन्द्रावह; स्वापक; गहन निद्रा लाने वाला

**Soporose.** Sleepy. तन्द्रालु; निद्रालु

**Soporous.** Relating to, or causing sopor. नींद सम्बन्धी अथवा नींद लाने वाला (कारक)

**Sorbefacient.** An agent producing absorption. अवशोषकर; अवशोषकारी; सोखने वाला

**Sorbent.** Absorbent. अवशोषक; सोखने वाला

**Sorbitol.** An alcohol; a sugar solution used in the treatment of patients whose skin is retaining too little oil. मद्यसार; सुरासार

**Sordes.** Small accumulation of debris on lips and gums in the last stages of serious illnesses. दन्तमल; मुखमल

**Sore.** A wound or ulcer. व्रण; क्षत; घाव; दाह; painful. दर्दनाक;

   **S.-throat,** any morbid or painful affection of the throat. कण्ठदाह; गलदाह;

   **Bed-s.,** decubitus. शय्या-क्षत;

   **Canker S.,** ulcerative stomatitis. सव्रण मुखपाक

**Soreness.** Pain; aching. दुखन; पीड़ा; कष्ट

**Sorghum.** A variety of cane-sugar. ज्वार; ज्वार वर्ग

**Soroche.** Mountain sickness. मेरु-रुग्णता; पर्वत-व्याधि

**SOS.** See **Si Opus Sit.**

**Souffle.** An auscultatory murmur; a bruit. सूफिल; मर्मर ध्वनि; ब्रूई; बिरुत;

   **Cardiac S.,** heart-murmur. हृद्-मर्मर;

   **Foetal S.,** an inconstant murmur heard during pregnancy. गर्भ-मर्मर;

   **Uterine S.,** a vascular sound in the pregnant uterus heard with the stethoscope. जरायु-मर्मर

**Sound.** Sensation produced in the ear when certain vibrations are caused in the surrounding air. ध्वनि; शब्द; आहट; a probe; an exploring instrument. गवेषिणी; प्रोब; healthy. स्वस्थ;

**Heart S.**, one of the sounds heard on auscultation over the heart. हृद्ध्वनि

**Soup.** A kind of broth. सूप; शोरबा

**Sour.** Having an acid taste. खट्टा; अम्लज

**Soyabean.** A highly nutritious legume used in Asiatic countries in place of meat. सोयाबीन; मांस के बदले खाई जाने वाली एक अति-पौष्टिक फली

**Space.** Any area or cavity in the body; spatium. स्थान; क्षेत्र; गह्वर; अन्तराल; अवकाश;

**Epidural S.**, the space around dura and brain. अधिदृढ़तानिका अवकाश;

**Episcleral S.**, the space between the sheath of the eyeball and the sclera. अधिश्वेतपटल अवकाश;

**Intercostal S.**, the space between two contiguous ribs. पर्शुकान्तराल;

**Interpleural S.**, the mediastinum; the median portion of the thoracic cavity. अन्तरापरिफुफ्फुस-अवकाश;

**Subarachnoid S.**, that between the arachnoid and the pia. अधोजालतानिका अवकाश;

**Subdural S.**, that between the dura and the arachnoid. अधोदृढ़तानिका अवकाश

**Spanemia.** Poverty of the blood. रक्ताल्पता; खून की कमी

**Spanish Fly.** Cantharis. कैंथरिस; स्पेन देश की एक मक्खी; एक चमकीला हरा कीड़ा

**Spasm.** An involuntary contraction of the muscles. आकर्ष; उद्वेष्ट; आक्षेप; ऐंठन; पेशियों की निरंकुश सिकुड़न;

**Clonic S.**, alternate involuntary contraction and relaxation of a muscle. अवमोटनाकर्ष;

**Tetanic S.**, spasm in which contractions continue for a time without interruption. धनुर्वाताकर्ष; हनुस्तम्भाकर्ष;

**Tonic S.**, continued involuntary contractions. तानिकाकर्ष;

**Torsion S.**, a spasmodic twisting of the body at the pelvis. मरोड़ आकर्ष

**Spasmatic.** See **Spasmodic**.

**Spasmodic.** Of the nature of a spasm; spasmatic; spasmodical. आकर्षी; उद्घ्रेष्टी; उद्घ्रेष्टकर; उद्घ्रेष्टकारी; ऐंठनयुक्त

**Spasmodical.** See **Spasmodic.**

**Spasmogenic.** Spasm-producing. आकर्षजन; उद्घ्रेष्टजन; ऐंठन पैदा करने वाला

**Spasmology.** A treastise on spasmodic troubles. आक्षेपविज्ञान; उद्घ्रेष्टप्रकरण

**Spasmolysis.** Arrest of a spasm or convulsion. उद्घ्रेष्टलयन; आक्षेपलयन

**Spasmolytic.** An agent allaying spasm. उद्घ्रेष्टहर; आक्षेपहर; ऐंठन कम करने वाला

**Spasmophilia.** A tendency to tetany and covulsions. हनुस्तम्भ तथा आक्षेप की प्रवृत्ति

**Spasmus.** A spasm. उद्घ्रेष्ट; आकर्ष; आक्षेप; ऐंठन;
   **S. Nutans,** nodding spasm; a nodding of the head from spasm of the sternomastoid muscle. शीर्षदोलन

**Spastic.** Spasticus; pertaining to spasm. संस्तम्भी; उद्घ्रेष्ट सम्बन्धी; rigid. कठोर; hypertonic. अतितानिक

**Spasticity.** The quality of being spastic. संस्तम्भता; कठोरता

**Spasticus.** See **Spastic.**

**Spatium.** See **Space.**

**Spatula.** A flexible flat blade with no sharp edges, used in pharmacy for spreading plasters and ointments. चमस; करनी; चपटा चिमटा; लेपनी

**Specialist.** One who treats the special kinds of diseases. विशेषज्ञ; दक्ष; विशेष प्रकार के रोगों की चिकित्सा करने वाला

**Specialization.** Confining one's practice to a particular branch of medicine or surgery. विशिष्टता; विशेषज्ञता

**Specialty.** The particular group of diseases or branch of medical science on which a physician or surgeon concentrates. विशेषता; विशिष्टता; दक्षता

**Species.** A subdivision of a genus. जाति; वर्ण; नस्ल

**Specific.** Of a definite character. विशिष्ट; एक निश्चित चरित्र का;
   **S. Gravity,** the weight of a substance compared with that of water. विशिष्ट गुरुत्व;
   **S. Remedy,** a remedy peculiarly curative of a disease. विशिष्ट औषधि; औषधि-विशेष

**Specificity.** Capable of being specific. विशिष्टता

**Specillum.** A button-shaped probe. क्षतदर्शीयंत्र; a lens. लेंस

**Specimen.** A sample of any substance or material obtained for testing. प्रतिदर्श; नमूना

**Spectacles.** Framed lense to correct metropia. चश्मा; ऐनक

**Spectra.** Plural of **Spectrum**.

**Spectral.** Pertaining to the spectrum. दृश्याभासी; प्रतिबिम्ब सम्बन्धी; चमक रेखा सम्बन्धी

**Spectrometer.** An instrument used in spectrum analysis or spectrometry. प्रतिबिम्ब-विश्लेषक

**Spectrometry.** Spectrum analysis; the process of determining the wavelength of light rays by using a spectrometer. प्रतिबिम्ब-विश्लेषण

**Spectrophotometer.** An instrument for spectral measurement of the light sense and/or for determining the amount of colour in spectrum analysis. प्रतिबिम्बमापी; प्रतिबिम्बमितिक

**Spectrophotometry.** The use of the spectrophotometer. प्रतिबिम्बमिति; प्रतिबिम्बमापन

**Spectroscope.** An instrument for observing spectra of light. प्रतिबिम्बदर्शी

**Spectroscopy.** The use of spectroscope. प्रतिबिम्बदर्शन

**Spectrum.** A colour-band from a ray of white or decomposed light; an illuminating ray. प्रतिबिम्ब; चमकरेखा; दृश्याभास

**Spectrums.** Plural of **Spectrum**.

**Specula.** Plural of **Speculum**.

**Speculum.** An instrument used to hold the wall of a cavity part so that the interior of cavity can be examined. वीक्षक; वीक्षणयंत्र

**Speech.** The use of the voice in conveying ideas; speaking; talk. वाक्; उच्चारण; भाषण

**Spell.** An attack; a paroxysm. दौर; दौरा

**Spend.** To ejaculate semen in coitus. शुक्रसेचन

**Sperm.** Semen containing protozoa; spermatozoon. शुक्राणु

**Spermacrasia.** Weakness of semen. शुक्रदौर्बल्य; वीर्यदौर्बल्य

**Spermatic.** Relating to the sperm or semen. वृषण, शुक्राणु अथवा वीर्य सम्बन्धी;

   **S. Artery,** a branch of the abdominal aorta. वृषण-धमनी;

   **S. Cord,** the suspensory cord of the testes. वृषण-रज्जु;

**S. Duct,** the seminal canal. शुक्रनलिका; शुक्रनली

**Spermaticidal.** Lethal to spermatozoa; spermatocidal; spermicidal. शुक्राणुनाशक; शुक्राणुनाशी; शुक्राणु नष्ट करने वाला

**Spermatid.** A cell produced by fission of a secondary spermatocyte. प्राक्शुक्राणु; शुक्राणुप्रसू

**Spermatism.** The emission of semen. शुक्राणुता; वीर्यस्खलनता

**Spermatitis.** Inflammation of the excretory duct of the testes. शुक्रवाहिकाशोथ; शुक्रनली का प्रदाह

**Spermatocele.** A spermatic cyst of the testicles. शुक्रपुटी

**Spermatocidal.** See **Spermaticidal.**

**Spermatocide.** An agent or substance destroying protozoa; spermicide. शुक्राणुनाशी; शुक्राणुनाशक

**Spermatocytal.** Relating to spermatocyte. शुक्राणुकोशिकीय; शुक्राणुकोशिका सम्बन्धी

**Spermatocyte.** Germinal cell of a spermatozoon. शुक्राणुकोशिका

**Spermatocytogenesis.** See **Spermatogenesis.**

**Spermatogenesis.** The production of spermatozoa; spermatocytogenesis; spermatogeny; spermiogenesis. शुक्राणुजनन

**Spermatogenic.** Sperm-producing. शुक्राणुजनक; relating to spermatogenesis. शुक्राणुजनन सम्बन्धी

**Spermatogeny.** See **Spermatogenesis.**

**Spermatogonium.** A formative seminal cell. शुक्राणुजन

**Spermatoid.** Resembling a spermatozoon. शुक्राणुवत्; शुक्राणु से मिलता-जुलता; शुक्राणु जैसा

**Spermatorrhea.** An involuntary discharge of semen; spermatorrhoea. शुक्रमेह; वीर्यपात; वीर्यस्खलनता

**Spermatorrhoea.** See **Spermatorrhea.**

**Spermatozoa.** Plural of **Spermatozoon.**

**Spermatozoon.** A mature, male reproductive cell; sperm. शुक्राणु; पुरुषों में एक परिपक्व प्रजनन-कोशिका

**Spermaturia.** The presence of semen in the urine; semenuria. शुक्रमेह; पेशाब में वीर्य जाना

**Spermicidal.** See **Spermaticidal.**

**Spermicide.** A agent that kills spermatozoa; spermatocide. शुक्राणुनाशी; शुक्राणुनाशक

**Spermiogenesis.** See **Spermatogenesis.**

**Spermolith.** A stone in the spermatic duct. शुक्रवाहिकाश्मरी; शुक्रनली की पथरी

**Sphacelation.** Gangrene; mortification; necrosis; sphacelism. कोथ; परिगलन

**Sphacelism.** See **Sphacelation**.

**Sphaceloderma.** Gangrene of the skin. त्वक्कोथ; चमड़ी का सड़ना-गलना

**Sphacelous.** Gangrenous. कोथज; necrotic or necrosed. परिगलित; sloughing. निर्मोकन

**Sphenocephaly.** Having a wedge-shaped head. शंकुशीर्ष; शंकुशीर्षता

**Sphenoconical.** Both spherical and conic. गोलशंक्वाकार; गोल तथा शंकु रूप

**Sphenoethmoidal.** Relating to the sphenoid and ethmoid bones. जतूक-झर्झरिकास्थिक; जतूकास्थि एवं झर्झरिकास्थि सम्बन्धी

**Sphenoid.** A bone in the skull and the sinuses it contains, located behind the nose in the centre of the head. जतूकाभ; जतूक जैसे फाने के आकार की (हड्डी);

**S. Bone,** one of the cranial bones at the anterior base of the skull articulating with all the other bones of the head. जतूकास्थि

**Sphenoidal.** Pertaining to sphenoid bone. जतूकास्थिक; जतूकास्थिज; जतूकास्थि सम्बन्धी; cuneiform or wedge-shaped. कीलाकार अथवा शंक्वाकार;

**S. Sinuses,** air sinuses that occupy the body of the sphenoid bone and connect with the nasal cavity. जतूक विवर

**Sphenoparietal.** Pertaining to the sphenoid and the parietal bones. जतूकपार्श्विकास्थि सम्बन्धी

**Sphere.** A ball or a globular body. गोल; कोई गोलाकार पिण्ड

**Spheric.** Like a sphere; spherical. गोलाकार; गोल; मण्डलाकार

**Spherical.** See **Spheric**.

**Spherocyte.** A small round blood cell. गोलककोशिका; गोलरक्तकोशिका

**Spherocytosis.** The condition of a cell being spherical. गोलककोशिकता

**Sphinter.** Muscle surrounding certain parts of the intestinal tract. संवरणी; अवरोधिनी; संकोचिनी; संकोची;

**S.-ani,** a muscle situated around the anus. गुदसंवरणी; गुदा-संकोचिनी; गुदा-संकोची (पेशी)

**Sphincteral.** Relating to a sphincter; sphincteric. गुदा-संकोचिनी (पेशी) सम्बन्धी

**Sphincteralgia.** Pain about the anus. गुदार्ति; मलद्वार की पीड़ा

**Sphincterectomy.** Excision of a portion of the iris, or of any sphincter muscle. उपतारा-उच्छेदन; परितारिका-उच्छेदन अथवा संवरणीपेशी-उच्छेदन

**Sphincteric.** See **Sphincteral**.

**Sphincteritis.** Inflammation of a sphincter. संवरणीशोथ

**Sphincteroplasty.** Plastic surgery of any sphincter muscle. संवरणीसंधान

**Sphincterotomy.** The surgical removal of the pyloric sphincter. संवरणी-उच्छेदन

**Sphygmic.** Pertaining to the pulse; sphygmical. नाड़ीस्पन्द अथवा स्पन्दन सम्बन्धी

**Sphygmical.** See **Sphygmic**.

**Sphygmocardiograph.** An apparatus for simultaneous graphic recording of the radial pulse and heart beat. स्पन्दनहृद्स्पन्दलेखी

**Sphygmograph.** An instrument for recording the differential features of the pulse in health and in disease. स्पन्दनलेखी

**Sphygmoid.** Resembling the pulse; pulse-like. नाड़ीस्पन्दाभ; नाड़ी जैसा

**Sphygmology.** The science of the pulse. स्पन्दनविज्ञान; नाड़ीविज्ञान

**Sphygmomanometer.** An instrument for measuring the arterial pressure; the blood pressure apparatus. रक्तदाबमापी; रक्तदाबमापकयंत्र

**Sphygmomanometry.** Determination of blood pressure by means of sphygmomanometer. रक्तदाबमिति

**Sphygmometer.** An instrument for measuring the pulse. स्पन्दनमापी; नाड़ीस्पन्दमापी

**Sphyrectomy.** Excision of the malleus of the foot. गुल्फोच्छेदन

**Spica.** A bandage applied in a figure of eight pattern. स्वास्तिक पट्टिका

**Spicula.** A small spike-shaped fragment of bone; spicule; spiculum. कंटिका; कण्टिका

**Spicule.** See **Spicula**.

**Spiculum.** See **Spicula**.

**Spina.** The spine. मेरुदण्ड; रीढ़; कण्टक; कंटक;

    **S. Bifida,** a congenital defect in which the vertebral neural arches fail to close; rachischisis. अयुक्त मेरुदण्ड; द्विमेरुता; द्विशाखीमेरुता;

    **S. Ventosa,** a tumour arising from the internal caries of a spinal bone. कण्टकार्बुद; कंटकार्बुद; मेरुदण्डार्बुद; रीढ़ की हड्डी की रसौली

M.D.F.-29

**Spinal.** Pertaining to the spine. मेरुदण्डीय; मेरुदण्डज; मेरुदण्ड अथवा रीढ़ सम्बन्धी;

**S. Anaesthetic,** a local anesthetic solution injected into the subarachnoid space so that it renders the area supplied by the selected spinal nerves insensitive. मेरु-संवेदनाहारी;

**S. Canal,** the central hollow throughout the spinal column. मेरु-नलिका;

**S. Caries,** disease of the vertebral bones. मेरु-क्षय; कशेरुकास्थियों का रोग;

**S. Column,** the back-bone. मेरु-दण्ड; पृष्ठवंश; रीढ़ की हड्डी;

**S. Cord,** the nerve structure running within the spinal canal of the spinal column. सुषुम्ना; मेरु-रज्जु;

**S. Marrow,** the spinal cord. मेरु-मज्जा;

**S. Nerves,** 31 pairs leave the spinal cord and pass out of the spinal canal to supply the periphery. मेरु-स्नायु; मेरु-तंत्रिकायें

**Spindle.** A tapering rod or pin. तर्कु;

**Neuromuscular S.,** small fusiform endorgans found in almost all the muscles of the body. तंत्रिकापेशी-तर्कु

**Spine.** The vertebral column. मेरुदण्ड; पृष्ठवंश; रीढ़; कण्टक

**Spinous.** Pertaining to the spine. मेरुदण्ड, पृष्ठवंश, कण्टक अथवा रीढ़ सम्बन्धी

**Spiradenoma.** A benign tumour of the sweat glands. स्वेदग्रन्थ्यर्बुद; स्वेद ग्रन्थियों की रसौली

**Spiral.** Screw-like; coiled. सर्पिल; चक्रिल

**Spirillum.** A bacterial germ. सर्पिल-दण्डाणु

**Spirit.** An alcoholic liquor stronger than wine; spiritus. सुरासार; स्पिरिट

**Spirituous.** Containing spirit or alcohol. सुरासारयुक्त; स्पिरिटयुक्त

**Spiritus.** See **Spirit.**

**Spirochaeta.** A bacterium having a spiral shape; spirochaete. सर्पकीट; चक्रकीट;

**S. Pallida,** the parasite that causes syphilis; treponema pallidum. पाण्डुर सर्पकीट; उपदंश पैदा करने वाला परजीवी

**Spirochaete.** See **Spirochaeta.**

**Spirochaetaemia.** Spirochaetes in the blood stream. सर्पकीटरक्तता

**Spirogram.** The tracing made by the spirograph. श्वसनलेख; श्वासलेख

**Spirograph.** An instrument for recording respiration. श्वसनलेख अथवा श्वासलेखयंत्र

**Spirometer.** An instrument for measuring respiration. श्वसनमापी; श्वासमापी

**Spirometry.** The measurement of breathing capacity. श्वसनमिति; श्वासमिति

**Spissated.** Thickened; inspissated. घनीभूत; सघन; गाढ़ा

**Spiteful.** Jealous. ईर्षालु; दुर्भावना से परिपूर्ण

**Spittle.** Saliva; sputum; that which is expectorated. थूक; लार

**Splanchnectopia.** Displacement of any of the viscera; splanchnodiastosis. अन्तरांगभ्रंश; आशयभ्रंश

**Splanchnic.** Pertaining to the viscera; visceral. अन्तरांगीय

**Splanchnicectomy.** Surgical removal of the splanchnic nerves. आशयानुकम्पीतंत्रिका-उच्छेदन

**Splanchnodiastosis.** See **Splanchnectopia.**

**Splanchnography.** A description of the viscera. अन्तरांगलेख; आशयलेख

**Splanchnology.** Science of the nature and functions of the viscera. आशयप्रकरण; अन्तरांगविज्ञान

**Splanchnopleure.** The wall of the alimentary tract of a vertebrae. आद्याशयास्तर; किसी कशेरुका की पोषण नली का पर्दा

**Splanchnoptosis.** Visceral prolapse; visceroptosis. आशयस्रंस; अन्तरांगच्युति

**Splanchnoscopy.** Examination of the viscera. आशयदर्शन; अन्तरांगदर्शन

**Splanchnotomy.** The dissection of the viscera. आशय-उच्छेदन

**Splay-foot.** A flat foot; talipes planus. सपाट-पाद; चपटा पैर

**Spleen.** A large vascular ductless gland lying in the upper part of the abdominal cavity on the left side, between the stomach and the diaphragm. प्लीहा; तिल्ली;

    **Floating S.,** one separated from its attachments; movable spleen. चल-प्लीहा; प्लवमान प्लीहा;

    **Movable S.,** see **Floating Spleen.**

**Splenalgia.** Neuralgia of the spleen. प्लीहार्ति; तिल्ली का दर्द

**Splenculi.** Plural of **Splenculus.**

**Splenculus.** Accessory spleen. उप-प्लीहा; अतिरिक्त प्लीहा

**Splenectomy.** Surgical removal of the spleen. प्लीहोच्छेदन; प्लीहा-उच्छेदन; प्लीहा काट कर हटा देना

**Splenetic.** See **Splenic.**

**Splenia.** Plural of **Splenium.**

**Splenic.** Relating to the spleen; splenetic; lienalis. प्लीहज; प्लीहा सम्बन्धी; तिल्ली का

**Splenisation.** Conversion of the lung, in inflammation, into a substance resembling the spleen. प्लीहाभवन; फेफड़ों का तिल्ली जैसा रूप लेना

**Splenitis.** Inflammation of the spleen. प्लीहाशोथ; तिल्ली का प्रदाह

**Splenium.** A bandage or compress. पट्टिका; पट्टी; सम्पीड

**Splenodynia.** Pain in the spleen. प्लीहार्ति; तिल्ली का दर्द

**Splenogram.** Radiographic picture of the spleen after injecting the radio-opaque medium. प्लीहाचित्र

**Splenography.** A description of the spleen. प्लीहाचित्रण

**Splenohepatomegaly.** Enlargement of both spleen and the liver. प्लीहायकृत्-बृद्धि; प्लीहायकृत्-अतिबृद्धि; तिल्ली और जिगर का अत्यधिक बढ़ जाना

**Splenoid.** Like spleen. प्लीहाभ; तिल्लीनुमा; तिल्ली जैसा

**Splenoma.** A tumour of the spleen; splenoncus. प्लीहार्बुद; तिल्ली की रसौली

**Splenomalacia.** Softening of the spleen. प्लीहामृदुता; तिल्ली की कोमलता

**Splenomegalia.** Enlargement of the spleen; splenomegaly. प्लीहाबृद्धि; प्लीहावर्धन; तिल्ली का बढ़ना

**Splenomegaly.** See **Splenomegalia.**

**Splenomyelomalacia.** Softening of the spleen and bone marrow. प्लीहा तथा अस्थि-मज्जा की कोमलता; प्लीहास्थिमज्जामृदुता

**Splenoncus.** See **Splenoma.**

**Splenopathy.** Any disease of the spleen. प्लीहाविकृति; तिल्ली की कोई बीमारी

**Splenopexy.** Surgical fixation of a movable spleen; splenorrhaphy. प्लीहा-स्थिरण

**Splenoportogram.** Radiographic picture of the spleen and portal vein after injection of radio-opaque medium. प्लीहाप्रतिहारचित्र

**Splenoptosis.** Downward displacement of the spleen. प्लीहापात

**Splenorrhaphy.** See **Splenopexy.**

**Splenotomy.** An incision of the spleen. प्लीहाछेदन

**Splenunculus.** A small spleen; any small, discrete mass of splenic tissue. लघुप्लीहा; क्षुद्रप्लीहा; सूक्ष्मप्लीहा

**Splint.** A rigid device for holding the broken bones in place or easing pain in certain rheumatic diseases. कुशा; कमची; कमठी

**Splinter.** A sharp piece of bone separated in a fracture or a small pointed piece of wood, penetrating the flesh. विभंगिका; कांटा

**Splitting.** In chemistry, the breaking up of complex molecules into two or more simpler compounds. खंडन; विपाटन

**Spondyl.** A vertebra; spondyle. केशरुकासन्धि

**Spondylalgia.** Pain in the vertebra. कशेरुकासंध्यार्ति; कशेरुकासंधिशूल

**Spondylarthritis.** Inflammation of the vertebral joint. कशेरुकासन्धिशोथ; कशेरुकासन्धि का प्रदाह

**Spondylarthrocace.** Caries of a vertebra. कशेरुकासंधिक्षय

**Spondyle.** See **Sondyl.**

**Spondylitis.** Inflammation of one or more vertebrae; spondylosis. कशेरुकासन्धिशोथ; कशेरुका-सन्धियों का प्रदाह;

   **Ankylosing S.,** a condition characterized by ossification of the spinal ligaments and ankylosis of sacroiliac joints; spondylitis ankylopoitica. बद्धकशेरुकासन्धिशोथ;

   **S. Ankylopoitica,** see **Ankylosing Spondylitis.**

   **S. Deformans,** vertebral arthritis deformans. विरूपक कशेरुकासन्धिशोथ;

   **S. Tuberculosa,** spinal caries; Pott's disease. मेरुक्षय

**Spondylodynia.** Pain in the vertebra. कशेरुकासन्धिपीड़ा

**Spondylolisthesis.** Vertebral dislocation. कशेरुकाग्रसर्पण; कशेरुकाओं का अपने स्थान से हट जाना

**Spondylopathy.** Any disease of the vertebras. कशेरुकाविकृति; कशेरुकासन्धिविकृति; कशेरुकासंधिरोग; कशेरुकासन्धियों की कोई बीमारी

**Spondylosis.** See **Spondylitis.**

**Spondylotomy.** Section of a vertebra. कशेरुका-उच्छेदन; कशेरुकासंधि-उच्छेदन

**Sponge.** A fibrous skeleton of a marine animal organism, used mainly as an absorbent. स्पंज; छिद्रिष्ट

**Spongel Seeds.** Isapgol; isapgula. ईसपगोल

**Spongioplasm.** The chromatin of a cell-nucleus. स्पंजीद्रव्य

**Spongiose.** See **Spongiosum**.

**Spongiosum.** Spongy; sponge-like; spongiose; porous. स्पंजी; स्पंजवत्; स्पंज जैसा

**Spongy.** See **Spongiosum**.

**Spontaneous.** Occurring without any external stimulation. स्वत:; स्वत:स्फूर्त

**Spoon-nail.** A nail with a concave outer surface. चमसनख; चम्मच जैसा गड्ढेदार नाखुन

**Sporadic.** Diseases, such as colds, as are neither endemic nor epidemic. विकीर्ण; किसी-किसी जगह पर होने वाला

**Spores.** Seed-bodies of fungi. बीजाणु; प्रांगारिक लघुपिण्ड

**Sporicidal.** An agent for destroying spores. बीजाणुनाशी; बीजाणुनाशक; बीजाणुघाती

**Sporiferous.** Producing spores. बीजाणुजनक

**Sporocyst.** The cyst containing spores. बीजाणुपुटी; बीजपुटी

**Sporogenesis.** Reproduction by means of spores; sporogeny. बीजाणुजनन

**Sporogenic.** Spore producing; sporogenous. बीजाणुजनक

**Sporogenous.** See **Sporogenic**.

**Sporogeny.** See **Sporogenesis**.

**Sporozoa.** Plural of **Sporozoon**.

**Sporozoon.** A member of the sporozoa; a class of protozoa. बीजाणु

**Sporulation.** The formation of the spores. बीजाणुजनन

**Sporule.** A small spore. सूक्ष्मबीजाणु

**Spot.** A macule; macula. बिन्दु; चित्ती; धब्बा;

    **Blind S.**, the optic disc where the optic nerve enters the retina; scotoma. अन्ध बिन्दु;

    **Corneal S.**, an opaque area on the cornea; leukoma. कनीनिका बिन्दु; श्वेत फुल्ली; स्वच्छ परान्धता;

    **Koplik's s.'s,** small red spots on the buccal mucous membrane, with a minute bluish white speck in the centre, regarded as a sign of measles. कोपलिक धब्बे

**Spotted.** Marked with maculas. चित्तीदार; कर्बुर; धब्बेदार;

**S. Fever,** cerebrospinal fever. कर्बुर ज्वर; मस्तिष्कमेरु-ज्वर; चित्तीदार बुखार

**Sprain.** A violent straining of ligament around a joint, often involving small fractures. मोच; मरोड़; to cause a sprain. मोच आना

**Spray.** Liquid vaporized by a strong air-current. फुहार; फुहारना

**Sprue.** Thrush; small white ulcers of the mouth. मुखव्रण; मुखक्षत; मुँह के अन्दर छोटी-छोटी सफेद फुन्सियाँ निकलना; a chronic malabsorption disorder associated with glossitis, indigestion, weakness, anaemia and stearrhoea. विद्र; स्रू

**Spur.** A projecting portion; calcar. प्रसर; नख; लांगूलिका; उपांगुष्ठ

**Spurious.** False; adulterated; not genuine; spurium. कूट; मिथ्या; कृत्रिम

**Spurium.** See **Spurious.**

**Sputa.** Spittle; secretion ejected from the mouth by spitting; expectorated matter; sputum. थूक; बलगम; कफ

**Sputum.** See **Sputa.**

   **Negative S.,** not containing the acid-fast bacillus. ऋण-थूक;

   **Positive S.,** contains the acid-fast bacillus. धन-थूक;

   **Rusty S.,** typical bloody sputum of the third stage of pneumonia. मंडूर कफ

**Squama.** Scaly eruption. पट्टक; शल्क; पपड़ीदार विस्फोट

**Squamae.** Plural of **Squama.**

**Squamate.** See **Squamous.**

**Squamosal.** See **Squamous.**

**Squamous.** Scaly; squamosal; squamate. पट्टकी; शल्की; शल्कीय; malignant. दुर्दम;

   **S. Carcinoma,** a carcinoma arising in squamous epithelium; epithelioma. दुर्दम उपकलार्बुद;

   **S. Cell Carcinoma,** malignant carcinoma arising in the squamous epithelium. दुर्दम कोशिका उपकलार्बुद

**Squint.** Strabismus; incoordinated action of the eyeball, so that the visual axes of the two eyes fail to meet at the objective point. तिर्यक्दृष्टि; तिरछी नजर; नेत्रबक्रता; दृष्टिबक्रता; बहंगापन

**S.S.** Abbreviation for **Statim Sumendum.**

**S.S.D.** Source skin distance. स्रोत त्वक् दूरी

**Stab.** To pierce with a knife. छुरा भोंकना; वेधना

**Stabile.** Unmoving; durable; stable; steady. स्थिर; दृढ़
**Stability.** The quality of being stable. स्थिरता; दृढ़ता
**Stable.** See **Stabile.**
**Staccato.** Intermittent. सविराम; सविरामी; रुक-रुक कर होने वाला; jerky. झटका मारती हुई
**Stactometer.** An instrument for measuring drops; stalagmometer. बिन्दुमापी; बूंदमापीयंत्र
**Stadium.** A stage or period, as of a disease. अन्तरावस्था
**Staff.** An instrument to guide the knife in lithotomy; director. खातयुक्तशलाका; स्टाफ्फ; डाइरेक्टर; a specific group of workers. कर्मचारी
**Stage.** A period of a disease, as first stage, pyogenetic stage, etc. अवस्था; हालत; a particular step, phase, or position in a developmental process. चरण; the part of a microscope on which the microslide bears the object to be examined. स्टेज; पटल; मंच
**Stagger.** To walk unsteadily. लड़खड़ाना; लड़खड़ाहट
**Staggers.** Dizziness; vertigo. भ्रमि; चक्कर
**Stagnate.** To cease to flow. निश्चल होना; स्थिर होना
**Stagnation.** Cessation of flow. निश्चलन; निश्चल; गतिहीनता
**Stain.** A dye. अधिरंजक; a discolouration. दाग; धब्बा
**Stalagmometer.** See **Stactometer.**
**Stalk.** The stem of a plant. डण्ठल; डांठ
**Stamina.** Vigour; inherent force. जीवट; ओजस्विता; ऐश्वर्य; दम
**Stammer.** To utter with hesitation and repetition. हकलाना; अटक-अटक कर बोलना
**Stammering.** Stuttering; an involuntary interruption or total inability to utter a letter or syllable. हकलाहट; अटक-अटक कर बोलने की आदत
**Stanch.** To check or stop a flow; staunch. स्तम्भन; प्रवाह रोकना
**Standardization.** Making any drug or other preparation conform to the type or standard. मानकीकरण
**Stand-still.** Arrest; cessation of activity. विराम; unchanged. अपरिवर्तित
**Stannic.** Pertaining to tin; stannous. त्र्यविक; टीनी; टीन सम्बन्धी
**Stannous.** See **Stannic.**
**Stannum.** Tin. टीन; टिन

**St. Anthony's Fire.** Erysipelas, and sometimes used for gangrene resulting from ergotism. विसर्प

**Stapedectomy.** Excision of the stapes. रकाब-उच्छेदन

**Stapedes.** Plural of **Stapes.**

**Stapedial.** Pertaining to the stapes. रकाब सम्बन्धी

**Stapes.** The stirrup-shaped medial bone of the middle ear. रकाब; छल्ला

**Staphyle.** The uvula. काकलक; कठोरतालु

**Staphylectomy.** Amputation of the uvula; uvulectomy. काकलक-उच्छेदन

**Staphyledema.** Edematous swelling of the uvula. काकलकशोफ; काकलक की पानी वाली सूजन

**Staphylion.** Median point of the posterior nasal spine. कठोरतालुबिन्दु

**Staphylitis.** Inflammation of the uvula. काकलकशोथ; कठोरतालु का प्रदाह

**Staphylium.** The mammary nipple. चूचुक

**Staphylococcal.** Relating to, or caused by any species of staphylococcus; staphylococcic. स्तवकगोलाणु सम्बन्धी अथवा स्तवकगोलाणुजनित

**Staphylococcemia.** Presence of staphylococcus in the circulating blood; staphylohemia. स्तवकगोलाणुरक्तता

**Staphylococci.** Plural of **Staphylococcus.**

**Staphylococcic.** See **Staphylococcal.**

**Staphylococcus.** A micrococcus; a genus of **Schizomycetes** in which the cocci are irregularly clustered like a bunch of grapes. स्तवकगोलाणु

**Staphylohemia.** See **Staphylococcemia.**

**Staphyloma.** A protrusion of the cornea or sclera. स्वच्छमण्डलार्बुद; अजका; स्फीति; उभार;

S. Corneae, see **Corneal Staphyloma.**

Annular S., one surrounded on all sides by atrophic choroid. वलयी अजका;

Anterior S., that with horny growths. अग्र-अजका;

Corneal S., bulging of the cornea; staphyloma corneae. स्वच्छमण्डलीय अजका;

Equatorial S., staphyloma in the equatorial region of the eye. निरक्षीय अजका;

**Posterior S.,** bulging backward of the sclerotica at the posterior pole. पश्च-अजका

**Staphyloncus.** A swelling of the uvula. काकलकस्फीति

**Staphyloplasty.** Plastic surgery of the uvula or the soft palate; palatoplasty. काकलकसंधान; कोमलतालुसंधान

**Staphyloptosis.** Abnormal relaxation or elongation of the uvula; staphyloptosia. काकलकदीर्घीभवन

**Staphylorrhaphy.** Suture of the cleft-patate; palatorrhaphy. तालुसीवन

**Staphylotomy.** Amputation of the uvula. काकलक-उच्छेदन

**Starch.** A substance obtained from vegetables and the grains of germinous plants. स्टार्च; मण्ड; श्वेतसार

**Startling.** Being moved suddenly from surprise, pain or other sudden feelings or emotions. चौंकना

**Starvation.** Long continued deprival of food; death from hunger. आहारहीनता; भुखमरी

**Starve.** To suffer from lack of food. भूखों मरना; to deprive of food. भोजन से वंचित करना

**Stases.** Plural of **Stasis.**

**Stasis.** Stagnation, as of blood-current. स्थैतिकता; स्थैर्य

**Stat.** Abbreviation for **Statim.**

**State.** Condition; situation; status. अवस्था; स्थिति; हालत

**Static.** At rest; in equilibrium; not in motion. स्थैतिक; स्थिर

**Statics.** The science of matter at rest. स्थैतिकी; स्थितिविज्ञान

**Statim.** Immediately; at once. तुरन्त;

   **S. Sumendum,** take immediately. तुरन्त लो

**Statistics.** A numeric collection of facts. सांख्यिकी

**Statometer.** An instrument for measuring amount of exophthalmos. नेत्रोत्सेधमापी

**Status.** A state; position; condition. परिष्ठा; स्थिति; सतत;

   **S. Arthriticus,** a gouty condition. सतत गठिया;

   **S. Asthmaticus,** a prolonged and refractory attack of asthma. सतत दमा;

   **S. Epilepticus,** a condition in which there occur successive spasms. अपस्मार; मिर्गी;

**S. Typhosus,** the typhoid condition. सतत आंत्रिक ज्वर; सतत आंत्रज्वर;

**S. Vertiginosis,** persistent vertigo. अविच्छिन्न भ्रमि; सतत भ्रमि

**Staunch.** See **Stanch.**

**Steam.** A vapour of water by heating it to the boiling point. वाष्प; भाप

**Steariform.** Resembling fat. वसाभ; वसारूप; चर्बी जैसा

**Stearrhoea.** The same as **Seborrhoea.**

**Steatomatosis.** Encystic condition of the skin. त्वक्सम्पुटमयता

**Steatopyga.** Possessing fat buttocks; steatopygia. नितम्बमेदुरता; नितम्बोनयन

**Steatopygia.** See **Steatopyga.**

**Steatorrhea.** See **Steatorrhoea.**

**Steatorrhoea.** Increased flow of sebaceous matter; steatorrhea. वसापुरीष; वसा पदार्थ का अत्यधिक बहाव

**Steatosis.** Fatty degeneration. वसापजनन; वसीय अपजनन

**Stella.** A star. तारा

**Stellae.** Plural of **Stella.**

**Stellate.** Star-shaped. ताराकार

**Stem.** The stalk of a plant or tree. तना; any stalk-like structure. स्तम्भ

**Steno-.** Prefix meaning narrowing or constriction. 'संकीर्ण' के अर्थ में प्रयुक्त उपसर्ग

**Stenocardia.** Angina pectoris. हृद्शूल; हृच्छूल; हृद्संकीर्णता

**Stenocephaly.** Narrowness of the head. संकीर्णकपालीयता

**Stenochoria.** Stenosis of the lacrimal pasages. अश्रुपथसंकीर्णता

**Stenopaic.** See **Stenopeic.**

**Stenopeic.** Provided with a narrow opening or slit; stenopaic. सूचीछिद्र

**Stenosed.** Narrowed or constricted. संकीर्ण

**Stenosis.** A narrowing, constriction or contraction. संकीर्णता; संकुचन; सन्निरोध;

**Aortic S.,** a narrowing of the aortic orifice at the base of the heart, or narrowing of the aorta itself. महाघमनी-संकीर्णता;

**Cardiac S.,** the decrease of the diameter of the arterial cones on each side of the heart. हृद्संकीर्णता; हृत्संकीर्णता;

**Mitral S.**, contraction of the mitral valves. हृदत्वक्कपाटीय संकीर्णता;

**Pulmonary S.**, narrowing of the opening into the pulmonary artery from the right ventricle. फुफ्फुसीकपाटिका; फुफ्फुस-संकीर्णता;

**Pyloric S.**, narrowing of the gastric pylorus. जठरनिर्गम-संकीर्णता

**Stenotic.** Contracted. संकीर्ण; संकुचित; सन्निरोधी; सन्निरोधयुक्त

**Stephanial.** Pertaining to the stephanion. किरीटबिन्दु सम्बन्धी

**Stephanion.** The point of intersection of the temporal ridge and coronal suture. किरीटबिन्दु

**Stercolith.** The faecal calculus. मलाश्मरी; मलपथरी

**Stercoraceous.** Faecal; consisting of excrementitious matter; stercoral; stercorous. पुरीषी; मलजात; बिष्ठायुक्त; बिष्ठा का; मल या गोबर सम्बन्धी

**Stercoral.** See **Stercoraceous.**

**Stercorous.** See **Stercoraceous.**

**Stercus.** Faeces; dung; excrement. बिष्ठा; मल; गोबर

**Stereognostic.** Pertaining to the shape and nature of the objects. आकृति-प्रकृति सम्बन्धी; रूपाकार सम्बन्धी

**Stereogram.** Picturing an object, stereograph. त्रिविमचित्र

**Stereograph.** See **Stereogram.**

**Stereoisomer.** A substance exhibiting stereoisomerism. त्रिविमसमावयवी

**Stereoisomerism.** Isomerism involving different structural arrangement of the same group. त्रिविमसमावयवता

**Sterile.** Free from germs or viruses. विसंक्रमित; निर्जीवाणुक; incapable of procreating; barren. बंध्य; बन्ध्या; बांझ; relating to sterility. निर्जीवाणुकता अथवा बंध्यता सम्बन्धी

**Sterility.** The condition of infertility or of being sterile. विसंक्रमणता; निर्जीवाणुकता; बन्ध्यता

**Sterilization.** The process of destructing germs or tissues of living microbes; rendering incapable of reproduction. निर्जीवाणुकरण; बन्ध्यीकरण

**Sterilize.** To produce sterility. निर्जीवाणुक कर देना या करना

**Sterilizer.** An instrument for sterilization. विसंक्रामकयंत्र; निर्जीवाणुकरणयंत्र

**Sterna.** Plural of **Sternum.**

**Sternal.** Connected with or relating to the breast-bone (sternum). उरोस्थिक; उरोस्थि सम्बन्धी

**Sternalgia.** Pain in the sternum; sternodynia. उरोस्थिशूल; उरोस्थिपीड़ा

**Sternebra.** Any one of the segments of the sternum. उरोस्थिखण्ड

**Sternebrae.** Plural of **Sternebra.**

**Sterno.** In the sternum. वक्ष में

**Sternoclavicular.** Pertaining to the sternum and the clavicle. उरोस्थिजत्रुकीय; उरोस्थि एवं जत्रुक सम्बन्धी

**Sternocostal.** Pertaining to the sternum and the ribs. उर:पर्शुकीय; छाती और पसलियों सम्बन्धी

**Sternodynia.** See **Sternalgia.**

**Sternoid.** Resembling the sternum. उरोस्थिवत्; उरोस्थ्याभ; उरोस्थि जैसा

**Sternomastoid.** Pertaining to the sternum and the mastoid process. उर:कर्णमूलीय

**Sternotomy.** Surgical division of the sternum. उरोस्थि-उच्छेदन; उरोस्थि को काट कर हटा देना

**Sternum.** The breast-bone; the narrow flat bone in the median line of the thorax in front. उरोस्थि; गर्दन से लेकर आमाशय तक की पसलियों का जाल

**Sternutament.** A substance causing sneezing. नस्य; नसवार; छींकें उत्पन्न करने वाला पदार्थ

**Sternutation.** The act of sneezing. छिक्का; छींक; छींकना

**Stertor.** The deep-snoring breathing which accompanies diseases, as apoplexy. घर्घराहट; श्वास की घर्घर ध्वनि

**Stertorous.** With deep snoring. घर्घराहटयुक्त; खर्राटेदार

**Stethogoniometer.** An apparatus for measuring the curvature of the thorax. वक्षबक्रतामापी

**Stethoscope.** A simple instrument used to carry sounds from within the chest or other parts of the body to the ears of the physician. परिश्रवणयंत्र; स्टेयोस्कोप

**Stethoscopy.** The use of stethoscope. परिश्रवणयंत्र-जांच

**Stethospasm.** Spasm of the chest. वक्ष-उद्वेष्ट

**Sthenia.** Strenghth; excessive force. बल; शक्ति; ओज; स्फूर्ति

**Sthenic.** Strong; active; powerful. सबल; प्रबल; ओजस्वी; स्फूर्त; शक्तिशाली; ताकतवर

**Stiff.** Not easily bent. कठोर; अकड़ा हुआ; अनम्य; ऐंठनयुक्त;
  **S.-joint,** fixation of joint; ankylosis. सन्धिग्रह; सन्धिस्तम्भ;
  **S.-neck,** twisted or wryneck; torticollis. मन्यास्तम्भ; गर्दन की अकड़न
**Stiffness.** The state of being stiff. अकड़न; कठोरता; अनम्यता; ऐंठन
**Stigma.** A red spot on the skin; marks of disease, or congenital abnormalities. लांछन; चमड़ी पर कोई लाल धब्बा
**Stigmas.** Plural of **Stigma.**
**Stigmata.** Plural of **Stigma.**
**Stigmatic.** Pertaining to stigma. लांछन सम्बन्धी
**Stigmatization.** Production of ecchymotic spots on the body. लांछनीकरण; लांछनीभवन
**Stigmatosis.** Ulceration of the skin. त्वग्व्रणता; चर्मव्रणता
**Stilet.** See **Stillette.**
**Still-birth.** See **Still-born.**
**Still-born.** Not born alive; still-birth. मृतजात; मृतजन्म; निष्प्राणजन्म
**Stillete.** A small, sharp-pointed instrument; stilet; style; stylet; styllete. अन्तःशलाका; स्टाइल; एक छोटा, तेज-नुकीला उपकरण
**Stimulant.** A drug or any other agent that raises the level of the body activity; stimulating; stimulator. उद्दीपक; उत्तेजक
**Stimulating.** See **Stimulant.**
**Stimulation.** A quickly diffused transient increase of vital energy and strength of action in the heart. उद्दीपन; उत्तेजना
**Stimulator.** See **Stimulant.**
**Stimuli.** Plural of **Stimulus.**
**Stimulus.** Anything which excites an organ. उद्दीपक; उत्तेजक; उत्तेजनाशील; उद्दीपन; दीपन
**Sting.** Sharp, smarting sensation. दंशानुभूति; a punctured wound made by an insect. दंश; डंक
**Stirrup.** The stapes. रकाब; छल्ला
**Stitch.** A suture. टांका; सीवन; a sharp sticking pain of momentary duration. सूचीवेधी (पीड़ा)
**Stitching.** Of the nature of piercing with a needle. सूचीवेधी; सुई चुभने जैसा;
  **S. Pain,** a sudden, sharp, darting pain. सूचीवेधी पीड़ा; सुई चुभने जैसा दर्द

**Stokes-Adams Syndrome.** Altered state of consciousness caused by decreased flow of blood to brain. स्टोक-एडम संलक्षण

**Stockholm Technique.** A method of treating carcinoma of the cervix by radium on three successive occasions at weekly intervals. विकिरण-चिकित्सा; स्टॉकहोम तकनीक

**Stoma.** The mouth; any opening. मुख; रन्ध्र; द्वार

**Stomacace.** Canker of the mouth, with blood-stained discharge from the gums; putrid sore mouth; stomatocace. मुखव्रण; मुँह के अन्दर होने वाला घाव

**Stomach.** The chief digestive organ. आमाशय; जठर; पेट

**Stomachache.** Pain in the stomach. जठरार्ति; जठरशूल; पेटदर्द

**Stomachal.** Relating to the stomach. आमाशय सम्बन्धी; stomachic. भूख बढ़ाने वाला; क्षुधावर्धक

**Stomachic.** Hunger-producing. क्षुधावर्धक; भूख बढ़ाने वाला; relating to stomach. आमाशय सम्बन्धी

**Stomas.** Plural of **Stoma**.

**Stomata.** Plural of **Stoma**.

**Stomatalgia.** Pain in the mouth; stomatodynia. मुखार्ति

**Stomatitis.** Inflammation of the mouth. मुखपाक; मुखशोथ; मुखार्ति; मुखकोथ;

**Aphthous S.,** see **Ulcerative Stomatitis**.

**Catarrhal S.,** a simple form marked by swelling of the mucous membrane, pain and salivation. प्रतिश्यायी मुखकोथ;

**Ulcerative S.,** a grave form of catarrhal stomatitis, marked by ulcers; aphthous stomatitis. सव्रण मुखकोथ

**Stomatocace.** See **Stomacace**.

**Stomatodynia.** See **Stomatalgia**.

**Stomatology.** The science of the mouth or the diseases of the mouth. मुखरोगविज्ञान; मुख अथवा मुख सम्बन्धी रोगों का विज्ञान

**Stomatomalacia.** Softening of any of the structures of the mouth. मुखमृदुता

**Stomatomycosis.** A fungal disease of the mouth. मुखकवकता

**Stomatopathy.** Any disease of the mouth. मुखविकृति

**Stomatoplasty.** Plastic operation on the mouth. मुखसंधान

**Stomatoscope.** An instrument for viewing the interior of the mouth. मुखदर्शी; मुख के अन्दरूनी भाग की जांच के लिये प्रयुक्त किया जाने वाला यंत्र

**Stone.** Calculus. अश्म; अश्मरी; पथरी;
    **Gall S.**, the calculus of the bile-duct. पित्ताश्मरी; पित्त-पथरी;
    **Renal S.**, the calculus of the kidneys or urinary bladder; urinary calculus. वृक्काश्मरी; मूत्राश्मरी; मूत्र-पथरी; गुर्दे की पथरी;
    **Urinary S.**, see **Renal Calculus.**
    **Tear S.**, dacryolith. अश्रुकोशाश्मरी

**Stool.** The alvine evacuation; the excrement from the bowels. मल; पुरीष; बिष्ठा; पाखाना

**Stooping.** Bending the head downward. अवनमन; नति; झुकना

**Storm.** Violence. उग्रता; तेजी

**Strabismal.** See **Strabismic.**

**Strabismic.** Pertaining to strabismus; strabismal. तिर्यकदृष्टि सम्बन्धी

**Strabismometer.** An instrument for measuring strabismus. तिर्यकदृष्टिमापी; तिर्यकदृष्टिमापकयंत्र

**Strabismus.** Squint, more commonly called crossed-eye; heterotropia. तिर्यकदृष्टि; बहंगापन; टेढ़ा देखना या दिखाई देना

**Strabotome.** A knife for performing strabotomy. तिर्यकदृष्टिसंधानक

**Strabotomy.** Operation for correting strabismus. तिर्यकदृष्टिसंधान

**Strain.** A sprain. मोच; tension. तनाव; pressure. दबाव; to filter. छानना

**Strait.** A narrow or constricted passage, as of the pelvic canal. परिवेष्टित; सीमित; एक तंग या सिकुड़ा हुआ पथ

**Stramonium.** Dhatura Stramonium, especially its dried leaves. धतूरा

**Strangle.** To suffocate; to choke. कण्ठघोटन; गला घोटना

**Strangulated.** Choked; compressed, so that the accumulation is arrested. विपाशित; सम्पीडित

**Strangulation.** Compression of a part by which it cannot return to its proper position and the blood cannot circulate freely through it. विपाशन; कण्ठघोटन; गला घोटना

**Strangury.** Difficult and painful expulsion of urine. बिन्दुमूत्रकृच्छ्; मूत्रकृच्छ्ता; अत्यन्त कठिनाई और दर्द के साथ पेशाब होना

**Strap.** The adhesive plaster for dressing of the wounds. पट्टी; चिपक-पट्टी

**Strapping.** The adhesive-paste for dressing of wounds. पट्टी चिपकाना

**Strata.** Plural of **Stratum.**

**Stratified.** Arranged in layers. अस्तरित

**Stratum.** A layer or lamina. अस्तर; तह; परत;

   **S. Cinereum,** the most superficial layer of the cortex of the cerebellum. भस्माभ अस्तर;

   **S. Corneum,** the outer epidermic layer. शल्क-अस्तर;

   **S. Granulosum,** the granular layer of the retina. कणमय अस्तर; परिडिम्ब-अस्तर;

   **S. Lucidum,** the transluscent layer of the epidermis. स्वच्छ अस्तर

**Strawberry Mark.** Naevus. न्यच्छ; तिल

**Strawberry Tongue.** The papillated tongue of scarlet fever. कणिकारक्तजिह्वा; हल्की-हल्की लाल दानेदार जीभ

**Streak.** Furrow, line, bend, or colour mark. रेखा; धारी; लकीर

**Strength.** Vitality; vigour. बल; शक्ति; सामर्थ्य

**Strengthening.** Making strong. शक्तिदायक; बलदायक; स्फूर्तिदायक

**Strephosymbolia.** Perception of objects reversed as if in a mirror. व्युत्क्रमदर्शनदोष

**Strepthroat.** A severe sore-throat due to infection with the streptococcus organism. उग्रकण्ठदाह

**Streptobacillus.** Gram positive, rod-shaped bacteria, that are parasitic to pathogenic for rats, mice and other mammals. ग्रामधन दण्डाणु

**Streptococcal.** Relating to, or caused by any organism of the genus streptococcus. मालाणुक; मालाणुज; गोलाणुक; गोलाणुज

**Streptococcemia.** Presence of streptococcus in the blood; streptosepticemia. मालाणुरक्तता; गोलाणुरक्तता

**Streptococci.** Plural of **Streptococcus.**

**Streptococcus.** A genus of micro-organisms. मालाणु; गोलाणु

**Streptosepticemia.** See **Streptococcemia.**

**Stress.** Circumstances which put a person under pressure which may have unfavourable influence on his mental or emotional health. दबाव

**Stretcher.** A portable cot for carrying the sick. बाही; पट्टी; मरीजों को इधर-उधर ले जाने के लिये प्रयुक्त की जाने वाली खाट; स्ट्रेचर

**Stria.** A streak or line. रेखा; लकीर; खरोंच; धारी;

   **S. Terminalis,** a narrow strip of white matter in the groove between the striate body and the optic thalamus. अन्त्य रेखा;

**S. Vascularis,** the vascular upper part of the spiral ligament of the vestibular membrane. वाहिका रेखास्तर

**Striae.** Plural of **Stria.**

**Striate.** See **Striated.**

**Striated.** Marked with furrows; striate; stripped. रेखित; रेखांकित; धारीदार;

    **S. Muscle,** stripped or voluntary muscle which is subject to control by will. रेखित पेशी

**Striation.** The state of being streaked. रेखन; रेखांकन

**Stricture.** Unnatural contraction of any part of the body. निकोचन; आकुंचन; निकुंचन; सन्निरोध;

    **Cicatricial S.,** a stricture due to cicatricial tissue. क्षतांकज निकोचन;

    **Impermeable S.,** one not permitting the passage of a bougie or catheter. अपारगम्य निकोचन

**Stridor.** A harsh grating sound. घर्घर; खर्वर

**Stridulent.** Making a grating sound; stridulous. खरखराती हुई; चर्र-मर्र, चर्र-मर्र करती हुई

**Stridulous.** See **Stridulent.**

**Stripe.** A streak. रेखा; धारी; लकीर

**Stripped.** See **Striated.**

**Stroke.** Brain injury from rupture; blocking or spasm of an artery; seizure. घात; आघात; प्रहार; धक्का;

    **Apoplectic S.,** apoplexy. रक्ताघात; अपसन्यास;

    **Heat S.,** caused by heat. आतपघात; तापाघात;

    **Sun S.,** caused due to heat of sun. सूर्याघात; लू लगना

**Stroma.** The tissue which forms the ground substance, or matrix of an organ. पीठिका; पंजर; अवर्णिका; घनांश

**Stromal.** Pertaining to the stroma; stromatic. पीठिकी; पंजरीय; अवर्णिकी; घनांशी

**Stromata.** Plural of **Stroma.**

**Stromatic.** See **Stromal.**

**Strongyloides.** Intestinal worms that can infest man. आन्त्रकृमि

**Strophulus.** An urticarial disease of the skin. शीतपित्त; छपाकी; जुलपित्ती

**Structural.** Pertaining to a structure. संरचनात्मक; रचना अथवा संरचना सम्बन्धी

**Structure.** Make-up of an organ. संरचना; रचना; विन्यास; बनावट

**Struma.** Scrofula. कण्ठमाला; simple goitre; bronchocele. सामान्य गलगण्ड; अवटुता

**Strumae.** Plural of **Struma.**

**Strumectomy.** Surgical removal of a goitrous tumour. गलगण्डार्बुद-उच्छेदन

**Strumiform.** Resembling a goitre. गलगण्डरूप; गलगण्ड जैसा

**Strumitis.** Inflammation of the thryroid body. अवटुशोथ; अवटु-पिण्ड का प्रदाह

**Strumous.** Pertaining to struma or scrofula. गलगण्ड अथवा कण्ठमाला सम्बन्धी

**Strychnia.** An alkaloid of **Strychnos nux vomica**; strychnine. कुचला; विषतुन्दुकी; कुचला का एक क्षार

**Strychnine.** See **Strychnia.**

**Strychninomania.** Delirium from the use of Strychnine. कुचलाविषोन्माद; कुचलाजनित प्रलाप

**Stump.** A part left after an aputation. स्थूणक; स्थूण; ठूंठ

**Stunned.** Confused and unconscious. स्तम्भित; अचेत; अशक्त

**Stupefacient.** Any narcotic. संज्ञाहारी; जड़िमाकारी; जड़िमाकारक

**Stupefaction.** Stupor; unconsciousness. संज्ञाहीनता; जड़ता; बेहोशी; निश्चेतना

**Stupefying.** That which stupefies. स्तम्भक; संज्ञाहीन करने वाला; चेतनाहारी

**Stupemania.** Mania with stupor. सोन्माद-जड़िमा

**Stupe.** A moist fomentation performed with a saturated flannel, or cloth. आर्द्रसेक; नमीदार सेक

**Stupor.** Insensibility; suppressed state of senses. जड़िमा; गहन तन्द्रा; the condition of unconsciousness. बेहोशी; निश्चेतना

**Stupration.** Rape; stuprum. बलात्कार

**Stuprum.** See **Stupration.**

**Stutter.** To hesitate and repeat in speech. हकलाना

**Stutterring.** A speech habit that is normal in children and is usually outgrown if not emphasized by parents. हकलाहट; हकलाना

**St. Vitus' Dance.** Chorea. लास्य; नर्तन रोग

**Sty.** Abbreviation for **Stye.**

**Stye.** An inflammatory condition of the eyelash; hordeolum; sty. अंजनी; विलनी; गुहेरी; गुहांजनी; वर्तिका

**Style.** See **Stillete.**

**Stylet.** See **Stillete.**

**Styllete.** See **Stillete.**

**Styloid.** Resembling a stylus; long and pointed. शर; शराभ; तीर जैसा लम्बा और नुकीला

**Stylomastoid.** Pertaining to the styloid and mastoid processes. शरकर्णमूलक; शर एवं कर्ण क्रियाओं सम्बन्धी

**Stylus.** An instrument for writing a pencil-shaped structure. शलाका; शर; लिखने के लिये प्रयुक्त किया जाने वाला एक लम्बा और नुकीला उपकरण; a probe or slender wire for stiffening or clearing a canal or catheter. स्टाइलस; सूचिका; एषणी

**Stype.** A cotton tampon. स्तम्भ; रक्तस्तम्भ

**Styptic.** An astringent; an application which restrains flooding. स्तम्भक; रक्तस्तम्भक; रक्तरोधक

**Sub-.** Prefix denoting under or beneath. 'उप', 'अव', 'अनु' के रूप में प्रयुक्त उपसर्ग

**Subacute.** Between acute and chronic. अनुतीव्र; अर्धजीर्ण

**Subarachnoid.** Under the arachnoid membrane; the space between the brain and its innermost covering. अवजालतानिका

**Subaural.** Beneath the ear. अवकर्णी; कान के नीचे

**Subaxillary.** Under the armpit. अवकक्षी; अनुकक्षी; कांख के नीचे

**Subclavian.** Beneath the clavicle; subclavicular. अवजत्रुकी; जत्रुक के नीचे

**Subclavicular.** See **Subclavian.**

**Subclinical.** Insufficient to cause the classical identifiable disease. लक्षणहीन

**Subconjunctival.** Beneath the conjunctiva. अवनेत्रश्लेष्मलीय; आँख की श्लैष्मिक झिल्ली के नीचे

**Subconscious.** Not wholly conscious. अर्धचेतन; अर्धमूर्च्छित

**Subconsciousness.** Partial unconsciousness. अर्धचेतना; आंशिक चेतना

**Subcortex.** Any part of the brain lying below the cerebral cortex. अवप्रान्तस्था

**Subcortical.** Beneath the cerebral cortex. अवप्रान्तस्थीय; मस्तिष्क-प्रान्तस्था के नीचे

**Subcostal.** Beneath the rib. अवपर्शुक्; अवपर्शुकी; पसली के नीचे

**Subculture.** A secondary bacterial culture. उपसंवर्ध

**Subcutaneous.** Under the skin. अवत्वचीय; अधस्त्वचीय; त्वचा के नीचे

**Subcuticular.** Beneath the epidermis. अधस्त्वचीय; अवत्वचीय; त्वचा के नीचे

**Subcutis.** The epidermis. अधस्त्वचा; अवत्वचा; उपत्वक्

**Subdural.** Beneath the dura mater. अवदृढ़तानिकी; दृढ़तानिका के नीचे

**Subendocardial.** Beneath the endocardium. अवअन्तर्हृदी; अन्तर्हृद्कला के नीचे

**Subendothelial.** Beneath an endothelial structure. अवअन्त:कलायज; अन्तर्कला के नीचे

**Subendothelium.** The connective tissue between the endothelium and inner elastic membrane in the intima of arteries. अवअन्त:कला

**Subepithelial.** Beneath the epithelium. अवोपत्वचीय; अवोपकलायज; उपकला के नीचे

**Subfascial.** Beneath the fascia. उपप्रावरणिक; प्रावरणी के नीचे

**Subglossal.** See **Sublingual.**

**Subhepatic.** Beneath the liver. अवयकृती; यकृत् के नीचे

**Subinfection.** A secondary infection. अवसंक्रमण; गौण संक्रमण

**Subinvolution.** Imperfect involution. अनुप्रत्यावर्तन; आंशिक प्रत्यावर्तन

**Subject.** A person. व्यक्ति

**Subjective.** Internal; pertaining to one's self. स्वप्रत्यय; स्वानुभूत

**Sublation.** Detachment, elevation or removal of a part. विच्छेदन; उच्छेदन; किसी अंश को काट देना या हटा देना

**Sublimate.** A solid deposit resulting from the condensation of a vapour. उत्साद; उत्सादित पदार्थ; ऊर्ध्वपातित द्रव्य; ऊर्ध्वपातज;

    **Corrosive S.,** mercuric chloride; an antiseptic. रस-कर्पूर; एक पारद विष; कोरोसिव सब्लीमेट

**Sublimation.** Vaporization and recondensation. उत्सादन व परिशोधन

**Subliminal.** Inadequate for perceptible response; subminimal. ऊनप्रभावी; अध:सांवेदनिक; ऊनालिप्ष्ठ

**Sublingual.** Beneath the tongue; subglossal; hypoglossal. अवजिह्वी; जीभ के नीचे

**Subluxation.** A partial dislocation. अपूर्णसन्धिभ्रंश; अनुसन्धिच्युति; आंशिक स्थानभ्रंश; a sprain or strain. मोच; मरोड़; दबाव

**Submandibular.** Below the mandible. अवअधोहनुज; अधोहनु के नीचे

**Submaxilla.** Mandibula. अधोहनु

**Submaxillaritis.** Inflammation affecting submandibular salivary gland. अवअधोहनुशोथ

**Submaxillary.** Under the jaw. अवऊर्ध्वहनुज; ऊर्ध्वहनु के नीचे

**Submental.** Under the chin. अवचिबुकीय; अधश्चिबुकीय; ठोढ़ी के नीचे

**Subminimal.** See **Subliminal.**

**Submucose.** The connective tissue beneath a mucosa, or mucous membrane. अवश्लेष्मकला; श्लेष्मकला के नीचे स्थित संयोजी ऊतक

**Submucous.** Below the mucous membrane. अवश्लेष्मकलायज; श्लेष्मकला के नीचे

**Subnation.** Under the nose. अवनासा; नाक के नीचे

**Subnormal.** Below the normal. अवसामान्य; सामान्य से कम

**Subnucleus.** A sub-division of a nerve-nucleus. अवकेन्द्रक; किसी स्नायु-केन्द्रक का उपविभाजन

**Suboccipital.** Beneath the occiput. अवपश्चकपालिक; पश्चकपाल के नीचे

**Suboperculum.** A part of an orbital gyrus that covers the insula. अवप्रच्छद

**Subpericardial.** Beneath the pericardium. अवपरिहृदीय; हृदयावरण के नीचे

**Subperitoneal.** Beneath the peritoneum. अवपर्युदर्यीय; उदरावरण के नीचे

**Subscapular.** Under the shoulder-blade. अवअंसफलकीय; अंसफलक के नीचे

**Subscription.** The part of the prescription containing directions to the pharmacists concerning the mixing of the ingredients. अवनिर्देश

**Subserous.** Beneath a serous membrane. अवसीरमी; सीरमी कला के नीचे

**Subside.** To disappear. लोप होना; उतर जाना

**Subsidence.** Gradual disappearance of a disease. लोप; उतार; उतराव

**Subsidiary.** Secondary. गौण

**Substance.** The material of which organ or body is made up. पदार्थ; वस्तु; द्रव; द्रव्य

**Substantia.** Substance. पदार्थ; द्रव; वस्तु; द्रव्य;

   **S. Alba,** the cerebral and the spinal white matter. श्वेत द्रव्य;

   **S. Cinerea,** the cerebral spinal gray matter; substantia grisea. धूसर द्रव्य; भूरा द्रव्य;

**S. Grisea,** see **Substantia Cinerea.**

**S. Nigra,** the dark area in the centre of a section of the leg-shaped structure of the cerebrum. श्याम द्रव्य; काला द्रव्य;

**S. Propria,** the essential tissue of an organ. मुख्य अस्तर

**Substantiae.** Plural of **Substantia.**

**Substernal.** Beneath the sternum. अवउरोस्थिज; उरोस्थि के नीचे

**Substitution.** Replacement of one thing by another. प्रतिस्थापन

**Substrate.** The substance acted upon and changed by enzymes. कार्यद्रव्य

**Substructure.** A tissue or structure wholly or partly beneath the surface. अवसंरचना

**Subsultus.** Any morbid tremor or twitching. कम्पन; स्फुरण; कम्प;

**S. Tendinum,** convulsive muscular twitching. पेशीकम्प; कण्डराकम्प; आक्षेपीपेशी-स्फुरण

**Subtarsal.** Beneath the tarsus or cartilage of the eyelid. अवनेत्रच्छदीय; नेत्रच्छद के नीचे

**Subtendinous.** Beneath the tendon. अवकण्डरीय; कण्डरा के नीचे

**Subthalamus.** A small yellow mass beneath the optic thalamus. अवचेतक; अक्षिचेतक के नीचे एक छोटा-सा पीला पिण्ड

**Subungual.** Beneath the nail; subunguial. अवनखी; नाखुन के नीचे

**Subunguial.** See **Subungual.**

**Subvaginal.** Below the vagina. अवयोनिज; योनि के नीचे

**Subvolution.** Turning over a flap of mucous membrane to prevent adhesion. अनुवर्तन

**Succenturiate.** Accessory. सहायक; अनुषंगी

**Succi.** Plural of **Succus.**

**Succus.** Juice; the fluid constituents of the body tissue. रस;

**S. Entericus,** the intestinal juice. आंत्र रस;

**S. Gastrium,** the gastric juice. पाचक रस

**Succusion.** The act of giving strong strokes in potentising a homoeopathic medicine by putting 1 part of medicinal substance and 9 or 99 part of alcohol in a vessel. आस्फालन; झटका; हल्लन; धूमन

**Suck.** To draw fluid into the mouth, especially milk from the breast. चूसना; स्तनपान करना

**Suckle.** To nurse; to feed by milk from the breast. स्तनपान कराना

**Suckling.** Unweaned infant or child. स्तनपायी (शिशु)

**Sucrose.** A complex sugar; common table sugar. इक्षुशर्करा; इक्षुसिता; चीनी

**Sucrosemia.** Presence of sucrose in the blood. शर्करारक्तता

**Sucrosuria.** The presence of sucrose in the urine. इक्षुशर्करामेह; पेशाब में चीनी जाना

**Sudamen.** Singular of **Sudamina.**

**Sudamina.** A disorder of the sweat glands with obstruction of their ducts; miliaria. स्वेदराजिका; श्वेतराजिका

**Sudation.** The act of sweating. स्वेदन; पसीना निकलना

**Sudatory.** See **Sudorific.**

**Sudomotor.** Denoting the nerves that stimulate the sweat glands to activity. स्वेदग्रन्थिप्रेरक

**Sudor.** Sweat; perspiration. स्वेद; स्वेदन; पसीना

**Sudoral.** Pertaining to sweat. स्वेद या पसीने सम्बन्धी

**Sudoriferous.** Sweat carrying, as of the glands of the skin. स्वेदोत्पादक; पसीना पैदा करने वाला

**Sudorific.** A medicine which produces perspiration; sudatory. स्वेदकारी; स्वेदजनक; पसीना लाने वाली औषधि

**Sudoriparous.** Secreting the perspiratory fluid. स्वेदजन; स्वेदस्रावी

**Sudorosis.** Profuse sweating. अतिस्वेदन; स्वेदाधिक्य

**Suet.** The fat from the belly-cavities of sheep or oxen. मेषवसा

**Suffocate.** To impede respiration; to asphyxiate. दम घुटना

**Suffocation.** Stoppage of respiration. घुटन; श्वासरोध; दम घुटना

**Suffusion.** Overspreading with a fluid or a colour. परिप्लावन; आप्लावन; फैलाव; भराव

**Sugar.** Sweet carbohydrates of various kinds. शर्करा; चीनी;

    **S. of milk,** lactose. दुग्ध-शर्करा;

    **Blood S.,** the carbohydrates in the blood, especially glucose. रक्त-शर्करा

**Suggestibility.** Capable of being suggested. संसूच्यता; सुझाने योग्य

**Suggestible.** Amenable to suggestion. संसूच्य

**Suggestion.** The production of psychic state in an individual in which he experiences sensations suggested to him. संसूचन; सुझाव

## Suggillation

**Suggillation.** A bruise; livid mark; ecchymosis. नील; नीलांछन; नीललांछन; त्वचा पर उभरे हुए नीले धब्बे

**Sulci.** Plural of **Sulcus**.

**Suicide.** The act of killing oneself; self-murder. आत्महत्या; आत्मघात

**Sulcus.** A furrow or groove. परिखा; खातिका;

    **S. Centralis,** the central sulcus. मध्यवर्ती परिखा;

    **S. Circularis,** the circular sulcus or fissure bounding the insula. वर्तुल परिखा;

    **S. Interpartietalis,** the interparietal or confluent group of fissures in the parietal lobe. अन्तःपार्श्विका परिखा;

    **S. Intertubercularis,** the intertubercular or bicipital groove. अन्तरागुलिका खातिका;

    **S. Lunatus,** the lateral occipital fissure. चन्द्राभ परिखा;

    **S. Olfactorius,** the olfactory fissure or the one occupied by the olfactory tract and bulb. घ्राण परिखा;

    **S. Spiralis,** the groove extremity of the cochlear spiral lamina. सर्पिल परिखा;

    **S. Temporalis,** the temporal fissure. शंख परिखा;

    **S. Tympanicus,** the tympanic membrane groove. मध्यकर्ण परिखा

**Sulfate.** See **Sulphate**.

**Sulfide.** See **Sulphide**.

**Sulfur.** See **Sulphur**.

**Sulfuring.** See **Sulphuring**.

**Sulphate.** A salt of sulfuric acid; sulfate. गन्धक अम्ल का लवण; सल्फेट

**Sulphide.** A combination of sulphur with a metal or other body; sulfide. गन्धक के साथ किसी तत्त्व का योगिक; सल्फाइड

**Sulphur.** An insoluble yellow powder once used extensively as **Sulphur Ointment** for scabies; sulfur. गन्धक; सल्फर

**Sulphuring.** Treatment with sulphur; sulfuring. गन्धकोपचार; सल्फर द्वारा की जाने वाली चिकित्सा

**Summer Cholera.** Diarrhoea occurring in summer; summer complaints. ग्रीष्म विसूचिका; शिशु-विसूचिका; ग्रीष्मातिसार

**Summer Complaints.** See **Summer Cholera**.

**Sunburn.** Dermatitis from exposure to sun. आतपदाह; सूर्यदाह; धूप की झुलसन

**Sunfever.** Severe tropical fever. आतप-ज्वर; धूप की तपन से होने वाला बुखार

**Sunstroke.** Heat-stroke from direct rays of the sun. आतपघात; सूर्याघात; घामाघात; लू लगना

**Super-.** Prefix denoting upon, above, or dorsad. 'ऊर्ध्व', 'उपरि', 'श्रेष्ठ', 'अधि', 'अति' के रूप में प्रयुक्त उपसर्ग

**Superacute.** Extremely acute. अत्युग्र

**Superalimentation.** Overfeeding. अत्याहार

**Supercilia.** Plural of **Supercilium.**

**Superciliary.** Relating to the eyebrows. अधिभ्रूज; ऊपर वाली भौंहों सम्बन्धी

**Supercilium.** The eyebrow. भ्रू; भौंह

**Superfecundation.** The fertilization of more than one ovum of the same ovulation by separate acts of coitus. अधिसंफलन; अतिप्रजनन

**Superfetation.** See **Superfoetation.**

**Superficial.** Situated on the surface; not deep, such as a wound, or cut; superficialis. उपरिस्थ

**Superficialis.** See **Superficial.**

**Superfoetation.** Conception by a pregnant woman; superfetation. अधिगर्भधारण

**Superior.** The upper of the two or more parts. ऊर्ध्व; more vital. उत्कृष्ट; प्रवर; वरिष्ठ

**Supermotility.** Excessive motility. अतिचरता

**Supernumerary.** Over the normal number. अधिसंख्य; अतिरिक्त; बहुसंख्यक

**Superscription.** The beginning of a prescription. अधिनिर्देश

**Superstructure.** A structure above the surface. अधिसंरचना

**Supination.** The attitude on lying upon the back. उत्तान; पीठ के बल लेटने की प्रवृत्ति

**Supine.** Lying flat or on the back. उत्तान; पीठ के बल लेटने की स्थिति

**Suppository.** A substance, medicinal or otherwise, in the form of a cone or cylinder, introduced into the rectum to favour or restrain evacuation, or to ease pain. वर्ति; वर्तिका; गुदवर्ति; पाखाना कराने के लिये गुदा के अन्दर डाली जाने वाली वैसलीन की बत्ती

**Suppress.** To conceal; to retain. दबाना; दमन करना; उपशमन करना

**Suppressed.** Stopped of natural, periodic or other evacuation. दमित; उपशमित; दबा हुआ या दबाया हुआ

**Suppression.** Stoppage of natural, periodic or other discharges. दमन; उपशमन; अधिलयन

**Suppurant.** See **Suppurative**.

**Suppurate.** To form pus. पूतिता होना; पीब बनना

**Suppuration.** Formation of pus. पूयता; पूतिता; पूयीभवन; पूतीभवन

**Suppurative.** Producing pus; promoting suppuration; suppurant. सपूय; पूतिज; पूतिवर्धक

**Supra-.** Prefix denoting over or above. 'अधि', 'उत्', 'उपरि', 'ऊर्ध्व' के रूप में प्रयुक्त उपसर्ग

**Supra-auricular.** Above the auricle. अधिकर्णी; कान के ऊपर

**Suprachoroid.** Above the choroid. अधिरंजितपटलीय; रंजितपटल के ऊपर

**Suprachoroidea.** The choroid layer next to the sclera. अधिरंजितपटल

**Supraciliary.** Above the cilia. अध्यक्षिक

**Supraclavicular.** Above the clavicle; supraclavicularis. अधिजत्रुकीय; जत्रुक के ऊपर

**Supraclavicularis.** See **Supraclavicular**.

**Supracolic.** Above the colon. अधिबृहदांत्रज; बृहदांत्र के ऊपर

**Supracondylar.** Above a condyle. अधिस्थूलकीय; किसी स्थूलक के ऊपर

**Supraglenoid.** Above the glenoid cavity; supraglenoidal. अध्यंसगर्तकी; अध्यंसगर्ती; अंसगर्त के ऊपर

**Supraglenoidal.** See **Supraglenoid**.

**Supragranular.** Above a granule. अधिकणिकीय; किसी कणिका के ऊपर

**Suprahyoid.** Above the hyoid bone. अधिकण्ठिकी; कण्ठिकास्थि के ऊपर

**Supramaxilla.** The upper jaw-bone. अधिऊर्ध्वहनु; ऊपरी हन्वस्थि

**Supramaxillary.** Pertaining to the upper jaw-bone. अधिऊर्ध्वहनुज; ऊर्ध्व-हन्वस्थि सम्बन्धी

**Supraoccipital.** Above the occiput. अधिपश्चकपालीय; पश्चकपाल के ऊपर

**Supraorbital.** Above the orbit. ऊर्ध्वाक्षिक

**Suprapleural.** Above the lung. अधिफुप्फुसी; अधिफुप्फुसीय; फेफड़े के ऊपर

**Suprapubic.** Above the pubis. अधिजघनिक; जघनास्थि के ऊपर

**Suprarenal.** Above the kidney. अधिवृक्कज; वृक्कोपरि; गुर्दे के ऊपर

**Suprascapular.** Above the shoulder-blade. अध्यंसफलकीय; अंसफलक के ऊपर

**Supraspinal.** Above a spine. अधिकण्टकीय; रीढ़ की हड्डी के ऊपर

**Suprasternal.** Above the sternum. अध्युरोस्थिक; उरोस्थि के ऊपर

**Supravaginal.** Above the vagina. अधियोनिज; योनि के ऊपर

**Supraventricular.** Above the ventricle. अधिनिलयी; निलय के ऊपर

**Supravesical.** Above the urinary bladder. अधिवस्तिक; मूत्राशय के ऊपर

**Sura.** The calf of leg. जंघापिण्ड; पिण्डली

**Sural.** Pertaining to the calf of leg; suralis. जंघापिण्ड अथवा पिण्डली सम्बन्धी

**Suralis.** See **Sural**.

**Surditas.** See **Surdity**.

**Surdity.** Deafness; surditas. बधिरता; बहरापन

**Surdomute.** A deaf and dumb person. मूकबधिर; गूंगा-बहरा

**Surface.** The outer part of a solid body. तल; पृष्ठ; सतह

**Surfactant.** Surface-active agent. पृष्ठसक्रियकारक; तलसक्रियकारक

**Surgeon.** One who practises surgery. शल्यचिकित्सक; शल्यकर्मी; सर्जन

**Surgery.** The branch of medicine which treats diseases by operative procedures. शल्यकर्म; शल्यक्रिया; शल्यचिकित्सा; शल्यविज्ञान; शस्त्रकर्म;

  **Ambulatory S.,** that performed on patients who are admitted to and discharged from the hospital on the same day. चल शल्यचिकित्सा;

  **Major S.,** major and serious operations involving a risk of life. बृहत् शस्त्रकर्म;

  **Minor S.,** simple operations not considered to involve a risk of life. लघु शस्त्रकर्म;

  **Open Heart S.,** direct vision correction of intracardiac disease. विवृतहृद् शस्त्रकर्म;

  **Plastic S.,** surgery concerned with the restoration, construction, reconstruction, or improvement in the shape and appearance of the body structures that are missing, defective, damaged, or misshapened. संधान शस्त्रकर्म; संधान शल्यविज्ञान

**Surgical.** Relating to surgery. शल्यक्रियात्मक; शल्यकर्म अथवा शल्यचिकित्सा सम्बन्धी

**Surrogate.** A medicine used as substitute. प्रत्यौषधि; किसी औषधि के बदले प्रयुक्त की जाने वाली अन्य औषधि

**Sursanure.** A lesion that has healed superficially with pus inside. अन्त:पूतिजक्षत; ऐसा घाव जो बाहर से ठीक दिखाई देता है लेकिन उसके अन्दर पीब भरी रहती है

**Survival**

**Survival.** The persistence of an individual or race after the general extinction of related form. अनुजीवन; जीवित रहना

**Susceptibility.** The opposite of resistance, usually refers to a disposition to infections. सुग्राह्यता; सुग्राहिता; संवेदनशीलता

**Susceptible.** Sensitive to an influence, liable to become affected with a disease. सुग्राह्य; सुग्राही; संवेदनशील

**Suspended Animation.** A temporary interruption of vital functions. जीवनीशक्ति की अस्थाई अवरुद्धता

**Suspension.** A temporary interruption of any function. निलम्बन

**Suspensory.** Serving to hold a part. निलम्बी; वृषणकोश को लटकाने वाला बन्धन

**Suspiration.** A sigh. उच्छ्वास; दीर्घनि:श्वास; लम्बी-लम्बी सिसकियाँ भरना

**Sustentaculum-tail.** The process of the calcaneum supporting the astragalus. घुटिका-धारक

**Sutura.** A suture. सीवन; टांका; रन्ध्र

**Suturae.** Plural of **Satura**.

**Sutural.** Relating to a suture. सीवनीय; सीवन सम्बन्धी

**Suturation.** The act of suturing. सीवन; घाव में टांका लगाने की प्रक्रिया

**Suture.** Line of joining or closure; the sewing up of a wound. सीवन; टांका; रन्ध्र;

   **Buried S.**, one in the depths of wounds, the skin completely covering it. गभीर सीवन;

   **Coronal S.**, the union of the frontal with the parietal bones transversely across the vertex of the skull. किरीट सीवन;

   **Frontal S.**, see **Metopic Suture**.

   **Lambdoid S.**, the union of the two superior borders of the occipital bone and the parietal bone; occipital suture. काकपद सीवन; पश्चक सीवन;

   **Mattress S.**, a continuous suture that is made back and forth through both lips of the wounds. मैट्रस सीवन;

   **Metopic S.**, one that at birth joins the two frontal bones from the interior fontanelle to the root of the nose, but that later becomes obliterated; frontal suture. ललाट सीवन;

   **Occipital S.**, see **Lambdoid Suture**.

   **Palatine S.**, the union of the palate bones. तालु सीवन

**Sutured.** Stitched or joined together. सिला हुआ; जोड़ा हुआ

**Swab.** A small piece of cotton wool or gauze used to collect material for bacteriological examination. फाहा; फुरेरी; स्वाब

**Swallow.** To perform deglutition. निगलना

**Swallowing.** The act of deglutition. निगरण; निगलना

**Sweat.** Perspiration; sweating. स्वेद; स्वेदन; पसीना; to perspire. पसीना आना

**Sweating Fever.** See **Sweating Sickness.**

**Sweating Sickness.** An old name for bad cases of congestive fever or fatal English cholera; sweating fever. स्वेदन रुग्णता; असाध्य रक्तसंलायी ज्वर अथवा सांघातिक विसूचिका का पुराना नाम

**Swelling.** Tumefaction. उत्सेध; सूजन; फुलाव; a morbid enlargement. असाधारण बृद्धि

**Swooning.** Syncope; fainting. सन्यास; सम्मूर्च्छी; मूर्च्छा; बेहोशी

**Sycoma.** A warty excrescence; a condyloma. मस्सा; मांसार्बुद

**Sycosis.** Figwart. अंजीरी मस्सा; a venereal disease. प्रमेह; सूजाक; barber's itch. लोमकूपशोथ; रोमपुटकशोथ

**Sycotic.** Affected with or relating to sycosis. प्रमेहग्रस्त; प्रमेहक; प्रमेहज; सूजाक सम्बन्धी

**Symbion.** Mutualist; an organism associated with another in symbiosis; symbiont; symbiote. सहजीवी

**Symbiont.** See **Symbion.**

**Symbiosis.** Mutualism; commensalism. सहजीविता; सहजीवन

**Symbiote.** See **Symbion.**

**Symbiotic.** Relating to symbiosis. सहजीविता सम्बन्धी

**Symblepharon.** Adhesion of the lid to eyeball. बद्धगोलकवर्त्म; पलकों का नेत्रगोलकों से चिपक जाना

**Symbol.** A sign or character significant of something else. चिन्ह; निशान

**Symbolism.** A mental state in which every occurrence is regarded by an individual as symbolic of his thoughts. प्रतीकता

**Symmetry.** A harmonious correspondence of parts. सममिति; सामंजस्य; संगति

**Sympathectomy.** Excision of a portion of the sympathetic nerve. अनुकम्पीतंत्रिकोच्छेदन; संवेदीतंत्रिका-उच्छेदन

**Sympathetic.** Relating to, or exhibiting sympathy; sympathic. अनुकंपी; संवेदी;

**S. Nerve,** that portion of the autonomic nervous system which stimulates the involuntary muscles of the body to activity. अनुकम्पी तंत्रिका; संवेदी तंत्रिका

**Sympathic.** See **Sympathetic.**

**Sympathicoblast.** See **Sympathoblast.**

**Sympathicomimetic.** See **Sympathomimetic.**

**Sympathoblast.** A primitive sympathetic nerve-cell; sympathicoblast. अनुकम्पीकोशिकाप्रसू

**Sympathomimetic.** Capable of producing changes similar to those produced by stimulation of the sympathetic nerves; sympathicomimetic. अनुकम्पी-अनुकारी; अनुकम्पीतंत्रिकानुकारी

**Symphyseal.** Relating to symphysis; symphysial. संधानक सम्बन्धी

**Symphyses.** Plural of **Symphysis.**

**Symphysial.** See **Symphyseal.**

**Symphysion.** The middle point of the outer border of the alveolar process of the inferior maxilla. संधानक-बिन्दु

**Symphysiotomy.** Section of the symphysis pubis. जघनसंधानक-उच्छेदन

**Symphysis.** A meeting point or union of bones or structures. अस्थि-संयोजिका;

**S. Pubis,** the line of the union of the pubic bones; pubic symphysis. जघन संधानक;

**Pubic S.,** see **Symphysis Pubis.**

**Symptom.** The manifestation of disease to the senses. It is by the aggregate and succession of the symptoms that disease is detected. लक्षण;

**Accessory S.,** a symptom that usually accompanies a certain disease; concomitant symptom. सहयोगी लक्षण; आनुषंगिक लक्षण;

**Cardinal S.,** the primary or major symptom. प्रमुख लक्षण;

**Concomitant S.,** see **Accessory Symptom.**

**Constitutional S.'s,** one produced by the effects of the disease on the whole body; general symptoms. सार्वदैहिक लक्षण; सर्वांगीण लक्षण;

**General S.'s,** see **Constitutional Symptoms.**

**Local S.,** one produced locally by the disease. स्थानिक लक्षण;

**Objective S.,** one observed by the physician and attendants, but not by the patient. परानुभूत लक्षण; चिकित्सक तथा परिचर्या करने वाले व्यक्तियों द्वारा रोगी में पाया जाने वाला लक्षण;

**Rational S.,** see **Subjective Symptom.**

**Reflex S.,** a disturbance of sensation or function in an organ or part not at the site of the morbid condition giving rise to it. प्रतिवर्त लक्षण;

**Subjective S.,** that observed by the patient himself; rational symptom. स्वानुभूत लक्षण; स्वयं रोगी को ही महसूस होने वाला लक्षण;

**Totality of s.,** see **Symptomatology.**

**S. Complex,** the totality of the symptoms of the disease; symptom grouping. लक्षण समूहन;

**S. Grouping,** see **Symptom Complex.**

**Symptomatic.** Pertaining to a symptom. लाक्षणिक; लक्षण सम्बन्धी

**Symptomatology.** The science of symptoms. लाक्षणिकी; लाक्षणिकता; लक्षणविज्ञान; the aggregate or symptoms of a disease, called totality of symptoms. लक्षण समष्टि

**Symptosis.** Wasting; collapse. क्षय; निपात

**Syn-.** Prefix denoting with or together. 'स', 'सह' के रूप में प्रयुक्त उपसर्ग

**Synaesthesia.** Sensation produced at one point arises from stimulation elsewhere. सहसंवेदन

**Synapse.** The entertwining of the terminal branches of the nervous system so that nerve impulses may pass from one to the other; synapsis. अन्तर्ग्रथन; गुणसूत्रीसंयोजन; सूत्रयुग्मन

**Synapses.** Plural of **Synapse** and **Synapsis.**

**Synapsis.** See **Synapse.**

**Synaptic.** Relating to synapse or synapsis. अन्तर्ग्रथन सम्बन्धी; अन्तर्ग्रथनीय

**Synarthrodia.** See **Synarthrosis.**

**Synarthrodial.** Relating to synarthrodia or synarthrosis. अचलसन्धि सम्बन्धी

**Synarthroses.** Plural of **Synarthrosis.**

**Synarthrosis.** An immovable articulation; synarthrodia. अचलसन्धि; न हिलने वाला जोड़

**Synchondroses.** Plural of **Synchondrosis.**

**Synchondrosis.** Union by intervening cartilage. उपास्थिसन्धि; उपास्थि का जोड़

**Synchronous.** Occurring at the same time. समकालिक; तुल्यकालिक; साथ-साथ प्रकट होने वाला

**Syncopal.** See **Syncopic.**

**Syncope.** Fainting or swooning. मूर्च्छा; सम्मूर्च्छा; बेहोशी;
   **S. Anginosa,** angina pectoris. हृच्छूल
**Syncopic.** Relating to syncope; syncopal. मूर्च्छा सम्बन्धी
**Syncytia.** Plural of **Syncytium.**
**Syncytial.** Relating to syncytium. संकोशिकीय; संकोशिका सम्बन्धी
**Syncytioma.** A tumour composed of syncytial tissue. संकोशिकार्बुद
**Syncytium.** A tissue in which no cell-boundaries can be recognized. संकोशिका
**Syndactylia.** See **Syndactylism.**
**Syndactylism.** The union of two or more digits; syndactylia; syndactylus; syndactyly. युक्तांगुलिकता; दो या दो से अधिक उँगलियों का जुड़ जाना
**Syndactylous.** Concerning syndactylism. युक्तांगुलिता सम्बन्धी
**Syndactylus.** See **Syndactylism.**
**Syndactyly.** See **Syndactylism.**
**Syndesis.** Artificial ankylosis; arthrodesis. सन्धिस्थिरीकरण; सन्धिसंसक्ति; कृत्रिम अस्थिसमेकन
**Syndesmitis.** Inflammation of ligaments. तन्तुसन्धिशोथ
**Syndesmologia.** See **Syndesmology.**
**Syndesmology.** The science of ligaments; syndesmologia. सन्धिप्रकरण
**Syndesmos.** A ligament. बन्धन; बन्धनप्रकरण
**Syndesmoses.** Plural of **Syndesmosis.**
**Syndesmosis.** Articulation by ligaments. तन्तुसन्धि
**Syndrome.** A commonly observed combination of symptoms. संलक्षण;
   **Adams-Stokes S.,** slow or absent pulse, vertigo, syncope or convulsions, usually due to heart block; Adams-Stokes disease; Stokes-Adams syndrome or disease; Morgagni's disease. एडम स्टोक संलक्षण;
   **Cushing's s.,** see under **Cushing.**
**Synechia.** A morbid union of parts. संसक्ति; अंगों का आपस में जुड़ जाना
**Synechiae.** Plural of **Synechia.**
**Synergia.** See **Synergy.**
**Synergic.** Exhibiting or relating to synergy. सहकारी; योगवाही
**Synergism.** See **Synergy.**

M.D.F.-30

**Synergist.** A supplementing agent or muscle; synergistic. सहकारी; योगवाही

**Synergistic.** See **Synergist**.

**Synergy.** Combined action; cooperation; synergia; synergism. योगवाहिता; सहकारिता

**Syngenesis.** Reproduction. पुनर्जनन

**Synocha.** Continued or inflammatory fever; synochus. सतत् ज्वर; प्रदाहक ज्वर

**Synochus.** See **Synocha**.

**Synopsis.** Abstract of matter so arranged as to exhibit a general view of the whole. झांकी; झलक

**Synosteotomy.** Dissection of joints; arthrotomy. सन्धि-उच्छेदन

**Synostosis.** Abnormal osseous union of bones. अस्थिसंयोजन; हड्डियों का अस्वाभाविक रूप से आपस में जुड़ना

**Synostotic.** Relating to synostosis. अस्थिसंयोजन सम्बन्धी

**Synovectomy.** Arthrectomy; the excision of a joint of the synovial membrane. सन्धि-उच्छेदन; श्लेषककला-उच्छेदन

**Synovia.** A lubricating fluid secreted in the joints of the bones. श्लेषक; स्नेहक

**Synovial.** Pertaining to the synovia. श्लेषक अथवा स्नेहक सम्बन्धी;
  **S. Membrane,** that lining a joint capsule. श्लेषक कला

**Synovioma.** A tumour of the synovial membrane. श्लेषककलार्बुद; स्नेहक झिल्ली की रसौली

**Synovitis.** Inflammation of the synovial membrane. श्लेषककलाशोथ; स्नेहक झिल्ली का प्रदाह

**Synovium.** The synovial membrane; membrana synovialis. श्लेषककला

**Syntaxis.** Articulation. सन्धि; जोड़

**Syntheses.** Plural of **Synthesis**.

**Synthesis.** The chemical building up of a complex substance from simple substance. संश्लेषण; संतुलन

**Synthetic.** Made by synthesis. संश्लिष्ट; कृत्रिम

**Syntonic.** Having even tone or temperament. समतानिक; समप्रकृति

**Syphilicoma.** A hospital for the syphilitics. उपदंश-उपचारगृह; उपदंश-चिकित्सालय

**Syphilid.** A syphilitic skin disease; syphilide. फिरंगचर्मता; सिफिलाइड

**Syphilide.** See **Syphilid**.

**Syphiliphobia.** A morbid fear of syphilis; syphilophobia. उपदंशभीति; उपदंश होने का डर

**Syphilis.** An infection with a spiral-shaped germ, spread by sexual or other personal contacts. उपदंश; आतशक; फिरंग रोग;

**Congenital S.,** one acquired by foetus in utero. सहज उपदंश;

**Constitutional S.,** hereditary syphilitic condition. वंशगत उपदंश; पैत्रिक उपदंश; खानदानी आतशक;

**Primary S.,** the first stage of the disease with the development of the chancre. प्राथमिक उपदंश;

**Secondary S.,** the second stage of the disease, characterized by slight fever and other constitutional symptoms. गौण उपदंश;

**Tertiary S.,** the final stage of the disease, characterized by formation of gammas, cellular infiltration and cardiovascular lesions. तृतीयक उपदंश

**Syphilitic.** Affected by syphilis. उपदंशग्रस्त

**Syphiloid.** Resembling syphilis. उपदंशवत्; फिरंगरोग जैसा

**Syphiloma.** A syphilitic tumour; gamma. उपदंशार्बुद

**Syphilophobia.** See **Syphiliphobia**.

**Syringe.** An instrument for injecting fluids. शृंगक; पिचकारी; सिरिंज

**Syringectomy.** Fistulectomy. नालव्रण-उच्छेदन

**Syringes.** Plural of **Syrinx**.

**Syringitis.** Inflammation of the Eustachian tube. कम्बुकर्णीनलीशोथ; कम्बुकर्णीनली का प्रदाह

**Syringotomy.** Fistulotomy. नालव्रणछेदन

**Syrinx.** A synonym for fistula. नालव्रण; नासूर; Eustachian tube. कम्बुकर्णीनली

**Syrup.** A concentrated solution of sugar in an aqueous fluid; syrupus. शर्बत; मिष्टोद

**Syrupus.** See **Syrup**.

**Systaltic.** Alternate contraction and dilatation. स्पन्दनशील; बारी-बारी से सिकुड़ने और फैलने वाला

**System.** The entire organism; methodic arrangement of the parts. तन्त्र; प्रणाली; जाल;

**Alimentary S.**, see **Digestive System**.

**Cardiovascular S.**, the heart and the blood vessels, comprising of aorta, arteries, arterioles, capillaries, venules, veins and venae cavae. हृद्वाहिका प्रणाली; हृद्वाहिका जाल;

**Central Nervous S. (CNS)**, consisting of the brain and spinal cord. केन्द्रीय स्नायु जाल; केन्द्रीय स्नायु तन्त्र;

**Circulatory S.**, the cardiovascular and lymphatic systems collectively; the system concerned with circulation of body fluids. संचार प्रणाली; संचार तन्त्र;

**Digestive S.**, the alimentary canal from mouth to anus with associated organs and glands concerned with ingestion, digestion and absorption of food-stuffs and nutrients; alimentary system. पोषण तन्त्र; पाचक तन्त्र;

**Genitourinary S.**, the organs involved in the formation and voiding of urine and in reproduction; urogenital system. जननमूत्र तन्त्र; जननमूत्र प्रणाली;

**Lymphatic S.**, the lymphatic vessels, lymph nodes and the lymphoid tissue. लसीका तन्त्र;

**Muscular S.**, all the muscles of the body, especially the voluntary skeletal muscles. पेशी तन्त्र; पेशी जाल;

**Nervous S.**, the entire neural apparatus, brain, spinal cord, nerve and ganglia. स्नायु-तन्त्र; स्नायु-जाल; तंत्रिका-तन्त्र;

**Reproductive S.**, the complex of male and female gonads, associated ducts and external genitalia concerned with procreation. जनन तन्त्र;

**Respiratory S.**, the air passages from the nose to the pulmonary alveoli. श्वास तन्त्र; श्वास प्रणाली;

**Urinary S.**, the kidneys, ureters, bladder and urethra. मूत्र तन्त्र;

**Urogenital S.**, see **Genitourinary System**.

**Systematic.** According to a system; methodic. तंत्रानुसारी; क्रमबद्ध; नियमबद्ध

**Systematized.** Arranged methodically. क्रमबद्ध; व्यवस्थित; नियमित

**Systemic.** Influencing or affecting the body as a whole. दैहिक; सर्वांगीण; relating to system. तन्त्रानुसारी

**Systole.** The act of contraction of the heart muscles to squeeze blood out. प्रकुंचन; सिकुड़न

**Systolic.** Concerned with the contraction of the cavities of the heart (diastolic is concerned with their dilatation). प्रकुंचनीय; हृत्प्रकुंचन सम्बन्धी

**Systolometer.** An instrument for estimating the intensity and quality of the cardiac murmur. प्रकुंचनमापी; हृत्प्रकुंचनमापी; हृद्कुंचनमापी; हृद्मर्मर की तीव्रता एवं गुण मापने के लिये प्रयुक्त किया जाने वाला उपकरण

# T

**Tabacosis.** Poisoning by tobacco. तम्बाकूविषण्णता; तम्बाकूविषाक्तता; तम्बाकूमयता; तम्बाकू से उत्पन्न होने वाली विषाक्त अवस्था

**Tabacum.** Tobacco. तम्बाकू

**Tabefaction.** Weakness; emaciation; debility. कृशता; क्षीणता; दुर्बलता: कमजोरी

**Tabella.** A troche; a medicinal tablet; a lozenge. टिकिया; वटी; गोली

**Tabellae.** Plural of **Tabella.**

**Tabes.** Consumption, or wasting away. अपजनन; अपघटन; यक्ष्मा; क्षय; शोष; क्षीणता; दुर्बलता;

**T. Diabetic,** peripheral neuritis affecting diabetics. परिसरीय तंत्रिकाशोथ, जो मधुमेहग्रस्त रोगियों में बहुतायत से पाया जाता है;

**T. Dorsalis,** wasting of the spinal marrow. मेरुरज्जु अपजनन; locomotor ataxia. गतिविभ्रम; चलनविभ्रम;

**T. Mesaraica,** see **Tabes Mesenterica.**

**T. Mesenterica,** consumption of the bowels; tabes mesaraica. आंत्रयोजनी यक्ष्मा; आंतों की टी० बी०;

**T. Urinalis,** wasting of the bladder. मूत्रमेह; diabetes. मधुमेह

**Tabetic.** Tabic; tabid; pertaining to tabes. शोर्ष सम्बन्धी; affected with tabes. शोषग्रस्त

**Tabetiform.** Resembling tabes. शोषवत्; शोषरूप; शोष से मिलता-जुलता

**Tabic.** See **Tabetic.**

**Tabid.** See **Tabetic.**

**Table.** A layer or plate of bone. पत्रक; आवरण; अस्थ्यावरण; अस्थिपत्रक; हड्डी का अस्तर; index of matter. सारणी

**Tablespoon.** A large-spoonful, i.e. half fluidounce or 15 milliliter. बड़ा चम्मच

**Tablet.** A troche or lozenge containing medicinal substance. टिकिया; गोली; वटी

**Taboo.** Restricted; prohibited or forbidden; tabu. वर्जित

**Tabu.** See **Taboo.**

**Tabular.** Having the form of a table. पत्राकार

**Tac.** Influenza. इंफ्लुएंजा; श्लैष्मिक-ज्वर

**Tache.** A spot; a colouration. धब्बा; रंजन

**Tachometer.** An instrument for measuring movements. परिक्रमणगणित्र; गतिमापकयंत्र; वेगमापीयंत्र

**Tachometric.** Pertaining to tachometer. त्वरमितिक; वेगमितिक; वेगमापीयंत्र सम्बन्धी

**Tachycardia.** Rapid heart; paroxysmal hurry of the heart; tachyrhythmia. क्षिप्रहृदयता; हृद्क्षिप्रता;

   **Paroxysmal T.**, recurring attacks of tachycardia. प्रवेगी हृद्क्षिप्रता

**Tachyphrenia.** Excessive mental activity. अतिमनोक्रियता; मानसिक अतिक्रियता; मन की अत्यधिक बढ़ी हुई क्रिया

**Tachypnea.** See **Tachypnoea.**

**Tachypnoea.** Abnormal frequency of respiration; tachypnea. क्षिप्रश्वसन; श्वासक्षिप्रता

**Tachyrhythmia.** See **Tachycardia.**

**Taciturn.** Reserve; silent; not talkative. मितभाषी; अल्पभाषी; कम बोलने वाला

**Tacky.** Adhesive. श्लेषी; आश्लेषी; चिपकने वाला

**Tactile.** Pertaining to the sense of touch or relating to touch. स्पर्शज्ञान अथवा विन्यासज्ञान सम्बन्धी;

   **T. Agnosia,** want of sense of touch. विन्यासज्ञानहीनता; स्पर्शज्ञानहीनता; स्पर्शज्ञान का अभाव होना

**Tactometer.** An instrument for measuring tactile sensibility. स्पर्शज्ञानमापी; विन्यासज्ञानमापी

**Tactual.** Relating to touch. स्पर्श सम्बन्धी; caused by touch. स्पर्शजनित

**Tactus.** Touch. स्पर्श

**Taenia.** A genus of flat, parasitic worms : cestodes or tapeworms. टीनिया; स्फीतकृमि; फीताकृमि; any bandlike structure. वेणी·

**Taenia**

**T. Saginata,** a hookless or unarmed tapeworm. सपाट कृमि; टीनिया सैजीनैटा; स्फीतकृमि अथवा फीताकृमि की एक जाति;

**T. Solium,** the common long tapeworms. टीनिया सोलियम; लम्बे आकार के फीताकृमि

**Taeniacide.** See **Teniacide.**

**Taeniafuge.** See **Teniafuge.**

**Tail.** The caudal extremity; cauda. पुच्छ; पूँछ;

**T.-bone,** the coccyx. पुच्छास्थि; उण्डुकपुच्छ; अनुत्रिक; रीढ़ की हड्डी का सबसे निचला भाग

**Taint.** An infection. रोग; a spot. धब्बा

**Talalgia.** Pain in the heel or ankle bone. पार्ष्णिकार्ति; एड़ी में दर्द होना

**Talc.** Powdered soapstone. टैल्क; साबुन बनाने के लिये प्रयुक्त किये जाने वाले पत्थर का चूर्ण (पावडर); talcum. टैल्कम

**Talectomy.** Surgical removal of the heel-bone. पार्ष्णिकास्थि-उच्छेदन; घुटिकास्थि-उच्छेदन; एड़ी की हड्डी काट कर निकाल देना

**Taleped.** A club-footed person; talepedic. मुद्गरपाद

**Talepedic.** See **Taleped.**

**Tali.** Plural of **Talus.**

**Talipes.** Club-foot, due to the contraction of certain muscles or tendons. मुद्गरपाद; टैलिपेस;

**T. Calcaneus,** club-foot, the heel alone touching the ground. पार्ष्णिकापाद;

**T. Cavus,** an increased curvature of the arch of the foot. अतिचापीपाद; बक्रपाद;

**T. Equinus,** club-foot, the patient walking on his toes. मुद्गरपाद;

**T. Planus,** flat-foot, a deformity marked by depression of the arch of the foot. सपाटपाद;

**T. Valgus,** club-foot, with eversion of the foot. बहिर्नतपाद;

**T. Varus,** club-foot, with inversion of the foot. अन्तर्नतपाद

**Talipomanus.** Club-hand. मुद्गरहस्त

**Talkative.** Loquacious. वाचाल; बातूनी; बहुत बोलने वाला

**Talkativeness.** Loquacity; loquaciousness. वाचालता; बातूनीपन

**Tallow.** The solid fat of cattle. पशुवसा; पशुओं की ठोस चर्बी सम्बन्धी

**Talma's disease.** Myotonia; delayed relaxation of a muscle after an initial contraction. पेशीतानता

**Talocalcaneal.** Relating to the ankle and the calcaneum; talocalcanean. घुटिका तथा पार्ष्णिका सम्बन्धी; टखने तथा एड़ी सम्बन्धी

**Talocalcanean.** See **Talocalcaneal.**

**Talpa.** A mole or wen. न्यच्छ; तिल

**Talus.** The second largest bone of the ankle; the astragalus. घुटिकास्थि; टखने की हड्डी

**Tamarind.** The tree **Tamarindus Indica;** also its cooling, laxative fruit. इमली; अम्लिका; चिंतपंडु

**Tamarindus Indica.** The tamarind tree. इमली-वृक्ष

**Tampon.** A plug of lint or cotton, used for plugging a bleeding orifice. पिचु; डाट; टैम्पन; रक्तस्राव रोकने के लिये किसी मुलायम कपड़े या रुई का डाट

**Tamponade.** The insertion of a tampon; tamponage. तीव्रसम्पीडन;

    **Cardiac T.,** compression of venous return to heart due to increased volume of fluid in the pericardium. हृद्-तीव्रसम्पीडन; हृद्-टैम्पोनेड

**Tamponage.** See **Tamponade.**

**Tantrum.** A fit of bad temper. आवेश

**Tap.** To perform paracentesis. वेध; वेधन; रेपण;

    **Spinal T.,** lumbar puncture. मेरु-वेध; रीढ़ की हड्डी में छेद करना

**Tapeinocephalic.** Characterized by tapeinocephaly; tapinocephalic. निम्नशीर्ष; छोटे चपटे सिर वाला

**Tapeinocephaly.** The condition of having a low, flat skull; tapinocephaly. निम्नशीर्षता; छोटा और चपटा सिर

**Tapeinocranic.** Characterized by a small skull. निम्नकरोटि; छोटी खोपड़ी वाला

**Tapeworm.** Tenia or taenia; an intestinal parasite; one of the cestoda, a class of worms parasitic in men and animals. स्फीतकृमि; फीताकृमि

**Tapinocephalic.** See **Tapeinocephalic.**

**Tapinocephaly.** See **Tapeinocephaly.**

**Tapping.** The operation for drawing off the effused fluid or water in dropsy. द्रवनिष्कासन; शोफ में पानी बाहर निकालने के लिये किया जाने वाला ऑपरेशन

**Tar.** A viscous mass obtained from the distillation of pine-wood. तारकोल; अलकतरा; बिरोजा

**Tarantism.** A dancing mania. नृत्योन्माद; नाचने का पागलपन

**Tardy.** Late. देरी से; रुक-रुक कर

**Target.** An object of fixation. लक्ष्य

**Tarsal.** Relating to tarsus. गुल्फ सम्बन्धी; वर्त्मपट्टिका सम्बन्धी;

    **T. Arches,** the arches of the palpebral arteries. गुल्फ चाप;

    **T. Cyst,** a chalazion; tarsal tumour. गुल्फ-पुटी; गुल्फार्बुद;

    **T. Tumour,** see **Tarsal Cyst.**

**Tarsale.** Singular of **Tarsalia.**

**Tarsalgia.** Pain in the tarsus; podalgia. गुल्फार्ति; गुल्फपीड़ा

**Tarsalia.** The tarsal bones. गुल्फास्थियाँ

**Tarsectomy.** Excision of the tarsal bones or the tarsus. गुल्फ-उच्छेदन; गुल्फोच्छेदन

**Tarsi.** Plural of **Tarsus.**

**Tarsomalacia.** Softening of the tarsus of the eyelid. वर्त्मगुल्फमृदुता

**Tarsometatarsal.** Pertaining to the tarsus and metatarsus. पदकूर्चप्रपदिक

**Tarsophyma.** Any tumour of the tarsus. गुल्फार्बुद

**Tarsoplasty.** Plastic reformation of an eyelid; blepharoplasty. वर्त्मसंधान

**Tarsorrhaphy.** An operation for lessening the size of the opening between the eyelids; blepharorrhaphy. वर्त्मसीवन

**Tarsotomy.** Removal of the tarsal cartilage of the foot by performing an operation. गुल्फास्थि-उच्छेदन; incision of the tarsal cartilage of an eyelid. वर्त्मोपास्थिछेदन; नेत्रच्छद-पट्टिकाछेदन

**Tarsus.** Instep. पदकूर्च; गुल्फ; cartilage of the eyelid. नेत्रच्छदपट्टिका; वर्त्मपट्टिका; वर्त्मगुल्फ; पलकों की उपास्थि

**Tartar.** The deposit which forms on the teeth; dental calculus. दन्तमल; दन्ताश्मरी

**Tartaric.** Relating to tartar. दन्तमल सम्बन्धी

**Taste.** The sense effected by tongue, the gustatory and other nerves. स्वाद;

    **T.-buds,** end-organs of the gustatory nerves; taste-bulbs; taste-ends. रसतंत्रिकान्त;

    **T.-bulbs,** see **Taste-buds.**

    **T.-ends,** see **Taste-buds.**

**Tatalgia.** Pain in the heel. पार्ष्णिकार्ति; एड़ी में दर्द

**Tattooing.** Production of permament colours in the skin by introducing foreign substance. गोदना; गोदन

**Tautomerism.** The attribution of two different formulas to one compound. चलावयवता

**Taxonomic.** Relating to taxonomy. वर्गिकी से सम्बन्धित; वर्गीकरणनियम सम्बन्धी

**Taxonomy.** The principles of classification. वर्गिकी; वर्गीकरणनियम

**T.B.** Tuberculosis. यक्ष्मा; क्षय

**T.D.S.** Ter in die sumendum; take three times a day. दिन में तीन बार लीजिये

**Tearing.** Like lacerating sensation. विदीर्णकारी

**Tears.** The drops of fluid secreted by the lachrymal glands. अश्रु; आँसू

**Teat.** The nipple. चूचुक

**Technic.** The method or procedure; technique. तकनीक; प्रविधि; प्रक्रिया

**Technique.** See **Technic.**

**Tecnology.** The science of childhood. बालविज्ञान

**Tecnotonia.** Child-murder; infanticide. शिशुहत्या

**Tecta.** Plural of **Tectum.**

**Tectal.** Relating to a tectum. आवरण या छद सम्बन्धी

**Tectorium.** An overlaying structure. आवरण; छद

**Tectum.** A roof or covering. आवरण; छद

**Tedious.** Tiresome. श्रमसाध्य; difficult. कठिन

**Teeth.** The organs of mastication; dentes. दन्त; दान्त;

    **Canine T.,** having sharp fang-like edge for tearing food; eye-teeth. रदनक दन्त;

    **Desiduous T.,** temporary teeth. अस्थायी दांत; अचिर दन्त; milk-teeth. दुग्ध-दन्त; दूध के दान्त;

    **Eye-t.,** see **Canine Teeth.**

    **Incisor T.,** having knife-like edge for biting food. कृन्तक दन्त;

    **Milk-t.,** those of the first dentition; opalescent teeth. अचिर दन्त; अस्थायी दान्त; दुग्ध-दन्त; दूध के दान्त;

    **Molar T.,** having a squarish termination for chewing and grinding food. चर्वणक दन्त;

**Opalescent T.**, see **Milk-teeth.**

**Permanent T.**, those of second dentition. स्थायी दान्त;

**Temporary T.**, milk-teeth. अस्थाई अथवा दूध के दांत;

**Wisdom T.**, the last molar-teeth. अन्त्यचर्वणक दन्त; अक्ल-दाढ़

**Teething.** Dentition; the eruption or cutting of the teeth. दन्तुरण; दन्तोद्गम; दन्तोद्भवन

**Tegmen.** A structure that covers or roofs over a part. छद; अन्तःबीजकवच; आवरण;

  **T. Tympani,** the roof of the tympanic cavity, or the tympanum. मध्यकर्णछद

**Tegmina.** Plural of **Tegmen.**

**Tegument.** The skin or covering of the body. त्वक्-आवरण; त्वचा; चर्म

**Tegumental.** See **Tegumentary.**

**Tegumentary.** Relating to the tegument; tegumental. त्वक्-आवरण अथवा त्वचा सम्बन्धी

**Teichopsia.** Temporary amblyopia with subjective images, often as accompaniment of migraine. प्रदीप्त रेखाभास

**Tela.** A web, or any web-like structure. टेला; कला; जाल; झिल्ली;

  **T. Araneae,** the spider's web; cobweb. लूता जाल; मकड़ी का जाल

**Telae.** Plural of **Tela.**

**Telangiectases.** Plural of **Telangiectasis.**

**Telangiectasia.** Dilatation of capillaries or smaller blood-vessels; telangiectasis. वाहिकास्फीति; कोशिकाओं अथवा रक्तवाहिनियों का फैलना;

  **Hereditary Haemorrhagic T.**, a disease with onset after puberty, marked by multiple small telangiectases and dilated venules that develop slowly on the skin and mucous membrane. आनुवंशिक रक्तस्रावी वाहिकास्फीति

**Telangiectasis.** See **Telangiectasia.**

**Telangiosis.** Any disease of the capillaries and terminal arterioles. कोशिकारुग्णता; कोशिकाओं का कोई रोग

**Telencephalon.** End-brain. उन्मस्तिष्क; मस्तिष्कान्त

**Teletherapy.** By custom refers to treatment with external radiation. दूरविकिरण-चिकित्सा

**Telophage.** The final stage of a cell-division. अंत्यावस्था; कोशिका-विभाजन की अन्तिम अवस्था

**Temper.** Mood; disposition. प्रकृति; स्वभाव; स्ववृत्ति; a display of irritation or anger. क्रोध

**Temperament.** Individual characteristics, manifested by acts, feelings, thoughts, etc.; temper. स्वभाव; प्रकृति

**Temperate.** Denoting temperance or moderation of all things. असंलयी क्रोध

**Temperature.** The degree of sensible heat or cold. ताप; तापमान

**Temple.** The flat portion between the forehead and occiput. कर्णपटी; कनपटी; शंख

**Tempora.** Plural of **Tempus.**

**Temporal.** Relating to, or connected with the temple; muscle of the temple. कर्णपटी अथवा कनपटी सम्बन्धी; शंखपेशीय; शंखास्थिक;

   **T. Bone,** situated on the lateral and inferior part of the cranium. शंखास्थि; कनपटी की हड्डी

**Temporary.** Not permanent. अस्थायी

**Temporomandibular.** Pertaining to the temple and the mandible. शंखअधोहनुज; कर्णपटी एवं अधोहनु सम्बन्धी

**Tempus.** The temple. कर्णपटी; कनपटी; time. समय

**Tenacious.** Sticky; adhesive; glutinous. चिपचिपा; तन्य; आश्लेषी; आश्लेषक

**Tenacity.** Cohesiveness; adhesiveness. चिपचिपापन; तन्यता

**Tenalgia.** See **Tenodynia.**

**Tendency.** Inclination. प्रवृत्ति; झुकाव

**Tender.** Sensitive. सम्वेदनशील; painful on pressure or contact. स्पर्शकातर; स्पर्शासह

**Tenderness.** Abnormal sensitiveness. सम्वेदनशीलता; painfulness on pressure or contact. स्पर्शकातरता; स्पर्शसह्यता; दाबवेदना;

   **Rebound T.,** tenderness felt when pressure, particularly abdominal pressure, is suddenly released. प्रच्छलन दाबवेदना

**Tendinitis.** Inflammation of the tendon; tendonitis. कण्डराशोथ; कण्डरा-प्रदाह

**Tendinous.** Relating to tendon. कण्डरीय; कण्डरा सम्बन्धी

**Tendo.** A tendon. कण्डरा; पुट्ठा;

   **T. Achilles,** the strong tendon of the heel; Achilles tendon. पार्ष्णिका-कण्डरा; एड़ी की कण्डरा

**Tendon.** A fibrous cord attached to the extremity of a muscle. कण्डरा; पुट्ठा

**Tendonitis.** See **Tendinitis.**

**Tendoplasty.** See **Tenoplasty.**

**Tendositis.** See **Tenositis.**

**Tendosynoitis.** See **Tenosynovitis.**

**Tendotomy.** See **Tenotomy.**

**Tenesmus.** Painful but useless urging to evacuate. कूथन; सपीडकुंथन; निस्तानिका

**Tenia.** The Same as **Taenia.**

**Teniacide.** An agent destroying tapeworms; taeniacide; tenicide. स्फीतकृमिनाशक; फीताकृमिनाशक; टीनियानाशक

**Teniafuge.** An agent expelling tapeworms; taeniafuge. स्फीतकृमिनिस्सारक; टीनियानिस्सारक

**Teniasis.** The presence of a tapeworm in the intestines. स्फीतकृमिरोग

**Tenicide.** See **Teniacide.**

**Tenodesis.** Fixation of a joint by shortening the tendons passing about the joint. कण्डरास्थिरीकरण

**Tenodynia.** Pain in a tendon; tenalgia. कण्डरार्ति

**Tenomyositis.** Inflammation of a muscle, or muscles and their tendons. कण्डरापेशीशोथ; किसी पेशी या पेशियों तथा उनकी कण्डराओं का प्रदाह

**Tenonectomy.** Excision of a tendon. कण्डरोच्छेदन; कण्डरा-उच्छेदन

**Tenontoplasty.** See **Tenoplasty.**

**Tenoplasty.** Plastic operation on a tendon; tenontoplasty; tendoplasty. कण्डरासंधान

**Tenorrhaphy.** The suturing of a tendon; tenosuture. कण्डरासीवन

**Tenositis.** Inflammation of a tendon; tendositis. कण्डराशोथ; कण्डरा-प्रदाह

**Tenosuture.** See **Tenorrhaphy.**

**Tenosynovitis.** Inflammation of the thin synovial lining of a tendon-sheath; tendosynovitis. कण्डरावरणशोथ; कण्डरावरण-प्रदाह

**Tenotomy.** Division of a tendon; tendotomy. कण्डरा-उच्छेदन; कण्डरोच्छेदन

**Tense.** Rigid; hard; stiff; drawn tightly. तना हुआ; दृढ़; कठोर; ठोस

**Tension.** Tenseness; the act or condition of being stretched or tense. तनाव;

**Arterial T.**, the blood pressure within an artery. धमनी तनाव;
**Intraocular T.**, the pressure of the fluid with in the eye-ball. अन्तरक्षि तनाव

**Tensor.** A muscle making a part firm and tense. तानिका

**Tent.** A small roll of lint or sponge. छदि; टेंट

**Tentorium.** A membranous cover or horizontal partition. छदि;
  **T. Cerebelli**, a fold of the dura mater roofing over the posterior cranial fossa; endocranium. अनुमस्तिष्क छदि

**Tephromyelitis.** Poliomyelitis. पोलियो

**Tephrosis.** Cremation. दाहसंस्कार

**Tepid.** Lukewarm; about blood heat. हल्का गरम; कोसा; अल्पोष्ण

**Ter-.** Prefix meaning three or three-fold. 'त्रि' अथवा 'त्रिगुण' के रूप में प्रयुक्त उपसर्ग

**Teratoblastoma.** See **Teratoma**.

**Teratogen.** Anything capable of disrupting foetal growth and producing malformation. अपरूपजन

**Teratogenesis.** The origin or mode of production of a malformed foetus; teratogeny. अपरूपजनन

**Teratogeny.** See **Teratogenesis**.

**Teratology.** The branch of embryology connected with the production, development, anatomy and classification of malformed foetuses. अपरूपविज्ञान; विरूपविज्ञान

**Teratoma.** A complex or congenital tumour; teratoblastoma. अपरूपार्बुद; कोई संकर अथवा जन्मजात अर्बुद

**Teratosis.** A congenital deformity. सहजदोष; कोई आजन्म अथवा जन्मजात दोष

**Terebinth.** The oil of turpentine; terebinthina. तारपीन का तेल

**Terebinthina.** See **Terebinth**.

**Teres.** Round and long; cylindrical. बेलनाकार; सिलिंड्राकार

**Teretes.** Plural of **Teres**.

**Ter in die.** Three times a day; abbreviated as **T.I.D.** दिन में तीन बार

**Ter in die sumendum.** Take three times a day; abbreviated as **T.D.S.** दिन में तीन बार लीजिये

**Term.** A definite or limited period, as full term of gestation, or pregnancy. अवधि

**Terminal.** Towards the extremity or terminus; ending; final. अन्त्य; अन्तस्थ; सीमान्त; अन्तिम

**Terminalis.** Terminal; ending. सीमान्त; अन्तिम; अन्त्य; अन्तस्थ

**Terminology.** The science of technical terms or words; nomenclature. शब्दावली; प्राविधिकशब्दविज्ञान

**Terms.** Menses. आर्तव; ऋतुस्राव; रजोधर्म; मासिक धर्म; माहवारी

**Terpentine Oil.** See **Terebinth.**

**Terra.** Earth. मृदा; मिट्टी;

　**T. Alba,** white clay. श्वेत मृदा; सफेद मिट्टी;

　**T. Japonica,** catechu. कत्था

**Terrific.** Dreadful. भयावह; भयानक; डरावना; causing terror. आतंकित करने वाला

**Terror.** Extreme fear. अतिभीति; अत्यधिक भय; आतंक

**Tertian.** Occurring every third day. तृतीयक; हर तीसरे दिन प्रकट होने वाला

**Tertiary.** Third in order. तृतीयक; तृतीय; क्रम में तीसरा या तीसरी;

　**T. Syphilis,** the third or the advanced stage of syphilis. तृतीयक उपदंश; उपदंश की तीसरी अथवा चरमावस्था

**Tertipara.** Pregnant for the third time. तृतीयगर्भा; त्रिगर्भा; तीसरी बार गर्भवती होने वाली स्त्री

**Tessellated.** Checkered. कुट्टिमचित्र; चतुष्कोणाकार; formed into little squares. खानेदार; वर्गाकार

**Test.** An examination or trial. परीक्षण; जांच;

　**T.-meal,** a meal given to test its action. परीक्षणाहार; प्रयोगाहार;

　**T.-tube,** a thin glass tube used for testing. परख नली; परीक्षण नली; जांच नली;

　**T.-types,** letters of different sizes to test the acuteness of vision. परीक्षण अक्षरमाला; परीक्षण अक्षरावली; परख अक्षरावली;

　**Agglutination T.,** a widely used test in which an antiserum containing antibodies to cells or bacteria causes them to agglutinate. समूहन परीक्षण;

　**Aschheim-Zondek T.,** test for pregnancy by injecting the patient's urine subcutaneously into immature female mice. If the patient is pregnant the ovaries of the mouse begin to mature prematurely. ऐशहाइम-जौंडेक परीक्षण (जांच);

**Benedict's T.**, a copy reduction test for glucose in urine. बेनीडिक्ट परीक्षण (जांच);

**Glucose Tolerance T.**, a test for diabetes, based upon ability of the normal liver to absorb and store excessive amounts of glucose as glycogen. शर्करा सह्यता परीक्षण (जांच);

**Mantoux T.**, tuberculin test. मांटू परीक्षण; टुबरकुलीन जांच;

**Tuberculin T.**, a test done for the diagnosis of tuberculosis in which tuberculin serves as an antigen; Mautoux test. टुबरकुलीन परीक्षण

**Testes.** Plural of **Testis**.

**Testis.** One of the two glandular organs of the male contained in the scrotum whose office is to secrete semen; testicle. वृषण; अण्ड; वृषणकोष अथवा अण्डकोष के अन्दर स्थित दो ग्रन्थिल पिण्ड, जिनका कार्य शुक्रस्राव होता है

**Testicle.** See **Testis**.

**Testicular.** Pertaining to, or like testes. वृषणों सम्बन्धी या वृषणों जैसा

**Testitis.** Inflammation of the testes. वृषणशोथ; वृषण-प्रदाह

**Tetanic.** Relating to tetanus. धनुस्तम्भी; धनुर्वाती; धनुस्तम्भ सम्बन्धी

**Tetaniform.** Resembling tetanus; tetanoid. धनुस्तम्भरूप; धनुस्तम्भाभ; धनुर्वाताभ; धनुर्वात से मिलता-जुलता

**Tetanigenous.** Causing tetanus or tetaniform spasm. धनुर्वाती; धनुर्वातजनक

**Tetanization.** The production of tetanus. धनुस्तम्भन; tetanizing the muscles. पेशीस्तम्भन

**Tetanoid.** See **Tetaniform**.

**Tetanus.** A rigid contraction of voluntary muscles; lock-jaw. धनुस्तम्भ; धनुर्वात; सततपेशीसंकुचन; हनुस्तम्भ

**Tetany.** Condition of muscular hyperexcitability in which mild stimuli produce cramps and spasms. अतिपेशी-उत्तेजना; पेशियों की अत्यधिक उत्तेजित अवस्था; अपतानिका

**Tetra-.** Prefix denoting four. 'चतु:' के रूप में प्रयुक्त अथवा चार का अर्थ देने वाला उपसर्ग

**Tetrad.** An element with the valency of four; quadrivalent; tetravalent. चतुष्टय; चतुष्क

**Tetradactyly.** Having only four fingers or toes on a hand or foot. चतुरंगुलिक; हाथ या पैर में केवल चार उँगलियों वाला व्यक्ति

**Tetralogy.** A collection of four things having something in common. चतुष्क

**Tetraplegia.** Peralysis of all four limbs; quadriplegia. चतुरांगघात; बाहों तथा टांगों का पक्षाघात

**Tetrapod.** Having four feet. चतुष्पाद; चौपाया; चार पैरों वाला

**Tetravalent.** See **Tetrad.**

**Tetter.** Herpetic eruption; ringworm; eczema. विसर्प; दाद; दद्रु; छाजन

**Text-blindness.** Word-blindness. शब्दान्धता

**Textiform.** Weblike. जालवत्; जालरूप; जाल जैसा

**Thalami.** Plural of **Thalamus.**

**Thalamic.** Relating to thalamus. चेतक सम्बन्धी

**Thalamocortical.** Pertaining to the optic thalamus and cerebral cortex. दृष्टि-चेतक तथा मस्तिष्क-प्रान्तस्था सम्बन्धी

**Thalamotomy.** Usually operative destruction of a portion of the thalamus. चेतक-उच्छेदन; चेतकोच्छेदन

**Thalamus.** The great posterior ganglion of the brain, the supposed origin of the optic nerve. चेतक; थैलेमस

**Thalassemia.** Any of a group of inherited disorders of haemoglobin metabolism in which there is a decrease in net synthesis of a particular globin change without change in the structure of that chain. थैलासीमिया

**Thanatoid.** Resembling death. मृत्युवत्; मौत से मिलता-जुलता

**Thanatology.** The branch of science concered with the study of death. मृत्युविज्ञान

**Thanatophobia.** Fear of death. मृत्युभीति; मौत का डर

**Thea.** Tea. चाय

**Theca.** A sheath investing membrane. पिधान; वेष्टन; थीका;

    **T. Cordis,** pericardium. परिहृद्; हृदयावरण;

    **T. Folliculi,** the wall of a vesicular ovarian follicle. पिधान पुटिका;

    **T. Vertebralis,** that of the spinal membranes. मेरुपिधान

**Thecae.** Plural of **Theca.**

**Thelalgia.** Pain in the nipples. चूचुकार्ति; चूचुकवेदना

**Thelitis.** Inflammation of the nipples. चूचुकशोथ; चूचुकों का प्रदाह

**Thenar.** The fleshy mass on the lateral side of the palm of hand, the ball of thumb, or sole of foot. करतल अथवा पदतल;

**T. Eminence,** the palmar eminence below the thumb. करांगुष्ठ उत्सेध; अंगूठे के नीचे हथेली पर उठा हुआ भाग

**Theomania.** Religious madness or melancholy. धार्मिक विक्षिप्ति अथवा विषाद

**Theory.** Principle. सिद्धान्त; वाद

**Therapeutic.** Concerned with the application of drugs to cure or relieve diseases. उपचारार्थ; चिकित्सार्थ; चिकित्सीय; उपचार सम्बन्धी औषधियों का प्रयोग

**Therapeutics.** The branch of medical science concerned with the application of remedies and treatment of diseases. चिकित्साशास्त्र; उपचारविज्ञान

**Therapeutist.** A person trained to give therapy by physical means; therapist. चिकित्सक; वैद्य; हकीम

**Therapia.** See **Therapy.**

**Therapist.** See **Therapeutist.**

**Therapy.** The medical word for treatment; therapia. चिकित्सा; उपचार; इलाज;

   **Occupational T.,** the use of work-related skills to treat or train the physically or emotionally ill-patients. व्यावसायिक चिकित्सा;

   **Physical T.,** treatment of diseases by using natural forces, massage, heat, radiation and other therapeutic exercises; physiotherapy. भौतिक चिकित्सा

**Theriaca.** Treacle; molasses. भेषज-योग

**Therm.** A heat unit. ताप

**Thermal.** Pertaining to heat. तापीय; ताप सम्बन्धी

**Thermalgesia.** Pain caused by heat. तापार्ति; तापवेदना; गर्मी से होने वाला दर्द

**Thermalgia.** Burning pain. ज्वलनार्ति; जलन के साथ दर्द

**Thermic.** Relating to heat. तापीय; ताप सम्बन्धी

**Thermo-.** Prefix meaning heat. 'ताप' अथवा 'ऊष्मा' के रूप में प्रयुक्त उपसर्ग

**Thermoanaesthesia.** Loss of heat-sense; thermoanalgesia; thermoanesthesia. तापसंवेदनाहरण; तापसंवेदनाभाव; तापज्ञान का अभाव

**Thermoanalgesia.** See **Thermoanaesthesia.**

**Thermoanesthesia.** See **Thermoanaesthesia.**

**Thermochemistry.** The science of the chemic action of heat. ऊष्मारसायन; गर्मी की रासायनिक क्रिया का विज्ञान

**Thermogenesis.** The production of heat. तापजनन

**Thermogenetic.** See **Thermogenic.**

**Thermogenic.** Producing heat; thermogenetic. तापजनक; relating to thermogenesis. तापजनन सम्बन्धी

**Thermograph.** An instrument for recording variations in heat. तापलेखी (यंत्र)

**Thermography.** A mode by which temperature differences throughout the body are recorded on photographic film for diagnostic purposes. तापलेखन

**Thermoinhibitory.** Inhibiting or arresting thermogenesis. तापजननरोधी; तापजननरोधक

**Thermolabile.** Capable of being changed by heat. तापपरिवर्ती

**Thermolysis.** Loss of heat. तापवियोजन; तापलयन

**Thermometer.** An instrument for ascertaining temperature. तापमापी (यंत्र); थर्मामीटर; ज्वरमापी (यंत्र);

  **Clinical T.,** a self-registering thermometer for taking the body temperature. नैदानिक ज्वरमापी;

  **Differential T.,** one for determining slight variations of temperature. ज्वरान्तरमापी;

  **Maximum T.,** one that registers the maximum heat to which it has been exposed. उच्चत्तम तापमापी;

  **Minimum T.,** one that registers the lowest temperature. निम्नतर तापमापी

**Thermometry.** Measurement of temperature. तापमापन; तापमिति

**Thermophilic.** Requiring great heat for growth. तापरागी

**Thermoplegia.** Heat-stroke. तापाघात

**Thermoregulation.** Temperature control. तापनियमन; तापनियंत्रण

**Thermostable.** Remaining unaltered at a high temperature, which is usually specified. तापस्थिर

**Thermostat.** A device, usually electronic, which controls temperature of air or water. तापस्थायी

**Thermotaxis.** Regulation of the temperature of the body. तापानुचलन

**Thermotherapy.** The treatment of diseases by heat. तापोपचार; ताप द्वारा की जाने वाली चिकित्सा

**Thiamin (e).** Vitamin B1; a heat-labile vitamin contained in milk, yeast, grain, etc., which is essential for growth. थायमिन; विटामिन बी१

**Thigh.** The upper leg, between the hip and knee. ऊरु; जांघ; रान; **T. Friction,** a form of masturbation. ऊरुघर्षण; ऊरुमैथुन

**Thigmotaxis.** The negative or positive response of certain motile cells to touch. स्पर्शानुचलन

**Thomson's disease.** Congenital myotonia. पेशीतानता; थामसन रोग

**Thorac.** See **Thoraci.**

**Thoracalgia.** Pain in the chest. वक्षार्ति; वक्षपीड़ा; वक्षवेदना; छाती में दर्द

**Thoracentesis.** Puncture of the thorax to withdraw an accumulation of fluid; paracentesis; thoracocentesis. वक्षवेधन

**Thoraci.** In the chest; thorac. वक्ष में; छाती में

**Thoracic.** Relating to, or connected with the chest or thorax. वक्ष सम्बन्धी

**Thoracocentesis.** See **Thoracentesis.**

**Thoracocyllosis.** Deformity of the thorax. वक्षविरूपता

**Thoracodynia.** Pain in the chest or thorax. वक्षवेदना; वक्षपीड़ा; छाती में दर्द

**Thoracolysis.** Breaking up of pleural adhesions. परिफुप्फुसवियोजन; परिफुप्फुसलयन

**Thoracopagus.** A double monster with fusion of the thoraces. बद्धवक्षयमल

**Thoracoplasty.** Plastic operation of the thorax. वक्षसंधान

**Thoracoscope.** A stethoscope. वक्षदर्शी; वक्षजांचयंत्र

**Thoracoscopy.** Examination of the chest. वक्षदर्शन; वक्षजांच

**Thoracostenosis.** Contraction of the chest. वक्षसंकीर्णन; छाती की सिकुड़न

**Thoracotomy.** An incision of the thorax; pleuracotomy; pleurotomy. वक्षछेदन

**Thorax.** The chest; the cavity above the abdomen. वक्ष; उर; छाती

**Thorium.** A radioactive metallic element. थोरियम

**Threadworm.** Oxyuris vermicularis, i.e. thread-like worm infecting man's intestine. सूत्रकृमि; धागे जैसा कृमि

**Three-day Fever.** Dengue. डेंगू; तीन दिन तक गतिशील रहने वाला ज्वर

**Threpsology.** The science of nutrition. पोषणविज्ञान; आहारविज्ञान

**Threshold.** The limit of perceptibilty of a stimulus. देहली; प्रभावसीमा

**Thrill.** A tremor; quiver; vibration as perceived by sense of touch. स्पृश्यतरंग; स्पर्शकम्प; कम्पन; कम्पकम्पी;

**Diastolic T.,** a thrill felt over the precordium or over a blood vessel during ventricular diastole. अनुशिथिलन स्पृश्यतरंग;

**Systolic T.,** a thrill felt over the precordium or over a blood vessel during ventricular systole. प्रकुंचन स्पृश्यतरंग

**Throat.** The interior part of the neck; jugulum. कण्ठ; गला;

**Sore-t.,** a condition characterized by pain or discomfort on swallowing due to any kind of inflammation. कण्ठदाह; गले में दर्द

**Throbbing.** Beating with unusual force. स्पन्दन; प्रस्पन्दन; तपकन; अस्वाभाविक शक्ति के साथ होने वाली धड़कन

**Thrombectomy.** Removal of a thrombus. घनास्र-उच्छेदन; घनास्रनिष्कासन; किसी थक्के या आतंच को काट कर हटा देना

**Thrombi.** Plural of **Thrombus**.

**Thromboangiitis.** Clot formation within an inflamed vessel. घनास्रवाहिकाशोथ; किसी रक्तवाहिनी के अन्दर थक्का बन जाने के कारण उत्पन्न होने वाला प्रदाह

**T. Obliterans,** an uncommon disorder of unknown cause. रोधक घनास्रवाहिकाशोथ

**Thromboarteritis.** Arterial inflammation with formation of a thrombus. घनास्रधमनीशोथ

**Thrombocyte.** Blood platelet. बिम्बाणु

**Thrombocythaemia.** See **Thrombocytosis**.

**Thrombocytopathy.** Any disease of the blood platelets. बिम्बाणु-विकृति

**Thrombocytopenia.** A reduction in number of platelets in the blood; thrombopaenia. बिम्बाणु-अल्पता; बिम्बाणुओं की कमी

**Thrombocytosis.** An increase in the number of platelets in the blood; thrombocythaemia. बिम्बाणुबहुलता; बिम्बाणुओं की अधिकता

**Thromboembolic.** Used to describe the phenomenon whereby a thrombus or clot detaches itself and is carried to another part of the body in the blood-stream to block a blood vessel there. घनास्रशल्य

**Thromboendarterectomy.** Removal of a thrombus from an artery following reboring. घनास्रअन्तर्धमनी-उच्छेदन; किसी धमनी के अन्दर से थक्का काट कर हटाना

**Thromboembolism.** Embolism from a thrombus. घनास्रअन्त:शल्यता

**Thromboendarteritis.** Inflammation of the inner lining of an artery with clot formation. घनास्रअन्तर्धमनीशोथ; थक्का बनने के साथ किसी धमनी की अन्दरूनी झिल्ली का प्रदाह

**Thrombogen.** Precursor of thrombus. घनास्रजन; थक्का बनाने वाला

**Thrombogenic.** Relating to thrombogen. घनास्रजन सम्बन्धी

**Thrombogenesis.** Formation of a thrombus. घनास्रजनन; रक्त में थक्के बनना

**Thromboid.** Resembling a thrombus. घनास्रवत्; घनास्र से मिलता-जुलता

**Thrombolytic.** Pertaining to disintegration of a blood clot. घनास्रलयी; खून का थक्का नष्ट करने सम्बन्धी

**Thrombopaenia.** See **Thrombocytopenia.**

**Thrombopenia.** The same as **Thrombopaenia.**

**Thrombophlebitis.** Phlebitis from the breaking down of a venous thrombus. घनास्रशिराशोथ; थक्का टूट कर बिखरने के कारण होने वाला शिरा का प्रदाह;

 **T. Migrans,** recurrent episodes of thrombophlebitis affecting short lenghts of superficial veins; migrating thrombophlebitis. चलघनास्रशिराशोथ;

 **Migrating T.,** see **Thrombophlebitis Migrans.**

**Thrombosis.** The complete or partial blocking of a blood vessel by clot-formation. घनास्रता; थक्का बनने से किसी रक्तवाहिनी की पूर्ण अथवा आंशिक अवरुद्धता;

 **Coronary T.,** coronary occlusion by thrombus formation. हृद्धमनी घनास्रता;

 **Mural T.,** formation of a thrombus in contact with the endocardial lining of a cardiac chamber. भित्तिक घनास्रता

**Thrombotic.** Relating to a thrombus. घनास्री; घनास्र सम्बन्धी; caused by a thrombus. घनास्रजन; characterized by thrombosis. घनास्ररूप

**Thrombus.** The presence of a clot in the blood vessels. घनास्र; श्राम्बस; रक्तवाहिनियों में थक्का विद्यमान रहना

**Thrush.** Aphthae; small white ulcers of the mouth. मुखव्रण; छाले

**Thumb.** The most external or nearly radial of the five digits of the hand. हस्तांगुष्ठ; हाथ का अंगूठा

**Thymectomy.** Surgical excision of the thymus. बाल्यग्रन्थि-उच्छेदन; बाल्यग्रन्थि को काट कर हटा देना

**Thymelcosis.** Suppuration of the thymus gland. बाल्यग्रंथिपूतिता

**Thymi.** Plural of **Thymus.**

**Thymic.** Relating to the thymus gland. बाल्यग्रंथि अथवा थाइमसग्रंथि सम्बन्धी

**Thymion.** A small wart on the skin. क्षुद्र मस्सा

**Thymitis.** Inflammation of the thymus gland. बाल्यग्रन्थिशोथ; बाल्यग्रन्थि का प्रदाह

**Thymol.** A phenol from the oil of the thyme. अजवायन का सत

**Thymoma.** A tumour arising in the thymus. बाल्यग्रन्थि-अर्बुद; बाल्यग्रन्थि में बनने वाली कोई रसौली

**Thymomata.** Plural of **Thymoma.**

**Thymopathy.** Any disease of the thymus gland. बाल्यग्रन्थिरोग

**Thymus.** A glandular structure lying beneath the breast which normally disappears at or about birth. थाइमस (ग्रंन्थि); बाल्यग्रन्थि

**Thymuses.** Plural of **Thymus.**

**Thyroadenitis.** See **Thyroiditis.**

**Thyroepiglottic.** Pertaining to the thyroid gland and epiglottis. अवटु-कण्ठच्छदीय; अवटुग्रन्थि एवं कण्ठच्छद सम्बन्धी

**Thyroglossal Duct.** A foetal passage between the thyroid gland and the tongue. अवटुजिह्वा-नली; अवटुग्रन्थि एवं जिह्वा के मध्य स्थित एक भ्रूण नली

**Thyroid.** A gland of internal secretion situated in the lower front region of the neck. अवटु; थाइराइड;

**T. Body,** see **Thyroid Gland.**

**T. Cartilage,** the largest cartilage of the larynx. अवटु-उपास्थि; स्वरयंत्र की सबसे बड़ी उपास्थि;

**T. Gland,** a butterfly shaped gland in front of the neck which regulates the body chemistry and helps control growth and maturing; thyroid body. अवटुग्रन्थि; गर्दन के आगे तितली के आकार की ग्रन्थि जो शारीरिक संतुलन बनाये रखती है

**Thyroidectomy.** Excision of the thyroid gland. अवटु-उच्छेदन; अवटुग्रन्थि-उच्छेदन; अवटुग्रन्थि को काट कर हटा देना

**Thyroidism.** Poisoning by thyroid extract. अवटुक्रियता; अवटुसार द्वारा होने वाली विषण्णता

**Thyroiditis.** Inflammation of the thyroid gland; thyroadenitis. अवटुशोथ; अवटुग्रन्थिशोथ; अवटुग्रन्थि का प्रदाह

**Thyroidotomy.** Incision of the thyroid gland. अवटुच्छेदन; अवटुग्रन्थिच्छेदन

**Thyrotomy.** Incision of the thyroid body of the cartilages; laryngofissure. अवटु-उपास्थिच्छेदन; अवटूपास्थिच्छेदन

**Thyrotoxic.** Designating the state produced by excessive quantities of endogenous or exogenous thyroid hormone. अवटुविषज

**Thyrotoxicosis.** One of the auto-immune thyroid diseases. अवटु-विषाक्तता; अवटुविषण्णता; एक स्वक्षम अवटु रोग

**Thyrotrophic.** A substance which stimulates the thyroid gland; thyrotropic. अवटुप्रेरक; अवटु-उद्दीपक; अवटुग्रन्थि को उद्दीप्त करने वाला पदार्थ

**Thyrotropic.** See **Thyrotrophic.**

**Tibia.** The inner and larger bone of the leg. अन्तर्जंघिका; अन्त:प्रकोष्ठिका; तिबिया; टांग की अन्दरूनी व सबसे लम्बी हड्डी;

  **T. Vara,** bow-leg. अन्तर्नत अन्तर्जंघिका; अन्तर्नत तिबिया

**Tibiae.** Plural of **Tibia.**

**Tibial.** Pertaining to tibia. अन्तर्जंघिकी; अन्त:प्रकोष्ठिकीय; अन्त:प्रकोष्ठिकापरक; तिबिया सम्बन्धी; टांग की अन्दरूनी व सबसे लम्बी हड्डी से सम्बन्धित

**Tibiofibular.** Pertaining to tibia and fibula. अन्तर्बहिर्जंघिकी; अन्त: एवं बाह्य जंघिकाओं सम्बन्धी

**Tic.** A twitching of the muscle. पेशीस्फुरण; स्वभावाकर्ष

**Tic-douloureux.** Violent neuralgia of the face. उग्राननार्ति; चेहरे की तंत्रिकाओं का तेज दर्द

**Tick.** A skin parasite common in wooded and bushy areas which infects animals and men. किलनी; टिक;

  **T. Fever,** an infectious spotted fever of high mortality caused by ticks. किलनी ज्वर; टिक ज्वर

**Tickling.** A peculiar sensation resulting from excitation of the cutaneous nerve; titillation. गुदगुदी; त्वक्-तंत्रिका की उत्तेजना के कारण होने वाली एक विशेष प्रकार की सम्वेदना

**T.I.D.** Ter in die; three times a day. दिन में तीन बार

**Tide.** An alternate rise and fall; ebb and flow; an increase or decrease. ज्वार;

  **Alkaline T.,** a period of urinary neutrality or alkanity after meals. क्षारीय ज्वार

**Tinctura.** See **Tincture.**

**Tincture.** An alcoholic solution of the medicinal substances; tinctura. मूलार्क; टिंचर

**Tinea.** Ringworm. दद्रु; मण्डलकुष्ठ; दाद; टीनिया;

    **T. Barbae,** ringworm of the beard; barber's itch; tinea sycosis. श्मश्रु-दद्रु; दाढ़ी का दाद;

    **T. Capitis,** ringworm of the head; scald-head. शीर्ष-दद्रु; सिर का दाद;

    **T. Circinata,** see **Tinea Corporis.**

    **T. Corporis,** ringworm of the body; tinea circinata. काय-दद्रु; बहुचक्री दद्रु;

    **T. Cruris,** ringworm of the crutch area; dhobie itch. वंक्षण-दद्रु;

    **T. Decalvans,** the same as **Alopecia Areata.**

    **T. Facei,** milk crust or scab. दुग्ध-निर्माक; आनन-दद्रु;

    **T. Imbricata,** a severe form of tinea. कुण्डलित दद्रु; दाद का एक उग्र रूप;

    **T. Pedis,** ringworm of the foot. पाद-दद्रु; पैरों का दाद;

    **T. Sycosis,** see **Tinea Barbae.**

    **T. Tarsi,** the same as **Blepharitis.**

    **T. Tonsurans,** ringworm of the scalp. करोटि-दद्रु; खोपड़ी का दाद;

    **T. Unguium,** ringworm of the nails. नख-दद्रु; नाखुनों का दाद;

    **T. Versicolor,** a funguous skin disease, characterized by patches of brown colour. बहुवर्णी दद्रु; एक कवक रोग, जिसमें चमड़ी पर कत्थई रंग के चकत्ते पड़ जाते हैं

**Tingling.** A peculiar pricking thrill caused by cold or mental shock. झुनझुनी; चुनचुनाहट; चुमचुमायन

**Tinnitus.** Ringing in the ear, or other ear noises. कर्णक्ष्वेड; कान के अन्दर घण्टी बजने जैसी या अन्य प्रकार की आवाजें सुनाई देना; टिनिटस

    **T. Aurium,** a subjective ringing in the ear. स्वानुभूत कर्णक्ष्वेड

**Tint.** Colour. वर्ण; रंग

**Tip.** Exremity; end. सिरा; छोर; किनारा

**Tire.** Weariness and exhaustion. थकना; थक जाना; थकान लगना तथा कमजोरी महसूस होना

**Tissue.** The various constituent parts of the body, such as muscular tissue, osseous tissue, etc. ऊतक;

    **Adenoid T.,** a form of connective tissue in which the meshes contain lymphoid cells. ग्रन्थि-ऊतक; ग्रन्थ्यूतक; lymphatic tissue; lymphoid tissue. लसीकोतक;

**Adipose T.**, areolar tissue with fat cells lodged in its meshes. वसा-ऊतक;

**Areolar T.**, a form of connective tissue made up of cells and delicate elastic fibres interlacing in every direction. अवकाशी ऊतक;

**Bone T.**, see **Osseous Tissue.**

**Cancellous T.**, a spongy osseous tissue. स्पंजी अस्थिऊतक;

**Chromaffin (e) T.**, a cellular tissue made up chiefly from chromaffine(e) tissue. वर्णरागी ऊतक;

**Connective T.**, a general name for all those tissues of the body that support the essential elements or parenchyma. संयोजी ऊतक;

**Elastic T.**, connective tissue composed of yellow elastic fibres. प्रत्यास्थ ऊतक;

**Embryonal T.**, see **Embryonic Tissue.**

**Embryonic T.**, connective tissue such as is present in the umbilical cord of the foetus; embryonal tissue; mucoid tissue; mucous tissue. भ्रूण ऊतक;

**Epithelial T.**, epithelium. उपकला ऊतक;

**Erectile T.**, a spongy tissue that becomes expanded and hard when filled with blood. उच्छ्रायी ऊतक;

**Fibrous T.**, the connective tissue of the body, consisting of white or yellow fibres. तन्तु-ऊतक;

**Granulation T.**, a new tissue, made up of granulations, repairing a loss of substance and becoming cicatrical tissue. कणिका ऊतक;

**Interstitial T.**, connective tissue that forms a network with the cellular elements of an organ. अन्तराली ऊतक;

**Lymphatic T.**, see **Adenoid Tissue.**

**Lymphoid T.**, see **Adenoid Tissue.**

**Mucoid T.**, see **Embryonic Tissue.**

**Mucous T.**, see **Embryonic Tissue.**

**Muscular T.**, that of the muscles. पेशी-ऊतक;

**Nerve T.**, see **Nervous Tissue.**

**Nervous T.**, tissue characteristic of the nervous system; nerve tissue. तंत्रिका-ऊतक; स्नायु-ऊतक;

**Osseous T.**, the bone tissue; a connective tissue whose matrix consists of collagen fibres and ground substance and in which are deposited calcium salts. अस्थि-ऊतक;

**Subcutaneous T.**, a layer of loose, irregular, connective tissue immediately beneath the skin. अधस्त्वकूतक;

**T. Remedies,** twelve salts, especially used in biochemical school of homoeopathy. ऊतक औषधियाँ

**Titer.** The standard of strength of a volumeric test solution; titre. अनुमापनांक

**Titillation.** See **Tickling.**

**Titration.** Volumeric analysis by the aid of standard solutions. अनुमापन

**Titre.** See **Titer.**

**Titthe.** The nipple. चूचुक

**Titubation.** The staggering gait of the diseased. प्रस्खलन; लड़खड़ाना; restlessness. बेचैनी; घबराहट

**Tobacco.** The dried leaves of nicotiana tabacum. तम्बाकू

**Tocology.** Midwifery. प्रसूतिविज्ञान; धात्रीविज्ञान

**Tocophobia.** A morbid fear of labour. प्रसवभीति; प्रसवसंत्रास; प्रसवातंक

**Tocus.** Childbirth. प्रसव; बच्चे का जन्म

**Toe.** A digit of the foot; digitus pedis. पादांगुलि; पैर की उँगली;

**Great T.,** the big-toe. पादांगुष्ठ; पैर का अंगूठा;

**Hammer T.,** permanent flexion at the midphalangeal joint of one or more of the toes. नखर पादांगुष्ठ

**Tolerance.** The tolerating power. सह्यता; सहनशक्ति;

**T. Test,** observation of the ability to take a large dose of sugar and utilize it effectively. सह्यता जांच;

**Immunologic T.,** acquired specific failure of the immunological mechanism to respond. रोगक्षम सह्यता

**-tomy.** Suffix denoting a cutting operation. '-उच्छेदन' अर्थात् आपरेशन द्वारा काट दिये जाने के रूप में प्रयुक्त प्रत्यय अथवा शब्दांत

**Tone.** The normal vigour or activity. तान; स्वर; स्वरक

**Tongue.** The organ of the taste and speech. जिह्वा; जीभ;

**Furred T.,** a coated tongue, the papillas of which are prominent, giving the mucous membrane the appearance of white fur. कुल्वक जिह्वा; फटी हुई जीभ;

**Geographical T.**, one with localized thickening of the epithelium. खर जिह्वा;

  **Straw-berry T.**, a hyperaemic tongue with the fungiform papillas very prominent. स्ट्राबेरी जिह्वा;

  **T. Depressor**, a spatula for depressing the tongue. जिह्वा अवनामक;

  **T.-tie**, a congenital shortening of the frenum of the tongue. जिह्वा-बद्धता

**Tonic.** Pertaining to, or producing normal tone or tension. तानिक

**Tonicity.** The normal condition of tone or tension. तानता; तनाव

**Tonics.** Medicines giving tone to the stomach and to increase the appetite. बल्य; टानिक; शक्तिवर्धक औषधियाँ

**Tonograph.** A recording tonometer. तनावअभिलेखी; तनावअभिलेखयंत्र

**Tonography.** Continuous measurement of blood, or intraocular pressure. तनावअभिलेखन

**Tonometer.** An instrument to measure tension. तनावमापी; तनाव मापने का यंत्र

**Tonometry.** Measuring the tension. तनावमिति; तनावमापन

**Tonsil.** Singular of **Tonsils.**

**Tonsilar.** See **Tonsillar.**

**Tonsillar.** Pertaining to the tonsils; tonsilar; tonsillary. गलतुण्डिकीय; गलतुण्डिकाओं सम्बन्धी

**Tonsillary.** See **Tonsillar.**

**Tonsillectomy.** Surgical removal of a tonsil. गलतुण्डिका-उच्छेदन; किसी गलतुण्डिका को काट कर हटा देना

**Tonsillitis.** Inflammation of the tonsils. गलतुण्डिकाशोथ; गलतुण्डिका-प्रदाह; टांसिल का प्रदाह;

  **Follicular T.**, a form especially involving the follicles. पुटकीय गलतुण्डिकाशोथ;

  **Pustular T.**, that marked by the formation of pustules, as in small-pox. पूयस्फोटक गलतुण्डिकाशोथ; पूयस्फोटी गलतुण्डिकाशोथ;

  **Suppurative T.**, quinsy. पूतिज गलतुण्डिकाशोथ

**Tonsillolith.** Concretion arising in the body of the tonsil; tonsolith. गलतुण्डिकाश्मरी

**Tonsillotome.** An instrument for excision of tonsils. गलतुण्डिका-उच्छेदक; गलतुण्डिका को काटने का यंत्र

**Tonsillotomy.** The cutting away of a portion of hypertrophied palatine tonsil. गलतुण्डिकाउच्छेदन; किसी गलतुण्डिका को काट कर हटा देना

**Tonsils.** Glands situated on each side of the throat. गलतुण्डिकायें; कण्ठ के दोनों ओर स्थित दो ग्रन्थियाँ

**Tonsolith.** See **Tonsillolith.**

**Tonus.** Tone; tonicity. तान; स्वरक

**Tooth.** Singular form of teeth. दन्त; दान्त; दांत

**Toothache.** Pain in the teeth; odontalgia. दन्तशूल; दन्तार्ति; दांत का दर्द

**Topectomy.** Modified frontal lobectomy. प्रमस्तिष्कप्रान्तस्था-अंशोच्छेदन; टोपेक्टोमी

**Topical.** Local; applied to the spot, as a topical application. स्थानिक

**Topography.** A description of the regions of the body. अंगरेखांकन; शरीर के क्षेत्रों का वर्णन

**Topophobia.** Morbid dread of places. स्थलभीति; स्थलसंत्रास; स्थलातंक; स्थानभीति

**Tormen.** A severe colicky pain. उग्रांत्रशूल; आन्तों में तेज दर्द

**Tormina.** Severe griping pains in the bowels. उग्रांत्रशूल; आन्तों में तेज बांयटेदार दर्द होना

**Torminal.** Affected with tormina; torminous. उग्रांत्रशूलग्रस्त; आन्तों के तेज दर्द से पीड़ित रोगी

**Torminous.** See **Torminal.**

**Torpent.** An agent modifying irritative action. उपशामक; उत्तेजित क्रिया को शान्त करने वाला पदार्थ

**Torpid.** Benumbed; inactive. सुन्न; जड़; निष्क्रिय

**Torpidity.** See **Torpor.**

**Torpor.** Numbness. सुन्नपन; inactivity. निष्क्रियता; loss of motion. गत्याभाव; torpidity. जड़ता; drowsiness. तन्द्रा

**Torrefaction.** Drying by means of high artificial heat. तापन; तपाना; उच्च कृत्रिम ताप देकर सुखाना

**Torrefy.** To dry over a fire. तपाना; आग के ऊपर सुखाना

**Torsion.** A twisting. मरोड़; ऐंठन

**Torso.** The trunk. धड़

**Torticollar.** Relating to, or marked by torticollis. मन्यास्तम्भ सम्बन्धी अथवा मन्यास्तम्भी

**Torticollis.** Twisted or wry-neck; stiff-neck. मन्यास्तम्भ; ग्रीवास्तम्भ; गर्दन की अकड़न

**Tortuous.** Twisted. कुटिल; मरोड़ा हुआ

**Torus.** A smooth rounded bulging. टोरस; पुष्पासन

**Total.** Complete; entire. पूर्ण

**Totality.** Completeness. समष्टि; पूर्णता;

   **T. of symptoms,** completeness of all symptoms. लक्षण-समष्टि; समस्त लक्षणों की पूर्णता

**Totipotence.** See **Totipotency.**

**Totipotency.** Ability of a cell to differentiate into any type of cell and thus form a new organism or regenerate any part of an organism; totipotence. पूर्णशक्तिमत्ता; पूर्णविभवता

**Totipotent.** Relating to totipotency. पूर्णशक्तिमान; पूर्णविभवी

**Touch.** The tactile sense. स्पर्श; स्पर्शानुभूति; digital examination. स्पर्श-जांच

**Toxaemia.** Poisoned state of blood; toxemia; toxicohemia. विषरक्तता; जीवविषरक्तता; रक्तविषण्णता

**Toxaemic.** Giving rise to blood poisoning; toxemic. विषाक्त; विषरक्तक; रक्तविषज; रक्तविषण्ण

**Toxamins.** Toxaemic substances. रक्तविषज पदार्थ

**Toxemia.** See **Toxaemia.**

**Toxemic.** See **Toxaemic.**

**Toxic.** Poisonous; toxicant. विषण्ण; विषाक्त; विषालु; विषैला

**Toxicant.** See **Toxic.**

**Toxicity.** The quality or degree of being poisonous. विषाक्तता; विषण्णता; विषालुता; विषैलापन

**Toxicogenic.** Producing or caused by a poison. विषजनक; विषोत्पादक; विषाक्त; विषण्ण

**Toxicohemia.** See **Toxaemia.**

**Toxicologist.** One versed in toxicology. जीवविषविज्ञ; विषविज्ञानी; अगदतंत्रविज्ञानी

**Toxicology.** The study of the detection, antidotes, action, and chemical composition of the poisons. जीवविषविज्ञान; विषविज्ञान; अगदतंत्र

**Toxicomania.** A morbid desire for poison. औषधिव्यसन; विभिन्न प्रकार की औषधियाँ लेते रहने का पागलपन

**Toxicophobia.** A morbid fear of poisoning. विषभीति; विषातंक; विष दिये जाने का भय

**Toxicosis.** Any disease due to poisoning. विषाक्तता; विषण्णता; विषालुता

**Toxiferous.** Carrying poison. विषवाहक

**Toxigenic.** See **Toxinogenic.**

**Toxigenous.** Producing poison. विषोत्पादक

**Toxin.** A poisonous albumin produced by the action of bacteria. विष; जीवविष; टॉक्सिन; जीवाणुओं की क्रिया द्वारा उत्पादित विषान्नसार

**Toxinemia.** Blood poisoning. रक्तविषण्णता; खून का जहर में बदल जाना

**Toxinic.** Relating to a toxin. विष अथवा जीवविष सम्बन्धी

**Toxinicide.** Any substance that destroys a toxin. विषनाशक; किसी विष को नष्ट करने वाला पदार्थ

**Toxinogenic.** Producing a toxin; toxigenic. जीवविषजनक

**Toxoid.** A toxin that has been deprived by power to injure but which still stimulates immunity formation. जीवविषाभ; रोगक्षम-क्रिया को उत्तेजित करने वाला विष पदार्थ

**Tr.** Symbol for tincture. 'मूलार्क' के लिये प्रयुक्त चिन्ह

**Trabecula.** Any one of the fibrous bands extending from the capsule into the interior of an organ. रज्जु; बन्धक; तन्तु-बन्ध; ट्रैबेकुला

**Trabeculae.** Plural of **Trabecula.**

**Trabeculotomy.** An operation on trabecula for glaucoma. बन्धकछेदन

**Trace.** A mark; a streak. चिन्ह; धारी; रेखा

**Tracer.** A substance or instrument used to gain information. अनुज्ञापक; सूचना प्राप्ति के निमित्त प्रयुक्त किया जाने वाला पदार्थ या यंत्र

**Trachea.** Wind-pipe in which air passes through the nose **via** larynx. श्वासप्रणाल

**Tracheal.** Pertaining to the windpipe. श्वासप्रणालीय; श्वासप्रणाल सम्बन्धी

**Tracheitis.** Inflammation of the trachea; trachitis. श्वासप्रणालशोथ; श्वासप्रणाल का प्रदाह

**Trachelagra.** Gout in the neck. गर्दन का गठिया; ग्रीवावात

**Trachelismus.** Spasm of the cervical muscles. ग्रीवापेशी-आकर्ष; गर्दन की पेशियों की अकड़न

**Trachelitis.** Inflammation of the cervix uteri; cervicitis. जरायुग्रीवाशोथ; गर्भाशयग्रीवाशोथ

**Tracheloplasty.** Plastic operation on the cervix uteri. जरायुग्रीवासंधान

**Trachelorrhaphy.** Suture of a laceration of the uterine cervix. गर्भाशयग्रीवासीवन

**Tracheobronchial.** Pertaining to the trachea and the bronchus. श्वासप्रणाल एवं श्वसनी सम्बन्धी

**Tracheobronchitis.** Inflammation of the trachea and the bronchus. श्वासप्रणालश्वसनीशोथ; श्वासप्रणाल तथा श्वसनी का प्रदाह

**Tracheolaryngeal.** Relating to the trachea and the larynx. श्वासप्रणाल एवं स्वरयंत्रपरक

**Tracheophony.** The hollow voice sound heard in auscultating over the trachea. श्वासप्रणालध्वनि

**Tracheoscopy.** Inspection of the trachea. श्वासप्रणालदर्शन; श्वासप्रणाल की जांच करना

**Tracheostenosis.** A narrowing of the trachea. श्वासप्रणालसंकीर्णन; श्वासप्रणाल की सिकुड़न

**Tracheostomy.** Surgical creation of an opening into the trachea or that opening. श्वासप्रणालछिद्रीकरण

**Tracheotome.** Instrument for opening the trachea. श्वासप्रणालछेदक; श्वासप्रणाल को खोलने का यंत्र

**Tracheotomy.** An incision of the trachea. श्वासप्रणालछेदन;
    **Inferior T.,** one performed below the isthmus of the thyroid gland. अधःश्वासप्रणालछेदन;
    **Superior T.,** one performed above the isthmus of the thyroid gland. ऊर्ध्वश्वासप्रणालछेदन

**Trachitis.** See **Tracheitis.**

**Trachoma.** Granular lids, as in a form of conjunctivitis. रोहे; ट्रैकोमा; infectious granular conjunctivitis. संक्रामक कणिकीय नेत्रश्लेष्मलाशोथ

**Trachomatous.** Relating to, or suffering from trachoma. ट्रैकोमा सम्बन्धी अथवा ट्रैकोमाग्रस्त

**Tracing.** Any graphic display of electrical or mechanical events. अनुरेखण

**Tract.** A track; tractus. पथ; मार्ग; a canal. नली;
    **Alimentary T.,** the digestive canal, extending from the mouth to anus; digestive tract. पोषण-पथ; पाचन-नली; पोषण-नली;

**Digestive T.**, see **Alimentary Tract**.

**Gastrointestinal T.**, the stomach, small intestine and large intestine. जठरांत्रपथ;

**Genital T.**, the genital passages of the urogenital system. जननांगी पथ;

**Olfactory T.**, the narrow portion of the olfactory lobe of the brain. घ्राणपथ; मस्तिष्क के घ्राण खण्ड का संकीर्ण भाग;

**Optic T.**, the fibres between the visual centre and the optic chiasma. अक्षिपथ;

**Respiratory T.**, the respiratory organs in continuity. श्वासपथ;

**Septomarginal T.**, a part of the descending posteromedial tract of the spinal cord. पटपरिसरपथ;

**Spinothalamic T.**, that part of the fibres in the anterior ascending cerebrospinal tract which goes to the lateral nucleus of the thalamus. मेरुचेतकपथ;

**Spinovestibular T.**, a tract of fibres in the posterior portion of the direct cerebral tract going to the vestibular nucleus. मेरुप्रघाण-पथ

**Traction.** A drawing or pulling. कर्षण; खिंचाव;

**Axis-t.**, traction in the direction or axis of a channel through which a body is to be drawn. अक्ष-कर्षण;

**External T.**, a pulling force created by using fixed anchorage outside the oral cavity. बाह्यकर्षण;

**Internal T.**, a pulling force created by the cranial bones, above the point of fracture for anchorage. अन्त:कर्षण;

**Skeletal T.**, traction pull on a bone structure mediated through a pin or wire inserted into the bone to reduce a fracture of long bones; skeletal extension. अस्थिकर्षण;

**Skin T.**, traction on an extremity by means of adhesive tape or other types of strapping applied to the limb. त्वचाकर्षण

**Tractotomy.** Incision of a nerve tract in the brain stem or spinal cord. पथछेदन; स्नायुपथछेदन

**Tractus.** See **Tract**.

**Tragacanth.** A gummy exudate. गोंदकतीरा

**Tragal.** Pertaining to the tragus. तुंगिकी; तुंगिका सम्बन्धी

**Tragi.** Plural of **Tragus**.

**Tragus.** The small prominence of cartilage projecting over the meatus of the external ear. तुंगिका

**Trait.** Any characteristic peculiar to an individual which distinguishes him from the others. विशेषक

**Trance.** An altered state of consciousness. उपसमाधि

**Tranquiliser.** Drug that calms distributed nervous reaction; tranquilizer. प्रशान्तक; विभाजित स्नायु-प्रतिक्रिया को शान्त करने वाली औषधि

**Tranquilizer.** See **Tranquiliser.**

**Trans.** Through; beyond. पार

**Transabdominal.** Through the abdomen. पार-उदरीय; पारौदरिक

**Transbronchial.** Through the bronchus. पारश्वसनीय; पारश्वसनिक

**Transection.** A cross-section; cutting across; transsection. पारपरिच्छेदन

**Transfer.** The passage of a symptom from one side of the body to the other; transference. स्थानान्तरण; अन्तरण; अन्यारोपण

**Transference.** See **Transfer.**

**Transfix.** To pierce through and through. पारवेध

**Transfixation.** Piercing through and through. पारवेधन

**Transformation.** See **Transmutation.**

**Transfusion.** Transfer of matching type of blood from one person into the veins of another; infusion. आधान; रक्ताधान;

    Arterial T., the transfusion of blood into an artery. धमनी-आधान;

    Blood T., the transfer of blood into a vein. रक्ताधान;

    Direct T., the transfusion of blood from one person to another without exposure to the air; immediate transfusion. प्रत्यक्ष रक्ताधान; प्रत्यक्ष आधान;

    Exchange T., removal of most of a patient's blood followed by introduction of an equal amount from donors; substitution or total transfusion. पूर्ण रक्ताधान;

    Immediate T., see **Direct Transfusion.**

    Indirect T., the introduction of blood that has first been drawn into a vessel; mediate transfusion. अप्रत्यक्ष रक्ताधान; अप्रत्यक्ष आधान;

    Mediate T., see **Indirect Transfusion.**

    Substitution T., see **Exchange Transfusion.**

    Total T., see **Exchange Transfusion.**

    Venous T., transfusion into a vein. शिरा-रक्ताधान

**Transient.** Not permanent; of short duration. अस्थायी; अल्पावधिक; थोड़े से समय के लिये

**Transillumination.** The lighting of a cavity by passing a strong light through its walls. पारप्रदीपन

**Translocation.** Transfer of a segment of a chromosome to a different life on the same chromosome or to a different one. स्थानांतरण; स्थलान्तरण

**Translucent.** Opaque; transparent. पारभासक; पारभासी

**Translucid.** Semi-transparent; partially admitting the passage of the rays of light. अर्धपारभासी

**Transmission.** Transfer, as of a disease. स्थानांतरण; संचरण; संचारण; प्रेषण

**Transmitter.** One who transmits. संचारक; प्रेषक

**Transmutation.** A change into another form; transformation. तवांतरण; रूपान्तरण

**Transnasal.** Through the nose. पारनासी; नाक से अथवा नाक द्वारा

**Transparent.** Admitting the passage of the rays of light. पारदर्शी; पारदर्शक

**Transplant.** To transfer from one part to another. प्रतिरोपण करना

**Transplantation.** The replacement of a diseased organ with a similar organ from another person. प्रतिरोपण

**Transposition.** An interchange of position; removal from one place to another. स्थिति-अन्तरण

**Transsection.** See **Transection.**

**Transthoracic.** Across or through the chest. पारवक्षीय

**Transudate.** A substance resulting from transudation. पारस्राव

**Transudation.** An oozing of a fluid through a membrane, especially of serum through vessel-walls. पारस्रवण

**Transverse.** Cross-wise; lying across the long axis of the body. अनुप्रस्थ

**Trapezium.** The first bone of the second carpal row. समलंबक (अस्थि)

**Trapezoid.** One of the bones of the wrist. समलंबिका

**Trauma.** A wound; an injury caused by a blunt instrument, or fall. अभिघात; गुमचोट; क्षति; घाव; चोट

**Traumatic.** Pertaining to a wound as a result of an internal injury or fall. अभिघातज; चोटमूलक

**Traumatism.** The condition of one injured. अभिघातता; चोट लगना

**Traumatology.** The branch of surgery dealing with injury from accidents. अभिघातविज्ञान; चोटविज्ञान

**Treatise.** A literary composition on a definite subject. ग्रंथ; किसी निश्चित विषय पर साहित्यिक लेख

**Treatment.** Therapy; the medical or surgical care of a patient; therapeutics. चिकित्सा; उपचार; उपचारण; इलाज

**Active T.,** treatment directed specifically toward cure of a disease. सक्रिय चिकित्सा;

**Domiciliary T.,** treatment given at home. गृह-चिकित्सा;

**Palliative T.,** treatment to alleviate symptoms without curing the disease. प्रशामक चिकित्सा;

**Preventive T.,** measures to be taken to protect a person from a disease to which he is liable to be exposed; prophylactic treatment. निरोधक चिकित्सा;

**Prophylactic T.,** see **Preventive Treatment.**

**Shock T.,** a form of psychiatric treatment used in certain types of mental disorders. आघातोपचार

**Trematode.** One of the trematoda; a class of worms. पर्णकृमि

**Trembles.** Milk-sickness. स्तन्यरुग्णता

**Trembling.** Tremor. कम्पन

**Tremor.** Involuntary shaking or trembling; tremour. कम्प; कम्पन;

**Intention T.,** one appearing on voluntary movement; volition or volitional tremor. चेष्टा-कम्प; ऐच्छिक कम्प;

**Volition T.,** see **Intention Tremor.**

**Volitional T.,** see **Intention Tremor.**

**Tremour.** See **Tremor.**

**Tremulous.** Trembling; quivering; shivering. प्रकम्प; कम्पायमान; कम्पमान

**Tremulousness.** The state of being tremulous. प्रकम्पता; कम्पमानता; कम्पन की अवस्था

**Trench Fever.** A fever with a sudden onset, with dizziness, headache, pains in lumbar region and legs, especially shins. खाई-ज्वर; खात-ज्वर

**Treponema-pallidum.** The parasite that causes syphilis. उपदंश-परजीवी

**Treponemacide.** Lethal to treponema. उपदंशपरजीवीनाशक; उपदंश पैदा करने वाले परजीवियों को नष्ट करने वाला

**Tri-.** Prefix denoting three. 'त्रि' अथवा तीन का अर्थ देने वाला उपसर्ग

**Tria.** Three. त्रि; तीन

**Triad.** A union of three. त्रिक

**Trial.** The act of testing. परीक्षा; जांच

**Triangle.** A space bounded by three lines or sides. त्रिभुज; त्रिकोण

**Triangular.** Any figure having three angles. त्रिभुजाकार; त्रिकोणक; त्रिकोणाकार

**Tribadism.** Unnatural intercourse between women. परस्परस्त्री-मैथुन; औरतों द्वारा आपस में मैथुन करना

**Triceps Muscle.** The three-headed muscle. त्रिशीर्षपेशी; तीन सिरों वाली पेशी

**Trichiasis.** Inversion of the eyelashes. पक्ष्मवर्तन; पक्ष्मकोप; पलकों का अन्तर्वर्तन

**Trichitis.** Inflammation of the hair bulbs. लोमकन्दशोथ; लोमकन्द का प्रदाह

**Trichocephalus.** Threadworm. सूत्रकृमि; धागाकृमि

**Trichology.** The science of the hair. लोमविज्ञान; केशविज्ञान

**Trichoma.** A fungus disease of the hair. लोमकवकता; बालों का एक कवक रोग

**Trichonosis.** Any disease of the hair; trichopathy; trichosis. लोमविकृति; केशविकृति; बालों का कोई रोग; ट्रिचिनोरुग्णता

**Trichopathy.** See **Trichonosis**.

**Trichosis.** See **Trichonosis**.

**Trichotillomania.** Morbid impulse to pull out one's hair. लोमकर्षणोन्माद; बाल नोचने का पागलपन

**Trichromate.** Possessing the quality of recognising the three primary colours, i.e. red, blue and green. त्रिवर्णदृष्टिक

**Trichromatic.** Trichromic; relating to three primary colours. त्रिवर्णदृष्टि; having normal colour vision. सामान्य वर्णदृष्टि

**Trichromatopsia.** Normal colour vision. सामान्य वर्णदृष्टिता; ability to perceive three primary colours, i.e. red, blue and green. त्रिवर्णदृष्टिता

**Trichromic.** See **Trichromatic**.

**Trichuriasis.** Infestation with whipworm. कशाकृमिरुग्णता

**Trichuricide.** Lethal to trichuris. कशाकृमिनाशक; चाबुककृमिनाशक

**Trichuris.** A genus of nematodes; whipworm. कशाकृमि; चाबुककृमि

**Tricuspid.** Having three cusps or points, as the right auriculoventricular valves of the heart; tricuspidal; tricuspidate. त्रिकपर्दी

**Tricuspidal.** See **Tricuspid**.

**Tricuspidate.** See **Tricuspid**.

**Trifacial Nerve.** See **Trigeminus**.

**Trigeminal.** Pertaining to trigeminus; the trifacial nerve. त्रिधारीय; त्रिधारा तंत्रिका सम्बन्धी

**Trigeminus.** The trifacial or the fifth cranial nerve. त्रिधारातंत्रिका

**Triginta.** Thirty. त्रिंशति; तीस

**Trigon.** A triangle; trigone; trigonum. त्रिकोण; त्रिकोणचर्वकशीर्ष; त्रिभुज;

    **Collateral T.,** a triangular area at the junction of the posterior horns of the lateral ventricles. समपार्श्वी त्रिकोण;

    **Habenular T.,** a depressed area on the postero-medial aspect of the thalamus; trigon habenae; trigon habenulae. पट्टिका त्रिकोण;

    **Inguinal T.,** the triangular area in the lower abdominal wall bounded by the inguinal ligament below; trigon inguinale. नाभि-त्रिकोण;

    **T. Habenae,** see **Habenular Trigon**.

    **T. Habenulae,** see **Habenular Trigon**.

    **T. Inguinale,** see **Inguinal Trigon**.

**Trigona.** Plural of **Trigon**.

**Trigone.** See **Trigon**.

**Trigonitis.** Inflammation of the trigone of the urinary bladder. मूत्राशयत्रिभुजशोथ

**Trigonum.** See **Trigon**.

    **T. Vesicae,** a triangular space on the inside of the bladder, immediately behind the surface of the urethra. मूत्राशय त्रिभुज

**Trimester.** A period of three months. त्रिमास; तीन महीने की अवधि

**Tripara.** A woman pregnant for the third time. त्रिगर्भा; तीसरी बार गर्भवती होने वाली स्त्री

**Triple.** Consisting of three. त्रिगुण; तिगुना; तीन गुना

**Triplets.** Three children born at one birth. त्रिज; एक साथ जन्म लेने वाले तीन बच्चे

**Triplex.** Three-fold. त्रिगुण; तिगुना

**Trismus.** Lock-jaw; spasm of the muscles of mastication. हनुस्तम्भ; चर्वणा-पेशियों की अकड़न

**Trisomy.** Division into three. त्रिविभाजन; त्रिगुणसूत्रता; तीन भागों में बांटना

**Trisplanchnic.** Pertaining to three visceral cavities: skull, thorax and abdomen. खोपड़ी (करोटि), छाती (वक्ष) एवं पेट (उदर); तीन अंतरांगी गह्वरों सम्बन्धी

**Tritanope.** Suffering from tritanopia. नीलवर्णान्ध

**Tritanopia.** A defect in the third constituent for colour-vision; blue-colour blindness; tritanopsia. नीलवर्णांधता; नीला रंग पहचानने की अक्षमता

**Tritanopsia.** See **Tritanopia.**

**Triticum Sativum.** Common wheat. धूम; गेहूँ का पौधा

**Triturable.** Susceptible of being triturated. अवपेषणीय; संपेषणीय; घोटने या पीस कर चूर्ण बनाने योग्य

**Triturate.** To make powder. अवपेषण करना; संपेषण करना; घोटना; पीस कर चूर्ण बनाना

**Trituration.** Substances prepared by fine subdivision with pestle and mortar and sugar of milk. अवपेषण; संपेषण; चूर्ण

**Trocar.** An instrument for withdrawing fluid from a cavity. ट्रोकार

**Trochanter.** One of the bony prominences developed from independent osseous centres near the upper extremity of the femur. ट्रोकेन्टर

**Troche.** See **Trochiscus.**

**Trochiscus.** A medicinal tablet; a lozenge; troche. चूष; चूषिका; चूषी जाने वाली गोली; लोजेंज

**Trochlea.** A pulley-like process. चक्रक

**Trochleae.** Plural of **Trochlea.**

**Trochlear.** Relating to trochlea. चक्रक सम्बन्धी

**Trochocephalia.** The state of being round-headed. चक्रकपालीयता; गोलकपालीयता; गोलाकार सिर होना

**Trochoid.** Denoting a revolving or wheel-like articulation. चक्रकाभ

**Trophic.** Pertaining to nutrition. पोषणज; पोषण सम्बन्धी

**Trophoblast.** Epiblast outside the germinal area that contributes to the formation of the placenta; trophoderm. बीजपोषक

**Trophoblastic.** Relating to the trophoblast. बीजपोषक सम्बन्धी;

   **T. Tissue,** cells covering the embedding ovum and concerning with the nutrition of the ovum. बीजपोषक ऊतक

**Trophoderm.** See **Trophoblast.**

**Trophoedema.** Localized permanent oedema. स्थानिक-स्थायीशोफ

**Trophology.** The science of nutrition. पोषणविज्ञान; आहारविज्ञान

**-trophy.** Suffix denoting food, nutrition. '-पुष्टि' का अर्थ देने वाला शब्दांत

**Tropical.** Pertaining to the tropics. ऊष्णकटिबन्धीय;

   **T. Chlorosis,** dochmiasis. उष्णकटिबंधीय अरक्तता

**True.** Conformable to fact; in accordance with reason. यथार्थ; वास्तविक; सत्य

**Truncus.** A trunk. प्रकांड; कांड; धड़; a large vessel. बृहत्वाहिका;

   **T. Arteriosus,** the large artery of the primitive heart giving off the two aortas. धमनी कांड

**Trunk.** The body, except the head, neck, arms and legs. धड़; प्रकाण्ड; कांड

**Truss.** A bent bar of the flexible steel covered with leather, to which a pad and strap are attached for retaining a rupture in its place. हर्निया-पेटी; ट्रस

**Trypsin.** A proteolytic enzyme present in the pancreatic juice. ट्रिप्सिन

**Tuba.** Tube. नली

**Tubae.** Plural of **Tuba.**

**Tubal.** Pertaining to the oviduct. डिम्बवाहिनीय; डिम्बवाहिनी सम्बन्धी;

   **T. Nephritis,** inflammation of the renal tubes. वृक्कनलीशोथ; गुर्दे की नलियों का प्रदाह

**Tube.** A pipe or hollow slender; tuba. नली; नाल; नलिका;

   **Auditory T.,** see **Eustachian Tube.**

   **Auscultation T.,** to test the acuteness of hearing. परिश्रवण नली;

   **Bronchial T.,** the smaller divisions of the bronchi. श्वसनी-नली;

**Drainage T.**, one of glass or rubber tubes to be inserted into a wound or cavity to allow the escape of fluids. निकास नली;

**Eustachian T.**, a tube from the tympanic cavity of the ear to nasopharynx; auditory tube. कम्बुकर्णी नली; श्रवण नली; यूश्टेशियन नली;

**Fallopian T.**, one of the two small tubes on each side of the uterus conveying the ova from the ovaries; oviduct; uterine tube. डिम्बवाहिनी नली; फैलोपी नली;

**Feeding T.**, one for introducing food into the stomach. पोषण नलिका; पोषण नली;

**Tracheotomy T.**, a curved tube for insertion into trachea, used to keep the mouth free after tracheotomy. श्वासप्रणालछेदन नली;

**Uterine T.**, see **Fallopian Tube.**

**Tuber.** A localized swelling. कन्द; गुलिका; स्थानिक सूजन

**Tubercle.** A pimple, swelling or small tumour; also applied to deposits in the lungs of consumptives; tuberculum. गुलिका; यक्ष्मिका; कन्दिलमूल; दण्डाणु;

**Adductor T.**, one at the lower end of the internal condylar line of the femur. अभिवर्तनी गुलिका;

**Genial T.**, one on each side of the median line on the inner surface of the lower maxilla. चिबुकान्त गुलिका;

**Supraglenoid T.**, one above the glenoid fossa of the scapula. अध्यंसगर्त गुलिका;

**T. Bacilli**, plural of **Tubercle Bacillus.**

**T. Bacillus**, mycobacterium. यक्ष्माणु; क्षयरोगाणु

**Tubercula.** Plural of **Tuberculum.**

**Tubercular.** Affected with, or pertaining to tuberculosis; tuberculated; tuberculous. यक्ष्माग्रस्त; यक्ष्मा सम्बन्धी

**Tuberculated.** See **Tubercular.**

**Tuberculin.** A preparation from the cultures of the tubercle bacillus used in the diagnosis of tuberculosis. टुबरकुलीन;

**T. Test**, a skin test which shows whether or not an individual has received tubercle bacillus in his body. टुबरकुलीन जांच

**Tuberculoid.** Resembling tuberculosis. यक्ष्माभ; गुलिकाभ; यक्ष्मा से मिलता-जुलता

**Tuberculoma.** A tuberculous tumour, usually in the lungs or brain. यक्ष्मिका गुल्म; यक्ष्मार्बुद

**Tuberculosis.** Any infection with the tubercle bacillus. यक्ष्मा; क्षय;
  **Miliary T.,** a rapidly fatal disease due to the general dissemination of tubercle bacilli in the blood. कंगु-यक्ष्मा;
  **Pulmonary T.,** that affecting the lungs. फुप्फुसीय यक्ष्मा; फुप्फुस-क्षय;
  **T. Larynx,** laryngeal tuberculosis. स्वरयंत्रजयक्ष्मा; स्वरयंत्रज-क्षय

**Tuberculostatic.** Inhibiting the growth of the tubercle bacillus. यक्ष्मास्तम्भी; यक्ष्मा-दण्डाणु (यक्ष्माणु) का विकास रोकने वाला; यक्ष्मारोधी

**Tuberculous.** Pertaining to, or resembling tuberculosis; tubercular. यक्ष्मज; यक्ष्मा सम्बन्धी; यक्ष्मा से मिलता जुलता; यक्ष्मा जैसा;
  **T. Adenitis,** tuberculous disease of the cervical glands; lymphadenitis. यक्ष्मज ग्रीवाग्रन्थिशोथ; गर्दन की ग्रन्थियों का यक्ष्मा

**Tuberculum.** See **Tubercle.**

**Tuberositas.** See **Tuberosity.**

**Tuberosity.** A bony protuberance; tuberositas. कन्दिलता; गण्डकता

**Tuberous.** Of the nature of tuberosity. कन्दिल

**Tubular.** Having the nature of a tube. नलिकीय; नलिकाकार

**Tubule.** A small tube; a minute tube-shaped structure; tubulus. नलिका; नली;
  **Seminiferous T.,** the tubular threads, arranged in fasciculi, that compose the substance of the testes. शुक्रजनक नलिका; शुक्रनली;
  **Uriniferous T.,** the urinary tube of the kidney. मूत्रनली

**Tubuli.** Plural of **Tubulus.**

**Tubulorrhexis.** Necrosis of the epithelial lining in localized segments of renal tubules. नलिकाभित्तिविलयन

**Tubulus.** See **Tubule.**

**Tubus.** Tube; canal. नली

**Tuft.** A small clump, cluster or coiled mass. स्तवक

**Tug.** To drag or pull. कर्ष; आकर्ष

**Tularaemia.** See **Tularemia.**

**Tularemia.** A disease by wild animals which infects man through breaks in the skin; tularaemia. टुलेरीमिया

**Tumefacient.** Swollen. सूजा हुआ; फूला हुआ

**Tumefaction.** A swelling of a part. उत्फुलन; फुलाव; सूजन; फूल जाना

**Tumescence.** To swell. फूलना; सूजना; a swelling. सूजन

**Tumescent.** See **Tumid.**

**Tumid.** Inflated; swollen; protuberant; tumescent. स्फीत; सूजा हुआ; फूला हुआ

**Tumor.** See **Tumour.**

**Tumour.** A swelling biggest or smaller, developed by a morbific cause in some parts of the body; tumor. अर्बुद; रसौली; गुल्म;

    **Benign T.,** one not giving rise to metastasis nor recurring after removal. सुदम अर्बुद; सौम्य अर्बुद;

    **Cystic T.,** one made up of cysts. पुटी-अर्बुद;

    **Fibroid T.,** a fibroma. तन्तु-अर्बुद; तन्त्वर्बुद;

    **Malignant T.,** one that is metastatic or recurs, and destroys life. दुर्दम अर्बुद; सांघातिक अर्बुद

**Tunic.** See **Tunica.**

**Tunica.** Lining membrane; a covering; tunic. कंचुक; आवरण; आवरक कला; झिल्ली;

    **T. Adenata,** the conjunctiva covering the eyeball. नेत्रश्लेष्मला; नेत्रगोलकों को ढक कर रखने वाली झिल्ली;

    **T. Adventitia,** the outermost fibrous coat of a vessel or an organ. बहि:कंचुक;

    **T. Albuginea,** a dense, white, collagenous sheath surrounding a structure. श्वेत कंचुक;

    **T. Mucosa,** mucous membrane. श्लेष्म कला;

    **T. Serosa,** serous membrane. सीरमी कला;

    **T. Vasculosa,** any layer well supplied with blood vessels. रक्तधर कंचुक

**Tunicae.** Plural of **Tunica.**

**Tuning-fork.** Device that when struck at, the forked-end vibrates and thus can be heard and felt. स्वरित्र

**Tunnel.** An elongated enclosed passage way, usually open at both ends. सुरंग

**Turbid.** In a general sense muddy; not clear. आविल; मृदावत्; मिट्टी जैसा; कीचड़ जैसा; cloudy. धुंधला; धूमिल

**Turbidity.** Cloudiness; muddiness. आविलता; धूमिलता

**Turbinal.** See **Turbinate.**

**Turbinate.** Shaped like a top or inverted cone; turbinal; turbinated. शंखाकार; शंकुरूप; लट्टूरूप; लट्टू के आकार का

**Turbinated.** See **Turbinate**.

**Turbinectomy.** Removal of the turbinate bone. नासाशुक्तिकोच्छेदन

**Turbinotome.** An instrument for excision of a turbinal. नासाशुक्तिकोच्छेदक

**Turbinotomy.** Incision of a turbinal. नासाशुक्तिकोच्छेदन

**Turgescence.** A swelling or enlargement of an organ. उच्छूनता; किसी अंग की सूजन या विबृद्धि

**Turgid.** Excessively full and distended; swollen. स्फीत; सूजा हुआ; फूला हुआ

**Turgidity.** Swollen up; growing large; distension of the blood vessels. स्फीति; फुलाव

**Turn of life.** Cessation of menstruation; change of life; the menopause. रजोनिवृत्ति; वय:सन्धि

**Tussal.** Of the nature of cough. कासवत्; खांसी से मिलता-जुलता

**Tussis.** A cough. कास; खांसी;

  **T. Convulsiva,** whooping cough. कूकर-कास; काली-खांसी

**Tussive.** Pertaining to cough. कास अथवा खांसी सम्बन्धी

**Twang.** Nasal quality of voice. अनुनासिका

**Twin.** One of the two individuals born at the same birth. यमल; युगल

**Twinge.** A sudden sharp pain. उग्र आकस्मिक पीड़ा; अचानक तेज दर्द उठना

**Twitch.** A short sudden pull or jerk. ऐंठन; मरोड़; स्फुरण

**Twitching.** A sudden, short pulling or jerking. स्फुरण; हल्का-सा आकस्मिक खिंचाव या झटका

**Tyloma.** A callosity. घट्टा; किण

**Tyloses.** Plural of **Tylosis**.

**Tylosis.** The formation of a callous thickening on the skin. त्वग्स्थूलता; चमड़ी मोटी होना; टाइलोसिस

**Tympanic.** Relating to the tympanum. मध्यकर्णिक; मध्यकर्णीय; मध्यकर्ण सम्बन्धी

**Tympana.** Plural of **Tympanum**.

**Tympanites.** A gaseous distension of the abdomen; meteorism. आध्मान; अफारा

**Tympanitic.** Drum-like; affected with tympanites. आध्मानयुक्त; आध्मानग्रस्त

**Tympanitis.** Inflammation of the tympanic membrane; myringitis. मध्यकर्णशोथ; मध्यकर्णीय झिल्ली का प्रदाह

**Tympanoplasty.** A plastic operation of the middle ear. मध्यकर्णसंधान

**Tympanum.** The tympanic cavity. मध्यकर्णगह्वर

**Tympany.** Tympanites. आध्मान; अफारा

**Type.** The usual form that all others of the class resemble, that is characteristic of the class. प्ररूप; प्रकार

**Typhlitis.** Inflammation of the caecum. अन्धान्त्रशोथ; अन्धान्त्र का प्रदाह

**Typhlosis.** Blindness. अंधता; अंधापन; दृष्टिहीनता

**Typhlostomy.** See **Caecostomy.**

**Typhoid.** Relating to, or resembling typhus. आंत्रिक; सावधिक; मियादी;
   **T. Fever,** enteric fever. आंत्रिक ज्वर; मियादी बुखार

**Typhous.** Having the nature of typhus fever. मोहज्वराभ; सन्निपात ज्वर की प्रकृति का

**Typhus.** An acute infectious and contagious disease caused by rickettsiae. टाइफस; सन्निपात;
   **T. Fever,** a form of low nervous fever, malignant infections, etc. मोहज्वर; सन्निपात ज्वर

**Typical.** Characteristic. प्ररूपी

**Tyriasis.** Elephantiasis. श्लीपद; हाथीपैर; हाथीपांव

**Tyroid.** Cheesy. पनीरी; पनीरयुक्त या पनीर जैसा

**Tyroma.** Alopecia; baldness. खल्वाटता; खालित्य; गंजापन

**Tyrranism.** Cruelty of morbid inception. क्रूरता

# U

**Ulcer.** A sore on any soft part of the body attended with discharge of pus. व्रण; घाव; फोड़ा;
   **Anastomotic U.,** ulcer of jejunum, after gastroenterostomy. सम्मिलिनी व्रण;
   **Chronic U.,** a long standing ulcer with fibrous scar tissue in its floor. चिरकारी व्रण; जीर्ण घाव; पुराना फोड़ा;

**Cold U.**, a small gangrenous ulcer on the extremities. शीत व्रण;

**Decubitus U.**, bed-sore. शय्या-व्रण; pressure sore. दाब-व्रण;

**Duodenal U.**, one originating from duodenum. ग्रहणी व्रण;

**Gastric U.**, an ulcer of the gastric or duodenal mucosa; stomach ulcer; peptic ulcer; ulcus ventriculi. उदर-व्रण; आमाशय-व्रण; पेप्टिक व्रण;

**Hard U.**, chancre. शैंकर; कठोर व्रण;

**Indolent U.**, one with an indurated elevated edge and a non-glanulated floor, usually occurring on the leg. मंदरोही व्रण;

**Peptic U.**, see **Gastric Ulcer**.

**Perforated U.**, an ulcer extending through the wall of an organ. बिद्ध व्रण; सछिद्र व्रण; छिद्रित व्रण;

**Phagedenic U.**, an ulceration in which the process extends insidiously, but obstinately; phagedaena. विनाशी व्रण; तीव्र विनाशी व्रण;

**Rodent U.**, a slowly enlarging ulcerated basal cell carcinoma, usually on the face; basal cell carcinoma. रोडेंट व्रण;

**Soft U.**, chancroid; venereal ulcer. शैंकराभ व्रण; कोमल व्रण; रतिज व्रण;

**Stercoral U.**, an ulcer of the colon. मलजात व्रण;

**Stomach U.**, see **Gastric Ulcer**.

**Trophic U.**, one due to impaired nutrition. अपोषणज व्रण;

**Tuberculous U.**, one due to tuberculosis. यक्ष्मज व्रण;

**Varicose U.**, one resulting from stasis or infection, usually in the leg. अपस्फीत व्रण;

**Venereal U.**, see **Soft Ulcer**.

**Ulcerate.** To produce an ulcer. व्रण अथवा घाव बनना

**Ulceration.** The process of ulcer formation. व्रण; व्रणोद्भव; व्रणोत्पत्ति

**Ulcerative.** Relating to, causing or marked by ulceration. व्रणमय; व्रणयुक्त; व्रणीय,

**Ulcerogenic.** Capable of producing an ulcer. व्रणजनक; व्रणोत्पादक; फोड़ा या घाव बनाने में सक्षम

**Ulcerous.** Pertaining to, or of the nature of an ulcer. व्रण सम्बन्धी अथवा व्रण जैसा

**Ulcus.** An ulcer. व्रण; घाव; फोड़ा

**Ulcuscle**

**U. Ventriculi,** see **Gastric Ulcer.**
**Ulcuscle.** A small ulcer. सूक्ष्मव्रण; लघुव्रण
**Ulcuscule.** The same as **Ulcuscle.**
**Uletic.** Pertaining to the gums. मसूड़ों सम्बन्धी
**Ulitis.** Inflammation of the gums. मसूड़ाशोथ; मसूड़ों का प्रदाह
**Ulna.** The medial and larger of the two bones of the forearms. अन्त:प्रकोष्ठिका; अलना
**Ulnae.** Plural of **Ulna.**
**Ulnar.** Relating to the ulna. अन्त:प्रकोष्ठिक; अन्त:प्रकोष्ठिका सम्बन्धी
**Ulotrichous.** Wooly-haired. संकुलित केशधारी; संकुलित केशधारक
**Ultracentrifuge.** A high speed centrifuge. द्रुत-अपकेन्द्रत्र
**Ultrafiltration.** Filtration through semi-permeable membrane or any filter that separates colloid solutions from crystalloids, etc. अतिसूक्ष्म-निस्यंदन
**Ultramicroscope.** A microscope for examining, by reflected light, objects beyond the power of ordinary microscope. अतिसूक्ष्मदर्शी
**Ultrasonic.** Relating to mechanical vibrations of very high frequency. पराध्वनिक; प्रतिध्वनिक
**Ultrasound.** Inaudible sound in the frequency range of more than 20,000 cycles per second. पराध्वनि; प्रतिध्वनि;
**Ultraviolet Rays.** Invisible actinic rays of the spectrum which are beyond the visible violet end; violet rays. पराबैंगनी किरणें; परानीललोहित किरणें
**Umbilectomy.** Excision of the umbilicus. नाभि-उच्छेदन; नाभ्युच्छेदन; नाभि को काटना
**Umbilical.** Relating to the navel. नाभि सम्बन्धी; नाभिपरक;
   **U. Cord,** the navel string. नाभि-रज्जु;
   **U. Hernia,** a hernia in the region of umbilicus. नाभि-हर्निया
**Umbilicate.** Umbilicated; navel-shaped. नाभ्याकार; नाभि के आकार का; pitlike. खाताकार; खड्ड जैसा; खड्डाकार
**Umbilicated.** See **Umbilicate.**
**Umbilicourinary.** Pertaining to the umbilicus and the urine. नाभि एवं मूत्र सम्बन्धी
**Umbilicus.** The navel. नाभि
**Umbo.** A boss; any central convex eminence. ककुद; अम्बो

**Umbones.** Plural of **Umbo.**

**Uncal.** Denoting or relating to uncus. अंकुश सम्बन्धी

**Unci.** Plural of **Uncus.**

**Unciform.** See **Uncinate.**

**Uncinaria.** The hookworm. अंकुशकृमि

**Uncinariasis.** Infection with hookworm. अंकुशकृमिरुग्णता; अंसीनेरिएसिस

**Uncinate.** Hooked; unciform. अंकुश; अंकुशित

**Unconscious.** Senseless. अचेत; मूर्च्छित; बेहोश

**Unconsciousness.** Loss of sense; the state of being without sensibility. अचेतनता; मूर्च्छा; बेहोशी; निश्चेतना

**Unctuous.** Greasy; oily. चिक्कण; चिकना

**Uncus.** A hook. अंकुश

**Undifferentiative.** Having no special structure or function. अविभेदित

**Undine.** A small, thin glass flask used for irrigating the eyes. अधिसेचनी

**Undulant Fever.** A widespread infectious febrile disease affecting principally cattle, swine, goats and sometimes man; brucellosis; Mediterranean fever; malta fever. माल्टा ज्वर

**Undulation.** A wave; a fluctuation. तरंगण; ऊर्मिलता

**Unendurable.** Intolerable. असह्य; सहन न होने वाला

**Unguent.** See **Unguentum.**

**Unguentum.** An ointment, medicated with certain tinctures; unguent. मरहम; मलहम; लेप; विलेपन

**Ungues.** Plural of **Unguis.**

**Unguis.** The nail of a finger or toe. नख; नाखुन

**Ungula.** A claw; an instrument for extracting a dead foetus. नखरक; धुरक; मृत भ्रूण को निकालने के लिये प्रयुक्त किया जाने वाला यंत्र

**Uni-.** Prefix signifying one or single. 'एक' का अर्थ देने वाला उपसर्ग

**Uniaxial.** Having only one axis. एकाक्षीय; एकाक्षिक; केवल एक अक्ष वाला

**Unicellular.** Composed of, but one cell. एककोशिक; एककोशिकी; केवल एक कोशिका वाला

**Unicorn.** Having a single horn; unicornous. एकशृंगी; केवल एक सींग वाला

**Unicornous.** See **Unicorn.**

**Unilateral. Affected, or confined to, but on one side. एकपार्श्वी; एकपार्श्विक; केवल एक पार्श्व को प्रभावित करने वाला

**Uniocular.** Having but one eye. एकनेत्री; केवल एक आँख वाला

**Union.** Joining; the process of healing. योग; जोड़; विरोहण प्रक्रिया

**Unioval.** See **Uniovular.**

**Uniovular.** Having but one egg; unioval. एकडिम्बज; केवल एक अण्डे वाला

**Unipara.** A woman who has born only one child. एकप्रसवा; केवल एक बच्चे को जन्म देने वाली स्त्री

**Uniparous.** Producing one child at a birth. एकजाता; एक समय में केवल एक बच्चे को जन्म देने वाली

**Unipennate.** Denoting a muscle with a lateral tendon to which the fibres are attached obliquely like one-half of feather. एकपक्षक

**Unipolar.** A cell with one process. एकध्रुवी; केवल एक ध्रुव वाली कोशिका

**Unit.** A single entity. मात्रक; एकक; यूनिट; कोई अकेली चीज;
    **Intensive Care U.** (ICU), a special unit for care of critically ill patients. गहन चिकित्सा यूनिट; गहन चिकित्सा एकक; इंटेंसिव केयर यूनिट

**Unsaturated.** Not saturated. असंतृप्त;
    **U. Fats,** fats having low contents of hydrogen than saturated fats, as vegetables in their origin. असंतृप्त वसायें

**Unstriated Muscle.** Involuntary muscle-fibres without transverse striations. अरेखित पेशी

**Unwell.** Sick; ill. अस्वस्थ; रुग्ण; बीमार; रोगी; मरीज

**Upper.** Higher in place; superior in rank. ऊर्ध्व; उपरि; उच्च;
    **U. Extremities,** comprising of arms, hands, etc. ऊर्ध्वांग, जैसे हाथ, भुजायें, आदि

**Uptake.** The absorption by a tissue of some substance. अवशोषण

**Uraemia.** Diseased state due to accumulation of wastes in the blood tissues consequent upon kidney failure; uremia. यूरीमिया

**Uraemic.** See **Uremic.**

**Uranium.** A feebly radioactive metallic element. यूरेनियम .

**Urate.** A combination of uric acid with a base. यूरेट (पदार्थ)

**Uratic.** Relating to, or characterized by urates. यूरेटी; यूरेट (पदार्थ) जैसा;
    **U. Diathesis,** the gouty tendency. गठियारोग-प्रवणता; यूरेट-प्रवणता

**Urea.** The chief solid constituent of urine and principal nitrogenous product of tissue catabolism. यूरिया; मिहेय

**Ureal.** Relating to urea. यूरियाई; यूरिया अथवा मिहेय सम्बन्धी

**Ureameter.** See **Ureometer.**

**Uremia.** See **Uraemia.**

**Uremic.** Due to or marked by uremia; uraemic. यूरीमियाजनित; यूरीमियायुक्त

**Ureometer.** An instrument for measuring the quantity of urea in the urine; ureameter. यूरियामापी

**Uresis.** The act of voiding urine; urination. मूत्रोत्सर्जन

**Ureter.** A tube carrying urine from the renal pelvis of the kidney to the bladder. मूत्रनली; गवीनी; गुर्दे से मसाने की ओर पेशाब ले जाने वाली नली

**Ureteral.** Pertaining to the ureter; ureteric. मूत्रनली अथवा गवीनी सम्बन्धी

**Ureteralgia.** Pain in the ureter. गवीनीशूल; मूत्रनली में दर्द होना

**Ureterectomy.** Excision of an ureter. गवीनी-उच्छेदन; मूत्रनली को काटकर निकाल देना

**Ureteric.** See **Ureteral.**

**Ureteritis.** Inflammation of an ureter. गवीनीशोथ; मूत्रनलीशोथ; मूत्रनली का प्रदाह

**Ureterocele.** Hernia of an ureter. गवीनीस्फीति; मूत्रनली का हर्निया

**Ureterocolostomy.** See **Ureterosigmoidostomy.**

**Ureterolithiasis.** Formation or presence of a calculus or calculi in one or both ureters. गवीनी-अश्मरी; मूत्रमार्गी-पथरी

**Ureterolithotomy.** Excision of an ureteral calculus. गवीनी-अश्मरीहरण; ऑपरेशन द्वारा मूत्रनली की पथरी निकाल देना

**Ureteropathy.** Any disease of the ureter. गवीनीरोग; मूत्रनली का कोई रोग

**Ureteroplasty.** A plastic operation on an ureter. गवीनीसंधान

**Ureterosigmoidostomy.** Surgical transplantation of the ureters from the bladder to the colon so that urine is passed by bowels; ureterocolostomy. गवीनी-अवग्रहान्त्रसम्मिलन

**Ureterostomy.** The formation of a ureteral fistula. गवीनीछिद्रीकरण

**Ureterotomy.** An incision of the ureter. गवीनीछेदन

**Urethra.** The excretory canal of the bladder. मूत्रमार्ग; मूत्रपथ; मूत्राशय की मूत्रनिस्सारक नली

**Urethral.** Pertaining to the urethra. मूत्रमार्गी; मूत्रमार्गीय; मूत्रमार्ग सम्बन्धी

**Urethralgia.** Pain in the urethra; urethrodynia. मूत्रमार्गशूल; मूत्रपथशूल

**Urethritis.** Inflammation of the urethra. मूत्रमार्गशोथ; मूत्रमार्ग का प्रदाह

**Urethrocele.** Prolapse of urethra. मूत्रमार्गभ्रंश; मूत्रपथभ्रंश; मूत्रमार्गविपुटी; मूत्रमार्गच्युति

**Urethrodynia.** See **Urethralgia.**

**Urethrometer.** An instrument for measuring the caliber of the urethra. मूत्रमार्गमापी; मूत्रपथमापकयंत्र

**Urethroplasty.** Any plastic operation upon the urethra. मूत्रमार्गसंधान

**Urethrorrhaphy.** The suturing of an abnormal opening into the urethra. मूत्रमार्गसीवन

**Urethroscope.** An instrument for examining the interior of urethra. मूत्रमार्गदर्शी; मूत्रमार्ग की जांच के लिये प्रयुक्त किया जाने वाला यंत्र

**Urethroscopy.** Inspection of the urethral mucous membrane. मूत्रमार्गदर्शन; मूत्रपथ की जांच करना

**Urethrotome.** An instrument used in urethrotomy. मूत्रमार्गछेदक; मूत्रमार्गछिद्रक

**Urethrotomy.** An incision of the urethra. मूत्रमार्गछेदन

**Urethrotrigonitis.** Inflammation of the urethra and trigone of the bladder. मूत्रमार्ग; मूत्राशयशोथ; मूत्रमार्ग एवं मूत्राशय का प्रदाह

**Uretic.** An agent promoting the flow of urine. मूत्रोत्सर्जक; मूत्र का बहाव बढ़ाने वाला पदार्थ

**Urging.** Desire. इच्छा; रुचि

**Uric.** Pertaining to the urine. मूत्र सम्बन्धी;

**U. Acid,** an acid formed in the break-down of nucleoproteins in the tissues and excreted in the urine. यूरिक अम्ल; यूरिक एसिड; मूत्राम्ल

**Uricolysis.** Decomposition of the uric acid. मूत्राम्ल-अपघटन; यूरिकाम्ल-अपघटन

**Uricolytic.** Relating to, or affecting the hydrolysis of uric acid. मूत्राम्ल-अपघटनी; यूरिकाम्ल-अपघटनी

**Uricosuria.** Excessive amount of uric acid in the urine. मूत्राम्लमेह; यूरिकाम्लमेह

**Uridrosis.** Excess of urea in the sweat, giving an urinous odour. मूत्रगन्धी स्वेदलता

**Urina.** Urine. मूत्र; पेशाब

**Urinal.** A vessel for receiving urine. मूत्रालय; पेशाब घर; मूत्रपात्र
**Urinanalysis.** The analysis of the urine. मूत्रविश्लेषण
**Urinary.** Relating to urine. मूत्र सम्बन्धी;
    **U. System,** the kidneys, ureters, bladder and urethra. मूत्र-प्रणाली
**Urinate.** To micturate. मूत्रत्याग करना; पेशाब करना
**Urination.** Micturition. मूत्रण
**Urine.** Water evacuated from the bladder. मूत्र; पेशाब
**Uriniferous.** Conveying urine. मूत्रजन
**Urinology.** A scientific study of the urine. मूत्रविज्ञान; मूत्र का वैज्ञानिक अध्ययन
**Urinometer.** An instrument for finding specific gravity of the urine; urometer. मूत्रगुरुत्वमापी; मूत्र के विशिष्ट गुरुत्व की जानकारी के लिये प्रयुक्त किया जाने वाला यंत्र
**Urinous.** Relating to, or of the nature of urine. मूत्रज; मूत्रल
**Urobilin.** A pigment from bilirubin. यूरोबिलिन
**Urobilinogen.** A pigment formed from bilirubin in the intestine by the action of bacteria. यूरोबिलिनोजन
**Urocele.** An effusion of urine in the scrotum. जलवृषण; वृषणकोष के अन्दर पेशाब का जमाव होना
**Urochrome.** A yellow urinary pigment. मूत्रवर्णक; यूरोक्रोम
**Urocystitis.** Inflammation of the bladder. मूत्राशयशोथ; मूत्राशय का प्रदाह
**Urodynia.** Pain on urination. मूत्रवेदना; दर्दनाक पेशाब होना
**Urogenital.** Pertaining to the urinary and genital organs. मूत्र तथा जननांगों सम्बन्धी; मूत्रजननांगी
**Urogenous.** Producing urine. मूत्रजनक; पेशाब पैदा करने वाला
**Urogram.** Radiograph of urinary tract. मूत्रपथचित्र
**Urography.** Radiographic description of the urinary tracts or x-ray examination. मूत्रपथचित्रण
**Urolith.** A calculus in the kidney, ureter, bladder or urethra. मूत्राश्मरी; मूत्रपथरी
**Urolithiasis.** The presence of urinary calculus in the urinary system. मूत्राश्मरता; मूत्रपथरी बनना
**Urologist.** A specialist concerned with the diseases of the urinary tract. मूत्रविशेषज्ञ; मूत्रविज्ञानी; मूत्र सम्बन्धी रोगों की चिकित्सा करने वाला विशेषज्ञ

**Urology.** The medical specialty in the diseases of the urinary system. मूत्रविज्ञान; मूत्र-प्रणाली के रोगों से सम्बन्धित विशिष्ट चिकित्सा

**Urometer.** See **Urinometer.**

**Uropathy.** Any disease of the urinary tract or urethra. मूत्रमार्गविकृति; मूत्रपथ का कोई रोग

**Urosis.** Any disease of the urinary organs. मूत्रांगविकृति; मूत्रांगों का कोई रोग

**Urostealith.** Fatty matter in the urinary calculi. वसाभ-मूत्राश्मरी; मूत्रपथरी में चर्बी विद्यमान रहना

**Urticaria.** Hives; nettle-rash; shingles. शीतपित्त; पित्ती; जुलपित्ती; छपाकी

**Urticarial.** Relating to, or resembling urticaria; urticarious. शीतपित्तज; शीतपित्ताभ; शीतपित्त, पित्ती, जुलपित्ती या छपाकी से सम्बन्धित या उसके जैसी

**Urticarious.** See **Urticarial.**

**Uteri.** Uterus; womb. जरायु; गर्भाशय; बच्चादानी

**Uterine.** Relating to the uterus. गर्भाशय, जरायु अथवा बच्चादानी सम्बन्धी

**Uteritis.** Inflammation of the womb; metritis. जरायुशोथ; गर्भाशयशोथ; बच्चादानी का प्रदाह

**Uteroplacental.** Pertaining to the uterus and the placenta. गर्भाशय एवं अपरा सम्बन्धी; गर्भाशय-अपरापरक

**Uteroplasty.** A plastic operation on the womb. जरायुसंधान; गर्भाशयसंधान

**Uterosalpingography.** X-ray by means of injection of contrast media (for patency of the Fallopian tube). गर्भाशयडिम्बवाहिनीचित्रण

**Uterovesical.** Pertaining to the uterus and bladder. गर्भाशय तथा मूत्राशय सम्बन्धी

**Uterus.** The female organ of gestation; the womb. जरायु; गर्भाशय; बच्चादानी;

**U. Bicornis,** one divided into two horns or compartments on account of arrested development; bicornuate uterus. द्विशृंगी गर्भाशय;

**U. Diadelphys,** a double or duplex uterus; diadelphys uterus. द्विगर्भाशय;

**U. Duplex,** see **Uterus Diadelphys.**

**U. Septus,** a uterus that is divided into two cavities by an anteroposterior septum; septate uterus. सम्पूर्ण-पटयुक्त गर्भाशय;

U. Unicornis, a one horned uterus with only one lateral half, the other being undeveloped or absent; unicorn uterus. एकशृंगी गर्भाशय;

**Bicornuate U.**, see **Uterus Bicornis.**
**Diadelphys U.**, see **Uterus Diadelphys.**
**Double U.**, see **Uterus Diadelphys.**
**Duplex U.**, see **Uterus Diadelphys.**
**Gravid U.**, a pregnant uterus. सगर्भ गर्भाशय;
**Septate U.**, see **Uterus Septus.**
**Unicorn U.**, see **Uterus Unicornis.**

**Utricle.** A little sac or pocket. लघुकोश; क्षुद्रकोश

**Uvea.** The pigmented layer of the eyeball; uveal tract; choroid. असितपटल; रंजितपटल

**Uveal Tract.** See **Uvea.**

**Uveitis.** Inflammation of uvea. असितपटलशोथ; यूवियाशोथ; रंजितपटल का प्रदाह

**Uveoparotitis.** Uveitis associated with parotitis. असितपटलकर्णपूर्वग्रंथिशोथ

**Uvula.** A soft spongy hanging body, situated above the tongue and between the tonsils; pendulum palati. काकलक; अलिजिह्वा;

**Vesical U.**, a small vesical prominence at the internal orifice of the urethra; uvula vesicae. वस्ति काकलक;

**U. Vesicae**, see **Vesical Uvula.**

**Uvular.** Pertaining to, or resembling uvula. काकलक सम्बन्धी या काकलक जैसा

**Uvulatomy.** Excision of the uvula; uvulectomy. काकलक-उच्छेदन; काकलक को काट कर हटा देना या अलग कर देना

**Uvulectomy.** See **Uvulatomy.**

**Uvulitis.** Inflammation of uvula. काकलकशोथ; काकलक-प्रदाह

**Uvulotomy.** Amputation of the uvula; staphylotomy. काकलक-उच्छेदन; काकलक को काट कर अलग कर देना या हटा देना

# V

**Vaccina.** See **Vaccinia.**

**Vaccinal.** Relating to vaccine or vaccination. टीका अथवा टीकाकरण सम्बन्धी

**Vaccinate.** To administer a vaccine. टीका लगाना; किसी टीके द्वारा रोगक्षमीकरण करना

**Vaccination.** Any immunisation by means of a vaccine. टीका; टीकाकरण

**Vaccinator.** One who inoculates with the cow-pox virus. वैक्सीनेटर; टीका लगाने वाला

**Vaccine.** A preparation of living, weakened or killed microorganisms or viruses, used in prevention of diseases through immunising of persons likely to be exposed; a genus of cowpox. वैक्सीन; टीका;

**Aqueous V.,** vaccine employing physiological salt solution as the vehicle. जल टीका;

**Bacterial V.,** a suspension of bacteria in saline solution. जीवणुजन्य टीका;

**BCG V.,** Bacillus Calmette-Guerin vaccine or tuberculous vaccine. बी०सी०जी० वैक्सीन अथवा टीका; यक्ष्मारोधक टीका;

**Cholera V.,** vaccine prepared from killed vibrio cholerae. विसूचिका वैक्सीन;

**DPT V.,** diphtheria and tetanus toxoid, plus pertussis vaccine; triple vaccine. डिफ्थीरिया (रोहिणी), टेटानस (धनुर्वात) एवं काली खांसी (कूकरकास) रोधक टीका;

**Live Virus V.,** one from living micro-organism. जीवित विषाणु टीका या वैक्सीन;

**Poliomyelitis V.,** see **Poliovirus Vaccine.**

**Poliovirus V.,** a vaccination for preventing polio; poliomyelitis vaccine. पोलियोरोधक टीका;

**Small-pox V.,** vaccinia virus suspensions. मसूरिकारोधी टीका; चेचकरोधी टीका;

**Tetanus V.**, see **DPT Vaccine.**

**Triple V.**, see **DPT Vaccine.**

**Tuberculous V.**, see **BCG Vaccine.**

**Vaccinella.** A secondary eruption sometimes following cow-pox. गोमसूरिकोत्तर-उद्भेद; गोशीतला के बाद प्रकट होने वाला उद्भेद

**Vaccinia.** Cow-pox; a contagious disease amongst cattle. गोशीतला; vaccina. गोमसूरिका; छोटी माता

**Vaccinial.** Relating to, or resembling vaccinia. गोशीतला सम्बन्धी या गोशीतला से मिलता-जुलता

**Vacciniform.** Resembling vaccinia. गोशीतलारूप; गोशीतला जैसा

**Vaccinin.** The inoculable principle of cow-pox. वैक्सीनिन

**Vacciniola.** A secondary vesicular vaccine eruption. टीकाजनित-उद्भेद

**Vaccinoid.** Like cow-pox. गोशीतलाभ; गोशीतला जैसा

**Vaccininum.** A homoeopathic attenuation of the virus of the cow-pox. वैक्सीनीनम; गोमसूरिका के विषाणु से तैयार किया गया एक होम्योपैथिक तनूकरण

**Vacuolation.** See **Vacuolization.**

**Vacuole.** A clear space in a cell filled with air or fluid. रिक्तिका

**Vacuolization.** The formation of vacuoles; vacuolation. रिक्तिकाभवन

**Vacuum.** An empty space exhausted of air or gas. निर्वात; वैक्यूम

**Vagabond's disease.** Discolouration of the skin from lice. यूकोपसर्ग; यूकाजनित त्वग्विवर्णता

**Vagi.** Plural of **Vagus.**

**Vagina.** The female genital canal extending from uterus to vulva. योनि; प्रजनन-नलिका; a sheath or any sheath-like structure. आवरण; पिधान; आच्छद

**Vaginal.** Relating to vagina, or to any enveloping sheath. योनि सम्बन्धी; आवरण सम्बन्धी

**Vaginismus.** A painful spasm of the vagina. योनि-आकर्ष; योनि की दर्दनाक ऐंठन

**Vaginitis.** Inflammation of the vagina. योनिशोथ; योनि-प्रदाह

**Vaginodynia.** Neuralgia of the vagina. योनिवेदना; योन्यार्ति; योनि-पीड़ा

**Vaginoperitonial.** Relating to the vagina and the peritoneum. योनि एवं उदरावरण सम्बन्धी

**Vaginotomy.** Incision of the vagina. योनिछेदन

**Vaginovesical.** Relating to the vagina and the bladder. योनि एवं मूत्राशय सम्बन्धी

**Vagitus.** The cry of an infant. शिशुक्रन्दन; शिशुरुदन

**Vagotomy.** Surgical division of the vagus nerve. वेगसतंत्रिका-उच्छेदन; अस्थिरतंत्रिका-उच्छेदन

**Vagus.** The pneumogastric or tenth cranial nerve. वेगस तंत्रिका; अस्थिर तंत्रिका

**Valence.** The combining power of an atom as compared with an atom of hydrogen; valency. संयोजकता

**Valency.** See **Valence**.

**Valgus.** Bent or twisted outward; talipes. बहिर्नत

**Vallate.** Cupped; surrounded with an elevation. परिवृत्त

**Vallecula.** A small depression or furrow. कन्दरिका

**Valleculae.** Plural of **Vallecula**.

**Vallum Unguis.** Fold of skin overlapping the nail; eponychium. अधिनख

**Value.** A particular quantitative determination. मान; मूल्य

**Valva.** See **Valve**.

**Valvae.** Plural of **Valva**.

**Valval.** Relating to a valve; valvar. कपाट अथवा कपाटिका सम्बन्धी

**Valvar.** See **Valval**.

**Valvate.** See **Valvular**.

**Valve.** A device permitting control of an opening so as to allow free passage one way, but not the other; valva. कपाट; कपाटिका;
Aortic V., the semilunar valve of three segments at the junction of the aorta with the heart. महाधमनी-कपाट;
Bicuspid V., the same as Mitral Valve.
Ileocaecal V., one consisting of two folds of mucosa that guards the passage between the ileum and caecum. शेषान्धान्त्र कपाटिका;
Ileocolic V., the same as Ileocaecal Valve.
Mitral V., one that controls the opening from the left auricle to the left ventricle. द्विकृपर्दी कपाटिका;
Semilunar V., one of the three valves of the aorta; also those of the pulmonary artery. अर्धचन्द्र कपाटिका;
Tricuspid V., that which controls the opening from the right auricle to the right ventricle. त्रिकृपर्दी कपाटिका

**Valvoplasty.** A plastic operation on a valve, usually reserved for the heart; valvuloplasty. कपाटिकासंधान

**Valvotomy.** An incision of a valve; valvulotomy. कपाटिकाछेदन

**Valvula.** A small valve. क्षुद्रकपाटिका; सूक्ष्मकपाटिका

**Valvular.** Relating to, or provided with a heart-valve; valvate. कपाटिकी; हृत्कपाटीय; हृत्कपाट सम्बन्धी

**Valvulitis.** Inflammation of a valve, especially the heart-valve. कपाटिकाशोथ; हृत्कपाट का प्रदाह

**Valvuloplasty.** See **Valvoplasty.**

**Valvulotomy.** See **Valvotomy.**

**Vapor.** A gaseous form assumed by a solid or liquid substance when sufficiently heated; vapour. वाष्प; भाप;

   **V.-bath,** steam-bath. वाष्प-स्नान; भाप के पानी से नहाना

**Vaporization.** The conversion of a substance into vapor. वाष्पन; किसी पदार्थ का भाप में बदलना; therapeutic application of a vapor. वाष्प-चिकित्सा; भाप द्वारा इलाज करना

**Vaporize.** To convert a solid or liquid into a vapor. वाष्पन करना; किसी ठोस अथवा तरल पदार्थ को भाप में बदलना

**Vapotherapy.** Therapeutic use of vapors. वाष्पोपचार; भाप द्वारा की जाने वाली चिकित्सा

**Variable.** Variate; inconsistant. परिवर्ती

**Variate.** See **Variable.**

**Variant.** Variable; having tendency to alter or change. प्रकारान्तर; रूपान्तर; परिवर्तन

**Variation.** Deviation from a given type. परिवर्तन; विभेद; परिवृत्ति

**Varicella.** Chicken-pox; varicelloid. लघु-मसूरिका; छोटी माता

**Varicelloid.** See **Varicella.**

**Varices.** Plural of **Varix.**

**Varicocele.** Abnormal enlargement of blood vessels of the spermatic cord; varicole. वृषण-शिरापस्फीति; अण्डकोष की रक्तवाहिनियों का बढ़ना

**Varicole.** See **Varicocele.**

**Varicose.** The dilated portion of a vein. अपस्फीत; किसी शिरा का फैला हुआ भाग;

   **V. Vein,** a varix. अपस्फीत शिरा; कुटिल शिरा

**Varicosity.** A varix or varicose condition. अपस्फीति

**Varicotomy.** Excision of a varicose vein. अपस्फीतशिरा-उच्छेदन; कुटिलशिरा को काट कर हटा देना

**Varicula.** A varix of the conjunctiva. अपस्फीतनेत्रश्लेष्मला; नेत्रों की श्लेष्मकला की फूली हुई शिरा

**Variety.** A term used in classifying individuals in a subpopulation of a species. भेद; अन्तर

**Variform.** Resembling a varix. कुटिलशिराभ; अपस्फीतशिराभ; कुटिलशिरावत्

**Variola.** Small-pox. मसूरिका; चेचक; बड़ी माता

**Variolar.** See **Variolous.**

**Variolation.** The inoculation of small-pox; variolization. मसूरिकाकरण; वैरियोलेशन

**Variolic.** See **Variolous.**

**Variolization.** See **Variolation.**

**Varioloid.** Attack of small-pox by previous vaccination. टीकाजन्य-मसूरिका; टीका लगने के कारण होने वाली चेचक; resembling small-pox. मसूरिकावत्; चेचक जैसा

**Variolous.** Having the nature of variola; variolar; variolic. मसूरिकाभ; चेचक की प्रकृति का

**Varix.** A venous dilatation, or an enlarged and tortuous vein. अपस्फीतशिरा; कुटिलशिरा; किसी शिरा का फूलना या बढ़ना

**Varus.** Displacement or angulation towards the midline of the body. अन्तर्नत; शरीर का मध्यरेखा की ओर झुकना

**Vas.** A vessel; duct; tube. वाहिका; नली; नलिका;

**V. Deferens,** the excretory duct of the testes. शुक्रनली; शुक्रवहानली; शुक्रवाहिका

**Vasa.** Plural of **Vas.**

**V. Afferentia,** lymphatics before they enter a lymph-gland. लस-अभिवाहिकायें;

**V. Brevia,** gastric branches of the splenic artery. लघुधमनी-वाहिकायें;

**V. Deferentia,** plural of **Vas Deferens.**

**V. Efferentia,** lymphatics after leaving a lymph gland. लस-अपवाहिकायें;

**V. Praevia,** umbilical vessels presenting in advance of the foetal head. सम्मुखी वाहिकायें;

**V. Recta,** the straight testicular tubules. ऋजु वाहिकायें;

**V. Vasorum,** the vessels supplying arteries and veins with blood. वाहिकावहाधमनियाँ; धमनियों तथा शिराओं में रक्त-संभरण करने वाली वाहिकायें

**Vasal.** Relating to a vas or vessel; vascular. वाहिकीय; वाहिका सम्बन्धी

**Vascular.** Full of blood vessels. रक्तधर; pertaining to vessels. वाहिकीय; वाहिकाओं सम्बन्धी;
> **V. Function,** blood circulation. वाहिकाक्रिया; रक्तसंचरण;
> **V. Reflex,** constriction or dilatation of vascular trunk or area; वाहिका-प्रतिवर्त; वाहिका प्रकाण्ड अथवा क्षेत्र का आकुंचन या विस्फार;
> **V. System,** the heart, blood vessels, lymphatics and their parts. वाहिका प्रणाली; हृदय, रक्तवाहिकाओं, लसीकावाहिकाओं तथा उनसे जुड़े अंगों का समुच्चय

**Vascularisation.** The acquisition of a blood supply; vascularization. वाहिकावर्धन

**Vascularity.** The quality of being vascular. वाहिकामयता; किसी रक्तवाहिका का प्रदाह होना

**Vascularization.** See **Vascularisation.**

**Vasculitis.** Inflammation of a blood vessel. वाहिकाशोथ; किसी रक्तवाहिका का प्रदाह

**Vasculomotor.** See **Vasomotor.**

**Vasculum.** A small vessel. क्षुद्रवाहिका; सूक्ष्मवाहिका

**Vasectomy.** Excision of the vas deferens. शुक्रवाहिकोच्छेदन; शुक्रवहानली को काट कर हटाना

**Vasiform.** Shaped like a tube. वाहिकारूप; वाहिकाभ; नलिकाभ; वाहिकाकार; नलिकाकार

**Vasitis.** Inflammation of ductus deferens; deferentitis. शुक्रवाहिकाशोथ; शुक्रवहानली का प्रदाह

**Vaso-.** Prefix denoting connection with blood. 'वाहिका' के रूप में प्रयुक्त उपसर्ग

**Vasoconstriction.** Narrowing of the blood vessels. वाहिकासंकीर्णन; रक्तवहनलियों की सिकुड़न

**Vasoconstrictive.** Promoting constriction of blood vessels; vasoconstrictor; vasohypertonic. वाहिकासंकीर्णक; वाहिकासंकोचक; वाहिकानिकोचक

**Vasoconstrictor.** See **Vasoconstrictive.**

**Vasodepressor.** An agent that lowers blood pressure. वाहिकादाबह्रासी; रक्तदाब घटाने वाला

**Vasodilatation.** Dilatation of blood vessels; vesodilation. वाहिकाविस्फार; रक्तवहानलियों का फैलना;
> **Antidromic V.,** resulting from stimulation of dorsal nerves, or inhibition of its constrictor substance or nerves. प्रतिवर्ती वाहिकाविस्फार

**Vasodilation. See Vasodilatation.**

**Vasodilator.** A drug that causes the smaller blood vessels to grow larger; vasohypotonic. वाहिकाविस्फारक; छोटी रक्तवाहिकाओं को बड़ा करने वाली औषधि

**Vasohypertonic. See Vasoconstrictive.**

**Vasohypotonic. See Vasodilator.**

**Vasomotion.** Increase or decrease of caliber of a blood vessel. वाहिकाप्रेरण; किसी रक्तवाहिका के तनाव की प्रेरकशक्ति बढ़ना या कम होना

**Vasomotor.** Regulating the tension of the blood vessels; vasculomotor. वाहिकाप्रेरक; रक्तवाहिकाओं के तनाव को नियमित करने वाला;

**V. Nerves,** the nerves which control the size of the blood vessels; vasculomotor; angiokinetic. वाहिकाप्रेरक तंत्रिकायें

**Vasopressor.** Producing vasoconstriction and a rise in blood pressure. वाहिकादाबवर्धी; रक्तवहानलियों की सिकुड़न एवं रक्तदाब बढ़ाने वाला

**Vasosection. See Vasotomy.**

**Vasospasm.** Constricting spasm of the vessel walls; angiospasm. वाहिकाकर्ष; वाहिका-उद्वेष्ट; वाहिका-प्राचीरों की सिकुड़नयुक्त ऐंठन

**Vasospastic.** Relating to, or characterized by vasospasm; angiospasm. वाहिकाकर्ष सम्बन्धी अथवा वाहिकाकर्षीय

**Vasotomy.** Incision into or division of the vas deferens; vasosection. शुक्रवाहिकाछेदन

**VCG.** Vectorcardiography; analysis of the direction and magnitude of the electrical forces of the heart's action. सदिशहृद्लेखन

**V.D.** Abbreviation for **Venereal Disease.**

**Vector.** An inveterate animal capable of transmitting an infectious agent among vertebras. रोगवाहक;

**Biological V.,** a vector essential in the life cycle of the pathogenic organism. जैव रोगवाहक;

**Mechanical V.,** a vector simply conveying pathogens to a susceptible individual without essential development of the pathogenic organisms in the vector. भौतिक रोगवाहक

**Vectorcardiography. See VCG.**

**Vegetable.** A plant specifically used for food. वनस्पति; शाक्; सब्जी

**Vegetarian.** On whose diet consists of foods of vegetable origin. शाकाहारी; शाकाहार पर अधिकाधिक निर्भर रहने वाला

**Vegetation.** A growth or excrescence of any kind. उद्भेद; किसी प्रकार का गुल्म या विवर्धन; inactive. निष्क्रिय; growing or functioning involuntarily. असंयत बृद्धि या क्रिया

**Vegetative.** Having the power of growth. वर्धी; वर्धन-शक्ति से सम्पन्न;

**Vehemence.** Violent; great force. प्रचण्ड; उग्र

**Vehicle.** Means of administering medicines. अनुपान; औषध-प्रयोग का माध्यम

**Veil.** That which intercepts view, as mist. धुन्ध

**Vein.** Vessel that receives blood from the arteries and returns it to the heart. शिरा; वह रक्तवाहिका जो धमनियों से रक्त लेकर हृदय को वापस करती है;

**Angular V.**, a continuation of the frontal vein downward to become the facial at the lower margin of the orbit; vena angularis. कोणीय शिरा; कोण-शिरा;

**Auricular V.**, the vein of the ear; vena auricularis. कर्ण-शिरा;

**Axillary V.**, a large vein formed by the junction of the inner branchial veins; vena axillaris. कक्षा-शिरा;

**Azygos V.**, one of the three veins situated toward the belly of the bodies of the thoracic vertebrae; vena azygos. अयुग्म-शिरा;

**Basilic V.**, one on the inner side of the arm; vena basilica. अन्तर्बाहु-शिरा;

**Brachial V.'s**, two veins in either arm accompanying brachial artery and emptying into the axillary vein. प्रगण्ड-शिरायें;

**Brachiocephalic V.**, one of the two large valveless veins returning the blood from head, neck and upper extremity; innominate vein. बाहुशीर्ष-शिरा;

**Cardiac V.**, one of the veins of the heart which drains blood from its tissues, circulates throughout the cardiac region and usually empties into the coronary sinus. हृद्-शिरा;

**Cephalic V.**, a large vein of the arm, formed by the union of the median cephalic and superficial radial, and empties into the upper part of the axillary vein. बहिर्बाहु-शिरा; प्रमस्तिष्कशिरा;

**Cerebellar V.'s**, veins draining the cerebellum. अनुमस्तिक शिरायें;

**Cerebral V.**, one relating to the cerebrum. प्रमस्तिष्क शिरा;

**Ciliary V.**, one of the several small veins, anterior and posterior, coming from the ciliary body. रोमक शिरा;

**Coronary V.**, the great cardiac vein opening into the coronary sinus of the heart. हृद्-शिरा;

**Emissary V.**, one of the small veins passing through the cranial foramens and connecting the cerebral sinuses with external veins. उद्गत शिरा;

**Facial V.**, a continuation of the angular vein. आनन-शिरा;

**Femoral V.**, accompanies femoral artery in the same sheath, being a continuation of the popliteal vein. और्वी-शिरा;

**Gastric V.**, one accompanying the gastric artery. जठर-शिरा;

**Hemiazygos V.**, one of the small accessory veins of the azygos veins. अर्धयुग्म-शिरा;

**Hemorrhoidal V.**, a plexus of veins surrounding the rectum; rectal vein. मलाशय-शिरा; मलांत्र-शिरा;

**Innominate V.**, see **Brachiocephalic Vein.**

**Lingual V.**, deep vein of tongue that receives blood from the tongue, sublingual and submandibular glands and muscles of the floor of the mouth. जिह्वा-शिरा; जीभ की गहन शिरा;

**Maxillary V.**, posterior continuation of the pterygoid plexus. ऊर्ध्वहनु-शिरा;

**Occipital V.**, drains the occipital region and empties into the internal jugular vein. पश्चकपाल-शिरा;

**Ophthalmic V.**, a short trunk carrying the blood from the eyes. नेत्र-शिरा;

**Pancreatic V.**, drains the pectoral muscles. अग्न्याशय-शिरा;

**Popliteal V.**, one formed by the accompanying veins of the anterior and posterior tibial arteries. जानुपृष्ठ-शिरा;

**Portal V.**, one formed by the junction of the superior mesenteric and splenic veins. प्रतिहारिणी शिरा;

**Pulmonary V.**, one of the four veins, i.e. two of each lung, returning the aerated blood from the lungs to the heart. फुप्फुस-शिरा;

**Radial V.**, one accompanying the musculocutaneous nerve. बहि:प्रकोष्ठिका-शिरा;

**Rectal V.**, see **Hermorrhoidal Vein.**

**Renal V.**, one accompanying the renal artery. वृक्क-शिरा;

**Splenic V.**, one returning the blood from the spleen and forming the portal vein by its union with the superior mesenteric vein. प्लीहा-शिरा;

**Subclavian V.**, a continuation of the axillary vein at the lateral border of the first rib. अधोजत्रुक-शिरा;

**Ulnar V.**, one extending up the anterior and inner surface of the forearm. प्रकोष्ठिका-शिरा;

**Umbilical V.**, one conveying the blood from the placenta to the foetus. नाभि-शिरा;

**Varicose V.**, one of many dilated veins, the valves of which become incompetent so that blood flow may be reversed. अपस्फीत शिरा;

**Vitelline V.**, one of the two veins conveying back the blood from the yolk-sac to the embryonic heart. पीतक-शिरा

**Vela.** Plural of **Velum.**

**Velum.** A veil or veil-like structure. छदन; छद;

**V.-palati,** the back part of the mouth; the soft palate. तालु-छद; मृदु अथवा कोमल तालु

**Vena.** A vein. शिरा; धमनियों से रक्त लेकर उसे हृदय की ओर वापस ले जाने वाली वाहिका;

**V. Angularis,** see **Angular Vein.**

**V. Auricularis,** see **Auricular Vein.**

**V. Axillaris,** see **Axillary Vein.**

**V. Azygos,** see **Azygos Vein.**

**V. Basilica,** see **Basilic vein.**

**V. Cava,** vein returning the blood to the heart. महाशिरा;

**V. Cava Anterior,** see **Vena Cava Superior.**

**V. Cava Inferior,** formed by the junction of the two common iliac veins, and empties into the right auricle of the heart. निम्नमहाशिरा;

**V. Cava Superior,** formed by the union of innominate veins, conveys the blood from the upper half of the body to the right auricle; vena cava anterior. ऊर्ध्वमहाशिरा

**Venae.** Plural of **Vena.**

**Venenata.** Poisoning. विषाक्तता; विषण्णता; विषालुता

**Venenatus.** Poisonous. विषाक्त; विषण्ण; विषालु

**Venene.** The snake-poison. सर्पविष; सांप का जहर

**Venenose.** See **Venenous.**

**Venenous.** Poisonous, venenose. विषाक्त; जहरीला

**Venepuncture.** Insertion of a needle into a vein; venipuncture. शिरावेध; शिरावेधन; किसी शिरा में सुई द्वारा छेद करना

**Venereal.** Concerned with diseases contacted by sexual intercourse. रतिज; सम्भोग के कारण होने वाले रोगों से सम्बन्धित;

   **V. Disease,** any disease due to venery; abbreviation: **V.D.** रतिज रोग; सम्भोग के कारण होने वाला रोग

**Veneriologist.** One who is versed in venereal diseases. रतिजरोगविज्ञानी: रतिजरोगविशेषज्ञ

**Veneriology.** The study and treatment of venereal diseases; venereology. रतिजरोगविज्ञान: रतिज रोगों का अध्ययन और उनकी चिकित्सा

**Venery.** Excessive sexual intercourse. अतिसम्भोग; अत्यधिक सम्भोग करना

**Venesection.** Bleeding by opening a vein; venisection; phlebotomy. शिरावेधन; किसी शिरा को छेद कर उससे खून निकालना

**Veniplexus.** A group of veins. शिरासमूह; शिरापुंज

**Venipuncture.** Needling of a vein; venepuncture. शिरावेधन; किसी शिरा को सुई द्वारा छेदना

**Venisection.** See **Venesection.**

**Venisuture.** Suture of a vein. शिरासीवन

**Venoclysis.** The introduction of nutrient or medicinal fluids into a vein. शिराधावन; किसी शिरा के अन्दर सूची द्वारा पौष्टिक या औषध-द्रव डालना

**Venoconstrictor.** An agent which constricts a vein. शिरासंकीर्णक; शिरा को सिकोड़ने वाला पदार्थ

**Venogram.** A radiograph of venous system after an opaque media injection. शिरालेख;शिराचित्र

**Venography.** X-ray examination of venous system by injection of opaque media. शिरालेखन; शिराचित्रण

**Venom.** The poisonous substance injected in bites by snakes, certain spiders, bees, wasps, etc. विष; जहर;

   **Snake V.,** the poisonous seretion of the labial glands of certain snakes. सर्प-विष; सांप का जहर

**Venomous.** Poisonous. विषाक्त; विष अथवा उन जीव-जन्तुओं सम्बन्धी, जिनके विष-निस्सारक ग्रन्थियां रहती हैं

M.D.F.-32

**Venous.** Relating to the veins. शिरापरक; शिराओं सम्बन्धी

**Vent.** An outlet, e.g. the anal opening. निकास अथवा द्वार, जैसे मलद्वार, गुदा, आदि

**Venter.** Belly or a belly-shaped part. उदर;पेट

**Ventilation.** The supplying of fresh air. संवातन; ताजी हवा का सम्भरण होना

**Ventilator.** A mechanical device for artificial ventilation of the lungs. संवातक

**Ventral.** Pertaining to the abdomen or the anterior surface of the body. अभ्युदरीय; उदर अथवा शरीर के अगले तल से सम्बन्धित; anterior. अग्र

**Ventricle.** A normal cavity in the brain or heart. निलय; मस्तिष्क अथवा हृदय के अन्दर स्थित गुहा;

    **Fourth V.,** the cavity above the pons and medulla of the brain. चतुर्थ निलय;

    **Lateral V.,** the cavity in each cerebral hemisphere. पार्श्व निलय;

    **Third V.,** the median cavity in the brain. तृतीय निलय

**Ventricular.** Pertaining to the ventricle. निलयी; निलय सम्बन्धी

**Ventriculitis.** Inflammation of the ventricles of the brain. मस्तिष्कनिलयशोथ; मस्तिष्कनिलयों का प्रदाह

**Ventriculocisternostomy.** Artificial communication between cerebral ventricles and subarachnoid space. मस्तिष्कनिलयकुंडसम्मिलन

**Ventriculography.** The localization of tumours by rediographs of the ventricles of the brain after replacing their fluid-contents. मस्तिष्कनिलयचित्रण

**Ventriculus.** Ventricle. निलय; stomach. उदर;पेट

**Ventrofixation.** The suture of a displaced viscus to the abdominal wall. उदराग्रस्थिरीकरण

**Ventrosuspension.** The fixation of the displaced uterus at the abdominal wall. गर्भाशय-अग्रनिलम्बन

**Venula.** See **Venule.**

**Venule.** A little vein; venula. तनुशिरा; शिरिका; क्षुद्रशिरा

**Verbigeration.** Repetition of words that are either meaningless or have no significance. निरर्थक-शब्दावृत्ति; अर्थहीन शब्दों की पुनरावृत्ति

**Verge.** An edge or margin. धार; किनारा; हाशिया

**Vermicide.** An agent which kills intestinal worms. कृमिनाशी; कृमिनाशक

**Vermicular.** That which resembles a worm. कृम्याभ; कृमिवत्; कृमि से मिलता-जुलता

**Vermiform.** Worm-like. कृम्याकार; कृमिवत्; कृमि जैसा;

   **V. Appendix,** a worm-shaped tube opening into the cecum. उण्डुकपुच्छ; उपांत्र

**Vermifugal.** Expelling worms; anthelmintic. कृमिनिस्सारक; कीड़े बाहर निकालने वाली (दवा)

**Vermifuge.** An agent expelling intestinal worms; anthelmintic. कृमिनिस्सारक; आंत्र-कृमियों को बाहर निकालने वाला पदार्थ

**Vermin.** A noxious or parasitic insect, or the one, destructive to crops, etc. अपकारी कीट; पीड़क जन्तु; फसलों को नष्ट करने वाला कीड़ा

**Verminal.** Concerning or caused by worms. कृमि सम्बन्धी; कृमिजनित

**Vermination.** The condition of one with worms. कृमिरुग्णता; कृमियों के कारण होने वाली रुग्णावस्था

**Verminous.** Relating to, caused by, or infested with worms, larvae, or vermin. कृमिरुग्ण; कृमिजन्य

**Vermis.** A worm. कृमि; the middle cerebellar lobe. मध्यशीर्षखण्ड; सिर का बिचला भाग

**Vernacular.** Indigenous. देशी; स्वदेशी

**Vernix Caseosa.** The fatty substance which covers the skin of the foetus at the birth and keeps it from becoming sodden by liquor amnii. भ्रूण-स्नेह

**Verruca.** A wart; verruga; a flesh-coloured growth characterized by circumscribed hypertophy of the papillae of the corium. मस्सा; अधिमांस;

   **V. Necrogenica,** a warty growth on the fingers of dissectors due to septic fluids of the cadaver. परिगलनी अधिमांस;

   **V. Vulgaris,** the common wart of the hands of brown colour and rough pitted surface. सामान्य अधिमांस

**Verruciform.** Wart-like; wart-shaped. अधिमांसवत्; मस्साभ; मस्से जैसा

**Verrucose.** See **Verrucuous.**

**Verrucuous.** Warty; resembling wart; verrucose; denoting wart-like elevations. अधिमांसी; अधिमांसल; मस्से जैसा

**Verruga.** See **Verruca.**

**Version.** Turning of the womb or the foetus in utero. गर्भवर्तन; गर्भाशय का मुड़ जाना;

   **Bimanual V.**, see **Bipolar Version.**

   **Bipolar V.**, version of acting upon both poles of the foetus; bimanual version. उभयध्रुवी गर्भवर्तन;

   **External V.**, version effected by external manipulation. बाह्य गर्भवर्तन;

   **Internal V.**, that effected by the hand within the uterus. आभ्यन्तर गर्भवर्तन;

   **Podalic V.**, bringing down one or both feet. गर्भपादवर्तन; पादगर्भवर्तन;

   **Spontaneous V.**, the process whereby a transverse position is, without external influence, changed into a longitudinal one. स्वत: गर्भवर्तन

**Vertebra.** One of the bony segments of the spinal column. कशेरुका; मेरुदण्ड का अस्थिखण्ड

**Vertebrae, Vertebras.** Plural of **Vertebra.**

**Vertebral.** Relating to the vertebra. कशेरुका सम्बन्धी;

   **V. Column,** the spinal column; back-bone. कशेरुका-खण्ड; मेरुदण्ड; रीढ़ की हड्डी

**Vertebras.** See **Vertebrae.**

   **Cervical V.**, the upper seven vertebrae of the neck. ग्रैव कशेरुकायें;

   **Coccygeal V.**, the rudimentary vertebrae of the coccyx. अनुत्रिक कशेरुकायें,

   **Dorsal V.**, twelve vertebral segments in the thoracic region to which the ribs are attached. अभिपृष्ठ कशेरुकायें; पश्च-कशेरुकायें;

   **False V.**, the sacral and coccygeal vetebrae that fuse; fixed vertebras. कूट कशेरुकायें;

   **Fixed V.**, see **False Vertebras.**

   **Lumbar V.**, the five vertebras adjoining the sacrum. कटि-कशेरुकायें;

   **Sacral V.**, the five fused vertabras forming the sacrum. त्रिक-कशेरुकायें;

   **Thoracic V.** the twelve vertebrae that connect the ribs and form part of the posterior wall of the thorax. वक्ष कशेरुकायें

**Vertebrarium.** The spinal column. कशेरुका-दण्ड; कशेरुकाखण्ड; मेरुदण्ड; रीढ़ की हड्डी

**Vertebrate.** Having a vertebral column. पृष्ठवंशी

**Vertebrosternal.** Extending, as a rib, from the spinal column to the sternum; sternovertebral. कशेरुका-उरोस्थिक; कशेरुका-उरोस्थीय; मेरुदण्ड से उरोस्थि की ओर फैला हुआ या फैली हुई, जैसे कोई पसली

**Vertex.** The crown of the head. कपालशीर्ष; शीर्ष; शिरोबिन्दु

**Vertical.** Perpendicular. लम्बरूप

**Vertiginous.** Relating to, or affected with vertigo. भ्रमि सम्बन्धी अथवा भ्रमिग्रस्त

**Vertigo.** Giddiness or swimming of the head; dizziness. भ्रमि; चक्कर; सिर चकराना;

    **Epileptic V.,** vertigo due to epilepsy. अपस्मारक भ्रमि;

    **Objective V.,** vertigo in which stationary objects appear to be moving. परानुभूत भ्रमि;

    **Positional V.,** see **Postural Vertigo.**

    **Postural V.,** vertigo which occurs with change of position; positional vertigo. स्थितिज भ्रमि;

    **Subjective V.,** vertigo in which the patient has the sensation of turning or rotating. स्वानुभूत भ्रमि

**Vesania.** Unsoundness of mind. मनोविक्षिप्ति; पागलपन

**Vesanic.** Relating to vesania or insanity. मनोविक्षिप्ति या पागलपन सम्बन्धी

**Vesica.** The bladder; vesicae. वस्ति; मूत्राशय;आशय

**Vesicae Urinaria.** The urinary bladder. वस्ति; मूत्राशय

**Vesical.** Pertaining to the bladder. मूत्राशयी; मूत्राशयिक; मूत्राशय सम्बन्धी

**Vesicant.** An agent producing a blister; vesicatory. जलस्फोट; स्फोटक; स्फोटकर

**Vesication.** The formation of blisters. स्फोटन; फफोले पैदा होना

**Vesicatory.** See **Vesicant.**

**Vesicle.** A little bladder of water formed under the skin; blister. जलस्फोट; पुटिका; फफोला;

    **Allantoic V.,** the internal or hollow portion of the allantois. अपरापोषिका-पुटिका;

    **Auditory V.,** the ectodermal sac from which is developed the membranous labyrinth ;otic vesicle. श्रवण-पुटिका;

    **Blastodermic V.,** the hollow sphere formed by the proliferation of the impregnated ovum. बीजजनस्तर-स्फोटिका;

    **Cerebral V.,** the division of the cephalic extremity of the primitive neural tube; encephalic vesicle. प्रमस्तिष्क-पुटिका;

**Encephalic V.**, see **Cerebral Vesicle.**

**Germinal V.**, the nucleus of the ovule. बीज-पुटिका;

**Lens V.**, the embryonic vesicle formed from the lens pit and develops into the lens of the eye. लेंस पुटिका;

**Ocular V.**, a protrusion of the anterior cerebral vesicle, the first indication of the eye; optic vesicle. नेत्र-पुटिका; अक्षि-पुटिका;

**Olfactory V.**, the primitive vesicle that develops into the olfactory lobe. घ्राण-पुटिका;

**Optic V.**, see **Ocular Vesicle.**

**Otic V.**, see **Auditory Vesicle.**

**Seminal V.**, one of the two lobulated pouches or sacs between the base of the bladder and the rectum that serve as reservoirs for the semen. शुक्राशय; वीर्य-पुटिका;

**Umbilical V.**, the largest of the two globes formed by the blastodermic membrane of the early development of the embryo. नाभि-पुटिका

**Vesicocele.** Hernia of the bladder. मूत्राशयस्रंस: मूत्राशयिक हर्निया

**Vesicula.** A vesicle or smalll bladder. पुटिका; जलस्फोट

**Vesicular.** Like, or pertaining to air vesicles, the ultimate structures of the lungs. वायुकोष्ठक जैसा या वायुकोष्ठक सम्बन्धी; कोष्ठकी; वायुकोषीय

**Vesiculation.** The formation of vesicles. जलस्फोटन

**Vesiculectomy.** Resection of a portion or all of each of the seminal vesicle. शुक्राशय-उच्छेदन

**Vesiculitis.** Inflammation of the seminal vesicles. शुक्राशयशोथ; शुक्राशय का प्रदाह

**Vessel.** Vas; a duct, tube or canal, conveying the fluids of the body. वाहिका; वाहिनी; शरीर के द्रव्यों को इधर-उधर ले जाने वाली नली;

**Blood V.**, any of the vessels carrying blood. रक्तवाहिका; रक्तवाहिनी

**Vestibula.** Plural of **Vestibulum.**

**Vestibular.** Relating to the vestibule. प्रघाणी; प्रघाणीय; प्रघाण सम्बन्धी

**Vestibule.** A porch or threshold. प्रघाण;

**Aortic V.**, the space formed by the left ventricle adjoining the root of the aorta. महाधमनी प्रघाण;

**V. of mouth**, the buccal cavity. मुख-प्रघाण; मुख-गह्वर;

**V. of vagina,** the space behind the clitoridis between the labia minora, consisting opening of the vagina, urethra and ducts of the greater vestibular glands; vestibule of vulva. योनि-प्रघाण;

**V. of vulva,** see **Vestibule of vagina.**

**Vestibulum.** Vestibule. प्रघाण; the cavity of the internal ear. अन्तर्कर्णगह्वर

**Vestige.** A remnant of something formerly present; vestigium. अवशेष

**Vestigial.** Forming a trace. अवशेषी; relating to vestige. अवशेष सम्बन्धी

**Vestigium.** See **Vestige.**

**Veta.** Mountain sickness. मेरु-रुणता

**Ve'erinarian.** One who practises veterinary medicine. पशुचिकित्सक; पशुवैद्य; जानवरों का इलाज करने वाला डाक्टर

**Veterinary.** Pertaining to the domestic animals; veternity. पालित-पशुओं सम्बन्धी

**Veternity.** See **Veterinary.**

**Viability.** Ability to live; the state of being viable. जीवनक्षमता; जीव्यता

**Viable.** Capable of living a separate existence. जीवनक्षम; स्वतन्त्र

**Vial.** Phial; a small glass bottle. छोटी शीशी

**Vibratile.** Swaying to and fro. कम्पशील

**Vibration.** A swinging back and forth or rapidly repeated oscillatory movement. कम्प; कम्पन

**Vibrative.** See **Vibratory.**

**Vibrator.** An apparatus for use in vibratory. कम्पित्र; कम्पक

**Vibratory.** Swaying ;vibrative. कम्पशील

**Vibrio.** A genus of micro-organisms. सूक्ष्माणु; विब्रियो

**Vibrissa.** One of the stiff hair within the nostrils. नासालोम; दृढलोम; नथुनों के अन्दर रहने वाले बाल

**Vicarious.** Taking the place of another; the assumption of the function of one organ by another. उन्मार्गी; अपथप्रवृत्त; अनुकल्प;

**V. Menstruation,** menstruation from a passage other than the uterus. अपथप्रवृत्तार्तव; उन्मार्गी-आर्तव; अनुकल्प रज:

**View.** Prospect, scene sight, intellectual or mental sight, display, show, appearance. दृश्य

**Vigil.** Insommia; wakefulness. अनिद्रा; नींद न आना;

**Coma V.,** muttering delirium. अस्फुट प्रलाप; नींद में बड़बड़ाना
**Viginti.** Twenty. विंशति; बीस
**Vigor.** Active force or strength of body or mind; vigour. शक्ति; ताकत
**Vigour.** See **Vigor.**
**Villi.** Plural of **Villus.**
**Villus.** A tuft. अंकुर
**Vincula.** Plural of **Vinculum.**
**Vinculum.** A ligament; a band. बन्धनी; बन्ध; पट्टी
**Vinegar.** A weak and impure dilution of acetic acid. सिरका
**Vinous.** Having the nature of wine. मदिराभ; शराब जैसा
**Vinum.** Wine; the femented juice of grapes. मदिरा; शराब
**Violation.** Rape. बलात्कार
**Violet Rays.** See **Ultraviolet Rays.**
**Viper.** Any venomous snake. व्याल; वाइपर
**Viraemia.** The presence of virus in the blood. विषाणुरक्तता; रक्त में विषाणुओं की विद्यमानता
**Viral.** Pertaining to, or caused by a virus. विषाणुज; विषाणु सम्बन्धी
**Virgin.** A woman who has had no sexual intercourse. कुमारी; कुँआरी
**Virginal.** Relating to virginity. कौमार्य सम्बन्धी
**Virginity.** Maidenhood; the condition of being virgin. कौमार्य; कुँआरापन
**Viricidal.** An agent which destroys virus. विषाणुनाशी; विषाणुनाशक: विषाणु नष्ट करने वाला पदार्थ
**Virile.** Pertaining to manhood; manly. पुंसत्व; पुरुषत्व अथवा पौरुष सम्बन्धी
**Virilism.** The appearance of secondary male characteristics in the female. स्त्रीपुंवत्ता; पुंवत्ता; पुंसत्व; स्त्रियों में पुरुषों जैसी विशेषतायें होना
**Virility.** The condition of mature manhood. पुंवत्ता; पुंसत्व
**Virologist.** One versed in virology. विषाणुविज्ञानी; वाइरसविज्ञानी
**Virology.** The study of viruses and the diseases caused by them. विषाणुविज्ञान; विषाणुओं तथा उनके द्वारा उत्पदित रोगों का अध्ययन
**Viropexis.** The fixation of a virus particle to a cell. वाइरसस्थिरण; विषाणुस्थिरण
**Virose.** Poisonous ; virous. विषाक्त

**Virous.** See **Virose.**

**Virtual.** Appearing to exist but not in actual fact or form. आभासी

**Virucide.** An agent which destroys virus. विषाणुनाशी; विषाणुनाशक; विषाणु नष्ट करने वाला पदार्थ

**Virulence.** Extremely poisonous. अतिविषण्ण; अत्यधिक विषाक्त

**Virulent.** Extremely injurious, malignant or poisonous. उग्र; दुर्दम; अति विषाक्त

**Virus.** An entity which grows only in living tissues, is too small to be seen by ordinary microscope, and is the cause of many diseases. विषाणु; वाइरस

**Viruses.** Plural of **Virus.**

**Vis.** Force or energy. शक्ति; बल;

   **V. Medicatrix Naturae,** instructive healing power of the body to correct itself; the power inherent in nature. जैवीशक्ति; प्राणशक्ति; प्रकृति-प्रदत्त शक्ति

**Viscera.** Plural of **Viscus.**

**Visceral.** Pertaining to viscera. अन्तरांगी; आशयी; आशयिक; अन्तरांगों सम्बन्धी

**Visceralgia.** Neuralgia of the abdominal viscera. अन्तरांगशूल; आशयशूल; औदरिक अन्तरागों का दर्द

**Visceroinhibitory.** Restricting or arresting the functional activity of the viscera. आशयसंवेदनासंदमी

**Visceroptosis.** Downward displacement or falling off of the abdominal organs. आशयभ्रंश; अन्तरांगभ्रंश; अंतरांगों की स्थानच्युति

**Viscerotome.** An instrument used at autopsy for obtaining a specimen of the liver for microscopic examination. आंशय-उच्छेदक

**Viscerotomy.** Excision of the viscera. आशयोच्छेदन

**Viscid.** Glutinous; sticky; tenacious; viscous; ropy. श्यान; चिपचिपा; रेशेदार

**Viscidity.** The adhering property. श्यानता; चिपचिपापन

**Viscometer.** See **Viscosimeter.**

**Viscose.** A gummy substance in viscous fermentation. गोंद

**Viscosimeter.** An instrument for measuring the viscocity of various liquids; viscometer. श्यानतामापीयंत्र; विभिन्न द्रव्यों में व्याप्त चिपचिपेपन को मापने का यंत्र

**Viscosity.** The state of being sticky or gummy. श्यानता; चिपचिपापन

**Viscous.** See **Viscid.**

**Viscus.** Any organ enclosed within the cranium, thorax, abdominal cavity or pelvis. अन्तरांग; आशय

**Visible.** That which can be seen or that which is capable of being seen. दृष्टिगत; जो दिखाई दे

**Visile.** Relating to vision. दृष्टि सम्बन्धी

**Vision.** Sight; the act of seeing. दृष्टि; नजर;

   **Binocular V.,** vision with a single image, with both eyes simultaneously. द्विनेत्री दृष्टि;

   **Chromatic V.,** pertains to the colour sense; colour vision. वर्णी-दृष्टि; रंग-दृष्टि;

   **Colour V.,** see **Chromatic Vision.**

   **Double V.,** diplopia. द्विगुण दृष्टि; बहुदृष्टि;

   **Field of v.,** the space within which an object can be seen while the eye remains fixed on one point. दृष्टि-क्षेत्र;

   **Half V.,** blindness in one or both eyes for half of the visual field; hemianopia. अर्ध-दृष्टि;

   **Multiple V.,** a condition of the eyes where more than one image of an object is formed upon the retina. बहुदृष्टि;

   **Photopic V.,** vision when the eye is light-adapted. प्रकाश-दृष्टि;

   **Scotopic V.,** vision when the eye is dark-adapted. तिमिर दृष्टि;

   **Solid V.,** see **Stereoscopic Vision.**

   **Stereoscopic V.,** the perception of relief or depth of objects obtained by bincoular vision; solid vision. त्रिविम दृष्टि

**Visit.** An encounter between the patient and doctor, either the former travels from his home to the latter's chamber or **vice versa.** निरीक्षण

**Visual.** Relating to the vision. दृष्टिपरक; दृष्टि सम्बन्धी;

   **V. Acuity,** a measure of the revolving power of the eye. दृष्टि-तीक्ष्णता;

   **V. Angle,** angle between the line of sight and the extremities of the object seen. दृष्टि-कोण;

   **V. Axis,** the line of vision from object seen through the pupil's centre to macula lutea (the yellow point). दृष्टि-अक्ष;

**V. Field,** the area within which objects can be seen when the eye is fixed. दृष्टि-क्षेत्र

**Visualization.** The act of viewing or sensing a picture of an object. वीक्षण

**Visuosensory.** Pertaining to the perception of visual stimuli. दृष्टि-सम्वेदी

**Vita.** Life. जीवन; प्राण

**Vital.** That which pertains to, or involves life. प्राणभूत; जीवनी; जैवी; जीवन सम्बन्धी; प्राण सम्बन्धी;

**V. Force,** the natural strength which keeps one alive. जीवनी-शक्ति; प्राणभूत शक्ति;

**V. Principle,** the force inherent in the constitution, during life, of maintaining and, to certain degree, controlling its operations. जैवशक्ति-सिद्धान्त; जैवी सिद्धान्त

**Vitalism.** The theory that bodily functions are due to a distinct vital principle. जीववाद; वह सिद्धांत जो व्याख्या करता है कि जैवीशक्ति के कारण ही शारीरिक क्रियायें गतिशील रहती हैं

**Vitality.** The vital principle of life; strength. प्राणशक्ति; जैवी शक्ति; ताकत

**Vitals.** The organs essential for life. जीवनदायी अंग; प्राणभूत अंग

**Vitamin.** The nutrient substance supplying no calories but essential to health and good nutrition, amply supplied to normal persons by well-chosen diet. विटामिन;

**Vitamin A,** essential for growth. विटामिन 'ए';

**Vitamin B** or **Vitamin B Complex,** a group of water soluble substance essential for growth; is antiberiberi, antineuritic and antiscorbutic. विटामिन बी अथवा विटामिन बी कॉम्प्लेक्स; बेरीबेरीरोगनिरोधक, तंत्रिकाशोथनिरोधक एवं स्कर्वीरोधक;

**Vitamin B1,** antineuritic; antiberiberi. विटामिन बी-१; स्नायुशोथरोधक; बेरीबेरीरोगरोधक;

**Vitamin B2,** antipellagric. विटामिन बी-2; पेलैग्रारोधक;

**Vitamin C,** antiscorbutic. विटामिन सी; स्कर्वीनिरोधक

**Vitamin D,** antirickets. विटामिन डी; रिक्केटनिरोधक

**Vitamin E,** presents sterility. विटामिन ई; बंध्यतापरक

**Vitamin F,** the same as **Vitamin B1**

**Vitamin G,** the same as **Vitamin B2**

**Vitamin K,** antihaemorrhagic factor. विटामिन के; रक्तस्रावरोधक तत्त्व;

**Vitamin PP,** the same as **Vitamin B2**

**Vitellin.** The chief protein of the yolks of the eggs. अण्डपीत; अण्डों की पीली जर्दी; विटेलिन

**Vitelline.** Pertaining to the vitellus or the yolk of an egg or the ovum. पीतक; अण्डपीतक; अण्डपीत सम्बन्धी

**Vitellus.** The yolk of an egg, especially a hen's egg. अण्डपीत; अण्डे की पीली जर्दी

**Vitiate.** To render impure. दूषित करना; अशुद्ध करना

**Vitiation.** Impuring, as of the blood. दूषण

**Vitiligo.** Acquired leucoderma. अर्जितश्वित्र; प्राथमिक श्वित्र

**Vitrea.** See **Vitreous.**

**Vitreous.** Like glass; vitrea. काचाभ; काच जैसा;

   **V. Humor,** the jelly-like substance in the posterior portion of the eye. नेत्रकाचाभ द्रव; आँख के पिछले भाग में लस्पी जैसा पदार्थ

**Vitritis.** Alternate name for **Glaucoma.**

**Vitu's Dance, St.** See **Chorea.**

**Vives.** Enlarged glands. विवर्धित ग्रन्थियाँ; बढ़ी हुई ग्रन्थियाँ

**Vividiffusion.** The arterial blood of a living animal is made to circulate out from and then back to another part of the body. जीवी-अपोहन

**Vivisection.** Scientific dissection of, or experimentation on living animals. अंगोच्छेदन; अंग-उच्छेदन

**Vocal.** Pertaining to, or connected with the voice. स्वर सम्बन्धी;

   **V. Bands,** see **Vocal Cords.**

   **V. Cords,** two transverse parallel folds of mucous membrane at the upper end of the larynx which can either be relaxed towards the sides of the larynx during soundless breathing or lightened or pulled towards each other to vibrate and produce sound; vocal bands. स्वर-रज्जु; स्वरयंत्र के ऊपरी अन्तिम भाग में श्लेष्मकला की दो अनुप्रस्थ सीधी तहें

**Vocalis.** A muscle of the vocal cord. स्वरपेशी

# Voice

**Voice.** Sound uttered by humen beings produced by vibration of the vocal cord. स्वर; आवाज; वाक्

**Void.** To evacuate; to cast, as waste matter. उत्सर्जन; उत्सर्ग

**Vola.** The palms or the soles; volaris. करतल अथवा पदतल

**Volaris.** See **Vola**.

**Volatile.** Tending to evaporate readily. वाष्पप्रवण

**Volatilisation.** The conversion of a substance into vapour; volatization. वाष्पीकरण; वाष्पीभवन; किसी पदार्थ का भाप में बदलना

**Volatilization.** See **Volatilisation**.

**Volition.** The will to act. संकल्प

**Volume.** The apparent space which a body occupies. आयतन;

    **Expiratory Reserve V. (ERV)**, the maximal volume of air that can be expelled from the lungs after a normal expiration. निःश्वसन आरक्षित आयतन;

    **Forced Expiratory V. (FEV)**, the maximal volume that can be expired in a specfic time interval when starting from maximal inspiration. बलात् निःश्वासी आयतन;

    **Inspiratory Reserve V. (IRV)**, the maximal volume of air that can be inspired after a normal inspiration. प्रश्वसन आरक्षित आयतन;

    **Mean Corpuscles V. (MCV)**, the average volume of red cells (corpuscles). कणिकामाध्य आयतन;

    **Packed Cell V. (PCV)**, the volume of blood cells in a sample of blood after it has been centrifuged in a hematocrit. संकुलित कणिका आयतन;

    **Residual V. (RV)**, the volume of air remaining in the lungs after a maximal expiratory effort. अवशिष्ट आयतन;

    **Tidal V. (TV)**, the volume of air inspired or expired in a single breath during regular breathing. श्वसन आयतन

**Voluntary.** Subjected to the will. ऐच्छिक; स्वैच्छिक; स्वायत्त; अपनी इच्छानुसार कार्य करने वाला;

    **V. Muscle**, a skeletal muscle, subject to the will. ऐच्छिक पेशी;

**Voluptuous.** Excessive excitement, especially sexual. कामुक; अतिकामोत्तेजक

**Vomer.** A bone forming the inferior and posterior portion of the nose. सीरिका; नाक की एक हड्डी; वोमर

**Vomit.** Ejection of the stomach contents through the mouth. वमन करना; the vomited matter. वमित पदार्थ

**Vomiting.** The forcible expulsion effort to vomit the contents of the stomach through the mouth. वमन; कै; उल्टी;

   **Dry V.,** retching; nausea without vomitus. शुष्क वमन;

   **Faecal V.,** see **Fecal Vomiting.**

   **Fecal V.,** ejection of fecal matter aspirated into the stomach from the intestine by repeated spasmodic contractions of the gastric muscle; stercoraceous vomiting; faecal vomiting. पुरीष वमन; बिष्ठा वमन; मल वमन;

   **Projectile V.,** expulsion of the contents of the stomach with great force. प्रक्षेपी वमन;

   **Stercoraceous V.,** see **Fecal Vomiting.**

**Vomiturition.** Retching; an ineffectual effort to vomit. उबकाई; वमन करने की निष्फल इच्छा

**Vomiturius.** Causing vomiting; emetic. वमनोद्रेकी; वामक; कै कराने वाला

**Vomitus.** Vomited matter. वमित पदार्थ; वमन

**Voracious.** Ravenous; insatiable. राक्षसी; अत्यधिक; अति;

   **V. Hunger,** an insatiable appetite. राक्षसी भूख; अतिक्षुधा; अत्यधिक भूख लगना

**Vox.** Voice. वाक्; स्वर; आवाज

**Vulnerable.** Easily injured or wounded. सुभेद्य

**Vulnerary.** A medicine good for wounds. क्षतरोधी; क्षतविरोहक (औषधि)

**Vulnus.** A wound or injury. घाव; क्षत

**Vulva.** The external famale genitalia. भग; स्त्री-बाह्यजननांग

**Vulval.** Pertaining to the vulva; vulvar. भग सम्बन्धी

**Vulvar.** See **Vulval.**

**Vulvectomy.** Excision of the vulva. भगोच्छेदन; भग-उच्छेदन

**Vulvitis.** Inflammation of the vulva. भगशोथ; भगप्रदाह; स्त्रियों के बाहरी जननांगों का प्रदाह;

   **Follicular V.,** inflammation of the hair follicles of the vulva. पुटिकामय भगशोथ; पुटिकीय भगशोथ;

   **Gangrenous V.,** necrosis and sloughing of the area of vulva. सकोथ भगशोथ

**Vulvouterine.** Relating both to the vulva and the uterus. भग एवं गर्भाशय सम्बन्धी

**Vulvovaginal.** Relating both to the vulva and the vagina. भग एवं योनि सम्बन्धी

**Vulvovaginitis.** Inflammation of the vulva and the vagina. भगयोनिशोथ; भग एवं योनि का प्रदाह

**Vulvovaginoplasty.** Recently devised operation for congenital absence of the vagina or acquired disabling stenosis. भगयोनिसंधान

# W

**Waist.** The part of the body between the thorax and the hips. कटि; कमर; शरीर का वक्ष तथा नितम्बों का मध्यवर्ती भाग;

   **W.- coat,** a jacket; straight coat. जैकेट; वेस्ट-कोट

**Wakeful.** Not able to sleep; sleepless. जागृत

**Wakefulness.** Absence of sleep; sleeplesness. अनिद्रा; जागृतावस्था; नींद का अभाव

**Walk.** The characteristic manner in which one moves on foot. चलना; घूमना-फिरना

**Walker.** A mobile device used to assist a person in walking. वाकर

**Walking.** Act of moving on foot; advancing by steps. भ्रमण; चलना-फिरना; टहलना;

   **W.-in sleep,** somnambulism. निद्राभ्रमण; नींद में चलना

**Wall.** An investing part enclosing a cavity, chamber, or any anatomical unit. प्राचीर; दीवार;

   **Cell W.,** the outer layer or membrane of some animal and plant cells. कोशिका प्रचीर;

   **Chest W.,** the thoracic wall, including rib cage, diaphragm, abdominal wall and abdominal contents; thoracic wall. वक्ष प्राचीर;

   **Thoracic W.,** see **Chest Wall**

**Wandering.** Moving freely about. भ्रमणकारी; भ्रमणशील; भ्रमी

**Wane.** To decrease; to decline; to fade. क्षय; ह्रास; उतार; कमी

**Wanton.** See **Lascivious.**

**Ward.** A room in hospital. कक्ष; वार्ड

**Warm.** Hot. उष्ण; गर्म; गरम

**Wart.** A virus infection of the skin; a small horny excrescence on the skin. मस्सा; अधिमांस

**Warty.** Resembling, or of the nature of warts. मस्साभ; मस्सों जैसा; अधिमांसल; मस्सों से मिलता-जुलता या उनकी प्रकृति का

**Wash.** To cleanse with a liquid. धावन; धोना; वाश;

   **Eye-w.,** a lotion for the eyes. नेत्रधावन; आई-वाश

**Wassermann's Reaction.** See **Wassermann's Test.**

**Wassermann's Test.** A serum-test used in the disgnosis of syphilis; Wasserman's reaction. वेसरमैन जांच; उपदंश के निदानार्थ की जाने वाली एक सीरमी जांच

**Wasting.** Destroying. क्षयकारी; नाशवान; atrophy; emaciation; marasmus. शोष; सुखण्डी

**Water.** A transparent, inodorous, tasteless fluid. जल; पानी;

   **W.-brash,** pyrosis; heart-burn. हृद्दाह;

   **W.-cure,** hydropathy. जलोपचार;

   **Distilled W.,** water that has been purified by distillation. आसुत जल;

   **Mineral W.,** water that contains appreciable amounts of certain salts which give to it therapeutic properties. खनिज-जल; मिनरल वाटर

**Waterbrash.** Regurgitation of watery fluid from stomach. मुखप्रसेक; आमाशय से पनीले द्रव्य का ऊपर उठ कर मुँह में भरना

**Waterpox.** A common name for the varicella. मोतियाशीतला; गोशीतला; लघुमसूरिका; छोटी माता

**Watersoluble.** Capable of being dissolved in water. जलविलेय; पानी में घुल जाने वाला

**Wave.** A movement of particles in an elastic body. लहर; तरंग;

   **Alpha W.,** oscillation in electric potential occurring at the rate of 8-½ to 12 seconds; alpha rhythm. ऐल्फा तरंग;

   **Beta W.,** wave ranging in frequency from 15 to 30 per second and lower voltage than alpha waves; beta rhythm. बीटा तरंग;

**Excitation W.**, alpha wave of altered electrical conditions propagated along a muscle fibre preparatory to its contraction. उत्तेजन तरंग

**Wave-length.** The distance from one point on a wave to the next point in the same phase. तरंग-दैर्घ्य

**Wax.** A thick, tenacious substance gathered by honey-bees. मोम; शहद की मक्खियों द्वारा संग्रहीत एक गाढ़ा, चिपचिपा पदार्थ

**Waxing-kernels.** Enlarged glands under the ears or in the groin in children. विवर्धित ग्रन्थियाँ; बढ़ी हुई गिल्टियाँ

**Waxy.** Like wax; resembling or pertaining to wax. मोमी; मोम जैसा

**Weak.** Debilitated; not strong. दुर्बल; कमजोर; अशक्त

**Weaken.** To reduce the strength. दुर्बल करना; अशक्त करना; कमजोर करना

**Weakness.** Loss of strength. दुर्बलता; कमजोरी; अशक्तता;

**Inward W.**, leucorrhoea. प्रदर; श्वेतप्रदर

**Weal.** Superficial blister. स्फोट; ददौड़ा; फफोला; छाला

**Wean.** To cease to give suck. स्तनापनयन; अपस्तनन; स्तनत्याग

**Weaning Brash.** See **Weaning Diarrhoea.**

**Weaning Diarrhoea.** Severe gastroenteritis; weaning brash. स्तन्यमोचन अतिसार; अपस्तन्यन अतिसार

**Weaver's bottom.** Chronic bursitis over the tuberosity of the ischium. बुनकर-नितम्ब; जीर्ण-जानुशोथ

**Weazand.** The trachea. श्वासप्रणाल

**Web.** A tissue or membrane bringing a space. जाली; झिल्ली

**Webbed.** Joined by a membrane. जालित; जालीदार; झिल्लीदार

**Weed.** The grass. घास

**Weeping.** The shedding of tears. रोदन; रुदनशील; exudation or leakage of a fluid; moist; dripping. सद्रव; नम; आर्द्र

**Weight.** Heaviness as determined by a given standard. भार; तौल; तोल; वजन

**Weil's disease.** Acute febrile icterus; infective jaundice. संक्रामी कामला; सज्वर पीलिया

**Wen.** A sebaceous cyst. त्वग्वसापुटी

**Wet.** Moist; not dry. आर्द्र; नम; गीला

**Wetnurse.** A woman who suckles the child of another. धात्री; दूसरे के बच्चे को स्तनपान कराने वाली स्त्री

**Wheezing.** A sibilant respiration in various diseases. खरखराहट; घरघराहट; विभिन्न रोगों में साँय-साँय करता हुआ श्वास

**Whelk.** Acne rosacea; a pimple. मुहासा; फुन्सी

**Whey.** The milk-serum separated from the curd in coagulation. तक्र; छाछ; मट्ठा; मस्तु; पनीरजल; छैने का पानी; घोल

**Whipworm.** A roundworm which infests the intestine of man in humid tropics. प्रदोतकृमि; कशाकृमि; एक गोलकृमि

**Whisper.** Speech without phonation. फुसफुसाहट; बिना आवाज बोलना

**Whistling.** Like a shrill sound with lips. सीटी बजने जैसी ध्वनि

**White.** The opposite of black. श्वेत; सफेद;

   **W. Cells,** minute bodies in the blood, about one-third larger than the red cells, which war against infection; white corpuscles. श्वेत कोशिकायें; श्वेतकोष;

   **W. Corpuscles,** see **White Cells.**

   **W. Fluid,** emulsion of tartaric acid and phenol in water, widely used for general disinfectant purposes. श्वेत द्रव; फेनौल;

   **W. Leg,** thrombophlebitis. घनास्रशिराशोथ

**Whites.** Leucorrhoea; fluor albus. प्रदर; श्वेतप्रदर

**Whitlow.** Felon; paronychia; abscess in the finger-ends. चिप्प; अंगुलबेढ़ा; उँगली की नोक पर फोड़ा बनना

**W.H.O.** World Health Organisation. विश्व स्वास्थ्य संगठन

**Whoop.** The sonorous inspiration with which the paroxysm of coughing terminates in pertussis. हूल; हूप

**Whooping Cough.** Pertussis; an acute infectious disease marked by recurrent attacks of spasmodic coughing. कूकर-कास; काली-खाँसी; हूल

**Willan's leprosy.** Psoriasis. विचर्चिका

**Wind.** Gas; flatulence. गैस; अधोवायु; आध्मान

**Windpipe.** The trachea. श्वासनली; वायुनली

**Wine.** A fermented juice of grapes. मदिरा; मद्य; शराब

**Wing.** Ala. पक्ष; पंख; विभाग

   **W.-shaped,** see **Pterygoid.**

**Wink.** To close and open rapidly, as of the eyes. उन्मीलन; झपकी लेना; झपकना, जैसे नेत्रोन्मीलन अर्थात् आँखे झपकना

**Winter Cough.** Chronic bronchitis. शीत-कास; जीर्णश्वसनिकाशोथ; श्वसनिका का जीर्ण प्रदाह

**Winter Itch.** Itching of the legs in winter. शीत-कण्डू; ठण्डियों मे टांगों को आक्रांत करने वाली खुजली

**Wire.** Metal drawn out into threads of varying thickness. तार; to join fracture fragments together by use of wire. तार बांधना अथवा तार से बांधना

**Wisdom Teeth.** The last molar teeth on each side of the jaw. अन्त्यचर्वक दन्त; अक्ल-दाढ़

**Withering.** Shrievelling atrophy of an organ. निस्तेज; म्लान; मुरझाया हुआ

**Woman.** A female. स्त्री; नारी; औरत; महिला

**Womb.** The uterus; female organ for protection and nourishments of the foetus. गर्भाशय; जरायु; गर्भकोष; बच्चेदानी

**Wood.** The main part of trees. काष्ठ; लकड़ी

**Woody.** Consisting of wood. काष्ठमय

**Wool-fat.** Linolin. ऊर्णवसा; लिनोलिन

**Word-blindness.** Inability to comprehend written words. शब्दांधता

**Word-deafness.** Inability to comprehend the sounds heard. शब्द-बधिरता

**Word-salad.** The use of words with no meaning; schizophasia. निरर्थक शब्दोच्चार

**Worm.** Any member of the vermin family, the common being hookworm, pinworm, roundworm and tapeworm. कृमि; कीड़ा;

   **W.-abscess,** an abscess due to the presence of worms. कृमि-विद्रधि;

   **W.- fever,** an infantile fever due to intestinal worms. कृमि-ज्वर; आंत्र-कृमियों के कारण बच्चों को होने वाला बुखार;

   **W.-wood,** absinthium. एक प्रकार का कड़वा पौधा; चिरायता;

   **Hook-w.,** a parasitic nematode belonging to **Ankylostoma duodenale** and **Necator Americanus.** अंकुशकृमि;

   **Pin-w.,** a parasitic nematode **Enterobius Vermicularis,** causing enterobiasis, infection of intestines and rectum. सूचीकृमि;

**Round-w.**, any member of the **phylum nemanthelminthes** belonging to class Nematoda. गोलकृमि;

**Tape-w.**, any of the species of parasitic worms belonging to the class **cestoda phylum platyhelminthes**. फीताकृमि;

**Thread-w.**, common name applied to pinworm, enterobius vermicularis. सूत्रकृमि

**Wormian Bone.** One of the small bones in the cranial suture. सीवनीअस्थि; वौर्मी-अस्थि; कपालसीवनी की एक छोटी हड्डी

**Wound.** An injury; break in continuity of a soft part from violence. क्षत; जख्म; घाव; चोट लगने के कारण शरीर में किसी प्रकार की टूट-फूट होना;

**Abraded W.**, caused or resulting from abrasion. खरोंचदार घाव;

**Contused W.**, a bruise or contusion. नील;

**Incised W.**, a clean cut as by sharp instrument. उत्कीर्ण क्षत;

**Lacerated W.**, caused by or resulting from laceration. विदीर्ण क्षत;

**Poisoned W.**, one depending on tearing of tissue. विषाक्त क्षत;

**Punctured W.**, a wound in which the opening is relatively small as compared to depth produced by a narrow pointed object. प्रकीर्ण क्षत; बिद्धक्षत

**Wrench.** A sprain. मोच; मरोड़; झटका; रेंच

**Wrick.** A sprain. मोच; मरोड़; झटका; a twist. ऐंठन

**Wrinkle.** A furrow; fold. वलय; झुरी; सिकुड़न

**Wrist.** The carpus; the part connecting the forearm and the hand. मणिबन्ध; कलाई; बाजू;

**W.-drop**, paralysis of the extensor muscle of wrist and fingers. मणिबन्धस्रंस; मणिबन्धघात; कलाई तथा उँगलियों की प्रसारक पेशी का पक्षाघात

**Writer's cramp.** Loss of power to perform certain movements required in writing, telegraphing, instrument playing, due to spasmodic action of the concerned muscle; writer's palsy. पेशी-उद्वेष्ट

**Writer's palsy.** See **Writer's cramp.**

**Wry-neck.** Torticollis. वक्र-ग्रीवास्तम्भ; अकड़ी हुई गर्दन

# X

**Xanthalin.** An alkaloid from opium. अफीम का क्षार

**Xanthein.** The yellow colouring matter of plants; xanthine. पीतरंजक; पौधों का एक पीला रंग

**Xanthelasma.** A variety of xanthoma. पीताबुर्द; जैंथिलास्मा

**Xanthic.** Yellow. पीत; पाण्डुर; पीला; ralating to xanthin. पीतरंजक सम्बन्धी

**Xanthine.** See **Xanthein**.

**Xanthochromia.** Yellow discolouration of the skin. पीतचर्मता; त्वचा की पीली विवर्णता; जैंथोक्रोमिया

**Xanthocronous.** Yellow-skinned. पीतचर्म; पीतत्वक्

**Xanthocyanopia.** A blindness for red-green colours. लोहितहरितवर्णान्धता; लाल और हरा रंग पहचानने की अयोग्यता

**Xanthoderm.** See **Xanthoderma**.

**Xanthoderma.** Yellowness of the skin. पीतत्वक्; पीतचर्मता

**Xanthodont.** Having yellow teeth. पीतदन्त

**Xanthodontous.** Yellow discolouration of teeth. पीतदन्तता; दान्तों का पीला पड़ना

**Xanthoma.** A new growth of the skin, flat or slightly raised, and yellow in colour. पीताबुर्द; कोई पीला चर्म-गुल्म;

**X. Diabeticorum,** a rare disease of the skin, usually associated with diabetes mellitus. मधुमेहज पीताबुर्द;

**X. Multiplex,** a form occurring usually in women about middle life. बहुपीताबुर्द; अधेड़ आयु की स्त्रियों में पाई जाने वाली अवस्था;

**X. Planum,** see **Xanthoma Palpebrarum**.

**X. Palpebrarum,** the commoner form of xanthoma, usually occurring on the eyelids; xanthoma planum. नेत्रच्छद-पीताबुर्द;

**X. Tuberosum,** a form marked by tubercular lesions on the extensor surfaces of the extremities and on parts exposed to pressure. कन्दिल पीताबुर्द

**Xanthomatosis.** Widespread xanthomas, especially on the elbows and knees. पीताबुर्दता;

**Biliary X.,** xanthoma resulting from biliary cirrhosis. पैत्तिक पीताबुर्दता

**Xanthopathy.** Morbid yellowness of the skin. पीतचर्मविकृति; त्वचा का विकारक पीलापन

**Xanthopia.** A condition of dryness of the skin. त्वग्रूक्षता; त्वचा का रूखापन

**Xanthopsia.** Yellow vision. पीतदृष्टि; पीला दिखाई देना

**Xanthous.** Having an yellow skin. पीतचर्म

**Xanthuria.** Excess of xanthin in the urine. पीतरंजकमेह

**Xenogenic.** See **Xeanogenous.**

**Xenogenous.** Caused by a foreign body; xanogenic. आगन्तुकशल्यजनित

**Xenomania.** An inordinate attachment to things foreign. विदेशमोह; विदेशी संस्कृति के प्रति मोह, प्यार या झुकाव

**Xenomenia.** Vicarious or supplementary menstruations. अपथ्यप्रवृत्तार्तव; उन्मार्गी-आर्तव; अनुकल्परज:

**Xenoparasite.** An ecoparasite that becomes pathogenic in consequence of weakened resistance on the part of its host. सम्भावीपरजीवी

**Xenophobia.** Morbid fear of unknown persons. अज्ञातव्यक्तिभीति; अपरिचित व्यक्तियों का भय

**Xerantic.** Causing dryness. शुष्ककर; सुखाने वाला

**Xerasia.** A morbid dryness of hair. केशरूक्षता; बालों का रूखापन

**Xero.** Dry; harsh. शुष्क; रूक्ष; खर

**Xeroderma.** A mild form of ichthyosis characterized by excessive dryness and harshness of the skin. त्वचाखरता; त्वग्रूक्षता; त्वचा का रूखापन और खुरदरापन;

**X. Pigmentosum,** a disease characterized by brown discolouration, cracking and ulceration of the skin. वर्णकित त्वचाखरता

**Xeroma.** See **Xerophthalmia.**

**Xeronosos.** A condition of the dryness of the skin. त्वग्रूक्षता; त्वचा का रूखा होना

**Xerophagy.** The use of dry aliments. शुष्कभोज्यता; सूखी चीजें खाना

**Xerophthalmia.** Dryness and ulceration of the cornea which may lead to blindness; xeroma. शुष्काक्षिपाक; कनीनिका की रूक्षता एवं व्रणग्रस्तता

**Xerosis.** Dryness. शुष्कता; रूक्षता; रूखापन

**Xerostomia.** Dryness of the mouth. मुखरूक्षता; मुखशुष्कता; शुष्कमुखता; मुख का रूखापन

**Xerotes.** Dry habit of the body; dryness. त्वग्रूक्षता; त्वग्शुष्कता; त्वचा का रूखापन

**Xerotic.** Marked by dryness. अतिरूक्ष; अतिशुष्क; अत्यधिक रूखा या रूखी

**Xerotripsis.** Dry friction. शुष्कघर्षण

**Xiphoid.** Sword-like structure, as sternum. असिरूप; खड्गवत्; खड्गाभ, जैसे उरोस्थि

**Xiphopagus.** A double monster united by the xiphoid cartilage or the epigastrium. बद्धउरोस्थियमल

**X-ray.** Roentgen rays. एक्स-रे; क्ष-किरण (चित्र)

**X-ray Therapy.** Treatment with roentgen-rays. क्ष-किरण चिकित्सा

**Xylem.** The inner part of the vascular bundle in a plant stem. दारू

**Xyster.** An instrument used to clean the bones by scrapping. निघर्षणी; खुर्चनी


# Y

**Yard.** A measure of three feet. गज; the penis. शिश्न; लिंग

**Yavaskin.** The same as **Elephantiasis.**

**Yawn.** To gape; to open the mouth widely. जम्हाई लेना; अंगड़ाई लेना

**Yawning.** Gaping; an involuntary opening of the mouth widely. जम्हाई; अंगड़ाई; जम्भाई

**Yaws.** A tropical disease which resembles raspberry-like tubercles. न्युपदंश; फफोले; याज

**Yeast.** A ferment; zyme; yest. खमीर; किण्व

**Yelk.** See **Yolk.**

**Yellow.** Pallid; jaundiced. पीत; पीला;

    **Y. Fever,** an epidemic disease with high fever, jaundice, black-vomit, etc. पीत-ज्वर;

**Y. Gum,** the jaundice of an infant. शिशु-कामला;

**Y. Marrow,** matter found in hollow centre shaft of bones. पीत-मज्जा;

**Y. Precipitate,** yellow oxide of mercury. पीत पारद;

**Y. Softening,** cerebral softening with yellow discolouration. पीतमस्तिष्क-मृदुता;

**Y. Spot,** yellow nodule of anterior end of vocal cord. पीत-बिन्दु; पीली चित्ती;

**Y. Vision,** condition in which objects are seen yellow in colour. पीतदृष्टि

**Yellows.** Jaundice. कामला; पीलिया

**Yest.** See **Yeast.**

**Yokebone.** The malar bone. गण्डास्थि

**Yolk.** The yellow portion of egg as distinguished from the white; yelk. अण्डपीत; अण्डे की पीली जर्दी; पीतक

**Youth.** Period between childhood and maturity. यौवन; जवानी

**Yucca.** A genus of plants of the Lily family. सितकुसुम; यक्का (कुमुदिनी जैसे फूल वाला एक पौधा)

# Z

**Z.A.R.** Zondek-Aschheim Reaction or Test; an urinary test to confirm pregnancy in women. जौंडक ऐश्चाइम जांच; सगर्भता के निदानार्थ की जाने वाली मूत्र-जांच

**Zeimus.** A skin disease caused by over-use of maize. जीमस; अधिक मात्रा में मक्की खाने से होने वाला एक चर्म रोग

**Zero.** The point from which thermometers are graded. शून्य; सिफर

**Zinc.** A metallic element; zincum. यशद; जस्ता; नीले-श्वेत रंग की एक धातु

**Zincum.** Zinc; Zincum Metallicum. यशद; जस्ता; नीले-श्वेत रंग की एक धातु

**Zingiber.** A genus of plant; zingr; dry ginger. सोंठ; शुण्ठी

**Zinn's artery.** The central artery of retina. जिन-धमनी; चक्षुपटल की केन्द्रीय अथवा प्रमुख धमनी

**Zoanotropy.** See **Zoanthropy.**

**Zoanthropy.** A maniacal condition in which the person believes himself an animal. स्वपश्वानुभूति; स्वयं को पशु महसूस करने का उन्माद

**Zoe.** Life. जीवन; जिन्दगी; प्राण

**Zoetic.** Pertaining to, or concerning life. जीवन सम्बन्धी

**Zoic.** Concerning animal life. पशुजीवन सम्बन्धी

**Zona.** A zone or girdle. क्षेत्र; मण्डल; अस्तर; बन्धन; herpes zoster. भैंसिया छाजन; भैंसिया दाद; shingles. शीतपित्त; छपाकी; जुलपित्ती; a segment. खण्ड;

**Z. Arcuata,** the inner zone of the basilar membrane; arcuate zone. चापाकार क्षेत्र;

**Z. Ciliaris,** the ciliary processes collectively. रोमक क्षेत्र;

**Z. Denticulata,** the inner zone of the basilar membrane together with the limbus of the spiral lamina. दन्तुर क्षेत्र;

**Z. Fasciculata,** the middle cortical layer of the suprarenal body. पूलिका अस्तर;

**Z. Glomerulosa,** the outer cortical layer of the suprarenal body. अस्तवकास्तर; अस्तवक-अस्तर;

**Z. Pellucida,** the thick, solid envelope of the ovum; zona striata; zona radiata. स्वच्छ अस्तर;

**Z. Radiata,** see **Zona Pellucida.**

**Z. Reticularis,** the inner cortical layer of the suprarenal body. जाल क्षेत्र; अधिवृक्क पिण्ड का अन्दरूनी प्रान्तस्था-अस्तर;

**Z. Striata,** see **Zona Pellucida.**

**Z. Verginitalis,** the hymen. कुमारीच्छद; योनिच्छद

**Zonae.** Plural of **Zona.**

**Zonal.** Relating to a zone; zonal; zonary. क्षेत्रीय; मण्डलीय

**Zonary.** See **Zonal.**

**Zondek Aschheim Test.** See **Z.A.R.**

**Zone.** See **Zona.**

Arcuate Z., see **Zona Arcuata.**

**Zonesthesia.** Sensation of a little zone or girdle about a part. बंधनानुभूति; किसी भाग के चारों ओर पट्टी बंधी होने जैसी अनूभूति

**Zonula.** A small zone. मंडलिका;

   **Z. Ciliaris,** suspensory ligament attaching periphery of the lens of eye to the cliliary body; ciliary zonule. रोमक मंडलिका

**Zonulae.** Plural of **Zonula.**

**Zonule.** A little zone, belt or girdle. मण्डलिका अथवा पट्टी;

   **Ciliary Z.,** See **Zonula Ciliaris.**

**Zoologist.** A biologist who specializes in the study of animal life. प्राणिविज्ञानी

**Zoology.** The science of animal life. प्राणिविज्ञान

**Zoonoses.** Plural of **Zoonosis.**

**Zoonosis.** A disease transmitted from animals to man and sometimes back again. पशुजन्य रोग

**Zooparasite.** An animal parasite. पशुपरजीवी

**Zoopathology.** Science of the diseases of animals. प्राणिरोगविज्ञान

**Zoophagous.** Living on animal food. पशुभोजी; मांसभोजी; मांसाहारी; मांसभक्षक

**Zoophobia.** Morbid fear of an animal. पशुभीति; जन्तुभीति; पशुओं का डर

**Zoophyte.** A plant-like animal. पौधाभ-पशु; पौधे जैसा जानवर

**Zootic.** Concerning animals. पशुओं सम्बन्धी

**Zoster.** An acute inflammatory painful disease of the skin consisting of grouped vesicles corresponding indistribution to the course of cutaneous nerves. छाजन; दाद;

   **Herpes Z.,** see **Herpes.**

**Z.-plasty.** A technique with a Z-shaped incision in plastic surgery to relieve tension in scar tissue. Z-संधान; Z-प्लास्टी

**Zuchar.** Sugar. शर्करा; चीनी

**Zygocyte.** See **Zygote.**

**Zygoma.** The arch formed by the union of zygomatic process of the temporal bone and the malar bone; cheek-bone. गण्ड; गण्डास्थि; कपोलास्थि; गाल की हड्डी

**Zygomatic.** Pertaining to zygoma. गण्डास्थिक; गण्डास्थीय; कपोलास्थि सम्बन्धी

**Zygomaticum.** The zygomatic bone. सृक्कोत्कर्षिका; कपोलास्थि

**Zygote.** The individual that develops from a fertilized ovum; zygocyte. युग्मनज; युग्मज; निषेचनज

**Zygotic.** Pertaining to zygote. युग्मनज सम्बन्धी

**Zyme.** A zyme or ferment. किण्व; खमीर

**Zymic.** Relating to zyme or ferment. किण्विक; खमीरी

**Zymin.** An organised ferment; yeast; a zyme. किण्व; खमीर

**Zymogen.** Producing the zyme. किण्वजन; खमीरजन; खमीर पैदा करने वाला

**Zymogenic.** Causing fermentation; zymogenous. किण्वजनक; खमीरजनक

**Zymogenous.** See **Zymogenic**.

**Zymosimeter.** An instrument for measuring the degree of fermentation. किण्वमापीयंत्र; खमीरमापीयंत्र

**Zymosis.** Fermentation. खमीरण; किण्वन; an infectious disease. संक्रामक रोग

**Zymotic.** Contagious; infectious. संक्रामक; संक्रामी; सांसर्गिक; relating to fermentation. किण्वन या खमीरण सम्बन्धी

**Zynoma.** Any ferment. किण्व; खमीर

# APPENDICES
## (परिशिष्ट)

# APPENDIX I
(परिशिष्ट १)

## RELATION OF FAHRENHEIT TO CENTIGRADE DEGREES AS REQUIRED IN CLINICAL PRACTICE
(चिकित्सा व्यवसाय में प्रयुक्त फाहरेनहाइट एवं सेन्टिग्रेड डिग्रियों का सम्बन्ध)

| Fahrenheit (फाहरेनहाइट) | Centigrade (सेन्टिग्रेड) |
|---|---|
| 97.7°F. | 36.5°C. |
| 98.6 | 37.0 |
| 99.5 | 37.5 |
| 100.4 | 38.0 |
| 101.3 | 38.5 |
| 102.2 | 39.0 |
| 103.1 | 39.5 |
| 104.0 | 40.5 |
| 104.9 | 40.5 |
| 104.9 | 40.5 |
| 105.8 | 41.0 |
| 107.6 | 42.0 |
| 109.4 | 43.0 |
| 111.2 | 44.0 |
| 113.0 | 45.0 |

(Continued)

Appendix 1 continued

| | |
|---|---|
| 122.0 | 50.0 |
| 131.0 | 55.0 |
| 140.0 | 60.0 |
| 149.0 | 65.0 |
| 158.0 | 70.0 |
| 176.0 | 80.0 |
| 185.0 | 85.0 |
| 194.0 | 90.0 |
| 203.0 | 95.0 |
| 212.0 | 100.0 |

**Conversion**
(रूपान्तरण)

1. To convert Fahrenheit into Centigrade, substract 32 from Fahrenheit, multiply the remainder by 5 and divide the result by 9.

2. To convert Centigrade into Fahrenheit, multiply centigrade by 9, divide by 5 and add 32.

१. फाहरेनहाइट को सेण्टिग्रेड में बदलने के लिये, फाहरेनहाइट से ३२ घटाइये, शेष को ५ से गुणा कीजिये तथा परिणाम अर्थात् गुणनफल को ९ से भाग कीजिये।

२. सेण्टिग्रेड को फाहरेनहाइट में बदलने के लिये, सेण्टिग्रेड को ८ से गुणा कीजिये, गुणनफल को ५ से भाग कीजिये और उसमें ३२ जोड़ दीजिये।

## APPENDIX II
(परिशिष्ट २)

### TEMPERATURE IN FAHRENHEIT AND PULSE RATE PER MINUTE
(फाहरेन्हाइट तापक्रम एवं नाड़ी दर प्रति मिनट)

| Temperature (तापक्रम) | Pulse Rate (नाड़ी दर) |
|---|---|
| 98° | 60 |
| 99° | 70 |
| 100° | 80 |
| 101° | 90 |
| 102° | 100 |
| 103° | 110 |
| 104° | 120 |
| 105° | 130 |
| 106° | 140 |

**Note :—** At the normal temperature of 98.4°F, the pulse rate remains between 60 to 70 per minute, but when the normal temperature rises by 1°F, the pulse rate also increases by 8-10 beats per minute in the same proportion.

टिप्पणी :- ९८.४° फाहरेन्हाइट के सामान्य तापक्रम पर नाड़ी-दर ६०-७० प्रति मिनट रहती है, लेकिन जब सामान्य तापक्रम १° फाहरेन्हाइट बढ़ जाता है तो नाड़ी दर भी उसी अनुपात से ८-१० स्पन्द प्रति मिनट बढ़ जाती है ।

# APPENDIX III
(परिशिष्ट ३)

## NORMAL CHARACTERISTICS OF BODY FLUIDS
(शारीरिक द्रव्यों के सामान्य लक्षण)

Figures having no marked units are based on milligrammes per 100 c.c. (जिन आंकड़ों के आगे कोई इकाई नहीं दी गई है वे प्रति १०० सी.सी.मि.ग्रा. पर आधारित है।)

**Blood** (रक्त)

| | |
|---|---|
| Acetone bodies (एसिटोन पिण्ड) | 0.5–1.0 |
| Albumin (अन्नसार) | 3.6–5.0 Gm. % |
| Albumin/globulin ratio (अन्नसार/ग्लोबुलिन अनुपात) | 1–3 |
| Amino acid, nitrogen (एमिनो एसिड, नाइट्रोजन) | 3.5–5.5 |
| Amino acid (एमिनो अम्ल) | 5.0–8.0 |
| Amylase (एमिलेज) | 50–160 Somoguy units (सोमोगी इकाइयां) |
| Ascorbic acid (एस्कॉर्बिक अम्ल) | 0.7–1.4 |
| Bilirubin (बिलिरुबिन) | 0.3–1.0 |
| Bromides (ब्रोमाइड) | 0.2–1.5 |
| Calcium (कैल्सियम) | 8.5–10.5 |
| Carotine (केरोटिन) | 0.1 |
| Cells (कोशिकायें) | 45–48 |
| Chlorides/Chloride ion (क्लोराइड/क्लोराइड आयन) | 350–380 |
| Chlorides/Sodium chloride (क्लोराइड/सोडियम क्लोराइड) | 570–620 |

(Continued)

## Appendix III continued

| | |
|---|---|
| Colesterol, total (कोलेस्ट्रॉल, कुल) | 140–270 |
| Chholoidal gold (कोलाइडल गोल्ड) | 0–1 Unit (इकाई) |
| Creatine (क्रिएटिन) | 0.2–0.8 |
| Creatinine (क्रिएटिनिन) | 1–2 |
| Erythrocyte Sedimentation Rate (E.S.R.) in first hour (रक्त अवसादन दर, पहले घण्टे में) : | |
| Men (पुरुष) | 3–5 mm fall, Westergren (3–5 मि. मी. जमाव, वेस्टरग्रेन) |
| Women (स्त्रियां) | 7–12 mm fall, Westergren (7–12 मि. मी. जमाव, वेस्टरग्रेन) |
| Newborn (नवजात शिशु) | 0.0–2.0 mm fall, Westergren (0.0–2.0 मि. मी. जमाव, वेस्टरग्रेन) |
| Children (बच्चे) | 9.0 mm fall, Westergren (90 मि. मी. जमाव, वेस्टरग्रेन) |
| Old age and pregnancy (वृद्धावस्था एवं गर्भावस्था) | Slightly increased (हल्की-सी बढ़ी हुई) |
| Fat, neutral (वसा, उदासीन) | 0–370 |
| Fatty acids (वसाम्ल) | 190–450 |
| Fibrinogen (फाइब्रिनजन) | 0.2–0.4 Gm. % |
| Globulin (ग्लोबुलिन) | 1.8–3.2 Gm % |
| Glucose (ग्लूकोज) | 70–120 |
| Guanidine (ग्वानिडीन) | 0.1–0.4 |
| Haemoglobin (रक्तकणरंजकद्रव्य) | 14.8 Gm. % = 100 % |
| Icterus index (कामला सूचकांक) | 4–6 units (4–6 इकाइयां) |
| Iodine (आयोडीन) | 3–13 micrograms (3–13 माइक्रोग्राम) |
| Iron inorganic (लौह, अजैवी) | 0.05–0.18 |

(Continued)

## Appendix III continued

| | |
|---|---|
| Lactic acid (दुग्धाम्ल) | 5–20 |
| Lipase (लाइपेज) | 0.2–1 c.c |
| Lipids, total (लाइपिड कुल) | 450–1000 |
| Magnesium (मैग्नीशियम) | 1.8–2.4 |
| Nitrogen, non-protein (नाइट्रोजन, प्रोटीनरहित) | 25–35 |
| Packed cell volume (संवेष्ठित कोषिका घनत्व) : | |
| Men (पुरुष) | 40–54% |
| Women (स्त्रियां) | 36–47% |
| Phenols, free (फिनोल, मुक्त) | 1–2 |
| Phosphatase, acids (फास्फोटेस, अम्ल) | 0.1–1.1 |
| Phosphatase, alkaline (फास्फोटेस, क्षार) : | |
| Adults (वयस्क) | 1–5.4 |
| Children (बच्चे) | 5–12 |
| Phosphate, inorganic (फॉस्फेट, अजैवी) | 2.5–4.5 |
| Phospholipids (फास्फोलाइपिड) | 150–300 |
| | 6–10 |
| | 2.5 |
| Phosphorus (फास्फोरस) | |
| Phosphorus, inorganic (फास्फोरस, अजैवी) : | |
| Adults (वयस्क) | 3.5–6.0 |
| Children (बच्चे) | 16–22 |
| Plasma (रक्तप्लाविका) | 52–55 |
| | (Continued) |

## Appendix III continued

| | |
|---|---|
| Platelets (बिम्बाणु) | 200000–500000/mm³ |
| Protein (प्रोटीन) | 6.2–8 Gm. % |
| Pyruvate, fasting (पायरूवेट, निराहार) | 0.4–0.7 |
| Red Cell Count, Total (लाल कोशिका गणन, कुल) | 4000000–6000000/mm³ |
| Sodium (सोडियम) | 19–23 |
| Solids (ठोस पदार्थ) | 1.055 |
| Specific gravity (विशिष्ट गुरुत्व) | 1.052–1.063 |
| Sugar, fasting (शर्करा, निराहार): | |
| Venous (शिराजन्य) | 55–90 |
| Capillaries (कोशिकाजन्य) | 60–95 |
| Sugar, PP (शर्करा, साहार) | 80–140 |
| Transferrin (ट्रांसफेरिन) | 120–200 |
| Triglyceride (ट्राइग्लिसराइड) | 2.5–15 |
| Urea (यूरिया) | 18–40 |
| Uric acid (यूरिक अम्ल) | 2.0–7.0 |
| **Volume (घनत्व) :** | |
| Part of body weight (शारीरिक भार का भाग) | 1 / 12th or 8% |
| Per sq. mt. of body surface (शरीर तल का प्रति वर्ग मीटर) | 2.5–4.0 litre (लिटर) |
| Water contents (जल पदार्थ) | 77–81 |
| White cell count (श्वेत कोशिका गणन) | |
| **Total (कुल)** | 4,000–10,000 / mm³ |

(Continued)

## Appendix III continued

**Differential (सर्पक) :**
(1) Polymorphonuclear cells (बहुकेन्द्रककोशिकायें) — 2500–7500/mm$^3$
(2) Eosinophils (इयोसिनरागीकोशिकायें) — 200–400/mm$^3$
(3) Basophils (क्षाररागीकोशिकायें) — 0–50/mm$^3$
(4) Lymphocytes (लसीकाकोशिकायें) — 1,500–2,500/mm$^3$
(5) Monocytes (एककेन्द्रककोशिकायें) — 400–800/mm$^3$

**Percentage (प्रतिशत) :**
(1) **Agranulocytes (अकणिकाकोशिकायें)**
  (i) Lymphocytes (लसीकाकोशिकायें) — 20–40%
  (ii) Monocytes (एकके-द्रककोशिकायें) — 4–8%
(2) **Granulocytes (कणिकाकोशिकायें) :**
  (i) Polymorphonuclear cells (बहुकेन्द्रककोशिकायें) — 50–90%
  (ii) Eosinophils (इयोसिनरागीकोशिकायें) — 1–3%
  (iii) Basophils (क्षाररागीकोशिकायें) — .05–1%

**Cerebrospinal fluid (मस्तिष्क मेरु-द्रव्य) :**
Colour (रंग) — Clear like water, colourless and without clot (पानी जैसा साफ, रंगहीन व थक्केहीन)
Protein (प्रोटीन) — 0.02%
Lymphocytes (लसीकाकोशिकायें) — 2–3 per field (प्रति क्षेत्र)
Polymorph (बहुकेन्द्रककोष) — 0

(Continued)

**Appendix III continued**

**Seminal fluid (वीर्य) :**
- Quantity (मात्रा) — 4 ml. approximately (लगभग ४ मि. लि.)
- Colour (रंग) — Whitish (सफेद-सा)
- Smell (गंध) — Typical seminal (विलक्षण वीर्य जैसा)
- Viscosity (चिपचिपापन) — Highly viscous (अत्यधिक चिपचिपा)
- Reaction (प्रतिक्रिया) — Slightly alkaline (हल्का-सा क्षारक)
- Total number of spermatozoa (शुक्राणुओं की कुल संख्या) — 150–200 million per cubic meter (१५०–२०० दसलक्ष प्रति घन मीटर)

**Sputum (थूक) :**
- Appearance and colour (रूप-रंग) — Transparent and colourless (पारदर्शक और रंगहीन)
- Odour (गंध) — Odourless (गंधहीन)

**Stool (मल) :**
- Quantity in 24 hours (२४ घण्टों में मात्रा) — 200 Gms. (२०० ग्राम.)
- Colour (रंग) — Paler due to milk diet (दुग्धाहार के कारण पीला)
  Black due to iron containing substances in diet (भोजन में लौह पदार्थ होने से काला)
  Dark green due to spinach (पालक खाने से हरा)
- Form and consistency (रूप तथा द्रढ़ता) — Semi-solid (अर्धठोस)
- Frequency in 24 hours (चौबीस घंटों में पुनराव‌ृत्ति) — Once or twice (एक–दो बार)

(Continued)

Appendix III continued
Urine (मूत्र) :

| | |
|---|---|
| Appearance (रूप) | Transparent (पारदर्शक) |
| Colour (रंग) | Amber, sometimes straw-like pale (अम्बर, कभी-कभी हल्का-सा पीला) |
| Odour (गंध) | Aromatic, later ammoniacal (भीनी-भीनी गन्ध वाला, बाद में तीखी गन्ध वाला) |
| Specific gravity (विशिष्ट गुरुत्व) | 1.015–1.025 |
| Average quantity in 24 hours (२४ घण्टे में औसत मात्रा) | 1200–1500 ml. (मि. लि.) |

## APPENDIX IV
(परिशिष्ट ४)
## BLOOD PRESSURE
(रक्त-दाब)

Normal (सामान्य) : Age (आयु) + 90

**Variation in different vessels per minute**
विभिन्न वाहिनियों में प्रति मिनट अन्तर

| Vessel (वाहिनी) | Systolic (प्रकुंचन) | Diastolic (अनुशिथिलन) |
|---|---|---|
| Left ventricle (वाम निलय) | 150 | — |
| Aorta (महाधमनी) | 150 | 100 |
| Brachial artery (भुजण्ड धमनी) | 120 | 80 |
| Radial artery (बहि:प्रकोष्ठिका धमनी) | 100 | 70 |
| Arterioles (धमनिकायें) | 80 | 60 |
| Capillaries (कोशिकायें) | 20 | 20 |
| Small veins (क्षुद्र शिरायें) | 15 | 15 |
| Femoral vein (और्वि शिरा) | 20 | — |
| Inferior vena cava (निम्न महाशिरा) | 3 | — |

**Note :–** The difference between systolic and diastolic pressures is equal to pulse pressure.

टिप्पणी :– प्रकुंचन एवं अनुशिथिलन दाबों के बीच का अंतर नाड़ी दाब के बराबर होता है।

# APPENDIX V
(परिशिष्ट ५)
## CONVERSION OF UNITS
(इकाइयों का रूपान्तरण)

| Unit (इकाई) | Inches to cms. (इंचो से सें.मि.) | Pounds to kg. (पौंड से कि.ग्रा.) | Tola to gms. (तोला से ग्रा.) | Seers to kg. (सेर से कि.ग्रा.) | Miles to kms. (मील से कि.मी.) | Yards to mtrs. (गज से मीटर) | Inches to m.m. (इंच से मि.मी.) | Tons to kilos (टन से किलो) | Gallons to litres (गैलन से लि.) |
|---|---|---|---|---|---|---|---|---|---|
| 1 | 2.54 | 0.45 | 11.66 | 0.93 | 1.61 | 0.91 | 25.40 | 1016.05 | 4.55 |
| 2 | 5.08 | 0.91 | 23.33 | 1.87 | 3.22 | 1.13 | 50.80 | 2032.09 | 9.09 |
| 3 | 7.62 | 1.36 | 34.99 | 2.80 | 4.82 | 2.74 | 76.20 | 3048.14 | 13.64 |
| 4 | 10.16 | 1.81 | 46.66 | 3.73 | 6.44 | 3.66 | 111.60 | 4046.19 | 18.18 |
| 5 | 12.70 | 2.27 | 58.32 | 4.67 | 8.05 | 4.57 | 127.00 | 5080.23 | 22.73 |
| 6 | 15.24 | 2.72 | 69.98 | 5.60 | 9.66 | 5.49 | 152.40 | 6029.28 | 27.28 |
| 7 | 17.78 | 3.18 | 81.65 | 6.53 | 11.27 | 6.40 | 177.80 | 7112.23 | 31.08 |
| 8 | 20.32 | 3.63 | 93.31 | 7.46 | 12.88 | 7.32 | 203.20 | 8128.38 | 36.37 |
| 9 | 22.86 | 4.08 | 104.97 | 8.43 | 14.48 | 8.23 | 228.60 | 9144.42 | 40.91 |
| 10 | 25.40 | 4.54 | 116.64 | 9.33 | 16.09 | 9.14 | 254.00 | 10160.47 | 45.46 |
| 20 | 50.80 | 9.08 | 233.32 | 18.77 | 32.18 | 18.30 | 508.00 | 20320.94 | 90.92 |
| 30 | 76.20 | 13.62 | 350.00 | 28.15 | 48.30 | 27.45 | 752.00 | 30481.41 | 136.38 |
| 40 | 101.60 | 18.16 | 466.64 | 37.54 | 64.40 | 36.60 | 1016.00 | 40641.88 | 18.84 |
| 50 | 127.00 | 22.70 | 583.32 | 46.93 | 80.53 | 45.74 | 1270.00 | 50802.35 | 227.30 |
| 100 | 254.00 | 45.40 | 1166.64 | 93.00 | 161.00 | 91.50 | 2540.00 | 101604.70 | 454.60 |

## APPENDIX VI
(परिशिष्ट ६)
## WEIGHTS AND MEASURES
(वजन तथा माप)

| English (अंग्रेज़ी) | Hindi (हिन्दी) |
|---|---|
| 1 grain = 0.0648 gms. | १ ग्रेन = 0.०६४८ ग्राम |
| 1 scruple = 20 gr. or 1.2959 gms. | १ स्कृपल = २० ग्रेन या १.२९५९ ग्राम |
| 1 drachm = 60 gr. or 3.8879 gms. | १ ड्राम = ६० ग्रेन या ३.८८७९ ग्राम |
| 1 ounce (avoirdupois) = 437 gr. or 28.3495 gms. | १ औंस (एवाइर्डुपोइस) = ४३७ ग्रेन या २८.३४९५ ग्राम |
| 1 ounce (apothecaries or troy) = 480 gr. or 31.1035 gms. | १ औंस (एपोथिकेरीज़ या ट्रॉय) = ४८० ग्रेन या ३१.१०३५ ग्राम |
| 1 pound = 7.000 gr. or 453.59 gms. or 0.4356 kgs. | १ पौंड = ७,००० ग्रेन या ४५३.५९ ग्राम या ०.४३५६ कि.ग्रा. |
| 1 minim = 0.0592 ml. | १ मिनिम = 0.०५९२ मि. लि. |
| 1 fluidrachm = 60 minims or 3.5515 ml. | १ फ्लुइड्राम = ६० मिनिम या ३.५५१५ मि. लि. |
| 1 fluidounce = 8 drachms or 28.4123 ml. | १ फ्लुइडऔंस = ८ ड्राम या २८.४१२३ मि. लि. |
| 1 pint = 20 ounces or 0.5682 litres | १ पिंट = २० औंस या ०.५६८२ लिटर |
| 1 gallon = 8 pints or 4.5459 litres | १ गैलन = ८ पिंट या ४.५४५९ लिटर |
| 1 metre = 39.3701 inches | १ मीटर = ३९.३७०१ इंच |
| 1 decimetre = 3.9370 inches | १ डेसिमीटर = ३.९३७० इंच |
| 1 centimetre = 0.3937 inches | १ सेंटिमीटर = ०.३९३७ इंच |
| 1 millimetre = 0.0393 inches | १ मिलिमीटर = ०.०३९३ इंच |

(Continued)

## TROY WEIGHT
(ट्रॉय भार)

1 Pound = 22.816 cubic inches of distilled water at 62°F.
(१ पौण्ड = ६२° फारेनहाइट पर आसुत जल का २२.८१६ घन इंच)

| Grains (ग्रेन) | Dwt. (पेनीवेट) | Ounces (औंस) | Pound (पौण्ड) |
|---|---|---|---|
| 24 = | 1 | | |
| 480 = | 20 = | 1 | |
| 5760 = | 240 = | 12 = | 1 |

## AVOIRDUPOIS WEIGHT
(एव्वाइर्डुपोइस भार)

1 Pound = 1.2153 pounds troy
(१ पौण्ड = १.२१५३ ट्रॉय पौंड)

| Grains (gr) (ग्रेन) | Drachms (dr.) (ड्राम) | Ounce (oz.) (औंस) | Pound (lb.) (पौण्ड) |
|---|---|---|---|
| 27.34375 = | 1 | | |
| 437.5 = | 16 = | 1 | |
| 7000.0 = | 256 = | 16 = | 1 |

## DOMESTIC DOSES AND THEIR APPROMIMATE EQUALS
(घरेलू मात्रायें तथा उनका निकटस्थ बराबरी का नाप)

| English (अंग्रेजी) | | Hindi (हिन्दी) | |
|---|---|---|---|
| 1 teaspoonful = | 1 drachms | १ चाय का चम्मच = | १ ड्राम |
| 2 desertspoondul = | 2 " | १ मझला चम्मच = | २ ,, |
| 1 tablespoonful = | 1/2 fluid ounce | १ बड़ा चम्मच = | १/२ फ्लुइड औंस |
| 1 wineglassful = | 1-2 fluid ounces or 3-4 tablespoonful | १ छोटा गिलास = | १-२ ,, ,, या ३-४ बड़े चम्मच |
| 1 teacupful = | 4-5 fluid ounces or 8-10 tablespoonful | १ चाय का प्याला = | ४-५ फ्लुइड औंस या ८-१० बड़े चम्मच |

(Continued)

Appendix VI continued

## CONVERSION OF POUNDS TO GRAMS AND KILOGRAMS
(पौण्ड को ग्रामों तथा किलोग्रामों में बदलना)

| Pound(s) (पौण्ड) | Grams (ग्राम) | Kilograms (किलोग्राम) |
|---|---|---|
| 1 | 453.59 | — |
| 2 | 907.18 | — |
| 3 | 1360.78 | 1.36 |
| 4 | 1814.37 | 1.81 |
| 5 | 2267.96 | 2.27 |
| 6 | 2721.55 | 2.72 |
| 7 | 3175.15 | 3.18 |
| 8 | 3628.74 | 3.63 |
| 9 | 4082.23 | 4.08 |
| 10 | 4535.92 | 4.54 |

## APOTHECHARIES' WEIGHT
(एपोथिकेरी भार)

| Grains (gr.) (ग्रेन) | Scruples (स्क्रुपल) | Drams ($\zeta$) (ड्राम) | Troy ounce ($\zeta$) (ट्राय औंस) | Pound (lb) (पौण्ड) |
|---|---|---|---|---|
| 20 | 1 | | | |
| 60 = | 3 = | 1 | | |
| 480 = | 24 = | 8 = | 1 | |
| 5760 = | 288 = | 96 = | 12 = | 1 |

## IMPERIAL MEASURE
(शाही माप)

| Minim (मिनिम) | Fluiddrams (फ्लुइडड्राम) | Fluidounces (फ्लुइडऔंस) | Pints (पिण्ट) | Gallons (गैलन) |
|---|---|---|---|---|
| 60 = | 1 | | | |
| 480 = | 8 = | 1 | | |
| 9,600 = | 160 = | 20 = | 1 | |
| 76,800 = | 1280 = | 160 = | 8 = | 1 |

## APPENDIX VII
(परिशिष्ट ७)

### NUTRIENTS IN FOODSTUFF (per 100 g. of edible portion)
(खाद्यानों में पोषक तत्त्व-आहार योग्य भाग का प्रति १०० ग्राम)

| Name of foodstuff (खाद्यान्न का नाम) | Proteen (g.) (प्रोटीन ग्रा.) | Fat (g.) (वसा ग्रा.) | Carbohydrates (g.) (श्वेतसार ग्रा.) | Energy cal. (ऊर्जा-कैलो.) | Calcium (mg.) (कैल्सियम मि. ग्रा.) | Iron (mg.) (लोहा मि. ग्रा.) |
|---|---|---|---|---|---|---|
| २ | ३ | ४ | ५ | ६ | ७ | |
| **Cereal grains and their products** (अनाज और उनके उत्पाद) | | | | | | |
| Bajra (बाजरा) | 11.6 | 5.0 | 67.5 | 361 | 42 | 5.0 |
| Jawar (ज्वार) | 10.4 | 1.9 | 72.6 | 349 | 25 | 5.8 |
| Maize, dry (मक्की, सूखी) | 11.1 | 3.6 | 66.2 | 342 | 10 | 2.0 |
| Ragi (रागी, जुन्हाई) | 7.3 | 1.3 | 72.0 | 328 | 344 | 6.4 |
| Rice parboiled handpounded (हाथ से कूटे गये, आधे उबले चावल) | 8.5 | 0.6 | 77.4 | 349 | 10 | 2.8 |
| Rice, parboiled milled (मिल के आधे उबले चावल) | 6.4 | 0.4 | 79.0 | 346 | 9 | 4.0 |
| Rice, raw, handpounded (हाथ से कूटे गये कच्चे चावल) | 7.5 | 1.0 | 76.7 | 346 | 10 | 3.2 |
| Rice, raw, milled (मिल के कच्चे चावल) | 6.8 | 0.5 | 78.2 | 345 | 10 | 3.1 |

(Continued)

## Appendix VII continued

| | | | | | |
|---|---|---|---|---|---|
| Rice puffed (चावल मुरमुरा) | 7.5 | 0.1 | 73.6 | 325 | 23 | 6.6 |
| Semolina (सूजी) | 10.4 | 0.8 | 74.8 | 348 | 16 | 1.6 |
| Wheat (गेहूँ) | 11.8 | 1.5 | 71.2 | 346 | 41 | 4.9 |
| Wheat flour (गेहूँ का आटा) | 12.1 | 1.7 | 69.4 | 341 | 48 | 11.5 |
| **Pulses and legumes (दालें और फलियाँ)** | | | | | | |
| Bengal gram (चना) | 17.1 | 5.3 | 60.9 | 360 | 202 | 10.2 |
| Bengal gram dal (दाल चना) | 20.8 | 5.6 | 59.8 | 372 | 56 | 9.1 |
| Black gram dal (उड़द) | 24.0 | 1.4 | 59.6 | 347 | 154 | 9.1 |
| Green gram, whole (साबुत मूंग) | 24.0 | 1.3 | 56.7 | 334 | 124 | 7.3 |
| Green gram dal (दाल मूंग) | 24.5 | 1.2 | 59.9 | 348 | 75 | 8.5 |
| Khesari dal (मल्का) | 28.2 | 0.6 | 56.6 | 345 | 90 | 6.3 |
| Lentil (मसूर) | 25.1 | 0.7 | 59.0 | 343 | 69 | 4.8 |
| Rajmah (राजमा) | 22.9 | 1.3 | 60.6 | 346 | 260 | 5.8 |
| Red gram dal (अरहर) | 22.3 | 1.7 | 57.6 | 335 | 73 | 5.8 |
| Soyabean (सोयाबीन) | 43.2 | 19.5 | 20.9 | 432 | 240 | 11.5 |
| **Leafy Vegetables (पत्तेदार सब्जियाँ)** | | | | | | |
| Amaranth, spined (कांटेदार चौलाई) | 3.0 | 0.3 | 7.0 | 43 | 800 | 22.9 |
| Amaranth, tender (चौलाई का साग) | 4.0 | 0.5 | 6.1 | 45 | 397 | 25.6 |
| Bathua leaves (बथुआ) | 3.7 | 0.4 | 2.9 | 30 | 150 | 4.2 |
| Bengal gram leaves (चने का साग) | 7.0 | 1.4 | 14.1 | 97 | 340 | 23.8 |
| Coriander leaves (हरा धनिया) | 3.3 | 0.6 | 6.3 | 44 | 184 | 18.5 |

(Continued)

## Appendix VII continued

| | | | | | |
|---|---|---|---|---|---|
| Drumstick leaves (सैजना का साग) | 6.7 | 1.7 | 12.5 | 92 | 440 | 7.0 |
| Methi or Fenugreek leaves (मेथी का साग) | 4.4 | 0.9 | 6.0 | 49 | 395 | 16.5 |
| Mint (पुदीना) | 4.8 | 0.6 | 5.8 | 48 | 200 | 15.6 |
| Mustard leaves (सरसों का साग) | 4.0 | 0.6 | 3.2 | 34 | 155 | 16.3 |
| Radish leaves (मूली का साग) | 3.8 | 0.4 | 2.4 | 28 | 265 | 3.6 |
| Spinach (पालक) | 2.0 | 0.7 | 2.9 | 26 | 73 | 10.9 |
| Tamarind leaves, tender (इमली) | 5.8 | 2.1 | 18.2 | 115 | 101 | 5.2 |
| **Radish and Tubers (मूली तथा गांठदार सब्जियाँ)** | | | | | | |
| Carrot (गाजर) | 0.9 | 0.2 | 10.6 | 48 | 80 | 2.2 |
| Colocasia (अर्वी) | 3.0 | 0.1 | 21.1 | 97 | 40 | 1.7 |
| Onion (प्याज) | 1.2 | 0.4 | 11.1 | 50 | 47 | 0.7 |
| Potato (आलू) | 1.6 | 0.1 | 22.6 | 97 | 10 | 0.7 |
| Radish, white (सफेद मूली) | 0.7 | 0.1 | 3.4 | 17 | 35 | 0.4 |
| Sweet potato (शकरकन्द) | 1.2 | 0.3 | 28.2 | 120 | 46 | 0.8 |
| Taplioca (कसावा, दक्षिणी मूल) | 0.7 | 0.2 | 38.1 | 157 | 50 | 0.9 |
| Turnip (शलगम) | 0.5 | 0.2 | 6.2 | 29 | 30 | 0.4 |
| Yam (जिमीकन्द, रतालू) | 1.4 | 0.1 | 26.0 | 111 | 35 | 1.3 |
| **Other Vegetables (अन्य सब्जियाँ)** | | | | | | |
| Beans (फलियाँ, सेम) | 7.4 | 1.0 | 29.8 | 158 | 50 | 2.6 |
| Bottle gourd (लौकी) | 0.2 | 0.1 | 2.5 | 12 | 20 | 0.7 |
| Brinjal (बैंगन) | 1.4 | 0.3 | 4.0 | 24 | 18 | 0.9 |

(Continued)

## Appendix VII continued

| | | | | | | |
|---|---|---|---|---|---|---|
| Cauliflower (फूलगोभी) | 2.6 | 0.4 | 4.0 | 30 | 33 | 1.5 |
| Cucumber (खीरा) | 0.4 | 0.1 | 2.5 | 13 | 10 | 1.5 |
| Ladies fingers (भिण्डी) | 1.9 | 0.2 | 6.4 | 35 | 66 | 1.5 |
| Mango, green (कच्चा आम) | 0.7 | 0.1 | 10.1 | 44 | 10 | 5.4 |
| Peas (मटर) | 7.2 | 0.1 | 15.9 | 93 | 20 | 1.5 |
| Pumpkin (सीताफल) | 1.4 | 0.1 | 4.6 | 25 | 10 | 0.7 |
| Tinda (टिण्डा) | 1.4 | 0.2 | 3.4 | 21 | 25 | 0.9 |
| Tomatoes, green (कच्चे टमाटर) | 1.9 | 0.1 | 3.6 | 23 | 20 | 1.8 |
| **Nuts and Oilseeds (गिरीदार पदार्थ एवं तेल-बीज)** | | | | | | |
| Coconut, dry (सूखा नारियल) | 6.8 | 62.3 | 18.4 | 662 | 40 | 2.7 |
| Coconut, fresh (कच्चा नारियल) | 4.5 | 41.6 | 13.0 | 444 | 10 | 1.7 |
| Gingelly seeds (तिल) | 18.3 | 43.3 | 25.0 | 563 | 1450 | 10.5 |
| Groundnut (मूंगफली) | 25.5 | 40.1 | 26.1 | 567 | 90 | 2.8 |
| Groundnut, roasted (तली हुई मूंगफली) | 26.2 | 39.8 | 26.7 | 570 | 77 | 3.1 |
| Mustard seeds (सरसों) | 20.0 | 39.7 | 23.8 | 541 | 490 | 17.9 |
| Sunflower seeds (सूरजमुखी के बीज) | 19.8 | 52.1 | 17.9 | 620 | 280 | 5.0 |
| Walnut (अखरोट) | 15.6 | 64.5 | 11.0 | 687 | 100 | 4.8 |
| **Condiments and Spices (मिर्च-मसाले)** | | | | | | |
| Chillies, green (हरी मिर्च) | 2.9 | 0.6 | 3.0 | 29 | 30 | 1.2 |
| Ginger, fresh (ताजी अदरक) | 2.3 | 0.9 | 12.3 | 67 | 20 | 2.6 |

(Continued)

Appendix VII continued

| | | | | | | |
|---|---|---|---|---|---|---|
| **Fruits** (फल) | | | | | | |
| Amla (आंवला) | 0.5 | 0.1 | 13.7 | 58 | 50 | 1.2 |
| Apple (सेब) | 0.2 | 0.5 | 13.4 | 59 | 10 | 1.0 |
| Banana, ripe (पका केला) | 1.2 | 0.3 | 27.2 | 116 | 17 | 0.9 |
| Dates, dried (छुवारे) | 2.5 | 0.4 | 75.8 | 317 | 120 | 7.3 |
| Guava (अमरूद) | 0.9 | 0.3 | 11.2 | 51 | 10 | 1.4 |
| Grapes (अंगूर) | 0.5 | 0.3 | 16.5 | 71 | 20 | 0.5 |
| Jack fruit (कटहल) | 1.9 | 0.1 | 19.8 | 88 | 20 | 0.5 |
| Limesweet (मौसम्बी) | 0.8 | 0.3 | 9.3 | 43 | 40 | 0.7 |
| Mango, ripe (पका आम) | 0.6 | 0.4 | 16.9 | 74 | 14 | 1.3 |
| Orange (संतरा) | 0.7 | 0.2 | 10.9 | 48 | 26 | 0.3 |
| Papaya, ripe (पपीता, पका हुआ) | 0.6 | 0.1 | 7.2 | 32 | 17 | 0.5 |
| Pears (नासपाती) | 0.6 | 0.2 | 11.9 | 52 | 8 | 0.5 |
| Phalsa (फालसा) | 1.3 | 0.9 | 14.7 | 72 | 129 | 3.1 |
| Pomegranate (अनार) | 1.6 | 0.1 | 14.5 | 65 | 10 | 0.3 |
| **Fish and other flesh foods** (मछली एवं अन्य मांसाहार) | | | | | | |
| Pomfrets, white (सफेद पाम्फ्रेट) | 17.0 | 1.3 | 1.8 | 87 | 200 | 0.9 |
| Rohu (रौ) | 16.6 | 1.4 | 4.4 | 97 | 650 | 1.0 |
| Egg (अंडा) | 13.3 | 13.3 | — | 173 | 60 | 2.1 |
| Fowl (मुर्गि का मांस) | 25.9 | 0.6 | — | 109 | 25 | |

(Continued)

Appendix VII continued

| | | | | | |
|---|---|---|---|---|---|
| Goat meat (बकरे का मांस) | 21.4 | 3.6 | — | 118 | 12 | — |
| Liver, goat (बकरे की कलेजी) | 20.0 | 3.0 | — | 107 | 17 | — |
| Pork, muscle (सुअर का मांस) | 18.7 | 4.4 | — | 114 | 30 | 2.2 |
| **Milk and milk products** (दूध और दूध से बने पदार्थ) | | | | | | |
| Buffalo milk (भैंस का दूध) | 4.3 | 8.8 | 5.0 | 117 | 210 | 0.2 |
| Cow milk (गाय का दूध) | 3.2 | 4.1 | 4.4 | 67 | 120 | 0.2 |
| Goat milk (बकरी का दूध) | 3.3 | 4.5 | 4.6 | 72 | 170 | 0.3 |
| Human milk (मां का दूध) | 1.1 | 3.4 | 7.4 | 65 | 28 | — |
| Curds (दही) | 3.1 | 4.0 | 3.0 | 60 | 149 | 0.2 |
| Buttermilk (छाछ) | 0.8 | 1.1 | 0.5 | 15 | 30 | 0.8 |
| Channa, buffalo milk (छन्ना, भैंस का दूध) | 13.4 | 23.0 | 7.9 | 292 | 480 | — |
| **Miscellaneous foodstuff** (विविध खाद्यान्न) | | | | | | |
| Bread, brown (भूरी, सिकी हुई रोटी) | 8.8 | 1.4 | 49.0 | 244 | 18 | 2.2 |
| Bread, white (सफेद रोटी) | 7.8 | 0.7 | 51.9 | 245 | 11 | 1.1 |
| Cane sugar (चीनी) | 0.1 | — | 99.4 | 398 | 12 | — |
| Sago (साबूदाना) | 0.2 | 0.2 | 87.1 | 351 | 10 | 1.3 |
| Butter (मक्खन) | — | 81.0 | — | 729 | — | — |
| Ghee, buffalo (भैंस का घी) | — | 100.0 | — | 900 | — | — |
| Cooking oil (खाने के तेल) | — | 100.0 | — | 900 | — | — |

(Continued)

Appendix VII continued

## CALCIUM RICH FOODS–PER 100 G. OF EDIBLE PORTION
(कैल्सियमयुक्त खाद्यान्न आहार योग्य भाग का प्रति १०० ग्राम)

| Foods (खाद्यान्न) | Calcium-mg (कैल्सियम मि. ग्रा.) |
|---|---|
| **Green leafy vegetables (हरी पत्तीदार सब्जियाँ)** | |
| Curry leaves (कड़ी पत्ते) | 830 |
| Amaranth spined (कांटेदार चौलाइ) | 800 |
| Amaranth tender (चौलाइ का साग) | 397 |
| Turnip leave (शलगम का साग) | 710 |
| Colocasia leaves (अर्बी का साग) | 460 |
| Methi leaves (मेथी का साग) | 395 |
| Beet greens (चुकन्दर की पत्तियां) | 380 |
| Radish leaves (मूली की पत्तियां) | 265 |
| Mint (पुदीना) | 200 |
| **Cereals and pulses (अनाज और दालें)** | |
| Ragi (रागी) | 344 |
| Rajmah (राजमा) | 260 |
| Soyabean (सोयाबीन) | 240 |
| Bengal gram, whole (चना साबुत) | 202 |
| **Fish, milk and other milk products** (मछली, दूध एवं अन्य दूग्ध पदार्थ) | |
| Small fish (छोटी मछली) | 790 |
| Milk, buffalo (भैंस का दूध) | 210 |
| Milk, cow (गाय का दूध) | 120 |
| Curds (दही) | 149 |

(Continued)

# ARTICLES OF FOOD RICH IN VITAMINS
(विटामिनों से परिपूर्ण खाद्यान्न)

| English (अंग्रेजी) | Hindi (हिन्दी) |
|---|---|
| **Vitamin A—** (Oil soluble). Essential to normal function of epithelial cells and prevention of eye and skin diseases. It is found in fish, liver, cod liver oil, milk, butter, green leafy vegetables, carrots, etc. | **विटामिन ए :** (तेल में घुलने वाले)। उपकला कोषों (epithelial cells) के साधारण कार्य करने तथा आँखों और चर्म रोगों की रोक-थाम के लिए आवश्यक है। मछली, यकृत्, मछली का तेल, दूध, मक्खन, हरी पत्तीदार सब्जियाँ, गाजर आदि खाद्य-पदार्थों में यह विटामिन होता है। |
| **Vitamin B 1 —** (Water soluble). Promotes growth, aids carbohydrate metabolism, promotes nerve function. It is found in yeast, cereals, meat, pork, egg, liver, egg yolk, nuts, vegetables, etc. | **विटामिन–बी १ :** (पानी में घुलनशील)। शरीर बढ़ाने में सहायक होता है। श्वेतसार के पाचन में सहायता देता है। स्नायु-कार्य गतिशील रखता है। खमीर, दाल, मांस, अण्डा, यकृत्, मेवे तथा हरी सब्जियों इस विटामिन से परिपूर्ण रहती है। |
| **Vitamin B 2 —** (Water soluble). Promotes growth, general health, essential to cellular oxidation. It is found in milk, cheese, meats, liver, organ meat, white egg, etc. | **विटामिन–बी २ :** (पानी में घुलनशील)। यह भी शरीर की बढ़ाने में सहायता देता है। शरीर स्वस्थ रहता है। यह कोशिकाक्षीकरण (cellular oxidation) के लिए आवश्यक है। दूध, पनीर, मांस, यकृत्, इन्द्रिय मांस सफेद अण्डा इस श्रेणी में आते हैं। |

(Continued)

Appendix VII continued

| | | | |
|---|---|---|---|
| **Vitamin B 6 –** | (Water soluble). Essential for cellular functions and metabolism of certain amino-acids. It is found in yeast, liver, meat, whole grain cereals, fish, vegetables, molasses, etc. | **विटामिन-बी ६** | (पानी में घुलनशील)। यह कोशिका-क्रियाओं (cellular functions) तथा कतिपय अमीनो-अम्लों (amino-acids) के पाचन में सहायक होता है। यह खमीर, यकृत, मांस, सभी प्रकार के अनाजों, दालों, मछली तथा हरी सब्जियों, आदि में मिलता है। |
| **Niacin or Nicotinic Acid-** | (Water soluble). Essential for health, tissue respiration, gastro-intestinal functions, prevention of pellagra and skin diseases. It is found in yeast, liver, organ meat, peanuts, wheat germ, etc. | **न्यासिन या निको-टिनिक अम्ल** | (पानी में घुलनशील)। यह स्वास्थ्य के लिए आवश्यक है। यह ऊतक-श्वसन (tissue respiration), जठर क्रिया (gastrointestinal function), पेलेग्रा (pellagra) तथा अन्य चर्म रोगों (skin diseases) की रोकथाम के लिए आवश्यक है। यह खमीर, यकृत, इन्द्रिय-मांस, मटर, नवासा, आदि से उपलब्ध होता है। |

Appendix VII continued

## CALCIUM RICH FOODS–PER 100 G. OF EDIBLE PORTION
(लौहयुक्त खाद्यान्न आहार योग्य भाग का प्रति १०० ग्राम)

| Foods (खाद्यान्न) | Iron-mg. (लोहा-मि. ग्रा.) |
|---|---|
| **Leafy vegetables (पत्तीदार सब्जियाँ)** | |
| Cauliflower (फूल गोभी) | 40.0 |
| Colocasia leaves (अर्बी का साग) | 38.7 |
| Turnip leaves (शलगम का साग) | 28.4 |
| Amaranth tender (चौलाइ का साग) | 25.5 |
| Bengal gram leaves (चने का साग) | 23.8 |
| Coriander (हरा धनियां) | 18.5 |
| Methi leaves (मेथी का साग) | 16.5 |
| Beet greens (चुकन्दर की पत्तियां) | 16.2 |
| Mint (पुदीना) | 15.6 |
| **Cereals (अनाज)** | |
| Whole wheat flour (गेहूं का चोकरयुक्त आटा) | 11.5 |
| Soyabean (सोयाबीन) | 11.5 |
| Bengal gram, whole (साबुत चना) | 9.5 |
| Bajra (बाजरा) | 5.0 |
| **Flesh foods (मांसाहार)** | |
| Liver, sheep (भेड़ की कलेजी) | 6.3 |
| Mutton, muscle (मांस, बोटी) | 2.5 |
| Egg, hen (मुर्गी का अण्डा) | 2.1 |

# APPENDIX VIII
(परिशिष्ट ८)

## DIETARY ALLOWANCES IN DIABETES
(मधुमेह में आहार की मात्रा)

| Height (ऊंचाई) | Calories per day (दैनिक कैलोरी) | Proteins (gm.) (प्रोटीन) (ग्रा.) | Fats (gm.) (वसा) (ग्रा.) | Carbohydrates (gm.) (श्वेतसार) (ग्रा.) |
|---|---|---|---|---|
| **To reduce weight (भार घटाने के लिये)** | | | | |
| Short (छोटा कद) | 800 | 60 | 15 | 100 |
| Medium (मझला कद) | 1,000 | 70 | 25 | 110 |
| Tall (लम्बा कद) | 1,200 | 80 | 35 | 125 |
| **To maintain ideal weight (उपयुक्त भार के लिये)** | | | | |
| Short (छोटा कद) | 1,800 | 80 | 85 | 180 |
| Medium (मझला कद) | 2,400 | 90 | 115 | 250 |
| Tall (लम्बा कद) | 2,700 | 100 | 120 | 300 |
| **To increase weight (भार बढ़ाने के लिये)** | 2,900 | 120 | 120 | 350 |

**N.B.** Fat contents of these diets should be reduced in case of acetonuria and arteriosclerotic patients.

टिप्पणी :— एसिटोन्यूरिया तथा धमनीकाठिन्य से पीड़ित रोगियों के लिये वसा की मात्रा कम कर देनी चाहिये ।

(Continued)

Appendix VIII continued

## DAILY DIET FOR THE DIABETICS
(मधुमेहग्रस्त रोगियों के लिये दैनिक आहार)

| For non-vegetarian patients (मांसाहारी रोगियों के लिये) | | | For vegetarian patients (शाकाहारी रोगियों के लिये) | |
|---|---|---|---|---|
| Atta (आटा) | 110 | G. (ग्रा.) | Atta (आटा) | 110 G. (ग्रा.) |
| Rice (चावल) | 60 | " | Rice (चावल) | 60 " |
| Pulse (दाल) | 60 | " | Pulse (दाल) | 60 " |
| Green leaf vegetables (हरी पत्तीदार सब्जियाँ) | 160 | " | Green leaf vegetables (हरी पत्तीदार सब्जियाँ) | 160 " |
| Other vegetables (अन्य सब्जियाँ) | 340 | " | Other vegetables (अन्य सब्जियाँ) | 340 " |
| Meat & fish (मांस-मछली) | 160 | " | Cheese (पनीर) | 110 " |
| Fats and oils (वसा और तेल) | 60 | " | Curds (दही) | 230 " |
| Brown bread slices (भूरी डबल रोटी के स्लाइस) | 2 | " | Fats and oils (वसा और तेल) | 60 " |
| Eggs (अण्डे) | 2 | " | Fruit (फल) | 1 " |
| Fruit (फल) | 1 | " | | |

**N.B.** 1. Other cereal preparations can be substituted for Atta. Rice and Brown bread.

2. Other vegetables should be of low carbohydrate value.

3. The diet prescribed above is meant for an adult diabetic of normal weight and height requiring 1800 calories.

टिप्पणी— १. आटा, चावल तथा भूरी डबल रोटी के स्लाइसों के बदले दूसरे अनाज भी दिये जा सकते है।

२. अन्य सब्जियों में श्वेतसार की कम मात्रा होनी चाहिये।

३. उपरोक्त आहार उस सामान्य शारीरिक भार तथा कद वाले व्यक्क रोगी के लिये निर्धारित किया गया है जिसे १८०० कैलोरियों की आवश्यकता होती है।

(Continued)

Appendix VIII continued

## DIVISION OF DAILY DIETETIC REQUIREMENT OF DIABETICS
(मधुमेहग्रस्त रोगियों के दैनिक आहार का विभाजन)

| For non-vegetarian (मांसाहारियों के लिये) | | For vegetarian (शाकाहारियों के लिये) | |
|---|---|---|---|
| **Breakfast** (सुबह का नाश्ता) | | **Breakfast** (सुबह का नाश्ता) | |
| Bread-slice (स्लाइस) | 1 | Bread-slice (स्लाइस) | 1 |
| Egg (अण्डा) | 1 | Fruit or Kheera (फल या खीरा) | 1 |
| Milk (दूध) | 1 | Milk (दूध) | 1cup (प्याला) |
| **Mid-day meal** (दोपहर का भोजन) | | **Mid-day meal** (दोपहर का भोजन) | |
| Roties/Chapaties (चपाती) | 2 | Roties/Chapaties (चपाती) | 2 |
| Dal (दाल) | 1 plate (प्लेट) | Curds (दही) | 1 plate (प्लेट) |
| Meat or fish (मांस-मछली) | 1 plate (प्लेट) | Green vegetables (हरी सब्जियाँ) | 1 plate (प्लेट) |
| Salad (सलाद) | 1 plate (प्लेट) | Salad (सलाद) | 1 plate (प्लेट) |
| **Tea** (चाय) | | **Tea** (चाय) | |
| Bread-slice (स्लाइस) | 1 | Bread-slice (स्लाइस) | 1 |
| Tea without sugar (बिना चीनी की चाय) | 2 cups (कप) | Tea without sugar (बिना चीनी की चाय) | 2 cups (कप) |
| **Dinner** (रात का भोजन) | | **Dinner** (रात का भोजन) | |
| Roties/Chapaties (चपाती) | 2 | Roties/Chapaties (चपाती) | 2 |
| Dal (दाल) | 1 plate (प्लेट) | Dal or curd (दाल या दही) | 1 plate (प्लेट) |
| Meat or fish (मांस-मछली) | 1 plate (प्लेट) | Green vegetables (हरी सब्जियाँ) | 1 plate (प्लेट) |

(Continued)

Appendix VIII continued

Salad with leafy vegetables (पत्तीदार सब्जियों का सलाद) 1 plate

Salad with tomatoes and leafy vegetables 1 plate (स्लेट)
(टमाटर सहित हरी पत्तीदार सब्जियों का सलाद)

टिप्पणी :-

उपर्युक्त आहार तालिका केवल ऐसी अवस्थाओं में जारी रखनी चाहिये जब रोगी का पेशाब शर्करारहित हो, उसमें रक्तशर्करा की मात्रा सामान्य हो और रोगी हृष्ट-पुष्ट रहे। परन्तु मूत्र में यदि शर्करा की मात्रा असामान्य हो जाये और रक्तशर्करा में बृद्धि हो जाये तो मधुमेहरोधक चिकित्सा दी जानी चाहिये।

N.B.:—

This menu of diet should be continued if the patient's urine is free from sugar, his fasting sugar is within normal limits and he feels energetic and fit. But if sugar in urine becomes abnormal and the fasting blood sugar rises, the antidiabetic treatment should be given to restore the patient to normal.

(Continued)

Appendix VIII continued

## DIETARY ACCORDING OF THE TYPE OF PATIENT
(रोगी के व्यक्तिगत स्वरूप पर आधारित भोजन)

| Type of patient (रोगी का स्वरूप) | Calories (कैलोरी) | Proteins (gm.) (प्रोटीन) (ग्राम) | Fats (gm.) (वसा) (ग्राम) | Carbohydrates (gm.) (श्वेतसार) (ग्राम) |
|---|---|---|---|---|
| Child 3 to 4 year (३-४ वर्ष का बच्चा) | 1,300 | 65 | 60 | 130 |
| Child 7 to 8 year (७-८ वर्ष का बच्चा) | 1,900 | 86 | 92 | 175 |
| Child 11 to 12 year (११-१२ वर्ष का बच्चा) | 2,200 | 103 | 99 | 220 |
| Child 14 to 17 year (१४-१७ वर्ष का बच्चा) | 2,400 | 110 | 109 | 240 |
| Young females (नवयुवतियाँ) | 2,200 | 107 | 97 | 225 |
| Women in later half of pregnancy (उत्तरार्ध गर्भावस्था में स्त्रियाँ) | 2,400 | 117 | 109 | 240 |
| Hardworking men (कठोर परिश्रम करने वाले पुरुष) | 2,600 | 121 | 121 | 225 |
| Middle-aged women (अधेड़ आयु की स्त्रियाँ) | 1,700 | 80 | 78 | 165 |
| Middle-aged men with sedentary occupations (अधेड़ आयु के पुरुष जो बैठे-बैठे काम करते है) | 2,000 | 99 | 95 | 180 |
| Obese women treated with diet alone (मोटी औरतें जिन्हें मात्र आहार-चिकित्सा दी जाती है) | 1,000 | 52 | 42 | 105 |
| Elderly diabetics treated with diet alone (वयोवृद्ध मधुमेहग्रस्त रोगी जिन्हें मात्र आहार-चिकित्सा दी जाती है) | 1,500 | 68 | 67 | 150 |

## APPENDIX IX
(परिशिष्ट ९)

## ABBREVIATIONS AND SYMBOLS USED IN PRESCRIPTIONS
(औषध-निर्देश पत्र में प्रयुक्त संक्षिप्त शब्द एवं चिन्ह)

| Abbreviations (संक्षिप्त शब्द) | Latin (लैटिन) | English (अंग्रेजी) | Hindi (हिन्दी) |
|---|---|---|---|
| aa | Ana | Of each | प्रत्येक का |
| Abs. febr. | Absente febre | In the absence of fever | अज्वरावस्था में |
| Ad. | Adde | Add | मिलाइये |
| Ad. 2 vic. | Ad daus vices | At twice taking | दो बार लेने पर |
| Aeq. | Aequales | Equal | बराबर |
| Admov. | Admove | Apply | प्रयोग कीजिये |
| Ad. us. ext. | Ad usum externum | For external use | बाह्री प्रयोग के लिये |
| Agit. | Agita | Shake or Stir | हिलाइये |
| Alt. noc. | Alternis nocte | Every other night | हर दूसरी रात |
| Aq. | Aqua | Water | जल, पानी |
| Aq. bull. | Aqua bulliens | Boiling water | उबलता पानी |

(Continued)

## Appendix IX continued

| Abbreviation | Latin | English | Hindi |
|---|---|---|---|
| Aq. com. | Aqua communis | Common water | सामान्य जल |
| Aq. dest. | Aqua destillata | Distilled water | आसुत जल |
| Aq. ferv. | Aqua fervens | Hot water | गरम जल |
| Aq. font. | Aqua fontana | Spring water | चश्मे का पानी |
| Aq. Pur. | Aqua pura | Pure water | शुद्ध जल |
| B.D. | Bis in die | Twice daily | दिन में दो बार |
| Bib. | Bibe | Drink | पीजिये |
| B.I.D. | Bis in die | Twice daily | दिन में दो बार |
| Bis in 7 d. | Bis in septem diebus | Twice a week | सप्ताह में दो बार |
| ℞ | Cum | with | साथ |
| C | — | Centesimal | शतमलव |
| C.M. | Cras mane | Tomorrow morning | कल सुबह |
| C.N. | Cras nocte | Tomorrow night | कल रात |
| C.N. | — | Common name | सामान्य नाम |
| Cochl. | Cochleare | Spoonful | चम्मच भर |
| Cochl. inf. (min.) | Cochleare infantin minimum | A teaspoonful | एक चाय का चम्मच भर |
| Cont. rem. | — | Let the medicine be continued | औषधि जारी रखिये |
| Crast | — | Tomorrow | कल |
| C.V. | Cras vespere | Tomorrow evening | कल शाम |
| Cyath. | Cyathus | A glassful | एक गिलास भर |
| D. | Dosis | A dose | एक मात्रा |

(Continued)

## Appendix IX continued

| | | | |
|---|---|---|---|
| D. | — | Decimal | दशमलव, दशमिक |
| d. | Da | Give | दीजिये |
| Det. | Detut | Let it be given | इसे देने दीजिये |
| Dieb. alt. | Diebus alternis | On alternate day | हर तीसरे दिन/एक दिन छोड़ कर |
| Dieb. tart. | — | Every third day | हर तीसरे दिन |
| Dim. | Dimiduis | One-half | आधा, अर्ध |
| Dil. | — | Dilution | तनूकरण |
| D.V. | — | Divide | बांट दीजिये |
| D.W. | Aqua destillata | Distilled water | आसुत जल |
| F. Mist. | Fiat mistura | Make a mixture | मिश्रण बनाइये |
| F. Pulv. | Fiat pulvis | Make a powder | विचूर्ण बनाइये |
| Fl. | — | Fluid | द्रव, तरल |
| Ft. | — | Let it be made | इसे बनने दीजिये |
| H.D. | Hora decubitus | At going to bed | सोते समय |
| G., Gm. | Gramme | Gram | ग्राम |
| Gr. | Granum | Grain | ग्रेन |
| G., Gtts. | Gutta or Guttage | Drop or drops | बूंद, बिन्दु या बूंदें |
| Garg. | Garagrisme | A gargle | गरारा |
| Hor. | Horis | Hour | घंटा |
| H.S. | Hora somni | Just before going to bed | सोने से ठीक पहले |
| H.S.S. | Hora somni sumendum | To be taken at bed time | सोते समय लीजिये |

(Continued)

## Appendix IX continued

| | | | |
|---|---|---|---|
| In. d. | In dies | Daily | रोज |
| M., Mist. | Misce | Mix | मिलाइये |
| m. | minim | A drop | एक बूंद |
| m. et n. | mane et nocte | Morning and night | सुबह और रात |
| Mg. | — | Milligram | मिलिग्राम |
| Ml. | — | Millilitre | मिलिलिटर |
| Ne tr. s. num | ne trades sine nummo | Deliver not without money | पैसे बिना मत दीजिये |
| n. r., non rep. | Non-repetatur | Let it not be repeated | इसे मत दुहराइये |
| O.H. | Omni horis | Every hour | प्रति घंटा, हर घंटे में |
| O.M. | Omni mane | Every morning | रोज सुबह, नित्य प्रात: |
| Omn. bih. | Omni bihora | Every two hours | हर दो घण्टे में |
| O.N. | Omni nocte | Every night | रोज रात को, नित्य राति |
| Om. 1/4h. | Omni quadrantee horis | Every 15 minutes | हर पन्द्रह मिनट बाद |
| P.C. | Post cibus | After food | खाने के बाद |
| Pr. C. | Prumis cibus | Before food | खाने से पहले |
| P. a.a. | Parti affectae applicetur | Let it be applied to the affected parts | रोगग्रस्त भाग पर इसे लगाइये |
| P., Pt. | Persteture | Continue | जारी रखिये |
| P.R. | Per rectum | By the rectum | मलांत्र द्वारा |
| P.V. | Per vaginum | By the vagina | योनि द्वारा |
| Q.I.D. | Quarter in die | Four times a day | दिन में चार बार |

(Continued)

## Appendix IX continued

| Abbr. | Latin | English | Hindi |
|---|---|---|---|
| Q.L. | Quantum libet | As much as required | आवश्यकतानुसार |
| Q.S. | Quantum sufficiant | Sufficient quantity | अपेक्षित मात्रा |
| ℞ | Recipe | Take | लीजिये |
| Stat. | Statim | Immediately | तुरन्त |
| Semi. h. | Semihora | Half an hour | आधे घण्टे में |
| Sol. | — | Solution | घोल |
| S.O.S. | Si-opus-sit | If necessary | यदि आवश्यक हो तो |
| SS | Semi or Semissis | A half | आधा, अर्ध |
| Syn. | — | Synonym | पर्यायवाची |
| T.D., T.I.D. | Ter in die | Three times a day | दिन में तीन बार |
| Tr. | — | Tincture | मूलार्क, अर्क |
| Trit. | — | Trituration | अवचूर्ण |
| Vac. Ven. | Vacuo ventriculo | On an empty stomach | खाली पेट |
| Ve. | Vel | Or | या |
| Wt. | — | Weight | भार |

## SOME IMPORTANT SIGNS (कुछ प्रमुख चिन्ह)

| | | |
|---|---|---|
| φ | Mother Tincture | मूलार्क, अर्क |
| X | Decimal | दशमलव, दशमिक |
| ℥i | A tea spoonful | चाय का चम्मच भर |
| ℥ii | A desert spoonful | मझला चम्मच भर |
| ℥iv or ℥ss | A table spoonful | बड़ा चम्मच भर |
| ℥ss | Half ounce | आधा औंस |
| ℥iss | One and a half ounce | डेढ़ औंस |

# SOME OF THE IMPORTANT
## ANATOMICAL CHARTS
### RELATING TO HUMAN BODY

# CHART NO. 1
# DIAGRAMMATIC REPRESENTATION OF SOME OF THE PARTS OF BODY
(शरीर के कुछ भागों का आरेखित चित्र)

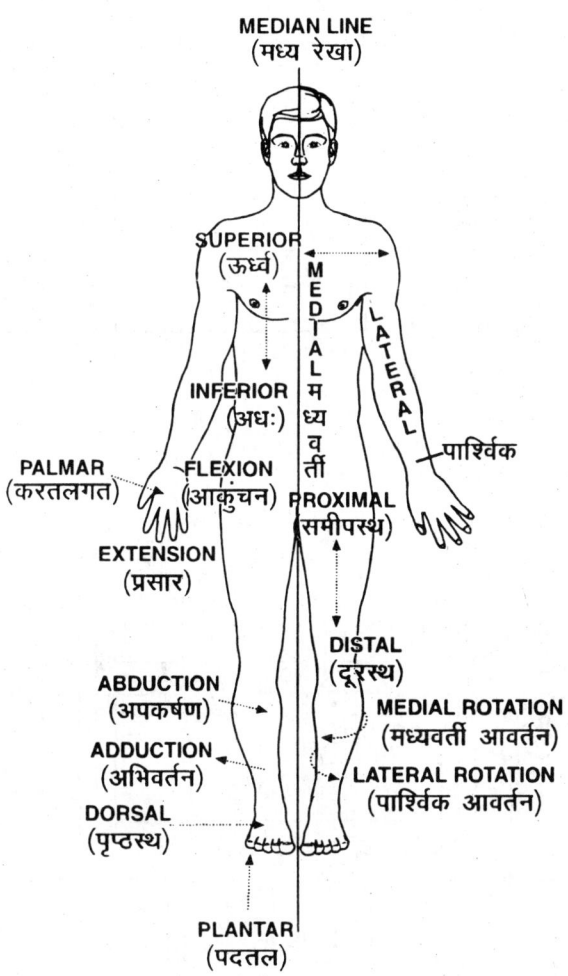

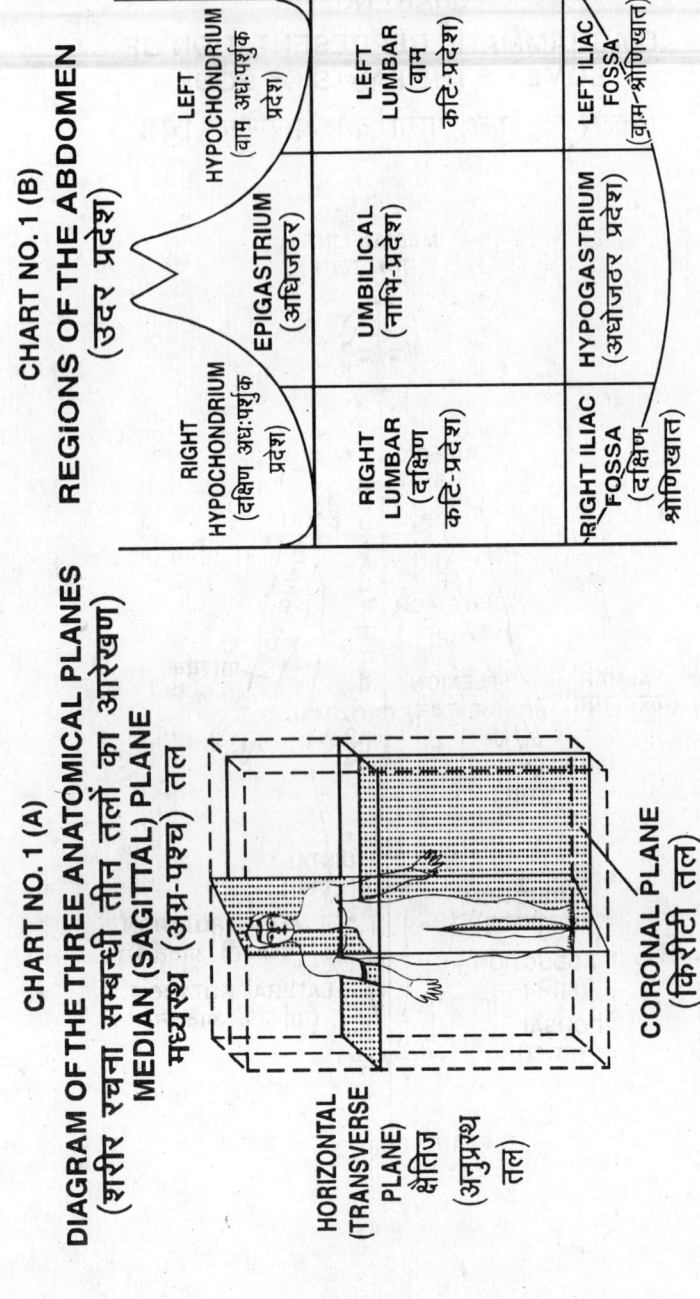

## CHART NO. 2
## THE SKELETON
(पंजर)

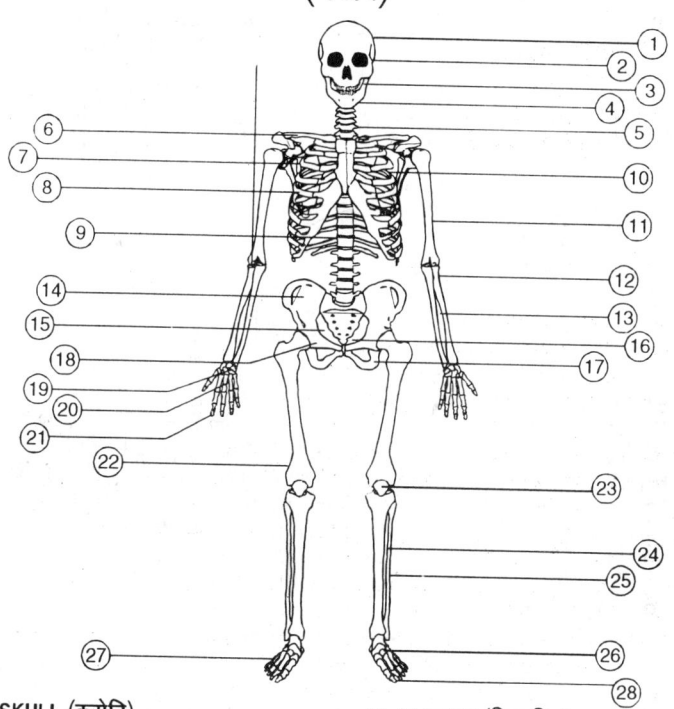

1. SKULL (करोटि)
2. ORBIT (नेत्रकोटर)
3. ZYGOMATIC ARCH (गण्ड-चाप)
4. MANDIBLE (अधोहनु)
5. CERVICAL VERTEBRAE (ग्रीवा-कशेरुकायें)
6. CLAVICLE (कण्ठास्थि)
7. SCAPULA (स्कन्ध/कंधा)
8. STERNUM (उरोस्थि)
9. THORACIC VERTEBRAE (वक्ष-कशेरुकायें)
10. RIBS (पर्शुकाएं)
11. HUMERUS (प्रगण्डिका)
12. RADIUS (त्रिज्या)
13. ULNA (अन्तःप्रकोष्ठिका)
14. ILIUM (श्रोणिफलक)
15. SACRUM (त्रिकास्थि)
16. COCCYX (पुच्छास्थि)
17. ISCHIUM (नितम्बास्थि)
18. PUBIS (जघनास्थि)
19. CARPALS (मणिबन्ध)
20. METACARPALS (करभिकास्थियाँ)
21. PHALANGES (अंगुल्यस्थियाँ)
22. FEMUR (ऊर्वस्थि)
23. PATELLA (जान्वस्थि)
24. TIBIA (अन्तर्जंघिका)
25. FIBULA (बहिर्जंघिका)
26. TARSALS (गुल्फ)
27. METATARSALS (प्रपदिकास्थियाँ)
28. PHALANGES (अंगुल्यस्थियाँ)

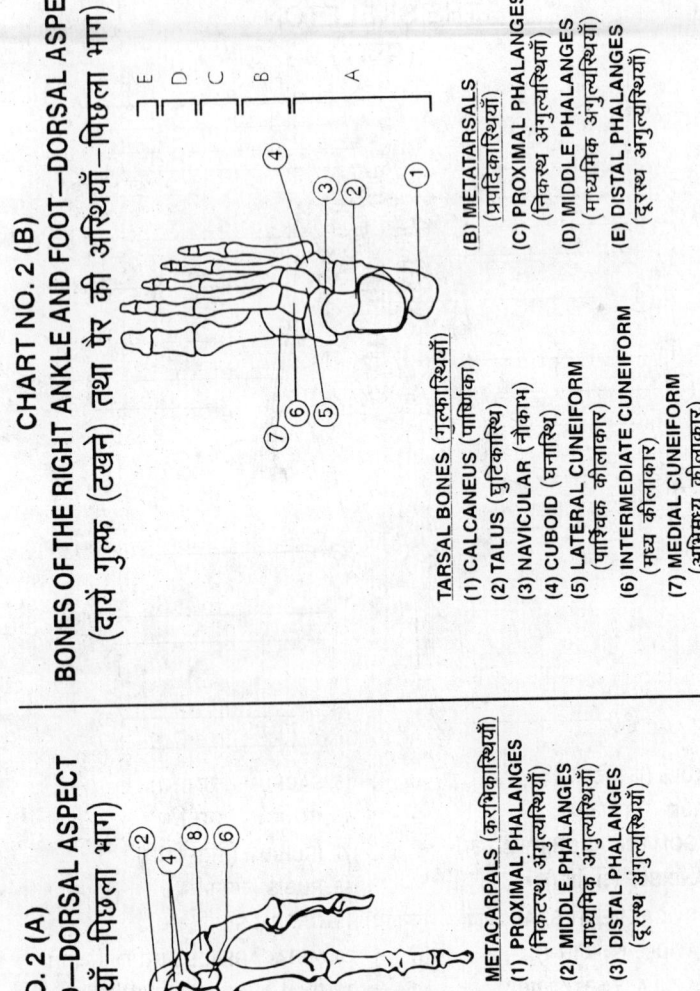

# CHART NO. 3
## THE MAIN ARTERIES OF HUMAN BODY
### (मानव शरीर की प्रमुख धमनियाँ)

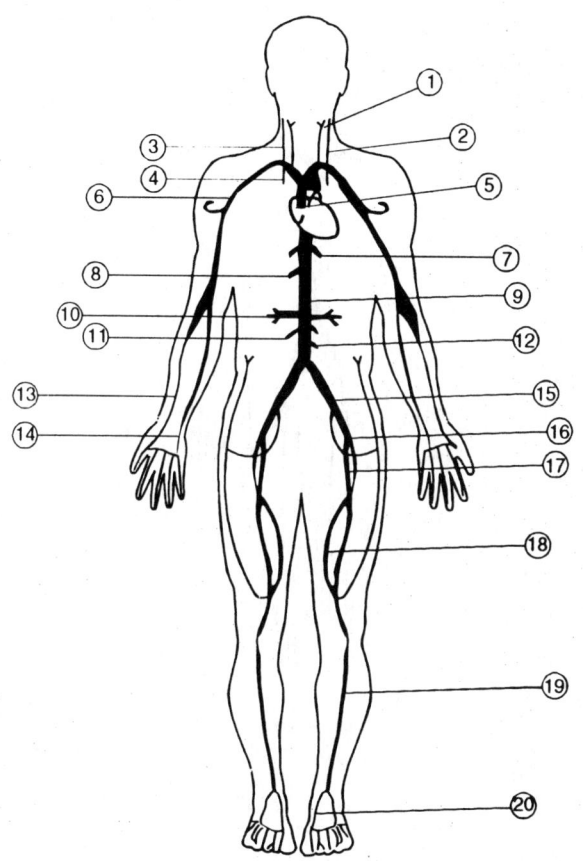

(1) COMMON CAROTID (सामान्य मन्या-)
(2) VERTEBRAL (कशेरुका-)
(3) SUBCLAVIAN (अधोजत्रुक-)
(4) LONG THORACIC (दीर्घवक्ष-)
(5) AORTA (महाधमनी)
(6) AXILLARY (कक्षा-)
(7) CELIAC (कुक्षि-)
(8) SUPERIOR MESENTERIC (ऊर्ध्व आंत्रयोजनी)
(9) ABDOMINAL AORTA (औदरिक महाधमनी)
(10) RENAL (वृक्क-)
(11) GONADAL (जननग्रंथि-)
(12) INFERIOR MESENTERIC (अघः आंत्रयोजनी)
(13) RADIAL (बहिः प्रकोष्ठिका-)
(14) ULNAR (अन्तः प्रकोष्ठिका-)
(15) COMMON ILIAC (सामान्य श्रोणिफलक-)
(16) INTERNAL ILIAC (अन्तः श्रोणिफलक-)
(17) FEMORAL (ऊर्वी-)
(18) PROFUNDA FEMORIS (गभीर ऊरु-)
(19) ANTERIOR TIBIAL (अग्रअंतर्जंघिका-)
(20) DORSALIS PEDIS (पादपृष्ठ-)

# CHART NO. 4

## THE MAIN VEINS OF HUMAN BODY
### (मानव शरीर की प्रमुख शिरायें)

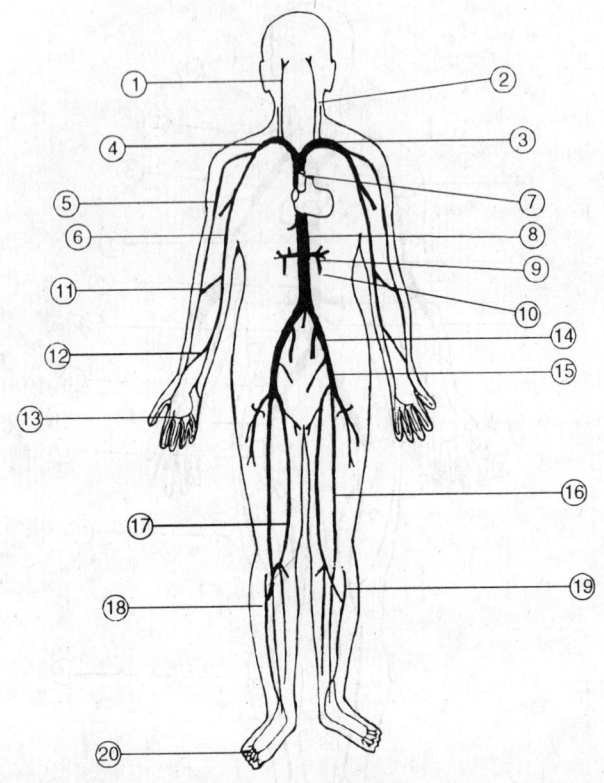

(1) INTERNAL JUGULAR (अन्तर्कण्ठ-)
(2) EXTERNAL JUGULAR (बहिर्कण्ठ-)
(3) SUBCLAVIAN (अधोजत्रुक-)
(4) BRACHIOCEPHALIC (बाहुशीर्ष-)
(5) CEPHALIC (प्रमस्तिष्क-)
(6) BRACHIAL (प्रगण्ड-)
(7) SUPERIOR VENA CAVA (ऊर्ध्व महाशिरा-)
(8) INFERIOR VENA CAVA (अधः महाशिरा-)
(9) RENAL (वृक्क-)
(10) GONADAL (जननग्रंथि-)
(11) MEDIAN CUBITAL (माध्यमिक प्रकोष्ठ-)
(12) BASILIC (अन्तःबाहु-)
(13) SUPERFICIAL PALMAR (उपरिस्थ करतल-)
(14) COMMON ILIAC (सामान्य श्रोणिफलक-)
(15) EXTERNAL ILIAC (बाह्य श्रोणिफलक-)
(16) FEMORAL (औरी-)
(17) GREAT SAPHENOUS (महा जतूक-)
(18) SMALL SAPHENOUS (लघु जतूक-)
(19) ANTERIOR TIBIAL (अग्र अन्तर्जंघिका-)
(20) DORSAL VENOUS ARCH (पृष्ठ-शिरा-चाप)

## CHART NO. 5

## DIAGRAMMATIC REPRESENTATION OF SOME OF THE IMPORTANT LYMPH NODES IN THE HUMAN BODY
(मानव शरीर में व्याप्त कुछ प्रमुख लसीका-पर्वों का आरेखण)

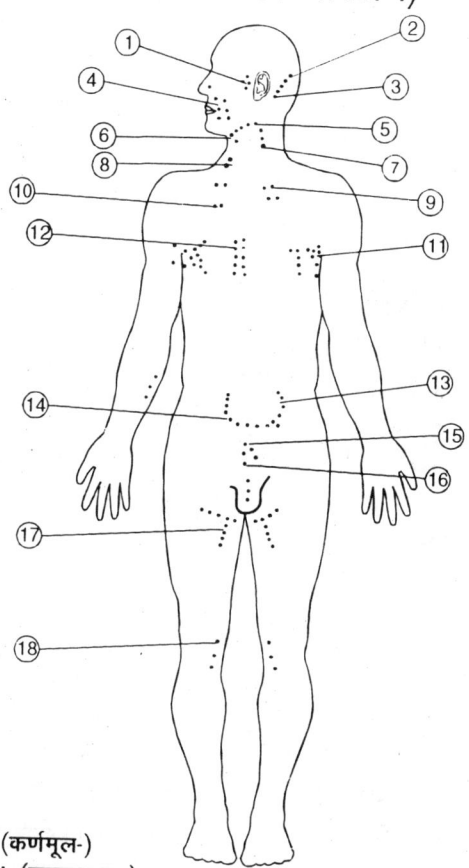

(1) PAROTID (कर्णमूल-)
(2) OCCIPITAL (पश्चकपाल-)
(3) POST AURICULAR (पृष्ठकर्ण-)
(4) FACIAL (आनन-)
(5) SUBMANDIBULAR (अवअधोहनु-)
(6) SUBMENTAL (अवचिवुक-)
(7) CERVICAL (ग्रीवा-)
(8) ANTERIOR CERVICAL (अग्रग्रीवा-)
(9) SUPRACLAVICULAR (अधिजत्रुक-)
(10) APICAL (शिखर)
(11) AXILLARY (कक्षा-)
(12) INTERCOSTAL (अन्तरापर्शुक-)
(13) SMALL INTESTINAL (लघ्वांत्र-)
(14) LARGE INTESTINAL (बृहदांत्र-)
(15) LUMBAR (कटि-)
(16) ILEAL (शेषांत्र-)
(17) SUPERFICIAL INGUINAL (उपरिस्थ वंक्षण-)
(18) POPLITEAL (जानुपृष्ठ-)

## CHART NO. 6

## LATERAL SIDE-VIEW OF THE SKULL
### (खोपड़ी के पिछले भाग का दृश्य)

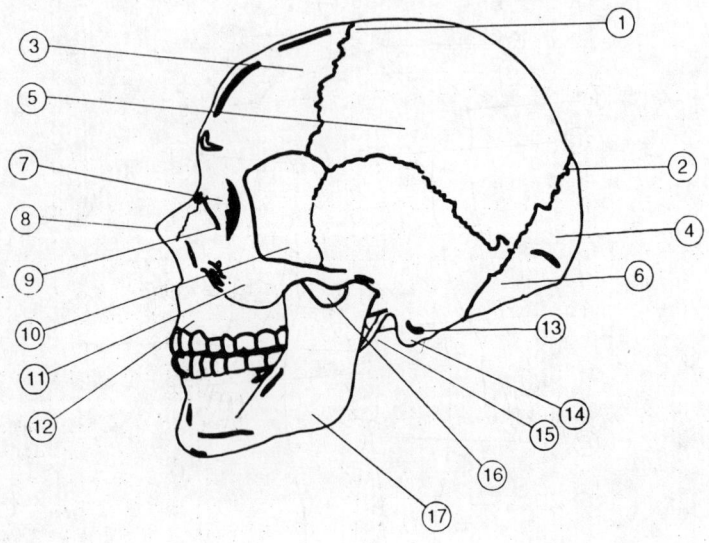

1. CORONAL SUTURE (किरीट सीवन)
2. LAMBDOID SUTURE (काकपद सीवन)
3. FRONTAL BONE (लटास्थि)
4. OCCIPITAL BONE (पश्च-कपालास्थि)
5. PARIETAL BONE (पाश्विकास्थि)
6. TEMPORAL BONE (शंखास्थि)
7. ETHMOID BONE (झर्झरिकास्थि)
8. NASAL BONE (नासास्थि/नासिकास्थि)
9. ORBIT (नेत्रकोटर)
10. SPHENOID BONE (जतूकास्थि)
11. ZYGOMATIC BONE (गण्डास्थि)
12. MAXILLA (ऊर्ध्वहन्वास्थि)
13. EXTERNAL ACOUSTIC MEATUS (बाह्य श्रवण कुहर)
14. MASTOID PROCESS (कर्णमूलास्थि)
15. STYLOID PROCESS (शलाखास्थि)
16. ZYGOMATIC ARCH (गण्ड-चाप)
17. MANDIBLE (अधोहन्वस्थि)

## CHART NO. 7
## DIAGRAM OF THE HEART
### (हृदय का चित्र)

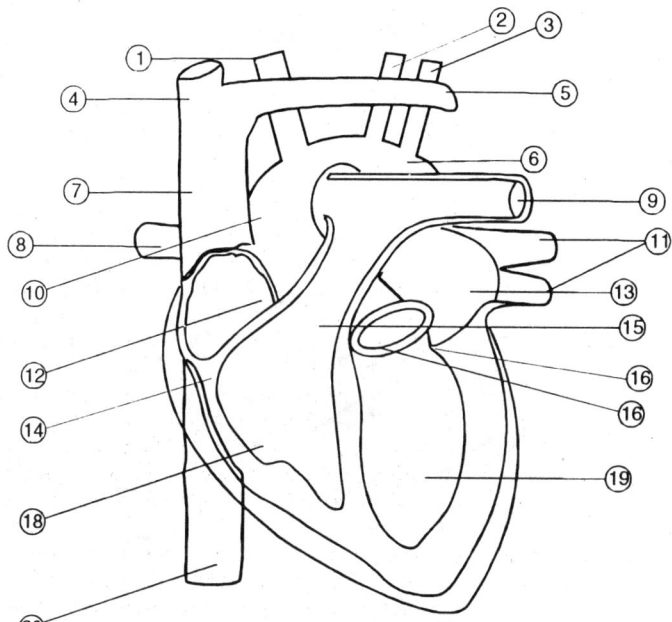

(1) BRACHIOCEPHALIC ARTERY (प्रगण्ड शीर्ष-धमनी)
(2) LEFT COMMON CAROTID ARTERY (वाम सामान्य मन्या-धमनी)
(3) LEFT SUBCLAVIAN ARTERY (वाम अवजत्रुक-धमनी)
(4) RIGHT BRACHIOCEPHALIC VEIN (दक्षिण प्रगण्डशीर्ष-शिरा)
(5) LEFT BRACHIOCEPHALIC VEIN (वाम प्रगण्डशीर्ष-शिरा)
(6) ARCH OF AORTA (महाधमनी-चाप)
(7) SUPERIOR VENA CAVA (ऊर्ध्व महाशिरा)
(8) RIGHT PULMONARY ARTERY (दक्षिण फुप्फुस-धमनी)
(9) LEFT PULMONARY ARTERY (वाम फुप्फुस-धमनी)
(10) ASCENDING AORTA (आरोही महाधमनी)
(11) PULMONARY VEIN (फुप्फुस-शिरा)
(12) RIGHT ATRIUM (दक्षिण अलिन्द)
(13) LEFT ATRIUM (वाम अलिन्द)
(14) TRICUSPID VALVE (त्रिकपर्दी कपाट)
(15) PULMONARY VALVE (फुप्फुस-कपाट)
(16) MITRDAL VALVE (द्विकपर्दी कपाट)
(17) AORTIC VALVE (महाधमनी-कपाट)
(18) RIGHT VENTRICLE (दक्षिण निलय)
(19) LEFT VENTRICLE (वाम निलय)
(20) INFERIOR VENA CAVA (निम्न महाशिरा)

# CHART NO. 8
## DIAGRAM SHOWING MID-SAGITTAL SECTION OF THE BRAIN
(मस्तिष्क के मध्यतल के अगले-पिछले अनुभाग का आरेखित दृश्य)

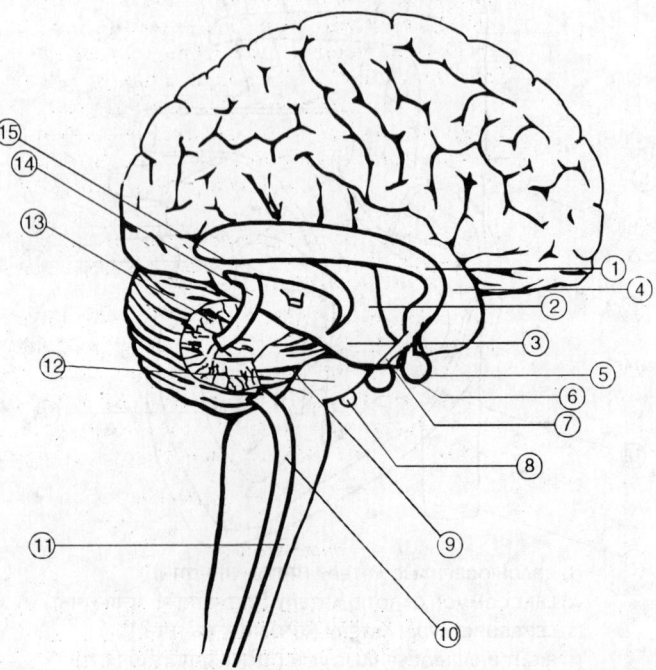

1. CORPUS CALLOSUM (महासंयोजक पिण्ड)
2. FORNIX CEREBRI (प्रमस्तिष्क चापिका)
3. THALAMUS (चेतक)
4. HYPOTHALAMIC SULCUS (अधःश्चेतक परिखा)
5. OPTIC CHIASMA (अक्षि-व्यत्यासिका)
6. INFUNDIBULUM (कीप)
7. PITUITARY BODY (पीयूषिका-ग्रन्थि)
8. MAXILLARY BODY (ऊर्ध्वहनु-ग्रन्थि)
9. CEREBRAL AQUEDUCT (प्रमस्तिक-कुल्या)
10. FOURTH VENTRICLE (चतुर्थ निलय)
11. MEDULLA OBLONGATA (पश्चकपाल-अन्तरथा)
12. PONS (संयोजक अंश)
13. CEREBELLUM (अनुमस्तिष्क)
14. CEREBRAL PEDUNCLE (प्रमस्तिष्क-वृन्तक)
15. PINEAL GLAND (पिनियल ग्रन्थि)

# CHART NO. 9
# DIAGRAM OF SAGITTAL SECTION OF THE EYEBALL
(नेत्रगोलक के अग्र-पश्च अनुभाग का आरेखण)

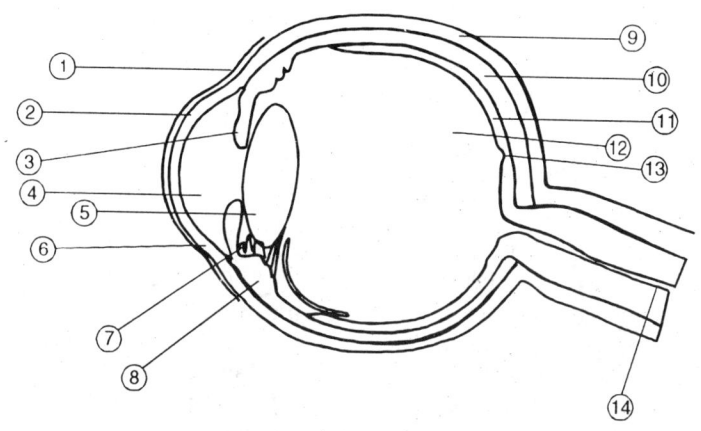

1. CONJUNCTIVA (नेत्रश्लेष्म-कला)
2. IRIS (परितारिका; उपतारा)
3. POSTERIOR CHAMBER (पश्च-कक्ष)
4. ANTERIOR CHAMBER (अग्र-कक्ष)
5. LENS (लेंस; वीक्ष)
6. CORNEA BODY (कनीनिका)
7. SUSPENSORY LIGAMENT (निलम्बी स्नायु)
8. CILIARY BODY (रोमक पिण्ड)
9. SCLERA (श्वेतपटल)
10. CHOROID (रंजितपटल)
11. RETINA (नेत्रपटल)
12. VITREOUS HUMOR (नेत्रकाचाभ द्रव)
13. FOVEA (लघुकोटर)
14. OPTIC NERVE (दृष्टि-तंत्रिका)

## CHART NO. 10

### DIAGRAM SHOWING STRUCTURE OF THE EAR
(कान की बनावट का आरेखण)

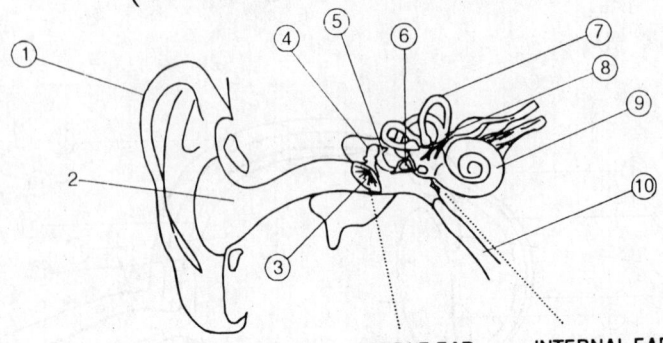

EXTERNAL EAR (बाहरी कान)  MIDDLE EAR (बिचला कान)  INTERNAL EAR (अन्दरूनी कान)

1. PINNA (कर्णपाली)
2. EXTERNAL AUDITORY MEATUS (बाह्य श्रवण-कुहर)
3. TYMPANIC MEMBRANE (मध्यकर्ण-कला)
4. MALLEUS (कर्णास्थि)
5. INCUS (स्थूलक)
6. STAPES (रकाब)
7. SEMICIRCULAR CANALS (अर्धवृत्ताकार-नलिकायें)
8. UTRICLE (क्षुद्रकोश)
9. COCHLEA (कर्णावर्त)
10. EUSTACHIAN TUBE (कम्बुकर्णीनली)

## CHART NO. 10 (A)

### DIAGRAM SHOWING LATERAL SURFACE OF PINNA
(कर्णपाली के एकपार्श्वी तल का आरेखण)

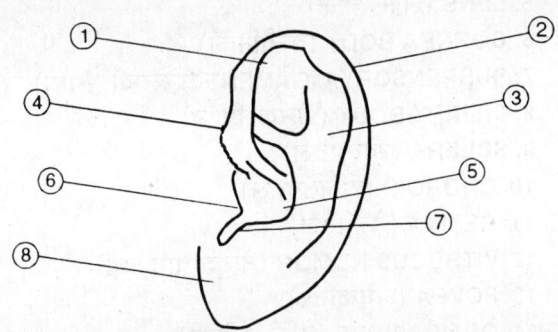

1. TRIANGULAR FOSSA (त्रिकोणक खात)
2. HELIX (कर्णकुण्डलिनी)
3. ANTIHELIX (प्रतिकर्णकुण्डलिनी)
4. CRUS OF HELIX (कर्णकुण्डलिनी-क्रस)
5. CONCHA (बाह्यकर्ण)
6. TRAGUS (तुंगिका)
7. ANTITRAGUS (प्रतितुंगिका)
8. LOBULE (खण्डक)

## CHART NO. 11
# DIAGRAM OF NOSE, MOUTH AND PHARYNX
(नाक, मुख और ग्रसनी का आरेखण)

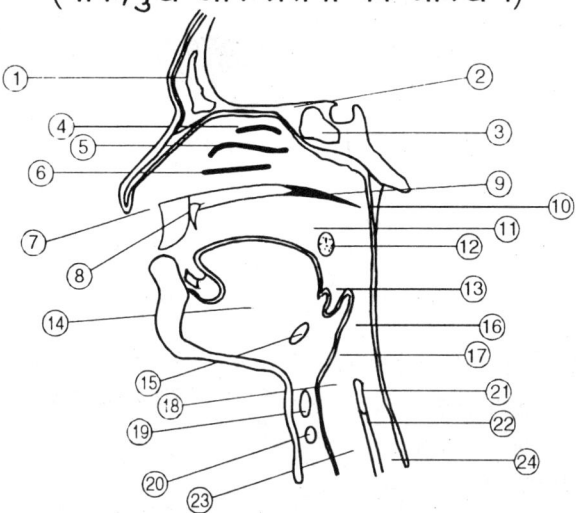

1. FRONTAL SINUS (अग्र-विवर)
2. ROOF OF NASAL CAVITY (नासाकोटरीय पटल)
3. SPHENOIDAL SINUS (जतूक विवर)
4. SUPERIOR CONCHA (उत्कृष्ट शुक्तिका)
5. MIDDLE CONCHA (माध्यमिक शुक्तिका)
6. INFERIOR CONCHA (निकृष्ट शुक्तिका)
7. ANTERIOR NARES (अग्र-नासारंध्र)
8. HARD PALATE (कठोर तालु)
9. SOFT PALATE (कोमल तालु)
10. POSTERIOR NARES (पश्च-नासारन्ध्र)
11. NASOPHARYNX (नासग्रसनी)
12. TONSIL (गलतुण्डिका)
13. OROPHARYNX (मुखग्रसनी)
14. TONGUE (जिह्वा)
15. HYOID BONE (कण्ठिकास्थि)
16. EPIGLOTTIS (कण्ठच्छद)
17. LARYNGOPHARYNX (स्वरयंत्रग्रसनी)
18. LARYNX (स्वरयंत्र)
19. THYROID CARTILAGE (अवटु-उपास्थि)
20. CRICOID CARTILAGE (मुद्रिका-उपास्थि)
21. ARYTENOID CARTILAGE (दर्वीकल्प-उपास्थि)
23. TRACHEA (श्वासप्रणाल)
24. OESOPHAGUS (ग्रासनली)

## CHART NO. 11 (A)
## DIAGRAM OF EXTERNAL NOSE
### (बाहरी नाक का आरेखण)

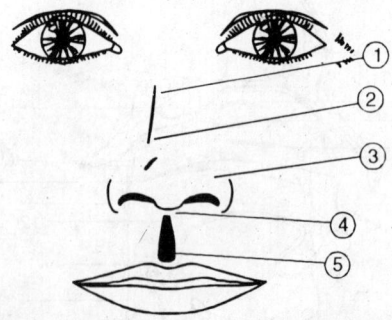

1. ROOT OF NOSE (नासा-पट)
2. DORSUM (पृष्ठतल)
3. ANTERIOR NARES
   (Nostrils) (अग्रनासारन्ध्र)
4. COLUMELLA (नासास्तम्भिका)
5. PHILTRUM (ओष्ठखात)

---

## CHART NO. 11 (B)
## THE UPPER SURFACE OF THE TONGUE
### (जीभ की ऊपरी सतह)

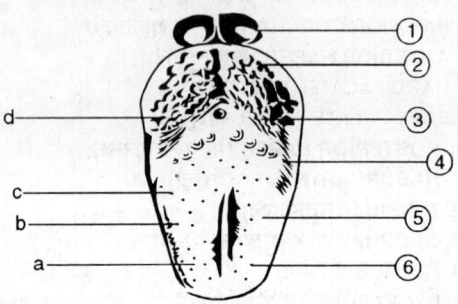

**TONGUE (जिह्वा)**
1. BASE OF TONGUE (जिह्वा-मूल)
2. SULCUS TERMINALIS (अन्त्य-परिखा)
3. VALLATE PAPILLAE (पृष्ठ-अंकुरक)
4. FOLIATE PAPILLAE (वलयी अंकुरक)
5. FILIFORM PAPILLAE (सूत्री अंकुरक)
6. FUNGIFORM PAPILLAE (कवकरूप अंकुरक)

**AREAS FOR TASTE**
**(स्वाद-क्षेत्र)**
(a) SWEET (मीठा)
(b) SOUR (खट्टा)
(c) SALTY (नमकीन)
(d) BITTER (कड़वा)

## CHART NO. 12
## PARTS OF A TOOTH
(दांत के भाग)

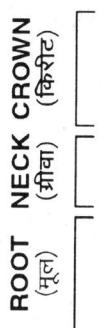
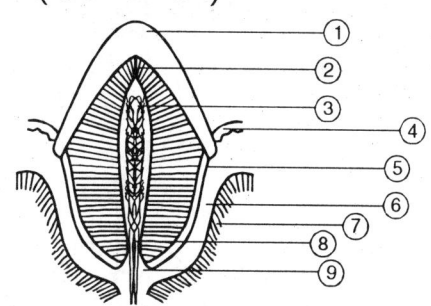

**CROWN** (किरीट)
**NECK** (ग्रीवा)
**ROOT** (मूल)

**PARTS OF A TOOTH**
(दांत के भाग)

1. ENAMEL (दन्तवल्क)
2. DENTINE (दन्तधातु)
3. PULP-CAVITY (मज्जा-कोटर)
4. GUM (मसूड़ा)
5. CEMENT (दन्तबज्र)
6. PERIODONTAL MEMBRANE (परिदन्त-कला)
7. ALVEOLAR BONE (दन्त-उलूखलास्थि)
8. BLOOD VESSELS (रक्त-वाहिनियाँ)
9. APICAL FORAMEN (शिखराग्र-रन्ध्र)

## CHART NO. 12 (A)
## ARRANGEMENT OF PERMANENT TEETH
(स्थायी दान्तों का विन्यासक्रम)

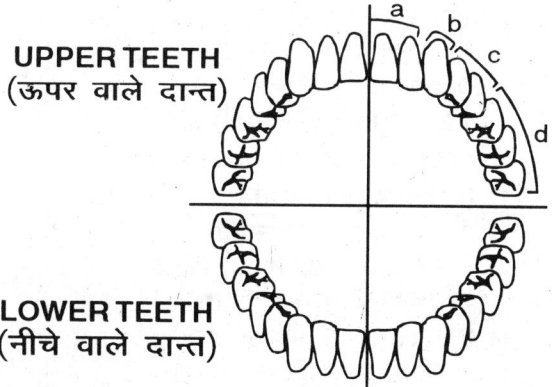

**UPPER TEETH**
(ऊपर वाले दान्त)

**LOWER TEETH**
(नीचे वाले दान्त)

SAME FOR EACH HALF OF EACH JAW
(हर जबड़े का आधा भाग समान)

a. INCISORS (2) : कृन्तक (२)
b. CANINE (1) : रदनक (१)
c. PREMOLARS (2) : अग्रचर्वणक (२)
d. MOLARS (3) : चर्वणक (३)

# CHART NO. 13
## DIAGRAM OF TRACHEA AND LUNGS
(श्वास प्रणाल और फुफ्फुसों का आरेखण)

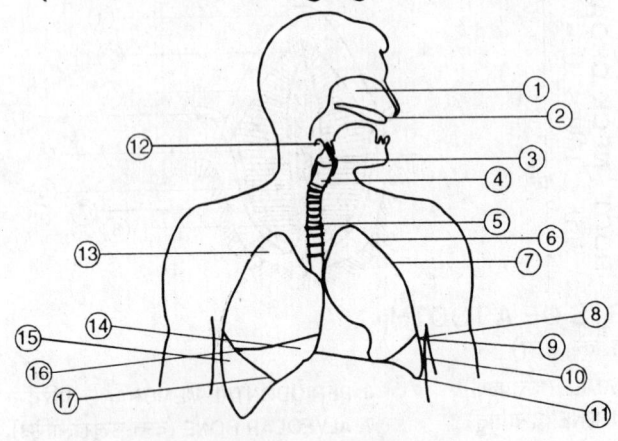

1. NASAL CAVITY (नासा-गह्वर)
2. ORAL CAVITY (मुख-गह्वर)
3. LARYNX (स्वरयंत्र)
4. THYROID (अवटुग्रन्थि)
5. TRACHEA (श्वासप्रणाल)
6. APEX (शिखर)
7. UPPER LOBE OF LEFT LUNG
   (बायें फुफ्फुस का ऊपरी खण्ड)
8. LOWER LOBE (निचला खण्ड)
9. CARDIAC NOTCH (हृद्-भंगिका)
10. OBLIQUE FISSURE (बक्र विदर)
11. DIAPHRAGM (मध्यच्छद)
12. OESOPHAGUS (ग्रासनली)
13. UPPER LOBE OF RIGHT LUNG
    (दायें फुफ्फुस का ऊपरी खण्ड)
14. MIDDLE LOBE (बिचला खण्ड)
15. LOWER LOBE (निचला खण्ड)
16. HORIZONTAL FISSURE (क्षैतिज विदर)
17. OBLIQUE FISSURE (बक्र विदर)

## CHART NO. 13 (A)
## DIAGRAM OF ALVEOLI

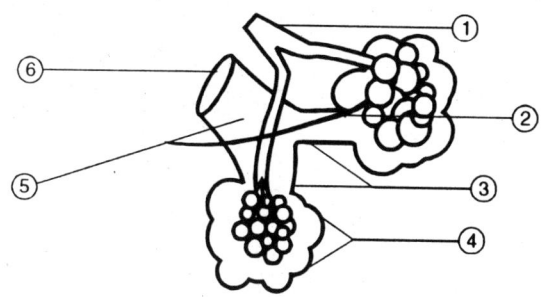

1. PULMONARY VEIN (फुप्फुस-शिरा)
2. PULMONARY ARTERY (फुप्फुस-धमनी)
3. ALVEOLAR DUCTS (वायुकोशीय नलिकायें)
4. ALVEOLI (वायुकोष्ठिकायें)
5. RESPIRATORY BRONCHIOLE (श्वसन-सूक्ष्मश्वासनलिका)
6. TERMINAL BRONCHIOLE (अन्त्य सूक्ष्मश्वासनलिका)

# CHART NO. 14

## DIAGRAM OF THE ALIMENTARY CANAL
## (भोजन नली का चित्र)

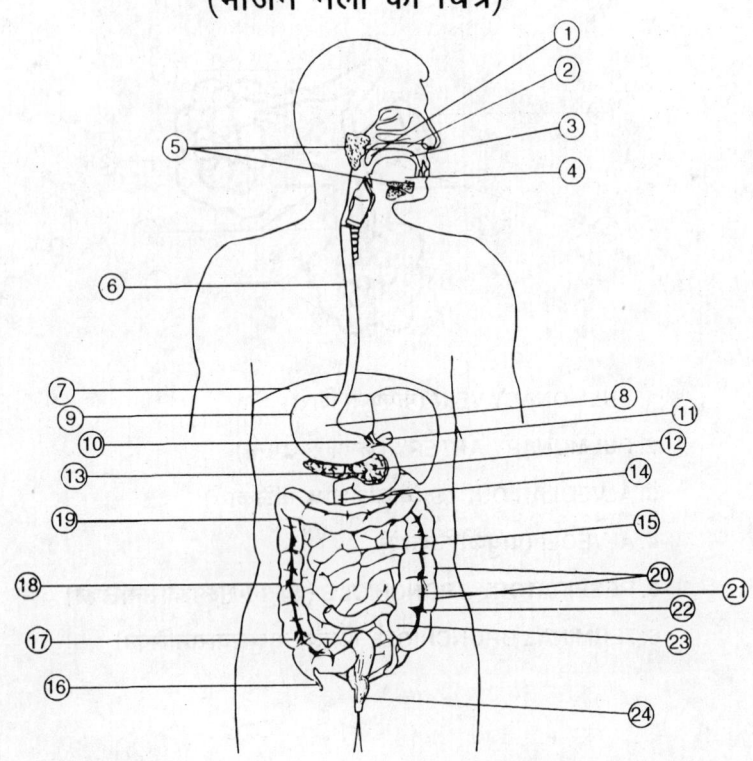

(1) **SOFT PALATE** (कोमल तालु)
(2) **HARD PALATE** (कठोर तालु)
(3) **MOUTH** (मुख)
(4) **TONGUE** (जिह्वा)
(5) **SALIVARY GLANDS** (लाला ग्रंथियाँ)
(6) **OESOPHAGUS** (ग्रासनली)
(7) **DIAPHRAGM** (मध्यच्छद)
(8) **STOMACH** (आमाशय)
(9) **LIVER** (यकृत्)
(10) **GALL BLADDER** (पित्ताशय)
(11) **BILE DUCT** (पित्त-नली)
(12) **PANCREAS** (क्लोमग्रन्थि/अग्न्याशय)
(13) **DUODENUM** (ग्रहणी)
(14) **JEJUNUM** (मध्यांत्र)
(15) **ILEUM** (शेषांत्र)
(16) **APPENDIX** (उपांत्र)
(17) **CAECUM** (अधांत्र)
(18) **ASCENDING COLON** (आरोही बृहदांत्र)
(19) **TRANSVERSE COLON** (अनुप्रस्थ बृहदांत्र)
(20) **HAUSTRA** (आवलियाँ)
(21) **DESCENDING COLON** (अवरोही बृहदांत्र)
(22) **SIGMOID COLON** (अवग्रहांत्र)
(23) **RECTUM** (मलांत्र)
(24) **ANUS** (गुदा/मलद्वार)

## CHART NO. 15
## EXCRETORY SYSTEM
(विसर्जन प्रणाली)

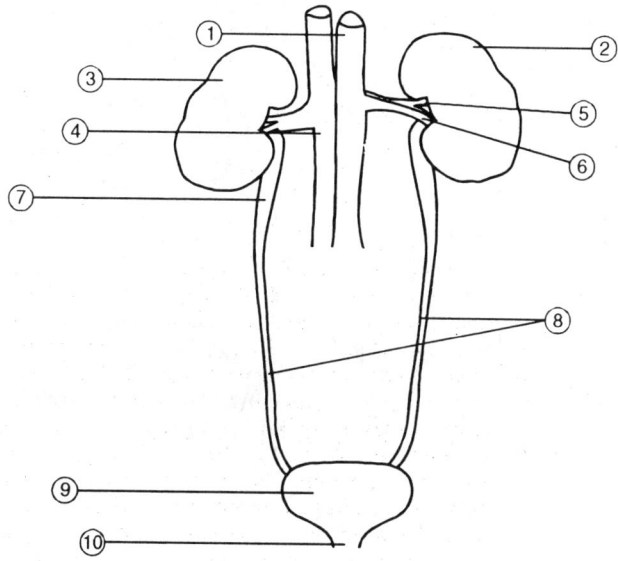

1. AORTA (महाधमनी)
2. LEFT KIDNEY (बांयाँ गुर्दा)
3. RIGHT KIDNEY (दांयाँ गुर्दा)
4. INFERIOR VENA-CAVA (निम्नमहाशिरा)
5. RENAL VEIN (वृक्क-शिरा)
6. RENAL ARTERY (वृक्क-धमनी)
7. PELVIC URETER (श्रोणि-मूत्रनली)
8. URETER (मूत्रनली)
9. URINARY BLADDER (मूत्राशय)
10. URETHRA (मूत्रमार्ग)

## CHART NO. 16

## DIAGRAM SHOWING CORONAL SECTION THROUGH KIDNEY
(गुर्दे द्वारा किरीटी अनुभाग का प्रदर्शन करता आरेखण)

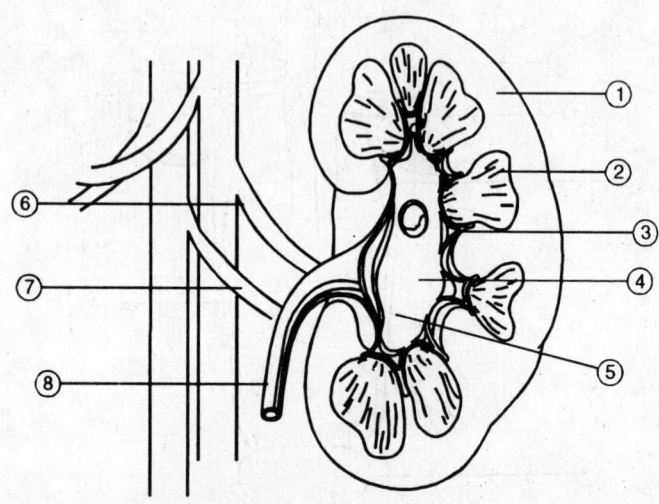

1. CORTEX (प्रान्तस्था)
2. MEDULLA (PYRAMID) (पिरामिद)
3. MINOR CALYX (लघु पुटक)
4. MAJOR CALYX (बृहत् पुटक)
5. RENAL PELVIS (वृक्क-गोणिका)
6. RENAL VEIN (वृक्क-शिरा)
7. RENAL ARTERY (वृक्क-धमनी)
8. URETER (मूत्रनली)

## CHART NO. 17
## VENTRAL VIEW OF A MALE PELVIS
### (पुरुष-गोणिका का अग्र दृश्य)

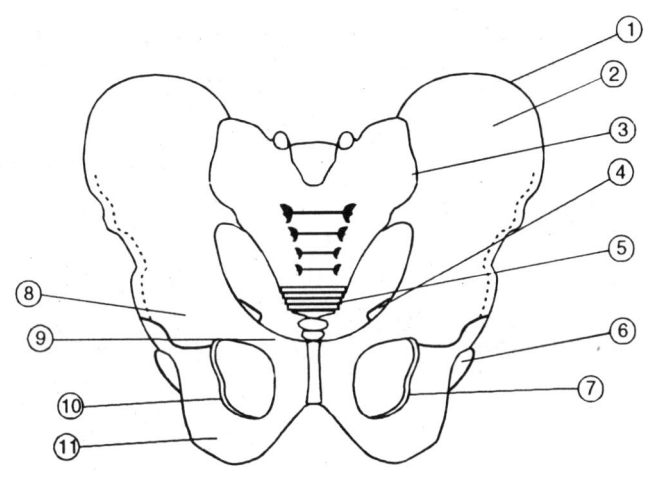

(1) ILIAC CREST (श्रोणिफलक शिखर)
(2) ILIUM (नितम्बास्थि)
(3) SACRUM (त्रिकास्थि)
(4) ISCHIAL SPINE (आसनास्थिक पृष्ठवंश)
(5) COCCYX (पुच्छास्थि)
(6) ACETABULUM (उलूखल)
(7) OBTURATOR FORAMEN (गवाक्ष रन्ध्र)
(8) PUBIS (जघनरोम)
(9) PELVIC TUBERCLE (श्रोणि गुलिका)
(10) SYMPHYSIS (जघन संधानक)
(11) ISCHIUM (आसनास्थि)

## CHART NO. 17 (A)
## VENTRAL VIEW OF A FEMALE PELVIS
### (स्त्री-गोणिका का अग्र दृश्य)

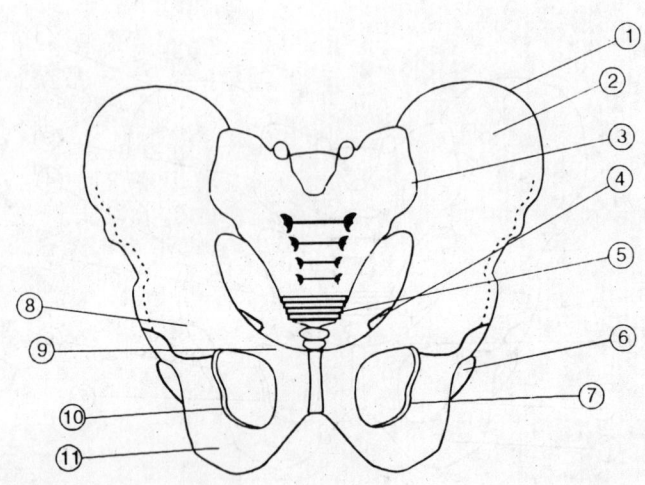

(1) ILIAC CREST (श्रोणिफलक शिखर)
(2) ILIUM (नितम्बास्थि)
(3) SACRUM (त्रिकास्थि)
(4) ISCHIAL SPINE (आसनास्थिक पृष्ठवंश)
(5) COCCYX (पुच्छास्थि)
(6) ACETABULUM (उलूखल)
(7) OBTURATOR FORAMEN (गवाक्ष रन्ध्र)
(8) PUBIS (जघनरोम)
(9) PELVIC TUBERCLE (श्रोणि-गुलिका)
(10) SYMPHYSIS (जघन संधानक)
(11) ISCHIUM (आसनास्थि)

# CHART NO. 18
## DIAGRAMMATIC REPRESENTATION OF VERTICAL SECTION OF TESTIS
(वृषण के लम्बरूप अनुभाग का आरेखित चित्र)

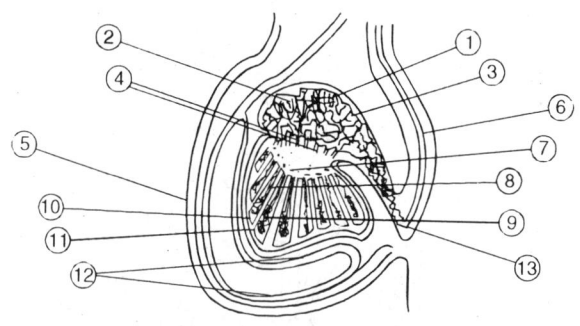

(1) EPIDIDYMIS (अधिवृषण)
(2) HEAD OF EPIDIDYMIS (अधिवृषण-शीर्ष)
(3) CONUS VASCULOSUS (वाहिका-शंकु)
(4) DUCTUS EFFERENTES (अपवाही नली)
(5) SCROTUM (वृषणकोश)
(6) VAS DEFERENS (शुक्र-नली)
(7) RETE TUBULE (वृषण-जालिका)
(8) STRAIGHT TUBULE (ऋजु नलिका)
(9) SEMINIFEROUS TUBULE (शुक्र-नली)
(10) TUNICA ALBUGINEA (श्वेत कंचुक)
(11) SEPTUM (पटल)
(12) TUNICA VAGINALIS (योनि-कंचुक)
(13) TAIL OF EPIDIDYMIS (अधिवृषण-पुच्छ)

# CHART NO. 19

## DIAGRAMMATIC (MEDIAN) VIEW OF MALE REPRODUCTIVE ORGANS
(पुरुष-जननांगों का आरेखित (माध्यमिक) दृश्य)

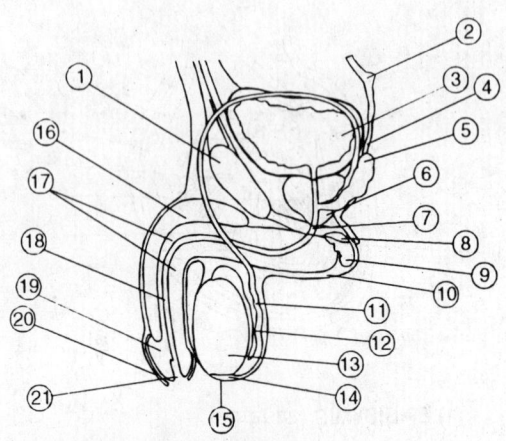

(1) SYMPHYSIS (जघन संधानक)
(2) URETER (मूत्रनली)
(3) URINARY BLADDER (मूत्राशय)
(4) AMPULLA OF VAS DEFERENS (शुक्रनलीय कलशिका)
(5) SEMINAL VESICLE (शुक्रपुटिका)
(6) UTRICULUS PROSTATICUS (पुरःस्थ-क्षुद्रकोश)
(7) EJACULATORY DUCT (वीर्यपाती नलिका)
(8) PROSTATE (पुरःस्थ-ग्रंथि)
(9) COWPER'S GLAND (कूपर ग्रंथि)
(10) BULBUS URETHRAE (मूत्रमार्गी कन्द)
(11) VAS DEFERENS (शुक्रनली)
(12) EPIDIDYMIS (अधिवृषण)
(13) TESTIS (वृषण)
(14) TUNICA VAGINALIS (योनि-कंचुक)
(15) SCROTUM (वृषणकोश)
(16) CORPUS CAVERNOSUM (रक्तधर पिण्ड)
(17) CORPUS SPONGIOSUM (स्पंजी पिण्ड)
(18) URETHRA (मूत्रमार्ग)
(19) GLANS PENIS (शिश्न-मुण्ड)
(20) PREPUCE (शिश्न-मुण्डच्छद)
(21) OPENING OF URETHRA (मूत्रमार्गी छिद्र)

# CHART NO. 19 (A)
## DIAGRAM OF FRONT OF A SPERMATOZOON
(शुक्राणु के अगले भाग का आरेखण)

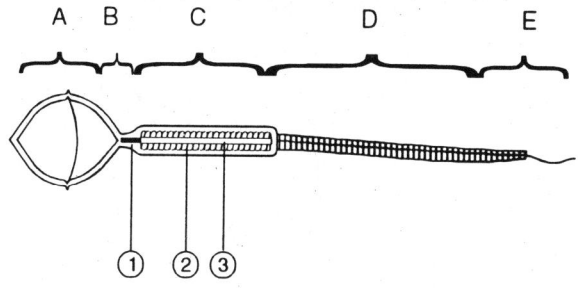

1. BASAL BODY (आधारी पिण्ड)
2. MITOCHONDRIAL SHEATH (सुक्ष्मतंतु-पिधान)
3. AXIAL FIBRES (अक्ष-तन्तु)

## PARTS (अंग)

A. HEAD (सिर)
B. NECK (गर्दन)
C. MIDDLE PIECE (बीच वाला अंश)
D. TAIL (पूंछ)
E. END PIECE OF TAIL (पूंछ का अन्तिम अंश)

## CHART NO. 20
## DIAGRAM OF VAGINA, UTERUS, FALLOPIAN TUBES AND OVARY
(योनि, गर्भाशय, डिम्बवाही नलियों तथा डिम्बाशय का आरेखण)

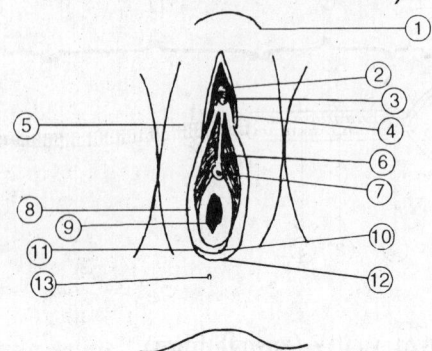

(1) MONS VENERIS (जघन-शैल)
(2) PREPUCE OF CLITORIS (भगशिश्निकाच्छद)
(3) CLITORIS (भगशिश्निका)
(4) FRENULUM (क्षुद्रबन्ध)
(5) LABIUM MAJUS (बृहत् भगोष्ठ)
(6) LABIUM MINORS (लघु भगोष्ठ)
(7) URETHRAL MEATUS (मूत्रमार्गी मुख)
(8) VAGINAL INTROITUS (मूत्रमार्गी-द्वार)
(9) HYMEN (योनिच्छद)
(10) VESTIBULE (प्रघाण)
(11) FOSSA NAVICULARIS (नौकाभ खात)
(12) FOURCHETTE (भगांजलि)
(13) PERINEUM (मूलाधार)
(14) ANUS (मलद्वार)

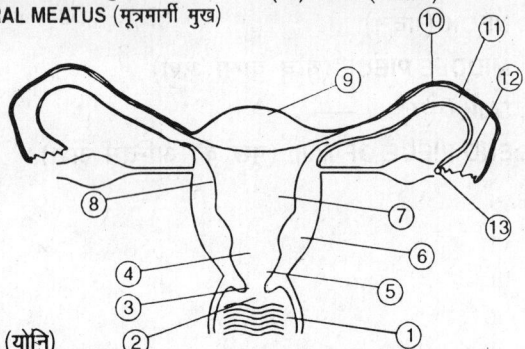

(1) VAGINA (योनि)
(2) CERVIX (जरायुग्रीवा)
(3) EXTERNAL OS (बाह्य मुख)
(4) INTERNAL OS (अन्तर्मुख)
(5) CERVICAL CANAL (गर्भाशय-ग्रीवा नली)
(6) UTERUS (जरायु/गर्भाशय)
(7) CAVITY OF UTERUS (गर्भाशय गह्वर)
(8) CORNU (शृंग)
(9) FUNDUS OF UTERUS (गर्भाशय-बुध्न)
(10) FALLOPIAN TUBE (डिम्बवाही नली)
(11) AMPULLA (कलशिका)
(12) FIMBRIAE (झालर)
(13) OVUM SHED FROM OVARY (डिम्बक्षरण पर डिम्बाशय से डिम्बनिर्गम)

## CHART NO. 20 (B)

### DIAGRAMMATIC REPRESENTATION OF UTERINE ENDOMETRIUM UNDERGOING CYCLE CHANGES DURING VARIOUS PHASES OF MENSTRUAL CYCLE
(ऋतुस्रावी चक्र के विभिन्न चरणों के दौरान अन्तर्गर्भाशय में होने वाले चक्र-परिवर्तनों का आरेखित प्रस्तुतीकरण)

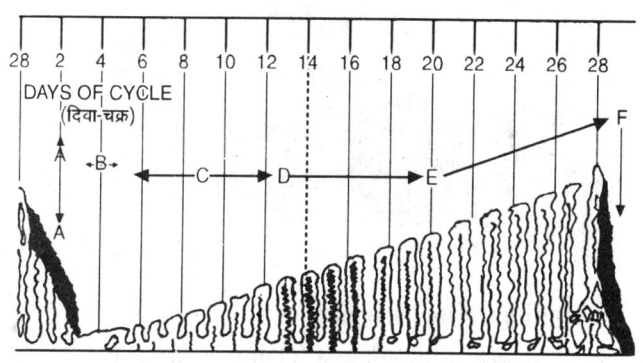

A- DEGENERATION AND SHEDDING (अपजनन और परित्यजन)

B- REPAIR (सुधार)

C- PROLIFERATIVE STAGES (प्रफलनात्मक चरण)

D. COILED BLOOD VESSELS (कुण्डलित रक्त-वाहिनियाँ)

E. SECRETORY PHASE (स्रावी चरण)

F. BLOOD AND MUCOUS DISCHARGED (स्रवित रक्त और श्लेष्मा)

## CHART NO. 21

## LONGITUDINAL STRUCTURE OF OVARY SHOWING VARIOUS STAGES IN MATURATION OF OVUM
(डिम्बाशय की अनुदैर्घ्य बनावट जो अण्डाणु-परिपक्वता की विभिन्न अवस्थाओं को बताती है)

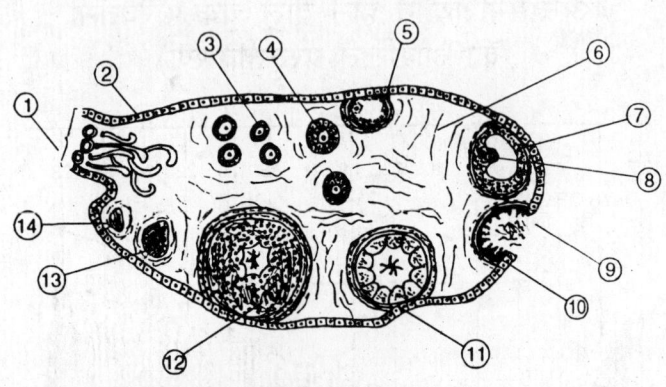

1. MESOVARIUM (डिम्बग्रन्थियोजनी)
2. GERMINAL EPITHELIUM (बीजांकुरक उपकला)
3. PRIMORDIAL FOLLICLE (मूल पुटक)
4. DOUBLE LAYERED FOLLICLE (द्विस्तरीय पुटक)
5. MATURING FOLLICLE (परिपक्वगामी पुटक)
6. CONNECTIVE TISSUE (संयोजक ऊतक)
7. MATURE GRAFFIAN FOLLICLE (परिपक्व ग्राफीपुटक)
8. OVUM (अण्डाणु)
9. RELEASED OVUM (विमुक्त पुटक)
10. RUPTURED FOLLICLE (विदरित पुटक)
11. YOUNG CORPUS LUTEUM (युवा पीत-पिण्ड)
12. MATURE CORPUS LUTEUM (परिपक्व पीत-पिण्ड)
13. DEGENERATING CORPUS LUTEUM (अपजननात्मक पीत-पिण्ड)
14. CORPUS ALBICANS (श्वेत-पिण्ड)

## CHART NO. 21 (A)
## LONGITUDINAL SECTION OF ADULT FEMALE BREAST
(वयस्क स्त्री-स्तन का अनुदैर्घ्य अनुभाग)

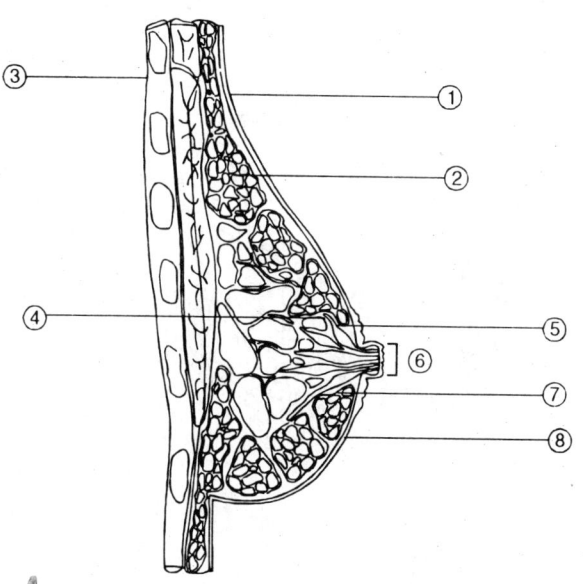

1. LIGAMENT OF COOPER (कूपर-बन्धन)
2. SUBCUTANEOUS FAT (उपत्वग्वसा)
3. PECTORAL FASCIA (वक्ष-प्रावरणी)
4. LOBULE (खण्डक)
5. LACTIFEROUS DUCT (दुग्ध-नली)
6. NIPPLE (चूचुक)
7. AREOLA (वृन्त)
8. SKIN (त्वचा/चर्म)

## CHART NO. 22

## DIAGRAM SHOWING SECTION OF THE SKIN
### (चर्म-अनुभाग का आरेखण)

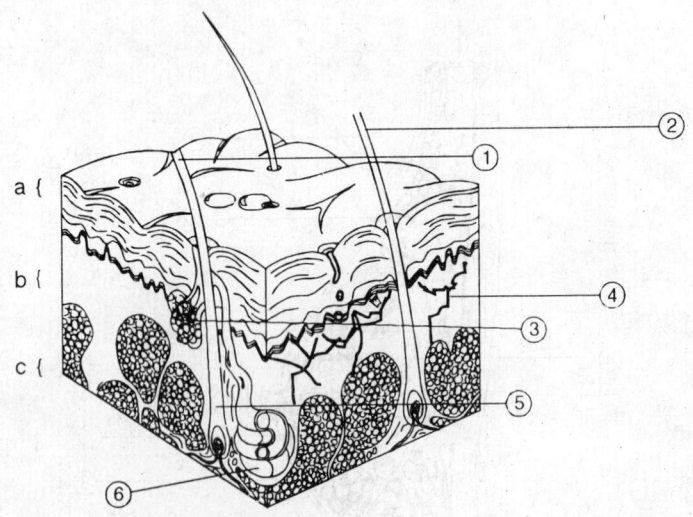

## SKIN (चर्म)

1. SWEAT PORE (स्वेद-छिद्र)
2. HAIR FOLLICLE (रोम-कूप)
3. SEBACEOUS GLAND (वसा-ग्रन्थि)
4. BLOOD CAPILLARIES (रक्त-केशिकायें)
5. SWEAT DUCT (स्वेद-नली)
6. SWEAT GLAND (स्वेद-ग्रन्थि)

## LAYERS OF SKIN (चर्म-पट)

(a) EPIDERMIS (उपत्वचा)

(b) DERMIS (अन्तस्त्वचा)

(c) SUBCUTANEOUS FAT
(अधस्त्वग्वसा)